Dominant Issues in Medical Sociology

Second Edition

Edited by
Howard D. Schwartz
Radford University

Ch. 2,4,15
p. 174 →

Random House
New York

5

**This Book Is Dedicated to
My Sister Suzanne,
Joyce Garber Gamse,
and
Catharine Cranford Mintzer, RN, MD**

Second Edition

98765432

Cover photo: Richard Wood/The Picture Cube

Library of Congress Cataloging-in-Publication Data

Dominant issues in medical sociology.

   Reprinted from various sources.
   Includes bibliographies and index.
   1. Social medicine.   I. Schwartz, Howard D.
[DNLM: 1. Social Medicine—collected works.
w. Sociology, Medical—collected works.   WA 31 D671]
RA418.D652   1987   362.1'042   86–31473
ISBN 0–394–36302–7

Manufactured in the United States of America

Preface

This book will always have a very strong hold on my heart since the material for the first edition was largely gathered at night in the Yale Medical Library at the time that my mother was dying of cancer in a room across the street. The effort allowed me to create something, which I now cherish, out of a great loss. That the book generated such a warm response and has become something of an "institution" to a generation of students is an extra bonus.

I believe the greatest improvement in this edition stems from my own growth as a sociologist during the time between editions. In that time, I returned to Yale in the School of Public Health. The end result of this very useful and invigorating experience has been a greater familiarity with the "macro" issues in the field. In addition, thanks to a grant from the Canadian government, I had an opportunity to spend considerable time viewing the Canadian health care system at close range. It is my firm belief that Part Four, in particular, is a most positive reflection of these experiences.

I hope, as with the first edition, the reader enjoys *Dominant Issues* because of its broad range of coverage and the readibility of its articles. As was the case with its predecessor, the second edition includes articles which were chosen with great care

from a uniquely wide variety of sources. These sources include the more traditional academic articles and books as well those written for wider audiences appearing in more popular publications and on best-seller lists. This edition also includes five key articles written especially for the second edition providing sociological perspectives on health care consumerism, the changing faces of nursing, the restructuring of the physician–hospital relationship, the "irrationality" embedded in the U.S. health care delivery system, and the link between social values and health care delivery in this country, Canada, and Great Britain.

For those who used the first edition, the format of this book will seem very familiar. On the other hand, the content has been substantially altered. In the last ten years, many things have changed in the health care field, and this edition takes note of those changes.

As regards the very practical concern of classroom use, a main strength of *Dominant Issues* continues to be its versatility. A large number of first edition adoptees employed *Dominant Issues* as the sole text in the course. For those who wish to use this volume in the same way, a very ample "introduction to the field" section has been added this time around. At the same time, the popularity of the format which explores issues from the individual to the system level makes *Dominant Issues* exceedingly compatible with several short, introductory texts that have recently emerged.

ACKNOWLEDGMENTS

A dept of gratitude is owed to my sister, Suzanne, who has always had a sympathetic ear, and to Larry and Cheryl Amy who took me on a walk in the Virginia woods when I needed it the most. In addition, I would like to express my appreciation to Stephen Lerch who, as department chairperson, provided as much support as one could possibly expect. Barbara Ewell, Bob Hyatt, Myrl Jones, Rita White, Larry Pollard, David Hayes, Susan Brown, and Gordon Darroch all responded when I needed them, and Machell Saunders and Carolyn Sutphin contributed, through their typing skills, to the completion of the book.

A very special thanks goes to Kay Alexander who was my left hand and who performed so admirably in so many "not-so-routine" routine functions that go into putting together a volume like this. She must be, quite literally, and for her young age, one of the truly gifted "cut and pasters."

Radford, Virginia H.D.S.
November, 1986

Introduction

Perhaps the most unusual aspect of this book is the degree to which it has been structured around the needs of a particular audience. It is explicitly directed to introductory students in medical sociology. The largest number of these are undergraduates, representing a wide variety of academic interests. I am convinced, however, that the graduate student and medical student being introduced to medical sociology will find *Dominant Issues* both challenging and interesting. One of the prime motivators of this edition and the previous one was the conviction that there now exists a virtually untapped, large and growing body of quality articles that can easily engage the student in his or her first exposure to the field. Although readability was an important criterion for selection, I had no intention to, and did not find it necessary to, sacrifice quality.

Old friends, and there are many of them who remember the first edition, will notice many structural similarities between this edition and the last one. In the first place, like its predecessor, this edition is very current and state-of-the-art. Almost ten years have elapsed between the two volumes. By any standard, that is an unusually long time between editions. But it seems particularly so in this case due to the dramatic changes that have occurred

in the realm of health care delivery. In the first edition, there was an article announcing the imminent arrival of national health insurance. We are now talking about health care in a competitive market place. In the first edition, Harvey Smith's classic article on the "two lines of authority" in the hospital—where physicians were more dominant than administrators—was appropriate in describing the essential character of the relationship at that time. In its place, this edition has an article by Bures and Bures, which was written specially for this book and deals with the important changes that are impacting upon the physician's role in the hospital. Two changes discussed are the corporatization of hospitals and the emergence of diagnostic related groups (DRGs) as a basis of payment. The piece on the explicit rationing of kidney dialysis in Great Britain deals with an issue that has become very "hot" as the costs of high-technology care in this country continue to rise. An article on the current state of nursing was written by me and two colleagues for this volume. At the same time, a piece has been included that discusses the possible consequences of the fact that more women than ever are training to become physicians. David Mechanic's concise but detailed description of the current structure of the American health care delivery system comes from a book that appeared in mid-1986. A number of articles deal with the implications of the increasing prominence of chronic disease and the related issue of the aging of the population for health care delivery in this country.

In addition to the above, some articles written earlier, but still relevant, have been updated. Arnold Relman, the editor of *The New England Journal of Medicine,* has written an update to his important and provocative article on the medical–industrial complex written in 1980. Regina Kenen and Robert Schmidt have added a section on the impact of labeling on those screened for AIDS as an update to their article on the same issue related to genetic screening in the 1970s. Paul Benson has written an overview of the last twenty-five years of the "deinstitutionalization" of mental patients from state hospitals into the community. This is an add-on to his article concerning the influence of labeling theorists like Scheff and Goffman on the California legislature's decision to embark on a program of deinstitutionalization in that state in the 1960s.

In a sense, this second edition, in keeping with my goal of making it current, is really a new book. The vast majority of the articles are new, although, in sum, they deal with many of the same topics as those in the first edition. The choice of such a complete revision was, in actuality, out of my hands due to the enormous changes that have occurred in the health care system and to the great amount of new material that has been published since the mid-1970s.

As with the first edition, *Dominant Issues* is not essentially polemical. While it certainly employs articles with points of view, I would hope that the overall feeling the reader will glean from this volume is that of a balanced presentation of what medical sociologists and others interested in the same issues are doing and thinking about health, health care, and illness. I would hope, for example, that even-handedness will be seen in the presentation of material dealing with "therapeutic nihilism"—the notion that modern medicine may not be all that effective. Although I include the well-known McKinley and McKinley article that takes this position, in my own article in Part Four, I discuss the recent work of Hadley and others who provide empirical support for the opposite conclusion. In Chapter 15, Waitz-

kin's article applying a Marxist critique to the development and use of coronary care units is followed by Bloom's response (just as the article and response appeared together in *The New England Journal of Medicine*).

Another major consideration shared by both volumes is a commitment to comprehensiveness. It is my feeling that there is an essential subject matter of which every student who has had the basic medical sociology course should have an understanding. As will be evident in an even casual perusal of the table of contents, *Dominant Issues* deals in depth with both micro and macro issues. In a sense, the even-handed emphasis on both sets of issues, which I have tried hard to achieve, stems from my training both as a doctoral student in medical sociology at Virginia and later at Yale in the Masters in Public Health program (in health services administration). The micro issues were the early focus of medical sociologists and relate to the interpersonal relationships between patients and health personnel in different medical settings. They are essentially social-psychological in nature. Of late, there has been an increasing emphasis on macro issues, which relate to the overall health of the nation and the provision of health care services. The work of David Mechanic shows this progression from an emphasis on micro issues to a later one on macro issues to the extent that Mechanic is now one of America's most prominent writers on health care policy. The articles in Parts One through Three deal with micro issues and those in Part Four, with macro issues.

An attempt was made to further insure that this edition would be comprehensive by including some very important review articles. Lois Verbrugge's extraordinary, and recent, overview of a wealth of material dealing with health differences between men and women is a case in point.

With the beginning student in mind, several articles will be found that provide straightforward and clear introductions to key concepts. Alexander Segall's study of the four characteristics of the sick role, Elizabeth Gustafson's summary of Julius Roth's ideas on the applicability of the concept of the career to the situation of the patient, and Nancy Waxler's overview of labeling theory and its relationship to definitions of health and illness are three that come immediately to mind.

Reflecting my own interest in the Canadian

health care system and my recent first-hand look at it, Part Four has a strong comparative flavor. Kaufmann, and to a lesser extent I, look at the U.S. health care system in a comparative perspective. As a result, the student should come away from *Dominant Issues* with a knowledge of health and health care in the United States as well as knowledge about Great Britain, Canada, and Sweden.

Many of the articles that appear in this volume have been tried and tested by my medical sociology students. If my experiences are repeated, students will find a number of these articles uniquely compelling. David Sudnow's discussion of DOAs (dead on arrivals) and their treatment in the emergency room has never failed to generate strong feelings. Such is also the case with the selections from Marcia Millman's *The Unkindest Cut*. Not only do my students have difficulty putting the book down once they have begun to read it, but they rarely ever sell it back to the bookstore, which is great praise indeed. I have, consequently, included two pieces from Millman's book. Other articles that I have found students to find highly absorbing are the Dowie and Johnston account of events surrounding the Dalkon Shield and David Hilfiker's account of his combat with medical mistakes in his practice of medicine.

As in the last volume, I have stayed with the traditional emergent levels separation of the four main parts of the book. Each part deals with health and health care on a more inclusive level than the previous one. I have found that this format and the use of broad sub-chapter categories provide more flexibility than other approaches, given the comprehensive nature of the book.

Two additional notes must be made here. First, because of the interrelatedness of many of the issues in this book, articles in various chapters may easily be related to one another. This is an act of creativity that I will leave to each individual instructor. In support of my point, however, I would suggest in passing that Glassman's article concerning the misdiagnosis of senile dementia is, in a number of its points, a very nice example of the limitations of the "biomedical model."

Second, and finally, there are a number of variables that determine the content of a course and how it is taught, among them, the interests of the instructor, the type of student, and the length of the term (semester or quarter). As has already been suggested, I intend to use *Dominant Issues* to provide my students with a more comprehensive view of medical sociology. However, it was also my intent that those with more limited aspirations for their course would, through a process of picking and choosing, find this volume very suitable to their needs. It is my firm conviction that they will.

Contents

ix

Introduction to Medical Sociology

The development of contemporary medical sociology has had a decidedly American flavor. A German medical sociologist writing in the mid-1970s stated that all publication and research in medical sociology comes from the United States. Although the United States still dominates the field, an increasing amount of important work is being done abroad. An international journal entitled *Social Science and Medicine* consistently publishes interesting and significant articles written by sociologists from around the world. With the advent of national health insurance in Canada, a great deal of work in medical sociology has been coming from, among others, a small group of researchers at the University of Toronto.

The field of medical sociology is very young as far as recognition within sociology is concerned. It was not until 1955 that an informal Committee on Medical Sociology was started within the American Sociological Association (ASA). A formal section was chartered within the ASA four years later. However, it wasn't until 1965 that the field gained a journal of its own, the *Journal of Health and Social Behavior,* which is now its official journal.

Since its founding in 1959, the section on medical sociology has grown by leaps and bounds. By 1980, its membership had grown to 1000, making it the ASA's largest and most active section.

The field of medical sociology has grown rapidly not just in numbers but also in domain. In the beginning, medical sociologists focused almost exclusively on microsociology—sociology at the social psychological (i.e., interpersonal) level. Although the doctor–patient relationship, the socialization and training of health professionals, and the like remain central issues, a great deal of interest in macro issues—relating to the health of Americans and provision of health-care services to the nation as a whole—has developed within medical sociology. Sociologists like Eli Ginzberg and David Mechanic have become important and prolific writers on a variety of health policy issues at the national level.

The first article in this chapter, by Frederick D. Wolinsky, focuses on a very important distinction between the sociologies *of* and *in* medicine. In many ways, this distinction parallels the micro (sociology *of*) and macro (sociology *in*) division just mentioned. Sociologists plying their trade in the sociology *of* medicine are most likely to be found in college and university sociology departments engaging in largely academic research (i.e., pure rather than applied research). Sociologists *in* medicine apply sociological methods to the applied problems of health care. They may work in such settings as medical schools, public health departments, or federal government agencies in such roles as statistician (e.g., a social epidemiologist studying the rate of disease in various groups), planner, or policy analyst. As Wolinsky observes, medical sociology work is increasingly being done in sociology *in* medicine. This is, to some extent, a reflection of changes in the job market for medical sociologists as college teaching jobs become more difficult to find.

The second article, by Renée C. Fox, is her presidential address to the ASA in 1985. To many, Fox is the "first lady" of American medical sociology. (This volume also includes her article "Training for Uncertainty" in a later chapter; most recently, she has written on applied aspects of medical ethics.) In her elegant piece in this chapter, Fox makes a number of suggestions as to the most useful directions in research that medical sociology could take in the future. Some of these are research in biomedical ethics, the emerging role of women in medicine, the role of nursing, the social world of the hospital, and the impact of the increasing numbers of elderly Americans. The reader will find most of the issues discussed by Fox addressed in this edition of *Dominant Issues in Medical Sociology*.

The Nature of the Field

Frederick D. Wolinsky

In order to examine the development of any scientific discipline, it is necessary to have a framework within which to organize the contributions to knowledge made by that discipline. An examination of the foundations of the sociology of health is no exception. About twenty-five years ago, when medical sociology was beginning to become an acceptable specialty area within sociology, Straus (1955) proposed such a framework for use in overviewing medical sociology. Straus's framework was neither elaborate nor revolutionary. It was readily accepted, however, and with some relatively minor changes it has stood the test of time. In this section, we shall trace the development of Straus's framework, and then use his framework to evaluate the present status of the sociology of health.

Straus's Sociologies *of* and *in* Medicine

Straus (1955, 1957) suggested two categories into which all efforts in medical sociology could be logically divided. These categories were the sociologies *of* and *in* medicine. He said (1957:203) that the subject matter of the sociology *of* medicine is ". . . concerned with studying such factors as the organizational structure, role relationships, value systems, rituals and functions of medicine as a system of behavior and that this type of activity can best be carried out by persons operating from independent positions outside the formal medical setting." In other words, Straus saw the sociology *of* medicine as the sociological study of medicine. These sociological studies should be conducted by professional sociologists whose employment is outside of the medical realm, such as academic sociologists housed in departments of sociology in universities.

At the heart of Straus's concept of the sociology

of medicine is the notion that it can provide an opportunity to apply, refine, and test sociological principles and theories. The particular arena or laboratory of medicine is not fundamentally important. The important point is the opportunity to submit existing sociological principles to empirical testing, and to use this new proving ground for the clarification of those principles.

The sociology *in* medicine category is quite different, according to Straus (1957:203), who stated it ". . . consists of collaborative research or teaching often involving the integration of concepts, techniques and personnel from many disciplines." Under this category, Straus placed all those efforts in which sociologists (and other social scientists) ply their skills within the realm of medicine. Those skills include the teaching of medical students, identifying differences in the definitions and reactions to health and illness, and social epidemiology. The primary concern of studies in this category is the introduction and use of sociological concepts, principles, and research in medicine.

At the heart of Straus's concept of the sociology *in* medicine is the opportunity it provides for sociologists to work within the medical world, as applied sociologists. (The important point here is the specification of the actual arena of medicine.) Its purpose is to make the medical world aware of the utility of sociological principles and concepts concerning social behavior, and the ability of sociologists to provide certain types of research within the realm of social medicine.

In addition to describing the two categories of the sociologies *of* and *in* medicine, Straus also identified their interrelationship. He suggested (1957:203) that the roles played by these two types of medical sociologists are incompatible: "[T]he sociologist of medicine may lose objectivity if he identifies too closely with medical teaching or clinical research while the sociologist in medicine risks a good relationship if he tries to study his colleagues." In this passage, Straus identified dilemmas that exist for

Reprinted by permission of the author from *The Sociology of Health* by Frederick D. Wolinsky (Boston: Little, Brown, 1980), pp. 38–53.

both the sociologist *of* medicine and the sociologist *in* medicine. According to Straus, the sociologist *of* medicine experiences difficulty having gained access to medical research sites, because the profession of medicine is not interested in being subjected to sociological scrutiny. This disinterest is especially salient when such scrutiny raises serious questions about the medical community, questions which may tend to diminish its power and prestige.

At the same time, the sociologist *in* medicine faces a perplexing dilemma as well. Using his sociological skills in an applied fashion, the sociologist *in* medicine easily gains access to valuable information and other resources, but in the process of serving the medical interests, he or she may find himself divested of his or her unique sociological perspective. This may occur primarily as a result of the secondary status accorded to the sociologist in medicine by most of the medical professionals with whom he or she works.

The noncompatibility between the roles of the sociologist *in* medicine and the sociologist *of* medicine may be abstracted to the more general level. There it can be recast in the form of the question that has interested many scientists in modern history. In order to advance the general discipline (in this case, sociology), which is more valuable, applied research or basic research? There are prestigious sociologists who would support the role of applied research, and there are those who would support the role of basic research. We shall withhold our support for either of these roles until the latter portions of this section. There, the ramifications of each of these roles will be discussed in terms of the future of medical sociology.

Elaborating on Straus's Distinctions

Straus's distinction between the sociologies *of* and *in* medicine was immediately recognized as a major contribution toward understanding not only this new specialty area, but also the directions in which it might develop. As medical sociology began to develop into a legitimate area within American sociology, however, the number of studies in this new specialty area increased exponentially. In a short period of time, the growing literature in medical sociology began to tax the simple distinction that Straus originally described, and a number of refinements were suggested that elaborated upon Straus's basic dichot-

omy (Kendall and Merton, 1958; Kendall, 1963; Suchman, 1967).

These refinements have been reviewed by Kendall and Reader (1972), who presented a useful elaboration of Straus's original distinction. Their paper provided a number of subclasses under which the growing numbers of studies in medical sociology might be classified, an elaboration that took form in the following outline.

I. Sociology in Medicine
   A. Ecology and etiology of disease
   B. Variations in attitude and behavior regarding health and illness
      1. Sociological continuities: the case of social class
      2. Reoriented sociological concerns: the cases of deviance, labeling and stigma
II. Sociology of Medicine
   A. Recruitment of physicians
   B. Training of physicians
   C. Relations of physicians to others in role-set
   D. Medical organization—the case of hospitals
   E. Development of community health

While Kendall and Reader's elaboration does permit more precise classification of studies within the two categories of medical sociology, the general theme of their framework is quite consonant with Straus's. According to Kendall and Reader, the sociology *of* medicine deals with

. . . questions which belong within the traditions of the sociology of the professions and organizational sociology. Relevant topics include recruitment into and training for the profession, the organization of the profession, and finally, its relations to external pressures and agencies.

Sociology *in* medicine, on the other hand, they describe as

. . . the application of sociological concepts, knowledge, and techniques in efforts to clarify medical and social-psychological problems in which the medical profession and its allied workers are interested. In this instance, sociological knowledge supplements medical knowledge, in order to find solutions to what are essentially medical problems.

Thus, although Kendall and Reader had elaborated upon the categorical nature of Straus's distinction, the basic decision criteria for the classification of studies remained the same. Studies that were conducted along the lines of traditional sociology belonged to the sociology *of* medicine. Studies that were conducted as an applied venture belonged to the sociology *in* medicine.

A Little Modernization

One might consider Kendall and Reader's framework suitable for evaluating existing contributions to medical sociology. But there is something missing, and that something is the scope of the framework and its concepts. Developing rather slowly at first, a new way of looking at health and health care has been emerging in the United States since the 1960s. There are at least two major factors that have stimulated this development.

The first factor has been the increasing role of the government, at the local, state, and federal levels, in providing health care to the population. Beginning with local governments in the early 1950s, the trend toward third-party payment or provision of health care has increased markedly. With the provision for Medicare, in 1965, followed by Medicaid and other programs, an ever growing portion of the population comes under the umbrella of health services provided by the government. This umbrella will certainly have wider coverage with the enactment of uniform and mandatory national health insurance.

As this umbrella of provided care expands, the nature of medicine becomes more social. This is particularly evident in the increasingly national nature of the health care delivery system. As the various levels of government become more and more involved in the health care enterprise, research addressing the many-faceted problems of comprehensive health care policy and planning becomes more and more important to them. Consequently, the various levels of government make available more and more financial and other support for such research. As a result, medical sociologists find, and are drawn to, new and nonmedical health research topics.

The second and somewhat related factor has been the growing redefinition of health and illness. Beginning with a classic essay by Dubos (1959), a

new orientation toward health has developed. Dubos argued that the traditional image of health as the absence of disease was merely a mirage. The conception of the established germ theory held that germs cause disease and that medicine's job was to eliminate germs, thus eliminating disease. Dubos argued that it is impossible to completely eliminate disease, especially in modern industrialized nations, where the process of living itself was constantly modifying the environment. For people, health consists of a relative state of adaptation to the environment. Because people constantly modify the environment, they are constantly in a relative state of maladaptation to it. Therefore, for Dubos and those that rallied to his position, the simplistic assumption that disease was something that could be totally eliminated by medical science became inappropriate. Rather, medicine should change its concentration of effort from strictly the elimination of disease to a balance that included the care and treatment of the sick. To do this, not only should physiological concerns be considered and treated, but so should social and psychological concerns.

As a result of the changing scope of medicine and the increasingly social nature of its delivery, sociological interest and research has gone beyond the general domain of medicine. Sociological studies now regularly report on a wide variety of health and health related issues. While *medicine* proper remains one of the major topics of theoretical and research interest, the allied fields and the general nature of *health* (in the broad sense consisting of physiological, social, and psychological adaptation) are being studied by many sociologists.

In order to modernize the original distinction between the sociologies *of* and *in* medicine, a number of medical sociologists have suggested that the distinction be modernized to the sociologies *of* and *in* health. Wilson (1970) has succinctly captured the meaning of this modernized distinction in writing that most sociological concerns with health may be characterized either as ". . . (1) detached observation and analysis, motivated primarily by a sense of *sociological* problem, or (2) more intimate, applied and conjoint research and teaching, motivated primarily by a sense of *health* problem." Those studies that fall under category one are studies in the sociology *of* health, while those falling under category two are studies in the sociology *in* health.

The Current Status
of the Sociology of Health

So far, we have developed and expanded Straus's initial concepts into the sociologies *of* and *in* health. It is now time to assess the current state of affairs in the sociology of health. The question of interest may be stated as follows: What is the current distribution of research efforts in the sociology of health in terms of the dichotomous distinction? In other words, what portion of the research currently being done may be classified as belonging to the sociology *of* health, and what portion may be classified as belonging to the sociology *in* health? We also want to know whether this proportion represents a change from the distribution of work done in this area during earlier periods.

To answer these questions, we must do two things. First, we must establish some benchmark for the distribution of work in medical sociology during its formative years. Second, we must survey current research efforts in the sociology of health. The first task, establishing a benchmark for purposes of comparison, is the easier of the two. Wilson has argued that in its formative years (approximately 1955 to 1964), most of the work done in medical sociology was clearly classifiable as sociology *of* medicine. In the years following this formative period (approximately 1965 to 1970), Wilson contends that efforts in medical sociology became rather evenly distributed. A review of the literature published during these periods provides a considerable amount of support for Wilson's evaluation.

A review of the state of medicine in these periods may provide an explanation for the changing distribution that Wilson describes. During the formative years of medical sociology, the invincible autonomy and private nature of medicine was reaching its peak, and starting on the rather rapid decline that it is currently experiencing. This decline was highly correlated with the increasing social nature of medicine, which was dramatically thrust upon the nation with the advent of Medicare, in 1965. As the social nature of medicine increased, the need for applied studies in the distribution and utilization of health services for use in planning new social programs and health care delivery systems also increased. The need for such applied studies was recognized, and research funds began to be earmarked more and more for

them (see Flook and Sanazarro, 1973). In addition to the social interest in health service studies, this helped to stimulate an increasing interest among sociologists for applied research. As a result of all this, research in the sociology *in* health soon became as common as research in the sociology *of* health.

Since 1970, popular and government interest in health and the health care system have become even more keen. It would seem reasonable to assume, therefore, that the distribution of research in medical sociology has continued to reflect the pattern that Wilson (1970) described. Our assumption is that this trend has continued to the point where most research in medical sociology may now be classified as sociology *in* health.

In order to test this assumption (the second task) we must survey the recent literature in the sociology of health. We can facilitate this survey by dividing the literature into the more or less natural categories of books and articles. Let us further limit our examination of articles to those published during a recent two-and-one-half-year period (1975 through 1977) in the *Journal of Health and Social Behavior* (the official medical sociology journal of the American Sociological Association). This should provide us with a rather representative example of the nature and distribution of articles published by sociologists of health.

Ninety articles were published in the issues of the *Journal of Health and Social Behavior* during this period. We reviewed these ninety articles using Wilson's distinction between the sociologies *of* and *in* health. Using what we considered to be a reasonable understanding of the sense of health problem versus the sense of sociological problem, we found a rather astonishing trend. Only about ten of the ninety articles could be classified as belonging to the sociology *of* health. The remaining eighty articles seemed rather clearly to belong to the sociology *in* health. Even more astonishing is the fact that this lopsided distribution may reflect a conservative bias favoring the sociology *of* health. This is because sociologists *in* health may seek to have their work published in journals that are more clearly oriented toward health service research. This would result in an underrepresentation of studies in the sociology *in* health appearing in the *Journal of Health and Social Behavior* (see Gold [1977] for an elaboration on this point).

An examination of books published during this period and falling into the general area of the sociology of health reveals a similar pattern. With the exception of a few new textbooks (such as Twaddle and Hessler, 1977) the majority of new books are primarily critiques of the political and economic aspects of health and medicine (including the following books by sociologists and nonsociologists: Illich, 1976; Carlson, 1975; Krause, 1977; Navarro, 1976; Mechanic, 1976; Gray, 1975). While this is a laudable topic, it is motivated primarily by a sense of the *health* problem. In fact, all too often these books are a reflection of their authors' outrage over the current status of the health care system. This frequently serves to reduce these books to the level of polemics, and in some cases to less than that (see especially Illich, 1976).

Ramifications of This Lopsided Distribution

What effect does this current concentration of research efforts in the sociology *in* health have upon the general development of the sociology of health? Has the lopsided distribution of efforts aided or hindered the growth of the sociology of health? This subject recently has been addressed in detail by Gibson (1972), Pflanz (1974, 1975), Johnson (1975) and Frankenberg (1974). In general, these authors believe that the dominance of the studies in the sociology *in* health has served to cultivate and perpetuate the atheoretical nature of the sociology of health. In all fairness to these authors, and to sociologists whom we would classify as health service researchers, we must point out that it is not our intent "to belittle the achievements, as far as they go, of empirical medical sociologists. It is medical sociology as integrative theory which is here under attack" (Frankenberg, 1974:426). Our primary concern is not to debunk the work of health service researchers. The quality and applicability of their research are not in question here. Our primary concern is with the adverse effect that the dominance of the sociology *in* health has had upon the development of the sociology of health as a *sociological enterprise,* and with the elimination of the adverse effects of what appears to be theoretical stagnation.

Much of the substance of Gibson's, Pflanz's, and Frankenberg's critiques must be taken with a grain of salt. Johnson, however, presents a realistic picture of the causes of the present atheoretical nature of the sociology of health, noting that the stunted theoretical growth of the sociology of health may be traced to three causal factors: ". . . (its) relative youth, financial and professional constraints and pressures on research, the apparent inability to challenge the fundamental precepts of society's dependence on medicine, and academic isolationism." These three factors . . . have resulted in the present concentration in the sociology *in* health rather than in the sociology *of* health. Being quite concerned that the stunted nature of theoretical development in the sociology of health would continue, Johnson proposed the following strategy:

> There must be an accommodation between the sociologies of *and* in *medicine, which allows their different perspectives to fertilize rather than antagonize each other. . . . It is suggested that a general pathway . . . is through the rediscovery of sociology as outlined earlier, and this can be divided into: (i) the widening of the sociological perspective in health and illness; (ii) becoming aware of and increasingly avoiding constraints on research; (iii) seeking firmer roots in mainstream sociology and (iv) reexcavating the theoretical tradition.*

Of these four routes to a sociology of health, the latter two are the most important. It is only through the medical sociologist's return to sociological training, especially its reliance upon the theoretical tradition, that a truly viable and useful *sociology* of health can be developed. This return to mainstream sociology within the sociology of health must not, however, ignore the contributions of sociologists *in* health. It should bring the distribution of efforts within the sociology of health back to the point where a more productive balance exists.

A SURVEY OF MEDICAL SOCIOLOGY

. . . We now turn our attention to the topic of what it is that medical sociologists are doing these days. Since its earliest days, medical sociology has been periodically surveyed, reviewed, and overviewed. Various of these "state of the field" pieces have been concerned with mapping out the early literature (Freeman and Reeder, 1957; Pearsall, 1963), the early research interests and priorities (Mangus, 1955; Jaco, 1958; Anderson and Seacat, 1958; Wallin and Seacat, 1962; Roemer and Elling, 1963; Medalia, 1964), the developing viewpoints (Bloom, 1965; Mechanic, 1966), the developing literature (Simmons and Berkanovic, 1972; Freeman, et al., 1972; Susser, 1974a, 1974b; Badgley, 1976; Litman, 1976), or concentrating on a specific topical area within medical sociology (McKinlay, 1972; Lorber, 1975). In addition to these and other individual efforts, the Medical Sociology Section of the American Sociological Association has recently prepared a monograph (Mechanic and Levine, 1977) which contains a series of state of the field papers for the major interest areas within medical sociology.

Rather than present yet another state of the field section, at this point, we shall briefly describe what medical sociologists are doing in the twelve special interest areas within which most contemporary medical sociology may be categorized. If, after reading the brief descriptions that follow, you find yourself developing an appetite for further information in any specific area, or for looking at the research literature in medical sociology firsthand, we suggest that you turn first to the *Journal of Health and Social Behavior*. It is the richest resource in all of medical sociology. Afterward, to find articles focusing on special topics you may want to thumb through the tables of contents in the more recent issues of these related journals: *Social Science and Medicine, Medical Care, Health Services Research*, the *American Journal of Public Health, Health and Society*, the *International Journal of Health Services*, the *Journal of Chronic Diseases*, the *Journal of Medical Education*, the *British Journal of Preventive and Social Medicine*, the *New England Journal of Medicine*, the *Journal of Human Stress*, and the *Journal of Behavioral Medicine*.

Social Epidemiology

Social epidemiology . . . involves studying the incidence, prevalence, and pattern of disease, disability, or mortality across a particular population. The social epidemiologist wants to: (1) determine on what basis a disease is distributed within the population; and (2) identify the social factors which may be among the causes of that disease. While social epidemiologists have traditionally been concerned with the social factors of age, sex, race, and social class, contemporary interest in the effects of attitudes and beliefs on the distribution of disease is increasing. Two examples of studies in social epidemiology are those studies that link social factors (such as the lifestyle trait of smoking) to the distribution of cancer and coronary heart disease. In these studies, higher incidence and prevalence rates for cancer and coronary heart disease are linked to cigarette smoking (showing how the disease is differentially distributed in the population). Then, the etiological or causal relationship is identified through controlled, longitudinal experiments. The most outstanding characteristic of social epidemiology is that it involves the application of the scientific method of investigation to trace the disease process. This investigation flows backwards from the end result or dependent variable (disease) through time to the social factors or independent variable (smoking) which occurred earlier in the patient's life. In essence, the social epidemiologist attempts to discover (much like a detective) what social factors are different in the life history of the disease-stricken individual from the life history of the general population.

Sociocultural Responses to Health and Illness

Studies that fall into this category of medical sociology are concerned with how people from different sociocultural heritages view their health, especially how their different sociocultural traditions affect their attitudes, beliefs, and behavior concerning health, illness, and death. At the moment, medical sociologists are especially interested in how and why people from different social groups respond differently to pain, and to the death and dying process. The underlying assumption here is that each sociocultural group has its own world view or philosophy. This world view is then manifested in the various typical behavior patterns that its members exhibit.

Patient–Practitioner Relationships

Studies in this category of medical sociology are primarily concerned with examining the social interactions that take place between the patient and the physician. Of special interest is the changing relationship between patient and physician in which the patient is becoming less dependent and more of an equal in these social interactions. This change from the traditionally physician-dominated patient–practitioner relationship may be traced to: (1) the rise of the consumer advocacy ethic; and (2) the growth of the women's equal rights movement in American society. Contemporary studies of the patient–practitioner relationships are showing much more of a negotiated-order process in medical care than ever before. The effects of this negotiated-order process on the traditional role of the patient and the physician are also of considerable interest. In fact, these effects serve as the motivation for several studies currently in progress.

The Sociology of the Hospital

In this area of medical sociology, the central theme concerns the organizational analysis of the hospital as a major component in the health care system. The most popular concepts or topics that are examined include: the bureaucratic structure of the hospital; intraprofessional relationships within the hospital; authority, power, and decision-making lines within the hospital; and the relationship of the hospital to the larger social community within which it exists. A particularly interesting phenomenon has been the changing nature of the hospital emergency room. The hospital emergency room was used in the past mainly for the intake of trauma or accident victims. It is now regularly used as the main source of primary care by the lower and lower-middle socioeconomic groups because: (1) they may not be able to afford private primary care (a function of insurance regulations which generally pay for emergency care but not office-related primary care); or, (2) they may not have access to primary care.

The Organization of Medical Care

Studies in this area of medical sociology are concerned with how differences in the organization of medical care and differences in the structure of the medical care system result in differences in the use of services by—and to the satisfaction of—the clientele. These studies typically examine the effects of differences in the delivery system such as method of payment (fee for service, prepaid, per capita) and type of practice setting (solo, partnership, group)

on outcome characteristics such as consumer satisfaction, surgical and hospital utilization, and the use of paraprofessionals. Most of these studies involve comparing these outcomes for individuals in one type of health care delivery system with the outcomes for similar individuals in a different type of health care delivery system. It was in studies such as these that the prepaid, group practice plans (health maintenance organizations) were shown to result in lower hospitalization rates, which meant a reduction in health care costs.

Health Service Utilization

Studies in health service utilization are concerned with finding out who uses (or does not use) health services (physicians, dentists, hospitals, clinics, and pharmaceuticals), how, when, where, and why. Most of these studies have emphasized two sets of individual characteristics, in addition to the nature and severity of the individual's illness, as the major causal factors. In the first set of characteristics are the sociodemographic variables such as age, sex, ethnicity, marital status, occupation, income, and education. In the second set of characteristics are the social psychological variables such as the individual's attitudes, beliefs, and orientation toward scientific medicine, and his or her perception of the marginal utility of health services to alleviate or prevent illness. These social psychological characteristics are viewed as determined in part by the sociodemographic characteristics. Health service utilization studies are concerned with the use of services for both restorative and preventive purposes.

The Sociology of Medical Education

The sociology of medical education has traditionally been one of the most popular areas in medical sociology. Most of the studies in this area have been concerned with how physicians are trained, how they come to be socialized into their role, and how they select a medical specialty. With the increasing societal concern and need for the production of more primary care physicians, studies concerned with the process of selecting a medical specialty have become quite popular. The major components in the causal process of medical specialty selection have been identified as the personal characteristics (past and present experiences and personality) of the medical student, the cognitive conception by the medical student of his or her environment, and the educational environment of the medical school attended (including reflected self-images, and refracted faculty images). Whether this information will be effectively used to increase the number of medical students opting for primary care specialties is not yet known.

The Sociology of Health Occupations

Interests in this area of medical sociology arise out of the general sociological concern with the study of occupations and professions. Studies of health occupations may be roughly divided into three groups. In the first group of studies, the central concern is with the profession of medicine, its development, growth, and continued autonomy as a true profession. Of particular interest here are the ramifications of the independence, autonomy, and dominance of physicians for the entire health care system. In the second group of studies, the general concern is with the development of the newer health occupations or the paraprofessionals (nurse practitioners, physicians' assistants, medical technologists). Of particular sociological interest here is the push for professional recognition by these occupations as evidenced in their increasing unionization, militancy toward physicians and health care administrators, and the changing nature of the assignments of health care tasks. The third group of studies is concerned with the relationships between the various health occupations, and how these relationships are changing. Of special interest here is the "pyramid" effect, in which, as the new health occupations are introduced at the patient contact level, the existing health occupations are pushed further away from the patient into bureaucratic, administrative, or consulting roles.

Medicalization of American Society

In this area of medical sociology, the major concern is with illness behavior as a form of deviance, generally studied with the theoretical perspective known as labeling or societal reaction. The particular sociological question that has been formulated is: How does deviant behavior become defined as a medical problem? The most widely known socially deviant behavior to be viewed in the context of medical problems have been, of course, certain forms of mental illness and homosexuality. Perhaps a less value-laden example of socially deviant behavior as an outcome of a medical problem would be hyperactivity (hyperkinesis). Although hyperactivity is recognized as a common medical illness among contemporary children, it did not exist a generation ago. In fact, the "hyperkinetic impulse disorder" was not recognized until 1957. While it is now a recognized disorder, no direct, organic causes of hyperactivity have yet been established. In essence, the medicalization of American society is concerned with how social control over socially deviant behavior is being transferred to the medical sector.

The Sociology of Stress and Coping Behavior

This area of medical sociology is concerned with studying (1) how social, organizational, and structural factors produce stress in our daily lives; (2) how social stress is related to illness; and (3) how individuals cope or adapt to their stressful environment. The major approaches in studying stress have their roots in social psychology. Some studies are concerned with how specific changes in our regular life events result in stress. Other studies are concerned with how these life change events are accumulated and increase the likelihood of illness and specific diseases (such as coronary heart disease, stomach ulcers, and schizophrenia). Some research focuses on the production of social stress from status inconsistency and downward occupational mobility. Medical sociologists appear to be divided on the issue of whether it is the life change events themselves, the individual's perceptions of these events, or the processes that produce the life change events that are the true causes of the social stress. In addition to studying how stress is produced and how it is related to illness, medical sociologists in this area are now working on models which explain how an individual copes with or adapts to social stress. A particular concern in this regard is whether or not the socialization process has provided the individual with the appropriate coping mechanisms or routines.

Social Psychiatry and Mental Health

One major result of research in this area of medical sociology has been the recognition that social factors affect the development, diagnosis, treatment, and duration of mental illness in the community. Much of this recognition has been the direct result of the earlier community psychiatry studies which were concerned with identifying the nature and prevalence of psychiatric impairment in the noninstitutionalized population. In these studies, the distribution of psychiatric disorders was found to be correlated with several social factors, especially social class position. Social class position was also found to play an important role in the differential treatment of psychiatric disorders. Of particular interest in recent years have been the social, legal, and ethical issues involved in defining mental illness and in the treatment of the mentally ill. In some respects, this concern with the treatment of the mentally ill has ceased to remain within the value-free orientation of sociology, and has taken on an ideological tone.

Social Policy and Health Care

Interest in this area of medical sociology is motivated by a desire to provide a better, or at least an equitable, health care delivery system. Accordingly, most of the studies that fall into this category suggest methods by which the alleged "crisis" in health care may be resolved. These studies and their proponents may be placed into three general groups. In the first group are those who suggest the crisis in the health care system may be fixed up or healed by minor adjustments to the existing delivery system. The second group of critics suggest that equitable and humane health care is just not feasible within a capitalistic system. They suggest that for the crisis in the health care system to be alleviated we must adopt a socialized medical subsystem within a larger socialized social system. The suggestions from the third group of critics are more devastating. They argue that we have misconceived the notions of health and illness, and have allowed our health to be expropriated by the established medical system. Their position is that we should increase self-care, assume more individual responsibility for our own health, and demystify medical care. . . .

References

ANDERSON, ODIN, and SEACAT, MILVOY
  1958 Behavioral science research in the health field: A statement of problems and priorities. *Social Problems* 6:268–71.

BADGLEY, ROBIN F., ed.
  1976 Social science and medicine in Canada. Special issue. *Social Science and Medicine* 10:1–68.

BILLINGS, JOHN S.
  1879 In *Treatise on Hygiene and Public Health,* edited by Henry Buck. New York: Wood.

BLOOM, SAMUEL
  1965 The sociology of medical education: Some comments on the state of the field. *Milbank Memorial Fund Quarterly* 43:143–84.

CARLSON, RICK
  1975 *The End of Medicine.* New York: Wiley-Interscience.

COCKERHAM, WILLIAM
  1978 *Medical Sociology.* New York: Prentice-Hall.

DENTON, JOHN
  1978 *Medical Sociology.* Boston: Houghton Mifflin.

DUBOS, RENE
  1959 *Mirage of Health.* New York: Doubleday.

FLOOK, EVELYN, and SANAZARRO, PAUL, eds.
  1973 *Health Services Research and R&D in Perspective.* Ann Arbor: Health Administration Press.

FRANKENBERG, RONALD
  1974 Functionalism and after? Theory and developments in social science applied to the health field. *International Journal of Health Services* 3:411–27.

FREEMAN, HOWARD, and REEDER, LEO
  1957 Medical sociology: A review of the literature. *American Sociological Review* 22:73–81.

FREEMAN, HOWARD, LEVINE, SOL, and REEDER, LEO, eds.
  1972 Present status of medical sociology. In *Handbook of Medical Sociology,* 2d ed., edited by Howard Freeman, Sol Levine, and Leo Reeder. New York: Prentice-Hall.

GIBSON, GEOFFREY
  1972 Theory vs. application at the ASA: A view of the issues. *Health Services Research* 7:243–53.

GOLD, MARGARET
  1977 A crisis of identity: The case of medical sociology. *Journal of Health and Social Behavior* 18:160–68.

GRAY, BRADFORD
  1975 *Human Subjects in Medical Experimentation: A Sociological Study of the Conduct and Regulation of Clinical Research.* New York: Wiley-Interscience.

ILLICH, IVAN
  1976 Medical Nemesis: The Expropriation of Health. New York: Pantheon.

JACO, E. GARTLEY
  1958 Areas for research in medical sociology. *Sociology and Social Research* 42:441–44.

JOHNSON, MALCOLM
1975 Medical sociology and sociological theory. *Social Science and Medicine* 9:227–32.

KENDALL, PATRICIA
1963 Medical sociology in the United States. *Social Science Information* 2:1–13.

KENDALL, PATRICIA, and MERTON, ROBERT
1958 Medical education as a social process. In *Patients, Physicians and Illness,* edited by E. G. Jaco. New York: Free Press.

KENDALL, PATRICIA, and READER, GEORGE
1972 Contributions of sociology to medicine. In *Handbook of Medical Sociology,* 2d ed., edited by H. E. Freeman, S. Levine, and L. Reeder. New York: Prentice-Hall.

KRAUSE, ELLIOTT A.
1977 *Power and Illness: The Political Sociology of Health and Medical Care.* New York: Elsevier.

LITMAN, THEODOR J.
1976 *The Sociology of Medicine and Health Care: A Research Bibliography.* San Francisco: Boyd and Fraser.

LORBER, JUDITH
1975 Women and medical sociology: Invisible professionals and ubiquitous patients. *Sociological Inquiry* 45:75–105.

McKINLAY, JOHN B.
1972 Some approaches and problems in the study of the use of services: An overview. *Journal of Health and Social Behavior* 13:115–52.

MANGUS, A. R.
1955 Medical sociology: Study of the social components of illness and health. *Sociology and Social Research* 49:158–64.

MECHANIC, DAVID
1966 The sociology of medicine: Viewpoints and perspectives. *Journal of Health and Human Behavior* 7:237–47.

1976 *The Growth of Bureaucratic Medicine: An Inquiry into the Dynamics of Patient Behavior and the Organization of Medical Care.* New York: Wiley-Interscience.

1978 *Medical Sociology: A Comprehensive Text,* 2d ed. New York: Free Press.

MECHANIC, DAVID, and LEVINE, SOL, eds.
1977 Issues in promoting health: Committee reports of the medical sociology section of the American Sociological Association. *Medical Care* 15 (supplement to issue 5):1–101.

MEDALIA, NAHUM Z.
1964 Foreword: The environmental health challenge to medical sociology. *Journal of Health and Human Behavior* 5:131–32.

NAVARRO, VICENTE
1976 *Medicine Under Capitalism.* New York: Prodist Press.

PEARSALL, MARION
1963 *Medical Behavioral Science: A Selected Bibliography.* Lexington: University of Kentucky Press.

PFLANZ, MANFRED
1974 A critique of Anglo-American medical sociology. *International Journal of Health Services* 4:565–74.

1975 Relations between social scientists, physicians and medical organizations in health research. *Social Science and Medicine* 9:7–13.

ROEMER, MILTON, and ELLING, RAY
1963 Sociological research on medical care. *Journal of Health and Human Behavior* 4:49–68.

SIMMONS, OZZIE, and BERKANOVIC, EMIL
1972 Social research in health and medicine: A bibliography. In *Handbook of Medical Sociology,* 2d ed., edited by Howard Freeman, Sol Levine, and Leo Reeder. New York: Prentice-Hall.

STRAUS, ROBERT
1955 The development of a social science teaching and research program in a medical center. Paper presented to the American Sociological Society.

1957 The nature and status of medical sociology. *American Sociological Review* 22:200–204.

SUCHMAN, EDWARD
1967 The survey method applied to public health and medicine. In *Survey Research in the Social Sciences,* edited by C. Y. Glock. New York: Russell Sage.

SUSSER, MERVYN
1974a Introduction to the theme: A critical review of sociology in health. *International Journal of Health Services* 4:407–409.

1974b A critical review of sociology in health. Special issue. *International Journal of Health Services* 4:403–578.

TWADDLE, ANDREW, and HESSLER, RICHARD
1977 *A Sociology of Health.* St. Louis: Mosby.

WELLIN, EDWARD, and SEACAT, MILVOY
1962 Social science in the health field: A review of research. *American Journal of Public Health* 52:1465–72.

WILSON, ROBERT N.
1970 *The Sociology of Health: An Introduction.* New York: Random House.

Reflections and Opportunities in the Sociology of Medicine

Renée C. Fox

. . . My wide-ranging experiences as a sociologist of medicine have been shaped, of course, by my background and training, interests and temperament, by my convictions, and by the mysterious forces of serendipity. But these experiences are also inherent in the place and meaning of health, illness, and medicine in society, and therefore, in principle, they are accessible to sociologists of medicine, whatever qualities, preferences, outlook, or style of work they bring to the field. Furthermore, in our own society since the 1950s, the scope of matters pertinent to the sociology of medicine has broadened and grown more inclusive as the health-illness-medicine complex has become a metaphorical language and a symbolic medium through which American society has been grappling with fundamental questions of value and belief, basic to our cultural tradition and collective conscience, that ramify far beyond medicine.

Here, in my view, we encounter a paradoxical feature of the way that the field of medical sociology has developed. Its sphere is potentially vast; the number of social scientists it has drawn into its orbit is impressively large; the literature it has generated is sizeable. And yet, on closer inspection, the phenomena, milieux, and themes with which sociologists of medicine have been concerned are relatively restricted and selective.

We sociologists have studied patients and patients' families less than we would like to believe, and medical professionals more than we would suppose, or probably consider appropriate. Within this framework, we have directed a large share of our attention to physicians, much less to nurses, and a negligible amount to the many other groups of professionals, semi-professionals, and non-professionals who do medical or medically associated work. By and large, we have been more concerned with mental than with physical illness, with sickness than with health, and only with a narrow cross-section of the array of diseases and disorders to which men, women, and children are subject. Over the course of three decades, we have devoted thousands of pages to debating the merits and demerits of the concepts of the sick role and of illness behavior. In our discussions about medical professionals, we have been preoccupied, if not obsessed with the professional dominance of physicians, their institutionalized individualism and autonomy, their insistence on self-regulation and self-control, their sense of hierarchy, their paternalism, and their power over patients' bodies, minds, and behavior, as well as their economic and political dominion.

In a somewhat different tone of voice, we have also written extensively about physicians' loss of idealism, their progressive cynicism, their problems of detached concern (particularly of over-detachment, distancing, and impersonality), their training for, and ways of coping with, uncertainty, limitation, and errors and mistakes at work.

We have focused mainly on medical professionals, especially the doctor, as he/she (more often, he) functions in medical training and hospital situations. Although we have been consistently interested in the culture as well as the social structure of medical schools, we have, with some classic exceptions, been more inclined to look at the hospital as a highly bureaucratized formal organization than as a social world with many distinctive features and much human pathos (Coser, 1962; Fox, 1959; Goffman, 1961; Stanton and Schwartz, 1954).

We have had a pronounced tendency to fixate on certain conceptual insights, and to use them rhetorically and ideologically, rather than as catalysts for detailed, first-hand empirical research. (If we continue in this fashion, then it is almost predictable

Reprinted from the *Journal of Health and Social Behavior,* vol. 26 (1985), pp. 6–14.

that phrases like "the coming of the corporation" in American medicine [Starr, 1982], and "the medical-industrial complex" [Relman, 1980] will soon replace the "professional dominance" theme [Freidson, 1970] that we have so continually invoked in recent years.) We have been social critics of medicine as much as, if not more than, we have been social observers of it. Particularly since the 1960s, it is striking how sparse the corpus of sociology of medicine studies we have conducted is in comparison with the copious, editorial-like commentary on undesirable aspects of the American medical profession and of health care in our society in which we have engaged. Searching social criticism and careful social research have not been joined in the way one would ideally hope, and partly as a consequence of the relative dearth of rich, new studies, in our teaching and writing, we still rely heavily (I would contend, too heavily) on medical sociological work that was done decades ago. Most of our research, analysis and interpretation is centered on health, illness, and medicine in American society. Our cross-cultural and comparative endeavors are thin in two senses: We do not do many studies of this sort, and when we do, they tend to be stronger in social structural than in cultural analysis.

SOME UNDERDEVELOPED DIRECTIONS OF INQUIRY

I hope that you do not consider my perspective on the current state of medical sociology unjust or unduly dolorous. My primary reason for sharing with you what seem to me to be some of the characteristic intellectual patterns in our field—its lacunae, as well as areas that are well-developed, and some that may even be overdeveloped—is to encourage you to undertake more research on some important and potentially engrossing medical sociological phenomena to which we have thus far paid relatively little attention. Let me identify a few such areas of inquiry that occur to me. I will simply mention some of these, and briefly discuss others.

The characteristics and implications of the greatly increased number of women who have been entering the medical profession in the past 15 years is an important subject for sociological research. Women make up almost 30% of students currently

in medical school, as compared to the less than 10% of the national medical student body that they constituted in the late 1960s. Who are these women, sociologically speaking? Why have they chosen medicine? How are they affected by the medical education and socialization process, and how, in turn, do they affect it? How do they relate to patients, patients' families, medical and nursing professionals, to each other, to family, friends and activities outside of, and beyond, their medical lives? What kinds of careers are they selecting and shaping, and why? In what ways are their experiences, reactions, and choices like and unlike those of male medical students, house officers, and physicians in practice? What short-term and long-term differences will the presence of a significant proportion of women in medicine make in the attitudes, values, patterns of work and interaction, ethos, atmosphere and style of the profession? Will a greater "feminization" of the medical profession take place, in the socio-cultural sense of the term and with what medical and social consequences?

Along with the altered sex ratio in medicine, another demographic shift has changed the age composition of patients. The aging of the American population has greatly increased the number of older persons now seeking and receiving medical care. This has modified the nature of the health problems with which medical personnel and institutions are being confronted, and the frequency with which certain medical problems come before them. For example, the greying of the patient population is significantly associated with the larger proportion of persons who are afflicted with chronic and degenerative diseases in general, and with the notable rise in the incidence of cancer and of Alzheimer's disease. This also means that medical and nursing caretakers are being brought into more continuous contact with what it is like to be elderly in our society, at our present stage of cultural, economic, political, and scientific development. They not only see many of the potentialities and special challenges of this stage of the life cycle, but they are confronted with all the painful, often tragic problems that it can entail, and with their own professional and human limitations in the face of them: problems of aloneness, retirement and idleness, financial difficulties, physical and/or mental incapacity, the spectre of a nursing home, and a prolonged, costly, anguishing process of dying sustained by technology, among others. We have only begun to grasp and to deal with such medically relevant aspects of growing old and being mortal in American society, and with their impact on the medical professionals and paraprofessionals responsible for the care of the elderly, as well as on these older patients themselves and their relatives. The cruelly desperate responses of house officers to hospitalized, elderly, chronically ill, demented patients, satirically described in Samuel Shem's notorious novel, *The House of God* (1978), on the one hand, and the development of the hospice as a new philosophical and organizational way of caring for dying patients, on the other, are both related phenomena that merit study in this and other connections. In any case, there is a great deal of needed and valuable research, writing, and teaching that sociologists can, and ideally ought to, undertake in this sphere.

In discussing women and the elderly in medicine, I have touched upon another set of concerns that I have long thought we sociologists have neglected. This is what I have termed in my own writing, "the human condition of health professionals" (Fox, 1980). By this I mean the ways in which the distinctive features of medical work, particularly its relationship to life, death and suffering, and to the human body and psyche, place demands and stresses on health professionals who, in response, tend to develop certain collective as well as individual defense mechanisms to cope with them. These characteristic modes of coming to terms have basic implications for the professional person's relationship to self, colleagues, patients, and patients' families, in ways that can powerfully affect the technical and the human quality of care that health professionals are and are not able to deliver and sustain. I am convinced that we should pay more systematic attention to these matters, including the phenomena of so-called "burnout" and "impairment" among health professionals about which there is increasing awareness and concern, and the question of whether and how the socialization of health professionals, their work situations, and their socially patterned defense mechanisms could be modified to make medicine more humane and humanizing, both for those who receive and those who deliver care.

I have alluded to the fact that, in my opinion, we have understudied nurses and nursing. There are at least three reasons why nursing ought to be of great interest to sociologists:

(1) It is a profession that always has been, and that continues to be, made up predominantly of women;

(2) It is an occupation that has been undergoing an extensive process of professional upgrading, sparked by a number of social developments (the women's movement among them), and accompanied by both internal and external struggles over such issues as hospital/diploma school versus baccalaureate training, unionization, and the emergence of nurse-practitioners;

(3) The nurse's professional role brings her more closely and continuously in contact with other members of the medical team, and with what it is like to be sick and a patient. As primary caretaker and observer-participant, she is a rich custodian and source of firsthand knowledge and understanding in this regard, from whom sociologists as well as physicians have a great deal to learn. In this connection, I can testify to the fact that in the kind of *in situ* medical sociological fieldwork I have done, whether in the United States, Europe, Africa or China, nurses have always been among my most important informants and valued teachers.

I have indicated that I think sociologists could do far more research on the social and cultural history and meaning of different diseases and disorders: how these conditions are thought about and what they signify in particular societies and time periods; how and why the conception and significance of these illnesses change; what persons with these conditions mutually experience as a consequence of the social and cultural as well as medical sense and import of their disease—the patterning of their symptoms and illness behavior, the kinds of personal, sociological stories they live out. Here, sociology of knowledge, science, and culture perspectives could be joined with sociology of medicine in an illuminating way. This perspective could also be brought to bear on sociological studies of the emergence of new disorders (the "battered child syndrome," for example, and AIDS—acquired immune deficiency syndrome): the processes by which they appear, are discovered, defined, explained, reacted to and handled. I have the general impression that medical anthropologists and medical historians, and certain European sociologists (Herzlich and Pierret, 1984) are more fruitfully involved in such studies of illness than we are. I do not think I am succumbing either to rancor about disciplinary turf or to intellectual chauvinism, when I say that there is no inherent reason why this should be so.

Nor is there any facile explanation for the fact that we no longer study patients in the hospital to the extent that we used to, and in the ways that we did in the 1950s and 1960s. In that period, we carried out and published an impressive array of studies—often ethnographic in nature, and more frequently set in mental hospitals than in those devoted to physical disease—in which we vividly described and systematically analyzed the social worlds of hospital patients, and both their separateness from, and interconnection with, the worlds of the hospital staff. Why do we now leave such accounts to novelists, writers of television scripts, and authors of eloquent personal testimony? For that matter, we have not been studying physicians and nurses at work in various hospital settings very much of late, either. Books like Charles Bosk's *Forgive and Remember* (1979), or Diane Scully's *Men Who Control Women's Health* (1980), are exceptions rather than the rule. And we have virtually never studied the occupational communities formed within the hospital by what we have treated as a gigantic residual category in medical sociology (made up of non-nurse, non-doctor, so-called "other members of the medical team," paramedical personnel, domestic, maintenance, transport, and business employees, and so on). No matter how well staffed a modern hospital may be with medical and nursing professionals, it could not function without all these other workers in whom we have never taken any real sociological interest.

There is a body of research in process that I hope will help to counterbalance our recent tendency to veer away from first-hand hospital studies. I refer here to doctoral and post-doctoral research being done by nurses with professional training in sociology and/or anthropology who are studying such things as the neonatal intensive care unit, the oncology ward, the nephrology service and the emergency room, from a combined nursing and social science point of view, using "thick descriptive," qualitative, as well as more quantitative methods to do so.

I am sure that every one of us here recognizes that whatever their genre or focus, our sociological studies of hospitals in the 1980s should include careful and extensive research on what Paul Starr, in *The Social Transformation of American Medicine* (1982), describes as "the coming of the corporation" to American health care in general, and to hospital care in particular. I have already stated how important I believe it to be that we not settle for judgmental stands, ideological positions, and Sinclair Lewis/ *Arrowsmith*-like moralizing about these developments, but that we base whatever evaluative, critical analyses we may eventually make on well-designed sociological studies of the forms that this ostensible growth of corporate medicine is taking, and of its planned and unplanned, manifest and latent, anticipated and unanticipated consequences. There is a certain irony in the fact that we have fewer ethnographic studies of the inner world of the hospital than we did two or three decades ago. For, they would provide valuable baseline data relevant to the microcosmic social, cultural, and human changes that this putative "transformation of American medicine" might effect, to place alongside of the macro-level kinds of political and economic data about its implications that are presently available.

CHANGES IN AMERICAN MEDICINE

These social organizational and political economic changes occurring in American medicine sharply remind us that, until now, we have confined our sociological studies of medicine, medical practice, medical professionals and practitioners, patients and clients to a restricted range of contexts. We have not even carried out many studies of physicians and patients in relatively ordinary, private practice settings. And we certainly did not have to wait until the present-day corporate developments in medicine had taken place to study medical professionals as they function in profit-making enterprises like the pharmaceutical industry, medical equipment manufacturing and supply firms, and health insurance companies. These, too, are studies we have neglected in the past that are worthy of future medical sociological attention, although because of the way that our field has been oriented, there is not much comparative, sociohistorically relevant data with which to work (Barber, 1967; Fox, 1961).[1]

I am not advocating that we only concentrate

on "establishment" and allopathic medicine, whether it takes individual, fee-for-service, group practice, health maintenance organization, or corporate form. Another whole set of developments into which we ought to inquire more vigorously and extensively are the many different kinds of alternative health movements present on the American scene. Such movements (both secular and religious in nature, and often complex mixes between the two) have always abounded in American society. But in certain historical periods—at the turn of the century, for example, and in the last twenty years as well, these movements have been especially prominent and plentiful. We need to know far more than we do about those that have developed since the 1960s: about the medical, social, and cultural factors that have been conducive to their florescence; about their leaders, members and practitioners; about the concepts, techniques, corpus of knowledge, values and beliefs, and in some cases, world view, around which they are organized; about their relationship to modern Western and/or other systems and professions of medicine, to the Malinowskian "three-cornered constellation" of science, religion, and magic (1948), and to the family, economy, and polity. Our studies of health and medicine-related movements of the past twenty years should include research on the variety of self-help and holistic medicine phenomena that are currently flourishing, whether these take the form of the collective effervescence around jogging and exercise regimes and diets and health foods, or the great interest in certain health situations and social settings in obtaining care without resort to a physician. The involvement of the women's movement in health and medical care rights, and the appearance of a whole series of movements concerned with the rights of patients, of handicapped persons, and of research subjects constitute another set of important, recent developments of considerable political and legal, as well as socio-cultural significance to which more serious medical sociological consideration ought to be given.

These social movements are related to a much larger and deeper societal happening: the fact that health, illness, and medicine have become media through which we are collectively struggling with issues that are integral to the value and belief systems of American society. Nowhere is this more evident than in the emergence and escalation of bioeth-

ics in the United States over the past 15 to 20 years: a new, interdisciplinary area, focused on what are considered to be serious problems associated with scientific and technological advances in biomedicine, that has now assumed great public and political as well as intellectual and professional importance. The limited participation of social scientists in this field troubles me.

Judith Swazey and I have indicated in our recent article, "Medical Morality Is Not Bioethics" (1984)[2]

In the prevailing ethos of bioethics, the value of individualism is defined in such a way, and emphasized to such a degree, that it is virtually severed from social . . . values concerning relationships between individuals; their responsibilities, commitments, and emotional bonds to one another; the significance of the groups and the societal community to which they belong; and the deep inward as well as outward influence that these have on the individual and his or her sense of the moral. Social dimensions of ethicality are largely compressed into and meted out through a "do good" and "avoid harm" idea of beneficence.

Bioethics is also inattentive to the social and cultural sources and implications of its own thought. Not only is this essentially unsocial and culturally near-sighted framework being brought to bear on ethical decision-making in medicine, but like Mr. Smith, it has "gone to Washington," where it has become the major grid within which bioethical issues are being deliberated in our courts, legislatures, and in the executive branch of our government. Furthermore, concentration on bioethics, defined and oriented in this way, has been progressively taking the social, the cultural and to some degree, the psychological, out of medical education. Increasingly, discussion of ethical issues and courses devoted to them are displacing teaching about what was termed, in a previous era of medical education, the behavioral science content of its curriculum and training.

These expansionary tendencies of bioethics, with their worrisome implications, constitute a veritable "ethics epidemic." I hope that I have said enough to indicate that the social significance of bioethics is neither trivial nor confined to medicine, and to persuade you that social scientists like ourselves ought to be more present and active in this field as conceptual, empirical, and social policy contributors to it, and analysts of it as a social and cultural phenomenon.

THE SOCIOLOGY OF BIOMEDICAL RESEARCH

There is one more item in my inventory of compelling medical sociological research that I would like to put before you. For many years, I have been amazed at the virtual absence of first-hand, sociology of medical science studies in our field—amazed, because I consider the study of how scientific discoveries are made and scientific work is done to be intellectually fascinating and socially important. As long ago as 1952, Robert K. Merton made the following statement about the general condition of the sociology of science:

> There already exists . . . a vast literature on "scientific method" and, by inference, on the "attitudes" and "values" of scientists. But this literature is concerned with what the social scientists would call ideal patterns, that is, with ways in which scientists ought to think, feel, and act. It does not necessarily describe, in needed detail, the ways in which scientists actually do think, feel, and act. Of these actual patterns, there has been little systematic study. . . . It is at least possible that if social scientists were to begin observations in the laboratories and field stations of physical and biological scientists, more might be learned, in a comparatively few years, about the psychology and sociology of science than in all the years that have gone before.

We have neither made such observations, nor learned very much about the sociology of science in the 32 years that have ensued since Merton wrote this. I am reminded of this fact continually in a variety of ways, as a consequence of some of the field observations I have made in connection with my interest in the sociology of medical research and of therapeutic innovation. For example, I have often been struck by the socially patterned array of game-like and humor-infused rituals that occur in many laboratories where medical investigators are engaged in path-making research that carries with it a high level of uncertainty and risk, especially when that research is related to an experimental therapy intended for patients. Under such circumstances, a highly structured "game of chance" is likely to develop between investigators through which they make playful predictions about, and take bets on, how certain of their experiments are likely to turn out. Not uncommonly, such research groups also name their laboratory animals in ways that make ironic or gallows-humor commentary on the experimental work in which they are involved: its meaning and justification, the hopes built into it, and the stresses that it entails. Considerable intellectual and emotional energy may be invested in choosing what the team considers to be an appropriate name for an animal, and in some instances there may even be something akin to a naming ceremony. We have scarcely begun to record such patterns of what I have come to think of as "scientific magic," much less interpret them and analyze their implications for the structure and dynamics of medical scientific work and its consequences.

Another, in some ways related, set of patterns shared by medical scientists concerns the nature of the technical vocabulary that they invent, adopt, and use in their published and oral communications. Many biomedical words and phrases have strong, more-than-scientific sentiments coded into them: the "dread graft-versus-host disease reaction" to bone marrow transplantation; for example, "harvesting" organs for human organ transplantation; "promiscuous DNA" (a term introduced into the molecular biology literature a year and a half ago); "recognition of self and not-self" in the language of immunology; and "searching for the Holy Grail" (i.e., for understanding of the structure of the "T cell"). There is cogent evidence to suggest that shared attitudes, values, beliefs, feelings, experiences, and something akin to a common metaphysical view are embedded in the inner-language messages that medical scientists' technical vocabulary contains. This is a tantalizing area for sociolinguistic analysis, from which (to reinvoke Merton's statement), we could learn much about "the ways in which scientists think, feel and act."

Finally, every time that I have read about and reflected on a case of scientific fraud that has come to light in the past few years, I am acutely reminded of the fact that because of the paucity of empirical social knowledge about how scientists work, we have very little data and only a few insights to offer that might help to answer the question of whether these forms of scientific deviance are happening more frequently than in the past, and to identify the phenomena that are contributing to their occurrence. It is striking, for example, that in several cases of biomedical fraud that have been publicly discussed, the chief investigator and director of the research team did not have the kind of direct, knowledgeable relationship to the work of his teammate who falsified data that could have prevented this deviant behavior from taking place, nipped it in the bud, or detected it quickly once it happened. One of the sets of factors to which this knowledge and communication gap may be related is the composition and organization of the modern scientific research team. Given the increasingly large size of the teams in which medical research, like other forms of scientific inquiry, is now done, with their complex, internal division of labor, of specialized knowledge, and of technical competence, it is difficult for even the most responsible and intelligent principal investigator to supervise or thoroughly understand all the work of all the colleagues doing research under his aegis. Having said this, however, it is difficult to find detailed, sociological studies that provide informative data on the social systems of present-day medical research teams, how they function and misfunction, and how they are perceived and experienced by the many persons in different statuses and roles who belong to them.

ZESTFUL DISCONTENTS

My criticism of the current state of the field of medical sociology and my dissatisfaction with it are, as I hope you have discerned, a form of divine sociological discontent. I like being a sociologist. That is plain. I not only believe in principle, but have found in fact, that working as a sociologist of medicine gives one the opportunity to study a variety of interesting and moving aspects of social and cultural life that are both basic and transcendent. It is also a meaningful way of contributing to sociological knowledge and understanding, to resonant teaching, and to humanely effective medical care and policy. This is not to say that my experience as a sociologist of medicine

has been devoid of doubt, anxiety, and sadness. The kind of intense, unrelenting, exposed field involvement with chronic and terminal illness, suffering, human comedy and tragedy, and with "experiment perilous" (Fox, 1959) medicine that my work as a sociologist has entailed, not only enriches, it also takes a toll. (This, too, is a matter that ideally ought to be studied: the long-term effect of working continually in a given sphere of society, using certain methods of inquiry, focusing on particular phenomena, issues, and themes—including how it looks and feels to the sociologist in different phases of one's personal and professional life cycle.)

In 1983, I wrote a paper reflecting on some of the exacting and depleting aspects of my long-term immersion as a participant observer in the medical and social evolution of dialysis and organ transplantation. Entitled "Leaving the Field," it was intended as an announcement that I was calling a personal moratorium on any further research and writing about dialysis and transplantation. In the last lines of the paper, I noted with some amusement that, my declaration notwithstanding, I was zestfully making plans for a field trip to Salt Lake City that spring to gather materials on the development of the Jarvik VII artificial heart and its implantation in Dr. Barney Clark. (Now, I would have to follow Dr. William De Vries, the Utah surgeon who performed that implant, to the Humana Heart Institute International in Louisville, Kentucky, with which he has become affiliated. This, in turn, would directly involve me in studying the role that such corporations currently play both in clinical research and in medical care.) I also noted at the time that my contemplated disengagement made me feel as though I were going through a divorce, leaving a religious order, and/or deserting comrades in crisis. It will not surprise you to learn that I am still "in the field" (Fox, 1984), and that the paper about leaving it has been relegated to my files.[3]

Notes

1. Bernard Barber's book, *Drugs and Society* (1967), took pioneering steps in exploring the drug industry, conceptually and empirically. Out of earlier, collaborative work that I did with him in the sociology of science, using the drug industry as one research site, I published an

article based on face-to-face interviews with all the physicians who were employed in a major pharmaceutical firm (Fox, 1961).

2. See especially pp. 352–360.

3. Judith Swazey and I are continuing our joint study of the development of the artificial heart, and have extended it from the University of Utah to the Humana Heart Institute in Louisville, Kentucky.

References

BARBER, BERNARD
1967 Drugs and Society. New York: Russell Sage Foundation.

BOSK, CHARLES L.
1979 Forgive and Remember: Managing Medical Failure. Chicago: University of Chicago Press.

COSER, ROSE L.
1962 Life in the Ward. East Lansing: Michigan State University Press.

FOX, RENÉE C.
1959 Experiment Perilous: Physicians and Patients Facing the Unknown. Glencoe, IL: Free Press.

1961 "Physicians on the drug side of the prescription blank." Journal of Health and Human Behavior 2:3–16.

1980 "The human condition of health professionals." Distinguished Lecture Series, School of Health Studies, University of New Hampshire, 1980.

1984 " 'It's the same, but different': A sociological perspective on the case of the Utah artificial heart." Pp. 68–90 in Margery W. Shaw (ed.), After Barney Clark: Reflections on the Utah Artifical Heart. Austin: University of Texas Press.

FREIDSON, ELIOT
1970 Professional Dominance. New York: Atherton Press.

GOFFMAN, ERVING
1961 Asylums. New York: Doubleday-Anchor.

HERZLICH, CLAUDINE, and JANINE PIERRET
1984 Malades d'hier, Malades d'aujourd'hui: De la mort collective au devoir de guerison (Patients of Yesterday, Patients of Today: From Collective Death to the Duty to Heal). Paris: Editions Payot.

MALINOWSKI, BRONISLAW
1948 Magic, Science and Religion. Glencoe, IL: Free Press.

MERTON, ROBERT K.
1952 "Foreword." Pg. xxii in Bernard Barber (ed.), Science and the Social Order. Glencoe, IL: Free Press.

RELMAN, ARNOLD S.
1980 "The new medical-industrial complex." New England Journal of Medicine 303:963–970.

SCULLY, DIANE
1980 Men Who Control Women's Health: The Miseducation of Obstetrician-Gynecologists. Boston: Houghton Mifflin Co.

SHEM, SAMUEL
1978 The House of God. New York: Richard Marek.

STANTON, ALFRED, and MORRIS S. SCHWARTZ.
1954 The Mental Hospital. New York: Basic Books.

STARR, PAUL E.
1982 The Social Transformation of American Medicine. New York: Basic Books.

SWAZEY, JUDITH P., and RENÉE C. Fox
1984 "Medical morality is not bioethics—medical ethics in China and the United States." Perspectives in Biology and Medicine 27:336–360.

PART ONE

The Client

CHAPTER 2

The Patient Status: The Sick Role Perspective

A central concern of sociologists studying the sick role has been the analysis of the expectations that society holds concerning the appropriate behavior for someone in that role. In 1951, Talcott Parsons presented his classic description of a set of four expectations that he felt were most commonly accepted by sick people. According to Parsons, the sick person typically understands that he or she (1) is relieved of normal duties, (2) is not responsible for the condition and cannot cure himself or herself, (3) is in an undesirable condition and must try to get better, and (4) must seek medical help. Parsons named this set of four expectations the "sick role," and it has become the most common view of the patient employed by sociologists. A person who accepts these expectations is said to have adopted the sick role. Studies have shown that people may accept some, but not necessarily all, of the four responsibilities.

Underlying the notion of a sick role is the recognition that an important distinction must be made between illness and sickness. Illness refers to the actual existence of ill health, whereas sickness refers to the behavior appropriate for one who is ill. Given this distinction, one can see the possibility of sickness without illness and illness without sickness. An example of the former would be a student who is not really ill but adopts the sick role when he or she wants to avoid taking a final exam. An article in this chapter suggests that some welfare mothers may accept the sick role without being ill in order to justify their dependence on society and their failure to support themselves. In contrast, not all persons who experience illness will adopt the sick role. There is some evidence, for example, that physicians find it difficult to accept the sick role for themselves. One writer cites the case of a middle-aged physician who had an acute coronary attack. His professional colleagues who diagnosed his illness advised immediate and absolute bed rest, quiet, and heavy sedation, all of which he refused. He maintained his normal routine of work and died suddenly in his office 20 hours later.

Critics of the sick-role model question what they see as its limited applicability. They maintain that it has much less relevance to those with chronic illnesses than to those with acute illnesses. Thus, a person with arthritis or multiple sclerosis cannot usually "get well" in the normal sense.

The first article in this chapter, by Alexander Segall, provides a clear introduction to Parsons' sick role within an empirical context. Segall looks at how cultural differences influence expectations related to each of the four sick-role obligations. In the following article (a study of welfare mothers), Stephen Cole and Robert Lejeune show that adoption of the sick role can sometimes be a response to the feeling that one is not fulfilling one's social obligations. David C. Stewart and Thomas J. Sullivan discuss the case of chronic illness and the problems it holds for the adoption of the sick role. In the case of patients suffering from multiple sclerosis, the difficulty in the diagnosis of the disease can lead to a substantial amount of distress, both physical and interpersonal. Finally, the article by Peter L. Heller and his colleagues explores the relationship between social class and perceptions of what constitutes mental illness and appropriate care.

Reference

PARSONS, T. 1951. *The Social System*. Glencoe, Ill.: The Free Press.

Sociocultural Variation in Sick Role Behavioural Expectations

Alexander Segall

SOCIOCULTURAL FACTORS AND ILLNESS BEHAVIOUR

The cultural approach to the analysis of health and illness involves the study of "the relationship between cultural content and cultural life styles on the one hand, and definitions of health and responses to illness on the other"[7]. The distinctive way of life which characterizes a particular group or subgroup of a society may influence illness behaviour in a variety of ways. For example, subcultural groups vary in the extent to which bodily conditions are perceived, evaluated and expressed as symptomatic of a state of illness. In other words, what is recognized as health or illness is largely a matter of cultural prescription. Furthermore, the cultural context also influences beliefs in regard to the cause of illness and the alternative forms of treatment considered.

There have been a number of empirical studies of the relationship between sociocultural factors and selected aspects of illness behaviour, including the following: (1) the meaning attached to the sensation of pain and the style of pain expression[20]; (2) the perception and reporting of symptoms[21]; (3) knowledge about the causes of various diseases and preventive medical behaviour[3,17]; and (4) willingness to consult a physician and to utilize health care facilities[8]. These studies all stress the importance of the influence exerted by sociocultural factors. However, this body of research provides very limited information regarding sociocultural variations in an extremely important aspect of the social process of

Reprinted from *Social Science and Medicine*, vol. 10 (1976), pp. 47–54.

"being sick," i.e. the perception of and willingness to adopt the sick role.

Sociocultural Differences and the Sick Role

A review of the literature reveals a lack of studies which have attempted, in a systematic and comprehensive fashion, to determine whether sociocultural differences exist in sick role behavioural expectations. The general tendency has been to accept uncritically the assumption that the pattern of expected behaviour described by Parsons is the same for all members of society. In fact, Gordon has argued that one effect of Parsons' original conceptualization "has been to draw investigators' attention away from sociocultural variations in illness behaviour"[4].

The role of the sick person was described by Parsons[11] in terms of two major rights and two major duties. Briefly, these four closely interrelated dimensions of the sick role are: (right one) the occupant of the sick role is exempt from responsibility for the incapacity, as it is beyond his control; (right two) he is also exempt from normal social role responsibilities; (duty one) the sick person is expected to recognize that illness is inherently undesirable and that he has an obligation to try to get well; and (duty two) he also has an obligation to seek technically competent help and to cooperate in the process of trying to get well.

The sick role concept has been widely utilized in the study of many different types of conditions. The Parsonian model (which is best typified by temporary, acute physical illness episodes) has been employed in the study of: chronic illness and physical disability[5,2]; aging[6]; pregnancy[15]; and alco-

25

holism[14]. All of these studies demonstrate that the dimensions of the sick role model (as originally acknowledged by Parsons) are relative to the nature and severity of the illness.

However, the sick role is not only affected by the nature of the illness, but also by social and cultural factors. "Consequently, it is necessary to determine the extent to which Parsons' description of sick role expectations is valid. Equally important is whether these expectations are affected by sociocultural variations"[4]. Indeed, one must ask to what extent the set of expectations described by Parsons is actually representative of different sociocultural groups. In view of the evidence provided by Mechanic, Suchman, Zola and others regarding the sociocultural patterning of conceptions of illness and help-seeking behaviour, it is also reasonable to anticipate the existence of a variety of subcultural beliefs regarding behaviour appropriate to the sick role.

In general terms, then, the objectives of the present study were to determine: (1) how closely actual perception of the rights and duties of the sick role correspond to the Parsonian model; (2) whether systematic sociocultural differences exist in the behavioural expectations held regarding the rights and duties of the sick role; and (3) whether systematic sociocultural differences exist in willingness to adopt the sick role.

RESEARCH DESIGN

Population Studied

The most frequently studied groups, in this area of research, have been Jewish, Italian Catholics, Irish Catholics and Anglo-Saxon Protestants. For the sake of comparison, this study focused upon the members of two of these groups, i.e. Jewish and Anglo-Saxon Protestants. Ethnic group affiliation was determined initially by the respondent's stated religious preference. Once the respondents had been categorized in terms of ethnic group affiliation they were chosen on the basis of the similarity of their illness and hospitalization experience. This step was necessary, in order for the study to be able to contribute to an increased understanding of how ethnic background may lead to different sick role behavioural expectations. The respondents who were included in this study were drawn from a population of hospitalized

patients who had undergone the same surgical procedure at either of two major Toronto hospitals.

In an effort to isolate the effects of ethnicity further, a number of restrictions were placed on the type of patients included in this study, i.e. only Anglo-Saxon Protestant or Jewish married housewives between 18 and 70 years of age were interviewed. The interviewing of patients began March, 1970 and concluded February, 1971. The present paper is based upon the information provided by 70 of these patients.

Data Collection

The interviews were conducted in the patients' hospital room and lasted on the average, approximately 45 min. Data were gathered regarding medical-hospital and personal-social factors, as well as the patients' sick role expectations and behaviour. Two Likert-type attitude scales were designed to get at the patients' perception of the kind of behaviour which would be appropriate for a person who was sick and their willingness to enter the role of the sick person.*

Perception of the Sick Role Scale consisted of eight items (one positive and one negative statement pertaining to each of the rights and duties of the sick role as outlined by Parsons). The four positive statements were presented first, followed by the four negative statements, so that the two complementary items for each right and duty would be evenly distributed. The patients responded to each of the eight attitudinal statements in the scale by indicating whether or not they agreed.† The Willingness to

---

* The statements included in these scales were adapted from the indices developed by Zola[21]; Mechanic[8]; and Suchman[17,18].

† The response categories for the positively stated items were scored 3 (agree), 2 (uncertain) and 1 (disagree), while the scoring for the four items stated in a negative sense was reversed. Those respondents who displayed an "ideal" perceptual pattern (according to the Parsonian model) agreed with the first statement and disagreed with the second statement for each of the four dimensions of the sick role. These respondents were assigned a score of six and were categorized as "positive" in Table 1. The opposite response pattern resulted in a score of two, which was interpreted as an indication of a "negative" perceptual pattern. All other combinations of responses (i.e., scores of 3, 4 and 5) were categorized as "uncertain."

TABLE 1 Respondents' perception of the rights and duties of the sick role

| | PERCEPTUAL PATTERN | | | | | |
| | NEGATIVE | | UNCERTAIN | | POSITIVE | |
RIGHTS AND DUTIES	NO.	%	NO.	%	NO.	%
Right 1—Exempt from responsibility for incapacity	6	8	48	69	16	23
Right 2—Exempt from normal role responsibilities	11	16	32	45	27	39
Duty 1—Obligation to try to get well	0	0	11	16	59	84
Duty 2—Obligation to seek competent help	4	6	37	53	29	41

Adopt the Sick Role Scale consisted of ten items, all negatively stated. Again, the respondents were asked to agree or disagree, and a high score on this scale was interpreted as a high willingness to adopt the sick role.*

Method of Analysis

The SPSS integrated system of computer programmes was used for the analysis of the data[10]. A two-way analysis was conducted to determine the nature of the relationship between ethnic group affiliation and the various indicators employed to gauge sick role expectations and behaviour.

PRESENTATION OF RESULTS AND RELATED DISCUSSION

The Hospitalized Patient: Some Characteristics

The Anglo-Saxon Protestant and Jewish female patients included in this study were found to be essentially similar in a number of respects, i.e. age, size of family, level of education and family income. Almost all of the patients reported that they have children, although very few reported having over four children. In addition, the majority of the patients had attended high school and reported a total family income for the preceding year in approximately the same range. All of the patients had been in a hospital

* Since all ten of the items were negatively stated, they were scored 1 (agree), 2 (uncertain) and 3 (disagree). The scores on this scale ranged from 10 to 30 and were categorized as: "low" willingness (10–18); "uncertain" (19–21); and "high" willingness (22–30).

before. The majority had been hospitalized four to six times and for most of the patients their last stay was within the past ten years. Both groups of patients, then, were quite similar in a variety of ways.

Variation in Perception of the Rights and Duties of the Sick Role

Few of the respondents interviewed in this study disagreed completely with Parsons' conception of the sick role. At the same time, the respondents' perception of the sick role did not overwhelmingly support the Parsonian model as many of the respondents were classified as "uncertain" due to their rather indefinite (or sometimes contradictory) responses. In fact, only one clear-cut area of agreement was found between Parsons' description of "ideal" sick role expectations and the respondents' perception of how a person should behave when sick, i.e. 84% of the respondents felt that a sick person has an obligation to try to get well. In other words, these patients would agree with Parsons that "to be ill is inherently undesirable"[11] and that the occupant of the sick role should strive to achieve a state of "good health." (See Table 1)

To understand why so many of the respondents fell into the "uncertain" category, the attitudinal statements included in this scale must be considered individually.† In investigating the first right of the

† The patients responses to each of the eight items were analyzed separately, as well as their combined responses to the complementary items pertaining to the four dimensions of the sick role. The findings have been summarized in the tables presented in an effort to make the paper more readable. For more detailed information about the results of the statistical analysis see Segall[16].

It should be acknowledged that the results may be partially explained in terms of the scaling procedure sick role, it was found that the majority of the women felt that a sick person cannot be "held responsible" for his condition. At the same time, only 31% of the patients agreed that "no matter how careful a person is, he can expect a good deal of illness in his lifetime." Many of the women said that an individual can take certain steps to minimize the occurrence of illness. What the patients seemed to be suggesting was that when a person becomes sick it is generally not "his own fault," although by being "careful" illness may be prevented.

Turning to the second right of the sick role, the majority of the women (69%) agreed that "when a person is sick, it is alright to have others do things for you," but were divided in regard to whether "one should try to keep up with the routine housework even when not feeling well." The respondents often qualified their answers by adding that it would "depend on how sick you are." Thus actual exemption from normal role responsibilities (e.g. child care, housework) depends upon the nature and severity of the illness.

The patients' perception of the sick person's obligation to try to get well and to seek technically competent help was much more consistent, than their perception of the other aspects of the sick role. As previously mentioned, the majority of the patients felt that "a person should try to get well as quickly as possible," and were very eager to terminate their dependency on others. Although the consensus was not as great, many of the respondents (65%) also believed that a sick person should seek technically competant help and cooperate in the process of trying to get well.

Although the present research evidence is somewhat limited and unclear, it offers little support for Parsons' general formulation of the rights and duties of the sick role (with the possible exception of the sick person's obligation to try to get better). These findings are consistent with the results of other recent attempts to examine empirically the validity of the sick role conceptualization. For example, Twaddle[19] found that many of the respondents he interviewed did not perceive the rights and duties

of the sick role in a manner consistent with Parsons' formulation. In a similar fashion, Berkanovic[1] interpreted his findings as evidence that the sick role is an inadequate conceptual tool.

Is the Parsonian model applicable to the members of different ethnic groups? In what way were the perceptual patterns described in the preceding section affected by the respondents' ethnic affiliation? In an attempt to answer these questions, the responses of the Anglo-Saxon Protestant and Jewish women were compared on each of the attitudinal items as well as the scale scores.

TABLE 2 Relationship between the respondents' ethnic group affiliation and a positive or "ideal" perception of the rights and duties of the sick role

| RIGHTS AND DUTIES | ETHNIC AFFILIATION | | | |
| | ANGLO-SAXON PROTESTANT | | JEWISH | |
	NO.	%	NO.	%
Right 1	6	15.0	10	33.3
Right 2	17	42.5	10	33.3
Duty 1	34	85.0	25	83.3
Duty 2	19	47.5	10	33.3

The two groups of patients were found to share basically the same expectations in regard to the sick role. Although the Anglo-Saxon Protestant patients generally perceived the sick role more in terms of the Parsonian ideal type model than the Jewish patients, the differences between the two groups were not statistically significant (i.e., $P > 0–05$). In one case (i.e., exemption from responsibility for the incapacity) the pattern was reversed. The Anglo-Saxon Protestant patients expressed the view that a person can do many things for him/herself to maintain a state of "good health." For these patients, the individual was viewed as capable of exercising a good deal of control over the state of his/her bodily condition.

Variation in Willingness to Adopt the Sick Role

In contrast to the very limited number of studies that have focused upon variation in the behavioural

---

employed. In Likert's method of summated ratings, differences may be masked by adding together the individual's scores on the items to arrive at a scale score.

expectations associated with the sick role, a great many research efforts have explored willingness to adopt the sick role[4,13,12]. Some studies have concentrated upon the relationship between ethnic and religious background and individual medical orientation, including factors such as acceptance of the sick role[8,17]. Generally, willingness to adopt the sick role has been operationalized as willingness to consult a doctor. A typical finding reported by these studies is that Jewish respondents display a greater willingness to consult a physician and more frequently utilize treatment facilities, than either Protestant or Catholic respondents.

A major weakness of this type of study is that only one dimension of the individual's willingness to adopt the sick role has been investigated. In addition to exploring "tendency" or "inclination" to visit a doctor, it is equally important to know if the person is actually ready to stop performing "normal" social roles and at the same time become dependent upon others for his well-being. Another limitation of research in this field is that attempts have been made to measure willingness to adopt the sick role, without first specifying the nature of the role expectations held by the respondents. Just what type of behavioural pattern is the individual willing to adopt when sick? The respondents' expectations in regard to the kind of behaviour perceived as appropriate for a sick person must first be understood if expressions of willingness to adopt the sick role are to be meaningfully interpreted.

In the present study, the respondents' willingness to adopt the sick role was measured by a Likert-type attitude scale. The patients' responses have been summarized in Table 3.

TABLE 3 Relationship between the respondents' ethnic group affiliation and willingness to adopt the sick role

| WILLINGNESS TO ADOPT | ETHNIC AFFILIATION | | | |
| | ANGLO-SAXON PROTESTANT | | JEWISH | |
	NO.	%	NO.	%
High	20	50	23	77
Uncertain	12	30	3	10
Low	8	20	4	13
Total:	40	100	30	100

Jewish patients displayed a greater willingness to adopt the sick role, while Protestant patients were more likely to be uncertain about their feelings rather than completely opposed to accepting the role of the sick person. Although the difference between the two groups of patients on their attitude scale scores was not statistically significant (i.e. $P > 0–05$), there was a clearly discernible trend in the way in which they responded to the scale items.

For instance, Protestant patients more frequently stated that they find it hard to give in and go to bed when sick, and hate to admit that they are not feeling well. To support her answer, one Anglo-Saxon Protestant patient emphatically stated "I like to be known as a healthy person." (A reference once again to the belief that the individual should be able to exert some influence or control over his "state of health"). In addition, Protestant patients agreed more readily than Jewish patients with the statement "If you ignore and don't worry about them, many physical symptoms will go away."

The reluctance of the Anglo-Saxon Protestant respondents to adopt the sick role was further illustrated by the fact that 55% (in contrast to only 27% of the Jewish respondents) agreed that when they think they are getting sick, they find it difficult to talk to others about their condition ($P \leq 0–05$). Based upon these findings, it may be concluded that what the Anglo-Saxon Protestant respondents were basically objecting to was the dependency upon others which accompanies the adoption of the sick role. They were, however, as willing as the Jewish respondents to accept the other dimensions of the sick role. For example, an equal proportion of the two groups of women expressed similar views about consulting a doctor and going to the hospital for medical care.

SUMMARY AND CONCLUSIONS

The fact that statistically significant differences were not found between these two groups in the present study does not necessarily indicate that there are no differences between Anglo-Saxon Protestant and Jewish respondents in their perception of and willingness to adopt the sick role. To understand the influence of sociocultural factors upon the sick role, more attention must be devoted to defining operationally the sick role concept and developing precise means of measurement.* The evidence seems to indicate that the sick role (as conceived by Parsons) is not a unitary concept and "empirically, the ideal model of the sick role is often not fully realized" [9].

Furthermore, ethnicity is a diffuse variable, which has been measured by a variety of indicators. For example, Mechanic[8] relied upon stated religious preference, and Suchman[17] utilized three characteristics (race, religion and country of birth). To what extent can variations in illness behaviour be explained in terms of these indicators of ethnicity? It is clear that the concept of ethnicity also requires further theoretical and methodological refinement if the nature of the relationship between ethnicity and illness behaviour is to be adequately understood.

Before the willingness of the members of different ethnic groups to adopt the sick role can be compared, their perception of the sick role must be understood. The range of behaviour perceived as appropriate for the sick person must be specified. Future attempts to measure willingness to adopt the sick role must also specify which dimensions of the role are being considered. All of these steps must be taken if the sick role concept is to have a meaningful relation to social reality, and the influence of ethnic group membership is to be understood as a determinant of whether a person will adopt the sick role, and if he/she does, in what manner.

References

1. Berkanovic E. Lay conceptions of the sick role. *Soc. Forces* **51**, 53, 1972.
2. Callahan E. M. *et al.* The sick role in chronic illness: some reactions. *J. Chron. Dis.* **19**, 883, 1966.
3. Croog S. H. Ethnic origins and responses to health questionnaires. *Hum. Org.* **20**, 65, 1961.
4. Gordon G. *Role Theory and Illness: A Sociological Perspective*. College and University Press, New Haven, CT, 1966.
5. Kassebaum G. G. and Baumann B. O. Dimensions of the sick role in chronic illness. *J. Hlth Hum. Behav.* **6**, 16, 1965.
6. Lipman A. and Sterne R. S. Aging in the United States: ascription of a terminal sick role. *Sociol. Soc. Res.* **53**, 194, 1969.
7. Mechanic D. *Medical Sociology*. Free Press, New York, 1968.
8. Mechanic, D. Religion, religiosity, and illness behaviour. *Hum. Org.* **22**, 202, 1963.
9. Mechanic D. and Volkart E. H. Stress illness behaviour and the sick role. *Am. Sociol. Rev.* **26**, 51, 1961.
10. Nie N., Bent D. H. and Hull C. H. *Statistical Package for the Social Sciences*. McGraw-Hill, New York, 1970.
11. Parsons T. *The Social System*. The Free Press, New York, 1951.
12. Petroni F. A. Social class, family size and the sick role. *J. Marriage Fam.* **31**, 728, 1969.
13. Phillips D. L. Self-reliance and the inclination to adopt the sick role. *Soc. Forces* **43**, 555, 1965.
14. Roman P. M. and Trice H. M. The sick role, labelling theory and the deviant drinker. *Int. J. Soc. Psychiat.* **14**, 245, 1968.
15. Rosengren W. R. The sick role during pregnancy: a note on research in progress. *J. Hlth Hum. Behav.* **3**, 213, 1962.
16. Segall A. Sociocultural Variation in Illness Behaviour. Unpublished Ph.D. dissertation. Department of Sociology, University of Toronto, 1972.
17. Suchman E. A. Sociomedical variations among ethnic groups. *Am. J. Sociol.* **70**, 319, 1964.
18. Suchman E. A. Social patterns of illness and medical care. *J. Hlth. Hum. Behav.* **6**, 2, 1965.
19. Twaddle A. C. Health decisions and sick role variations: an exploration. *J. Hlth Hum. Behav.* **10**, 195, 1969.
20. Zborowksi M. *People in Pain*. Jossey-Bass, San Francisco, 1969.
21. Zola I. K. Culture and symptoms—an analysis of patients presenting complaints. *Am. Sociol. Rev.* **31**, 615, 1966.

---

* For a more detailed assessment of the present status of this conceptual model and implications for future research see A. Segall, "The Sick Role Concept: Understanding Illness Behaviour," forthcoming in the *Journal of Health and Social Behaviour* 1976.

Illness and the Legitimation of Failure

Stephen Cole
Robert Lejeune

Illness exempts individuals from their normal role obligations. Most of us are sick on occasion. Some, however, see themselves as permanently sick. Generally, we associate this adjustment with a serious physiological or psychological breakdown; rarely do we view sociological variables as prompting chronic illness. It is the central hypothesis of this paper that people who come to view themselves as unable to fulfill their normal roles will be motivated to define themselves as permanently sick to legitimize their self-defined failure.[1]

Sociologically, a person is sick when he acts sick. Thus, the conditions that motivate people to view themselves as sick or healthy are important. Clearly, the "objective" physiological condition of one's body plays a major part in self-definition of health. Both medical doctors and social scientists, however, have become increasingly aware that physiological and social-psychological forces intertwine in determining objective and subjective states of health. (Crandell and Dohrenwend 1967; Hinkle et al. 1956; Mechanic and Volkart 1961; Wolff 1958; Zola 1966). In this paper, we shall discuss one social-psychological determinant of one's subjective health definition. Our data treat the hypothesis that inability to fulfill their role obligations is one factor leading people to define their health as poor. To explore this hypothesis, we shall examine how definition of health relates to a mother's adjustment to being on welfare. We shall also analyze the relationship between definition of health and performance of roles as wives and mothers among a sample of working-class black women.

The data derive from three studies: The first was conducted in New York City in the summer of 1966. The National Opinion Research Center interviewed a probability sample of 2179 female heads of households receiving family public assistance in New York City in April, 1966.[2] The second study was conducted in New York City in the summer of 1968. National Analysts interviewed a quota sample of 412 working-class black mothers living in public housing projects.[3] The final study was conducted in Camden, New Jersey, in the summer of 1969. The Center for Research on the Acts of Man, University of Pennsylvania, interviewed a quota sample of 447 women recipients of Aid to Dependent Children.[4]

The dependent variable in this study is one's subjective health definition. We asked: "In general, would you say your own health is excellent, good, fair, or poor?" A major problem in the analysis is empirically separating the physiological and social psychological components of health definition. If people fail to fulfill their role obligations because they are physiologically ill, it would make little sense to say they are defining themselves as sick to legitimize failure. In clear-cut cases of physical breakdown, such as terminal cancer, heart attacks, or tuberculosis, almost everyone will act ill. However, since practically all respondents in the three surveys are women under fifty, and most are under forty, the frequency of such illness among the respondents would not be high. In less than clear-cut cases, individuals having similar physiological conditions may behave quite differently. Most people have some health problems and some aches and pains; yet they continue to function adequately. Others magnify their aches and pains until they dominate their lives.

Even if we assume that a small minority suffered from clear-cut physiological breakdown, we are still faced with the problem of causal order. Without longitudinal data we do not know if taking the sick role proceeds or precedes a self-definition of failure.

Reprinted from the *American Sociological Review*, vol. 37 (1972), pp. 347–356.

Hence, our study is exploratory rather than conclusive. The best we can do to handle the problem of causal order is to show that the relationship between self-defined failure and health persists even when we control for a few relatively more objective indicators of health such as symptoms, number of doctor-patient contacts, and number of reported illnesses. Our analysis begins with a discussion of the meaning of being on welfare in America.

WELFARE AS FAILURE

One reason why the United States has had a weak socialist movement and a relatively conservative working class is that Americans typically see social status as a result of personal success or failure. If someone is socially mobile, it is because he is talented and works hard. If someone is not socially mobile, it is thought to be a result of his personal shortcomings. The individual's location in the social structure is not viewed as a prime determinant of his fate. It is for this reason that many Americans look down on welfare recipients. Many welfare recipients themselves believe that being on welfare signifies personal rather than societal failure.[5]

What evidence is there that welfare recipients accept that stigma attached to their status by the dominant culture? Most welfare recipients have been repeatedly exposed to the view that they are immoral and undeserving. The data indicate that a large number of AFDC mothers share this view. Seventy-one percent of the New York welfare sample agreed with the statement, "A lot of people getting money from welfare don't deserve it." Another ten percent did not know or would not reply and only 19 percent disagreed.[6] If it is objected that some welfare mothers merely wanted to give the "expected" or "right" answer, this confirms our point: that welfare recipients know that the dominant culture defines their status as illegitimate. While we cannot tell from these replies to what extent and with what intensity welfare mothers view themselves as undeserving, they are very likely aware of the stigma attached to their status and probably prone to question the claims of need of other welfare recipients. Thus, it is not surprising that 55 percent of the New York welfare mothers agreed that "getting money from welfare makes a person feel ashamed." And fully 87 percent agreed that "people should be grateful for the money they get from welfare."

The Camden welfare mothers expressed similar views on receiving public assistance. Fifty-seven percent said it was more often true than false that "people I know look down on welfare," and 34 percent admitted that "there are times when I have been embarrassed in front of my family or friends because of being on welfare." Another indicator of whether or not the welfare mothers think of being on welfare as a type of personal failure is provided by their opinions about the conditions under which welfare should be available. For example, 84 percent of the Camden mothers believed that welfare should not be available "if there is one parent (female) and she does not try to keep up her home." We can conclude that at least a substantial proportion of mothers on welfare accept the stigma attached to the status by the general culture. These data indicate that a majority of welfare recipients do not share the attitudes of welfare rights organizations. We wish to make explicit at this point that we do not consider welfare mothers to be failures; rather this is the view of many Americans and the data show that many welfare mothers internalize this view.

How do people who define themselves as failures cope with the knowledge of their stigma? One technique of handling this problem is to believe that things will be better in the future. Welfare clients may reduce the conflict between their need for welfare and their perception of their status as an undesirable and degrading one by believing in a welfare-free future for themselves. Only 25 percent of the New York women thought they would "surely be on welfare" and another thirty-three percent thought they would "probably be on welfare" a year from the time of the interview. Forty-two percent either did not know or thought they would not be on welfare.[7] Sixty-one percent said yes to the question: "Do you think you will ever (again) work for pay?" While work is not their only way to economic independence, it is certainly the most important for the majority who are husbandless or whose husbands' earnings cannot support the family. Given the poor objective chances for most welfare mothers to succeed in an economy demanding ever higher levels of training, we would expect most of them to abandon hope.

That the opposite is true attests to the continued strength of the dominant goal of success. Seventy percent of both the New York and Camden welfare samples say they would rather work than remain home.[8]

THE LEGITIMATION OF DEPENDENCY

A woman who sees being on welfare as a personal failure but views her own welfare status as temporary may feel no need to justify her dependency; but a woman who has abandoned hope of escape from this position of self-defined failure will probably have a strong need to justify it. Thus, we hypothesize that mothers who no longer think of welfare as a temporary status will be the most likely to use illness to justify their self-defined social failure. We do not argue that welfare mothers consciously use poor health as an excuse for remaining on welfare. Although some may do this, we do not think them typical. More probably, a woman who feels the need to justify her status to herself, gradually adopts the sick role. Over time, she comes to feel and act as if she were in fact sick.[9] She is likely to develop a series of psychosomatic symptoms.

Margaret Olendzki (1965), who studied 1976 applicants for public assistance in Manhattan, collected data to support this view.[10] As part of that study, a checklist of medical conditions was presented to each applicant. The most often mentioned health complaint was "nerves," reported by 45 percent of the women respondents who were heads of families and thus correspond most closely to the respondents in our samples. We cross-tabulated the "suffering from nerves" complaint with Olendzki's question on self-defined health. It turns out that defining one's health as poor is highly associated with the presence of emotional complaints. Sixty-nine percent who said their health was poor also said they "suffered from nerves." Sixty-one percent who viewed their health as fair made the same complaint. The proportion who said they were in good and excellent health yet suffered from nerves was smaller, though not unsubstantial: 35 percent and 27 percent respectively.[11] We conclude that welfare mothers who claim to be sick are probably so; however, sociopsychological factors may play at least as great a role as physiological factors in the development of their illness.

We can now present the data bearing on our main hypothesis—that women who have abandoned hope of getting off welfare will be more likely than those who maintain hope to define their health as poor. The New York survey showed that expectation not to work was correlated ($r = 0.22$) with definition of health.[12] Women who did not expect to work were more likely to define their health as poor. This correlation would be spurious if it disappeared when we controlled for background variables affecting work expectations such as education, age, and a more objective indicator of health. This does not happen. When we remove the variance due to education, the partial correlation of work expectations and definition of health is $p/r = 0.18$. Similarly, removing the variance due to age only slightly reduced the relationship between work expectation and definition of health ($p/r = 0.17$). Though we have no adequate measure of objective health, we did have data on the number of times the respondent reported she was ill during the preceding year. This health indicator is also a subjective measure. It is far from perfectly correlated with definition of health ($r = 0.49$) and thus probably measures at least a different aspect of health conception. When the variance due to this variable was removed, the correlation between work expectation and health definition was hardly changed ($p/r = 0.20$). Tabular presentation of the data indicates that in each category of number of illnesses, women who do not expect to work in the future are more likely than those who do to define their health as fair or poor.

The Camden survey had similar results. Here we used two questions to measure welfare mothers' attitudes toward their health. Women not currently working were asked why. One choice was that they were "not interested in working at present time—health reason or handicap." Women who did not expect to work in the future were more likely to give this reason ($r = 0.27$).[13] We also asked: "What part does your health play in your decision not to work or in the kind of work you can take?" Women who did not expect to work were more likely to say that health played a part in their decision ($r = 0.20$).

The Camden data allow us to test several hypotheses concerning the conditions under which welfare mothers are likely to use poor health to legitimize their dependency. We have suggested that welfare mothers view being on welfare as a type of failure and that when they give up hope of leaving welfare they develop a need to justify their permanent dependency. Some welfare recipients, however, do not accept the stigma generally attached to their position. We would expect to find that among women who do not view welfare as a temporary status, those who accept the stigma should be more likely to take the sick role. As an indicator of attitudes towards welfare, we used the score on an index of questions concerning the conditions under which welfare should be available.[14] Those who believe that welfare should not be available unless the recipient lives up to rigorous moral standards are more likely to define welfare as an illegitimate status. As Table 1 indicates, among mothers who expect to get off welfare, attitudes towards welfare have little effect on adopting the sick role. Among mothers not expecting to work, however, those who accept the dominant cultural view of welfare (in the table those who have "strict" attitudes towards the availability of welfare) are more likely than those who reject it (in the table those who have "lenient" attitudes towards the availability of welfare) to adopt the sick role. Clearly both conditions, defining one's status as illegitimate and viewing that status as permanent, contribute to one's adopting the sick role.

TABLE 1 Percentage giving health as reason for preferring not to work by attitudes toward welfare and expectation to work in the future (Camden Welfare Sample)

AVAILABILITY OF WELFARE		LENIENT	STRICT
Expect to be work-	Yes	10 (106)	12 (137)
ing in the future	No	15 (88)	26 (94)

A counter theory to explain the data of Table 1 would be that poor health leads a woman to give up hope of working. Collapsing Table 1 we find that 42 percent of people with poor health and 60 percent of those without poor health, expect to work. While poor health may lead women to give up hope of working, this does not explain why women who accept the dominant view of welfare are more likely to view their health as poor than those who reject that view.[15]

FAMILY CYCLE, AGE, AND LEGITIMATION OF DEPENDENCY

Welfare mothers can use mechanisms other than illness to legitimize failure. One condition influencing the type of mechanism adopted is the family-life cycle. AFDC's primary rationale is that women without husbands should be supported so they can stay home and care for their children. A woman with a preschool child can easily legitimize her dependency. Indeed, 77 percent of the New York women who preferred not to work gave child care as a reason. It is initially surprising to find that only 19 percent of those who prefer not to work gave illness as a reason. We must remember, however, that the respondents were women. Their primary obligations center around expressive family rather than instrumental work roles.[16] We would therefore expect them to be more likely to define their health as poor when they no longer have preschool children.

In both the New York and Camden samples the age of a mother's youngest child was associated with citing health as a reason for preferring not to work. (See Table 2.) Hardly any mothers with preschool children, but a substantial proportion of those with school age children gave poor health as a reason for preferring not to work. Whereas the age of the youngest child is positively associated with giving poor health as a reason for preferring not to work, it is negatively associated with giving child care as a reason. Thus, of the Camden women not expecting to work, 72 percent with children under six and 42 percent with children six or over gave child care as their reason for preferring to stay at home. As long as a mother has young children, she can view her dependency as an objective necessity.

A possible source of error in our interpretation of the data of Table 2 could be the correlation between the mother's age and the age of the youngest child. Women who have no preschool children are generally older than those who do. The results in Table 2 might be an artifact of the "self-evident" fact that older people are more likely to be sick and "therefore" less employable. Actually "employability" is a culturally defined state. There are probably few disabilities which restrict work under all circumstances and in all social contexts. The sociologist must therefore view the system's classification of

TABLE 2 Percentage giving health reasons for preferring not to work by age of youngest child (only those preferring not to work)

	N.Y. WELFARE SAMPLE		
Age of youngest child	0–5	6–10	11 or older
	9 (401)	20 (143)	53 (120)

	CAMDEN WELFARE SAMPLE	
Age of youngest child	Under 6	6 or older
	14 (145)	42 (38)

some welfare recipients as "totally and permanently disabled" as providing a socially acceptable rationale for the limited opportunities such persons have in the labor market. As in many other areas of social life the labeling process functions to tidy up the bookkeeping of a society riddled with value inconsistencies. That those excluded from participation would seek these labels is a natural outcome of the process.

As a more conclusive test of the family cycle hypothesis it is necessary to see if the relationship between age of youngest child and definition of health persists with the mother's age controlled. (See Table 3.) In Table 3, the age of the youngest child is used as an indicator of the extent of child-rearing responsibilities. It turns out that even with mother's age controlled, the age of the youngest child is associated in the expected direction with giving health as a reason for preferring not to work. The association is particularly strong for those over forty. Women over 40 with no children under the age of 11 are almost three times more likely than any other group to give health reasons for preferring not to work. The decline of child-rearing functions, as one aspect

TABLE 3 Percentage giving health reasons for preferring not to work by age and age of youngest child (only those preferring not to work) (New York Welfare Sample)

AGE OF YOUNGEST CHILD	AGE		
	UNDER 30	30–39	40 AND OVER
0 to 5	8 (202)	9 (165)	15 (34)
6 to 10	13 (16)	14 (64)	27 (63)
11 or over	* (2)	21 (24)	63 (94)

* Too few cases.

of aging, leads to an increasing tendency to legitimize welfare dependency by evoking the sick role. The issue here is not whether older respondents are "sicker" than younger ones. Even if they were, only among those whose children are growing up does poor health become salient as their reason for welfare dependency. We would guess that even middle-class women would be more likely to take the sick role as they age and their child-rearing function declines in significance. A middle-class woman who has devoted her life to rearing children might find poor health an acceptable way of legitimizing to herself her failure to find another socially acceptable status when her children have grown up.

Thus it is evident that though illness plays a small part in legitimizing dependency for the total family welfare population, it becomes one of the primary bases for legitimizing a claim to welfare support among women over 40 whose youngest child has reached adolescence. As these women end their child-rearing years, their chance for economic independence is highly limited. They are over forty, lack a recent job history, and have limited marketable skills. If at the same time they are black or Puerto Rican (as most are) their realistic opportunities for independence are further restricted. The sick role may provide one "substitute" status for the lack of any other socially approved positively evaluated statuses.

In Table 3 it is evident that the mother's age has a strong independent effect on adopting the sick role. Is this predominantly the result of a genuine decline in health with age, or can the finding be explained sociologically? It is necessary to separate the physiological and social components of aging. Although this is impossible given our data, we can control for some relatively more objective indicators of health. In Table 4 the relation between age and giving poor health as a reason for preferring not to work is shown, with the number of reported illnesses in the past year held constant.[17] Table 4 shows once again that with increasing age, welfare mothers are more likely to give poor health as a reason for preferring not to work. This association is found even among women who had reported earlier in the interview that they had not been sick at all in the past year. Thus, even though the number of reported illnesses in the past year may itself have been affected by subjective considerations, older respondents who

TABLE 4 Percentage giving health reasons for preferring not to work by age and number of illnesses in the past year (only those preferring not to work) (New York Welfare Sample)

NUMBER OF ILLNESSES IN PAST YEAR	AGE		
	UNDER 30	30–39	40 AND OVER
None	1 (86)	3 (93)	24 (63)
1 or more	4 (52)	9 (75)	37 (51)
3 or more	18 (80)	21 (84)	62 (76)

TABLE 5 Percentage giving health reasons for preferring not to work by age and number of doctor-patient contacts in the past year (only those preferring not to work) (N.Y. Welfare Sample)

NUMBER OF DOCTOR-PATIENT CONTACTS IN PAST YEAR:	AGE		
	UNDER 30	30–39	40 AND OVER
None or 1	5 (88)	7 (118)	30 (84)
2 to 6	4 (72)	13 (79)	38 (69)
7 or more	12 (60)	18 (57)	66 (53)

by their own account had not been ill were nonetheless more likely than younger respondents to give poor health as a reason for preferring not to work.

Chronological age and number of illnesses have both independent and interactive effects on mentioning poor health as a reason for preferring not to work. Thus, among women under 30, the number-of-illnesses variable accounts for a 17 percentage-point difference in the first column of Table 4. There is a similar difference (18 percentage points) in the 30–39 age group. In the 40 and over group, the difference is 38 percentage points, indicating that not only illness per se but more importantly illness combined with aging increases the likelihood that illness will become a basis for legitimizing dependency. Not only does taking the sick role legitimize being on welfare, but age legitimizes taking the sick role.[18] A young person who complains of aches and pains calls forth negative sanctions; an older person calls forth sympathy.

In Table 4, one cannot distinguish between "serious" and "nonserious" illnesses by simply counting the number of self-reported illnesses for the year. It was beyond the scope of the study to measure how seriously ill the women were. This can be approximated, however, by the number of doctor-patient contacts in the past year. We may assume that the sicker respondents would on the average contact physicians more often. Table 5 shows of those women with at least seven doctor-patient contacts in the last year, only 12 percent of the youngest and fully 66 percent of the oldest gave poor health as the reason for preferring not to work. Also, 30 percent of women over 40 who saw the doctor once or not at all during the year made the poor health claim.

GENERALIZATION OF THE HYPOTHESIS

Thus far we have presented data illustrating how some welfare mothers use illness to legitimize self-defined failure. We believe that this practice is a widespread phenomenon in achievement-oriented societies like ours.[19] Health is perceived as physiologically determined and therefore basically beyond individual control. If one fails to fulfill a socially defined role expectation, he is not to be blamed if he has poor health.

We decided to test the validity of this generalization on another set of data. We were interested in whether or not mothers and wives who defined their own role performance as below par would be more likely to define their health as poor. As part of the New York study of welfare mothers, we interviewed a "control" sample of 412 nonwelfare black mothers. These working class women lived in several public housing projects. In this questionnaire were a series of questions designed to measure the degree of self-defined success which the women had as wives and mothers. The data are presented in Table 6. For all five questions, those women who defined themselves as relative failures in their roles as wives and mothers were more likely to define their health as fair or poor than women who felt they adequately performed these roles.[20] For example, of those women who judged their marriage "average or unhappy," 40 percent defined their health as fair or poor; but only 22 percent of those who judged their marriage "happy" defined their health negatively. Though we have no data to measure the intervening mechanisms, we would guess that many women who view themselves as failures as mothers and wives develop a need to legitimize their failure and a

TABLE 6 Percentage defining health as fair or poor by self-defined role performance (New York working-class sample)

Compared with your friends would you say that you are an:	
Excellent cook	20 (54)
Good cook	31 (169)
Average or below cook	33 (187)
How often do you feel that you can't control your children:	
Frequently or sometimes	38 (125)
Rarely	34 (86)
Never	24 (200)
How often do you feel that you are not as good a mother as you would like to be:	
Frequently or sometimes	38 (155)
Rarely	29 (98)
Never	24 (159)
Would you say that your marriage has been:	
Happy	22 (214)
Average or unhappy	40 (132)
Compared with your friends would you say that you and your husband get along:	
Very well	23 (188)
About average or not so well	36 (160)

substantial minority use poor health to do this.

It is, of course, possible that the associations reported in Table 6 could be spurious. It could be that women who are older, have little education, low income, and are physiologically in poor health might be more likely to see themselves as failures as wives and mothers and define their health negatively. Were we to control for these variables and eliminate the effect of self-defined role performance, then our interpretation of Table 6 would be incorrect.

To analyze this possibility, we combined the answers to all five questions on role performance in an index. Women scoring high on this index (defining their role performance favorably) were least likely to define their health as fair or poor. Whereas 18 percent of the high scorers defined their health as fair or poor, 45 percent of the low scorers viewed their health as fair or poor (see Column (1) of Table 7). Age, education, income, and objective health were correlated with scores on the role performance index and definition of health. The association between these latter variables could therefore be spurious. To test this possibility we have used the technique of test-factor standardization.[21] The results presented in Table 7 are equivalent to three-variable tables in which we examine the effect of role performance on definition of health, controlling separately for age, education, income, and objective health.

Standardizing separately for age, education, and income did not substantially reduce the effect of the role-performance index on definition of health. Thus, for example, although older women were likely to score low on the role-performance index and to define their health as fair or poor, within each age category role-performance was still associated with definition of health. The results obtained when we standardized on objective health were not as clear. Objective health was measured by the number of symptoms reported. The interviewer read a list of 28 symptoms ranging from "Have you lost a lot of weight recently without dieting?" to "Have you recently been very depressed and blue?" Those reporting no symptoms were considered to be in excellent health, one or two symptoms good health, three or four symptoms fair health, and five or more symptoms poor health. This measure of objective health is, of course, not an indicator of the respondent's physiological condition. Many of the symptoms were psychosomatic.

TABLE 7 Percentage defining health as fair or poor by self-defined role performance—standardized by age, education, income, and "objective" health (New York working-class sample)

		STANDARDIZED ON			
ROLE PERFORMANCE		AGE	EDUCATION	INCOME	OBJECTIVE HEALTH
Low	(4,5) 45 (109)	46	44	45	35
Medium	(2,3) 28 (193)	28	28	27	29
High	(0,1) 18 (108)	19	19	20	22

Also, people who define their health as poor are more likely to search for symptoms to justify their taking the sick role. Furthermore, as we observed above, it is almost impossible to separate physiological from sociopsychological determinants of many physical symptoms. As the standardized data of Table 7 indicate (see last column of Table 7), the objective health measure does reduce the relationship between role performance and self-defined health. When the data are standardized on objective health, 35 percent of mothers scoring low on the role-performance index and 22 percent scoring high called their health fair or poor. Since the objective and subjective health measures probably measure only marginally different aspects of the same phenomenon, we conclude that the data are supportive and the hypothesis merits further consideration.

CONCLUSION

How an individual defines his health influences many areas of his life. People who think they are unhealthy act as if they were ill and may in fact become so. In this paper we analyzed some sociological determinants of definition of health. We argued that in the United States people use poor health to legitimize a sense of failure to fulfill socially prescribed roles. In America the cultural values stress the importance of maintaining economic independence and striving to move up the social hierarchy. As Merton (1957) observed, not trying to better oneself is a form of deviance.

Welfare recipients occupy a stigmatized status in America. A substantial proportion of welfare recipients themselves define being on welfare as a type of failure; yet many have given up hope of becoming independent. When people occupy a self-defined illegitimate status and have little expectation of leaving this status, they feel a need to legitimize their failure. We have shown that defining one's health as poor is one way that welfare mothers have of legitimizing their status. Drawing on data from another study we showed that women who defined their performance as wives and mothers as being less than adequate were more likely than those who were satisfied with their performance to define their health as poor. We would hypothesize that wherever there are high rates of self-defined failure there will be high rates of self-defined poor health.

Notes

1. Two decades ago, Parsons, following the psychoanalytic model, noted that sick people sometimes become unconsciously motivated to retain the "privileges and exemptions of the sick role" (Parsons 1951:437). In a subsequent examination of the problem, Parsons hypothesized that the high level of achievement demanded in America might accentuate the unconscious desire to use ill health to exempt oneself from role obligations (Parsons 1958).

2. For a detailed description of this sample, see Richard Pomeroy in collaboration with Robert Lejeune and Lawrence Podell, *Studies in the Use of Health Services by Families on Welfare,* The Center for the Study of Urban Problems, Baruch College, The City University of New York, 1969; also Robert Lejeune, *Illness Behavior among the Urban Poor,* unpublished doctoral dissertation, Columbia University, 1968.

3. For a detailed description of this sample see Lawrence Podell and Richard Pomeroy, *Studies in the Use of Health Services by Families on Welfare: Special Population Comparisons,* The Center for the Study of Urban Problems, Baruch College, The City University of New York, 1969.

4. For a detailed description of this sample see Samuel Z. Klausner *et al., The Work Incentive Program: Making Adults Economically Independent,* Center for Research on the Acts of Man, Philadelphia, Pennsylvania, 1970.

5. As long as a low-status group like welfare recipients blame themselves for this misfortune, there will be little pressure to change society; and organizations like the welfare rights groups will fail to attract mass support.

6. In their responses to this question, welfare mothers may, in part, be invidiously comparing their own financial status and that of other welfare mothers. Each respondent may think that she deserves welfare more.

7. The question was: "Do you think that a year from now you will *surely be* on welfare, *probably be* on welfare, *probably not be* on welfare?" As it turned out, one year from the time of the interview, 89% of the respondents were still receiving public assistance in New York City. Furthermore, it is likely that the majority who left the rolls in the one year period—judging from case histories—will be back on again.

8. For an analysis of the determinants of work expectations see Stephen Cole and Robert Lejeune, "Illness, Welfare Retreatism and the Legitimation of Failure," project report, Center for Research on the Acts of Man, Philadelphia, Pennsylvania. The key variables are edu-

cation, previous job experience, race, intelligence, "objective health," and age.

9. It is also possible that the poverty which attends welfare life may contribute to physiological deterioration.

10. We thank Dr. Olendzki for making her data available.

11. Suffering from nerves was highly correlated with other psychosomatic symptoms such as: "Do you have trouble sleeping?" "Are you continually troubled by aches and pains?" "Do you feel tired all the time for no special reason?" "Have you recently been very depressed and blue?"

12. The question was worded: "Do you think you will ever again work for pay?" Here, for simplicity of presentation we have used correlation coefficients rather than tables. We do this despite the fact that at times the data do not meet all the assumptions necessary for statistical analysis. None of our variables explained a great deal of variance. It is not the size of the associations but their consistency that gives us confidence in the plausibility of our conclusions. The hypotheses were developed on the basis of the New York welfare sample and we were able to test them on the other two surveys.

13. The question was worded: "In the near future (whether or not you are working now) would you prefer a full time job or would you prefer to stay at home?"

14. The index was composed of the following questions: "Assuming jobs are available, do you think that welfare should be available to families in the following situations? a) If there are a lot of children and the parent cannot support them adequately. b) If the parent is able bodied and will only work if she can get the type of work desired. c) If the parent is able bodied and simply does not feel like working. d) If there is one parent (female) and she does not want to work (for any reason). e) If there is one parent (female) and she feels that the mother's place is at home. f) If there is one parent (female) and she does not try to keep up her home." Those women who said that welfare should *not* be available in five or six of these situations are classified as having "strict" attitudes towards its availability. Those saying that welfare should *not* be available in four or less of these situations were classified as having "lenient" attitudes toward its availability.

15. Another plausible explanation for Table 1 would be that those who have lenient attitudes towards welfare become casual about their continuing dependence. In contrast, those who have strict attitudes are more reluctant to rely on welfare and tend to do so only when genuinely ill. We thank the ASR reader for pointing out this possibility.

16. Much ambivalence exists about the role of the working woman in America. Though women are sometimes expected to work, they are not expected to achieve too much. Whereas middle-class women may be urged to stay home and tend their children, welfare mothers are "lazy boondogglers" if they don't work. On the cultural ambivalence towards working women see Coser and Rokoff (1971).

17. Though "the number of reported illnesses in the past year" is not an adequate measure of the "physiological component of aging," it is the best measure we have and provides at least a tentative test.

18. For a similar analysis, see Coser (1961).

19. We do not mean that most people who define themselves as failures use ill health as a means of self-legitimation; but that a substantial minority use ill health to legitimize failure in a wide variety of situations. Clearly other techniques are used to legitimize failure. Detailed investigations of these are likely to be theoretically fruitful.

20. One could interpret the data in this table to mean that all responses result from a general negative self-image. Women who view themselves as bad mothers are also likely to have a low evaluation of their bodies and health. To further test our hypothesis would require data to show more specifically that women who define themselves as failures take the sick role in attitude and behavior.

21. For a description of the technique of test factor standardization see Morris Rosenberg, "Test Factor Standardization as a Method of Interpretation," *Social Forces*, 41 (1962–63), 53–61.

References

COSER, ROSE LAUB
    1961 Life in the Ward. East Lansing, Michigan: Michigan State University Press.

COSER, ROSE LAUB, and GERALD ROKOFF
    1971 "Women in the Occupational World: social disruption and conflict." Social Problems 18 (Spring):535–554.

CRANDELL, DEWITT L., and BRUCE DOHRENWEND
    1967 "Some relations among psychiatric symptoms, organic illness, and social class." American Journal of Psychiatry 123 (June):1527–1537.

HINKLE, L. E., JR., R. H. PINSKY, I. D. J. BROSS, and N. PLUMMER
    1956 "The distribution of sickness disability in a homogeneous group of 'healthy' adult men." American Journal of Hygiene 64 (September):220–242.

MECHANIC, DAVID, and EDMUND H. VOLKHART
1961 "Stress, illness behavior and the sick role." American Sociological Review 26 (February):51–58.

MERTON, ROBERT K.
1957 "Social structure and anomie." Pp. 131–160 in Robert K. Merton, Social Theory and Social Structure. Glencoe, Illinois: The Free Press.

OLENDZKI, MARGARET
1965 Welfare Medical Care in New York City: A Research Study. Unpublished Ph.D. dissertation, University of London.

PARSONS, TALCOTT
1951 The Social System. Glencoe, Illinois: The Free Press.
1958 "Definitions of health and illness in the light of American values and social structure." Pp. 165–187 in E. Gartly Jaco (ed.), Patients, Physicians, and Illness. Glencoe, Illinois: The Free Press.

ROSENBERG, MORRIS
1962–63 "Test factor standardization as a method of interpretation." Social Forces 41:53–61.

WOLFF, HAROLD
1958 "Disease and Patterns of Behavior." Pp. 54–61 in E. Gartly Jaco (ed.), Patients, Physicians, and Illness. Glencoe, Illinois: The Free Press.

ZOLA, IRVING KENNETH
1966 "Culture and symptoms: an analysis of patients presenting complaints." American Sociological Review 31 (October):615–630.

Illness Behavior and the Sick Role in Chronic Disease: The Case of Multiple Sclerosis

David C. Stewart
Thomas J. Sullivan

Illness behavior has been a focus of theoretical development and empirical research in the behavioral sciences for several decades. Illness behavior refers to "the ways in which symptoms are perceived, evaluated and acted upon by a person who recognizes some pain, discomfort, or other signs of organic malfunction" [1]. Most studies in this area have focused on individuals with acute organic illnesses, while chronic illnesses have received less

Reprinted from Social Science and Medicine, vol. 16 (1982), pp. 1397–1404.

attention. In many studies, in fact, the focus of research has been on not a particular type of disease but rather on response to any symptoms. In addition, virtually all studies focus only on certain phases of the illness behavior process, especially lay definitions of illness and the doctor-patient relationship after a diagnosis has been made.

It has long been recognized that the findings and concepts deriving from studies of patients' responses to acute diseases may not be applicable to the experiences of individuals with chronic illnesses [2]. The typical biomedical characteristics of these two types of diseases differ considerably. Most acute illnesses are self-limiting; the individual is sick for a short period of time and then either recovers or dies. Furthermore, the classic symptoms of these illnesses (e.g. fever, nausea, chills, pain) are, from their onset, serious, incapacitating and to most Americans, highly recognizable. Finally, since acute illnesses have been the focus of scientific attention, successful diagnostic techniques and treatments are available. In contrast, most chronic diseases are characterized by their permanent and continuing nature; the initial symptoms are often mild, nondisabling and vague; the symptoms are often not easily recognizable by lay people or most physicians; and effective diagnostic and treatment strategies do not exist for many chronic diseases. Given these differing biomedical characteristics, it can be assumed that patients' responses will also vary. Thus, existing findings and concepts focusing on symptom recognition, help-seeking behavior, and the therapeutic encounter among the acutely ill may not be directly relevant to the prediagnosis behavior of the chronically ill.

While these differences have been recognized for at least two decades, little has been done to document them or to delineate their theoretical implications. These issues are addressed in this paper, using findings from an investigation of the prediagnosis illness behavior of individuals with one chronic illness—multiple sclerosis. On the basis of these findings, the applicability of prior research findings and concepts to the experiences of individuals with chronic illnesses such as multiple sclerosis will be assessed.

ILLNESS BEHAVIOR IN ACUTE ILLNESS

Beginning with Talcott Parsons' model of illness behavior, the illness experience has commonly been viewed as socioculturally controlled; the individual's responses to illness and the doctor-patient relationship are viewed as governed by explicit normative expectations [3, 4]. The sick person's response to illness is to adopt the societally recognized and defined 'sick role' and to contact a physician to legitimize his action. The doctor-patient relationship is generally viewed as functional, predictable, and harmonious because each of the parties is assumed to know and understand what behavior is expected of both themselves and the other. While the doctor-patient relationship involves reciprocity in the form of behavioral expectations, the power of the parties is not equal. Due primarily to their technical expertise, physicians are the dominant and active participants, determining whether it is appropriate that a person adopt the sick role, whereas the patient is expected to be subordinate and relatively passive.

The limitations of Parsons' structural-functional model have been widely recognized, especially its simplicity and failure to account for variations in the behavior of both patients and physicians [5–8]. At each stage of the illness behavior process, the patient's decisions, actions and interactions are not uniform, as Parsons appeared to suggest, but highly variable. Many variables—the nature of the illness, psychological social, cultural and situational factors—have been analytically delineated that might produce variation in the sick person's responses [9–13]. However, most empirical research on illness behavior supports the basic assumptions of the model [14]. In most studies, the process beginning with symptom recognition and ending with diagnosis is described as rapid and straightforward and the decisions, actions and interactions of participants in episodes of illness are described as culturally or normatively determined. This is well illustrated in the conclusions of Edward Suchman's study of illness behavior [15]. First, most afflicted individuals self-diagnosed their symptoms as illness and contacted a physician within one week after their recognition. Second, most patients obtained an acceptable professional diagnosis and began a successful treatment regimen following their first visit to a physician. Third, nearly all patients cooperated with their physicians in carrying out their prescribed regimen and, consequently, returned to health. Finally, at each stage, most patients received support for their decisions and actions from their lay associates. These findings led Suchman [16] to conclude that:

> *In general, the description of the 'natural history' of illness in our society would support a positive appraisal of the pathways and routines established by the medical system for the care of the ill . . . the seeking and finding of the medical care appears to take place without too much difficulty.*

Put another way, Suchman's findings, along with the findings of most other empirical studies, suggest that the illness experience is governed by well-defined behavioral expectations, as Parsons indicated.

ILLNESS BEHAVIOR AMONG MULTIPLE SCLEROSIS PATIENTS

The investigation of pre-diagnosis illness behavior among people with multiple sclerosis enables us to assess the impact of the biomedical characteristics of disease on patients's and physicians's behavior. It also provides further documentation for the manner in which illness behavior in chronic disease varies from the Parsonian model. Given the biomedical characteristics of multiple sclerosis described above, we would expect the illness behavior process to be more complex. More specifically, we would expect that:

(1) Defining the symptoms will be a more difficult process for individuals with the symptoms of multiple sclerosis, and definitional disagreements between afflicted individuals and their relatives and physicians will be more common.

(2) Help-seeking behavior, sick role adoption, doctor-patient and patient-significant other relationships will be complicated due to the physicians' difficulties in diagnosing the disease.

(3) The social and emotional impact of the pre-diagnosis period will be greater for individuals with multiple sclerosis.

Such variations in the illness behavior of the chronically ill have been suggested in the literature. However, research, and most analytical assessments on chronic illness, have focused on the post-diagnosis doctor-patient relationship, the post-diagnosis sick role, and the post-diagnosis coping mechanisms of patients—not on the social processes beginning with symptom recognition and ending with the diagnosis [17–19]. This period—a time of contact with medical professionals but without authoritative legitimation for the sick role—has been virtually ignored. The stages that are most often the focus of research are precisely the stages at which social consensus and definitional clarity are likely to exist. The focus on

these stages has led investigators to ignore the process by which normative consensus is achieved, the role of both physicians and patients in that process, and the consequences of the failure to achieve consensus. Thus, the research on the prediagnosis behavior of multiple sclerosis patients has important theoretical implications for traditional models of illness behavior. When illnesses are acute, adoption of the sick role appears to be a straightforward process and patient-practitioner relationships are governed by explicit normative expectations. Definitional and role clarity, consensus and harmony do appear to exist. The experiences of multiple sclerosis patients and other chronically ill individuals, however, suggest that illness behavior can be, and often is, less normatively controlled, rigid, and static. Situational and interactional processes influence the actors' decision-making more than has been previously recognized. Symptom definition, help-seeking behavior, and role consensus and legitimation are problematical processes that are 'worked on' by the participants. In short, illness behavior is often shaped as much by a negotiation process as by normative restraints.

RESEARCH QUESTIONS AND METHODOLOGY

The study described in this paper sought to discover how multiple sclerosis patients responded to the biomedical characteristics of their disease and to use these findings to compare their behavior to reports of the behavior of the acutely ill. The focal research questions were:

(1) How do patients and their family members interpret and respond to the initial symptoms?

(2) What criteria are used by lay individuals in defining their symptoms as indicative of illness or wellness?

(3) What is the nature of interaction between afflicted individuals and their lay associates concerning the symptoms?

(4) At what point and for what reasons do patients consult physicians?

(5) How do physicians interpret the symptoms?

(6) What is the nature of doctor-patient relationships over time?

The data on these questions presented in this paper were obtained as a part of a larger study that the senior author conducted on the adjustment of multiple sclerosis patients and their families throughout the course of their disease. The study was done in the San Francisco Bay Area over an 18-month period from 1975 to 1977.

The data were gathered through in-depth interviews with 60 patients and many of their immediate family members. The interview schedule included a series of standardized, open-ended questions focusing on the individuals' interpretations of symptoms and their actions and interactions in response to them during the pre-diagnosis period. Since all the individuals in this study were diagnosed as having multiple sclerosis, the data obtained on the pre-diagnosis period were entirely retrospective. The inherent limitations of retrospective data were minimized somewhat by cross-checking the patients' reconstructions of this period with the reconstructions of their close relatives.

The sample consisted of 20 white men, 20 white women and 20 black women [20]. These persons, whose average age was 42 years, had suffered from multiple sclerosis for an average of 14 years. Forty-eight were married, 11 were divorced and 1 was single. In terms of religious affiliation, 39 were Protestants, 16 were Catholics and the remaining five indicated no affiliation. Fifty-eight patients had graduated from high school and 9 were also college graduates. The primary economic providers in the patients' families were employed in white-collar occupations, skilled trades, or semi-skilled trades.

RESULTS

Among the patients in this study, the diagnosis of multiple sclerosis was seldom easily or rapidly reached. It took an average of 5½ years for the individuals to be correctly diagnosed. During this time, the illness behavior of the patients could be divided into three distinct temporal phases, based on the patients' self-diagnoses and the actions they produced. These phases, through which almost all individuals passed, were termed the *nonserious phase,* the *serious phase* and the *diagnosis phase.* During the nonserious phase, the patients did not define their symptoms as illness and took minimal actions in response to them. The serious phase, which is emphasized in this paper, began with the patients'

re-definition of their symptoms as illness and ended with their tentative diagnosis of multiple sclerosis. This was the main period of medical care contacts. The diagnosis phase is the period in which the patients underwent the final tests that resulted in their multiple sclerosis diagnosis.

The great duration of the pre-diagnosis period (the nonserious and serious phases) and the patients' changing interpretations of their conditions during this time resulted largely from the vague and mild nature of their symptoms and the lack of specific medical diagnostic tests for the disease. The most common symptoms individuals experienced were numbness and tingling sensations, coordination problems, double or blurred vision and general fatigue. The mild and invisible nature of these symptoms resulted in the patients' defining them as nonserious and, thus, not contacting a physician, for a considerable length of time. The lack of medical diagnostic tests resulted in their having difficulties obtaining correct diagnoses once they defined their symptoms as serious and began contacting physicians.

The Nonserious Phase

Interpreting the Symptoms. Nearly all patients (85%) viewed their initial symptoms as 'nonserious.' They maintained this outlook for an average of 3 years. Such persons saw little reason to be concerned because their symptoms were not greatly discomforting, persistent, visible, or disabling and most importantly, could usually be explained in nonmedical terms. For example, Franklin's [21] lack of concern about his initial symptoms, and his belief that his job (installing radios in airplanes) was the cause of his symptoms, was typical of patients' interpretations:

> When I was diagnosed, my doctor told me that I had probably had MS for five years. He said that the numbness in my ankles and the early bouts of double vision and clumsiness were my first symptoms . . . At the time, I never thought much about them at all. They came and then they'd go away and I'd forget about them. I just thought they were a side effect of my work, I did precision work in cramped spaces in airplanes and it had always been hard on my legs and eyes. All the guys who did this complained of the same types of things.

Instead of seeing their symptoms as indicative of serious illness, these patients viewed them as *ailments, minor illness,* or as *symptoms of other treated illnesses, injuries* or *pregnancies*. They used one, two, or all three of these rationales to explain their different symptoms or to explain the same symptom at different periods.

The first and most common explanation for symptoms given by patients was that they were simply ailments, i.e. slight changes in health status caused by nonmedical conditions. Symptoms were attributed to: personal situations (e.g. 'overwork,' 'social stress'); personal limitations, such as an innately weak constitution (e.g. 'I've always been sickly'); poor personal health care (e.g. 'out of shape,' 'rundown'); or simply 'getting older'. Ailments were perceived as within the range of normal bodily functioning, and it was assumed that most adults had some type of ailment (e.g. chronic headaches or backaches). They were felt to be largely incurable and, hence, simply to be lived with.

Second, patients often explained their symptoms as being minor illnesses. Minor illnesses were similar to ailments in that they were assumed to be within the range of normal adult health. They differed from ailments since they were defined as actual illnesses, although illnesses so mild and commonplace that a physician was usually not needed. Patients and their relatives or friends typically diagnosed these problems as 'arthritis,' 'iron deficiency,' 'poor circulation,' 'a pinched nerve,' 'bursitis,' 'inner ear problems,' 'ulcer,' or 'poor weakening vision.'

The final common explanation for their symptoms was that they were a side effect of other illnesses, injuries, or pregnancies for which they were being treated. Included were such medically defined afflictions as joint problems, tendonitis, bursitis, arthritis, high blood pressure, influenza, bad teeth, eye cold, eye strain, trick knee and injuries to various bones, muscles, or the eyes.

Response to the Symptoms. Most patients did take some action to alleviate their nonserious symptoms. The action taken most frequently was home treatments: simple procedures deriving from popular beliefs about the treatment of mild afflictions. These included behavioral changes (e.g. increased or decreased physical activity), over-the-counter medications (e.g. aspirin, eye drops, rubbing alcohol) and vitamins. Half of the individuals also consulted a physician. In nearly all cases, they discussed their symptoms with a physician with whom they were already having treatment for other illnesses. The physicians either supported the patients' self-diagnoses or could find nothing physically wrong. At this point in the disease trajectory, such diagnoses were acceptable because patients also believed that nothing was seriously wrong. Normative consensus was easily accomplished because both physician and patient accepted the same definition of the patient's condition.

The Serious Phase

All patients eventually rejected their initial interpretations and began to view their symptoms as representing acute physical illness. Typically, symptomatic changes (i.e. increased severity, persistence, or visibility) were the main reasons for this definitional shift. This began the primary period of medical care contacts. Most patients went to several physicians and were misdiagnosed a number of times before eventually receiving a correct diagnosis of multiple sclerosis. The misdiagnoses naturally produced uncertainty, confusion, and frustration and often caused strain in the patients' relationships with physicians and with relatives and friends.

Response to Symptoms: Medical Care Contacts. Once they considered their symptoms to be serious, the patients visited physicians. Although uncertain about their illness, they initially assumed that it could be readily diagnosed and cured. One patient confessed:

> I didn't think I had any disease that doctors didn't know much about. . . . I guess I was naive. When this all began, I thought doctors knew about most all diseases and could cure them.

This assumption rarely proved to be correct. In the aggregate, the patients spent an average of almost 2½ years before receiving an accurate diagnosis. During this time, they consulted 227 different physicians for a total of 407 diagnostic appointments, not counting follow-up appointments for treatments and tests.

The outcome of most (75%) patients' trips to physicians were ultimately unacceptable and inaccurate diagnoses. Most patients were often variously diagnosed during the serious phase. The most common types of physical illnesses attributed to the victims were neurological diseases and muscle, bone, and joint diseases. Generally, less serious diagnoses (e.g. eye infection, bursitis, inner ear infection, neuritis) preceded the more severe misdiagnoses (e.g. brain tumor, myasthenia gravis, muscular dystrophy and arthritis). Patients misdiagnosed as psychosomatically ill usually received vague diagnoses, such as nervousness, anxiety, depression or stress.

Patients underwent a wide assortment of therapeutic regimens based upon their misdiagnoses. Prescription drugs such as tranquilizers, cortisone-like drugs (prednisone, ACTH), pain pills and antidepressants were the main treatments they received from physicians. Other treatments included physical therapy or traction, psychotherapy, vitamins and minerals and even surgery.

Impact of the Serious Phase.   Since the symptoms did not respond to treatments, the patients' faith in their physicians' diagnoses were usually short-lived. This placed them in the difficult position of viewing themselves as sick but not being socially defined as such. This not only heightened their diagnostic uncertainties, but also produced alterations in their relationships with their physicians and relatives. Physicians and relatives seldom supported the patients' self-diagnoses as sick. This definitional conflict produced a stressful situation for patients which had important health consequences. Symptoms of stress often became more troublesome to the patients than the MS-related symptoms. The problems could only be resolved by obtaining an acceptable diagnosis and for most of the patients this became a focus of their thoughts and actions.

The patients' response to their physicians' unacceptable diagnoses and treatments was to view their physicians in increasingly negative terms. Their initial positive views of their physicians changed over time. As their initial confidence in the physician's skills waned, they began to see them as 'evasive,' 'nonsupportive,' 'insensitive,' 'uncaring,' and 'dishonest.' Mrs. Harmon reflects the views of many patients:

I went to seven or eight doctors in less than two years. I'd tell them about my pins-and-needles feelings, or my numbness, or my weak arms and they'd all do the same thing—nothing. I really

got upset with those doctors. They'd usually just say that my problems were normal for a woman my age (25) and things like that. And I'd get really uptight because they would just give me a valium and not try to find out what was really wrong. Some of them thought I was going off my rocker. They thought I was imagining the problems. . . . One of them just threw up his arms and said he didn't know what was wrong with me. Now isn't that some way for a doctor to act. I got so I didn't believe any of them. I knew something was wrong and felt they could find out if they would just try.

Physicians simply were not meeting the patients' expectations of caring and curing. Physicians appeared not to be concerned about them or to have the skills to ameliorate their physical problems. As a consequence, patients changed their expectations of themselves as patients. They viewed it as necessary to take a more active role in defining what the problem was and in deciding what should be done. No longer passively accepting their physicians' assessments, they felt their own diagnostic participation was essential. To this end, they encouraged their physicians to take further action; they 'shopped' for concerned and skilled physicians; and they attempted systematically to diagnose themselves.

The basic way that patients displayed their more active role in the therapeutic relationship was by returning to their physicians after they had been initially (and incorrectly) diagnosed and treated. Fifty-seven of the 60 patients eventually rejected their initial diagnoses and returned to their physician desiring further actions. Implicitly or explicitly, the patients were challenging their physicians' diagnoses and encouraging and sometimes demanding further tests and new diagnoses. Furthermore, for 42 of the patients this became a long-term process in which they repeatedly visited their physician to question the latest in a series of diagnoses they had received. While each encounter often produced further actions on the part of physicians, these actions seldom led to a diagnosis that was satisfactory to the patients. Only 15 patients were diagnosed as having multiple sclerosis by their original physician or by a physician they were referred to by their original physician. The remainder felt it necessary to 'shop' for a new physician.

The second way patients displayed autonomy and aggressiveness in therapeutic encounters was to search for a new physician who they felt could resolve their problems. Forty-five patients went to at least three different physicians and 23 went to six or more before finding one who acceptably and accurately diagnosed them. On the average, these patients contacted 6½ physicians. While each visit produced increasingly negative feelings towards physicians, most remained convinced throughout that they could find a 'good' physician.

During this phase, most patients also tried to diagnose themselves. They began reading popular and scientific medical books and consulting friends and relatives with medical or nursing training hoping to find an illness that fit their symptoms. Interestingly, 10 patients self-diagnosed themselves as having multiple sclerosis. This was done to assist physicians and also to relieve anxieties. While in a few cases self-diagnoses did produce the desired results, in most it did not. Physicians usually did not take their diagnoses seriously. Many patients were told by physicians that they were 'reading too much' or that they should 'leave their medical care to them.'

This self-diagnosis is an interesting 'move' in the negotiation process because it violates a very powerful normative expectation held by physicians—namely, that it is physicians alone who have the technical expertise to diagnose illness. Physicians respond very strongly to this normative violation because it threatens the very foundation of their authority. This dimension of the doctor-patient relationship is, for most physicians, an absolutely 'nonnegotiable' item.

In addition, the patients' self-diagnoses often increased their uncertainties and stress. The reason for this was that most patients changed their initial interpretations of their symptoms from curable acute illnesses to more severe or often life threatening illnesses (e.g. multiple sclerosis, cancer, myasthenia gravis, amyotrophic lateral sclerosis). These definitions were based not only on their self-diagnoses, but also their negative evaluations of physicians' evasiveness and lack of explicit diagnoses. As one patient stated:

> For the last year I thought I was dying of stomach cancer. I thought the numbness and tingling feelings in my stomach and my big loss of weight (45 pounds in nine months) were sure signs of cancer. I told my doctor but he wouldn't say or do nothing. I thought he knew it was cancer but was afraid to tell me.

In terms of the doctor-patient relationship and sick role adoption, the process characterized by these MS patients in the serious phase is quite different from what occurs with most acute illnesses. The seriousness and persistence of the symptoms motivate patients to refuse to accept the physician's judgment regarding their condition. They continue to pursue a definition of the situation consistent with their interpretation of their symptoms. They pester physicians to change their diagnosis and even bring in supporting medical information to bolster their position. The rapid emergence of social consensus and legitimacy that underlies the functional approach to the sick role is not present. In fact, quite the reverse, MS patients commonly take a more active and aggressive stance in their efforts to get their definition to prevail.

Following the physicians' unacceptable diagnoses, changes also occurred in the patients' relationships with their relatives and friends. At the beginning of the serious phase, patients reported discussing their symptoms frequently with immediate family members (i.e. spouses and parents) and a few of their closest friends. However, this level of interaction was maintained throughout the serious phase by only one-third of the patients. The remaining patients discussed their symptoms less frequently with their relatives and friends as the phase progressed. The reason for this was that the patients assumed that everyone was tired of constantly hearing their same complaints.

Most patients also felt they received less support from their relatives and friends over the course of the serious phase. Compared with the patients, relatives and friends accepted the physicians' diagnoses much more frequently and viewed the patients' conditions as mild physical or psychosomatic illnesses. As a result, the patients had as much difficulty convincing their relatives and friends that they really were sick as they did their physicians. When they complained about their symptoms or took it easy on days when their symptoms were particularly severe, they felt that others viewed them as hypochondriacs or as malingerers.

The changes in the patients' interaction with and support from their relatives and friends are illustrated in the following statement by Mrs. Willis:

I discussed my problems quite a bit at first with my husband, and my mother and a few friends. But after awhile, I got tired of complaining and they were getting tired of hearing the same old things, so I just kept it to myself. Other people think you're crazy when you're always complaining about strange things and the doctors can't find nothing wrong. I know my husband and most of the rest of them thought it was all in my head. They usually wouldn't say that to my face, but I knew what they were thinking. . . . When I'd say something to my husband, he'd say all you do is complain, you've always been a complainer—so I quit complaining.

The Emotional Impact of Role Negotiation

It has been well documented that the social environment can have substantial impact on one's health status (see Refs [22, 23] for summaries). One element of this social environment is the role structure surrounding the individual. Beginning with Durkheim's investigation of suicide and continuing to the present, there is substantial evidence that the ambiguity and the degree of integration in a person's role structure can have an effect on health status. Other studies have focused on the degree to which uncertainty in defining situations can produce physiological arousal that may have detrimental health consequences (e.g. [24]).

The multiple sclerosis victims in this study found themselves—until they were finally diagnosed—in a very ambiguous situation in which they were unable to accomplish social consensus and an integrated role structure. They were pushed, on the one hand, by the increasing seriousness and discomfort of their symptoms toward an effort to adopt the sick role. They were prevented from successfully adopting the sick role, on the other hand, by the diagnostic uncertainties, the refusal of physicians to legitimize their sick role adoption and the negative reactions of relatives and friends. They found themselves in an ambiguous and uncertain limbo—they were not allowed to assume the social role that their physical symptoms seemed to propel them toward.

The outcome was abnormal amounts of emotional conflicts and tensions for almost all the patients. Feelings of frustration, worry and intermittent periods of depression were nearly universal. Over half of the patients also reported experiencing more severe psychological problems. Their most common symptoms were frequent periods of depression, anxieties, moodiness, and irritability. Less frequent emotional problems—or side effects—included social withdrawal (9 patients), difficulty falling asleep (7 patients), weight loss of more than 30 pounds (7 patients), regressive behavior (4 patients), mental confusion and memory loss (3 patients), increased alcohol consumption (3 patients), suicidal thoughts (2 patients) and stomach aches (1 patient). The types of problems these patients reported experiencing are illustrated in the following statement by Mrs. Adams:

I was in bad shape emotionally. I got so I was depressed and worried all the time. I thought for sure it was a brain tumor, and I didn't know if others were hiding it from me or if they just didn't care enough to believe me. I turned into a child. I was totally wrapped up in myself and my problems. I didn't want to see other people. I just wanted to be alone. At the same time, I started getting terrible stomach aches that were diagnosed as colitis.

Eventually, some physicians began to suspect that the patients had multiple sclerosis or a related neurological disease. This suspicion resulted either from the patient contacting a physician during a dramatic acute attack of symptoms suggestive of multiple sclerosis, or simply by the patient consulting a physician experienced with multiple sclerosis. At this point, nearly all the patients were hospitalized (for an average of 3 weeks) for a final series of tests that within 6 months usually resulted in a multiple sclerosis diagnosis.

During this diagnosis period, nearly all the patients reported a reduction in stress. Even the diagnosis of multiple sclerosis and the realization that they were permanently ill produced little immediate emotional impact on the patients. They gave four reasons for their positive reactions. First, they were pleased to finally have a name for their symptoms. Second, the patients received greater social support from their relatives, friends, and physicians who, often for the first time, indicated that they were entirely certain the symptoms were real. Third, for patients who had thought they were terminally ill, the diagnosis of multiple sclerosis relieved their fears that they were going to die. Finally, most were very optimistic about the future course of their illness. This resulted from their physician's unrealistically optimistic prognoses. According to patients, physicians stressed the possibility of remissions, mild cases, and the development of a cure for multiple sclerosis. Mrs. Irving's reaction was typical:

> I was so glad to find out I had MS. . . . Then I knew I wasn't dying and knew what I had to cope with. . . . I could also finally say ha-ha to all these people who thought it was all in my head. . . . MS didn't frighten me because I thought my condition would never get any worse. My doctor told me a lot of research was being done to find a cure. . . . I was just waiting for the cure to be discovered.

The experience of these MS patients during the pre-diagnosis and diagnosis phases suggests the importance of a type of iatrogenic disease not frequently discussed: disease resulting from the stress of a doctor-patient relationship that is characterized by ambiguity and a lack of integration. Iatrogenic disease is commonly limited to physical conditions caused by the *treatment process*. Our study suggests that behavioral scientists might fruitfully investigate the dimensions of the *social relationship* between patient and doctor that contribute to a diminution in the patient's health status. Although we were unable to quantitatively measure the extent of this impact, it seems clear from our interviews that it occurred with almost all patients.

CONCLUSION

Summary

This study demonstrates some of the specific variations in illness behavior due to the biomedical characteristics of chronic illnesses such as multiple sclerosis. Compared to prior studies, defining symptoms, help-seeking, sick role adoption and the doctor-patient relationship were more complex for multiple sclerosis patients and as a result, they suffered more emotional and social conflicts. To include chronic

illnesses such as multiple sclerosis within the domain of illness behavior, a wider range of symptom definitions and the potential for definitional and role disagreements must be considered.

The major findings of this study that are different from much existing research on illness behavior are the following:

1. Due to the relatively mild and vague nature of the initial symptoms of multiple sclerosis, a great deal of diversity and conflict occurs in lay and professional interpretations of the symptoms.
2. Lay individuals recognize an intermediate state between health and illness which might be termed 'pseudo illness' (i.e. ailments and minor illnesses) that does not usually lead to medical care contacts.
3. While virtually all patients view physicians positively and seek them out as soon as they define themselves as ill, patients will reject physicians' diagnoses and treatments when they appear ineffective to them.
4. The result of this is a lack of diagnostic consensus between the doctor and patient, and this typically extends to the sick individual's relationships with relatives who usually accept the physicians' assessments.
5. The patient's response to this dissensus is typically to take a more active role in the diagnostic process which changes the nature of the doctor-patient relationship. Their aim is to assist the physician in diagnosing their condition.
6. The situation of definitional and role conflict is very stressful for most patients and often leads to a variety of psychosomatic symptoms. These symptoms are ameliorated when the patient is acceptably and accurately diagnosed as having multiple sclerosis which also resolves the social conflict. Thus, surprisingly, the diagnosis of multiple sclerosis usually resolves more psychological stress than it creates.

Theoretical Implications

Conceptualizations of illness behavior have assumed that, once people recognize they are ill and seek medical attention, the physician quickly diagnoses the illness, the patient receives authoritative legitimation for the sick role and treatment is initiated. Because of the nature of acute illness which has been the focus of most studies, this view of illness behavior appears to be accurate. Normative clarity and consensus are assumed to exist in the doctor-patient relationship and social interaction is assumed to flow smoothly.

These assumptions do not appear to pertain to some aspects of illness behavior among multiple sclerosis patients or, we suggest, the illness behavior of patients with many other chronic illnesses, especially during the period we termed the 'serious phase' (when patients defined themselves as sick and sought out physicians to obtain an acceptable diagnosis that would legitimize their claim to the sick role). Prior research on these processes, in support of the structural-functional perspective, has suggested that professional legitimation of the sick role is straight-forward and that the physician-patient relationship is characterized by a high degree of definitional and role consensus and harmony. The underlying reason for this is that physicians can readily diagnose and treat the types of illnesses that have been studied—acute illnesses. In contrast, when physicians have difficulty diagnosing and treating the illness, as is the case in multiple sclerosis and many other chronic illnesses, the entire process is more problematic and cannot be explained solely in structural-functional terms. The situation is less normatively controlled and as a result social dissensus and disharmony occur. The therapeutic encounter clearly involves a process downplayed by structural-functional theorists: role negotiation. The behavior of patients and physicians is shaped as much by a situational bargaining process as by normative expectations. The legitimation of the sick role and patient-practitioner consensus emerge only after a lengthy bargaining process. The physicians's ultimate legitimation of the patient's claim to the sick role was in part dependent on the patient's ability to negotiate effectively.

The theoretical perspective that appears best suited to the study of illness behavior among the chronically ill is not structural-functionalism, but instead the 'negotiated order theory.' In this view, the role relationship between a physician and patient is not a static, rigid element of social interaction determined by sociocultural learning (although it is clearly influenced by that learning). Rather, it is a problematic relationship that must be continuously 'worked on' by the participants. As Day and Day have stated:

> In contrast to the structural-functional and rational-bureaucratic theories . . . , the negotiated order theory downplays the notion of organizations as fixed, rather rigid systems which are highly constrained by strict rules, regulations, goals, and hierarchical chains of command. Instead, it emphasizes the fluid, continuously emerging qualities of the organization, the changing web of interactions woven among its members, and it suggests that order is something at which the members of the organization must constantly work [25].

In our investigation of patients with multiple sclerosis, we were able to observe the manner in which this role negotiation occurred between patient and physician. Each person was attempting to maintain the definition of the situation they felt to be appropriate, and ultimate legitimation and consensus arose in part because of the negotiation process.

Physicians are in an extremely powerful position in the therapeutic encounter because of their ultimate control of legitimation and thus, consensus. This control rests on the physician's ability to diagnose and treat the symptoms presented. In illnesses such as multiple sclerosis where the diagnosis is problematic and effective treatments do not exist, physician's position is threatened. They may not recognize the symptoms and thus, be incapable of legitimizing the patient's claim to the sick role. Even if physicians suspect multiple sclerosis, they may be unwilling to legitimize the patient's claim because they are uncertain of the correctness of the diagnosis due to the lack of specific diagnostic tests. In this situation, physicians may opt to delay informing the patient until more clinical evidence is collected. Delaying the diagnosis appears to have several benefits from the physician's point of view, and in fact, this strategy is routinely suggested in medical texts on multiple sclerosis. Thus, in one text, the author states:

> Even if MS is considered possible, there is a natural reluctance to make the diagnosis because no-

*body likes to be the bearer of bad news and, in
any case, there is no certain way of confirming
it. Nearly always everything soon subsides and
is forgotten or ignored. At present, there is no
particular virtue in establishing an early diagnosis [26].*

The most obvious benefit of delaying the diagnosis to physicians is that it allows them to collect
more data and consequently, decrease the risk of
misdiagnosis. At the same time, physicians also postpone the difficult personal and professional task of
bearing the bad news that the individual has a severe
illness that medical science can do little about therapeutically.

What is not clearly indicated in the medical literature on multiple sclerosis is when the physician
should inform the patient. This decision appears to
be left largely to the physician's discretion. Clearly,
the quantity of clinical evidence and the severity
of the patient's symptoms are important considerations. However, as our study has indicated, it also
depends, in part, on the patient's interactional skills.
The patient's ability to negotiate can play a role in
convincing the physician that symptoms are severe
or that the costs of not legitimizing the sick role
will be high. Patients can assist the physician by
gaining knowledge that allows them to present their
symptoms in a way that makes them more recognizable to the physician. Patients also control costs in
this situation in a number of ways: their persistence
can be very time-consuming and aggravating to physicians; they can hint that legal action might result
if a physician misses or withholds a diagnosis; or
they can seek diagnoses from other physicians with
the implied threat that the previous physician's inadequate diagnostic skills will be discovered. These
factors clearly seem to play a role in the physician's
decision to diagnose multiple sclerosis and thus, legitimize the patient's claim to the sick role.

These conclusions also have applied implications
for medical practice. When physicians assume that
there is no advantage in providing an early diagnosis,
they are ignoring the social and personal implications of the situation from the patient's point of view.
They are placing the patients in the difficult position
of feeling very sick, but not being socially recognized
as such. As we have illustrated, this situation is
productive, in many cases, of severe stress for patients that may lead to serious emotional problems.
Physicians should consider this when deciding
whether or not to delay informing a patient of their
tentative diagnosis.

References

1. Mechanic D. and Volkart E. Stress, illness behavior
and the sick role. *Am. Sociol. Rev.* **25,** 52, 1961.
2. Kassebaum G. and Bauman B. Dimensions of the sick
role in chronic illness. *J. Hlth Soc. Behav.* **6,** 16, 1965.
3. Parsons T. *The Social System.* The Free Press, Glencoe,
IL.
4. Parsons T. and Fox R. Illness, therapy and the modern
urban American Family. *J. Soc. Issues* **8,** 31, 1952.
5. Suchman E. Stages of illness and medical care. *J. Hlth
Hum. Behav.* **6,** 114, 1965.
6. Kasl L. and Cobb S. Health behavior, illness behavior,
and sick role behavior. *Archs Envir. Hlth* **12,** 246, 1966.
7. Twaddle A. Health decisions and sick role variations:
An exploration. *J. Hlth Soc. Behav.* **10,** 105, 1969.
8. Fabrega H. Toward a model of illness behavior. *Med.
Care* **6,** 470, 1973.
9. Bauman B. Diversities in conceptions of health and
physical illness. *J. Hlth Soc. Behav.* **2,** 39, 1969.
10. Szasz T. S. and Hollender M. H. A contribution to the
philosophy of medicine: The basic models of the doctor-
patient relationship. *Archs Intern. Med.* **97,** 585, 1956.
11. Kasl L. and Cobb S. *op. cit.*
12. Mechanic D. *Medical Sociology,* 2nd Edition. The Free
Press, New York, 1978.
13. Twaddle A. and Hessler R. *A Sociology of Health.* C. V.
Mosby Co., St Louis, MO, 1977.
14. Arluke A., Kennedy L. and Kessler R. C. Re-examining
the sick role concept: An empirical assessment. *J. Hlth
Soc. Behav.* **20,** 30, 1979.
15. Suchman E. *op. cit.*
16. *Ibid.,* p. 171.
17. Szasz T. S. and Hollender M. H. *op. cit.*
18. Kassebaum G. and Bauman B. *op. cit.*
19. Gallagher E. Lines of reconstruction and extension in
the Parsonian sociology of illness. In *Patients, Physicians, and Illness* (Edited by Jaco E. G.), 3rd Edition,
pp. 162–182. The Free Press, New York, 1979.
20. This sample was drawn to assess sex and ethnic differences in the impact of multiple sclerosis. Data on these
topics are not presented in this paper because significant differences did not occur in the patients' general
patterns of prediagnosis illness behavior.

21. All personal names in this paper are pseudonyms.

22. Kaplan H. B. Social psychology of disease. In *Handbook of Medical Sociology* (Edited by Freeman H. E. *et al.*), 3rd Edition, pp. 53–70. Prentice-Hall, Englewood Cliffs, NJ, 1979.

23. Graham S. and Reeder L. G. Social epidemiology of chronic diseases. In *Handbook of Medical Sociology* (Edited by Freeman H. E. *et al.*), 3rd Edition, pp. 71–96. Prentice-Hall, Englewood Cliffs, NJ, 1979.

24. Kaplan H. B. Studies in sociophysiology. In *Patients, Physicians and Illness* (Edited by Jaco E. G.), 2nd Edition, pp. 86–96. The Free Press, New York, 1972.

25. Day R. A. and Day J. V. A review of the current state of negotiated order theory: An appreciation and a critique. *Sociol. Q.* **18,** 132, 1977.

26. Mathews B. *Multiple Sclerosis: The Facts*, pp. 35–36. Oxford University Press, Oxford, 1978.

Socioeconomic Class, Classification of 'Abnormal' Behavior and Perceptions of Mental Health Care

Peter L. Heller
Maria del Carmen Rivera-Worley
H. Paul Chalfant

Since the earliest studies in 1917, a massive amount of research concerning the relationship between lower-class status and mental illness has been reported. While this research suffers from a multitude of conceptual and methodological problems, the findings do strongly suggest that lower-class populations have disproportionately high rates of mental illness. Investigators have offered a number of explanations for this higher rate without any definite conclusion concerning cause being made (Mishler and Scotch, 1963; Roman and Trice, 1967; Kohn, 1978; Dohrenwend and Dohrenwend, 1969;

Fried, 1969; Riessman *et al.*, 1964; Chalfant, 1974; Warheit *et al.*, 1973; Andersen *et al.*, 1977; Myers *et al.*, 1975; Liem and Liem, 1978).

Two of the suggested explanations, psychiatric or diagnostic bias and the labeling approach, suggest that mental health is basically a middle-class concept and that lower-class individuals are more frequently defined as mentally ill because they do not behave in middle-class ways (Strauss, 1969; Gursslin *et al.*, 1959; Scheff, 1968). Hollingshead and Redlich, and Langner and Michael (Hollingshead and Redlich, 1958; Langner and Michael, 1963), for example, suggest that feeling state changes such as depression are likely to be defined as indicators of poor mental health among middle-class populations, while lower class respondents focus upon behavioral problems

Reprinted from the *Sociology of Health and Illness*, vol. 1 (1979), pp. 108–121.

such as aggression in assessing a person's mental health. Following this lead, we propose to investigate the relationship between socioeconomic status and rates of mental illness in terms of lower-class perceptions of certain disordered behaviors and the sources of help, if any, thought relevant to these behaviors.

Certainly there is no lack of research findings and theorizing which suggest that the lower-classes in society differ from the middle statuses in both life style and perception of the social environment (Rainwater et al., 1959). The middle-class world is seen as more predictable and middle-class children tend to be socialized into the expectation of such predictability. Middle-class 'members' participate in community life because such participation makes sense in a stable world that implies an identification of oneself in terms of others within the system, and a perception of a stable and ongoing set of roles defined as legitimate within the community itself (Farber, 1971).

Depending upon the particular circumstances, working- or lower-class individuals tend not to have such a life view, at least not to the same extent. Their social universe is more unpredictable and life is not generally perceived in career terms; at least for the unskilled and semiskilled families, it is seen as a series of jobs interspersed by periods of unemployment and crisis. Rainwater et al. (1959:45) have stated one view of the lower-class woman's perception of herself in the world:

> A central characteristic of the working class wife is her underlying conviction that most significant action originates from the world external to herself rather than within herself. For her, the world is largely unchangeable, a kind of massive, immovable apparatus that is simply there.

And again:

> This feeling of smallness before the world is not restricted to a specific context, but is pervasive . . . she tends to see the world beyond her doorstep as fairly chaotic, and potentially catastrophic (1959:325).

The research findings from several studies also suggest that, regardless of the culture studied, people located in the lower strata of society tend to share a number of central characteristics (Roman and Trice, 1967; Prince, 1969). Of special interest here are the cross-cultural findings that lower-class members tend to: define the entire social world outside peer group and family as 'them,' with a concomitant distrust of all 'them' and 'their' institutions; perceive the outer world as chaotic and fear its unpredictable and catastrophic qualities; seldom participate in community life; and surround themselves with a family circle consisting of both immediate and secondary relatives. While such typifications of working- class individuals clearly do not apply to all such persons, varying certainly with the nature of the world, they have been established as sufficiently adequate descriptions that some generalization can be made.

We argue, then, that working-class people less often participate in community life, and more frequently surround themselves with a family circle consisting of both immediate and secondary relatives because such *behavior patterns make sense, given the nature of the environment in which they live.* There is less perceived reward for participation in community life, and the unpredictable nature of a world ruled by the out-group, middle class, as well as the lesser prestige associated with working-class occupations and stress of residence lead to a shunning of community involvement. In an unstable social structure, positions frequently do not endure, and those that do endure are not legitimated so that community participation would be a painful reminder of one's inferior status. To the extent that activities are perceived to be 'community' organized and run, lower- or working-class populations will hold their involvement to a minimum. Thus, emotional and physical needs will be satisfied where possible on an informal basis through interaction with kin and friends—people with whom the individual has sentimental attachments and has established trust relationships.

HYPOTHESES

Our formal hypotheses are derived from this attempt to look at disordered behavior from the perspective of the lower-class individual and view the behavior in terms of the conditions of their life. We hypothesize then that certain types of behavior and perceptions of the environment which could be abnormal in middle-class society are perceived as quite normal in the lower class or working class world, and that lower class respondents will tend to describe such behaviors and perceptions as normal or only slightly extreme. Further, we hypothesize that lower class living conditions lead to the development of an informal network of mutual aid relationships and a tendency to seek formal, professional mental health care facilities only for concrete and extreme examples of abnormal behavior. Specifically, our hypotheses are:

H_1: The extent to which a deviant behavior will be defined as a 'mental health problem' is positively related to class.

H_2: The extent to which a person who manifests a 'deviant' behavior pattern will be said to need therapy from a professional health worker is positively related to class.

H_3: The extent to which an individual would turn to a professional mental health worker for an emotional problem is positively related to class.

H_4: The extent to which an individual would turn to a professional mental health worker for information concerning a source of treatment is positively related to class.

DATA AND MEASURES

Data for this study are taken from interviews with 36 working- and 37 middle-class female respondents. Interviews were conducted in two small West Texas towns during the summer and fall months of 1975. Placement of respondents in socioeconomic strata was determined exclusively by husband's occupational role. The lower-class sample includes all respondents whose husbands were in occupational categories of wage workers in unskilled, semi-skilled or skilled jobs. 'Middle-class' refers to respondents whose husbands were employed in entrepreneurial, managerial, or professional occupations. Excluded from analysis are respondents from lower-middle class occupations such as clerical, or owners of extremely small businesses.

Perceptions of mental illness and care for such illness were elicited by seeking response to five examples of behavior patterns considered indicative of mental disorder by mental health professionals:

'Mental Health' Stories Told to Respondents

Story 1—Frank Jones

I'm thinking about a man . . . let's call him Frank Jones . . . who is very suspicious. He doesn't trust anybody and he's sure that everybody is against him. Sometimes he thinks that people he sees on the streets are talking about him or following him. A couple of times now, he has beaten up his wife terribly and threatened to kill her, because he said, she was working against him, too, just like everyone else.

Story 2—Betty Smith

Betty Smith is a young woman in her twenties. She hasn't had a job, and she doesn't seem to want to go out and look for one. She is a very quiet girl, she doesn't talk much to anyone except her own family, and she acts like she is afraid of people, especially young men her own age. She won't go out with anyone and when someone comes to visit her, she stays in her own room until they leave. She just stays by herself and daydreams all the time, and shows no interest in anything or anybody.

Story 3—Bill Williams

For another example of different types of people, here is a man named Bill Williams. He never seems to be able to hold a job very long because he drinks so much. Whenever he has money in his pocket, he goes on a spree; he stays out till all hours drinking, and never seems to care what happens to his wife and children. Sometimes, he feels very bad about the way he treats his family; he begs his wife to forgive him and promises to stop drinking, but he always goes off again.

Story 4—Patricia Brown

Mrs. Patricia Brown is a middle-aged mother of seven who never leaves the house. Until recently, she was always considered a 'good mother and housewife' and her children always looked clean and neat. Lately, she has been quite nervous and touchy. She says that she is killing herself working for nothing, that nobody cares and that the family will only realize her efforts after she dies or leaves home for good.

Story 5—James Arnett

My last example is James Arnett. James, a young high school dropout, simply doesn't care about anything. He says that the future is for the birds and that life must be lived now. He started to experiment with drugs and left home shortly thereafter. He is now hooked on hard drugs, although he denies it.

Examples ranged from withdrawal and depression to 'excessive' drug and alcohol use. Respondents were asked two questions regarding each of the five behavior examples. The first question involved respondent's classification of the behavior patterns: 'What do you think is wrong with ——?' Responses were coded into one of two response categories, *light symptoms* or *mental incapacity*.[2] The second question concerned the type of help the respondent felt was needed by the person in the example. This two-part question was asked as follows: 'Do you think—— needs some kind of help?'; and if yes, 'What kind of help do you think——needs?' Responses to the two-part second question were coded as 'doesn't need help'; 'informal therapy,' such as talking to a family member of clergyman; or professional mental health worker.

Two other dependent variables were measured. The source of treatment the respondent would use if he developed an emotional problem was measured by the question, '. . . let's suppose you had a lot of personal problems and you're very unhappy most of the time. Let's suppose you've been that way for a long time and it isn't getting any better. What do you think you'd do about it?' Answers to this question were coded: 'informal source,' 'medical doctor' or 'professional mental health source' (see Table 11 footnotes 'b' and 'c' for classification schema). The last question concerned the source of information the respondent would use to decide where to find help for an emotional problem. The question asked was, 'Suppose you didn't know of any places yourself. Do you know of anywhere you might go to find out about where help is available?' Responses to this question were coded into three categories: 'informal source,' 'medical doctor,' or 'professional mental health source.'

FINDINGS

Tables 1 through 5 show the relationship between respondent's definition of a given behavior pattern and class. In three out of five behavior examples, the two variables are significantly associated. In the Frank Jones example (Table 1) a strong association (gamma = 0.72) exists between response classification and class. Moderately strong to strong associations are also found for the Betty Smith example (gamma = 0.58, Table 2), and the Patricia Brown story (gamma = 0.89, Table 4).

Behavioral definitions and class are not significantly related in the Bill Williams and James Arnett

TABLE 1 Classifications of Frank Jones'[a] behavior by class

	RESPONSE CLASSIFICATIONS					
	LIGHT SYMPTOMS[b]		MENTAL INCAPACITY[c]		TOTAL[d]	
RESPONDENT'S CLASS	N	%	N	%	N	%
Lower	15	44	19	56	34	100
Middle	4	11	31	89	35	100
	gamma = 0.72; z = 2.75; p < 0.01					

[a] See p. 53 for Frank Jones example.

[b] Response examples would be nervous, shy, unfriendly, etc.

[c] Response examples would be mentally ill, emotionally disturbed, paranoid, crazy, losing his mind, etc.

[d] Each class is represented by 36 respondents. In this and other tables, totals will fall short of 36 because of 'don't know' or answers irrelevant to the question.

TABLE 2   Classification of Betty Smith's[a] behavior by class

| | RESPONSE CLASSIFICATIONS | | | | | |
| | LIGHT SYMPTOMS | | MENTAL INCAPACITY | | TOTAL | |
RESPONDENTS' CLASS	N	%	N	%	N	%
Lower	21	72	8	28	29	100
Middle	14	41	20	59	34	100
	gamma = 0.58; z = 2.23; p < 0.05					

[a] See p. 53 for Betty Smith example.

TABLE 3   Classification of Bill Williams'[a] behavior by class

| | RESPONSE CLASSIFICATION | | | | | |
| | LIGHT SYMPTOMS | | MENTAL INCAPACITY | | TOTAL | |
RESPONDENTS' CLASS	N	%	N	%	N	%
Lower	2	6	32	94	34	100
Middle	2	6	32	94	34	100
	gamma = 0; p > 0.05					

[a] See p. 53 for Bill Williams example.

TABLE 4   Classification of Patricia Brown's[a] behavior by class

| | RESPONSE CLASSIFICATIONS | | | | | |
| | LIGHT SYMPTOMS | | MENTAL INCAPACITY | | TOTAL | |
RESPONDENT'S CLASS	N	%	N	%	N	%
Lower	27	96	1	4	28	100
Middle	21	60	14	40	35	100
	gamma = 0.89; z = 3.05; p < 0.001					

[a] See p. 53 for Patricia Brown example.

TABLE 5   Classification of James Arnett's[a] behavior by class

| | RESPONSE CLASSIFICATIONS | | | | | |
| | LIGHT SYMPTOMS | | MENTAL INCAPACITY | | TOTAL | |
RESPONDENT'S CLASS	N	%	N	%	N	%
Lower	7	21	27	79	34	100
Middle	13	38	21	62	34	100
	gamma = 0.41; z = 1.32; p > 0.05					

[a] See p. 54 for James Arnett example.

examples (Tables 3 and 5, respectively). It should be noted that these behavior examples involve 'excessive' alcohol consumption and use of drugs. The other three examples (Tables 1, 2, and 4) relate to suspiciousness, withdrawal and nervousness or depression. These findings directly support the Hollingshead and Redlich, and Langner and Michael suggestions noted above that lower-class residents are more prone, than their middle-class counterparts, to focus on concrete behavior problems rather than mental states in determining the state of an individual's mental health.

Tables 6 through 10 summarize the association between type of help respondent feels is needed by the person in the story, and class. Once again, the same three behavior stories (Frank Jones, Betty Smith, and Patricia Brown) involve significant degrees of association between suggested therapy and class. It should again be noted that significant degrees of association found in Tables 1, 2 and 4 (Jones, Smith, and Brown examples) demonstrate the relative unwillingness of lower-class respondents to perceive emotional problems such as 'extreme' suspiciousness, withdrawal or depression as important enough to need formal treatment. Behavioral extremes such as excessive drinking or drug addiction are seen by both classes as 'abnormal' to an extent where some type of professional treatment is necessary.

Table 11 presents data designed to test Hypothe-

TABLE 6 Suggestions for therapy for Frank Jones[a] by class

RESPONDENT'S CLASS	DOESN'T NEED THERAPY		INFORMAL THERAPY		PRO- FESSIONAL THERAPY		TOTAL	
	N	%	N	%	N	%	N	%
Lower	1	3	4	14	24	83	29	100
Middle	0	0	2	6	33	94	35	100
	gamma = 0.55; z = 1.88; p < 0.05							

[a] See p. 53 for Frank Jones example.

TABLE 7 Suggestions for therapy for Betty Smith[a] by class

RESPONDENT'S CLASS	DOESN'T NEED THERAPY		INFORMAL THERAPY		PRO- FESSIONAL THERAPY		TOTAL	
	N	%	N	%	N	%	N	%
Lower	11	33	11	33	11	33	33	99
Middle	3	9	9	26	22	65	34	100
	gamma = 0.56; z = 3.86; p < 0.001							

[a] See p. 53 for Betty Smith example.

TABLE 8 Suggestions for therapy for Bill Williams[a] by class

RESPONDENT'S CLASS	DOESN'T NEED THERAPY		INFORMAL THERAPY		PRO- FESSIONAL THERAPY		TOTAL	
	N	%	N	%	N	%	N	%
Lower	0	0	2	6	31	94	33	100
Middle	0	0	1	3	34	97	35	100
	gamma = 0.33; z = 0.34; p > 0.05							

[a] See p. 53 for Bill Williams example.

TABLE 9 Suggestions for therapy for Patricia Brown[a] by class

RESPONDENT'S CLASS	DOESN'T NEED THERAPY		INFORMAL THERAPY		PRO- FESSIONAL THERAPY		TOTAL	
	N	%	N	%	N	%	N	%
Lower	15	50	9	30	6	20	30	100
Middle	9	27	11	33	13	39	33	99
	gamma = 0.40; z = 3.37; p < 0.001							

[a] See p. 53 for Patricia Brown example.

TABLE 10 Suggestions for therapy for James Arnett[a] by class

RESPONDENT'S CLASS	DOESN'T NEED THERAPY		INFORMAL THERAPY		PRO- FESSIONAL THERAPY		TOTAL	
	N	%	N	%	N	%	N	%
Lower	1	3	3	10	27	87	31	100
Middle	2	6	4	12	27	82	33	100
	gamma = −0.20; p > 0.05							

[a] See p. 54 for James Arnett example.

TABLE 11 Source respondent would use for treatment of emotional problem[a] by class

RESPONDENT'S CLASS	SOURCE						TOTAL	
	INFORMAL SOURCE[b]		MEDICAL DOCTOR[c]		PRO- FESSIONAL MENTAL HEALTH SOURCE			
	N	%	N	%	N	%	N	%
Lower	18	69	6	23	2	8	26	100
Middle	12	44	5	18	10	37	27	99
	gamma = 0.51; z = 3.15; p < 0.001							

[a] See text for specific question.   [b] Relative, friend or clergyman.   [c] Not including psychiatrist.

TABLE 12 Source of information for treatment source by class

RESPONDENT'S CLASS	SOURCE						TOTAL	
	INFORMAL SOURCE		MEDICAL DOCTOR		PRO- FESSIONAL MENTAL HEALTH SOURCE			
	N	%	N	%	N	%	N	%
Lower	10	62	4	25	2	12	16[a]	99
Middle	10	40	12	48	3	12	25	100
	gamma = 0.32; z = 2.24; p < 0.05							

[a] Twenty lower-class respondents (about 55 per cent of the lower-class sample) did not know of any source of information concerning mental health care.

sis 3. As predicted, middle-class respondents would be more prone than are their lower-class counterparts to use professional mental health sources for treatment of an emotional problem. A moderately strong association (gamma = 0.51) is found between health treatment and respondent's class.

Finally, middle-class respondents show a significantly greater tendency (Table 12) than lower-class respondents, to use a non-informal source for information concerning where to go for problem related treatment. Hypothesis 4 is thus supported.

DISCUSSION

It is not possible to generalize these rural West Texas research findings to all of middle- and lower-class America. Still, our findings do point to a number of conclusions and suggestions for further research. First, the study's general theoretical hypotheses are supported. Lower-class respondents, more frequently than middle-class respondents, tend not to define certain forms of deviant behavior as mental or emotional incapacities; tend to suggest informal rather than formal sources of help for these deviant behaviors; tend not to suggest using professional mental health specialists for treatment of emotional disorders; and use informal sources for information concerning treatment of emotional problems.

We can also make a tentative suggestion concerning the finding that lower-class respondents were less likely than their middle-class counterparts to consider three of the five behavior patterns summarized on pp. 53–54 to be indicators of mental or emotional incapacity. It has been suggested in the literature that one factor influencing this type of finding could be lack of education (or inappropriate socialization). It has been suggested that lower-class people have been differentially socialized (in families and/or through lack of formal schooling) to perceive these behavior patterns as 'abnormal' in a psychiatric sense. Also, a 'culture of poverty' approach might predict these findings in terms of lower-class values. We disagree with both these explanations. It should be noted that among both lower- and middle-class respondents, excessive alcohol and drug use were considered to be disordered forms of behavior. Both groups, in fact, suggested formal, professional sources of treatment for these types of problems.

We suggest an alternative explanation to the differential socialization and/or culture of poverty arguments. A number of authors including Goffman (1967) have noted that every behavior defined as 'mentally ill' may be considered appropriate in other situations. Says Goffman,

> I know of no psychiatric misconduct that cannot be matched precisely in everyday life by the conduct of persons who are not psychologically ill nor considered to be so; and in each case, one can find a host of different motives for engaging in the misconduct . . . (1967:147)

Most researchers have at least provisionally accepted the fact that mental illness occurs disproportionally among lower-class people. Research has tended to focus either on the mechanisms that lead to this disproportionate amount of mental illness, or reasons why lower-class people are more prone to come into contact with authorities who have the power to label behavior 'abnormal.' If Goffman's message is taken literally, it could be hypothesized that much of the behavior which is defined as abnormal may indeed be normal given the exigencies of the individual's situation. Noted above are the cross-cultural findings that lower-class populations in general: define the entire social world outside peer group and family as an alien environment; perceive the outer world as chaotic, unpredictable and potentially catastrophic; seldom participate in community life; and surround themselves with people whom they feel can be trusted. In such an environment, are the 'suspicious' and aggressive behaviors of Frank Jones, the withdrawn behavior of Betty Smith, and the nervousness and depression of Patricia Brown 'abnormal,' given the nature of lower-class environment? Lower-class respondents may see these behaviors as mild, rather than extreme symptoms of abnormal behavior because such behavior is commonly witnessed in day-to-day interactions. It is the middle-class sample[3] that interprets these mental states and behaviors as abnormal, because such feelings and behaviors would indeed be abnormal in an environment which is stable and predictable.

The findings presented in Tables 6, 7 and 9 can likewise be explained in this light. If the behaviors exhibited by Frank Jones, Betty Smith and Patricia Brown are only mildly different from those exhibited by others adapting to the catastrophic world associated with lower-class existence, it does not make sense to advise formal, professional treatment for these people. This type of advice is even more irrelevant if professional treatment centers are perceived as part of the formal and alien world connected with lower-class life. Informal help from family or friends, or perhaps a talk with a clergyman, should be enough to help the individual cope with his day-to-day living conditions.

It should be noted that alcoholism (Bill Williams) and drug addiction (James Arnett) are fully considered to be pathological behavior by members of each class—behaviors which perhaps cannot be handled informally. Such behaviors, in fact, may lead to family and peer group disruption to the extent that the very ability of the group to survive is threatened. Under such conditions, the individual and his family and friends are better off if the offending individual is removed from the group for therapy.

The study's final conclusion focuses upon findings presented in Tables 11 and 12, that lower-class respondents would not tend to use professional mental health sources for help with an emotional problem. Again, among lower class respondents, existence in general tends to isolate and alienate the individual from middle-class bureaucratic life. Especially interesting here is the extent to which our lower-class respondents were completely lacking in knowledge about mental health information. About 55 per cent of our lower-class sample (see footnote a, Table 12) simply had no idea of where they would go for advice concerning help for a mental health problem.

We have tried in this paper to demonstrate that behavior labeled 'mentally ill' by middle-class professionals in the mental health field will be perceived to be normal or only slightly extreme by a sample of lower-class respondents. It is further suggested that these behavior patterns are normal or only slightly extreme by a sample of lower-class respondents. It is further suggested that these behavior patterns are normal reactions to general structural conditions associated with lower- and (to a lesser extent) working-class life. In behavior stories representing paranoia, withdrawal and nervousness, lower-class people were significantly less likely than their middle-class counterparts, to perceive these patterns as constituting extreme behavior aberations, or to proscribe a need for formal treatment.

In overt drunkenness and drug addiction, the two classes were close together in perceptions and proscriptions.

The alienating and mean nature of lower-class life depicted above would appear to indicate a need for suspiciousness, nervousness, and at times withdrawal, as normal adaptive behaviors. It would indeed be 'abnormal' to trust and openly participate in an environment which is hostile and unpredictable. It would also make sense to turn toward informal sources for treatment of all but the most extreme examples of overt behavior. Formal sources, after all, are directly associated with the world outside the neighborhood—the unpredictable and hostile world rules by 'them' and 'their' impersonal bureaucratic institutions.

Notes

1. Reprint requests should be directed to H. Paul Chalfant, Professor and Chair, Department of Sociology, Texas Tech University, Lubbock, Texas 79409.

2. Statements made by respondent which indicated that the behavior exemplified in the behavior example is at most a fairly minor deviation from normal behavior. Examples of such statements are, 'He (she) is just nervous,' 'he (she) is an unfriendly person,' 'he (she) is shy around other people.' Responses such as 'He (she) is crazy,' 'he (she) is mentally ill,' 'he (she) is losing his (her) mind,' or '. . . is paranoid,' or '. . . emotionally disturbed' were coded as definitions of the behavior exemplified as a type of mental incapacity. In short, coding for Tables 1 through 5 was based upon respondent's propensity to share (albeit in lay person's language) or not to share, the professional's definition of behaviors typified by the five behavior stories presented on pp. 53–54.

3. It should be noted that in the Patricia Brown example (Table 4) 60 per cent of the middle-class respondents considered this behavior pattern as consisting of light symptoms. On the other hand, 72 per cent of these respondents felt Ms. Brown needed some sort of therapy for her behavior (Table 9).

References

ANDERSEN, RONALD, FRANCIS, ANITA, LION, JO-ANNA and DAUGHERTY, VIRGINIA S. 1977 'Psychologically related illness and health services utilization.' *Medical Care* 15 (May):59–73.

CHALFANT, H. PAUL 1974 'Mental health and the poor.' Pp. 218–33 in Joan Huber and H. Paul Chalfant (eds.), *The Sociology of American Poverty.* Cambridge, Mass.: Schenkman.

DOHRENWEND, B. P. and DOHRENWEND, B. S. 1969 *Social Status and Psychological Disorder.* New York: Wiley-Interscience.

FARBER, B. 1971 *Kinship and Class: A Midwestern Study.* New York: Basic Books.

FRIED, M. 1969 'Social differences in mental health.' Pp. 113–67 in J. Kosa, A. Antonovsky and I. K. Zola (eds.), *Poverty and Health: A Sociological Analysis.* Cambridge, Mass.: Harvard University Press.

GANS, H. 1962 *The Urban Villagers: Groups and Class in the Life of Italian-Americans.* New York: Free Press.

GOFFMAN, E. 1967 *Interaction Ritual: Essays on Face-to-Face Behavior.* New York: Ancho Books.

GURSSLIN, O. R., HUNT, R. G. and ROACH, J. L. 1959 'Social class and mental health movement.' *Social Problems* 7:210–18.

HOLLINGSHEAD, A. and REDLICH, F. 1958 *Social Class and Mental Illness.* New York: Wiley.

KOHEN, M. L. 1968 'Social class and schizophrenia: a critical review.' In D. Rosenthal and S. S. Kety (eds.), *The Transmission of Schizophrenia.* London: Pergamon Press.

LANGNER, T. and MICHAEL, S. 1963 *Life Stress and Mental Health.* New York: Free Press.

LIEM, RAMSAY and LIEM, JOAN 1978 'Social class and mental illness reconsidered: The role of economic stress and social support.' *Journal of Health and Social Behavior* 19 (June): 139–56.

MISHLER, E. G. and SCOTCH, N. 1963 'Sociocultural factors in the epidemiology of schizophrenia: a review.' *Psychiatry* 26:315–51.

MYERS, JEROME K., LINDENTHAL, JACOB J. and PEPPER, MAX P. 1975 'Life events, social integration and psychiatric symptomatology.' *Journal of Health and Social Behavior* 16 (Dec.):421–29.

PRINCE, R. 1969 'Psychotherapy and the chronically poor.' Pp. 20–41 in J. C. Finney (ed), *Culture Change, Mental Health and Poverty.* New York: Simon & Schuster.

RAINWATER, L., COLEMAN, R. P. and HANDEL, C. 1959 *Workingman's Wife.* New York: Oceana.

RIESSMAN, F., COHEN, J. and PEARL, A. (eds.) 1964 *Mental Health and the Poor.* New York: Free Press.

ROMAN, P. M. and TRICE, H. M. 1967 *Schizophrenia and the Poor.* Ithaca, New York: Cayuga Press.

SCHEFF, T. J. 1968 *Being Mentally Ill.* Chicago: Aldine.

STRAUSS, A. 1969 'Medical organization, medical care and lower income groups.' *Social Science and Medicine* 3:143–77.

WARHEIT, GEORGE, HOLZER III, CHARLES E. and SCHWAB, JOHN J. 1973 'An analysis of social class and radical differences in depressive symptomotology: A community study.' *Journal of Health and Social Behavior* 14 (Dec.):421–9.

_____

CHAPTER 3

The Patient Status: The Career Perspective

While a great deal of research has been focused on why people accept the sick role, surprisingly little attention has been paid to what follows the acceptance. The career perspective follows the patient through the stages of illness.

Two of the more prominent applications of the career perspective have been to the cases of the terminally ill patient and the patient in the mental hospital. Elizabeth Kübler-Ross (1969) has presented a classification of five stages through which terminal patients go. These include (1) denial of the illness and isolation from others, (2) anger, (3) bargaining with medical personnel and/or God for additional time, (4) depression, and (5) acceptance. Although there is general agreement about the earlier stages, there is considerable disagreement concerning the extent to which terminal patients accept the nature of their illness.

In his book *Asylums* (1961), Erving Goffman discusses the "moral career" of individuals confined to total institutions such as prisons and mental hospitals. The moral career is defined as the process "through which a progressive change occurs in the belief system of the individual concerning himself and others." Goffman is not very clear about the exact stages of the moral career with the exception of his description of the first stage of mortification. During the period of mortification the individual is stripped of his or her previous identity by several means. This stripping process is seen by the staff of the mental hospital as a way of getting the mental patient to accept his or her illness and as a necessary condition for eventual rehabilitation.

It is important to note that it is unrealistic to conceive of most patients as moving in a completely linear fashion through the stages of their careers. It is more likely, as Gustafson shows in relation to the nursing home patient in this chapter, that a patient's progress in his or her career will occur in a back and forth movement. That is, at any point, a movement to an earlier stage is just as possible as a movement to a later one.

In the lead article in this chapter, Elizabeth Gustafson describes the career perspective and applies it to the case of the nursing home patient. The unique nature of the nursing home patient's career is brought out by comparing it with the career of the TB patient. A major point that Gustafson makes is that a major fear of the nursing home patient concerns one's social death preceding one's biological death. In the following article, Jean Comaroff and Peter Maguire discuss the indeterminacy of the careers of children afflicted with leukaemia. Employing the terminology from the previous article by Gustafson (although Comaroff and Maguire do not do this), the careers of these children are marked both by progressive elements (the disease seems to be in remission) and regressive elements (the disease reappears). Once again, the role of the uncertainty of medicine is examined—here, in terms of its effects on child and family.

References

GOFFMAN, E. 1961. *Asylums*. New York: Doubleday-Anchor.
KÜBLER-ROSS, E. 1969. *On Death and Dying*. New York: Macmillan.

Dying: The Career of the Nursing Home Patient

Elizabeth Gustafson

In this study, the "career timetables" format developed by Julius Roth in *Timetables: Structuring the Passage of Time in Hospital Treatment and Other Careers* (1963) is applied to the experience of elderly persons in convalescent hospitals and nursing homes. One theoretical objective of the paper is to demonstrate that analytical sets appropriate for the study of young and middle-aged Americans can be useful in the study of the aged. Another is to study the concept of careers in a different setting. The analysis of the degree to which careers of nursing home patients fit Roth's paradigm throws light on their social and psychological problems. The conclusions indicate that nursing home staffs should develop ways of helping their patients to live fully and die gracefully.

This paper presents an hypothesis about life in the nursing home which may be amenable to partial empirical substantiation. It is based on an informed but informal study of events in one nursing home where the author was employed for one year. Visits in other nursing homes and familiarity with the literature suggest that the hypothesis has merit. Fortunately, there is no chance that a systematic bias was built into the observations because all experience in the nursing home preceded exposure to Roth's theory.

The development and uses of a career timetable are the subject of Roth's book. Roth claims that "when many people go through the same series of events, we speak of this as a career and of the sequence and timing of events as their career timetable"

Reprinted from the *Journal of Health and Social Behavior*, vol. 13 (1972), pp. 226–235.

(1963:93). Roth uses the institutionalized TB patient as his model. According to his definition, a career is

> *a series of related stages or phases of a given sphere of activity that a group of people goes through in a progressive fashion (that is, one step follows another) in a given direction or on the way to a more or less definite and recognizable end-point or goal. (1963:94)*

Roth found that people involved in a career try to define when certain salient things will happen to them. By pooling their observations in an unsystematic way, career participants develop time norms against which to measure their individual progress. The benchmarks on this timetable are the significant events that occur in the average career.

When the career is "part of a service or authority relationship," each of the two groups establishes a timetable for the same set of events. The norms of the two groups are bound to be somewhat different because their criteria for progress and their idea of proper timing are different (Roth 1963:107). Bargaining occurs when the career participant tries to bring the judgment of the authority figure into line with his own more optimistic view of his status on the timetable.

Roth's paradigm consists of these three aspects. The career is a series of commonly defined stages on the way to a recognizable end point. The timetable consists of benchmarks which identify these stages. Bargaining between the career participants and figures in authority occurs when their respective opinions as to the patient's position on the timetable are not compatible.

THE CAREER

A majority of patients in a nursing home for old people are, more or less actively, dying. Except in cases where the patient is severely incapacitated intellectually, patient, relatives, and staff almost always know that, generally speaking, this is a "terminal case." So there exists what Glaser and Strauss (1965) call "an open awareness context." This is true whether the patient is suffering from a rapidly progressive disease of which he will soon die or from the general deterioration of old age, in which case he may linger indefinitely. He may not know which is his situation, and he may deny the fact that his days are numbered, but he does know that he has come to stay until he dies.

The nursing home is the last resource for old people and their families (if they have any), who have tried to maintain their social independence as long as possible (Kahana 1971; Jacobs 1969). Admission to a nursing home is widely considered the ultimate failure in one's social career. Roth himself perceives the nursing home patient as a "chronic side-track" (1963:105). He claims that life in such a cul-de-sac is not a career because it moves in no direction. It is marked only by a "failure timetable," which serves the most limited function: "to split long blocks of time into smaller, more manageable units" (Roth 1963:12).

Our interpretation of the picture, however, is that the simple facts of advanced debility and chronological age prevent the nursing-home patient from fitting into the "side-tracked" category. It may be that the TB or mental patient or the prisoner with a life sentence at age thirty also has nothing to look forward to but death, but it is still so far away that he and his peers do not associate it with their present existence. For the aged patient, the passage of days of itself brings him noticeably closer to the end of the road. Admission to the nursing home immediately launches him into a new, regressive career ending in death.

Although in common parlance the term "career" signifies a forward or upward progress of some sort, Roth's definition (see page 63) clearly can include the regressive experience of the nursing home patient. Group definitions of timetable benchmarks and end points of the careers are the crucial factors, not the positive or negative nature of the goal. (Erving Goffman, whose book *Asylums* is the source of many of Roth's concepts, also defines career as "any social strand of any person's course through life. . . . Such a career can no more be a success than a failure" (1961:127). There is a universal acknowledgment that death is the end of the nursing home career and there is a generally accepted timetable which will be described in this paper.

The fact that the nursing home patient's career is regressive instead of progressive constitutes the important difference between this career and the career of TB patients and others. In the case of the TB patient, minimizing treatment time constitutes success. For the nursing home patient, success is the maximum delay of passage from one stage to the next. This contrast is pictured in Fig. 1.

In the TB patient's career, passage of significant events and bargaining efforts move in the same direction, towards recovery. In the nursing home patient's career, events progress in one direction (towards death) and bargaining efforts pull in the other direction, back towards health. This tension makes life very difficult, but it may be essential to the maintenance of any kind of life at all. This idea is considered in more detail later.

Before we go on with the discussion, it will be useful to elaborate briefly on the nature of death. Death includes both physical termination and a final social separation. The ordinary person does not conceptualize these aspects separately. Therefore the scheme in Fig. 1 represents well enough the view of dying held by the ordinary patient and staff mem-

Fig. 1. Schematic View of TB and Nursing Home Patient Careers

TB Hospital	Timetable of events[a]	Recovery
Health	Bargaining	
Nursing home	Timetable of events[a]	
	Bargaining[b]	Death

[a] The time which elapses between any two benchmarks is fairly regular in the TB treatment career and is often very irregular in the nursing home career.

[b] The discontinuation of bargaining by the nursing home patient is discussed in the paper.

ber: it is one continuous and irreversible process of physical deterioration and social loss. A more careful scrutiny suggests a breakdown of the total career into social dying—progressive separation—and biological or psychological death, both of which imply total psychic separation from the environment. (See Fig. 2.)

This scheme makes it clear that during most of his career, the patient is really fighting social death, the increasing degrees of separation. In the ideal scheme, only the onset of the terminal phase signifies the appropriate end of social life and of efforts to maintain it.

THE CAREER PARTICIPANTS

It will be clear at once that not all patients in a nursing home are involved in the establishment of the timetable and bargaining efforts. Some patients are out of touch with reality before they are admitted. Others are too depressed or severely ill at admission to take part in bargaining behavior. Some patients once active in these matters have become senile, psychotic, or very ill. A very few may have been able to give up bargaining behavior consciously (more on this later) but it seems unlikely that there are any mentally competent patients who *never* take part in this activity simply because they "don't fear death" (cf. Kastenbaum 1967). Patients may welcome a prospective end to physical fatigue and pain but the bargaining behavior we will discuss is a response to social death. Moreover, it seems probable that ambivalent feelings are common in this matter. Even if one is not afraid, surely one might be glad to delay the event as long as possible. Schneidman claims that "psyde (death)-postponing is the habitual, indeed the unthinking, orientation of most humans towards cessation . . . the psyde-postponer is one who . . . wishes it would not occur for as long as possible" (1963:218). The disinclination of the patient

to give up this life-long stance we feel is reinforced by the fact that life in the nursing home puts pressure on him to give it up prematurely.

THE TIMETABLE

A person moves through his career as a nursing home patient according to a timetable informally defined by the patients and their caretakers. The timetable may be said to consist of four overlapping categories of benchmarks on a regression scale. Physical deterioration is measured by degrees of social activity, mobility, and functional control. Mental deterioration is measured by declining mental control. (See Fig. 3.)

This informal timetable of overlapping scales stands in marked contrast to the formalized system of classification and status-identifying privileges that Roth reports from TB hospitals (1963:101). The fact that these reference points are not formally defined means that the discrepancy between functional and status positions, which confuses the scene at the TB hospital (Roth 1963:19), is hard to perceive in the nursing home.

An additional difference between this and the TB treatment scheme is that there is no standard duration for each stage of the nursing home career (cf. Roth 1963:22) and there is no guarantee that every patient will move in an orderly way through this regressive scheme. Improved health and relapses occur frequently and cause constant shifts in the patient's time perspective.

One reason why the benchmarks on these scales are so general is that considerably limited communication in the nursing home situation makes it difficult to construct a more elaborate scheme. The top medical staff, of course, has a different and more detailed set of norms by which to judge a patient's position. The patient has little access to these reliable medical clues, however. Strauss and Glaser point

Fig. 2. Components of death

| Health | Social phase Timetable of social death ————————————→ Bargaining ←———————————— | Terminal phase Bodily death ————————————→ No bargaining | Biological or psychological } DEATH |

Fig. 3.   Timetable Scales in Nursing Home Career

PHYSICAL DETERIORATION SCALE		MENTAL DETERIORATION SCALE	
SOCIAL ACTIVITY	MOBILITY	FUNCTIONAL CONTROL	MENTAL CONTROL
1. Passes to "outside"	1. Walks	1. Continent	1. Occasional forgetfulness
2. Responsibility for own affairs; social contacts			
3. Meaningful hobby or job	3. Hobbles		
4. Physical recreation			4. Occasional incoherence
5. Spectator recreation	5. Wheelchair	5. Incontinent	5. Considerable disorientation
6. Minimal activity	6. Bed		
7. Lassitude[b]	7. Extreme weakness[b]		7. Totally *non compos mentis*[a]
8. Coma	8. Transfer to general hospital		

[a] Persons who have regressed to this point are too far out of touch to take any part in the definition and accomplishment of their careers. Their progress is of interest only to the medical staff and other people.

[b] These symptoms often signify the onset of the "terminal phase." (See Fig. 2.)

out that, for medical personnel, "the highest professional reward is in the patient's recovery and return to his normal personal and social life" (1965:178). In order to uphold staff morale, in most general hospitals in "wards that contain dying patients there is some typical ratio of both certain and uncertain death" (Glaser and Strauss 1965:179). The nursing home cannot provide this balance and as a result is the most demoralizing (and least prestigious) setting for medical personnel to work in. Doctors feel justified in giving first priority to patients elsewhere who show some promise of recovery, and therefore they visit nursing home patients only rarely and briefly as a rule. Often, his own unresolved anxieties about death prevent the doctor from participating in an honest discussion with the patient of his condition (Kübler-Ross 1969; Strauss and Glaser 1965; Quint 1967).

The staff of a nursing home consists mainly of minimally trained nurses' aides, who rarely know anything useful to the patient and even more rarely give up the cheerful, noncommittal, and evasive line used with aged and dying patients. Friends and relatives are usually in the same self-protective situation as the nurses' aides. The chief nurse is the staff member most often in a knowledgeable position and may occasionally provide a useful clue for the patient.

Communication among patients also tends to be minimal. There are a number of explanations for the striking lack of interaction among patients. Although public opinion lumps all old persons into one social class, they are not of course a homogeneous group. Even within one nursing home, especially if it serves both welfare and private patients, the variety of experiential backgrounds is likely to be great. Therefore patients may simply find that they have very little in common, very little to talk about, with one another. The disengagement theory of Cumming and Henry (1961) offers another explanation for the lack of communication. However, in this situation as in the outside world, disengagement may not be voluntary. Although no staff member or relative will directly discourage the patient from making new friends in the nursing home, he is often not expected or encouraged to do so. As we have mentioned earlier, admission to the home is usually treated as the end of one's useful social career. A clear correlation between degree and duration of institutionalization and lack of communication has been found in several studies (Rosenfelt and Slater 1964; Coe 1965; Kahana 1971; and others).

Erving Goffman describes withdrawal behavior as characteristic of the newcomer to the mental hospital ward. The function of withdrawal is to deny the new identity of self with inmates (1961:146). Admission to a nursing home often follows rapidly upon the occurrence of a paralyzing stroke, amputation, or similar trauma to both body and psyche. Thus, withdrawal may understandably be pronounced. Moreover, the nursing home patient may remain in this stage longer than the mental patient because there is no progressive career for him to enter.

Another possible explanation for isolationist behavior is that many patients are already bearing such a "grief load," including grief over their own imminent deaths (Wiesner 1968; Birren 1964; Feifel 1959), that they are not willing to take the emotional risk of establishing a friendship with yet another person who may well die soon.

In most cases, a combination of all of these factors is probably involved in the low level of communication among nursing home patients. The most interesting hypothesis from the point of view of this study is that the patients are intuitively conniving to minimize the exchange of information about timetable norms so that they can more easily delude themselves that they are holding out against death better than they really are.

Just as the incomplete exchange of information about timetable norms may have a function in a regressive career, perhaps the obviously limited dependability of the reference points also has some use. The scales are approximate at best and in any case are not really a reliable indicator of the approach of death, which could unexpectedly overtake the patient at any time. However, there is a utility in this kind of timetable for a regressive career. When things look bad, one can find fault with the benchmarks. When things look good, one ignores the fact that death does not always "follow the rules" implied by the timetable. Objectively speaking, the norms are not reliable, but psychologically speaking, they are comforting. Working out one's position on a career timetable is in itself a lively, hopeful, social activity.

At the end of the regression, the reality is harder to avoid. Confinement to bed accompanied by extreme lassitude or coma are pretty sure signs. And transfer to a general hospital, except for repair of fractures or routine treatments, suggests that the end is near. (For this reason, routine trips to the general hospital can be very traumatic for the patient who has not been helped to understand the reason

for the trip.) There is an obvious utility in this scheme. Early in his career, norms are vague and the patient is kept busy evaluating his status and bargaining for a sense of social viability. At the end of the career, perhaps within a week or two of death, the signs are much more dependable and the imminence of death cannot be avoided. At this point the patient enters the terminal phase (see Fig. 2) and is encouraged by unavoidable signs to "let go" all social ties and bargaining effort, to resign himself to death.

BARGAINING

Bargaining is as important an aspect of life in a nursing home as it is in the TB hospital, but it has a subtly different meaning. Goffman has commented that the concept of career is two-sided: it refers both to such internal matters as one's "image of self and self-identity" and also to one's public status and official position (Goffman 1961:127). The TB patient bargains for a change in his official position: he wants those in authority to do something to change his status. Patients in nursing homes are not assigned to any official position. Therefore the nursing home patient bargains for moral and social support for his self-image: he wants both authorities and peers to do and say things assuring him that he is maintaining a "lively" status, that he is important to other people, and that his social death will not precede his physical death. Thus the objectives of bargaining in the nursing home are harder to define but easier, if tact outweighs strict honesty, to confer.

Patterns of bargaining in the nursing home are similar to those in the sanatorium, but of course they work in reverse. While the TB patient increases his bargaining activity as he moves towards the end of his hospital career (Roth 1963:40), the nursing home patient starts out actively bargaining and often gives up this effort towards the end of his career. In both cases, the change in bargaining intensity is related to a changing time perspective. Both TB and nursing home patients commonly start their careers with the idea that it won't take long—to get cured, or to die (Roth 1963:104). In almost all cases, the patient soon learns that the goal is much further away than he thought at first. This realization discourages the TB patient from bargaining hard until the chances for success seem greatest: at the end of his progressive career. But the realization is a kind of reprieve for the nursing home patient and encourages him to fight for the maintenance of his social life. When the end does come into sight, it is not worth the effort to bargain any more.

For patients suffering primarily from impairment of intelligence, all socially coherent bargaining will take place before they move into level seven of the mental control scale. (See Fig. 3.) Patients located at an earlier point on this scale may be aware of the timetable and make efforts to control their status on it. They try hard to control their intellectual processes—by moving and talking with deliberation, by cooperating with staff in matters of rest, diet, drugs, and activities, and by conserving their energies to make special efforts for the doctor and family when they visit. They are well satisfied when they succeed in persuading everyone that they are doing very well, even if they "crash" afterwards.

Bargaining on the physical deterioration scales is easy but so unsophisticated that the patient may have trouble fooling even himself. Patients attach great importance to such signs of timetable status as personal social contacts, participation in recreational activities, ability to walk, and to control bladder and bowels. The patient avoids admitting that his rating according to some indicators may be determined less by his own vigor than by the enthusiasm of staff and relatives to help him (Roth 1963:50). Passes to visit away from nursing home, participation in social activities, provision with "nonessential" physical aids and therapies, and retraining in bladder control are all areas in which the contribution of other people is important. (The exception to this rule is seen in cases where the patient stubbornly gets into bed and refuses to do things that he could and should do. This can be interpreted as a perverse kind of disease-defying behavior in which the patient says, "I will not allow this disease to limit my activities: I will limit them right now of my own free will!" This is as effective a way as any of handling the timetable.)

When there is no escaping a clear symptom of debility, the patient may prefer to interpret it as a minor temporary ailment: the stroke patient denies the permanent paralysis of his arm and hand by saying he "sprained his wrist last week." Another avoidance technique is finding fault with the nursing home. Petty complaints about the staff arise from a deep underlying grievance: the staff resists bargaining efforts. The patient with means transfers from one institution to another in a hopeless and unconscious search for a place with a different kind of timetable on which he will rate higher.

Patients in the nursing home use another bargaining trick found in the TB hospital (Roth 1963:36–39): they choose inappropriate models for themselves. In a common example, the patient classifies himself with persons of similar socioeconomic background when this gives him confidence about his timetable status, instead of with other patients suffering from the same type of disease. The usual presence of both physically and mentally ill patients in the same facility is well used. The physically ill patient chooses to compare himself (to obvious advantage) with senile or other confused patients. On the other hand, the mentally ill patient often categorizes himself with the physically ill group, for the obvious reason that he is in reassuringly better physical health than they. By using this device, he not only puts death far away but avoids facing the probability of his own decline into incoherence and social incompetence, which is as unacceptable to many as physical death.

In the nursing home, as in the TB hospital, patients sometimes use extraneous criteria to improve their bargaining position. Provision with glasses, hearing aids, dentistry, occupational and physical therapy, and other aids and services which staff may consider nonessential are often highly valued by patients mainly as status symbols indicating that they have social value and possibly a long future. The old lady never reads but indignantly fights for new glasses: by getting them for her the staff shows that they consider her to have a future. Private possessions assume great importance as signs of viable social life for some patients; this accounts for the compulsive hoarding of "junk" such as Bingo prizes, greeting cards, holiday decorations, and items made in craft programs.

Like TB patients (Roth 1963:38), nursing home patients introduce moral criteria sometimes: "I have led an honest, hard-working life and therefore should be spared longer than that no-good Charlie." (People who use this approach often have doubts about the actual uprightness of their lives which they constantly beg friends and staff to allay.)

CONCLUSIONS

The unreliable nature of the career timetable of the nursing home patient and the type of unrealistic bargaining that it provokes are basic factors underlying the social scene in the nursing home. There are always some patients who are pitifully hopeful about their bargaining position until they die. A larger number drop out of the bargaining scene, especially towards the end of the career, as Fig. 1 indicates. Some of these have become too ill to maintain bargaining behavior. For others, it becomes impossible to avoid the fact that one is "serving an indeterminant sentence on death row." This has been called a perfect hell, and it is indeed for many aged persons. The stress of this situation contributes to the depression-apathy-passivity syndrome in many and may play a causative role in some kinds of senility and psychosis. Some patients whose personalities survive this test soon come to prefer death itself to this torture and attempt suicide or try to will themselves to death (Glaser and Strauss 1965; among others). An emotionally exhausted patient often gives up bargaining attitudes for a period, only to return to them when his emotional strength has returned and it becomes clear that his will to die is not yet going to be effective.

It is our hypothesis that this most unsatisfactory bargaining situation is partially caused by the fact that the career of the nursing home patient is perceived by patient and staff alike to follow an undifferentiated regressive trend as represented by the diagram in Fig. 1. The most difficult thing about the nursing home career as so defined is that there is no one but God—or death—to bargain with. In most careers, including TB treatment, the authority figure has only incomplete control over the passage of events; for example, the response of an individual case to treatment. In the case of the nursing home patient, however, medical authorities influence appearances but exert *no* real control over events. The timetable norms are irrelevant to the actual approach of death, which could "jump the gun" and occur at any time. The patient really bargains for more time directly with his disease, or death, or God.

Dealing with an opponent who is not human is terribly frustrating, for we do not know his norms.

The fact that people keep on bargaining in this situation when almost all other social activity is discontinued suggests that this is a primary form of social behavior. Gregory Rochlin goes so far as to suggest that the process (career?) of becoming civilized is a lifetime bargaining process that starts when the child (at around three years of age) perceives that he has limitations, including mortality. His life from this point on is dedicated to resolving (by bargaining tactics?) the conflicts with others and within himself that constitute limitations on his potential (Rochlin 1967:62–63). Insofar as these limitations are symbols of, or perhaps in a philosophical sense even derive from, his mortality, the whole process of becoming civilized and mature involves a constant bargaining with death. Conflict with others over his needs and desires is a constant in the life of the individual virtually from birth. Skills in bargaining for his various career interests are among the first a child learns and are so basic to social existence that he uses them even when they are ineffectual, just to assure himself that he is still socially alive.

Is it necessary that this desperate and ineffectual bargaining be the main source of social life for the nursing home patient? The popular concept of the dying career as a simple case of physical deterioration allows no hope to patient or staff, even when the patient's life stretches out over months or years. The staff attempts half-heartedly to keep up the patient's false hopes and to maintain his comfort. The patient, finding the staff unresponsive to the real meaning of his bargaining, becomes frantic and eventually lapses into despair (or senility or psychosis).

The differentiated view of death as including a social phase and a terminal phase before the final separation caused by psychological or biological death (Fig. 2) puts things into a different perspective. In this light it becomes clear that during the social stage, which includes most of the career, the patient is putting up a justifiable fight against the tendency of society (as represented by relatives, staff, visitors, and peers) to force him into premature social death. This kind of bargaining will and should continue in the best of institutions. But it will become effective and wholesome when the staff members and visitors respond by doing all they can to facilitate the preservation of the patient's maximum status according to the timetable scales. The staff member with this positive goal will find it easier to acknowledge (sometimes directly to the patient) that death is the inevitable end of the career. The patient who feels he has been valued and respected during this phase will find it easier to approach the end of his life willingly.

Only when the patient moves into the terminal phase should he feel he is bargaining directly with God for more time. Staff personnel can be trained to deal honestly with the patient in this phase and to help him move beyond the bargaining process in a positive way before he dies. A number of experts have discussed—and some have practiced—ways in which medical staff and relatives can be helped to accept the patient's death and become a source of strength to him. (See especially Kübler-Ross 1969; Quint 1967; Glaser and Strauss 1965; and Weisman and Kastenbaum 1968). The abandonment of bargaining signifies that the patient is ready to give up both social and biological life, willing to accept death graciously. It is important to note the fine psychological line between this patient and the suicidal patient who wants to be spared the torture of bargaining with death. The suicide's intention is to take the initiative into his own hands, to take the control of time and place and manner of death, at least, away from his Opponent (Schneidman 1970:40). The accepting patient lays down his arms, literally lays down his life, and takes up death in a positive and willing frame of mind. Only persons who can do this will "die happy," will die "in a state of grace." It should become the common goal of staff and patients that each dying career should end in this positive way.

SUMMARY

This analysis of the nursing home patient's experiences supports and extends Julius Roth's examination of human experience in terms of career timetables. The last phase of life, when it takes place in an institution, can be considered a career as appropriately as any other phase of life.[1] Nursing home patients and their overseers establish timetables by which to measure the status of individuals in the dying career. The vague and unreliable nature of the benchmarks, which would make the timetable of a progressive career close to useless, serves a function in this case where success consists of moving,

or appearing to move, from one stage to the next as slowly as possible.

Medical staff, friends, and relatives, and often patients themselves think of the patient career as an unbroken decline towards death. Instinct and will-to-live cause the patient to fight against the premature social death forced upon him in this situation. The increasing tension makes this a hellish existence for the patient. The social instinct to bargain for one's career interests is so strong, however, that patients often maintain this behavior, despite the pain it causes, after most other social behavior has been given up. Thus bargaining alone sustains social life.

It is suggested that a differentiated view of the dying career as consisting of a social stage and a terminal stage would be useful to nursing home staff and others concerned with the aged patient. A staff with this view would endeavor to extend the patient's social life for as long as possible, thus introducing vitality and honesty into the inevitable conflict between patient and staff interests during this phase; and to support the patient during the transition (the terminal phase) to an accepting and acceptable death.

Note

1. The effects of different environments (for example, community, open institution, total institution) and of relative duration of the career of the dying patient would make a useful study. Other studies are needed to elucidate the ways in which such variables as sex, education, wealth, fulfillment of life expectations, mental health, and family relations influence the bargaining behavior of aged dying patients.

References

BIRREN, JAMES.
1964 The Psychology of Aging. New Jersey: Prentice-Hall.
BRIM, FREEMAN, LEVINE & SCOTCH (eds.).
1970 The Dying Patient. New York: Russell Sage Foundation.
COE, RODNEY.
1965 "Self-conception and institutionalization." Pp. 225–243 in Arnold Rose and Warren Peterson, (eds.),

Older People and Their Social World. Philadelphia: Davis Company.

CUMMING, E. and W. HENRY.
1961 Growing Old. New York: Basic Books.

DUFF and HOLLINGSHEAD.
1968 Sickness and Society. New York: Harper & Row.

FEIFEL, H.
1959 The Meaning of Death. New York: McGraw-Hill.

GLASER, BARNEY G. & ANSELM L. STRAUSS.
1965 Awareness of Dying. Chicago: Aldine Publishing Company.
1968 Time for Dying. Chicago: Aldine Publishing Company.

GOFFMAN, ERVING.
1961 Asylums. New York: Doubleday and Sons (Anchor Books).

JACOBS, RUTH.
1969 "Adjustment to a home for the aged." The Gerontologist 9, (Winter):268–275.

KAHANA, EVA.
1961 "Emerging issues in institutional services for the aging." The Gerontologist 11 (Spring):51–58.

KASTENBAUM, ROBERT (ed.).
1964a New Thoughts on Old Age. New York: Springer.
1964b "The interpersonal context of death in a geriatric institution." Paper presented at Seventeenth Annual Scientific Meeting, Gerontological Society: Minneapolis.
1967 "The mental life of dying patients." The Gerontologist 7, (June):97–100.

KÜBLER-ROSS, ELISABETH.
1969 On Death and Dying. London: Macmillan.

QUINT, JEANNE.
1967 The Nurse and the Dying Patient. New York: Macmillan.

ROCHLIN, GREGORY.
1967 "How young children view death and themselves." Pp. 51–87 in Earl Grollman (ed.), Explaining Death to Children. Boston: Beacon Press.

ROSENFELT, R., R. KASTENBAUM, and P. SLATER.
1964 "Patterns of short-range time orientation in geriatric patients." Pp. 291–299 in Robert Kastenbaum (ed.), New Thoughts on Old Age. New York: Springer.

ROTH, JULIUS.
1963 Timetables: Structuring the Passage of Time in Hospital Treatment and Other Careers. Indianapolis: Bobbs-Merrill.

ROTH, JULIUS and ELIZABETH EDDY.
1967 Rehabilitation for the Unwanted. New York: Atherton Press.

SCHNEIDMAN, EDWIN.
1963 "Orientations towards death." Pp. 200–227 in Robert White (ed.), Study of Lives. New York: Atherton Press.
1970 "The enemy." Psychology Today (August):37ff.

WEISMAN, A. D. and T. HACKETT.
1961 "Predilection to death." Psychosomatic Medicine 23, (May-June):232–256.

WEISMAN, A. D. and R. KASTENBAUM.
1968 The Psychological Autopsy. Community Mental Health Monograph #4.

WODINSKY, ABRAHAM.
1964 "Psychiatric consultation with nurses on a leukemia service." Mental Hygiene 48, (April):282–287.

Ambiguity and the Search for Meaning: Childhood Leukaemia in the Modern Clinical Context

Jean Comaroff

Peter Maguire

The real hell of this illness is that you just don't know!

Parent of a leukaemic child

The immediate concerns of this paper are the changing social and experiential implications of childhood leukaemia under conditions of modern medical management [1]. In the last decade, developments in the clinical context of the disease have significantly altered its course in most sufferers. Remissions of five or more years are now secured for up to 50% of children in many treatment centres, and a small proportion have survived much longer [2]. Inevitably, such changed patterns of intervention have significant psychological and socio-cultural implications: the very meaning of the disease is undergoing revision, both among clinicians and laypeople. Ironically, apparent clinical gains have heightened immediate medical and experiential uncertainties. Insight into etiology and into variation in response to treatment have not kept pace with chemotherapeutic advance, and prognosis in individual cases remains relatively unpredictable. In fact, knowledge has advanced in piece-meal fashion, its gains highlighting the vastness of remaining ignorance.

The condition of childhood leukaemia is a graphic instance of the state of knowledge on the margins of bio-medical science, of the manner in which the known becomes distinguished from the unknown in this domain. Our concern in this paper is the effect of this process upon the experience of those to whom such changing knowledge is applied. The case of childhood leukaemia shows clearly how advances in empirical knowledge may occur in seemingly uneven fashion—as when, for example, modes of intervention precede knowledge of etiology. These developments imply specific reformulation of the contrast between the certain and the uncertain, the predictable and the random, and the relevant and the irrelevant. . . .

Our study of the impact of childhood leukaemia revealed this process in clear detail; the experience of uncertainty and the search for meaning were *the* characteristic features of the impact of the disease upon sufferers and their families. While these features are inherent in the experience of threatening illness itself, their striking form in this case was clearly the result of a particular set of developments in treatment. In this paper, we examine this relationship between advancing medical knowledge, its clinical application and its effects upon the sick. We place this process in its total socio-cultural context, and then discuss its implications for the social role of medical knowledge in general. . . .

THE STUDY

The data drawn upon here were collected as part of a study of the families of 60 children with acute

Reprinted from *Social Science and Medicine*, vol. 15B (2), 1981, pp. 115–123.

myoloblastic or lymphoblastic leukaemia, admitted to a regional pediatric oncology unit in England between January 1976 and April 1977 [3]. Research focussed on the psychological and social implications of the disease for close kin and significant others associated with the afflicted children. Of particular concern was the relationship between the disease and its socio-cultural context. We wished to examine both how pre-existing socio-economic and cultural factors contributed to its impact and management and how the challenge of the condition itself, the confrontation with suffering, grief and death, articulated collective conceptions and values.

In this paper we discuss the normal, i.e. typical features of the illness process observed, rather than the minority of cases (some 25%) in which reactions were definable in terms of psychiatric morbidity. However, the structure of the situation described here applied to all families in our study, and focusses doubt on the appropriateness of established criteria for assessing its impact criteria of psycho-social 'normality,' 'coping' and 'adjustment.'

IMPLICATIONS OF THERAPEUTIC ADVANCE: CRISIS AND REMISSION

. . . Our own observations reinforced [the] view [that there are] social and psychological effects of improved prognosis. For the most striking feature of the condition is now the *unpredictability* of its course and outcome, which turns upon the starkest of alternatives—life or death. In fact, overall improvement in the length of survival of victims dramatically heightens the perceptions of uncontrollable threat in particular cases. Thus the hope of long-term (perhaps complete) remission becomes the preoccupation of all families [4], despite their awareness that the odds are unfavourable; and this hope is poignantly maintained against counter evidence. The course of the disease now becomes extremely difficult to define and classify. The significance of remission is not easily interpretable at any point in a particular survivor's career; comprehending clinical predictions and translating them into conventional cultural terms is problematic. While the longer the child survives, the better his chances, relapse *can* occur at any time; and statistical attempts to factorize the risk of such occurrence are as yet of

little help in particular cases. Hence prognosis is difficult to fix, and the illness is neither clearly 'acute' nor 'chronic' for much of its course, a pattern which does not fit established cultural categories. Like other forms of 'acute' illness, this one is threatening on impact; yet no defined phase of resolution follows. For the very meaning of the term 'remission' (i.e. the retreat of symptoms) is profoundly ambiguous, both clinically and experientially. Is it partial or total? When does long-term survival become apparent 'cure'? Periods of remission in leukaemia and related malignant disease combine both the everpresent threat of relapse with the more mundane uncertainties of chronic illness (such as how to manage the sufferer's ambiguous blend of 'illness' and 'normality'). The condition thus raises problems of meaning, management and communication, both in face-to-face and in less bounded social contexts.

CRISIS: THE EARLY PHASE OF IMPACT

While the 'typical' course of childhood leukaemia today is difficult to define in clinical and cultural terms, as a social phenomenon it displays regularities which serve to organize our present discussion. The first of these deals with the phase of impact [5], during which the disease is clinically diagnosed and the diagnosis is communicated to close adult kin, and sometimes, to the victim himself. Some aspects of this phase are a function of the impact of threatening disease everywhere; others are more specifically linked to current advances in leukaemia treatment.

The onset of leukaemia is often insidious. The child displays symptoms—e.g. lack of appetite, tiredness and aches and pains—which are easily attributable to trivial illnesses. Only when these persist, or there is a dramatic change in the child's physical and/or psychological disposition, is the possibility of serious disease usually recognized. Other more distinctive clinical features—pallor, bruising and petechiae, or bone pain—may also be misread by parents; and lack of first-hand knowledge of the condition by the primary practitioner may further impede diagnosis.

Such procrastination has distressing consequences once the nature of the disease becomes known. Parents who delay consulting a doctor feel guilt. If the primary practitioner initially misdiagnoses the condition, parents are resentful and may impugn his clinical judgement. The apparent deficiencies in the primary physician's competence are often heightened by the seemingly dramatic and specialist intervention which follows referral to a hospital. Once the child has been discharged, the problem of primary care is often exacerbated by a lack of confidence (both by the parents and the physician himself) in his ability to treat so special a case. Thus, while the hospital specialist becomes the object of optimistic faith, the primary doctor is frequently devalued, or made the target of anger and guilt. Here the effects of the moving margin of specialist knowledge upon perceptions and social relationships is clearly seen.

INTERPRETING THE DIAGNOSIS

We have suggested that in our culture malignant disease in childhood has particularly distressing emotive connotations, due not only to its inherent implications, but also, to its symbolic marking of the critical frontier of medical science. The most cogent initial response to clinical identification of the disease among the families observed was that they had been singled out to suffer the kind of irreversible misfortune that usually seemed "only to happen to others." Davis [6], in his classic account of the 'passage through crisis' of childhood polio victims, makes a similar observation: such threatening information taxes a family's sense of sharing in a common universe or experience and implies a position of marginality and collective stigma.

Among the families of leukaemic children, the isolating effects of receiving the diagnosis were modified once contact was made with a new group of reference, comprising others similarly afflicted. Here constructions of the event were reappraised in relation to a universe of comparable experience. As one mother put it:

> When you first learn that your child has such a disease, your world collapses. You think: 'It can't happen to us? It only happens to other people!' Then you get to the hospital and learn that there are others like you and that helps. Not that you are pleased by their suffering; it's just

> that you're not alone in it. They've been through the same, or worse sometimes. . . . But when you go home again, it's difficult. You feel different, and people avoid you. I suppose it's because they don't know how to take you. But it's upsetting—like you've all got the plague or something!

Sociological observations show that participants in ordeals of apparently uncertain course and duration (such as periods of imprisonment and hospitalization) seek to systematize information and construct norms against which to gauge their present state and future prospects [7]. The parents of leukaemic children performed similar activities. It was here that the implications of therapeutic advance and changing prognosis were clearly seen, for predicting the course of the disease in particular cases has become increasingly difficult. Families discovered that 'leukaemia' comprised a category of related clinical conditions, with differing individual implications for treatment and outcome. Moreover, within this category knowledge and technical control were unevenly distributed. . . .

The case of childhood leukaemia is an instance of Durkheim's classic assertion that science, inherently fragmentary and incomplete, cannot provide an 'impetus' to everyday action. The theories which make it possible for men to 'live and act' are thus 'obliged to pass science and complete it prematurely' [8]. Doctors in our study were seldom able, on the basis of available knowledge, to provide clear biomedical guidelines for parents facing the uncharted course of the illness. Thus parents (and frequently, sick children) set about collating all available information in the attempt to formulate timetables and statements of probability for themselves. In doing this, they drew heavily upon knowledge of other laymen with more experience of the disease, and from the case-histories of other victims. A subtle process of cross-referencing occurred whereby parents sought to systematize the range of differing types of data at their disposal. In their efforts, however, they tried to maintain an optimistic definition of their case for as long as possible. They would thus stress similarities between their child and others who appeared to be doing well, and avoid identification with those who appeared to be failing. Significantly, the quest was not only for prognostic certainty, but for an extension of clinical definitions to include psychological, social and moral dimensions. As time passed, progress of the condition itself often narrowed the limits of expectation; a relapse dispelled the hope of further long-term remission. But the process of classification, and the search for meaning in carefully collated bodies of evidence persisted for as long as the illness lasted. And each case of relapse and death occurring within the reference group presented a fresh challenge to survivors and their families.

The process of systematization also varied with the progress of the disease. At points of crisis—initial diagnosis, relapse and death—there was an expressed need to identify with others who had experienced the same affliction, to ease the isolation of being picked out to suffer irreversible tragedy. But when individual and collective definitions had reached relative stability, referencing often declined and other sufferers were avoided as possible sources of disorienting information.

The attempt to manage communication so as to maintain fragile optimism also reflects another feature of the changing relationship between what is formally 'known' and what is 'unknown'—i.e. the discontinuity between widely held lay images of leukaemia and those current in clinical oncology. In this case, rapid therapeutic advance in recent years has resulted in a significant gap. Lay people generally continue to perceive leukaemia as intractable, short-lived and fatal. Clinical diagnosis presents contrary, but bewildering information about variations in types of disease and treatment and about unpredictable possibilities of survival. Those afflicted now attempt to construct and maintain expectations which counter their own previously pessimistic, common-sense views (still shared by many others in the wider community, including some health care professionals outside the field of oncology).

In assessing how those involved seek a stable understanding of the illness and its implications, we are not dealing with unambiguous, uniform states of awareness, definable as 'realistic acceptance' or 'irrational denial.' States of knowledge which follow in the wake of such crises often display contradiction and situational variation, suggesting that the perception of threat to life (whether in the victim or those close to him) is a developing consciousness. Parents showed that this process often involved oscillation between contradictory responses: repugnance,

guilt, optimism and despair. It follows that such processes are not easily reducible to stable descriptive models such as 'awareness context' [9], or to finite and unambiguous communications (often implied in the classic cancer literature on 'telling' or 'not telling' fatal prognoses). The referencing activities through which constructions of the illness process are formed by those caught up in it are expressions of the need to 'complete' seemingly inadequate clinical knowledge—to bring its definitions into line with everyday experience, and to transcend the stark and apparently arbitrary boundary between the formally 'known' and the 'unknown.'

THE MEANING OF AFFLICTION

An interrelated and crucial feature of the early phase of leukaemia (but one which recurred throughout its course) was the attempt to explain *why* it happened. Again, other sociological accounts of the experience of crisis suggest that this 'stock-taking' (what Davis calls the 'inventory stage') generally occurs once the critical peak and initial shock have passed. However, studies of the social role of Western medicine have not been particularly concerned with this quest for meaning, except to note that our medical knowledge addresses a relatively limited range of causal explanations of disease—the 'how' rather than the 'why' of illness; or its proximate 'cause' rather than its 'meaning' [10]. In the literature on childhood leukaemia all that emerges is that in the post-crisis period, self-searching and guilt give way to resigned acceptance if feelings of personal culpability are effectively allayed [11].

Our observations indeed confirmed that perceptions of guilt were significant in parents' attempts to impose meaning on the illness. The identity of children is generally regarded as a function of that of their parents, who feel practical and moral responsibility for their well-being and their suffering. Threatening illness is frequently seen as an assault on childrearing capacities [12]. Hence the quest for cause and meaning in such illness is closely tied to the attempt to allocate responsibility for its occurrence.

But the search for meaning also reflects the widely observed effects of threatening and seemingly random events upon everyday assumptions and modes of knowledge. All cultures provide repertoires of explanation—theories—to account for and manage such events [13]. We, in the Western industrialized societies, have come to think increasingly in the idiom of 'scientific' explanation, in which 'objective' and 'neutral' principles serve to order the elements of a materially constituted world. Such theories are explicitly impersonal and amoral. They do not relate specific physical causes to more embracing social, moral or spiritual orders. Scientific explanation fails to account for the seeming random occurrence of a wide range of 'natural' events (such as the onset of disease). However, where such affliction strikes to the heart of everyday realities and resists control, it calls into question tacit assumptions about reality and the nature of human control. And it is in such cases—of which childhood leukaemia is typical—that the ambiguities of current bio-medical knowledge are most keenly perceived.

Parents in our study typically tried to bring the stunning diagnosis of leukaemia into relation with perceived medical facts, the experience of others and their own biographies and world-view. While the process was most intense during the initial phase of impact, the quest for a satisfactory explanation was, by its nature, inconclusive and continuous, often asserting itself strongly after relapse and bereavement. One mother remarked after the death of her child:

> Well, now it's all over, and I have time to think again. I find myself going over and over the problem in my mind, just like I did at the beginning: 'Why did he get it? How does it start?' You can drive yourself crazy with those sort of questions! Could it happen to the other children too? I want to ask the hospital to let us know if they find that out—how it starts. Even if it's in 15 years, I'll still want to know.

In their search for an explanation for the onset of the disease, parents generally sought knowledge at two interrelated levels: first, that of proximate biological and medical cause (what has happened in the child's body?) and second, that of more ultimate cause (Why us? Why now?). In our society, bio-medical science and practice may provide satisfactory explanation and resolution for a wide range of afflictions, often (but not always) seeming to render more thoroughgoing metaphysical speculation re-

dundant. But precisely *because* of its apparent wide applicability in everyday life, particularly in the wake of the decline of overarching cosmological systems, we are especially bereft when we have to face events for which no rational explanation or remedy is forthcoming. The search for meaning, in short, becomes a conscious problem under such conditions. Threatening illness strikes at personal identities and challenges everyday realities, calling for an interpretive framework to order fragmented experience; but the process of 'completing' scientific etiologies is not as automatic as Durkheim [8] and others have suggested. It founders on the essential Western cultural opposition between material and moral realities.

Precisely because this is so, both medical and popular speculation about possible psychological and environmental components in malignant disease serve as a bridge for moving from proximate (clinically framed) explanations to encompassing (cosmologically ordered) explanations. Despite the lack of clinical concern with psycho-social factors, the parents we observed reviewed their own biographies, passing from questions like: "Should I have breast-fed?" and "Could one X-ray in pregnancy have done it?," to more diffuse issues: "Could it be that I work with chemicals?" or "Perhaps it's because we live in such a filthy industrial environment?" The incidence of disease at present suggests no regional or socio-economic bias. Social and environmental factors in etiology were a concern of both working-class and middle-class families. About 10% of parents tentatively invoked metaphysical explanations: "It's a punishment for something we've done." Those who held strong beliefs in divine causation were less concerned with other aspects of etiology. But few found such encompassing reassurance, either from the doctrines or the representatives of the church. For most, nagging concerns about 'hidden' carcinogenic features in the everyday environment remained strong. Problems raised by this search for meaning reveal fundamental features of the structure of knowledge in our culture, and derived from the contradictions which characterize its social role. Parents' reactions express the dilemma of relating the complexity of what is known about the disease to what remains stubbornly unknown, of reconciling, for example, how etiology can remain almost a total mystery while progress is made at the level of intervention (many perceived this as an inversion of common-sense as-

sumptions about the logical priority of causal knowledge). Their problems also stress the contradictory
detachment of bio-medical knowledge from the
multi-faceted contours of illness experience. And,
most fundamentally, they express ambiguous perceptions about efficacy and the absence of control
in the everyday exercise of knowledge. Not surprisingly, physicians aware of problems in fixing the
cause of the illness found it very difficult to confront
them within the parameters of established clinical
practice.

THE SOCIAL IMPLICATIONS
OF UNCERTAIN PROGNOSIS

The uncertain prognosis of leukaemia victims has
considerable impact upon the social relationships
which surround them. In the first instance, the symbolic associations of the disease have patent effects
upon everyday encounters for the families affected.
As Strauss has pointed out, knowledge of potential
fatality is disrupting of ordinary social encounters
[14]. Others often reacted with embarrassment or
emotion when confronting the leukaemic child or
his family after hearing of the illness. This could
be misinterpreted by the family, who resented being
treated as 'contagious' or being patronized with sympathy. And these more usual components of threatening illness were complicated by the uncertain definition of the child's condition.

At the heart of the drama was the relationship
between the sick child and his parents, often a source
of agonizing difficulty. For parents generally felt it
important to conduct as 'normal' a mode of domestic
existence as possible and were strongly encouraged
by the clinicians to do so. Yet such 'normality' was
maintained in a domestic context whose meaning
for them had been tragically redefined. Hence, apart
from having to deal with the child's own perceptions
of the illness and treatment [15], they had to face
dilemmas in their relationship to him which
stemmed from his own uncertain future [16]. How
far a child should be made to conform to normal
expectations (based on the premise of socialization
of adulthood) or how far he (rather than the disease
and treatment) was responsible for his behaviour
was not easily resolved. As one mother put it:

They say: "Take him home and treat him as
normal." But it's hardly a normal situation, is
it? I mean, he's a different child, for a start.
He throws tantrums for the least thing. He can't
bear to be crossed. What I don't know is how
much of this is due to the treatment and the
leukaemia. So, do I punish him? It's hard when
you think that it might not be his fault, and
when you think of what he's got and all. If he's
not going to grow up, what does it matter? But
if we don't check him and he pulls through this,
he'll be a little monster one day!

Indeed, a series of situational and cultural constraints (such as the child's ignorance of the condition, and the diffuse but widespread sanction in our
society against dwelling on issues deemed 'morbid')
tend to result in families striving to stifle any overt
acknowledgement of the illness. Yet most reveal
clearly that the illness radically alters the meaning
of their lives, their values and their expectations
for the future. And, while most faced the ordeal without manifest sign of collapse, the child's suffering,
and the disruption of familial relations and quality
of life, raised searching questions about the meaning
of survival. Moreover, as noted above, at least one
longitudinal study of survivors suggests that these
disruptions are a continuing source of emotional distress for children and their families [17].

REMISSION

Unlike the classic model of acute illness, malignancies such as leukaemia do not, under modern clinical
conditions, entail an explicit stage of 'recovery' or
resolution after initial crisis. Rather, early crisis is
usually followed by a remission phase of uncertain
length and status, during which major symptoms
of the disease are in abeyance, but its clinical definition remains tentative. The family of the sufferer
now has to reconcile their knowledge of the possible
future implications of the illness with the seeming
absence of serious symptoms. Many of the problematic features of this stage are in the uncertain
nature of chronic illness itself—i.e. its protracted
course, uncertain outcome and oscillation between
apparent 'health' and 'illness' [18]. But the more
usual stresses are here exacerbated by the ever-
present threat of fatal relapse, a threat whose likeli-

hood does not simply diminish with the passage of time. As one father remarked:

> It's on your mind all the time. In fact, it's worse once the first panic is over and everything is more-or-less back to normal. The heat is off, and other people now have their own lives to lead. And you sit here, when you're alone and wonder: "How is it going to turn out? Will she make it?" The real hell of this illness is that you just don't know. They can be fine for two years and then suddenly relapse.

In fact, the notion of 'remission' as the first clinical hurdle which victims must reach has come to symbolise the fragile balance of threat and hope which their survival connotes. The terms itself, widely associated with the clinical battle against disease which remains fundamentally intractable, entails a range of meanings which combine the notion of divine pardon with the retreat of symptoms. It represents in condensed form the entanglement of control and chaos at the frontiers of medical knowledge.

THE THREAT OF UNCERTAIN OUTCOME

The phase of remission entails the process of learning to live with the uncertain status and outcome of the illness. Here again, the changing prognosis of leukaemia is important. For the dramatic risks that this represents have to be reconciled with the apparent normality of everyday existence while the child remains symptom free. In theory, the longer the child survives, particularly after the suspension of chemotherapy, the better his overall chances. But, in fact, the proportion who remain in remission after three years remains very small [19]. Relapses thus continue within the reference group, some well after the suspension of active treatment. This, plus the fundamental clinical uncertainties as regards etiology and the effects of treatment mean that the therapy itself comes to be viewed by the families as rather unspecific or 'hit and miss.' It is generally understood as not yet capable of striking at the origins of the disease itself. While these ambiguities become more clearly delineated in parents' perceptions, clinicians and other agents of care tend to encourage short-

term optimism. Thus the overall contradictions in the predicament of family and victim become more marked over time, typically inducing oscillations in perception and mood from unreflective hope to fear and depression. As a result, at least one set of recent observers of this situation have characterized the experience in terms of the 'double-bind' hypothesis [20].

Both agents of care and most lay confidantes project strongly positive definitions of the illness and discourage speculation about possible loss. Families in our study perceived strong taboos against raising these issues in clinical encounters. Thus, while it was usually not the result of concerted strategy, both clinicians and lay people systematically deflected the expression of basic anxieties. Those seeking to reconcile the profound ambiguities inherent in the remission phase found little opportunity for ventilating these concerns. Even when parents' discussion groups were formally instituted by clinicians after our observations had ceased, initial reactions of those questions suggested that here too they felt constrained not to "upset those who were more hopeful by dwelling on morbid things." Family practitioners were turned to by some, but most responded by prescribing psychotropic drugs, which were regarded by parents as distressingly inappropriate. Here again, an existing cultural bias within our wider society and our medical practice discourages overt acknowledgement of mortality and related fears. The ambiguous definition of modern childhood leukaemia make projection of unquestioned optimism by doctor and lay person the predictable course of action.

The lack of opportunities for addressing these uncertainties in remission is heightened by the absence of markers intrinsic to illness and treatment which might signal longer-term prospects. The only 'bench-marks' which punctuate the protracted period of remission are regular clinical check-ups, which assume symbolic significance as hurdles, or pointers with which to map out the disease's uncharted course. At such points, families look hopefully toward the doctors for an indication of the relationship between the child's present state and longerterm outcomes.

> I don't sleep before bone marrow day [21]. I still can't get used to it, and it's over a year now that he's been in remission. Even when they tell

me that it's all O.K., I'm still down, because I keep hoping to hear more about his real progress. They say it like this: "He's fine at the moment!" And I think: "Dear God, but for how long? What does it mean for his chances?"

Families raised the problems of uncertainty and disorientation during the phase of remission with distressing regularity and symptoms of depression (feelings of despair, helplessness and hopelessness), had not abated in the majority of this 'typical' population eighteen months after the onset of the disease. Attempts to deflect doubt about treatment and concern about outcome exacerbate the effects of uncertainty. In our society, explicit avoidance of the practical and conceptual implications of death coexists with a stress on rational life-planning—both arguably the outcome of our perception of ourselves as self-determining corporeal individuals. But these cultural values appear to be tragically at odds with certain forms of experience, such as imperfectly controlled, life-threatening illness. The ambiguities of protracted remission are thus the outcome of deeper contradictions which shape the overall predicament: the contrast between the perception of illness and clinical definition; between the values of planning and predictability and seemingly random uncertainty; between technical control and chaos and between an ideology or rational meliorism and the 'meaninglessness' of suffering and mortality. While these contradictions are written into the very structure of our socio-cultural system, they are realized particularly acutely in the context of affliction and serious illness. And the increasingly aggressive intervention of modern bio-medicine in the course of malignant disease has served to sharpen these oppositions, rendering more explicitly problematic both the experience and the management of clinical treatment.

CONCLUSION: ILLNESS, UNCERTAINTY, AND THE PROVISION OF CARE

The situation of clinicians and patients in the treatment of childhood leukaemia is an expression of fundamental features of our society and culture, which themselves shape the direction and implications of technical advance in this domain. Because the form

and direction of clinical knowledge is part and parcel of a more encompassing system of thought and action, it cannot be either evaluated or transformed in any simple, decontextualized manner. Thus, while it is now quite widely acknowledged in the social and health sciences that bio-medical criteria fail in themselves to define and manage the experience of illness, the implications of this for medical research and practice are more complex than is often supposed. As is increasingly being realized, the meaning of illness and medicine—if not defined merely as physical disease and neutral technical intervention—becomes profoundly problematic. It is then open to essential dilemmas of human value and meaning, which exist currently both in applied science and in other spheres of our formal and popular knowledge.

In relation to the predicament of childhood leukaemics and their families, simple remedies are likely to be merely palliative; the etiology of the more thoroughgoing malaise it represents lies in the very logic of our social and cultural forms. It is with the form and function of medical knowledge in our wider society that real consideration of the problems expressed in this study must begin. Like a host of previous social science investigations, the study of childhood leukaemia reveals the contrast between the meanings and values attached to illness by the sufferers and by clinical definitions. But this account suggests also that this relationship is not static; it is not dictated by an unavoidable or constant gap between formal and lay knowledge, a gap clearly justified by the efficacy of the former. It suggests, rather, that the moving frontier of bio-medical science rests upon a set of contradictions that increasingly widens the gulf, *opposes* formal and lay knowledge and raises basic questions about the meaning and value of biomedical science itself. Thus for parents in our study, uncertain physical survival (often at the cost of pain, confusion and distress) gave rise to persistent doubt, not only about the nature of clinical intervention, but also about established professional definitions of health and well-being.

The reality of these concerns has to be acknowledged by those working for clinical progress, if the meaning of hard-won advance is not to become dangerously irrelevant to our perceptions of need. The important implications of intervention in malignant disease cannot merely be defined as 'psychological maladjustments' or failure to 'cope' on the part of a few unfortunate victims. Neither can they be delegated to agents of care ancillary to somatic medicine, such as psychiatrists or social workers, who are expected to assist sufferers in adapting to clinically defined realities. For it is precisely these realities which such illness experience calls into doubt. And failure to recognise this merely aggravates the victim's dilemma.

In practical terms, no neat professional solutions are at hand for the problems discussed here—either those of the sick, or those of the specialists who work to extend biomedical knowledge and advance their treatment. Yet, in an important sense, the solutions to both orders of problem are entailed in one another. For evaluations of technical developments should begin by acknowledging the ambiguous experience of the recipients of new modes of intervention. In the process of understanding the shape and origins of their distress, we gain insight into the complex social effects of uneven shifts in medical knowledge. It is only in this manner that we become aware of the multi-faceted implications of particular courses of technical advance, and the contradictions attendant upon all 'discoveries' in applied science. At the very least, this must engage the specialist in a process of self-consciousness—of seriously questioning whether current bio-medical definitions adequately reflect the parameters of human distress and suffering, and whether current clinical knowledge might not in fact exacerbate problems central to the experience of health and illness.

References

1. The research upon which this paper is based was made possible by the interest and cooperation of the doctors, children and families associated with the regional oncology centre upon which the project focussed. Research was funded by the Leukaemia Research Fund of Great Britain, and preparation for publication was assisted by Bio-Medical Research Support Grant (PHS 5 SO7 RR-07029-14) from the Division of Social Science of the University of Chicago.

2. Simone J., Rhomes M. A. A., Husto H. O. and Pinkel D. 'Total therapy' studies of acute lymphocytic leukaemia in children. *Cancer* 30, 1488, 1972; Till M. M., Hardisty R. M. and Pike M. C. Long survivals in acute leukaemia. *Lancet* I 534, 1973; Li F. P. and Stone R. Survivors of cancer in childhood. *Ann. Intern. Med.* 84, 551, 1976.

3. A total of 82 children in these categories were admitted during the period, 9 of whose parents refused to participate in the study, 9 who died before we were able to establish contact with their families, and 4 whose families left the region while the research was in progress. Of the 60 children included in the study, 50 were A.L.L. cases and 10 were A.M.L. cases, roughly the ratio of incidence in the general population. The data were collected largely by means of semi-structured interviews with parents in their homes, first shortly after diagnosis, and then some 18 months later. Initial contact included an interview with both parents, and one with the mother alone. During home visits, it was possible to observe the ambience of family life, the relationship of the family to the immediate neighborhood, and so on. On-going contact was maintained with families in the clinical setting, where interaction between doctors and patients was observed. A series of lengthy, semi-structured interviews were also conducted with different categories of clinical staff during the research period.

4. This is true only for the families of children with Acute Lymphoblastic Leukaemia, the commonest form of the disease in childhood and the form most responsive to current treatment regimes. It is in this category that dramatic increase in length and overall rate of survival has been achieved.

5. We use the notion of 'impact' in a similar sense to Davis in his discussion of polio in childhood as an existential and social process [6]. However, the obvious differences in the course of the two diseases renders his overall classification (of the structure of *acute* illness) inappropriate here. While leukaemia presents a particularly stark instance of the lack of fit between illness form and conventional cultural categories—both in sociology and everyday life—it is obviously not unique to this disease. All inherently uncertain conditions (and hence much so-called 'chronic' illness) pose similar sorts of problems of classification.

6. Davis F. *Passage Through Crisis*. Bobbs Merrill, New York, 1963.

7. See Roth J. A. *Timetables*. Bobbs Merrill, New York, 1963 and Fox R. C. *Experiment Perilous*. The Free Press, New York, 1959. The construction of interpretations of the illness by clinicians and lay people is examined in detail elsewhere. (Comaroff J. The symbolic constitution of Western medical knowledge. Forthcoming in *Cult. Med. Psychiat.*).

8. Durkheim E. *Elementary Forms of the Religious Life*, trans. by Swain J., 4th edn, p. 431. Allen & Unwin,

London, 1915. One parent provided a particularly graphic example of the attempt to 'complete' available information: as a life-insurance broker, he attempted to collate relevant data on the course of the disease from all available sources—doctors, paramedical personnel and other parents. He devised a multifactorial model of risk and survival for the population at hand, against which he plotted his son's prognosis.

9. See Glaser B. and Strauss A. *Awareness of Dying.* Wiedenfeld & Nicholson, London, 1965.

10. See Powles J. On the limitations of modern medicine. *Sci. Med. Man* 1, 1, 1973; Horton R. African traditional thought and Western science. *Africa* 31, 50, 155, 1969; Crick N. *Explorations in Language and Meaning: Towards a Semantic Anthropology.* Malaby Press, London, 1976.

11. See Natterson J. M. and Knudson A. G. Observations concerning fear of death in fatally ill children and their mothers. *Psychosom. Med.* 22, 456, 1960.

12. See *Pediatrics* 515 1967.

13. See Horton *op. cit.* [11].

14. Strauss A. L. (Ed.), *Chronic Illness and the Quality of Life,* p. 59. Mosby, St. Louis, 1975.

15. While our study did not focus directly upon the perceptions of the sick children, all of the victims over the age of 10 presented direct or indirect signs of anxiety about their condition. However, only in eleven cases did one or both parents suggest that the child might be expressing concern about survival, and in only six cases (all involving children over the age of four) had the full known implications of the child's condition been discussed with him/her.

16. C.f. Bluebond-Langner M. *The Private World of Dying Children.* Princeton Univ. Press, Princeton, 1978.

17. O'Malley J. E. Long-term follow-up of survivors of childhood cancer: psychiatric sequalae. Paper presented to the *85th Annual Convention of the American Psychiatric Association,* San Francisco, 1977.

18. Strauss (Ed.) *op. cit.* [15].

19. See Li and Stone, *op. cit.* [2].

20. Longhofer J. with the collaboration of Floersch J. E. Dying and living: the double bind. *Cult. Med. Psychiat.* 4, 119, 1980.

21. Bone-marrow aspirations are performed at regular intervals to detect whether leukaemic cells are present, or whether the disease remains in remission.

CHAPTER 4

The Nature and Consequences of Labeling

What is a schizophrenic and how does a person become identified as one? The following statement from a book by Dorothy Tennov (1975) is directed to these questions:

Schizophrenia is the diagnostic term applied to the largest category of hospitalized mental patients. One quarter of all mental patient beds throughout the world belong to persons so classified. Common, often severe, more often so mild it goes unrecognized, it is also baffling. Absence of expression of emotionality, poor insight, the feeling that thoughts are being broadcast to others, free and spontaneous flow of incoherent speech, and bizarre, nihilistic, and widespread delusions are some of the criteria on which a diagnosis of schizophrenia is based. There are many theories, and much controversy; nothing one could say about it would not be disputed in some corner. There are those who would abandon use of the term as a diagnostic category altogether, claiming that the criteria are not only vague but favor certain social groups over others, and that stigmatization has evolved around the very term.

This statement describes the controversy over schizophrenia and expresses the view and concerns of those who adhere to a labeling perspective of mental illness. These labeling theorists do not see mental illness as resulting from an individual's inability to cope with life. They propose that the designation of mental illness is often given to behavior which does not threaten the welfare of oneself and others but which a society, at a given time, deems inappropriate. The labeling theorists draw support from many sources. They note that definitions of mental illness change and that many behaviors, such as masturbation, which were once considered mental aberrations, are now considered perfectly normal. Thomas Szasz (1970), a psychiatrist himself and a harsh critic of psychiatry, notes the case of a woman who as late as 1860, under Illinois law, was committed to a Jacksonville mental hospital for disagreeing with her husband. It is also pointed out by labeling theorists that a higher percentage of individuals of certain groups seem to be labeled as mentally ill although several studies have shown that a sizeable proportion of the so-called normal society could be so defined.

Labeling theorists express particular concern over the effect that labeling has on those who are labeled. Frequently, victims of labeling may perceive themselves differently from the way they did before being labeled. Thus, older people who exhibit a loss of memory may be labeled as senile and may begin to see themselves this way. This, despite the fact that the same loss of memory by a 25-year-old would be seen as denoting nothing out of the ordinary. Often, labeled persons are unable to shed their labels. For example, former mental patients frequently continue to be viewed as mentally ill. This continuing stigma may account, in part, for a high rate of recidivism among mental patients. Finally, the process of labeling may result in a masking of the real causes of a behavioral disorder. In the case of schizophrenia this may mean that attempts are made to restructure patients' behavior while the root causes of their problems, such as a poor family situation, are ignored.

In the lead article, Nancy E. Waxler presents a comprehensive overview of labeling as it relates to health and health care. The article begins with a revealing description of the myriad social factors that influence whether or not a label of mentally retarded is imposed on a child. It also touches on several issues already mentioned in this introduction. In the next article, Catherine Kohler Riessman explores the ways in which aspects of women's health, which might be viewed as normal aspects of life, are "medicalized"—that is, defined as medical problems. Among Riessman's major points is the belief that, for a variety of reasons, women are more likely to be labeled than men. Her paper is more provocative than others on the same general issue in that she focuses not only on the role of physicians in the process of medicalization but also on the role of a certain stratum of women who are pictured as serving as physicians' willing accomplices. Also employing the medicalization theme, Peter Conrad, in the following article, covers some of the same territory as Riessman. However, his gaze is focused on the "discovery," made about 25 years ago, of a disease in children called hyperkineses. The major thrust of his argument lies in the identification of those groups in society, like the pharmaceutical companies, whose vested interests were served by the appearance of this medical label. Conrad, like Riessman, also looks at the link between "medicalization" and social control over those labeled.

Perhaps nowhere is the uncertainty of medicine greater than in the area of psychiatry, as indicated in the quote from Tennov that begins this introduction. This uncertainty gives psychiatrists a great degree of discretion in their decisions about who to define as mentally ill. In a portion of one of the most famous articles in the literature, D. L. Rosenhan discusses a study that clearly shows just how much diagnostic discretion mental health professionals have and how difficult it is to get rid of a label once it has been attached. Next, Marjorie Glassman provides evidence that the elderly are very vulnerable to being incorrectly labeled by doctors as suffering from senile dementia. This is partly due to the existence of many pervasive and stereotypical notions of what it is to be old. In the next to last article, Regina Kenen and Robert Schmidt analyze the consequences of screening programs for those labeled as carriers of genetic diseases and AIDS. There has been increasing concern in many quarters that, although we have become more sophisticated in our diagnostic testing, we are nowhere near as sophisticated in terms of understanding the socioemotional consequences of these tests for those labeled by them. Finally, Paul R. Benson looks at how labeling theory has impacted on public policy surrounding the "deinstitutionalization" of many mentally ill persons from state hospitals to the community. Citing historical documents, he makes a persuasive argument that the testimony of leading labeling theorists before the California state legislature in the 1960s helped convince that body to institute a deinstitutionalization program. Within less than a decade of its inception, this legislation caused the number of residents in California state mental hospitals to decrease by two-thirds. Benson follows his original article with an update summarizing the overall consequences for the nation of over two decades of deinstitutionalization.

References

SZASZ, T. 1970. *The Manufacture of Madness*. New York: Dell.
TENNOV, D. 1975. *Psychotherapy: The Hazardous Cure*. New York: Abelard-Schuman.

The Social Labeling Perspective on Illness

Nancy E. Waxler

Recent research has turned up some rather puzzling findings. For example, in California a child's "failure" on the school psychologist's IQ test does not insure a diagnosis of "mental retardation"; in fact, whether a child is diagnosed as mentally retarded and referred to special classes is more closely associated with whether he is Mexican-American or Black than with his score on an IQ test (Mercer 1973). Or, persons who think they have heart disease but in fact do not often alter their lives on the basis of their beliefs about themselves, not on the basis of presence or absence of symptoms (Eichorn and Anderson 1962). The psychiatric patients who feel that they are "back to normal" one month after their first hospitalization are no different, diagnostically, from the "still sick" group; instead, their better clinical outcome can be explained by the greater power certain hospitals give patients to renegotiate their legal status, treatment plans and diagnoses with hospital staff (Waxler et al. 1979). Whether a hospitalized tuberculosis patient gets well quickly is partly explained by whether he has cooperated with the ward staff; those who cooperate stay sick longer, those who do not cooperate get well more quickly (Calden et al. 1960).

None of the above findings is easily explained by reference to medical textbooks nor to the ways physicians have been taught to apply the biomedical model of disease. The patient's diagnosis, not his ethnic group, should determine his referral and treatment. Outcome for treated disease should be predictable from diagnosis and treatment, not from the bureaucratic organization of the treating hospital. Patients who cooperate with treatment are expected to do better and certainly not expected to do worse than non-cooperative patients.

All of these findings, however, can be explained by an alternate sociological theory, the theory of social labeling (Schur 1971; Scheff 1966; Gove 1975). For labeling theory who is to be called "ill" is determined by the individual's social position and society's norms rather than by universal and objectively defined signs and symptoms. Further, a person is labeled as "ill" in the course of social negotiations between himself, his doctor, his family, sometimes ward staff and others. The outcome of such social negotiations is influenced by each person's beliefs and training and also by the social and organizational contexts in which the negotiation occurs. Once labeled as "ill" the individual may find himself caught in the midst of a self-fulfilling prophecy. Depending upon his social position he may find that de-labeling is difficult, that continued illness is expected and therefore that his symptoms continue.

These examples contrast two perspectives on illness and treatment, the biomedical and social labeling perspectives. Each perspective uses a conceptual model to organize an abundant array of small facts, to weigh, select, discard, and integrate facts about disease, illness and treatment; neither model is coterminous with the facts themselves. While both the biomedical and social labeling models are used to analyze medical phenomena they do not compete directly with each other in an attempt to better explain or predict these phenomena. Instead, the biomedical model of disease is used by practitioners in their everyday work to understand a client's symptoms and to make decisions about etiology, diagnosis, prognosis and treatment. Balint (1957), for example, shows how the general practitioner questions and listens, selecting from a patient's report certain facts that "fit" his biomedical conception of disease, thus

Reprinted from *The Relevance of Social Science for Medicine*, edited by Arthur Kleinman and Leon Eisenberg, pp. 283–306. Copyright © 1981 by D. Reidel Publishing Company, Dordrecht, Holland.

providing him with a particular diagnosis and treatment plan. This model of disease underlies all that doctors are taught in medical school.

The sociologist using a social labeling model to understand disease, illness and medical practice stands outside the doctor-patient interview and asks how the social context, the social roles and relationships, the application of the biomedical model of disease itself, influence what the doctor does and what happens to the patient. A social labeling theorist looking at the general practitioner's interview might ignore altogether the patient's report of physical symptoms but attend, instead, to the relative power and control exerted by physician and patient, and use these selected bits of data to predict whether the sick person will remain "ill" or return to his normal routine.

AN INTRODUCTION TO SOCIAL LABELING

Mercer's study of mental retardation (1973) shows how the social labeling model can be used to analyze diagnostic and treatment practices and thus the careers of children who may or may not be called "retarded." The biomedical model, followed by physicians, most teachers and school psychologists, assumes that "mental retardation is a pathological condition" and that "although organic involvement cannot be established in cases classified as undifferentiated, familial or sociocultural, it is assumed that 'minimal brain dysfunction' exists but cannot be detected because of the inadequacy of diagnostic tools" (Mercer 1973:7–8). Intelligence tests are the usual diagnostic tools and special education and training for those who can respond is the normal treatment. One might expect, then, that the diagnosis of a mentally retarded child follows quite routine and universal medico-psychological procedures.

Using social labeling theory as a guide Mercer traced this diagnostic process, one in which children in a California community were referred for IQ testing, evaluated, diagnosed and sent to special classes within the public school system. While all children who were diagnosed as retarded did, indeed, have IQ scores lower than 80, her investigation of the series of steps leading to this diagnosis shows clearly that many children with equally low IQ scores were never so diagnosed. In fact it is the social characteristics of the children, their families, the schools they go to, that are better predictors of who, out of the pool of all low IQ students, are to be treated as "retarded."

A brief description of this social labeling process will introduce some of the ways in which labeling theory examines all medical questions.[1] Think of the diagnosis of mental retardation as the end-point in a series of decisions; at each decision point it is possible for some low IQ children to be returned to the pool of "normal" children, thus never to be called "retarded." The very first sorting point is at school enrollment itself. Children enrolled in private schools (mostly Catholic parochial schools in this case) are immediately saved from the diagnosis of retardation, not because these children have higher IQ's (1.1% had IQ's less than 80), but because parochial schools do not have school psychologists, testing programs, nor procedures for referrals. Since, by law, a child must be tested before being sent to special classes, no child in the private school system is diagnosed as "retarded" nor "treated." Teachers perceive most of the low IQ students as simply poor in their academic work. Thus, the organizational structure of the parochial schools serves as a social context in which no diagnosis of retardation can occur.

Public schools, however, do have psychologists, special classes and formal procedures for making decisions about who is to be called "retarded." The first step in this procedure consists of "failing" or "keeping the child back" a grade. The elementary school teacher is the prime decision-maker and uses his/her norms as a basis for this decision; many children are initially labeled as retarded at this point because they are poor in social and academic skills. However it is the family background that profoundly distinguishes between children "held back" and children promoted. The former are much more likely to be Spanish-speaking Mexican-Americans of low socioeconomic status. At this very early stage in the sorting process, then, students from certain backgrounds have a much greater likelihood of being provisionally labeled as "retarded."

If a child is held back in school he may, next year, be referred by the school principal for psychological testing. This decision is not affected by the child's family background but it is influenced by an organizational characteristic of the school system. A school policy protects overburdened psychologists by imposing a quota on referrals for psychological testing; each school is allocated an equal number of psychologist-days, regardless of the size of the school. Thus, children tentatively labeled by teachers as retarded are much more likely to be sent on to the next labeling stage if they go to a small school. Children of equally low levels of academic and social performance escape the next diagnostic stage because school principals must limit the numbers of children they refer. Again, an organizational constraint has an impact on who is to be called retarded.

Referrals from the school principal do not necessarily insure that the child will actually be tested, however. Since psychological testing is a legal requirement for "treatment" (i.e., referral to special classes) it is apparent that the psychologist's decision to test or not is a crucial one for the child's career. While the child's family background has no bearing on the psychologist's decision, that is, he/she does not choose to test proportionately more Mexican-Americans or children from middle class families, the decision to test is highly related to the principal's reason for referral, mentioned in his/her referral statement. Those children presented as "possibly retarded" were tested 90% of the time. Thus, the psychologist chooses most often to "rubber stamp" the provisional label of mental retardation made by the principal and teacher. Children referred for academic difficulties, but in which no mention of retardation is made, are not as likely to be tested.

Of the children who are referred and actually tested by the psychologist, some "pass," that is, have IQ scores greater than 80, while others "fail." "Once tested, a child's IQ becomes the most critical variable determining whether he retains the status of 'normal' student or moves closer to the status of 'mental retardate'" (Mercer 1973:114). The children who were referred for testing were similar to the whole population of the school district; those who "failed" were significantly more likely to be from poor and minority, Mexican-American or Black, homes. Failure of larger proportions of Mexican-Americans is probably not due to a lower level of intelligence in that group but is more reasonably explained by the middle class biases of intelligence tests which rest heavily on verbal skills. Many of the Mexican-American children

come from Spanish-speaking homes but are taught and tested in English.

Diagnoses of "mental retardation" are applied by the school system to a selected sample of children, but that is not the end of selective processing. In fact, some children who are called retarded are never referred to special classes; these non-referred children are significantly more often from white or middle-class families. The children who are selected for special classes have scores similar to the non-referred group but are significantly more likely to be Mexican-American, from poor families and to have been provisionally labeled as retarded by their classroom teachers. Further selection is apparent when Mercer examines which children actually appear in the special classes, the final decision point. Ten of the 81 referred children escaped the label of "retarded" by not going to these classes; these tended to be younger girls from Anglo families. Two remained in their original classrooms; one transferred to a parochial school where she was not considered retarded; seven moved out of the community. There is the hint here that middle class white families may be more able to resist labeling of their child by negotiating alternative arrangements.

Thus, Mercer has shown that while one might assume that the diagnosis of mental retardation is an objective judgement based on IQ scores derived from a standard intelligence test, the actual operation of this process is systematically influenced by a number of social and organizational factors that have nothing to do with the child's basic intelligence. One result of the selective labeling is examplified in the segment of Mercer's Table 7 (1973:112) which appears at the top of the next page.

After examining Mercer's data, then, some might recommend that the California school system "tighten up," "systematize" and "make more objective" the procedures for identifying the "truly retarded" so that no child in that category slips through the net and remains "untreated." Implicit in this recommendation are the assumptions of the biomedical model of disease.

Social labeling theory makes quite different assumptions, however, some of which are implicit in our discussion of Mercer's findings. First, there is no universal definition of "illness." Whether an individual is to be called "ill" is relative to the society or organization in which he is found; poor academic/

		CHARACTERISTICS OF PUBLIC SCHOOL POP. (6–15 YEARS AGE) IN %'s (N = 1565)	CHARACTERISTICS OF CHILDREN IN SPECIAL CLASSES FOR RETARDED IN %'s (N = 71)
Sex:	Male	50.4	69.1
	Female	49.6	30.9
Ethnic group:	Anglo	81.0	32.1
	Mex-Amer.	11.0	45.3
	Black	7.9	22.6
Social status:	Poor housing	36.1	74.6

social performance in parochial schools or in lower class Mexican-American families is believed to be just that, not evidence of mental retardation. Organizational practices as well constrain the definition of illness; only if the society or organization has procedures for defining or labeling illness does the illness exist. Thus, illness is a social fact, one that cannot be separated from the processes through which it is socially identified and labeled. From this perspective there are no "truly retarded" children waiting to be discovered.

This then leads to the second principle, that whether symptoms, unusual behavior, poor performance are to be called "illness" is the result of a social negotiation process among interested parties. Clearly many people—teachers, students, families, psychologists—have contributed to the final label or lack of it and each has brought to that negotiation process his own assumptions about mental retardation as well as his own interests in the child, the process, or the diagnostic outcome. Social labeling theory focuses much of its attention on the relative power of "labelers" and "labeled" and assumes that the negotiation process and its outcome can often be predicted from the interests of those in power. The fact that it is children from middle class white families who are more likely to escape the label "retarded" is thus consistent with social labeling hypotheses.

Since labels of "illness" result from social negotiations in certain social and organizational contexts, the theory also assumes that "de-labeling" occurs within these contexts. That is, whether a person who has been called "ill" returns to "normal" is predictable from his social characteristics, the expecta-

tions that others have for him, the interests of all parties, and the nature of the treatment organization itself. For some, returning to "normal" is easily done; this may have been true for some of the young, white girls from middle-class families in Mercer's sample. For others, the label of illness and involvement in the treatment process may so delimit the range of normal interactions and relationships that the individual has only one available role, as a "sick person." Our classes, schools, and homes for the mentally retarded which are organized to "treat" or "train" children for participation in normal society may have the unintended effect of prolonging "illness" or of leading to what labeling theory calls "secondary deviant roles." Some of the children who are labeled as retarded in the school system may have been given a label that sticks for life, and that has profound implications for jobs, marriage, and future social relationships.

SOME EVIDENCE FOR SOCIAL LABELING THEORY

Mental retardation is a "fringe" disease. It is quite easy to see how social factors might become involved in decision-making in the face of symptoms that are unclear and thus difficult to evaluate. But social labeling theory is used to analyse the selection, negotiation and treatment of all sorts of illnesses including those diseases that one might assume are objectively defined and routinely processed.[2] It assumes, then, that the process of becoming ill, being treated and getting well is a social process. It also allows for, and even predicts, that some patients who are treated within a medical system may, from the biomedical perspective, have no "true" disease (for example, the "crocks" whom physicians feel get in the way of treating the "truly ill") and that some "truly diseased" people never appear in any medical system (for example, the Indian woman who sees her pregnancy as a normal phenomenon, the busy mother who ignores her headaches, the man who attributes his shortness of breath to old age). For social labeling theory the "crock" and the old man who has difficulty breathing are not evidence that the medical system is not working well but instead are predictable in terms of how the social processes of identification, selection and negotiation actually work.

We will look here at three general stages of illness labeling. The first is the initial decision that something is wrong that should be called "illness." The second stage involves the negotiation among interested parties regarding what sort of illness it is and what should be done about it. Finally, the third stage is one in which the negotiated label (which, in reality, may change several times) influences social relationships and symptoms, and thus affects whether the labeled individual is able to "de-label" and return to normal. We have selected a few empirical studies relevant to each of the stages to provide concrete examples of the ways in which labeling theory examines the career of the ill person. These examples are not meant to provide a survey of empirical support for the theory since empirical evidence varies considerably, depending on the particular hypothesis; there is much more evidence for the initial selective labeling of ill people than for the later stages of labeling. Instead we use the examples to clarify the labeling hypotheses themselves.

SOME CONDITIONS UNDER WHICH "ILLNESS" IS IDENTIFIED AND LABELS OF ILLNESS ARE GIVEN

The first stage in social labeling of illness usually occurs when someone, often the individual himself, thinks that "something is wrong." Neither he nor his family may know what it is, even whether it is an illness; they may simply decide that things are not normal. There are, however, many social conditions under which the same individual feeling or behaving in the same way may never label himself nor be labeled by others as ill. Whether initial labeling occurs depends on the norms of the society in which he lives, his own social position within the society, and the characteristics of organizations with which he may be involved. We will look briefly at each of these three factors.

Cultural and Social Norms

Each society has its own peculiar definitions for the kinds of behaviors, dysfunctions, even feelings, that are to be called and treated as "illnesses." We see these culturally specific definitions of illness most clearly if we look across time within our culture or if we compare across cultures. For example, just recently in many places in the West the set of behaviors we call "alcoholism" has been legally shifted from the category of "crime" to the category of "illness," leading to new types of decisions about who is an "alcoholic" and to profound changes in the career of the labeled person. Definitions of other illnesses have also changed. Homosexuality is, formally, no longer an illness according to the American Psychiatric Association but "lack of sexual desire" now is, at least, as it is represented in textbooks describing specific etiologies and treatment strategies (Kaplan 1979). Further, in the West if a person does not go to work our first thought is that he might be "ill." This is not true in peasant Sri Lanka (Ceylon), for example, where "not working," while often deviant, is not necessarily a sign of illness. In Sri Lanka, too, the Western psychiatrist's cues for "depression"—withdrawal, lack of communication, lethargy—are seldom thought of as illness by the individual or his family (Waxler 1974a, b). One might also expect that in societies where diseases such as malaria, leprosy, hookworm, and schistosomiasis are highly prevalent they are less likely to be called "illness" than to be seen as "problems in daily living." For example, Indian mothers traditionally have not defined the high rate of infant death (often due to tetanus from the use of cowdung to treat the umbilical cord) as a problem of "illness" but instead have understood the repeated loss of their babies in religious terms. Thus, cultures vary in the extent to which a specific set of behaviors or feelings is judged to be deviant (e.g., "depression" in Sri Lanka is "normal"); cultures vary as well in terms of the type of deviance ("illness," "crime," "sin," etc.) the behavior is believed to represent.

Available Treatment Systems

Beliefs and norms within a specific culture allow for selective decisions about what phenomena are to be called "illnesses." But just as important in the labeling decision are the characteristics and capacities of available treatment organizations. Thus, whether an individual is to be called "ill" or "ill in a certain way" depends very clearly on the existence and kind of treatment and treatment systems that the society provides.

Hospital administrators have long had the uneasy feeling that the more beds they provide the more sick people there are to fill them. Recently Harris (1975) has shown that this is, indeed, probably true. Examining 56 counties in New York State he showed that increases in the number of hospital beds per 1000 population is associated with increases in the use of these beds, not because there was an initial demand or need, but because physicians respond to the new, and empty, beds by increasing admissions and lengthening patient stays. Thus, the availability of hospital services has a direct effect upon the norms of medical practice which, in turn, affects the number of individuals who will be labeled as "sick enough to be in a hospital." The fact of being so defined and treated may, according to labeling theory hypotheses, have important implications for the future of these hospitalized individuals.

We see just that in D'Arcy's analysis (1976) of changes in the health services in the Province of Saskatchewan during the period 1946–70. These changes led for a time to a startling increase in the numbers of older people labeled as "mentally ill." The high in 1950s for people over 70 was 600 per 100,000 people in Saskatchewan as compared with all-Canada rate for the same age group of 250 per 100,000.

The introduction of a program of free hospitalizations for mental illness interacting in the context of a rapidly increasing older age component in the population and the lack of facilities for the care of the aged had the effect of dramatically increasing the rate of mental illness . . . (D'Arcy 1976:5)

Free care for those old people who have no place to go was associated, then, with an enormous increase in psychiatric morbidity. A decrease in psychiatric hospitalization that was just as dramatic occurred in the early 1960s associated with changes in the delivery of health and welfare services, including

. . . increased old age allowance . . . the shift in the basis of allocating monies from a 'means test' to a 'needs' test, increased provincial funding for low cost housing . . . hostels, nursing homes . . . and the making of mental hospital admission discretionary (by the medical officer in charge of the hospital). (D'Arcy 1976:11)

Thus, by 1965 the psychiatric admission rates for patients over 70 years was down to 250 per 100,000. As D'Arcy suggests, changes in the availability of alternative social and health services clearly contribute to the "manufacture and obsolescence of madness." If the label of mental illness were benign and/or transitory one might view these changes as vagaries of the health bureaucracy but labeling theory hypothesizes that the label of mental illness in itself has significant and often negative effects on the social relationships of the labeled person. Thus, the increase in hospitalization rates has results that are not entirely benign.

Whether "trouble" is called "illness" is sometimes also dependent upon other characteristics of the practice of medicine, including whether an effective treatment is at hand to deal with it. For example, not until specific drugs were available to give to hyperactive children did "hyperkinesis" become a disease category that physicians and others attended to (Conrad 1978). Not until lithium became known as an effective agent for endogenous depression did manic-depressive psychosis come to be something other than an unusual disease, seldom seen in Western psychiatric hospitals (Kendell et al. 1971). Readily available treatments "create" diseases that might otherwise, and have in the past, not been called disease at all.

The decision to label some sort of "trouble" as "illness" is exceptionally common if the individual lives within the context of a "total institution" such as a prison or on a Navy ship. When all aspects of one's life occur within the boundaries of the prison walls the rate of labeled illness is four times the national average; that is, prisoners are four times as likely to make visits to the prison clinic requesting treatment (Twaddle 1976). Characteristics of institutional life and the ways in which medical systems have been organized in response to them have the ultimate effect of producing large numbers of people labeled "ill." Some prisoners, called "skaters," label themselves as ill in order to use the clinic to meet friends; others appear often in the clinic due to the organizational policy that prescription drugs are given only one week at a time. Clinic physicians are also arbiters of who is allowed to purchase "civilian" shoes. Even when these unique characteristics are accounted for the rate of labeled illness is three times the national average.

These unique characteristics are important to social labeling theory. They appear clearly in the prison data but they illustrate a phenomenon that is more general. Whether an individual labels himself as "sick" occurs within and is affected by the norms of the society around him. Physicians following the biomedical model might say that some of these prisoners are not "really" sick; social labeling theory takes a different view, that all are labeled and processed as "ill" and that the very processing has important implications for the individual and the organization.[3]

What we have shown so far are some of the contextual factors that impinge on the labeling of illness. Cultural as well as treatment system variables have very clear and selective effects on whether the individual who feels or thinks that "something is wrong" is labeled as "ill."

The Characteristics of the Individual

Selective labeling is also contingent on characteristics of the individual himself, upon his position in the family and the society. For example, Campbell (1975) has shown that mothers are more likely to see their children as "ill" than themselves as "ill" even when the symptoms are identical. Two-thirds of a list of common symptoms (headaches, fever, toothache, sore throat, etc.) were judged by mothers to be "illnesses" in children while only one-half were believed to be illnesses if the mother had them. Further, mothers are twice as likely to call a doctor for a child's illness than for the same illness in themselves. Thus, the decision about whether "something is wrong" depends upon age and family position;

the decision of mothers to normalize their own symptoms removes them from the set of labeled and treated patients.

Self-selection by the person who has symptoms is also often contingent, not on the symptoms or presence of "disease," but on the individual's social and economic background. The way in which social background impinges on these self-labeling decisions is apparent among physically handicapped individuals who drop out of a rehabilitation program before the prescribed regimen is completed (Ludwig and Adams 1968). Drop-outs are more likely to be men, white, in middle-age groups, and to have had previous employment; those who complete the program are women, the very old and very young, blacks, and the unemployed. If the handicapped person has a job to return to he will redefine himself as "normal" and leave the rehabilitation program; this definition takes precedence over the physician's judgement that the individual has not yet returned to a normal physical state. It is those handicapped individuals who are in the relatively more powerful social positions (men, whites, but especially the employed) who can and do choose to think of themselves as "normal" rather than "sick" and who can and do act on this decision by dropping out of the treatment system.

LABELING AND DE-LABELING: A NEGOTIATED PROCESS

Cultural norms, the presence or absence of particular treatment systems and the social position of individuals within their social group are all variables significant in the initial decision about whether an individual is "ill" or not. If that decision is affirmative then the troubled individual often finds himself in a doctor's office or hospital emergency room. It is here that the "trouble" is transformed into a specific "illness" through a process of negotiation, often between professionals, family members and the sick person. The illness label, whether it is "pneumonia," "fatigue," "too much drinking," "just being ornery," is affected by the social positions and interests of all the parties involved.

Considerable research has focused on this negotiation stage, often following the biomedical perspective on disease. Many of these studies of physician-patient interactions look at communication and emotional and social-class barriers that prevent the physician from obtaining diagnostic information, making a correct decision about treatment and getting the patient to follow, or comply with, his recommendations (Hauser 1979). Social labeling theory examines the same negotiations but follows quite different assumptions. It says that what the "trouble" is called is constructed within the interaction and is dependent, not on how accurately the physician can use interview and examination data to match the reported symptoms with a textbook description, but instead on social characteristics of the professionals and the patient and the social contexts in which they meet.

Characteristics of the Individual

What the trouble is to be called, and what is done about it is often predictable from the interests and relative social position of the troubled individual himself. For example, some individuals learn through experience with particular treatment systems how to state their case (regardless of their symptoms) in order to get what they want, either hospital admission or discharge. Those who want admission to a very selective psychiatric ward, for example, know that mention of suicidal tendencies is the key to admission since the law requires that; being "hospital-wise" tips the balance in the emergency room negotiations. A similar phenomenon occurs in a chronic care hospital (Roth and Eddy 1967) where the very small proportion of individuals who are informed about the variety of services are able to negotiate or to have others act on their behalf in order to be admitted to the most desirable "rehab" service. "Nearly always these knowledgeable individuals are chosen even though the physician may feel that little can be done to help them and may only take them to prevent their 'rotting away' on the less desirable wards" (1967:16).

The social and economic position of the potentially "ill" person along with that of his family or spokesman may have a significant impact on the negotiation of the problem. This is often apparent in the negotiations around psychiatric hospitalization where the decision to label someone as "mentally ill" may have long-term negative effects. Some of these negotiations take place in commitment hearings where physicians, lawyers, prospective pa-

tients, sometimes family members, meet to consider whether the individual should be hospitalized against his will. One group of investigators systematically examined 81 hearings held in an Ohio state psychiatric hospital (Wenger and Fletcher 1969). In every one of these hearings the court-appointed referee (fulfilling the functions of a judge) rubber-stamped the recommendation made by the psychiatrist. Yet the psychiatrist's recommendation was not systematically based on the seriousness of the individual's symptoms nor the threat of his behavior to himself or others. Instead, recommendations were strongly related to the presence of a lawyer representing the individual's interests. If a lawyer were present not only was the hearing longer and less perfunctory but also the psychiatrist was significantly less likely to recommend hospitalization. Thus, only 26% of those with lawyers were involuntarily committed while 92% of those not legally represented were committed. This significant difference held true for individuals whose symptoms and behaviors met the legal criteria for admission as well as for those whose symptoms were less serious. While the lawyer's presence was a significant predictor of the recommended course, psychiatrists making the recommendations were not aware of that effect; one said, "Legal counsel has no effect on my decision. . . . If the patient is sick, he's sick" (1969:71).

If we looked at these negotiation processes we would probably see a cluster of characteristics that are correlated with the "non-commitment" decision; the 18% of individuals who have lawyers are probably middle class with educational and economic resources that give them power. Even if they are not economically or socially "equal" to the examining physicians, the fact that they have a professional speaking for them (since legal counsel is sometimes available free through Legal Aid) means that the label of illness (or lack of it) is negotiated between professionals of equal status. The investigators suggest that there exists "an uneasy peace which is sustained between the two professions, partly on the basis of the psychiatrists' unintended and unwitting trade-off of effective authority to the lawyers, in exchange for the privilege of ostensible authority in the carefully staged setting of the admission hearings" (1969:72). Thus, whether an individual is to be called "mentally ill" and to be involuntarily hospitalized is the result of a complex set of social relationships between several professionals and the prospective patient.

Characteristics of the Institution

The ways in which the institution operates has an important and selective effect on the negotiation of illness as well. Certain hospitals, dependent upon patient fees, may organize admission procedures in such a way as to produce the numbers of "ill" people that are required to keep the system going. For example, one private psychiatric hospital, in its brochure searching for "moonlighting" physicians to work at night, offers $125 per night *plus* $25 for each patient admitted. While we have no empirical evidence that the additional payment increases admissions, the incentive for admissions is an incentive to define individuals as "ill enough to need hospitalization."

More systematic investigation has been done linking the workings of treatment systems to the negotiation processes that result in someone being called "ill." In a study of 269 consecutive decisions for or against hospital admission to the psychiatric division of the Los Angeles County-U.S.C. Medical Center, it was discovered that the severity of the prospective patient's symptoms played no part in the outcome of negotiations (Mendel and Rapport 1969). However, the time of day and the day of the week that an individual appeared in the admissions office had a significant effect on the negotiation. Of those who appeared during regular working hours, 9–5, Monday through Friday, only 32% were admitted; of the others who showed up at night or on weekends, 51% were admitted, even though they were no different from the former group in severity of symptoms. A major factor in the increased admissions at night/weekends was the way the hospital organized its work-load, putting social workers and senior psychiatrists (who tend not to hospitalize) on duty during the day and residents on night duty. The resident on duty tended "to hospitalize patients to be 'safe' because he is unsure of his evaluation and is far less resourceful in planning and implementing an alternative to hospitalization" (1969:326). The resident's conservative stance interacts with the fact that individuals who request admission at odd hours are less likely to have or bring with them an interested family member who might provide an alternative to hospitalization. The way

the hospital organization works, then, produces labeled illnesses that might not exist if, for example, social workers did night duty.

Similar institutional effects on negotiated illnesses appear in social agencies. For example, a person who becomes blind often voluntarily consults an agency for the blind and soon finds that "not all people who have been labeled 'blind' can follow a course entirely of their own choosing" (Scott 1969:73). Agency staff may negotiate an illness label with the individual that has little or nothing to do with the degree to which vision is impaired but is dependent instead on the ideology of the agency. A blind person who has residual vision (this is the most common form of blindness) is under strong pressure to think of himself as blind in the way which the agency happens to define it. For example, blind people who select one type of agency find that they are expected to "accommodate" to what the agency defines as a debilitating and life-long handicap. In these settings blind people are provided with extensive substitutes for sight, for example, tape recordings in the elevators to announce the floors; cafeterias that serve food easily eaten by blind people; sheltered workshops geared to special handicaps of the blind rather than to training for regular jobs. The implicit assumption of these agencies is that blindness makes one incompetent and thus dependent (Scott 1969:85).

But some agencies take a different stand, that a blind person can be restored to quasi-normal life, provided he accepts the fact he is blind and receives training/counseling. Blind individuals who appear in these agencies are encouraged to think of themselves as going through an emotional crisis in which personal independence and self-esteem has been lost with the loss of sight and in which reintegration of the personality involves pain. Stress, then, is on psychological rather than physical adaptation to poor vision. This "total psychological change" ideology contrasts with a third sort of ideology, represented by the Veterans' Administration, in which re-training of the blind is limited in time and the agency's expectation is that the individual will return to the normal community with the help of physical devices and some income maintenance.

The expectations of each type of agency for the blind are evident in the ways in which they negotiate with, or train, the blind person. Thus, one might expect that these varied negotiations produce blind persons whose lives follow quite different pathways. And this seems to be true. Compared with blind men treated in the V.A. program, blind civilians who receive services from other agencies "are less active in nonblindness-related clubs and organizations . . . they visit less; they have fewer sighted friends; they do not engage in social activities to the same degree; and they tend to be more isolated" (Scott 1969:116). Institutions such as agencies for the blind have a significant impact upon the kind of illness label that the sick person will take on and, in the long run, a significant impact on his social relationships.

Thus, what kind of illness an individual is believed to have, and what he and others expect of him is not a cut and dried affair dependent simply on the physician's diagnosis. Instead, illness labels are created in social negotiations between several parties, including professionals and the troubled individual, and they occur within institutional and social contexts that play an important part in the negotiation. Ideologies and organizational procedures as well as the relative power and interests of the negotiating parties contribute to the label of illness. Further, illness labels are often changed as the negotiation process continues. Thus, there is not only an on-going process of labeling, but also of re-labeling and de-labeling.

THE EFFECTS OF ILLNESS LABELS ON SOCIAL RELATIONSHIPS AND SYMPTOMS

Illness labels, we have seen, are given selectively, the result of negotiation between physician, patient and others, often in an institutional context. That these labels are not simply generated in a social exercise that is irrelevant to the individual's life situation is evident when we examine what happens to labeled individuals.

Someone who has been labeled as having cancer, who has been successfully treated, and who returns to work often finds that the label "sticks." Further, the label of "cancer" is a stigmatizing one (perhaps because of its equation with death) that often generates significant changes in the individual's social and work life. For example, in a recent study,

Many recovered patients complained of feeling isolated at work because their co-workers acted as though cancer was contagious. . . . Over 80 percent of the blue-collar workers and 50 percent of the white-collar workers surveyed encountered some form of job discrimination relating to the fact that they had been successfully treated for cancer. (New York Times 1979)

Discrimination with regard to promotions, work assignments, access to health insurance, etc., is common although illegal. Illness labels, therefore, are often difficult to discard, even when the disease has disappeared; it is the label itself that has impact on the individual's life.

An illness label may, as well, mean that the individual so labeled becomes enmeshed within certain institutions that sustain the label rather than encourage its discard. Certain illness organizations seem to have this function. For example, the Diabetes Clubs for adolescent diabetics, whose explicit function is to educate and support the patient so that he can take on a "normal" role, may, in reality, encourage the diabetic to spend more and more time in the company of others just like himself, thus sustaining the label of illness. Alcoholics Anonymous is a prime example of an institution that prolongs the illness label in its formal ideology (the requirement that individuals publicly confirm that they are "alcoholics") as well as in its function. A large percentage of AA members' social lives centers on the organization and other members, thus isolating them from normal relationships and further strengthening their role as "alcoholics."

Labels of "Illness" Affect Social Relationships

Whether and what kind of illness label one has, then, may have a profound effect upon one's social relationships, irrespective of whether the symptoms or the disease itself have disappeared. Others (and the labeled person) may continue to think of the individual as "a diabetic," "having cancer," "mentally ill" or "a heart patient"; further, organizational norms and functions may sustain the label and set limits on the role the individual can take.

The effect of a label on one's work is apparent in Eichorn and Anderson's (1962) comparison of farmers with labeled and unlabeled heart diseases. Two sets of farmers labeled themselves as having "heart disease," but only one set actually had, upon medical examination, any evidence of the disease. The group of farmers that mistakenly believed themselves to have diseased hearts, but in fact were well, received the label "through improper diagnosis or failure to understand the doctor's diagnosis" (Eichorn and Anderson 1962:242–243). The third and fourth sets of farmers did not label themselves as having heart disease but one group of them, upon examination, were found to have diseased hearts.

Comparison of the four sets provides for a test of the relative effects of disease and illness label on social role and findings show that both variables have some effect on the individual's life. Farmers with true heart disease, whether they were labeled or not, are more likely to cut down on the amount of work that they do; they reduce their hours of work, sell off some land, or take easier jobs in town. "Even though 'hidden cardiacs' did not believe they had heart disease they, like the true cardiacs, tended to report chest pains" (1962:246). Thus, the symptoms themselves, whether labeled as "heart disease" or not, may have had some effects on the farmers' decisions to cut down on work.

But labels have an effect on role, too, regardless of the presence of disease. If a farmer believes himself to have a diseased heart he will take more heart-related precautions than will the farmer who labels himself as "normal." Those who mistakenly labeled themselves or had been labeled as "heart diseased" chose to take naps, to use sun-shades on their tractors and to stop smoking just as did those who were "true cardiacs." The label itself—what the farmer or his family *believes* to be the case—has an important effect upon his behavior, even when he has no symptoms and no heart disease.

Another result of illness labeling may be longer or more frequent hospitalizations; once an individual is labeled as "ill" he is likely to be labeled again. For example, in the Los Angeles psychiatric service the one factor that residents, social workers and staff psychiatrists uniformly took into account in making a decision about hospital admission was whether the person had been admitted in the past, even though the decision-makers were unaware that they attended to this phenomenon (Mendel and Rapport 1969:325). In fact, sixty percent of previously hospi-

talized individuals were readmitted while only 11% of those not previously hospitalized were admitted, even though the two groups were almost identical in the severity of their symptoms. The implication of this tendency to re-label is important since in the course of re-hospitalizations the individual may become further and further removed from the normal world of work and his normal social relationships. Psychiatric patients who are removed from the labor market for considerable periods of time by virtue of their hospitalization have difficulty in finding jobs. Lack of work after discharge from psychiatric hospitalization is an excellent predictor of further re-hospitalizations, even when severity of symptoms is controlled for (Maisel 1967).

Some institutions, in fact, create and/or sustain lifelong roles for people labeled as "ill," roles that far outlast the disease itself. The Public Health Service leprosy hospitals, for example, accept the ideology that leprosy is socially stigmatized and thus provide patients with a small but isolated society in which they can remain for life. Houses, jobs, recreation, are all available on the grounds of the hospital. Thus, rather than discarding the label of "leper" once the disease is arrested ex-patients retain that label and are removed from society with the assistance of the institution whose goal is "cure" (Waxler 1979).

Similarly, some agencies for the blind offer broad services and encourage dependency such that some blind people become what Scott (1969) calls "professional blind men." These are blind individuals whose whole lives are organized around the fact of their blindness, and who are retained in the role partly as a result of their having been hired to work in such activities for the blind as sheltered workshops, home-teaching and counseling programs and residential schools.

Labels of Illness Affect Symptoms

To this point we have presented labeling theory as a conceptual model in which the label of illness is selectively applied to an individual, often on the basis of his social characteristics and the social context in which he lives, and in which labels are negotiated and re-negotiated, often within treatment institutions. The result of illness labeling is an alteration, temporary or permanent, in the individual's social relationships.

Nothing has been said about possible effects of labeling on the disease process or on symptoms themselves.[4] Yet this is probably the question of most interest to physicians. Practitioners are likely to ask, "Does the social labeling process impinge on the patient's illness and therefore on my job, the treatment of diseased individuals?"

The crucial question here is this: are labels of illness the result of disease or do they cause disease? Which comes first? The layman's assumption (and probably most physicians' as well) is that if one experiences symptoms then one labels oneself as ill. In this case labels are simply ways of conceptualizing a more basic biological process; they have no impact upon that process. Labeling theory hypothesizes just the opposite, that if one is labeled as "ill" this label has an effect upon disease; in this case we cannot conceive of the label simply as a cognitive phenomenon but must see it as having a direct impact on the illness itself.

Longitudinal studies of labels and disease and/or well-controlled analyses are required in order to sort out this "chicken-egg" phenomenon and few studies attempt to test these alternate hypotheses directly. However, there is considerable evidence that labels of illness and the expectations that others have of labeled individuals do have an impact on the disease process, particularly on prognosis. Often the mediating process is one in which the labeled person or the system around him comes to reject or to re-negotiate the label of illness and thus the individual drops the "sick role." He thinks of himself as "well," others treat him as "well" and expect him to be so and the organized, well-defined package of symptoms becomes diffuse, is not attended to, not rewarded, and may be redefined as "normal." Ultimately, as symptoms are socially redefined they disappear as significant biomedical phenomena as well.[5]

For example, acceptance of the label of "tuberculosis" as defined by a particular TB hospital is significantly associated with the rate of recovery from the disease itself. Calden et al. (1960) followed a cohort of newly admitted TB patients through the initial four months of hospitalization and classified them as having a relatively "fast" or "slow" recovery rate, relative to each patient's own initial condition. While very few of the medical/psychological variables were predictive of recovery rate, there was a "significant relationship between the patient's ward behavior and his rate of recovery" (1960:352). Patients who cooperated with the institutional regime—who accepted the label of "illness"—recovered slowly. Those who did not conform to the rules about bed rest and who were aggressive about getting what they wanted—that is, who rejected the label—recovered more quickly. It was the "good patient," the one who internalized the institution's label of illness, whose symptoms lasted longer.

A similar link between the label of illness and the retention of symptoms is apparent in psychiatric illness. Doherty (1975) looked at the acceptance and rejection of illness labels by psychiatric patients in the first four weeks of their hospitalization. In this hospital one of the major staff goals was to socialize patients to accept the fact that they were indeed "ill." The staff reasoned that not until one sees oneself as "ill" can the psychotherapeutic treatment orientation ("working out one's problems") be effective. Thus, one staff goal is to make sure that all patients label themselves as "mentally ill." In fact, some patients immediately so labeled themselves and retained that label of mental illness throughout the four-week period. Another group initially labeled themselves but quickly rejected the label and thought of themselves as "not mentally ill." A third group never did accept the label of illness. They denied that they were ill.

The three groups did not differ initially in overall psychopathology ratings by the staff; thus, whether one's symptoms were severely disturbing or only moderately so did not determine the initial label. But once the individual had taken on (or not taken on) a particular illness label, that label predicted two things: one, the extent to which the individual's global symptom level improved and, two, the length of time he stayed in the hospital. It was only the group of individuals who, at first, thought of themselves as "mentally ill" but then rejected that label who improved significantly in terms of symptoms. Further, this group (along with the "label deniers") stayed in the hospital a shorter period of time. The crucial group, those patients who accepted the label of "mental illness," were significantly less likely to improve and significantly more likely to stay in the hospital longer.

A comparison of individuals labeled as "ill" in different cultures is another way of examining the effects of labels on symptoms and prognosis. By varying cultures we also often vary beliefs about illness, expectations for the labeled person and modes of social processing. For example, in Sri Lanka (Ceylon) mental illnesses are commonly believed to be supernaturally caused and easily and quickly cured. Further, the availability of multiple types of treatments (Western as well as Ayurvedic medicine, exorcism, several religion-based methods, astrology, etc.) leave the power over the labeling and de-labeling processes and the ill individual's life in his own and his family's hands. In contrast, in many industrialized societies mental illnesses are believed to involve serious personality change for which the individual is held responsible and which may last a lifetime. Further, treatment agents work in large bureaucratically organized hospitals or clinics that often take power and responsibility for de-labeling from the ill person (Waxler 1977).

Social labeling theory predicts that these culturally based beliefs and expectations and the modes of social processing will produce illness outcomes congruent with cultural expectations. Evidence suggests that this may be true for individuals labeled as "schizophrenic" (Waxler 1979). A five year follow-up of diagnosed schizophrenics living in Sri Lanka shows that social adjustment and clinical state at the end of five years is remarkably good. The findings for Sri Lankan patients are consistent with similar individuals in other traditional societies such as Nigeria and India and consistently different from outcome for schizophrenia in patients followed in industrial societies. For example, the proportion of individuals labeled "schizophrenic" who have no further episodes of illness after the first one ranges from 58% in Nigeria, 51% in India, 40% in Sri Lanka to 7% in USSR and 6% in Denmark. These large and consistent differences suggest that industrial societies process psychiatric patients such that large proportions are alienated from their normal roles and continue to have symptoms. In contrast, beliefs and practices in nonindustrial societies encourage short-term illness and quick return to normality. Cultural differences in prognosis, then, may be the result of culturally based labeling and de-labeling processes.

Physicians have always known that if they treat an individual as if he were "ill" they may encourage illness rather than health. Administrators of old-style state psychiatric hospitals saw new symptoms of withdrawal and regression develop when patients were transferred to "chronic-care" wards (Wing and Brown 1970). Our examples from tuberculosis and psychiatric patients in our own and other societies have shown that the everyday work of the treatment system, designed to foster recovery, may instead encourage the "sick role" and even sustain symptoms. There is evidence, then, that the labeling process is not simply a social phenomenon that is superimposed on the real work of diagnosing and treating biomedical phenomena but that labeling has an impact on disease and/or its symptoms. Labeling theory speaks of this phenomenon in terms such as "sick role" and "secondary deviance." The biomedical model refers to "iatrogenesis." The contribution that labeling theory makes to physicians' understanding of iatrogenesis is to broaden the range of iatrogenic variables and to specify just how the social processing of ill people contributes to the maintenance of or recovery from disease.

EFFECTS OF LABELING ON MEDICAL PRACTICE

We have shown how the social processing of people labeled as "ill" impinges on the lives of "ill" persons. Those who are selected into the domain of illness and medicine may find that the label of illness is not always benign nor temporary. Some illness labels are stigmatizing and some lead to social isolation. In some instances treatment systems are so structured that they unintentionally sustain labels and even symptoms.

These social labeling processes also have significant effects on the everyday practice of medicine. For example, the kinds of illnesses physicians and other health workers find they are called upon to treat are profoundly affected by the early stages of labeling. The large numbers of geriatric patients in Saskatchewan psychiatric hospitals (D'Arcy 1976) were admitted presumably because alternative services for old people were not available; the fact that they were selected into the hospital and given psychiatric diagnoses meant that physicians and others were obligated to treat them. Thus, physicians come to be specialists in geriatric psychiatry in response to the "new" illness. Similarly, medical practitioners have recently been called upon to treat such new problems as hyperkinesis, sexual desire disorders and alcoholism that now fall into the realm of "illness." Practitioners, then, often deal with illness or with ill people who are defined and selected by others (families or the individual himself) for reasons that have little to do with biomedical processes.

Labeling and social processing of sick persons, we have seen, sometimes even prolongs or creates symptoms that physicians are then asked to treat. Just as psychiatrists now must deal with the iatrogenic phenomenon of tardive dyskinesia they were also, in the past, called upon to treat symptoms of withdrawal and regression that resulted from prolonged psychiatric hospitalization on "back wards."

Selective labeling and social processing of ill people also impinges on the physician's practice in a somewhat more subtle way. These social processes provide most physicians with a very selected sample of patients, those who have been sorted into the "ill" category at several previous decision points. This pool of highly selected labeled individuals may serve as "data" for physicians' hunches about disease process and the effectiveness of treatment. Even the information from hospital or clinic records that we tend to think of as "hard" data can also be conceived as the product of social processing. Labeling theory suggests that facts such as diagnosis, length of stay, prognosis, may tell us much more about the social characteristics of selected patients and the workings of the treatment system than about a biomedical process. Highly selective diagnoses reported by physicians for medical insurance purposes are one example of this phenomenon.

But physicians and health workers do not stand entirely outside of the health system, prepared to treat or handle individuals who have been labeled as "ill" by family, self or society. They are active participants in the labeling and de-labeling processes; in fact, making decisions about who is to be called "ill" and who is "well" is central to a doctor's job. Labeling theory suggests that very often this labeling process is not entirely beneficial to the ill person and that medical personnel, in spite of their intentions, may process ill people in ways that prolong symptoms, socially isolate, or stigmatize. For example, psychiatrists working in a small ward in which demands for beds are very great and thus patient turnover rapid and length of stay short, find that they must continually argue that their patients

are "still sick" if they are to retain patients long enough to gain their cooperation in taking medication and to make sure that their acute symptoms are controlled. This argument for "illness" is communicated to staff, family and often the patient himself and it may become a self-fulfilling prophecy (Howard, et al. 1979). Medical professionals' tendencies toward caution and conservatism may also often be a tendency to prolong the label of illness and thus to encourage the sick role, isolate individuals from normal social relationships and, perhaps, encourage secondary symptoms.

CONCLUSION

We have introduced some of the ways in which labeling theory is used to understand illness by looking at studies that examine specific segments of that process. Findings suggest that labels of illness are applied selectively, and that the physician's criteria for disease (symptoms, signs, severity, etc.) are only one of several factors that predict who is to be called "ill." Social characteristics of the individual (his family position, his socioeconomic status, etc.) or of his society (beliefs about illness, etc.) and the existence of and kind of treatment system available (how many beds, whether alternative services are present, etc.) are significant to the initial labeling decision. If the "trouble" is labeled as "illness" then the selected group of labeled individuals may appear in a treatment system where further negotiation and renegotiation of the "illness" occurs. At this stage, too, whether an individual remains "ill" is associated with his background (his social position, how powerful he is, etc.) as well as with the organizational operation of medical practice and treatment systems (who selects, the predominant ideology of the system, etc.). Finally, the selected group of labeled individuals may, as a result of social processing, find that they remain "ill" and that their symptoms are sustained. A selected group drops through this net and returns to "normal." The highly selected group of "ill" individuals appears in that category, not simply because they had the most severe or intransigent symptoms, but because they have been involved in a series of social processes that have led to their selection into the role of "ill person." Thus, whether an individual is called "ill" and remains "ill" is a social, not simply a biomedical, phenomenon.

In contrast, the biomedical model of disease assumes that whether a person is "ill" is an objective fact, whether and how he is to be treated is a technical decision and whether he "gets well" is related to the state of technical treatment and the patient's compliance with it. We have seen that this model does not always accurately predict the realities of illness careers and treatment system operations.

Labeling theory suggests that it is not simply that treatment systems and medical practices need "tinkering with" in order to get them to work more objectively and effectively but that the very selective way that individuals are defined as "ill" is inherent in our society's processing of all sorts of deviant people and fulfills more general social functions. For example, those who end up in prison are highly selected samples of the population of people who break the law. Police interrogation, court hearings and prison life then isolate the selected individuals from normal society and serve as training grounds for the "hardened criminal." In this system police, lawyers, judges, and court psychiatrists act as agents of social control, often removing and/or punishing selected individuals in ways that the society demands. Thus, formal law does not predict who will be labeled a "criminal."

Similar phenomena occur with regard to illness; physicians, social workers, even family members serve as agents of social control. They negotiate labels of illness that justify temporary (or sometimes permanent) isolation and abrogation of normal responsibilities on the part of the ill person. And they negotiate illness labels in a systematic way, based on our society's norms and beliefs, so that some individuals are more likely to be called "ill" and removed from society than are others. The biomedical theory of disease, then, does not always predict who is "ill." Some labeling theorists suggest that selective labeling of "illness" has little to do with disease itself but much more to do with the relative status, power and role of the individual. The illness labeling process, like the labeling of criminals, may, when seen in its broadest sense, simply be another way of removing society's unwanted.

Notes

1. Mental retardation is, of course, not an illness that ordinary physicians often treat. Instead, it has been handed over to psychologists and special teachers, probably because the most effective current "treatment" involves social/educational training rather than physical/medical "cure." However, the cause of mental retardation is explained in biomedical terms (as the result of minimal brain damage, etc.) and thus it falls within the biomedical theory of disease. We present Mercer's investigation of mental retardation because it is currently the most complete and systematic examination of the social labeling of a biomedical phenomenon.

2. Social labeling theory takes several forms. The most radical version questions the biomedical model of disease itself by stating that the labeling process "creates" the disease, that sick people are "sick" only because they have been so labeled. This leads very easily to a conclusion that physicians and other labelers are malevolent and motivated to cause trouble for people who would otherwise be well. If Mercer had followed this perspective she might have concluded that teachers and principals knowingly select Mexican-Americans and Blacks and call them retarded. Or that psychiatrists ignore real symptoms and selectively choose to recommend for long-term hospitalization and/or commitment only patients who are lower class or socially isolated.

A more conservative version of the theory, represented here, assumes that the labeling of illness usually begins when there are a set of diffuse or disorganized signs or symptoms, that is, when an individual evidences some sort of personal or behavioral deviation; whether these deviations are caused by genetic, biochemical, psychological, etc., factors is of no interest to the theory. Much of the time these signs and symptoms are ignored or explained away; only a small proportion are labeled and thus become grist for the medical negotiation process. In this version of the theory then there is no need to deny the presence of or significance of biomedical factors; these factors along with social characteristics of the individual and his social context contribute to the ways in which he is labeled or not labeled.

3. Waitzkin and Waterman (1974) suggest that the high rates of "sick call" in prisons may function to drain off tension that otherwise might take less controllable forms.

4. Some proponents of labeling theory would say that this question is irrelevant since "illness" is a social role and whether someone is called "diseased" is the result of a negotiation or decision in a social context. They say that "disease" is a concept of the biomedical model, a distinctly separate conceptual system.

5. Some authors call for an integration of the biomedical and social labeling perspectives when dealing with the hypothesis that predicts a causal effect of labels on symptoms or disease. Townsend (1978) discusses these re-

lationships in some detail, pointing out that medicine's concern with psychosomatic illness, for example, already assumes that "role expectations mobilize organic systems of the body. . . . A person's biology *interacts* with his social experience; each influences the other" (1978:97).

Thus, the dichotomy between social processes and biomedical processes may be quite artificial and more a matter of relative emphasis than of competing explanations.

References

BALINT, M.
1957 The Doctor, His Patient and The Illness. New York: International Universities Press.

CALDEN, G., W. DUPERTUIS, J. HOKANSON, and W. LEWIS
1960 Psychosomatic Factors in the Rate of Recovery From Tuberculosis. Psychomatic Medicine 22:345–355.

CAMPBELL, J. D.
1975 Attribution of Illness: Another Double Standard. J. of Health and Social Behavior 16:114–126.

CONRAD, P.
1978 Identifying Hyperactive Children: The Medicalization of Deviant Behavior. Lexington, Mass.: D.C. Heath.

D'ARCY, C.
1976 The Manufacture and Obsolescence of Madness: Age, Social Policy and Psychiatric Morbidity in a Prairie Province. Social Science and Medicine 10:5–13.

DOHERTY, E.
1975 Labeling Effects in Psychiatric Hospitalization. Archives of General Psychiatry 32:562–568.

EICHORN, R. and R. ANDERSON
1962 Changes in Personal Adjustment to Perceived and Medically Established Heart Disease: A Panel Study. J. of Health and Human Behavior 3:242–249.

GOVE, W., ed.
1975 The Labeling of Deviance. New York: Wiley.

HARRIS, D.
1975 An Elaboration of the Relationship Between General Hospital Bed Supply and General Hospital Utilization. J. of Health and Social Behavior 16:163–172.

HAUSER, S. T.
1979 Physician-Patient Relations. *In* Social Contexts of Health, Illness and Medical Care. E. G. Mishler, L. AmaraSingham, S. Hauser, R. Liem, S. Osherson and N. E. Waxler: Cambridge University Press.

HOWARD, L., S. ROSES, N. WAXLER, and J. WELSH
1979 Environmental Constraints, Occupational Conflict, and Patient Definitions in Three Psychiatric Settings. Unpublished paper.

KAPLAN, H. S.
1979 Disorders of Sexual Desire. New York: Brunner/Mazel.

KENDELL, R. E., J. COOPER, A. GOURLEY, and J. COPELAND
1971 Diagnostic Criteria of American and British Psychiatrists. Archives of General Psychiatry 25:123–130.

LUDWIG, E. and S. ADAMS
1968 Patient Cooperation in a Rehabilitation Center: Assumption of the Client Role. J. Health and Social Behavior 9:328–336.

MAISEL, R.
1967 The Ex-Mental Patient and Rehospitalization: Some Research Findings. Social Problems 15:18–24.

MENDEL, W. and S. RAPPORT
1969 Determinants of Decision for Psychiatric Hospitalization. Archives of General Psychiatry 20:321–328.

MERCER, JANE
1973 Labelling the Mentally Retarded. Berkeley: University of California Press.

ROTH, J. and E. EDDY
1967 Rehabilitation for the Unwanted. New York: Atherton Press.

SCHEFF, T.
1966 Being Mentally Ill. Chicago: Aldine.

SCHUR, E.
1971 Labeling Deviant Behavior. New York: Harper and Row.

SCOTT, R.
1969 The Making of Blind Men. New York: Russell Sage Foundation.

NEW YORK TIMES
1979 August 26, 1979.

TOWNSEND, J. M.
1978 Cultural Conceptions and Mental Illness: A Comparison of Germany and America. Chicago: University of Chicago Press.

TWADDLE, A. C.
1976 Utilization of Medical Services by a Captive Population: An Analysis of Sick Call in a State Prison. J. of Health and Social Behavior 17:236–248.

WAITZKIN, H. and B. WATERMAN
1974 The Exploitation of Illness in Capitalist Society. Indianapolis: Bobbs-Merrill Co.

WAXLER, NANCY E.
1974a The Domain Called "Madness" in the Peasant Villages of Ceylon. Unpublished paper.

1974b Culture and Mental Illness: A Social Labeling Perspective. J. of Nervous and Mental Disease 159:379–395.

1977 Is Mental Illness Cured in Traditional Societies? A Theoretical Analysis. Culture, Medicine and Psychiatry 1:233–253.

1979 Is Outcome for Schizophrenia Better in Nonindustrial Societies: The Case of Sri Lanka. J. of Nervous and Mental Disease 167:144–158.

In press Learning to Be a Leper: A Case Study in the Social Construction of Disease. *In* Social Contexts of Health, Illness and Medical Care. E. G. Mishler, L. AmaraSingham, S. Hauser, R. Leim, S. Osherson, and N. E. Waxler: Cambridge University Press.

WAXLER, NANCY E., L. HOWARD, S. ROSES, and J. WELSH
1979 Does Hospital Organization Facilitate De-Labeling? Unpublished paper.

WENGER, D. and C. R. FLETCHER
1969 The Effect of Legal Counsel on Admissions to a State Mental Hospital: A Confrontation of professions. J. of Health and Social Behavior 10: 66–72.

WING, J. and G. BROWN
1970 Institutionalism and Schizophrenia. Cambridge, England: Cambridge University Press.

Women and Medicalization: A New Perspective

Catherine Kohler Riessman

Illness expands by means of two hypotheses. The first is that every form of social deviation can be considered an illness. Thus, if criminal behavior can be considered an illness, then criminals are not to be condemned or punished but to be understood (as a doctor understands), treated, cured. The second is that every illness can be considered psychologically. Illness is interpreted as, basically, a psychological event, and people are encouraged to believe that they get sick because they (unconsciously) want to, and that they can cure themselves by the mobilization of will; that they can choose not to die of the disease. These two hypotheses are complementary. As the first seems to relieve guilt, the second reinstates it. Psychological theories of illness are a powerful means of placing the blame on the ill. Patients who are instructed that they have, unwittingly, caused their disease are also made to feel that they have deserved it.

Susan Sontag, 1979

Reprinted from *Social Policy*, vol. 14 (Summer, 1983), pp. 3–18. Copyright © 1983 by Social Policy Corporation, New York, New York, 10036.

It is widely acknowledged that illness has become a cultural metaphor for a vast array of human problems. The medical model is used from birth to death in the social construction of reality. Historically, as a larger number of critical events and human problems have come under the "clinical gaze" (Foucault, 1973), our experience of them has been transformed. For women in particular, this process has had far-reaching consequences.

Feminist health writers have emphasized that women have been the main targets in the expansion of medicine. These scholars have analyzed how previous religious justifications for patriarchy were transformed into scientific ones (Ehrenreich and English, 1979). They have described how women's traditional skills for managing birth and caring for the sick were expropriated by psychomedical experts at the end of the nineteenth century (Ehrenreich and English, 1973). Feminist writers have described the multiple ways in which women's health in the contemporary period is being jeopardized by a male-controlled, technology-dominated medical-care system (Dreifus, 1978; Frankfort, 1972; Ruzek, 1978; Seaman, 1972). These critics have been important voices in changing women's consciousness about their health. They have identified the sexual politics embedded in conceptions of sickness and beliefs about appropriate care. In addition, they have provided the analytic basis for a social movement that has as its primary goal the reclaiming of knowledge about and control over women's bodies.

However, in their analyses, feminists have not always emphasized the ways in which women have simultaneously gained and lost with the medicalization of their life problems. Nor have the scholars always noted the fact that women actively participated in the construction of the new medical definitions, nor discussed the reasons that led to their participation. Women were not simply passive victims of medical ascendancy. To cast them solely in a passive role is to perpetuate the very kinds of assumptions about women that feminists have been trying to challenge.

This paper will extend the feminist critique by emphasizing some neglected dimensions of medicalization and women's lives. I will argue that both physicians and women have contributed to the redefining of women's experience into medical categories. More precisely, I will suggest that physicians seek to medicalize experience because of their specific beliefs and economic interests. These ideological and material motives are related to the development of the profession and the specific market conditions it faces in any given period. Women collaborate in the medicalization process because of their own needs and motives, which in turn grow out of the class-specific nature of their subordination. In addition, other groups bring economic interests to which both physicians and women are responsive. Thus a consensus develops that a particular human problem will be understood in clinical terms. This consensus is tenuous because it is fraught with contradictions for women, since, as stated before, they stand both to gain and lose from this redefinition.

I will explore this thesis by examining five conditions that pertain to women. An examination of childbirth and reproductive control will ground the analysis historically. Premenstrual syndrome and weight will be considered in order to illustrate present-day manifestations of medicalization. Finally, I will present some beginning thoughts on the ways the analysis might be applied to mental health.

At the outset I want to state that this represents my early thinking about an interactional model that can explain the medicalization of women's lives. It is not a final analysis of the problem, but rather represents work in progress. I invite responses from readers to the ideas I have developed thus far.

THE MEDICALIZATION FRAMEWORK

The term medicalization refers to two interrelated processes. First, certain behaviors or conditions are given medical meaning—that is, defined in terms of health and illness. Second, medical practice becomes a vehicle for eliminating or controlling problematic experiences that are defined as deviant, for the purpose of securing adherence to social norms. Medicalization can occur on various levels: conceptually, when a medical vocabulary is used to define a problem; institutionally, when physicians legitimate a program or a problem; or on the level of doctor-patient interaction, when actual diagnosis and treatment of a problem occurs (Conrad and Schneider, 1980a).

Historically, there has been an expansion of the spheres of deviance that have come under medical social control (Freidson, 1970; Zola, 1972; Ehrenreich and Ehrenreich, 1978). Various human conditions such as alcoholism, opiate addiction, and homosexuality—which at one time were categorized as "bad"—have more recently been classified as "sick" (Conrad and Schneider, 1980). Currently, more and more of human experience is coming under medical scrutiny, resulting in what Illich has called "the medicalization of life." For example, it is now considered appropriate to consult physicians about sexuality, fertility, childhood behavior, and old-age memory problems. It is important to note that the medical profession's jurisdiction over these and other human conditions extends considerably beyond its demonstrated capacity to "cure" them (Freidson, 1970).

There is disagreement about what causes medicalization. Some have assumed that the expansion of medical jurisdiction is the outcome of "medical imperialism"—an effort on the part of the profession to increase its power (Illich, 1976). Others have argued that an increasingly complex technical and bureaucratic society has led to a reluctant reliance on scientific experts (Zola, 1972; 1975). Other scholars have stressed the ways in which the medical establishment, in its thrust to professionalize, organized to create and then control markets (Larson, 1977). In order for the occupational strategy of this emerging professional class to succeed, it was necessary to control the meaning of things, including interpretations of symptoms and beliefs about health care. Stated differently, professional dominance could be achieved only if people could be convinced of the medical nature of their problems and the appropriateness of medical treatment for them. Thus physicians, as part of an occupational strategy, created conditions under which their advice seemed appropriate (Starr, 1982).

In spite of the disagreement about what motivates medicalization, there is a consensus that it has mixed effects. Greater humanitarianism, tolerance, and other benefits associated with "progress" may be more likely with medical definitions than with criminal ones. Yet medical labeling also has negative social consequences. Far from reducing stigma, the label of illness may create deviance. For example, the career of a psychiatric patient begins with a diagnosis of schizophrenia. As a result, family and friends perceive and interpret the patient's behavior in light of the illness, even after the acute symptoms subside (Mills, 1962). Another consequence of medicalization is that the shroud of medical language mystifies human problems, and thus removes them from public debate (Conrad and Schneider, 1980). A deskilling of the populace takes place when experts manage human experiences. The application of medical definitions makes it more likely that medical remedies will be applied, thereby increasing the risk of iatrogenic disease. In addition, both the meaning and interpretation of an experience is transformed when it is seen as a disease or syndrome (Freidson, 1970). For example, the meaning of murder is significantly altered when the label of "sociopathic personality" is used to account for the behavior. In this way, moral issues tend not be be faced and may not even be raised (Zola, 1975). Finally and most important, awareness of the social causes of disease is diminished with medicalization. As Stark and Flitcraft state:

> Medicine attracts public resources out of proportion to its capacity for health enhancement, because it often categorizes problems fundamentally social in origin as biological or personal deficits, and in so doing smothers the impulse for social change which could offer the only serious resolution.

Medicalization is a particularly critical concept because it emphasizes the fact that medicine is a social enterprise, not merely a scientific one. A biological basis is neither necessary nor sufficient for an experience to be defined in terms of illness. Rather, illness is constructed through human action—that is, illness is not inherent in any behavior or condition, but conferred by others. Thus, medical diagnosis becomes an interpretive process through which illnesses are constructed (Mishler, 1981).

Not only is illness a social construction, but so is science itself. Although medicalization theorists have tended to stop short of a critique of science, there are at least three ways in which scientific ideology plays a role in the medicalization process. First and most obviously, the production of scientific knowledge is a historically determined social activity, rather than what it is commonly assumed to be—the abstract, value-free pursuit of truth. Certain problems are selected for study, others are not. Certain phenomena are embraced by scientific theory, others are not. Social agenda are embedded in these choices. Thus, for example, sexist beliefs about the biological roots for gender roles formed the basis for endocrinology research in the 1920s (Hall, 1980), as did racist beliefs about the genetic basis for intelligence in the 1970s (Herrnstein, 1971). To the extent that clinical practice is rooted in science, these social agenda are incorporated by physicians in their ways of thinking about the problems of their patients. Second, in the scientific mentality, complex, dynamic, and organic processes are reduced to narrow cause-and-effect relationships. Clinical science locates the problem of disease in the individual body (Crawford, 1980). As a consequence, physicians use a particular framework in both seeing and solving human problems (Bell, forthcoming). Social and emotional aspects of illness that do not fit a physiological model are likely to be ignored, and uncertainty is excluded (Plough, 1981). Third, the assumption is that medical practice is based on scientific knowledge. In other words, science legitimates the power of physicians over definitions of illness and the form of treatment. Yet historical and contemporary evidence reveals that the assertion of therapeutic efficacy has frequently been sufficient to justify medical intervention, even when evidence was shaky (Reverby, 1981; Banta and Thacker, 1979). In sum, scientific "facts" themselves are socially constructed. Clinical practice is founded as much on ideas and beliefs as it is on hard, objective evidence. These ideological components drive the process of medicalization.

The social nature of medicine is clarified further when we note that deviance is implicit in medical definitions. Parsons made this point long ago, but failed to emphasize the negative consequences of this fact. As Hubbard states, "Medical norms don't describe what is, but rather what should be." Thus, physicians create and reinforce social norms when they define behaviors or conditions as pathological, such as hyperactivity in children or childlessness in women. A particular behave in certain ways and when women have babies.

Finally, the medicalization framework emphasizes that the power of physicians to define illness and monopolize the provision of treatment is the outcome of a political process. It highlights the ways in which medicine's constructions of reality are related to the structure of power at any given historical period. The political dimension inherent in medicalization is underscored when we note that structurally dependent populations—like children, old people, racial minorities, and women—are subject disproportionately to medical labeling. For example, childrens' behavior is medicalized under the rubric of juvenile delinquency and hyperkenesis (Conrad and Schneider, 1980). Old people's mental functioning is labeled organic brain syndrome or senility. Racial minorities, when they come in contact with psychiatrists, are more likely than whites to be given more severe diagnoses for comparable symptoms and to receive more coercive forms of medical social control, such as psychiatric hospitalization (Gross et al., 1969). Women, as I will argue, are more likely than men to have problematic experiences defined and treated medically. In each of these examples, it is important to note that the particular group's economic and social powerlessness legitimates its "protection" by medical authorities. Of course, physicians act on behalf of the larger society, thus further reinforcing existing power relations.

Although medicalization theory has emphasized power, it has tended to minimize the significance of class. Historically, as I will suggest, the medicalization of certain problems was rooted in specific class interests. Physicians and women from the dominant class joined together—albeit out of very different motives—to redefine certain human events into medical categories. Women from other class groups at times embraced and at other times resisted these class-based definitions of experience.

In sum, the medicalization framework provides useful analytic categories for examining the medicalization of women's problems as a function of (1) the interests and beliefs of physicians; (2) the class-specific needs of women; and (3) the "fit" between these, resulting in a consensus that redefines a human experience as a medical problem. As stated before, I will use this framework to explore five areas that are especially germaine to women's experience: childbirth, reproductive control, premenstrual syndrome, weight, and psychological distress. Clearly, because of space considerations, it is impossible to discuss each example in depth. Instead, I hope to provide a fresh look at each problem and lay out the issues as I perceive them at this point.

CHILDBIRTH

Today, pregnancy and birth are considered medical events. This was not always the case. Moreover, there is nothing inherent in either condition that necessitates routine medical scrutiny. In fact, birth is an uncomplicated process in roughly 90 percent of cases (Wertz and Wertz, 1979). In order to understand the medicalization of childbirth, it must be analyzed as the outcome of a complex sociopolitical process in which both physicians and women participated.

In mid-nineteenth-century America, virtually anyone could be a doctor. As a result, there was an oversupply of healers—a series of competing sects with varying levels of training. These included "regular" college-trained physicians, physicians trained by apprenticeship, homeopaths, botanic physicians, male accoucheurs, midwives, and other healers (Drachman, 1979). The "regular" physicians—white, upper-class males—struggled to achieve professional dominance as boundaries between professional and lay control shifted. It is important to emphasize that this group sought control over the healing enterprise at a time when they were not more effective than their competitors in curing disease. As Larson (1977) has noted, the diffusion of knowledge about scientific discoveries in microbiology that revolutionized medical care occurred only after medicine successfully gained control over the healing market. Thus, in the absence of superior skill, it was necessary to convert public perceptions. In order to gain "cultural authority" (Starr, 1982) over definitions of health and disease and over the provision of health services, "regular" doctors had to transform general human skills into their exclusive craft. Social historians of medicine have documented the political activities that succeeded in guaranteeing a closed shop for "regular" doctors in late nineteenth- and early twentieth-century America (Reverby and Rosner, 1979; Walsh, 1977).

A central arena for the struggle over professional dominance was childbirth. In colonial America, this event was handled predominantly by female midwives who, assisted by a network of female relatives and friends, provided emotional support and practical assistance to the pregnant woman both during the actual birth and in the weeks that followed. Over

a period of more than a century, "social childbirth" was replaced (Wertz and Wertz, 1979). The site of care shifted from the home to the hospital. The personnel who gave care changed from female midwives to male physicians. The techniques changed from noninterventionist approaches to approaches relying on technology and drugs. As a consequence, the meaning of childbirth for women was transformed from a human experience to a medical-technical problem.

A crucial historical juncture in the medicalization of childbirth occurred in the second decade of the twentieth century. In 1910, about 50 percent of all reported births were attended by midwives. The medical profession and the laity generally believed that the midwife—essentially a domestic worker—was an adequate birth attendant. Nature was thought to control the process of birth. As a result, there was little to be done in case of difficulty. The teaching of obstetrics in medical schools was minimal, and direct experience with birth by medical students was rare (Kobrin, 1966).

Beginning around 1910, a contest began between the emerging specialty of obstetrics, the general practitioner, and the midwife. Although seemingly about issues of science and efficacy, this struggle was also about class and race. Obstetricians were from the dominant class, whereas midwives were mostly immigrant and Black women. Struggling to differentiate themselves from general practitioners, obstetricians fought to upgrade the image of their field. They searched for a respectable science to legitimate their work. They argued that normal pregnancy and parturition were an exception rather than the rule. Because they believed that birth was a pathological process, obstetricians often used surgical interventions as well as instruments, such as high forceps previous to sufficient dilation. These approaches, used routinely and often unnecessarily, frequently had deleterious effects on both mother and child. Over a period of several decades, obstetricians were successful in persuading both their physician colleagues and the general public of the "fallacy of normal pregnancy," and therefore of the need for a "science" of obstetrical practice. Their political activities, coupled with changing demographic trends, resulted in the demise of midwifery (Kobrin, 1966).

It is important to note that the medical management of childbirth did not result in greater safety for women, at least in the short run. The evidence suggests that both maternal and infant mortality rates actually rose during the period between 1915 and 1930 when midwives' attendance at birth abruptly declined (Wertz and Wertz, 1979). In the long run, there has been a steady decline in death rates, which has coincided with modern childbirth practice. However, it is not clear how much of this decline is due to improved environmental circumstances and nutrition and how much to medical care.

In light of these facts, what motivated women to go along with the medicalization of childbirth? Because childbirth is an event that occurs without complications in most cases, it is tempting to emphasize the many losses that accompanied its medicalization. In modern birth, the woman is removed from familiar surroundings, from kin and social support, and subjected to a series of technical procedures—many of which are dehumanizing and others of which carry significant health risks (Shaw, 1974; Rothman, 1982). A woman's experience of birth is alienated because the social relations and instrumentation of the medical setting remove her control over the experience (Young, forthcoming). Because of these negative consequences of modern birth, there is a tendency to romanticize the midwife and pretechnological childbirth and fail to consider the contradictory nature of the process.

Women participated in the medicalization of childbirth for a complex set of reasons. First, nineteenth-century women wanted freedom from the pain, exhaustion, and lingering incapacity of childbirth. Pregnancy every other year was the norm for married women, and this took a significant toll on the reproductive organs. Contraception was not a viable alternative, for reasons I will discuss shortly. For working-class women, the problems of maternity were intensified by harsh working and housing conditions. The letters of early twentieth-century working-class women vividly portray the exhaustion of motherhood (Davies, 1978). Albeit for different reasons, women from different class groups experienced birth as a terrifying ordeal (Dye, 1980).

In the early decades of the twentieth century, relief from the pain of childbirth was promised with "twilight sleep," a combination of morphine and scopolamine, which European physicians had begun to use. Historical analysis of the twilight sleep movement in the United States reveals that it was women who demanded it, frequently pitting themselves against the medical profession who both resented lay interference and feared the dangers of the drug (Leavitt, 1980). These women—middle- and upper-class reformers with a progressive ideology—wanted to alter the oppressive circumstances of women's lives. Thus, the demand for anesthesia in childbirth was part of a larger social movement. Pregnancy was no longer seen as a condition to be endured with fatalism and passivity (Smith-Rosenberg and Rosenberg, 1973). As Miller argues, people believed that civilization had increased the subjective experience of pain in childbirth, and that anesthesia would once again make childbirth natural. The upper class experienced greater pain than working-class women, who were thought to be more like primitive peoples. People believed that upper-class women had been particularly warped by civilization. (The corset also may have distorted their internal organs.) In other words, pain had accompanied the progress of civilization. If freed from painful and exhausting labor, women could (the reformers felt) more fully participate in democratic society (Miller, 1979).

Second, because of declining fertility in upper- and middle-class women at the end of the nineteenth century, the meaning of birth was particularly significant to them. Because childbirth was a less frequent event, concern about fetal death was greater. In addition, women were fearful because it was common to have known someone who had died in childbirth (Dye, 1980). Thus, well-to-do women wanted to be attended by doctors not only because they were of higher social status compared to midwives but also because they possessed the instruments and surgical techniques that might be beneficial in cases of prolonged labor, toxemia, fetal distress, and other abnormal conditions. Of course, physicians used these fears to gain control over the entire market, including routine births.

Thus, the demise of midwifery and the resultant medicalization of childbirth were consequences of forces within the women's community as well as from outside it. Furthermore, it was a class-specific process. Well-to-do women wanted to reduce the control that biology had over their lives. They wanted freedom from pain. Because of their refinement, medical ideology of the period insisted that well-to-do women were more delicate and hence, were more likely to experience pain and complications. By contrast, working-class women were believed to be inherently stronger (Cott, 1972). Perhaps as a way of resisting these ideological assumptions, well-to-do women wanted control over the birthing process—the right to decide what kind of labor and delivery they would have. The contradiction was that the method these women demanded—going to sleep—put them out of control (Leavitt, 1980).

Obstetricians also wanted control. They believed that birth was a pathological process and that "scientific birth" would result in greater safety for affluent women especially. In addition it was in the interest of physicians to capture the childbirth market, because this event provided a gateway to the family, and hence the entire healing market (Wertz and Wertz, 1979). Physicians were particularly anxious to attend the births of well-to-do women, because the social status of these women lend legitimacy and respectability to the shift from midwifery to obstetrics (Drachman, 1979). In order to control childbirth, physicians needed drugs and technology to appear indispensable (Miller, 1979). Therefore, they went along with twilight sleep, at least for a time. The irony for women was that this approach to the pain of childbirth served to distance women from their bodies and redefine birth as an event requiring hospitalization and physician attendance (Leavitt, 1980).

Currently, the medicalization of childbirth is taking new forms. First, there is a trend toward more cesarean births. Although some of these are necessary for maternal health as well as infant survival, evidence suggests that many cesareans are unnecessary (O'Driscoll and Folcy, 1983). In view of medicalization, it is important to point out that the potential need for a cesarean places childbirth squarely and exclusively in the hands of the physician. Vaginal delivery, by contrast, can be the province of nonphysician experts, such as nurse–midwives.

Second, there is a trend to make the birth experience more humane, for both mother and baby. Hospitals are developing "birthing rooms" and other alternatives to the usual delivery room atmosphere of steel tables, stirrups, and bright lights. After birth, maternal-infant contact is permitted so as to foster "bonding." Pediatricians believe that a critical period exists for the development of an optimal relationship between mother and newborn (Klaus and Kennell,

1976).* Thus, pediatricians are joining obstetricians in medicalizing the childbirth experience. By defining what should be (and therefore what is) deviant, pediatricians create social norms for parenting.

The contradiction is that the recent changes in the hospital environment of birth have both helped and hurt women. Birthing rooms and early contact between mother and newborn are a welcome change from previous oppressive obstetrical and pediatric practices (which poor women still face because these reforms are more characteristic of elite hospitals than of public ones). Yet the contemporary feminist critique of childbirth practice has been cut short by these reforms. As in many reform movements, larger issues are silenced. Challenges to the medical domination of pregnancy and demands for genuine demedicalization have been co-opted by an exclusive focus on the birth environment. Even when "natural" childbirth occurs in birthing rooms, birth is still defined medically, is still under the control of physicians, and still occurs in hospitals (Rothman, 1981).

Moreover, the social meaning of parenting changes when scientific rationales such as "bonding" and "attachment" are used to justify mothers being near their babies after giving birth (Arney, 1980). In addition, sex roles are reinforced when it is mothers and not fathers who need to be "bonded" to their infants.

REPRODUCTIVE FREEDOM

Abortion

Today, abortion is treated as a medical event. Yet in previous historical periods, it was defined in nonmedical terms. Physicians brought specific professional and class interests to the abortion issue in the nineteenth century. To realize their interests, they needed to alter public beliefs about the meaning of unwanted pregnancy. Well-to-do women formed an alliance with doctors in this redefinition process because of their own needs.

As Mohr documents, abortion before quickening (the perception of fetal movement) was widely prac-

* The ideological assumptions and methodological flaws of this research tradition have been well described by Arney (1980).

ticed in the mid-nineteenth century and was not seen as morally or legally wrong. Information on potions, purgatives, and quasi-surgical techniques was available in home medical manuals. As auto-abortive instruments came on the market, women became skillful in performing their own abortions, and they shared information with one another. In addition, midwives, herbal healers, and other "irregular" doctors established lucrative practices in the treatment of "obstructed menses." It is estimated that by 1878 one in five pregnancies was intentionally aborted. The growing frequency of abortion was particularly evident in the middle and upper classes (Mohr, 1978).

"Regular" physicians were central figures in redefining abortion as a social problem. The practice of abortion was leading to a declining birth rate, especially among the middle and upper classes who feared that this could lead to "race suicide" (Smith-Rosenberg and Rosenberg, 1973). One physician warned that abortion was being used "to avoid the labor of caring for and rearing children" (Silver as quoted in Mohr, 1978). In other words, women were shirking the responsibilities of their seemingly biologically determined role.

Mohr (1978) argues that physicians led the moral crusade against abortion not so much out of these antifeminist feelings, but primarily in order to restrict the practice of medicine. They wanted to get rid of competitors ("irregulars" and "doctresses") and gain a monopoly over the practice of medicine. By altering public opinion and persuading legislators, they succeeded in establishing their code of ethics (which specifically excluded abortion) as the basis for professional practice. These actions limited the scope of medicine's competitors, especially women doctors whose practices were devoted to the care of female complaints. By the late 1870s, anti-abortion statutes were on the books. Professional dominance was further strengthened in the 1880s when physicians became more organized. They used the scientific paradigm to force more and more folk practitioners from the field.

It is interesting to note the social relations at work in the nineteenth-century abortion struggle. First, the "regulars"—upper- and middle-class men—had natural allies in the state legislators, who were also men from prosperous families. Second, patriarchal class interests in general and nativism in particular provided the racist and sexist ideology for the anti-abortion movement. Physicians, legislators, and other well-to-do men wanted their women to reproduce the species, or, more specifically, the dominant class of the species. These groups, fearing the increasing numbers of the foreign-born, were concerned that the upper classes would be out-bred. Finally, the conflict between the "regular" doctors and their competitors was not only about issues of science and professional control but also about the issues of class and patriarchy. The "irregular" doctors were, in general, not from families of the dominant class. In addition, these practitioners were more likely to be female. Thus social characteristics provided the rationale for exclusion, further reinforcing patriarchal class relations.

Women's participation in the anti-abortion crusade of the 1870s also was class-specific. Feminists of the period—well-to-do women—came out against abortion, arguing instead for voluntary motherhood. These early feminists recommended periodic or permanent abstinence as methods of birth control because they did not approve of contraceptive devices (Gordon, 1976).

It is obvious that women lost significant freedoms when abortion was defined as a medical procedure and ruled illegal. Yet, from the perspective of the sexual politics of late nineteenth-century America, it is significant that women favored abstinence over abortion. Abstinence was a more radical response to the power relations in the patriarchal family than a pro-abortion stance would have been.

Well-to-do women of the late nineteenth century had a level of hostility toward sex, both because it brought unwanted and dangerous pregnancy and because it was a legally prescribed wifely duty. Even more important, Gordon argues that these women resented the particular kind of sexual encounter that was characteristic of American Victorian society: intercourse dominated by the husband's needs and neglecting what might bring pleasure to a woman. Men's style of lovemaking repelled women. They felt that men were oversexed and violent. Furthermore, because men visited prostitutes, marital sex for women not infrequently resulted in venereal disease. Under these conditions, a woman's right to refuse was central to her independence and personal integrity.

In sum, the termination of an unwanted pregnancy underwent a series of changing definitions: it went from a human problem to a topic of medical concern to a crime. With the 1973 Supreme Court decision, it was remedicalized, but this time with the support of the medical profession. Physicians no longer needed this issue to advance their sovereignty.

Contraception

In the twentieth century, well-to-do women joined physicians again in the medicalization of reproduction with the issue of contraception. These women struggled to define a "new sense of womanhood" that did not require sexual passivity, maternity, domesticity, and the absence of ambition. In order to achieve these goals, feminists overcame their scruples against artificial contraception. Importantly, women ultimately won the battle of reproductive freedom. Technology to limit family size was developed in response to the social demand for it (Gordon, 1976).

But as women gained from this newly won independence, they also lost. Birth control technology is not without problems, both in its female centricity and its risk. Furthermore, as Gordon argues, the professionalization and medicalization of birth control stripped it of its political content. As a result of its definition as a health issue, contraception became somewhat separate from the larger social movement that gave rise to the demand for birth control in the first place. Finally, the battle over medicalization was lost again when birth control methods went in the direction of high technology. The pill, the IUD, and injectable contraceptives are forever in the hands of medicine, because access to these drugs and devices is legally controlled. In contrast, the low-technology barrier methods—the condom, cervical cap, or diaphragm—require little medical intervention or control.

These historical examples underscore the fact that women's experience was a site for the initial medicalization effort. Medicine "staked claims" for childbirth, abortion, and birth control and secured them as "medical turf" by altering public beliefs and persuading the state of the legitimacy of their claim. (For further elaboration of the metaphor of prospecting applied to medicine, see Conrad and Schneider, 1980.) Physicians used science as the rationale for professional dominance. As I have suggested, women's participation in the redefinition of each experience was the result of complex historical and class-specific motives, and they not only gained but lost with the medicalization of each area.

MEDICALIZATION OF WOMEN'S LIVES

Because women's health was a site for professional monopolization in the past, it is not surprising that medicine has continued to focus on women in the effort toward medicalization. A plethora of female conditions has come to be either reconceptualized as illnesses or, if they escape medical labeling, understood in ways that connote deviation from some ideal biological standard. Because they are seen as biological events, medical solutions are applied. For example, "sexual dysfunctions" are defined in terms of health and illness, and an industry of sex clinics and counselors offers treatment. Pregnancy care has been broadened to include fetal as well as maternal health, which has resulted in diagnostic procedures aimed at the fetus as well as experimental treatments, such as fetal surgery (Hubbard, 1982). Fertility is seen as a medical issue, and the production of the "custom-made child" (Holmes et al., 1981) has become the focus of a reproductive engineering industry. Menopause is understood and treated medically, with far-reaching consequences for women's health and self-esteem. Aging has spawned a new specialty—gerontology—for which women are the primary market. Teen-age pregnancy and wife battering are being conceptualized increasingly in psychiatric terms. The medicalization of women's lives can be examined by way of two other examples—premenstrual syndrome and weight.

Premenstrual Syndrome

Premenstrual syndrome (PMS) has found a place among the medical maladies of our culture. Although PMS lacks a firm definition and a base of rigorous scientific research (Parlee, 1973; Friedman et al., 1980), specific premenstrual signs and symptoms have come under medical scrutiny. These include physical manifestations such as edema (resulting in weight gain and bloatedness), breast swelling and tenderness, backache, and acne. Mood changes also may occur, including increased tension and irritability, depression and lethargy. As evidence of medicalization, both medical and lay health journals are dealing with the topic with greater frequency, and a number of self-help guides written by physicians have appeared (Reid and Yen, 1981; Gonzales, 1981; Burd, 1982; Harrison, 1982). Significantly, the diagnosis of PMS was used successfully by the defense in several recent legal cases (Newsweek, 1982).

Despite the lack of solid evidence linking psychological changes in the premenstrual period with endocrinological events, the American Psychiatric Association has proposed that a new diagnostic category—premenstrual dysphoric disorder—be added to the revised version of the *Diagnostic and Statistical Manual of Mental Disorders,* or DSM-III-R (Holden, 1986). At the same time, other medical investigators are more cautious about adopting a medical vocabulary to understand and to treat the premenstrual period. This caution is especially warranted in light of the history of the medicalization of menopause; the conceptual transformation which made it possible also brought in its stead a series of iatrogenic consequences for women, most notably increased risk of reproductive tract cancer from hormone therapy (Bell, forthcoming).

What are the interests and beliefs that physicians currently bring to this new disease construction of PMS? Clearly, it is more risky to analyze motives for the medicalization of contemporary problems than it is for those of the past (such as childbirth and abortion), where the historical record can provide supporting evidence. Nevertheless, market conditions exist that suggest some reasons as to why the medical profession might be prospecting for new turf at this time. First, there is a declining birth rate. With fewer babies to be delivered, gynecologists must develop other areas in order to guarantee a successful practice. Second, there are more gynecologists per capita than ever before. As a result of federal programs in the 1960s, medical schools expanded and more physicians graduated. Consequently, the supply of obstetrician/gynecologists in the United States increased from 15,984 in 1966 to 25,215 in 1979 (Theodore and Sutler, 1966; Wunderman, 1980)—an increase of 64 percent. Finally, there are more women in the population in their thirties, as a result of the postwar baby boom. Given these conditions—lower demand, increased supply, and a pool of appropriately aged women—it is not unreasonable to hypothesize that gynecologists would actively seek out new "disease" entities to which they could apply their skills. Premenstrual syndrome, as well as endometriosis, may represent new disease constructions that are a response to these conditions.

In addition, physicians hold beliefs about women that are likely to influence the disease construction of PMS, especially when they are joined with economic interests. In medical education, physicians are trained to think about women in ways that are anything but neutral and value-free (Howell, 1974). Medical textbooks describe women's sexuality in terms that vary from most women's experience and that reinforce male opinions of sexual pleasure (Scully and Bart, 1981). Physicians are taught psychiatric theories about the development of gender identity that reinforce existing power relations between the sexes. No doubt these beliefs also influence physicians' understanding of menstruation, although the particular ways that sexist ideology is embedded in current scientific thought about the premenstrual period needs further study.

Other communities also influence the clinical scrutiny of menstruation. The drug industry is actively looking for new markets. Corporations shape physicians' perceptions through drug advertising, personal contacts, and free samples of their products. Research has shown that physicians' behavior is remarkably sensitive to the "educational" efforts of the pharmaceutical houses (Christensen and Bush, 1981). In addition to the drug industry, other parties that can affect physicians' perceptions include the legal profession (which has found the diagnosis of PMS useful in adjudicating clients) and the insurance industry (which will have to contend with this new diagnostic category in their reimbursement policies). As Bell has demonstrated in her case study of DES, these communities are functionally interdependent. They interact in complex ways with one another and with physicians in the creation of new technologies and disease entities.

From the perspective of women, the medicalization of the premenstrual experience is filled with contradictions. On the positive side, physicians' recognition of women's experience with menstruation is important, for it legitimates an important aspect of women's lives. Women have often observed that their moods varied over the course of their menstrual cycle and shared their observations with one another, but until recently they were discounted by the medical establishment. Doctors responded either by dismissing women's premenstrual complaints or by ascribing them to unresolved problems with their femininity. The clinical construction of PMS acknowledges the cyclic nature of women's lives and opens up the possibility that attention will be paid to other phases of the menstrual cycle. For example, some suggest that a "Menstrual Joy Questionnaire" be created, using the model of the "Menstrual Distress Questionnaire" (Moos, 1963), in order to document the pleasurable feelings, increased energy, and creativity that are experienced during the cycle (Delaney et al., 1976).

Women in certain economic groups are currently seeking out physicians regarding problems with menstruation just as an earlier, similar class group sought physicians for care during pregnancy. These women are actively participating in the construction of the new medical syndrome of PMS just as they were in creating the "new childbirth." Of course, feminists are ambivalent about the new diagnostic category of PMS, for reasons I will discuss shortly. In light of this, it is interesting to note that the contemporary feminist movement is responsible for a new consciousness that, in some ways, encourages women to be assertive regarding discomfort in menstruation, just as a previous social movement encouraged women to seek relief from pain in childbirth. This is not to deny that physicians do not also have an interest in creating a market and exploiting women for economic gain. But for the small group of women who have premenstrual problems that severely interfere with functioning, relief is possible with medical treatment (Dalton, 1977). It is also possible that scientific research can supply knowledge that might be used in nutritional, exercise, and other treatment approaches.*

On the negative side, the medicalization of menstruation has disturbing implications for women's lives. Most obviously, it reinforces the idea that

women are controlled by biology in general and their reproductive systems in particular. This has been used to legitimate the exclusion of women from positions of power because of supposed emotional instability and irrationality due to "raging hormonal imbalances" (Romey, 1973). It has also been used to suggest that women are violent as a result of their biology, because of the apparent correlation between PMS and crimes committed by women. Thus, medical scrutiny of the premenstrual period serves to emphasize cyclic phenomena in women when, in fact, hormonal blood levels are episodic in both men and women (Hoffman, 1982). In addition, medical scrutiny also reinforces scientific assumptions about the existence of universal norms, or a "natural" menstrual history. This has been refuted by anthropological evidence, which demonstrates considerable cross-cultural variation in all aspects of menstrual cycling (Hubbard, 1981). Further, labeling hormonal changes as a syndrome implies a pathological condition—something to be controlled—rather than suggesting that mood shifts and bodily changes are a normal part of everyone's life. Thus, there is a danger that medical treatments will be applied routinely to women, as estrogen replacement therapy has been for menopause. In other words, insufficiently tested, ineffective, or dangerous pharmaceutical remedies and surgical interventions may be used to treat premenstrual problems. Finally, medical labeling may create cultural beliefs and attitudes about the premenstrual period. It may create suffering in women who were previously asymptomatic. It may encourage them to perceive fluctuating bodily and emotional states differently, simply because a medical explanation for them exists. Support for this hypothesis was found in an experimental study conducted prior to the development of the diagnostic category of PMS. Women who were told they were premenstrual reported more severe physical symptoms than women who believed they were simply between periods (Ruble, 1977).

Most important, the medicalization of PMS deflects attention from social etiology. Rather than looking at the circumstances of women's lives that may make them irritable, depressed, or angry, their strong feelings can be dismissed ("You'll feel better when you get your period"). The contradiction lies in the fact that the label of PMS allows women to

* See Michelle Harrison (1982) for a model of such an approach.

be angry and say what's on their minds at a certain time each month, while at the same time it invalidates the content of their protest.

The Medical Beauty Business: Getting Thin

Like menstruation, women's physical appearance has come under the lens of the medical establishment. Cosmetic surgeons treat everything from facial wrinkles to breast size. The medical beauty business has concentrated with special intensity on the bodily changes associated with women's aging. Another subject of medical scrutiny is weight. "Obesity" is now a medical condition.

Although weight is not exclusively a women's issue, it is an excellent example of the medicalization of women's experience for a number of reasons. It highlights the relationship between the social norms for femininity and medical social control. By medicalizing weight, medical science participates in programming aesthetics for women's bodies. This has far-reaching consequences for self-esteem, as women are evaluated on the basis of personal appearance more than men (Millman, 1980). Weight is also a good example of medicalization because it illustrates in a most graphic form how power relations are maintained through medical social control, how women internalize their oppression by desiring to be thin and turning to doctors for help.

As background, let me review briefly some basic information about weight. Adult weight is the outcome of the interplay of a complex of factors including heredity, body type, childhood eating patterns, and metabolism. Although amount of food intake is clearly relevant, its causal significance appears to lie in its interaction with these other factors (Mann, 1974). The most recent evidence suggests that genetic influences play a strong role in determining human fatness (Stunkard et al., 1986). Also it appears that obesity is more prevalent in lower socioeconomic groups. This is true for both children and adults (Goldblatt et al., 1972). . . .

. . . therapies for weight control are far from efficacious and, in some cases, are dangerous. Dietary treatment rarely works, and recidivism rates are high (Mann, 1974). Drug treatments have also failed to demonstrate efficacy and have a definite potential for dependence (FDA, 1972). Surgical treatments such as ileal bypass surgery, have been called hazardous by some medical evaluators (Mann, 1974). More successful are self-help groups and behavior modification approaches to weight loss (Stunkard, 1970). In general, however, the pattern for most individuals is a cycle of weight loss followed by weight gain, which is repeated over and over. The cyclical process further undermines the metabolic system's ability to regulate body weight (Beller, 1977).

In light of these facts, it is not surprising that physicians now consider obesity "a relatively incurable disorder" (Mann, 1974). Hence the medicalization of weight is a clear example of the extension of medicine into an area where it lacks the demonstrated capacity to cure (Freidson, 1970).

Weight was not always considered a medical problem, or even a liability. Renoir and other nineteenth-century artists idealized women with round, soft, voluptuous bodies. Physicians of the nineteenth century did not define excess weight as something to be treated. Even in the twentieth century, popular cultural heroines such as Mae West and Marilyn Monroe had ample bodies. My research suggests that it was not until the late 1960s and the 1970s that medicine began to deal with the topic of weight with such intensity.

It was in the interest of physicians to define weight as a medical problem for a number of reasons. Its apparent association with chronic disease legitimated its clinical scrutiny. More important, a market for weight control opened up as the sedentary life and associated weight gain came to characterize postindustrial society. In addition, particular medical specialties had specific reasons for going into the weight business. Surgeons, for example, facing conditions of oversupply, needed to create markets for their services. The development of surgical approaches to obesity was a logical outcome. Other specialties also needed to generate demand, as the care of infectious diseases took less and less of physicians' time. Here was a potential pool of patients who were concerned about weight and who were so desperate that they were willing to try anthing to bring it under control.

Nevertheless, physicians did not act in a vacuum. The medicalization of weight graphically illustrates how medical definitions, cultural ideology, and corporate interests work hand in hand.

Although the struggle to dominate the body may

be endemic to patriarchal culture, Chernin argues that the preoccupation with women's slenderness has been particularly intense in the last 20 years. This "tyranny of slenderness" coincided with the feminist movement. A contradictory cultural process was taking place: on the one hand was the emergence of a women's movement that emphasized release of power, freeing of potential, and shaking off restraints; and on the other hand was the emergence of the self-help diet groups that emphasized keeping watch over appetites, controlling impulses, and restraining hunger. Women confronted two opposing mandates, one calling for self-control and the other for release (Crawford, forthcoming). Thus, an ideology of slenderness emerged during a historical period when women were growing in their sense of themselves as autonomous, independent beings. Chernin argues that this reflects a fear of women's power. The covert advice to women is not to grow too large or too powerful for the culture. Medical control of weight became a tool for implementing this ideology.

In my research on the clinical construction of obesity, I found a relationship between the extent of the medical literature on the topic and the growth of the women's movement. Reviewing the number of citations in *Index Medicus* by year, I found obesity to be an insignificant topic in 1960, warranting only slightly more than a page of entries. By 1981, more than seven pages were devoted to citations on the topic. Interestingly, articles referring to surgical remedies for obesity were insignificant in 1970 (only 8), rose to a high in 1976 (of 73), and declined thereafter.

In their research on cultural "ideals" of feminine beauty, Garner and his colleagues also found a shift in norms that coincided with the growth of the women's movement. They studied the weights of *Playboy* magazine centerfolds and contestants and winners of the Miss America Pageant from 1959 through 1978. They found that in both contexts the women selected as exemplars of feminine beauty were significantly thinner than the norm for comparable women in the population. More important, they found that when age and height were controlled, weight declined over the 20-year period they studied. Ideal body shape became progressively thinner in spite of the fact that the average weight of women in the general population grew slightly during the same period (Garner et al., 1980).

In addition to cultural ideals and medical definitions, once again other communities shape beliefs about weight. Several industries profit from the cultural preoccupation with women's size. Pharmaceutical companies market anorectic drugs, including amphetamines and other appetite suppressants. The food industry markets low-calorie foods and artificial sweeteners; in advertising, it depicts attractiveness in terms of weight. The fashion industry simultaneously creates and reflects images of the cultural ideal—the thin woman. The beauty business provides places to realize this ideal—the health spa and figure salon.

In this context, it is not surprising that some women have gone along with the medicalization of weight. They believe it is in their interest to be thin. Yet at the same time that they have internalized this dominant value, women have also resisted it—they gain weight. This contradiction further drives the process of medicalization. Thus, economically advantaged women become the major market for a series of weight control industries. The data uniformly show that, compared to men, women are more likely to have ileal bypass surgery, to receive prescriptions for weight-related drugs, to undertake "scientifically based" diets, and to read the physician-authored diet books on the market. Women are also the primary participants in self-help groups such as Weight Watchers, TOPS (Take Pounds Off Sensibly), and Overeaters Anonymous (Millman, 1980).*

These women want to be thin. Some think of themselves primarily in terms of their size. They develop an identity as a "fat person"; everything else becomes secondary. They feel intense psychological pain when their weight is high (Millman, 1980). They are responsive to cultural messages that suggest that they can be in control of how they look in

---

* Fox has stated that these approaches that rely on mutual aid, as opposed to professional intervention, are examples of the "demedicalization" of a human problem in contemporary society. However, as Conrad and Schneider note, deprofessionalization is not the same thing as demedicalization. More specifically, many of the self-help groups oriented toward weight loss share medicine's disease orientation to the problem of weight. Because many of these peer approaches to behavior change do not challenge medicine's assumptions, they do not "demedicalize" human problems, but rather medicalize under lay auspices.

part because of the powerlessness they feel in other areas of their lives. Yet, paradoxically, the feeling of being out of control ultimately takes over, as women discover they cannot really be successful in controlling weight through diet. Women may generalize this sense of lack of control to the rest of their lives. In despair, they collaborate willingly with surgeons and drug-oriented physicians who offer external solutions, further reinforcing their feelings of powerlessness.

Ironically, medical science has given women some tools for understanding the psychological determinants of eating. Psychiatric thought has provided insight into the meaning that food has in their lives and the conflicts that lead them to overeat. However, with the exception of therapies and diet groups with a feminist perspective, psychological approaches rarely question the cultural ideal of slenderness. Nor do they help women see that the internalization of this value reflects alienation from the natural self and the feminine nature of their bodies (Chernin, 1981).

It is clear that the medicalization of physical appearance has had many negative effects on women. Medical science, in collaboration with a series of industries, participates in creating social norms for physical appearance in the guise of supposedly neutral, objective, scientific standards for "ideal" body weight. These standards are based on white, middle-class norms and neglect the diversity of women's bodies. Further, these standards do not take into account the fact that certain cultural groups value women with substantial bodies (Millman, 1980). Further damage results when a woman feels personally to blame when her body fails to measure up to the ideal. In sum, medical scrutiny of weight can create a "spoiled identity" (Goffman, 1964; Courtot, 1982) for fat women. In addition, it may prompt a lifelong pattern—a seesaw of weight gain and weight loss—that has deleterious health consequences.

In light of the class and racial bias in medical norms for weight, it is significant that resistance has tended to come from poor and working-class women, as well as from women of color. While listening respectfully to physicians' admonitions about their weight, some of these women persist in their own beliefs about appropriate body size for themselves. As a result, they are likely to be labeled noncompliant by their doctors.

Most important, by treating weight as a medical problem, medicine diverts attention away from the social causes of poor nutrition and an obsession with thinness. Obesity is correlated with poverty. In poor communities, food preparation has been commercialized in particular ways that undermine health. Poor neighborhoods are focal markets for fast-food chains, because there is a need for high caloric, relatively inexpensive convenience meals. Nutritional status has been compromised further by junk food; especially problematic for weight is the high sugar and salt content. Thus, the food industry has played a major role in generating poor eating habits and, as a result, disease (McKinlay, 1981). In this context, the medicalization of weight is a classic case of blaming the victim.

Furthermore, by individualizing the problem of weight, crucial questions are never asked. Why is it that women are more likely than men to be defined as overweight? Why is anorexia almost exclusively a women's health issue? What is the connection between nutritional malaise and the problems of women in this culture? Does the source of the problem lie in women's roles? Or is the problem with the norms that define appropriate appearance for men compared with women? Why should women be thin anyway? So they can take up less space?*

MEDICALIZATION AND PSYCHIATRY

In addition to weight, women's psychological problems are also a central focus for the drug and medical industries. Women receive more prescriptions for valium and other psychotropic drugs than do men (Cooperstock and Parnell, 1982; Koumjian, 1981). They receive more outpatient psychotherapy (NIMH, 1981). These facts need to be analyzed in terms of the diverse interests of the various medical industries, as well as the diverse needs of women from different class groups that bring them into contact with psychiatry. In the context of this article, I can only introduce some of the issues related to this topic.

Middle-class women have been influenced in major ways by psychiatric thought. Psychiatrists as well as other mental-health professionals view emotional

---

* For thoughtful discussions of these questions, see Chernin, 1981; Crawford, (forthcoming); and Schwartz et al., 1980.

pain as a symptom of an illness. Middle-class women have tended to internalize these sentiments, whereas working-class women have been more likely to resist them.

In the late fifties and early sixties, many middle-class women went into psychotherapy with a series of concerns about their lives—"the problem with no name," in the words of Betty Friedan. But in therapy, these women came to understand their feelings as depression. They learned to examine their early childhood for the origins of their problems. They learned to examine the ways in which they continued self-defeating behaviors in their present-day lives. Paradoxically, many highly educated women found support in psychoanalytic therapy for their private despair at being expected to find fulfillment in marriage and suburban living. The process of introspection helped individual women to voice their concerns and to act to improve their lives. At the same time, these women were subjected to an ideology of femininity that made it difficult for them to realize their ambitions outside of traditional marriage. They needed the emerging contemporary women's movement to redefine their experience in structural terms.

But there is a contradiction in this, in that presenting complaints to psychotherapists is more progressive than keeping problems behind closed doors; but then issues are depoliticized (Stark, 1982). There is an ever-present danger that feminist content will be diminished with medicalization. This can occur not only with psychological problems but with physical ones as well.

For example, Stark and Flitcraft found that when battered women came in contact with hospitals, their problems were exacerbated by physicians and nurses. A purely medical definition of the situation prevailed, replacing any alternative understanding of the problem. Social workers further colluded by seeing the problem as part of a larger issue of the "multiproblem family." Note also how feminist content is further undermined with the term "family violence."

THE FIT BETWEEN WOMEN'S INTERESTS AND PHYSICIANS' INTERESTS

These examples illustrate a general point about medical social control: there are times when the interests of women from the middle and upper classes are served by the therapeutic professions, whose political and economic interests are in turn served by transforming these women's complaints into illnesses. In other words, both historically and currently, there has tended to be a "fit" between medicine's interest in expanding its jurisdiction and the need of women to have their experience acknowledged. I have emphasized that this "fit" has been tension-filled and fraught with contradictions for women, who have both gained and lost with each intrusion medicine has made into their lives.

While necessary, the particular interests of women and physicians do not alone explain the expansion of the clinical domain. Other communities also influence what occurs in the doctor's office. In the context of a capitalist economy and a technologically dominated medical-care system, large profits accompany each redefinition of human experience into medical terms, since more drugs, tests, procedures, equipment, and insurance coverage are needed. As mentioned before, specific medical industries have played a direct role in influencing both physicians' and women's perceptions of reproductive control, premenstrual syndrome, and weight. Yet it is important to emphasize that corporations, in their effort to maximize profits, work *through* both physicians and women.

Implicit in my analysis is the assumption that women's experience has been medicalized more than men's.* Yet it could be argued instead that medicine has encroached into men's lives in a different but equal fashion. For example, medicine has focused on childhood hyperactivity and the adult addictions—problems more common in males than females (Conrad and Schneider, 1980). Occupational medicine has tended to focus on male jobs. In particu-

---

* Conrad and Schneider correctly identify children as another "population at risk" for medicalization. As they describe it, medical jurisdiction has expanded to cover more and more issues of childhood (normal child development, learning disabilities, child abuse, et cetera). It would be interesting to relate this expansion to the internal politics and economic issues faced by pediatrics and its subspecialties. The field needed new turf as childhood infectious diseases could be prevented or controlled. Further, the 1960s and 1970s saw a declining birth rate and an increase in the supply of pediatricians. A logical strategy for the field was to focus on "behavioral pediatrics."

lar, "stress management" programs are targeting male executives. However, while not to diminish these examples, I believe that women's lives have undergone a more total transformation as a result of medical scrutiny. Medicalization has resulted in the construction of medical meanings of *normal* functions in women—experiences the typical woman goes through, such as menstruation, reproduction, childbirth, and menopause. By contrast, routine experiences that are uniquely male remain largely unstudied by medical science and, consequently, are rarely treated by physicians as potentially pathological. For example, male hormonal cycles and the male climacteric remain largely unresearched. Less is known about the male reproductive system than about that of the female. Male contraceptive technology lags far behind what is available for women. Baldness in men has not yet been defined as a medical condition needing treatment, even though an industry exists to remedy the problem of hair loss. Men's psychological lives have not been subjected to psychiatric scrutiny nearly to the degree that women's emotions have been studied. As a result, male violence, need for power, and over-rationality are not defined as pathological conditions. Perhaps only impotence has been subject to the same degree of medical scrutiny as women's problems.

Why has women's experience been such a central focus for medicalization? In addition to the complex motives that women bring to each particular health issue, physicians focus on women as a primary market for expansion for a number of reasons. First, there is a good match between women's biology and medicine's biomedical orientation. External markers of biological processes exist in women (menstruation, birth, lactation, and so forth), whereas they are more hidden in men. Given modern medicine's biomedical orientation, these external signs make women easy targets for medical encroachment. A different medical paradigm (one that viewed health as the consequence of harmony between the person and the environment, for example) might have had less basis for focusing on women.

Second, women's social roles make them readily available to medical scrutiny. Women are more likely to come in contact with medical providers because they care for children and are the "kin keepers" of the family (Rossi, 1980). In concrete terms, women are more likely to accompany sick children and aged relatives to the doctor.

Third, women have greater exposure to medical labeling because of their pattern of dealing with their own symptoms, as well as medicine's response to that pattern. Women make more visits to physicians than men, although it is not clear whether this is due to the medicalization of their biological functions, "real" illness, behavior when ill, or cultural expectations (Nathanson, 1977). When they visit the doctor for any serious illness, they are more likely than men to be checked for reproductive implications of the illness. They are more subject to regular checks of their reproductive systems, in the form of yearly PAP smears or gynecological exams. Importantly, whenever they visit the doctor there is evidence that they receive more total and extensive services—in the form of lab tests, procedures, drug prescriptions, and return appointments—than do men with the same complaints and sociodemographic risk factors (Verbrugge and Steiner, 1981). Thus, a cycle of greater medical scrutiny of women's experience is begun with each visit to the doctor.

Finally, women's structural subordination to men has made them particularly vulnerable to the expansion of the clinical domain. In general, male physicians treat female patients. Social relations in the doctor's office replicate patriarchal relations in the larger culture, and this all proceeds under the guise of science. (Patriarchal control is most evident when physicians socialize young women regarding appropriate sexual behavior, perhaps withholding contraceptive advice, or lecturing them about the dangers of promiscuity.) For all these reasons, it is not surprising that women are more subject to medical definitions of their experience than men are. In these ways, dominant social interests and patriarchal institutions are reinforced.

As a result, women are especially appropriate markets for the expansion of medicine. They are suitable biologically, socially, and psychologically. The message that women are expected to be dependent on male physicians to manage their lives is reinforced by the pharmaceutical industry in drug advertisements and by the media in general. Yet it is far too simple to portray the encroachment of medicine as a conspiracy—by male doctors and the "medical industrial complex"—to subordinate women further. Although some have argued that medicine is the scientific equivalent of earlier customs like marriage laws and kinship rituals that controlled women by controlling their sexuality, such an analysis is incomplete. As I have stressed, medicalization is more than what doctors do, although it may be through doctors that the interests of other groups are often realized. Nor does a conspiracy theory explain why, for the most part, women from certain class groups have been willing collaborators in the medicalization process. Rather than dismissing these women as "duped," I have suggested some of the complex motives that have caused certain classes of women to participate with physicians in the redefinition of particular experiences.

In addition, a conspiracy theory does not explain why medicalization has been more virulent in some historical periods and in some medical specialties than in others. For example, gynecologists initially trivialized menopausal discomfort, only to reclaim it later for treatment. At the same time that gynecologists were unwilling to acknowledge the legitimacy of women's complaints, the developing specialty of psychiatry moved in with the psychogenic account. I have argued that these shifts and interprofessional rivalries over turf are explained by internal issues facing each specialty at particular points in history. Thus, an analysis of the market conditions faced by physicians in general, and certain specialties in particular, is necessary to explain the varying response of medicine to women's problems.

Further research is needed to capture more fully the historical aspect of these shifts in medical perception. Such an analysis needs to focus in depth on specific events in women's experience and trace their medicalization in historical and class context: the issues brought in turn by groups of women, by the particular medical specialties, by the pharmaceutical industry, and by the "fit" between these that resulted in a redefinition. A conspiracy theory fails to capture the nuances of this complex process.

CONCLUSION

The medicalization of human problems is a contradictory reality for women. It is part of the problem and of the solution. It has grown out of and in turn has created a series of paradoxes. As women have tried to free themselves from the control that biologi-

cal processes have had over their lives, they simultaneously have strengthened the control of a biomedical view of their experience. As women visit doctors and get symptom relief, the social causes of their problems are ignored. As doctors acknowledge women's experience and treat their problems medically, problems are stripped of their political content and popular movements are taken over. Because of these contradictions, women in different class positions have sought and resisted medical control.

I have argued that the transformation of such human experiences as childbirth, reproduction, premenstrual problems, weight, and psychological distress into medical events has been the outcome of a reciprocal process involving both physicians and women. Medicine, as it developed as a profession, was repeatedly redefined. The interest of physicians in expanding jurisdiction into new areas coincided with the interest of certain class groups in having their experience in those areas understood in new terms. In other words, physicians created demand in order to generate new markets for their services. They also responded to a market that a class of women created.

This analysis suggests that women have played and may continue to play a major role in stabilizing medicine in American society. Historically, establishing childbirth, abortion, and birth control as medical events were critical junctures on the road to professional dominance. New areas of medical domain are needed because old ones have become saturated. Thus, expansion is occurring in such areas as menstruation, physical appearance, emotional distress, fertility, sexuality, and aging. Furthermore, we can expect the medicalization of women's experience to increase as the supply of physicians increases. In fact, the federal government estimates that the supply of obstetrician/gynecologists will increase from the 1970 figure of 9.3 per 100,000 population to 13.6 per 100,000 in 1990 (DHEW, 1974).

As Conrad and Schneider note, the potential for medicalization increases as science discovers the subtle physiological correlates of human behavior. A wealth of knowledge is developing about women's physiology. As more becomes known, the issue will be how to acknowledge the complex biochemical components that are related to menstruation, pregnancy, weight, and the like without allowing these conditions to be distorted by scientific understanding. The issue will be to gain understanding of our biology, without submitting to control in the guise of medical "expertise." The answer is not to "suffer our fate" and return exclusively to self-care, as Illich recommends, thereby turning our backs on discoveries and treatments that may ease pain and suffering. To "demedicalize" is not to deny the biological components of experience but rather to alter the *ownership, production,* and *use* of scientific knowledge.

Ultimately, however, demedicalization may involve profound questions about the nature of science itself. The very structure of science—its system of beliefs, assumptions, methods, and the description of "reality" it offers—is problematic for understanding women's experience. As scholars have argued, and as my analysis has illustrated, science is neither objective, neutral, nor value-free. Furthermore, feminist scientists have stressed that there is an intrinsic masculine bias in Western scientific thought: an emphasis on power and control, a separation between knower and known, a distinction between objectivity and subjectivity, and an emphasis on reason rather than feeling (Fee, 1982; Hubbard, 1979; Arditti, 1980; Keller, 1978). Particularly significant for women's health is the emphasis on domination over nature that characterizes the entire scientific enterprise, especially in light of the fact that nature is seen as female (Merchant, 1980). As Keller has eloquently stated, the quest is for a different science, undistorted by masculinist bias and characterized instead by "a conversation with nature," rather than domination over nature (McClintock, as quoted in Keller, 1982).

In sum, women's health is faced by a series of challenges. We need to expose the "truth claims" (Bittner, 1968) of medical entrepreneurs who will seek to turn new areas of experience into medical events, and instead introduce a healthy skepticism about professional claims. We need to develop alternatives to the masculinist biomedical view and place women's health problems in the larger context of their lives. Specifically, it is not at all clear what form pregnancy, menstruation, weight, sexuality, aging, or other problems would take in a society "that allowed women to normally and routinely express anger, drive, and ambition, a society in which women felt more empowered" (Harrison, 1982). We need to reconceptualize our whole way of thinking about biology and explore how "natural" phenomena are, in fact, an outgrowth of the social circumstances of women's lives (Hubbard, 1981).

In the meantime, because we will continue to need health care, the challenge will be to alter the terms under which care is provided. In the short term, we need to work for specific reforms and gain what we can while, at the same time, acknowledging the limitation of reform. As I have argued, reform is not what we want in the long run. For certain problems in our lives, real demedicalization is necessary; experiences such as routine childbirth, menopause, or weight in excess of cultural norms should not be defined in medical terms, and medical-technical treatments should not be seen as appropriate solutions to these problems. For other conditions where medicine may be of assistance, the challenge will be to differentiate the beneficial treatments from those that are harmful and useless. The real challenge is to use existing medical knowledge selectively and to extend knowledge with new paradigms so as to improve the quality of our lives.

References

R. ARDITTI, "Feminism and Science," in R. Arditti, P. Brennan, and S. Cavrak (eds.), *Science and Liberation* (Boston, Mass: South End Press, 1980), pp. 350–368.

W. R. AMEY, "Maternal-Infant Bonding: The Politics of Falling in Love with Your Child," *Feminist Studies,* vol. 6, (1980), pp. 547–570.

D. BANTA and S. B. THACKER, "Policies Toward Medical Technology: The Case of Electronic Fetal Monitoring," *American Journal of Public Health,* vol. 69 (1979), pp. 931–935.

S. E. BELL, "A New Model of Medical Technology Development: A Case Study of DES," in J. Roth and S. Ruzek (eds.), *Research in the Sociology of Health Care,* vol. 4 (Greenwich, Conn.: JAI Press, forthcoming).

———"PMS and the Medicalization of Menopause: Sociological Perspectives," in B. Ginsburg and B. Frank Carter (eds.) *The Premenstrual Syndrome: Legal and Ethical Implications* (New York: Plenum Press, forthcoming).

A. S. BELLER, *Fat and Thin: A Natural History of Obesity* (New York: Farrar, Straus and Giroux, 1977).

E. BITTNER, "The Structure of Psychiatric Influence," *Mental Hygiene,* vol. 52 (1968), pp. 423–430.

R. BURD, "Dealing with Premenstrual Syndrome," *Medical Self-Care,* vol. 17 (1982), pp. 46–49.

Characteristics of Admission to Selected Mental Health Facilities, National Institute of Mental Health, Series CN, no. 2 (Washington, D.C.: U.S. Printing Office, 1981).

K. CHERNIN, *The Obsession: Reflections on the Tyranny of Slenderness* (New York: Harper & Row, 1981).

D. B. CHRISTENSEN and P. J. BUSH, "Drug Prescribing: Patterns, Problems and Proposals," *Social Science and Medicine,* vol. 15A (1981), pp. 343–355.

P. CONRAD and J. W. SCHNEIDER, *Deviance and Medicalization: From Badness to Sickness* (St. Louis, Mo.: C. V. Mosby, 1980).

———"Looking at Levels of Medicalization: A Comment on Strong's Critique of the Theses of Medical Imperialism," *Social Science and Medicine,* vol. 14A (1980a), pp. 75–79.

R. COOPERSTOCK, and P. PARNELE, "Research on Psychotropic Drug Use: A Review of Findings and Methods," *Social Science and Medicine,* vol. 16 (1982), pp. 1179–1196.

N. F. COTT (ed.), *Root of Bitterness: Documents of the Social History of American Women* (New York: E. P. Dutton, 1972).

M. COURTOT, "A Spoiled Identity," *Sinister Wisdom,* vol. 20 (1982), pp. 10–15.

R. CRAWFORD, "A Cultural Account of 'Health': Self-Control, Release and the Social Body," in J. B. McKinlay (ed.), *Issues in the Political Economy of Health Care* (New York: Methuen, forthcoming).

R. CRAWFORD, "Healthism and the Medicalization of Everyday Life," *International Journal of Health Services,* vol. 10 (1980), pp. 365–389.

K. DALTON, *The Premenstrual Syndrome and Progesterone Therapy* (Chicago, Ill.: Year Book Medical Publishers, 1977).

M. L. DAVIES, *Maternity: Letters from Working Women* (New York: Norton, 1978).

M. DELANEY, J. LUPTON, and E. TOTH, *The Curse* (New York: E. P. Dutton, 1976).

V. G. DRACHMAN, "The Loomis Trial: Social Mores and Obstetrics in the Mid-Nineteenth Century," in S. Reverby and D. Rosner (eds.), *Health Case in America: Essays in Social History* (Philadelphia, Pa.: Temple University Press, 1979), pp. 67–83.

C. DREIFUS, (ed.), *Seizing Our Bodies: The Politics of Women's Health* (New York: Vintage, 1978).

N. S. DYE, "History of Childbirth in America," *Signs,* vol. 97 (1980), pp. 97–108.

B. EHRENREICH and J. EHRENREICH, "Medicine and Social Control," in J. Ehrenreich (ed.), *The Cultural Crisis of Modern Medicine* (New York: Monthly Review Press, 1978).

B. EHRENREICH and D. ENGLISH, *Complaints and Disorders: The Sexual Politics of Sickness* (Old Westbury, N.Y.: Feminist Press, 1973).

———*For Her Own Good: 150 Years of the Experts' Advice to Women* (Garden City, N.Y.: Anchor, 1979).

FDA Drug Bulletin, Food and Drug Administration (Rockville, Md.: 1972).

E. FEE, "A Feminist Critique of Scientific Objectivity," *Science for the People,* vol. 14 (1982), pp. 5–32.

M. FOUCAULT, *The Birth of the Clinic: An Archeology of Medical Perception* (New York: Pantheon, 1973).

R. FOX, "The Medicalization and Demedicalization of American Society," *Daedalus,* vol. 106 (1977), pp. 9–22.

E. FRANKFORT, *Vaginal Politics* (New York: Quadrangle Books, 1972).

E. FREIDSON, *Profession of Medicine* (New York: Dodd, Mead, 1970).

B. FRIEDAN, *The Feminine Mystique* (New York: Dell, 1963).

R. C., FRIEDMAN, S. W. HURT, M. S. ARONOFF, and J. CLARKIN, "Behavior and the Menstrual Cycle," *Signs,* vol. 5 (1980), pp. 719–738.

D. M. GARNER, P. E. GARFINKEL, D. SCHWARTZ, and M. THOMPSON, "Cultural Expectations of Thinness in Women," *Psychological Reports,* vol. 47 (1980), pp. 483–491.

E. GOFFMAN, *Stigma: Notes on the Management of Spoiled Identity* (Englewood Cliffs, N.J.: Prentice-Hall, 1964).

P. B. GOLDBLATT, M. E. MOORE, and A. J. STUNKARD, "Social Factors in Obesity," *Journal of American Medical Association,* vol. 192, (1972) pp. 1039–1044.

E. R. GONZALES, "Premenstrual Syndrome: Ancient Woe Deserving of Modern Scrutiny," *Journal of American Medical Association,* vol. 245 (1981), pp. 1393–1396.

L. GORDON, *Woman's Body, Woman's Right: A Social History of Birth Control in America* (New York: Penguin, 1976).

H. S. GROSS, M. R. HERBERT, G. L. KNATTERUD, and L. DONNER, "The Effect of Race and Sex on the Variation of Diagnosis and Disposition in a Psychiatric Emergency Room," *Journal of Nervous and Mental Disease,* vol. 148 (1969), pp. 638–643.

D. L. HALL, "Biology, Sex Hormones and Sexism in the 1920's" in C. C. Goud and M. W. Wartofsky (eds.), *Women and Philosophy: Toward a Theory of Liberation* (New York: G. P. Putnam's, 1976).

J. HANMER and P. ALLEN, "Reproductive Engineering: The Final Solution?" *Feminist Issues,* vol. 2 (1982), pp. 53–74.

M. HARRISON, *Self-Help for Premenstrual Syndrome* (Cambridge, Mass.: Matrix Press, 1982).

R. HERRNSTEIN, "IQ," *Atlantic Monthly,* vol. 228 (1971), pp. 43–64.

J. C. HOFFMAN, "Biorhythms in Human Reproduction: The Not-So-Steady States," *Signs,* vol. 7, (1982), pp. 829–844.

C. HOLDEN, "Proposed New Psychiatric Diagnoses Raise Charges of Gender Bias," *Science,* vol. 231 (1986), pp. 327–328.

H. HOLMES, B. HASKINS, and M. GROSS (eds.)., *The Custom-Made Child? Women-Centered Perspectives* (New York: Humana, 1981).

M. C. HOWELL, "What Medical Schools Teach about Women," *New England Journal of Medicine,* vol. 291 (1974), pp. 304–307.

R. HUBBARD, "Have Only Men Evolved?" in R. Hubbard, M. S. Henifin, and B. Fried (eds.), *Women Look at Biology Looking at Women* (Cambridge, Mass.: Schenkman, 1979).

———"The Politics of Women's Biology" (Lecture given at Hampshire College, October 1981).

———"Legal and Policy Implications of Recent Advances in Prenatal Diagnosis and Fetal Therapy," *Women's Rights Law Reporter,* Rutgers, vol. 7 (1982), pp. 201–218.

———"Women and Biology" (Lecture at annual conference, New England Women's Studies, Keene State College, Keene, N. H., 1983).

I. ILLICH, *Medical Nemesis: The Expropriation of Health* (New York: Pantheon, 1976).

E. F. KELLER, "Gender and Science," *Psychoanalysis and Contemporary Science,* vol. 1 (1978), pp. 409–433.

———"Feminism and Science," *Signs,* vol. 7 (1982), pp. 589–602.

M. H. KLAUS and J. H. KENNELL, *Maternal-Infant Bonding: The Impact of Early Separation or Loss on Family Development.* (St. Louis, Mo.: C. V. Mosby, 1976).

F. E. KOBRIN, "The American Midwife Controversy: A Crisis of Professionalization," *Bulletin of the History of Medicine,* vol. 40 (1966), pp. 350–363.

K. KOUMJIAN, "The Use of Valium as a Force of Social Control," *Social Science and Medicine,* vol. 15E (1981), pp. 245–249.

M. S. LARSON, *The Rise of Professionalism: A Sociological Analysis* (Berkeley: University of California Press, 1977).

J. W. LEAVITT, "Birthing and Anesthesia: The Debate over Twilight Sleep," *Signs,* vol. 6 (1980), pp. 147–164.

G. MANN, "The Influence of Obesity on Health: Part I," *New England Journal of Medicine,* vol. 291, no. 4 (1974), pp. 178–185.

———"The Influence of Obesity on Health: Part II," *New England Journal of Medicine,* vol. 291, no. 5 (1974), pp. 226–232.

J. MCKINLAY, "A Case for Refocussing Upstream: The Political Economy of Illness," in P. Conrad and R. Kern (eds.), *The Sociology of Health and Illness* (New York: St. Martin's Press., 1981), pp. 613–633.

C. MERCHANT, *The Death of Nature: Women, Ecology and the Scientific Revolution* (New York: Harper and Row, 1980).

L. G. MILLER, "Pain, Parturition, and the Profession: Twilight Sleep in America," in S. Reverby and D. Rosner (eds.), in *Health Care in America: Essays in Social History* (Philadelphia, Pa.: Temple University Press, 1979), pp. 19–37.

M. MILLMAN, *Such a Pretty Face: Being Fat in America* (New York: Berkley Books, 1980).

E. MILLS, *Living with Mental Illness: A Study of East London* (London: Routledge and Kegan Paul, 1962).

E. G. MISHLER, "The Social Construction of Illness" in E. G. Mishler, et. al., *Social Contexts of Health, Illness, and Patient Care* (Cambridge: Cambridge University Press, 1981), pp. 141–168.

J. C. MOHR, *Abortion in America: The Origins and Evolution of National Policy, 1800–1900* (New York: Oxford University Press, 1978).

R. H. MOOS, "The Development of a Menstrual Distress Questionnaire," *Psychosomatic Medicine,* vol. 30 (1963), pp. 853–867.

C. NATHANSON, "Illness and the Feminine Role: A Theoretical Review," *Social Science and Medicine,* vol. 9 (1975), pp. 57–62.

Newsweek, "Not Guilty Because of PMS?" (Nov. 8, 1982), p. 111.

K. O'DRISCOLL and M. FOLEY, "Correlation of Decrease in Perinatal Mortality and Increase in Caesarean Section Rates," *Obstetrics and Gynecology,* vol. 61 (1983), pp. 1–5.

M. B. PARLEE, "The Premenstrual Syndrome," *Psychological Bulletin,* vol. 80 (1973), pp. 454–465.

T. PARSONS, "Definitions of Illness and Health in Light of American Values and Social Structure," in E. G. Jaco (ed.), *Patients, Physicians and Illness,* 2nd ed. (New York: Free Press, 1951).

A. L. PLOUGH, "Medical Technology and the Crisis of Experience: The Cost of Clinical Legitimation," *Social Science and Medicine*, vol. 15F (1981), pp. 89–101.

R. L. REID and S. S. C. YEN, "Premenstrual Syndrome," *American Journal of Obstetrics and Gynecology*, vol. 139 (1981), pp. 85–104.

S. REVERBY, "Stealing the Golden Eggs: Earnest Amory Codman and the Science and Management of Medicine," *Bulletin of the History of Medicine*, vol. 55 (1981), pp. 156–171.

S. REVERBY, and D. ROSNER (eds.), *Health Care in America: Essays in Social History* (Philadelphia, Pa.: Temple University Press, 1979).

E. R. ROMEY, "Sex Hormones and Executive Ability," *Annals of the New York Academy of Science*, vol. 308 (1973), pp. 237–245.

S. ROSE and H. ROSE, "The Myth of the Neutrality of Science," in R. Arditti, P. Brennan, and S. Cavrak (eds.), op.cit, pp. 16–32.

A. ROSSI, "Life Span Theories and Women's Lives," *Signs,* vol. 6 (1980), pp. 4–32.

B. K. ROTHMAN, "Awake and Aware, or False Consciousness: The Cooptation of Childbirth Reform in America," in S. Romalis (ed.), *Childbirth: Alternatives to Medical Control* (Austin, Tex.: University of Texas Press, 1981), pp. 150–180.

———*In Labor: Women and Power in the Birthplace* (New York: Norton, 1982).

D. RUBLE, "Premenstrual Symptoms: A Reinterpretation," *Science,* vol. 197 (1977), pp. 291–292.

S. B. RUZEK, *The Women's Health Movement: Feminist Alternatives to Medical Control* (New York: Praeger, 1978).

D. M. SCHWARTZ, M. G. THOMPSON, and C. L. JOHNSON, "Anorexia Nervosa and Bulimia: The Sociocultural Context," *International Journal of Eating Disorders,* vol. 1 (1980), pp. 20–36.

D. SCULLY and P. BART, "A Funny Thing Happened on the Way to the Orifice: Women in Gynecology Textbooks," in P. Conrad and R. Kern (eds.), *The Sociology of Health in Illness: Critical Perspectives* (New York: St. Martin's Press, 1981).

B. SEAMAN, *Free and Female* (New York: Coward, McCann, and Geoghegan, 1972).

N. S. SHAW, *Forced Labor: Maternity Care in the United States* (New York: Pergamon Press, 1974).

C. SMITH-ROSENBERG and C. ROSENBERG, "The Female Animal: Medical and Biological Views of Woman and Her Role in Nineteenth-Century America," *Journal of American History,* vol. 60 (1973), pp. 332–355.

S. SONTAG, *Illness as Metaphor* (New York: Vintage, 1979).

E. STARK, "What Is Medicine?" *Radical Science Journal,* vol. 12 (1982), pp. 46–89.

E. STARK and A. FLITCRAFT, "Medical Therapy As Repression: The Case of Battered Women," *Health and Medicine,* vol. 1 (1982), pp. 29–32.

P. STARR, *The Social Transformation of American Medicine* (New York: Basic Books, 1982).

A. STUNKARD, H. LEVINE, and S. FOX, "The Management of Obesity," *Archives of Internal Medicine,* vol. 125 (1976), pp. 1067–1072.

A. J. STUNKARD, T. I. A. SORENSEN, C. HANIS, T. W. TEASDALE, R. CHAKRABORTY, W. J. SCHULL, and R. SCHULSINGER, "An Adoption Study of Human Obesity," *New England Journal of Medicine,* vol. 314 (1986): 193–201.

C. N. THEODORE and G. E. SUTTER, *Distribution of Physicians in the U.S.,* Department of Survey Research, Management Services Division, American Medical Association, 1966.

U.S. DEPARTMENT OF HEALTH, EDUCATION, and WELFARE, *The Supply of Health Manpower: 1970 Profiles and Projections to 1990,* DHEW Publications No. (HRA) 75–38, (1974).

L. M. VERBRUGGE and R. P. STEINER, "Physician Treatment of Men and Women Patients: Sex Bias or Appropriate Care?" *Medical Care,* vol. 19 (1981), pp. 609–632.

M. R. WALSH, *Doctors Wanted: No Women Need Apply* (New Haven, Conn.: Yale University Press, 1977).

R. W. WERTZ and D. C. WERTZ, *Lying In: A History of Childbirth in America* (New York: Free Press, 1979).

L. E. WURDERMAN, *Physician Distribution and Medical Licensure in the U.S., 1979,* Center for Health Services Research and Development, American Medical Association (1980).

I. M. YOUNG, "The Pregnant Body: Subjectivity and Alienation," *Journal of Medicine and Philosophy,* vol. 9 (forthcoming).

R. M. YOUNG, "Science Is Social Relations," *Radical Science Journal,* vol. 5 (1977), pp. 65–131.

I. K. ZOLA, "Medicine as an Institution of Social Control," *Sociological Review,* vol. 20 (1972), pp. 487–504.

———"In the Name of Health and Illness: On Some Sociopolitical Consequences of Medical Influence," *Social Science and Medicine,* vol. 9 (1975), pp. 83–87.

The Discovery of Hyperkinesis: Notes on the Medicalization of Deviant Behavior

Peter Conrad

The increasing medicalization of deviant behavior and the medical institution's role as an agent of social control has gained considerable notice (Freidson 1970; Pitts 1971; Kitterie 1971; Zola 1972). By medicalization we mean defining behavior as a medical problem or illness and mandating or licensing the medical profession to provide some type of treatment for it. Examples include alcoholism, drug addiction and treating violence as a genetic or brain disorder. This redefinition is not a new function of the medical institution: psychiatry and public health have always been concerned with social behavior and have traditionally functioned as agents of social control (Foucault 1965; Szasz 1970; Rosen 1972). Increasingly sophisticated medical techology has extended the potential of this type of social control, especially in terms of psychotechnology (Chorover 1973). This approach includes a variety of medical and quasi-medical treatments or procedures: psychosurgery, psychotropic medications, genetic engineering, antibuse, and methadone.

This paper describes how certain forms of behavior in children have become defined as a medical problem and how medicine has become a major agent for their social control since the discovery of hyperkinesis. By discovery we mean both origin of the diagnosis and treatment for this disorder; and discovery of children who exhibit this behavior. The first section analyzes the discovery of hyperkinesis and why

Reprinted from *Social Problems*, vol. 23 (October, 1975), pp. 12–21 by permission of the Society for the Study of Social Problems. Copyright © 1975 by the Society for the Study of Social Problems.

it suddenly became popular in the 1960's. The second section will discuss the medicalization of deviant behavior and its ramifications.

THE MEDICAL DIAGNOSIS OF HYPERKINESIS

Hyperkinesis is a relatively recent phenomenon as a medical diagnostic category. Only in the past two decades has it been available as a recognized diagnostic category and only in the last decade has it received widespread notice and medical popularity. However, the roots of the diagnosis and treatment of this clinical entity are found earlier.

Hyperkinesis is also known as Minimal Brain Dysfunction, Hyperactive Syndrome, Hyperkinetic Disorder of Childhood, and by several other diagnostic categories. Although the symptoms and the presumed etiology vary, in general the behaviors are quite similar and greatly overlap.[1] Typical symptom patterns for diagnosing the disorder include: extreme excess of motor activity (hyperactivity); very short attention span (the child flits from activity to activity); restlessness; fidgetiness; often widly oscillating mood swings (he's fine one day, a terror the next); clumsiness; aggressive-like behavior; impulsivity; in school he cannot sit still; cannot comply with rules, has low frustration level; frequently there may be sleeping problems and acquisition of speech may be delayed (Stewart 1966; 1970; Wender 1971). Most of the symptoms for the disorder are deviant behaviors.[2] It is six times as prevalent among boys as among girls. We use the term hyperkinesis to present all the diagnostic categories of this disorder.

THE DISCOVERY OF HYPERKINESIS

It is useful to divide the analysis into what might be considered *clinical factors* directly related to the diagnosis and treatment of hyperkinesis and *social factors* that set the context for the emergence of the new diagnostic category.

Clinical Factors

Bradley (1937) observed that amphetamine drugs had a spectacular effect in altering the behavior of school children who exhibited behavior disorders or learning disabilities. Fifteen of the 30 children he treated actually became more subdued in their behavior. Bradley termed the effect of this medication paradoxical, since he expected that amphetamines would stimulate children as they stimulated adults. After the medication was discontinued the children's behavior returned to premedication level.

A scattering of reports in the medical literature on the utility of stimulant medications for "childhood behavior disorders" appeared in the next two decades. The next significant contribution was the work of Strauss and his associates (Strauss and Lehtinen 1947) who found certain behavior (including hyperkinesis behaviors) in postencephaletic children suffering from what they called minimal brain injury (damage). This was the first time these behaviors were attributed to the new organic distinction of minimal brain damage.

This disorder still remained unnamed or else it was called a variety of names (usually just "childhood behavior disorder"). It did not appear as a specific diagnostic category until Laufer *et al.* (1957) described it as the "hyperkinetic impulse disorder" in 1957. Upon finding "the salient characteristics of the behavior pattern . . . are strikingly similar to those with clear-cut organic causation" these researchers described a disorder with no clearcut history of evidence for organicity (Laufer *et al.* 1957).

In 1966 a task force sponsored by the U.S. Public Health Service and the National Association for Crippled Children and Adults attempted to clarify the ambiguity and confusion in terminology and symptomology in diagnosing children's behavior and learning disorders. From over three dozen diagnoses, they agreed on the term "minimal brain dysfunction" as an overriding diagnosis that would include hyperkinesis and other disorders (Clements 1966). Since this time M.B.D. has been the primary formal diagnosis or label.

In the middle 1950s a new drug, Ritalin, was synthesized, that has many qualities of amphetamines without some of their more undesirable side effects. In 1961 this drug was approved by the F.D.A. for use with children. Since this time there has been much research published on the use of Ritalin in the treatment of childhood behavior disorders. This medication became the "treatment of choice" for treating children with hyperkinesis.

Since the early sixties, more research appeared on the etiology, diagnosis and treatment of hyperkinesis (cf. DeLong 1972; Grinspoon and Singer 1973; Cole 1975)—as much as three-quarters concerned with drug treatment of the disorder. There had been increasing publicity of the disorder in the mass media as well. The *Reader's Guide to Periodical Literature* had no articles on hyperkinesis before 1967, one each in 1968 and 1969 and a total of forty for 1970 through 1974 (a mean of eight per year).

Now hyperkinesis has become the most common child psychiatric problem (Gross and Wilson 1974:142); special pediatric clinics have been established to treat hyperkinetic children, and substantial federal funds have been invested in etiological and treatment research. Outside the medical profession, teachers have developed a working clinical knowledge of hyperkinesis' symptoms and treatment (cf. Robin and Bosco 1973); articles appear regularly in mass circulation magazines and newspapers so that parents often come to clinics with knowledge of this diagnosis. Hyperkinesis is no longer the relatively esoteric diagnostic category it may have been twenty years ago, it is now a well-known clinical disorder.

Social Factors

The social factors affecting the discovery of hyperkinesis can be divided into two areas: (1) The Pharmaceutical Revolution; (2) Government Action.

The Pharmaceutical Revolution. Since the 1930s the pharmaceutical industry has been synthesizing and manufacturing a large number of psychoactive drugs, contributing to a virtual revolution in drug making and drug taking in America (Silverman and Lee 1974).

Psychoactive drugs are agents that affect the central nervous system. Benzedrine, Ritalin, and Dexedrine are all synthesized psychoactive stimulants which were indicated for narcolepsy, appetite control (as "diet pills"), mild depression, fatigue, and more recently hyperkinetic children.

Until the early sixties there was little or no promotion and advertisement of any of these medications for use with childhood disorders.[3] Then two major pharmaceutical firms (Smith, Kline and French, manufacturer of Dexedrine and CIBA, manufacturer of Ritalin) began to advertise in medical journals and through direct mailing and efforts of the "detail men." Most of this advertising of the pharmaceutical treatment of hyperkinesis was directed to the medical sphere; but some of the promotion was targeted for the educational sector also (Hentoff 1972). This promotion was probably significant in disseminating information concerning the diagnosis and treatment of this newly discovered disorder.[4] Since 1955 the use of psychoactive medications (especially phenothiazines) for the treatment of persons who are mentally ill, along with the concurrent dramatic decline in inpatient populations, has made psychopharmacology an integral part of treatment for mental disorders. It has also undoubtedly increased the confidence in the medical profession for the pharmaceutical approach to mental and behavioral problems.

Government Action. Since the publication of the U.S.P.H.S. report on M.B.D. there have been at least two significant governmental reports on treating school children with stimulant medications for behavior disorders. Both of these came as a response to the national publicity created by the *Washington Post* report (1970) that five to ten percent of the 62,000 grammar school children in Omaha, Nebraska were being treated with "behavior modification drugs to improve deportment and increase learning potential" (quoted in Grinspoon and Singer 1973). Although the figures were later found to be a little exaggerated, it nevertheless spurred a Congressional investigation (U.S. Government Printing Office 1970) and a conference sponsored by the Office of Child Development (1971) on the use of stimulant drugs in the treatment of behaviorally disturbed school children.

The Congressional Subcommittee on Privacy chaired by Congressman Cornelius E. Gallagher held hearings on the issue of prescribing drugs for hyperactive school children. In general, the committee showed great concern over the facility in which the medication was prescribed; more specifically that some children at least were receiving drugs from general practitioners whose primary diagnosis was based on teachers' and parents' reports that the child was doing poorly in school. There was also a concern with the absence of follow-up studies on the long-term effects of treatment.

The H.E.W. committee was a rather hastily convened group of professionals (a majority were M.D.s) many of whom already had commitments to drug treatment for children's behavior problems. They recommended that only M.D.s make the diagnosis and prescribe treatment, that the pharmaceutical companies promote the treatment of the disorder only through medical channels, that parents should not be concerned to accept any particular treatment and that long-term follow-up research should be done. This report served as blue ribbon approval for treating hyperkinesis with psychoactive medications.

DISCUSSION

We will focus discussion on three issues: How children's deviant behavior became conceptualized as a medical problem; why this occurred when it did; and what are some of the implications of the medicalization of deviant behavior.

How does deviant behavior become conceptualized as a medical problem? We assume that before the discovery of hyperkinesis this type of deviance was seen as disruptive, disobedient, rebellious, antisocial or deviant behavior. Perhaps the label "emotionally disturbed" was sometimes used when it was in vogue in the early sixties, and the child was usually managed in the context of the family or the school or, in extreme cases, the child guidance clinic. How then did this constellation of deviant behaviors become a medical disorder?

The treatment was available long before the disorder treated was clearly conceptualized. It was 20 years after Bradley's discovery of the "paradoxical effect" of stimulants on certain deviant children that Laufer named the disorder and described the characteristic symptoms. Only in the late fifties were both the diagnostic label and the pharmaceutical treatment available. The pharmaceutical revolution in mental health and the increased interest in child psychiatry provided a favorable background for the dissemination of knowledge about this new disorder. The latter probably made the medical profession more likely to consider behavior problems in children as within their clinical jurisdiction.

There were agents outside the medical profession itself that were significant in "promoting" hyperkinesis as a disorder within the medical framework. These agents might be conceptualized in Becker's terms as "moral entrepreneurs," those who crusade for creation and enforcement of the rules (Becker 1963).[5] In this case the moral entrepreneurs were the pharmaceutical companies and the Association for Children with Learning Disabilities.

The pharmaceutical companies spent considerable time and money promoting stimulant medications for this new disorder. From the middle 1960s on, medical journals and the free "throw-away" magazines contained elaborate advertising for Ritalin and Dexedrine. These ads explained the utility of treating hyperkinesis and urged the physician to diagnose and treat hyperkinetic children. The ads run from one to six pages. For example, a two-page ad in 1971 stated:

MBD . . . MEDICAL MYTH OR DIAGNOSABLE DISEASE ENTITY What medical practitioner has not, at one time or another, been called upon to examine an impulsive, excitable hyperkinetic child? A child with difficulty in concentrating. Easily frustrated. Unusually aggressive. A classroom rebel. In the absence of any organic pathology, the conduct of such children was, until a few short years ago, usually dismissed as . . . spunkiness, or evidence of youthful vitality. But it is now evident that in many of these children the hyperkinetic syndrome exists as a distinct medical entity. This syndrome is readily diagnosed through patient histories, neurologic signs and psychometric testing—has been classified by an expert panel convened by the United States Department of Health, Education and Welfare as Minimal Brain Dysfunction, MBD.

The pharmaceutical firms also supplied sophisticated packets of "diagnostic and treatment" information on hyperkinesis to physicians, paid for professional conferences on the subject, and supported research in the identification and treatment of the disorder. Clearly these corporations had a vested interest in the labeling and treatment of hyperkinesis; CIBA had $13 million profit from Ritalin alone in 1971, which was 15 percent of the total gross profits (Charles 1971; Hentoff 1972).

The other moral enterpreneur, less powerful than the pharmaceutical companies, but nevertheless influential, is the Association for Children with Learning Disabilities. Although their focus is not specifically on hyperkinetic children, they do include it in their conception of Learning Disabilities along with aphasia, reading problems such as dyslexia and perceptual motor problems. Founded in the early 1950s by parents and professionals, it has functioned much as the National Association for Mental Health does for mental illness: promoting conferences, sponsoring legislation, providing social support. One of the main functions has been to disseminate information concerning this relatively new area in education, Learning Disabilities. While the organization does have a more educational than medical perspective, most of the literature indicates that for hyperkinesis members have adopted the medical model and the medical approach to the problem. They have sensitized teachers and schools to the conception of hyperkinesis as a medical problem.

The medical model of hyperactive behavior has become very well accepted in our society. Physicians find treatment relatively simple and the results sometimes spectacular. Hyperkinesis minimizes parents' guilt by emphasizing "it's not their fault, it's an organic problem" and allows for nonpunitive management or control of deviance. Medication often makes a child less disruptive in the classroom and sometimes aids a child in learning. Children often like their "magic pills" which make their behavior more socially acceptable and they probably benefit from a reduced stigma also. There are, however, some other, perhaps more subtle ramifications of the medicalization of deviant behavior.

THE MEDICALIZATION OF DEVIANT BEHAVIOR

Pitts has commented that "medicalization is one of the most effective means of social control and that it is destined to become the main mode of *formal* social control" (1971:391). Kitterie (1971) has termed it "the coming of the therapeutic state."

Medicalization of mental illness dates at least from the 17th century (Foucault, 1965; Szasz, 1970). Even slaves who ran away were once considered to be suffering from the disease *drapetomania* (Chorover 1973). In recent years alcoholism, violence, and drug addiction as well as hyperactive behavior in children have all become defined as medical problems, both in etiology or explanation of the behavior and the means of social control or treatment.

There are many reasons why this medicalization has occurred. Much scientific research, especially in pharmacology and genetics, has become technologically more sophisticated, and found more subtle correlates with human behavior. Sometimes these findings (as in the case of XYY chromosomes and violence) become etiological explanations for deviance. Pharmacological technology that makes new discoveries affecting behavior (e.g., antibuse, methadone, and stimulants) are used as treatment for deviance. In part this application is encouraged by the prestige of the medical profession and its attachment to science. As Freidson notes, the medical profession has first claim to jurisdiction over anything that deals with the functioning of the body and especially anything that can be labeled illness (1970:251). Advances in genetics, pharmacology, and "psychosurgery" also may advance medicine's jurisdiction over deviant behavior.

Second, the application of pharmacological technology is related to the humanitarian trend in the conception and control of deviant behavior. Alcoholism is no longer sin or even moral weakness, it is now a disease. Alcoholics are no longer arrested in many places for "public drunkenness," they are now somehow "treated," even if it is only to be dried out. Hyperactive children are now considered to have an illness rather than to be disruptive, disobedient, overactive problem children. They are not as likely to be the "bad boy" of the classroom; they are children with a medical disorder. Clearly there are some real

humanitarian benefits to be gained by such a medical conceptualization of deviant behavior. There is less condemnation of the deviants (they have an illness, it is not their fault) and perhaps less social stigma. In some cases, even the medical treatment itself is a more humanitarian social control than the criminal justice system.

There is, however, another side to the medicalization of deviant behavior. The four aspects of this side of the issued include (1) the problem of expert control; (2) medical social control; (3) the individualization of social problems; and (4) the "depoliticization" of deviant behavior.

The Problem of Expert Control.   The medical profession is a profession of experts; they have a monopoly on anything that can be conceptualized as illness. Because of the way the medical profession is organized and the mandate it has from society, decisions related to medical diagnoses and treatment are virtually controlled by medical professionals.

Some conditions that enter the medical domain are not ipso facto medical problems, especially deviant behavior, whether alcoholism, hyperactivity, or drug addiction. By defining a problem as medical it is removed from the public realm where there can be discussion by ordinary people and put on a plane where only medical people can discuss it. As Reynolds states,

> The increasing acceptance, especially among the more educated segments of our populace, of technical solutions—solutions administered by disinterested politically and morally neutral experts—results in the withdrawal of more and more areas of human experience from the realm of public discussion. For when drunkenness, juvenile delinquency, sub par performance, and extreme political beliefs are seen as symptoms of an underlying illness or biological defect the merits and drawbacks of such behavior or beliefs need not be evaluated (1973:220–221).

The public may have their own conceptions of deviant behavior but that of the experts is usually dominant.

Medical Social Control.   Defining deviant behavior as a medical problem allows certain things to be done that could not otherwise be considered; for example, the body may be cut open or psychoactive medications may be given. This treatment can be a form of social control.

In regard to drug treatment Lennard points out: "Psychoactive drugs, especially those legally prescribed, tend to restrain individuals from behavior and experience that are not complementary to the requirements of the dominant value system" (1971:57). These forms of medical social control presume a prior definition of deviance as a medical problem. Psychosurgery on an individual prone to violent outbursts requires a diagnosis that there was something wrong with his brain or nervous system. Similarly, prescribing drugs to restless, overactive and disruptive school children requires a diagnosis of hyperkinesis. These forms of social control, what Chorover (1973) has called "psychotechnology," are very powerful and often very efficient means of controlling deviance. These relatively new and increasingly popular forms of social control could not be utilized without the medicalization of deviant behavior. As is suggested from the discovery of hyperkinesis, if a mechanism of medical social control seems useful, then the deviant behavior it modifies will develop a medical label or diagnosis. No overt malevolence on the part of the medical profession is implied; rather it is part of a complex process, of which the medical profession is only a part. The larger process might be called the individualization of social problems.

The Individualization of Social Problems. The medicalization of deviant behavior is part of a larger phenomenon that is prevalent in our society, the individualization of social problems. We tend to look for causes and solutions to complex social problems in the individual rather than in the social system. This view resembles Ryan's (1971) notion of "blaming the victim;" seeing the causes of the problem in individuals rather than in the society where they live. We then seek to change the "victim" rather than the society. The medical perspective of diagnosing an illness in an individual lends itself to the individualization of social problems. Rather than seeing certain deviant behaviors as symptomatic of problems in the social system, the medical perspective focuses on the individual diagnosing and treating the illness, generally ignoring the social situation.

Hyperkinesis serves as a good example. Both the school and the parents are concerned with the child's behavior; the child is very difficult at home and disruptive in school. No punishments or rewards seem consistently to work in modifying the behavior; and both parents and school are at their wits' end. A medical evaluation is suggested. The diagnoses of hyperkinetic behavior leads to prescribing stimulant medications. The child's behavior seems to become more socially acceptable, reducing problems in school and at home.

But there is an alternate perspective. By focusing on the symptoms and defining them as hyperkinesis we ignore the possibility that behavior is not an illness but an adaptation to a social situation. It diverts our attention from the family or school and from seriously entertaining the idea that the "problem" could be in the structure of the social system. And by giving medications we are essentially supporting the existing systems and do not allow this behavior to be a factor of change in the system.

The Depoliticization of Deviant Behavior. Depoliticization of deviant behavior is a result of both the process of medicalization and individualization of social problems. To our western world, probably one of the clearest examples of such a depoliticization of deviant behavior occurred when political dissenters in the Soviet Union were declared mentally ill and confined in mental hospitals (cf. Conrad 1972). This strategy served to neutralize the meaning of political protest and dissent, rendering it the ravings of mad persons.

The medicalization of deviant behavior depoliticizes deviance in the same manner. By defining the overactive, restless and disruptive child as hyperkinetic we ignore the meaning of behavior in the context of the social system. If we focused our analysis on the school system we might see the child's behavior as symptomatic of some "disorder" in the school or classroom situation, rather than symptomatic of an individual neurological disorder.

CONCLUSION

I have discussed the social ramifications of the medicalization of deviant behavior, using hyperkinesis as the example. A number of consequences of this medicalization have been outlined, including the depoliticization of deviant behavior, decision-making power of experts, and the role of medicine as an agent of social control. In the last analysis medical social control may be the central issue, as in this role medicine becomes a de facto agent of the status quo. The medical profession may not have entirely sought this role, but its members have been, in general, disturbingly unconcerned and unquestioning in their acceptance of it. With the increasing medical knowledge and technology it is likely that more deviant behavior will be medicalized and medicine's social control function will expand.

Notes

1. The U.S.P.H.S. report (Clements, 1966) included 38 terms that were used to describe or distinguish the conditions that it labeled Minimal Brain Dysfunction. Although the literature attempts to differentiate M.B.D., hyperkinesis, hyperactive syndrome, and several other diagnostic labels, it is our belief that in practice they are almost interchangeable.

2. For a fuller discussion of the construction of the diagnosis of hyperkinesis, see Conrad (forthcoming), especially Chapter 6.

3. The American Medical Association's change in policy in accepting more pharmaceutical advertising in the late fifties may have been important. Probably the F.D.A. approval of the use of Ritalin for children in 1961 was more significant. Until 1970, Ritalin was advertised for treatment of "functional behavior problems in children." Since then, because of an F.D.A. order, it has only been promoted for treatment of M.B.D.

4. The drug industry spends fully 25 percent of its budget on promotion and advertising. See Coleman *et al.* (1966) for the role of the detail men and how physicians rely upon them for information.

5. Freidson also notes the medical professional role as moral entrepreneur in this process also:

   The profession does treat the illnesses laymen take to it, but it also seeks to discover illness of which the laymen may not even be aware. One of the greatest ambitions of the physician is to discover and describe a "new" disease or syndrome. . . . (1970:252)

References

BECKER, HOWARD S.
  1963 The Outsiders. New York: Free Press.

BRADLEY, CHARLES
  1937 "The behavior of children receiving Benzedrine." American Journal of Psychiatry 94 (March): 577–585.

CHARLES, ALAN
  1971 "The case of Ritalin." New Republic 23 (October): 17–19.

CHOROVER, STEPHEN L.
  1973 "Big brother and psychotechnology." Psychology Today (October): 43–54.

CLEMENTS, SAMUEL D.
  1966 "Task force I: Minimal brain dysfunction in children." National Institute of Neurological Diseases and Blindness, Monograph no. 3. Washington, D.C.: U.S. Department of Health, Education, and Welfare.

COLE, SHERWOOD
  1975 "Hyperactive children: The use of stimulant drugs evaluated." American Journal of Orthopsychiatry 45 (January): 28–37.

COLEMAN, JAMES, ELIHU KATZ, and HERBERT MENZEL
  1966 Medical Innovation. Indianapolis: Bobbs Merrill.

CONRAD, PETER
  1972 "Ideological deviance: An analysis of the Soviet use of mental hospitals for political dissenters." Unpublished manuscript.

  Forthcoming "Identifying hyperactive children: A study in the medicalization of deviant behavior." Unpublished Ph.D. dissertation, Boston University.

DELONG, ARTHUR R.
  1972 "What have we learned from psychoactive drugs research with hyperactives?" American Journal of Diseases in Children 123 (February): 177–180.

FOUCAULT, MICHAEL
  1965 Madness and Civilization. New York: Pantheon.

GRINSPOON, LESTER and SUSAN SINGER
  1973 "Amphetamines in the treatment of hyperactive children." Harvard Educational Review 43 (November): 515–555.

GROSS, MORTIMER B. and WILLIAM E. WILSON
  1974 Minimal Brain Dysfunction. New York: Brunner Mazel.

HENTOFF, NAT
  1972 "Drug pushing in the schools: The professionals." The Village Voice 22 (May): 21–23.

KITTERIE, NICHOLAS
  1971 The Right to Be Different. Baltimore: Johns Hopkins Press.

LAUFER, M. W., DENHOFF, E., and SOLOMONS, G.
  1975 "Hyperkinetic impulse disorder in children's be-

havior problems." Psychosomatic Medicine 19 (January): 38–49.

LENNARD, HENRY L. and ASSOCIATES
1971 Mystification and Drug Misuse. New York: Harper and Row.

OFFICE OF CHILD DEVELOPMENT
1971 "Report of the conference on the use of stimulant drugs in treatment of behaviorally disturbed children." Washington, D.C.: Office of Child Development, Department of Health, Education and Welfare, January 11–12.

PITTS, JESSE
1968 "Social control: The concept." In David Sills (ed.), International Encyclopedia of the Social Sciences, Volume 14. New York: Macmillan.

REYNOLDS, JANICE M.
1973 "The medical institution." Pp. 198–324 in Larry T. Reynolds and James M. Henslin, American Society: A Critical Analysis. New York: David McKay.

ROBIN, STANLEY S. and JAMES J. BOSCO
1973 "Ritalin for school children: The teachers perspective." Journal of School Health 47 (December): 624–628.

ROSEN, GEORGE
1972 "The evolution of social medicine." Pp. 30–60 in Howard E. Freeman, Sol Levine, and Leo Reeder, Handbook of Medical Sociology. Englewood Cliffs, N.J.: Prentice-Hall.

RYAN, WILLIAM
1970 Blaming the Victim. New York: Vintage.

SILVERMAN, MILTON and PHILIP R. LEE
1974 Pills, Profits and Politics. Berkeley: University of California Press.

SROUFE, L. ALAN and MARK STEWART
1973 "Treating problem children with stimulant drugs." New England Journal of Medicine 289 (August 23): 407–421.

STEWART, MARK A.
1970 "Hyperactive Children." Scientific American 222 (April): 794–798.

STEWART, MARK A., A. FERRIS, N. P. PITTS and A. G. CRAIG
1966 "The hyperactive child syndrome." American Journal of Orthopsychiatry 36 (October): 861–867.

STRAUSS, A. A. and L. E. LEHTINEN
1947 Psychopathology and Education of the Brain-Injured Child. Vol. 1. New York: Grune and Stratton.

U.S. GOVERNMENT PRINTING OFFICE
1970 "Federal involvement in the use of behavior modification drugs on grammar school children of the right to privacy inquiry: Hearing before a subcommittee of the committee on government operations." Washington, D.C.: 91st Congress, 2nd session (September 29).

WENDER, PAUL
1971 Minimal Brain Dysfunction in Children. New York: John Wiley and Sons.

ZOLA, IRVING
1972 "Medicine as an institution of social control." Sociological Review 20 (November): 487–504

On Being Sane in Insane Places

D. L. Rosenhan

I f sanity and insanity exist, how shall we know them?

The question is neither capricious nor itself insane. However much we may be personally convinced that we can tell the normal from the abnormal, the evidence is simply not compelling. It is commonplace, for example, to read about murder trials wherein eminent psychiatrists for the defense are contradicted by equally eminent psychiatrists for the prosecution on the matter of the defendant's sanity. More generally, there are a great deal of conflicting data on the reliability, utility, and meaning of such terms as "sanity," "insanity," "mental illness," and "schizophrenia."[1] Finally, as early as 1934, Benedict suggested that normality and abnormality are not universal.[2] What is viewed as normal in one culture may be seen as quite aberrant in another. Thus, notions of normality and abnormality may not be quite as accurate as people believe they are.

To raise questions regarding normality and abnormality is in no way to question the fact that some behaviors are deviant or odd. Murder is deviant. So, too, are hallucinations. Nor does raising such questions deny the existence of the personal anguish that is often associated with "mental illness." Anxiety and depression exist. Psychological suffering exists. But normality and abnormality, sanity and insanity, and the diagnoses that flow from them may be less substantive than many believe them to be.

At its heart, the question of whether the sane can be distinguished from the insane (and whether degrees of insanity can be distinguished from each other) is a simple matter: do the salient characteristics that lead to diagnoses reside in the patients themselves or in the environments and contexts in which observers find them? From Bleuler, through Kretchmer, through the formulators of the recently revised *Diagnostic and Statistical Manual* of the American Psychiatric Association, the belief has been strong that patients present symptoms, that those symptoms can be categorized, and, implicitly, that the sane are distinguishable from the insane. More recently, however, this belief has been questioned. Based in part on theoretical and anthropological considerations, but also on philosophical, legal, and therapeutic ones, the view has grown that psychological categorization of mental illness is useless at best and downright harmful, misleading, and pejorative at worst. Psychiatric diagnoses, in this view, are in the minds of the observers and are not valid summaries of characteristics displayed by the observed.[3-5]

Gains can be made in deciding which of these is more nearly accurate by getting normal people (that is, people who do not have, and have never suffered, symptoms of serious psychiatric disorders) admitted to psychiatric hospitals and then determining whether they were discovered to be sane and, if so, how. If the sanity of such pseudopatients were always detected, there would be prima facie evidence that a sane individual can be distinguished from the insane context in which he is found. Normality (and presumably abnormality) is distinct enough that it can be recognized wherever it occurs, for it is carried within the person. If, on the other hand, the sanity of the pseudopatients were never discovered, serious difficulties would arise for those who support traditional modes of psychiatric diagnosis. Given that the hospital staff was not incompetent, that the pseudopatient had been behaving as sanely as he had been outside of the hospital and that it had never been previously suggested that he belonged in a psychiatric hospital, such an unlikely outcome would support the view that psychiatric

Reprinted from *Science*, vol. 179 (January 9, 1973), pp. 250–258. Copyright © 1973 by the American Association for the Advancement of Science.

diagnosis betrays little about the patient but much about the environment in which an observer finds him.

This article describes such an experiment. Eight sane people gained secret admission to 12 different hospitals.[6] Their diagnostic experiences constitute the data of the first part of this article; the remainder is devoted to a description of their experiences in psychiatric institutions. Too few psychiatrists and psychologists, even those who have worked in such hospitals, know what the experience is like. They rarely talk about it with former patients, perhaps because they distrust information coming from the previously insane. Those who have worked in psychiatric hospitals are likely to have adapted so thoroughly to the settings that they are insensitive to the impact of that experience. And while there have been occasional reports of researchers who submitted themselves to psychiatric hospitalization,[7] these researchers have commonly remained in the hospitals for short periods of time, often with the knowledge of the hospital staff. It is difficult to know the extent to which they were treated like patients or like research colleagues. Nevertheless, their reports about the inside of the psychiatric hospital have been valuable. This article extends those efforts.

PSEUDOPATIENTS AND THEIR SETTINGS

The eight pseudopatients were a varied group. One was a psychology graduate student in his 20s. The remaining seven were older and "established." Among them were three psychologists, a pediatrician, a psychiatrist, a painter, and a housewife. Three pseudopatients were women, five were men. All of them employed pseudonyms, lest their alleged diagnoses embarrass them later. Those who were in mental health professions alleged another occupation in order to avoid the special attentions that might be accorded by staff, as a matter of courtesy or caution, to ailing colleagues.[8] With the exception of myself (I was the first pseudopatient and my presence was known to the hospital administrator and chief psychologist and, so far as I can tell, to them alone), the presence of pseudopatients and the nature of the research program were not known to the hospital staffs.[9]

The settings were similarly varied. In order to generalize the findings, admission into a variety of hospitals was sought. The 12 hospitals in the sample were located in five different states on the East and West coasts. Some were old and shabby, some were quite new. Some were research-oriented, others not. Some had good staff-patient ratios, others were quite understaffed. Only one was a strictly private hospital. All of the others were supported by state or federal funds or, in one instance, by university funds.

After calling the hospital for an appointment, the pseudopatient arrived at the admission office complaining that he had been hearing voices. Asked what the voices said, he replied that they were often unclear, but as far as he could tell they said "empty," "hollow," and "thud." The voices were unfamiliar and were of the same sex as the pseudopatient. The choice of these symptoms was occasioned by their apparent similarity to existential symptoms. Such symptoms are alleged to arise from painful concerns about the perceived meaninglessness of one's life. It is as if the hallucinating person were saying, "My life is empty and hollow." The choice of these symptoms was also determined by the *absence* of a single report of existential psychoses in the literature.

Beyond alleging the symptoms and falsifying name, vocation, and employment, no further alterations of person, history, or circumstances were made. The significant events of the pseudopatient's life history were presented as they had actually occurred. Relationships with parents and siblings, with spouse and children, with people at work and in school, consistent with the aforementioned exceptions, were described as they were or had been. Frustrations and upsets were described along with jobs and satisfactions. These facts are important to remember. If anything, they strongly biased the subsequent results in favor of detecting sanity, since none of their histories or current behaviors were seriously pathological in any way.

Immediately upon admission to the psychiatric ward, the pseudopatient ceased simulating *any* symptoms of abnormality. In some cases, there was a brief period of mild nervousness and anxiety, since none of the pseudopatients really believed that they would be admitted so easily. Indeed, their shared fear was that they would be immediately exposed as frauds and greatly embarrassed. Moreover, many of them had never visited a psychiatric ward; even those who had, nevertheless had some genuine fears about what might happen to them. Their nervousness, then, was quite appropriate to the novelty of the hospital setting, and it abated rapidly.

Apart from that short-lived nervousness, the pseudopatient behaved on the ward as he "normally" behaved. The pseudopatient spoke to patients and staff as he might ordinarily. Because there is uncommonly little to do on a psychiatric ward, he attempted to engage others in conversation. When asked by staff how he was feeling, he indicated that he was fine, that he no longer experienced symptoms. He responded to instructions from attendants, to calls for medication (which was not swallowed), and to dining-hall instructions. Beyond such activities as were available to him on the admissions ward, he spent his time writing down his observations about the ward, its patients, and the staff. Initially these notes were written "secretly," but as it soon became clear that no one much cared, they were subsequently written on standard tablets of paper in such public places as the dayroom. No secret was made of these activities.

The pseudopatient, very much as a true psychiatric patient, entered a hospital with no foreknowledge of when he would be discharged. Each was told that he would have to get out by his own devices, essentially by convincing the staff that he was sane. The psychological stresses associated with hospitalization were considerable, and all but one of the pseudopatients desired to be discharged almost immediately after being admitted. They were, therefore, motivated not only to behave sanely, but to be paragons of cooperation. That their behavior was in no way disruptive is confirmed by nursing reports, which have been obtained on most of the patients. These reports uniformly indicate that the patients were "friendly," "cooperative," and "exhibited no abnormal indications."

THE NORMAL ARE NOT DETECTABLY SANE

Despite their public "show" of sanity, the pseudopatients were never detected. Admitted, except in one case, with a diagnosis of schizophrenia,[10] each was discharged with a diagnosis of schizophrenia "in remission." The label "in remission" should in no way

be dismissed as a formality, for at no time during any hospitalization had any question been raised about any pseudopatient's simulation. Nor are there any indications in the hospital records that the pseudopatient's status was suspect. Rather, the evidence is strong that, once labeled schizophrenic, the pseudopatient was stuck with that label. If the pseudopatient was to be discharged, he must naturally be "in remission"; but he was not sane, nor, in the institution's view, had he ever been sane.

The uniform failure to recognize sanity cannot be attributed to the quality of the hospitals, for, although there were considerable variations among them, several are considered excellent. Nor can it be alleged that there was simply not enough time to observe the pseudopatients. Length of hospitalization ranged from 7 to 52 days, with an average of 19 days. The pseudopatients were not, in fact, carefully observed, but this failure clearly speaks more to traditions within psychiatric hospitals than to lack of opportunity.

Finally, it cannot be said that the failure to recognize the pseudopatient's sanity was due to the fact that they were not behaving sanely. While there was clearly some tension present in all of them, their daily visitors could detect no serious behavioral consequences—nor, indeed, could other patients. It was quite common for the patients to "detect" the pseudopatients' sanity. During the first three hospitalizations, when accurate counts were kept, 35 of a total of 118 patients on the admissions ward voiced their suspicions, some vigorously. "You're not crazy. You're a journalist, or a professor [referring to the continual note-taking]. You're checking up on the hospital." While most of the patients were reassured by the pseudopatient's insistence that he had been sick before he came in but was fine now, some continued to believe that the pseudopatient was sane throughout the hospitalization.[11] The fact that the patients often recognized normality when staff did not raises important questions.

Failure to detect sanity during the course of hospitalization may be due to the fact that physicians operate with a strong bias toward what statisticians call the type 2 error.[5] This is to say that physicians are more inclined to call a healthy person sick (a false positive, type 2) than a sick person healthy (a false negative, type 1). The reasons for this are not hard to find: it is clearly more dangerous to mis-diagnose illness than health. Better to err on the side of caution, to suspect illness even among the healthy.

But what holds for medicine does not hold equally well for psychiatry. Medical illnesses, while unfortunate, are not commonly pejorative. Psychiatric diagnoses, on the contrary, carry with them personal, legal, and social stigmas.[12] It was therefore important to see whether the tendency toward diagnosing the sane could be reversed. The following experiment was arranged at a research and teaching hospital whose staff had heard these findings but doubted that such an error could occur in their hospital. The staff was informed that at some time during the following three months, one or more pseudopatients would attempt to be admitted into the psychiatric hospital. Each staff member was asked to rate each patient who presented himself at admissions or on the ward according to the likelihood that the patient was a pseudopatient. A 10-point scale was used, with a 1 and 2 reflecting high confidence that the patient was a pseudopatient.

Judgments were obtained on 193 patients who were admitted for psychiatric treatment. All staff who had had sustained contact with or primary responsibility for the patient—attendants, nurses, psychiatrists, physicians, and psychologists—were asked to make judgments. Forty-one patients were alleged, with high confidence, to be pseudopatients by at least one member of the staff. Twenty-three were considered suspect by at least one psychiatrist. Nineteen were suspected by one psychiatrist *and* one other staff member. Actually, no genuine pseudopatient (at least from my group) presented himself during this period.

The experiment is instructive. It indicates that the tendency to designate sane people as insane can be reversed when the stakes (in this case, prestige and diagnostic acumen) are high. But what can be said of the 19 people who were suspected of being "sane" by one psychiatrist and another staff member? Were these people truly "sane," or was it rather the case that in the course of avoiding the type of 2 error the staff tended to make more errors of the first sort—calling the crazy "sane"? There is no way of knowing. But one thing is certain: any diagnostic process that lends itself so readily to massive errors of this sort cannot be a very reliable one.

THE STICKINESS OF PSYCHODIAGNOSTIC LABELS

Beyond the tendency to call the healthy sick—a tendency that accounts better for diagnostic behavior on admission than it does for such behavior after a lengthy period of exposure—the data speak to the massive role of labeling in psychiatric assessment. Having once been labeled schizophrenic, there is nothing the pseudopatient can do to overcome the tag. The tag profoundly colors others' perceptions of him and his behavior.

From one viewpoint, these data are hardly surprising, for it has long been known that elements are given meaning by the context in which they occur. Gestalt psychology made this point vigorously, and Asch[13] demonstrated that there are "central" personality traits (such as "warm" versus "cold") which are so powerful that they markedly color the meaning of other information in forming an impression of a given personality.[14] "Insane," "schizophrenic," "manic-depressive," and "crazy" are probably among the most powerful of such central traits. Once a person is designated abnormal, all of his other behaviors and characteristics are colored by that label. Indeed, that label is so powerful that many of the pseudopatients' normal behaviors were overlooked entirely or profoundly misinterpreted. Some examples may clarify this issue.

Earlier I indicated that there were no changes in the pseudopatient's personal history and current status beyond those of name, employment, and, where necessary, vocation. Otherwise, a veridical description of personal history and circumstances was offered. Those circumstances were not psychotic. How were they made consonant with the diagnosis of psychosis? Or were those diagnoses modified in such a way as to bring them into accord with the circumstances of the pseudopatient's life, as described by him?

As far as I can determine, diagnoses were in no way affected by the relative health of the circumstances of a pseudopatient's life. Rather, the reverse occurred: the perception of his circumstances was shaped entirely by the diagnosis. A clear example of such translation is found in the case of a pseudopatient who had had a close relationship with his mother but was rather remote from his father during his early childhood. During adolescence and beyond, however, his father became a close friend, while his relationship with his mother cooled. His present relationship with his wife was characteristically close and warm. Apart from occasional angry exchanges, friction was minimal. The children had rarely been spanked. Surely there is nothing especially pathological about such a history. Indeed, many readers may see a similar pattern in their own experiences, with no markedly deleterious consequences. Observe, however, how such a history was translated in the psychopathological context, this from the case summary prepared after the patient was discharged.

This white 39-year-old male . . . manifests a long history of considerable ambivalence in close relationships, which begins in early childhood. A warm relationship with his mother cools during his adolescence. A distant relationship to his father is described as becoming very intense. Affective stability is absent. His attempts to control emotionality with his wife and children are punctuated by angry outbursts and, in the case of the children, spankings. And while he says that he has several good friends, one senses considerable ambivalence embedded in those relationships also. . . .

The facts of the case were unintentionally distorted by the staff to achieve consistency with a popular theory of the dynamics of a schizophrenic reaction.[15] Nothing of an ambivalent nature had been described in relations with parents, spouse, or friends. To the extent that ambivalence could be inferred, it was probably not greater than is found in all human relationships. It is true the pseudopatient's relationships with his parents changed over time, but in the ordinary context that would hardly be remarkable—indeed, it might very well be expected. Clearly, the meaning ascribed to her verbalizations (that is, ambivalence, affective instability) was determined by the diagnosis: schizophrenia. An entirely different meaning would have been ascribed if it were known that the man was "normal."

All pseudopatients took extensive notes publicly. Under ordinary circumstances, such behavior would have raised questions in the minds of observers, as, in fact, it did among patients. Indeed, it seemed so certain that the notes would elicit suspicion that elaborate precautions were taken to remove them from the ward each day. But the precautions proved needless. The closest any staff member came to questioning these notes occurred when one pseudopatient asked his physician what kind of medication he was receiving and began to write down the response. "You needn't write it," he was told gently. "If you have trouble remembering, just ask me again."

If no questions were asked of the pseudopatients, how was their writing interpreted? Nursing records for the three patients indicate that the writing was seen as an aspect of their pathological behavior. "Patient engages in writing behavior" was the daily nursing comment on one of the pseudopatients who was never questioned about his writing. Given that the patient is in the hospital, he must be psychologically disturbed. And given that he is disturbed, continuous writing must be a behavioral manifestation of the disturbance, perhaps a subset of the compulsive behaviors that are sometimes correlated with schizophrenia.

One tacit characteristic of psychiatric diagnosis is that it locates the sources of aberration within the individual and only rarely within the complex of stimuli that surrounds him. Consequently, behaviors that are stimulated by the environment are commonly misattributed to the patient's disorder. For example, one kindly nurse found a pseudopatient pacing the long hospital corridors. "Nervous, Mr. X?" she asked. "No, bored," he said.

The notes kept by pseudopatients are full of patient behaviors that were misinterpreted by well-intentioned staff. Often enough, a patient would go "berserk" because he had, wittingly or unwittingly, been mistreated by, say, an attendant. A nurse coming upon the scene would rarely inquire even cursorily into the environmental stimuli of the patient behavior. Rather, she assumed that his upset derived from his pathology, not from his present interactions with other staff members. Occasionally, the staff might assume that the patient's family (especially when they had recently visited) or other patients had stimulated the outburst. But never were the staff found to assume that one of themselves or the structure of the hospital had anything to do with a patient's behavior. One psychiatrist pointed to a group of patients who were sitting outside the cafeteria entrance half an hour before lunchtime. To a group of young residents he indicated that such behavior was characteristic of the oral-acquisitive nature of the syndrome. It seemed not to occur to him that there were very few things to anticipate in a psychiatric hospital besides eating.

A psychiatric label has a life and an influence of its own. Once the impression has been formed that the patient is schizophrenic, the expectation is that he will continue to be schizophrenic. When a sufficient amount of time has passed, during which the patient has done nothing bizarre, he is considered to be in remission and available for discharge. But the label endures beyond discharge, with the unconfirmed expectation that he will behave as a schizophrenic again. Such labels, conferred by the mental health professionals, are as influential on the patient as they are on his relatives and friends, and it should not surprise anyone that the diagnosis acts on all of them as a self-fulfilling prophecy. Eventually, the patient himself accepts the diagnosis, with all of its surplus meanings and expectations, and behaves accordingly.[5]

The inferences to be made from these matters are quite simple. Much as Zigler and Phillips have demonstrated that there is enormous overlap in the symptoms presented by patients who have been variously diagnosed,[16] so there is enormous overlap in the behaviors of the sane and the insane. The sane are not "sane" all of the time. We lose our tempers "for no good reason." We are occasionally depressed or anxious, again for no good reason. And we may find it difficult to get along with one or another person—again for no reason that we can specify. Similarly, the insane are not always insane. Indeed, it was the impression of the pseudopatients while living with them that they were sane for long periods of time—that the bizarre behaviors upon which their diagnoses were allegedly predicated constituted only a small fraction of their total behavior. If it makes no sense to label ourselves permanently depressed on the basis of an occasional depression, then it takes better evidence than is presently available to label all patients insane or schizophrenic on the basis of bizarre behaviors or cognitions. It seems more useful, as Mischel[17] has pointed out, to limit our discussions to *behaviors,* the stimuli that provoke them, and their correlates.

It is not known why powerful impressions of personality traits, such as "crazy" or "insane," arise.

Conceivably, when the origins of and stimuli that give rise to a behavior are remote or unknown, or when the behavior strikes us as immutable, trait labels regarding the *behavior* arise. When, on the other hand, the origins and stimuli are known and available, discourse is limited to the behavior itself. Thus, I may hallucinate because I am sleeping, or I may hallucinate because I have ingested a peculiar drug. These are termed sleep-induced hallucinations, or dreams, and drug-induced hallucinations, respectively. But when the stimuli to my hallucinations are unknown, that is called craziness, or schizophrenia—as if that inference were somehow as illuminating as the others. . . .

· · ·

SUMMARY AND CONCLUSIONS

It is clear that we cannot distinguish the sane from the insane in psychiatric hospitals. The hospital itself imposes a special environment in which the meanings of behavior can easily be misunderstood. The consequences to patients hospitalized in such an environment—the powerlessness, depersonalization, segregation, mortification, and self-labeling—seem undoubtedly countertherapeutic.

I do not, even now, understand this problem well enough to perceive solutions. But two matters seem to have some promise. The first concerns the proliferation of community mental health facilities, or crisis intervention centers, of the human potential movement, and of behavior therapies that, for all of their own problems, tend to avoid psychiatric labels, to focus on specific problems and behaviors, and to retain the individual in a relatively nonpejorative environment. Clearly, to the extent that we refrain from sending the distressed to insane places, our impressions of them are less likely to be distorted. (The risk of distorted perceptions, it seems to me, is always present, since we are much more sensitive to an individual's behaviors and verbalizations than we are to the subtle contextual stimuli that often promote them. At issue here is a matter of magnitude. And, as I have shown, the magnitude of distortion is exceedingly high in the extreme context that is a psychiatric hospital.)

The second matter that might prove promising speaks to the need to increase the sensitivity of mental health workers and researchers of the *Catch 22* position of psychiatric patients. Simply reading materials in this area will be of help to some such workers and researchers. For others, directly experiencing the impact of psychiatric hospitalization will be of enormous use. Clearly, further research into the social psychology of such total institutions will both facilitate treatment and deepen understanding.

I and the other pseudopatients in the psychiatric setting had distinctly negative reactions. We do not pretend to describe the subjective experiences of true patients. Theirs may be different from ours, particularly with the passage of time and the necessary process of adaptation to one's environment. But we can and do speak to the relatively more objective indices of treatment within the hospital. It could be a mistake, and a very unfortunate one, to consider that what happened to us derived from malice or stupidity on the part of the staff. Quite the contrary, our overwhelming impression of them was of people who really cared, who were committed and who were uncommonly intelligent. Where they failed, as they sometimes did painfully, it would be more accurate to attribute those failures to the environment in which they, too, found themselves than to personal callousness. Their perceptions and behavior were controlled by the situation, rather than being motivated by a malicious disposition. In a more benign environment, one that was less attached to global diagnosis, their behaviors and judgments might have been more benign and effective.

Notes

1. P. Ash, *J. Abnorm. Soc. Psychol.* 44, 272 (1949); A. T. Beck, *Amer. J. Psychiat.* 119, 210 (1962); A. T. Boisen, *Psychiatry* 2, 233 (1938); N. Kreitman, *J. Ment. Sci.* 107, 876 (1961); N. Kreitman, P. Sainsbury, J. Morrisey, J. Towers, J. Scrivener, *ibid.,* p. 887; H. O. Schmitt and C. P. Fonda, *J. Abnorm. Soc. Psychol.* 52, 262 (1956); W. Seeman, *J. Nerv. Ment. Dis.* 118, 541 (1953). For an analysis of these artifacts and summaries of the disputes, see J. Zubin, *Annu. Rev. Psychol.* 18, 373 (1967); L. Phillips and J. G. Draguns, *ibid.,* 22, 447 (1971).

2. R. Benedict, *J. Gen. Psychol.* 10, 59 (1934).

3. See in this regard H. Becker, *Outsiders: Studies in the Sociology of Deviance* (Free Press, New York, 1963); B. M. Braginsky, D. D. Braginsky, K. Ring, *Methods of Madness: The Mental Hospital as a Last Resort* (Holt,

Rinehart & Winston, New York, 1969); G. M. Crocetti and P. V. Lemkau, *Amer. Sociol. Rev.* 30, 577 (1965); E. Goffman, *Behavior in Public Places* (Free Press, New York, 1964); R. D. Laing, *The Divided Self: A Study of Sanity and Madness* (Quadrangle, Chicago, 1960); D. L. Phillips, *Amer. Sociol. Rev.* 28, 963 (1963); T. R. Sarbin, *Psychol. Today* 6, 18 (1972); E. Schur, *Amer. J. Sociol.* 75, 309 (1969); T. Szasz, *Law, Liberty and Psychiatry* (Macmillan, New York, 1963); *The Myth of Mental Illness: Foundations of a Theory of Mental Illness* (Hoeber Harper, New York, 1963). For a critique of some of these views, see W. R. Gove, *Amer. Sociol. Rev.* 35, 873 (1970).

4. E. Goffman, *Asylums* (Doubleday, Garden City, N.Y., 1961).

5. T. J. Scheff, *Being Mentally Ill: A Sociological Theory* (Aldine, Chicago, 1966).

6. Data from a ninth pseudopatient are not incorporated in this report because, although his sanity went undetected, he falsified aspects of his personal history, including his marital status and parental relationships. His experimental behaviors therefore were not identical to those of the other pseudopatients.

7. A. Barry, *Bellevue Is a State of Mind* (Harcourt Brace Jovanovich, New York, 1971); I. Belknap, *Human Problems of a State Mental Hospital* (McGraw Hill, New York, 1956); W. Caudill, F. C. Redlich, H. R. Gilmore, E. B. Brody, *Amer. J. Orthopsychiat.* 22, 314 (1952); A. R. Goldman, R. H. Bohr, T. A. Steinberg, *Prof. Psychol.* 1, 427 (1970); unauthored, *Roche Report* 1 (No. 13), 8 (1971).

8. Beyond the personal difficulties that the pseudopatient is likely to experience in the hospital, there are legal and social ones that, combined, require considerable attention before entry. For example, once admitted to a psychiatric institution, it is difficult, if not impossible, to be discharged on short notice, state law to the contrary notwithstanding. I was not sensitive to these difficulties at the outset of the project, nor to the personal and situational emergencies that can arise, but later a writ of habeas corpus was prepared for each of the entering pseudopatients and an attorney was kept "on call" during every hospitalization. I am grateful to John Kaplan and Robert Bartels for legal advice and assistance in these matters.

9. However distasteful such concealment is, it was a necessary first step to examining these questions. Without concealment, there would have been no way to know how valid these experiences were; nor was there any way of knowing whether whatever detections occurred were a tribute to the diagnostic acumen of the staff or to the hospital's rumor network. Obviously, since

my concerns are general ones that cut across individual hospitals and staffs, I have respected their anonymity and have eliminated clues that might lead to their identification.

10. Interestingly, of the 12 admissions, 11 were diagnosed as schizophrenic and one, with the identical symptomatology, as manic-depressive psychosis. This diagnosis has a more favorable prognosis, and it was given by the only private hospital in our sample. On the relations between social class and psychiatric diagnosis, see A. deB. Hollingshead and F. C. Redlich, *Social Class and Mental Illness: A Community Study* (Wiley, New York, 1958).

11. It is possible, of course, that patients have quite broad latitudes in diagnosis and therefore are inclined to call many people sane, even those whose behavior is patently aberrant. However, although we have no hard data on this matter, it was our distinct impression that this was not the case. In many instances, patients not only singled us out for attention, but came to imitate our behaviors and styles.

12. J. Cumming and E. Cumming, *Community Ment. Health*, 1, 135 (1965); A. Farina and K. Ring, *J. Abnorm. Psychol.* 70, 47 (1965); H. E. Freeman and O. G. Sim-mons, *The Mental Patient Comes Home* (Wiley, New York, 1963); W. J. Johannsen, *Ment. Hygiene* 53, 218 (1969); A. S. Linsky, *Soc. Psychiat.* 5, 166 (1970).

13. S. E. Asch, *J. Abnorm. Soc. Psychol.* 41, 258 (1946); *Social Psychology* (Prentice-Hall, Englewood Cliffs, 1952).

14. See also I. N. Mensh and J. Wishner, *J. Personality* 16, 188 (1947); J. Wishner, *Psychol. Rev.* 67, 96 (1960); J. S. Bruner and R. Tagiuri, in *Handbook of Social Psychology*, G. Lindzey, Ed. (Addison-Wesley, Reading, Mass., 1954), vol. 2, pp. 634–654; J. S. Bruner, D. Shapiro, R. Tagiuri, in *Person Perception and Interpersonal Behavior,* R. Tagiuri and L. Petrullo, Eds. (Stanford Univ. Press, Stanford, Calif., 1958), pp. 277–288.

15. For an example of a similar self-fulfilling prophecy, in this instance dealing with the "central" trait of intelligence, see R. Rosenthal and L. Jacobson, *Pygmalion in the Classroom* (Holt, Rinehart & Winston, New York, 1968).

16. E. Zigler and L. Phillips, *J. Abnorm. Soc. Psychol.* 63, 69 (1961). See also R. K. Freudenberg and J. P. Robertson, *A.M.A. Arch. Neurol. Psychiatr.* 76, 14 (1956).

17. W. Mischel, *Personality and Assessment* (Wiley, New York, 1968).

Misdiagnosis of Senile Dementia: Denial of Care to the Elderly

Marjorie Glassman

Older persons who, for a variety of physical and psychological reasons, become confused, disoriented as to time and place, forgetful, and sometimes delusional, are frequently diagnosed as being senile or having senile dementia. This can sometimes become a "wastebasket" diagnosis that serves to deny adequate medical care to the confused elderly, the implication being that their situation is hopeless anyway. For that reason, senile dementia is one of the most serious medical diagnoses possible. It implies gradual, unrelenting, irreversible deterioration of the mind resulting from brain damage or atrophy of unknown origin.

In spite of the implications of this prognosis, older people are often called senile without the benefit of even routine medical tests. Although mental failure can be caused by brain damage, it can also be the result of reversible medical and psychiatric conditions, such as anemia, malnutrition, depression, reactions to medication, hypothyroidism, congestive heart failure, and many others.[1] Research has indicated widespread failure to diagnose and treat causes of reversible acute brain syndrome and symptoms of mental failure. When conditions causing such acute brain syndrome are not treated, they can become chronic and irreversible.[2]

This article will discuss a series of clients seen by social workers who are geriatric specialists in the Service for Older People of the Family Service Association of Greater Boston. Some of these clients were erroneously labeled senile under circumstances that had serious effects on their life and health. They

were receiving substandard medical care in a community in which high-quality medical care was available through home medical teams, primary care clinics, and neighborhood health centers.

These cases are presented to show that social workers have to function as both skilled clinicians and forceful advocates for clients who are deprived of adequate medical care. The social workers in these cases recognized the importance of psychosocial factors in the differential diagnosis of senile dementia. They took complete psychosocial histories, evaluated the clients' current social functioning, and looked for factors in the clients' life that could cause symptoms of mental failure. Sharing this vital information with physicians and hospital staff was insufficient in many cases to obtain adequate medical care for the client. The workers' clinical assessments frequently had to be combined with advocacy, including filing complaints with hospitals and helping the clients find other sources of medical care. The social workers had to function as independent professionals rather than follow medical orders. Several cases also illustrated how teamwork between physician and social worker resulted in the development of a comprehensive care plan and facilitated accurate diagnosis.

Butler feels that medical neglect and disinterest in the elderly reflect society's negative attitudes about old people. In a medical context, this attitude manifests itself as lack of interest and understanding of the special medical and psychiatric problems of the aged, denial of access to emergency care, careless prescribing of medication, and inadequate diagnostic procedures for the confused client.[3] Findings from the cases handled by the geriatric social workers in the Service for Older People illustrate the problems that Butler outlined, and several examples are presented in this article. Many of these incidents of misdiagnosis illustrate serious neglect of clients' medical needs. The staff also share Wershow's conclusion that

> it is little short of criminal to casually dismiss an aged patient as senile or arteriosclerotic without careful and thorough medical-social evaluation, and to "put him/her away" in the socially unstimulating and medically nihilistic environment of the average nursing home where untreated pathology is more likely to reach a stage of irreversibility.[4]

However, the picture is not entirely bleak. The number of excellent medical facilities for older clients are increasing, particularly in urban areas. Home medical teams with geriatric specialists, primary care centers in hospitals, and clinics specializing in the diagnosis of senile dementia are being developed. Although social workers assist clients in need of care by making referrals, they also need to be involved in mobilizing the community to help older people gain access to good medical care.

PSYCHOSOCIAL EVALUATION

Geriatric social workers have specialized skills in understanding the interplay of psychological, social, and biological factors that might cause the client to manifest symptoms of mental failure. These workers have an important role in the differential diagnosis of senile dementia. A team approach is one of the best ways to evolve both a correct diagnosis and a comprehensive treatment plan. Diagnostic errors are rarely found among home medical teams or hospital-based primary care programs, in which the staff take care to obtain a meaningful history and give attention to psychological and social factors that can cause problems in the client's mental functioning.

A vital role for the social worker is compiling the necessary information and making a careful evaluation of emotional, cultural, reality, and socioeconomic factors affecting the client, including both the present situation and past history of social functioning. Detailed information in some of the following areas is particularly relevant to the differential diagnosis of senility: client's nutritional habits, types and use of medication, social and personal network, quality and quantity of medical care, and circumstances surrounding the onset of symptoms. Older people who have several different medical specialists are particularly at risk because of the danger of taking conflicting medications. The experience of the Service for Older People indicates that one of the most important factors to consider is the symptoms' abruptness of onset. Sudden onset appears to indicate the client's behavior is due to causes other than senile dementia.

Neighbors, family, and friends can sometimes supply information that the confused client is unable to remember. Social workers in this program have found, however, that the client is usually the best source of information about psychological and social factors that may relate to his or her behavior. A warm, trusting relationship, patience, and frequent contact with the client can provide diagnostic material and also be therapeutic in improving the client's social functioning.

Butler has described the "emergency room hustle" as a way for medical personnel to avoid dealing thoroughly with the problems of older persons.[5] This involves giving clients a cursory examination, deciding there is nothing drastically wrong with them, and sending them home. Because clients' symptoms are often blamed on senility, the social worker has to become a strong advocate for the client. The following case is an example of the interplay between psychological, social, and medical factors that cause confused behavior.

> Mrs. A, 89 years old and housebound with arthritis, congestive heart failure, and hypertension, requested counseling to help her decide whether to enter a nursing home. She was deeply depressed because her two brothers, now in their nineties, could no longer travel the twenty miles to see her. In the previous few months she had lost weight and was periodically troubled by diarrhea. In the worker's estimation, Mrs. A's intellect was intact, but she had multiple-risk factors for developing acute brain syndrome. Mrs. A's depression and loneliness caused loss of appetite and probable malnutrition, a common cause of confused behavior among the elderly who are misdiagnosed as being senile. She was taking diuretics, the standard treatment for her congestive heart failure and hypertension. Prolonged

diarrhea can be a serious problem for the elderly who take diuretics because of the danger of dehydration and chemical imbalance.

Mrs. A's source of medical care was a clinic where she rarely saw the same doctor. The social worker's plan was to provide Mrs. A with counseling for her depression and the opportunity to decide about placement. Arrangements were made for a hot lunch program, a home medical team, and a friendly visitor. Before these plans were put into effect, Mrs. A had a sudden episode of confusion, disorientation, and general weakness and went to the emergency room of the hospital. She was examined briefly and sent home with an appointment at the medical clinic in two weeks. She was seen as just a lonely, senile old lady looking for attention.

The worker intervened by calling the hospital's emergency department. She provided information about factors that could have caused Mrs. A's confused state. She then called the hospital social worker to meet the client, who was sent back to the emergency room. The hospital social worker acted as an advocate for the client in obtaining a complete medical evaluation. Mrs. A was admitted to the hospital and treated for a severe case of dehydration, which could have been fatal. The client was kept in the hospital until it was possible to place her in a nursing home near her brothers, who now could visit her several times a week.

EFFECTS OF MEDICATION

Prescribing medication for the elderly is particularly difficult, and their use of drugs should be rigorously monitored. Medications that are effective and safe with younger people may cause serious side effects in older people, who metabolize drugs at a different rate. Problems with medication become particularly serious when additional drugs are given to treat symptoms that are side effects of the original medication.

The geriatric social worker therefore needs to be knowledgeable about drugs and their side effects. Part of the assessment of elderly clients should include a list of drugs they take and the dosages,

whether they take the medication as prescribed, and if it is used in combination with alcohol. Medications should be checked in the *Physician's Desk Reference* and any side effects reported to the physician.[6] Particular attention must be given to the client who combines alcohol with barbituates, tranquilizers, or antidepressants. These combinations cause serious side effects and can be fatal.

For the elderly, confusion is a common side effect of antidepressants. When this results, the benefits of the drug may be nullified by the client's anxiety about memory loss and fears of "going crazy." The following case example illustrates the chain of events that can result from improper use of medication.

Mrs. D, age 76, was an intelligent, able person who had had an active life. However, she was beginning to slow down with advancing age and verbalized feelings of depression. Mrs. D refused to see a social worker for counseling. At the request of the family, her physician prescribed an antidepressant drug for her, although the social worker warned them about the potential side effects.

Several months later the family called the worker in a state of panic. Although initially Mrs. D had responded to the medication with slight decrease in depression, she also experienced mild forgetfulness that began to frighten her. She then developed dizziness and episodes of hypotension alternating with hypertension. The physician placed her on medication for high blood pressure. Although previously healthy, Mrs. D began to feel that she was "falling apart" and became very depressed. The final blow came when she fell, breaking her finger, and needed help to care for herself. She became agitated and could not sleep, so the physician prescribed sleeping pills. Mrs. D became so confused that she had to be hospitalized and then transferred to a nursing home. She had to be tied to the bed at night or she would wander and end up in another patient's bed. All the medical tests were negative.

The worker felt the client's problems were related to the medication, complicated by an acute reactive depression. She recommended a psychiatric consultation. The consulting psychiatrist diagnosed the problem as senile dementia but felt that Mrs. D's condition could be improved with changes in medication and with counseling, which was provided at the nursing home. After several months of treatment, Mrs. D went home. She no longer took any antidepressant medication, blood pressure drugs, or sleeping pills. She was completely independent and showed no symptoms of senile dementia, although she continued to manifest a mild chronic depression. Mrs. D's family was referred to the agency's family life education group, called "Understanding Your Aging Parent," to help them become more competent in dealing with Mrs. D's medical and psychological problems.

INADEQUATE DIAGNOSIS

Many of the case examples presented in this article of misdiagnoses of senile dementia were the results of poor or incomplete medical workups. Diagnoses were often based on impressions or observation of behavior without case histories or medical or neurological examinations. The social workers had to advocate vigorously for the necessary medical evaluation. A common excuse for inadequate treatment was that the client was "old and senile anyway," as in the following case history.

Mrs. G, age 72, was a community leader, with good coping abilities in times of stress. Over a period of six weeks she became confused and delusional. In view of the client's history of good social functioning and the abruptness of the symptoms' onset, the social worker contacted Mrs. G's physician to request psychiatric and neurological consultation. The doctor refused, saying that Mrs. G was probably just getting a little senile. The worker then convinced Mrs. G to get a complete medical evaluation at the medical center, where it was discovered that she had an active case of syphillis. After treatment, her delusions disappeared, and she returned to normal functioning.

The devastating effect of poor medical care is illustrated in the following cases. The physicians did not carry out even the most routine tests normally included in a general physical examination, although the elderly patients showed marked symptoms of serious illness.

Miss K, age 83, had become completely disoriented and incontinent and was unable to tolerate any solid food for two months. Her physician made the diagnosis of senile dementia. Miss K's decline in health had begun the previous year with weight loss and general debilitation. She had been to her physician at least five times during the previous year. On each visit the doctor took her blood pressure and consoled her sister about the increasing symptoms of mental failure, but not once performed even a routine physical examination or gave any treatment to alleviate the client's acute discomfort.

This case was referred for social work intervention to provide concrete help and emotional support for the sister, who was Miss K's caretaker. When the worker saw Miss K, she was partly naked, lying on her bed. She appeared emaciated, and there was tumorous mass the size of a grapefruit protruding from her abdomen. The worker immediately called for medical assistance. That night Miss K began to hemorrhage and was taken to the hospital, where she died of cancer three days later.

Miss S, age 62, began to show symptoms of memory loss, confusion, and disorientation. The worker was called in to provide counseling and contacted Miss S's physician. The physician was reluctant to examine Miss S, who, he felt, was becoming prematurely senile due to alcohol abuse. He finally saw her at the request of the worker and spent the time lecturing Miss S on the evils of alcohol.

The worker made a careful assessment, determining that the client occasionally went on a binge but was not a serious alcohol abuser. The worker arranged for a medical evaluation at another facility, where they found Miss S had hypothyroidism. Her face had the characteristic appearance of a person affected with myxedema. Miss S's confusion completely disappeared after replacement therapy with thyroid preparation. The worker continued counseling with the client concerning her drinking problem, and a change in medical care was made.

HOSPITALIZATION

Many older people have adverse reactions to hospitalization. Separated from their familiar surroundings and in heightened states of anxiety, they become more easily confused and disoriented and sometimes become delusional. The sequelae to many illnesses and medical procedures, particularly prostate problems, heart conditions, and surgery, may leave elderly people in agitated, depressed states. During hospital stays, when the elderly are at their most disoriented, it is easy to make inappropriate plans, such as nursing home placements, that lead to irreversible life decisions.

Adverse reactions among the elderly are especially common in newer hospitals that emphasize privacy in accommodations for patients. The social work department in these institutions can help alleviate such stress reactions by providing supportive group work and reality orientation. The staff of the Service for Older People has observed that elderly patients in large, old-fashioned wards, which offer stimulation, emotional support, and companionship, rarely develop the typical symptoms of confusion and disorientation from the stress of hospitalization that the following case example illustrates.

Miss J, an 84-year-old woman, was terrified of entering the hospital for treatment of an ulcerated foot because she feared it would be amputated and she would be placed in a nursing home. She had almost died of a diabetic coma in a previous temporary placement. The worker discussed Miss J's situation with the hospital staff and alerted them that Miss J, who was usually a capable and intelligent person, might react in a disoriented manner under the stress of hospitalization. In fact, Miss J became so anxious, confused, and delusional that the hospital staff tried to persuade her to enter a nursing home. This only caused Miss J more anxiety. The worker intervened and accepted the responsibility for a home care plan for Miss J. The confusion ended as soon as Miss J returned home.

Miss J was so angry about her treatment that she changed doctors and hospitals. During a subsequent hospitalization, the staff was sensitive in dealing with her anxieties and never suggested placement, and Miss J did not exhibit confused behavior.

IMPROVING ACCESS TO CARE

Elderly clients can receive substandard medical care in a community where excellent facilities are available for them. The older client may be unaware of medical resources or may reject them because of their size or location or fear of change.

After Miss K died of cancer, her sister recognized the poor quality of care that her sister had received and was very angry with the family physician. However, she forgave him and continued to see him for her own personal medical care. Her choice to continue with him was based on what she perceived as a lack of medical alternatives in her neighborhood. The physician, however lax, was the last of the neighborhood family practitioners. There was no nearby health center, and going to the large teaching hospital down the street meant seeing a different physician every time. The home medical team did not serve her section of the city. Seeking medical care outside her own neighborhood was not an acceptable option from her viewpoint.

Although the Family Service worker failed to help Miss K or her sister find adequate medical care, part of the problem of poor access to adequate medical care for the elderly in that section was resolved through community action. The social worker organized a task force of health and social agencies serving the elderly in the area. The task force set up an outreach program to find elderly people who needed social services and medical care. The home medical team was contacted and agreed to provide regular service to clients referred by members of the task force. Staff of a nearby hospital attended meetings and established close ties that helped task-force members refer their clients to qualified physicians from the hospital's ambulatory care center. Arrangements could be made through the social service department at the hospital for volunteers to escort elderly clients to the physicians' offices in the building. The task force continues to meet on a regular basis to insure the existence of coordinated social service and health care in the community.

A typical case uncovered during the outreach program was that of a married couple, Mr. and Mrs. M, ages 88 and 86. They were a reclusive, isolated couple, with no friends or family in the community. Mr. M was hesitant about allowing the outreach worker past the door. However, he accepted informational pamphlets, and when the worker discovered they had no regular source of medical care, she explained the couple's options.

The next week, when Mrs. M appeared to be acutely ill, Mr. M called the home medical team, who came immediately. Mrs. M was hospitalized for malnutrition and congestive heart failure. Mr. M had previously been hesitant to seek any medical care for Mrs. M. Her medical problems made her appear confused and feeble, and Mr. M was afraid people might discover that his wife was "crazy" and put her in a nursing home. This is a common reason for older people's failure to seek medical attention.

After treatment Mrs. M's mental functioning improved. Through team efforts of the Home Care Corporation, which provided homemaker services, the home medical team, the Visiting Nurse Association, and the Family Service social worker, the couple was able to remain in the community. The care plan included homemaker and home health aide service, physicians' visits, visiting nurse supervision, and supportive counseling.

TEAMWORK

Although this article has been critical of physicians in their care of the elderly, a growing number of physicians are becoming more skilled and sensitive to the needs of older persons and the benefits of working with a team. As geriatric medicine becomes a real specialty, the author hopes this trend will continue.

The following case posed a difficult diagnostic problem for the social worker and the physician. Close teamwork allowed them to find the cause of the client's symptoms, make an accurate diagnosis, and plan appropriate treatment. Intervention with this client may have saved her life, since her judg-

ment was so impaired at this time that she had continual accidents.

Mrs. H, an 80-year-old client, was successfully treated for a reactive depression following a mastectomy and a heart attack in close succession. A year later, she contacted the worker for assistance. She was having episodes of falling, dizziness, confusion, and disorientation and was both frightened and depressed about the situation. The worker talked to her physician, who was concerned about the possibility of either metastatic cancer or the onset of senile dementia. He gave Mrs. H a battery of medical tests, which were inconclusive.

The worker consulted with the physician, and they developed a plan that included counseling and treatment with a mild antidepressant medication. Household help was obtained for the client's apartment, which was in shambles. The client made no progress for the first three counseling sessions, until the worker uncovered the fact that Mrs. H's closest friend, a younger woman who had been taking her out every week, had moved to Florida. At the same time, Mrs. H's other helpful friend was so preoccupied with the care of her own mother that she had little time for Mrs. H. Mrs. H was then able to talk about her grief and anger about her losses. Within ten sessions her symptoms disappeared and she made arrangements to visit her friend in Florida. During the worker's follow-up visit a year later, Mrs. H appeared in good health with no signs of confusion.

Although all depressed elderly people do not develop symptoms of senility, depression in an elderly person is the most frequent cause of pseudodementia. The incidence of depression in the general population is about 10 percent but may run as high as 50 percent among elderly people who have physical illnesses.[7]

Unfortunately, many social workers play only a limited role with the confused elderly client. Frequently, they are assigned to the task of making a nursing home placement. However, such placements should not be made automatically without doing a careful, detailed psychosocial evaluation. As the cases in this article illustrate, the worker can sometimes uncover psychological and social factors in the client's life that may be the cause of behavior diagnosed as senile dementia. Social workers can help improve service to the elderly by functioning as independent professionals who can make a detailed psychosocial evaluation, question standards of medical care, act as advocates for older clients in obtaining the best possible medical attention, and provide leadership for the community action necessary to help older people gain access to good medical care.

Notes and References

1. Jacob B. Fox, Jordan L. Topel, and Michael Hackman, "Dementia in the Elderly, A Search for Treatable Illnesses," *Journal of Gerontology,* 30 (September 1975), pp. 557–564; Robert N. Butler, *Why Survive? Being Old in America* (New York: Harper & Row, 1975), p. 176; and Leslie Lebow, "Pseudosenility: Acute and Reversible Organic Brain Syndromes," *Journal of the American Geriatrics Society,* 21 (1973), pp. 112–120.

2. Butler, op. cit., pp. 175–176.

3. Ibid., pp. 178–182.

4. Harold Wershow, "Comment: Reality Orientation for Gerontologists," *Gerontologist,* 17 (1977), pp. 297–298.

5. Butler, op. cit., p. 188.

6. *Physicians' Desk Reference* (Oradell, N.J.: Medical Economics Co., 1979).

7. Thomas A. Ban, "Aspects and Treatment of Organic Brain Syndrome," *Journal of Geriatric Psychiatry,* 11 (1978), pp. 143–148.

Social Implications of Screening Programs for Carrier Status: Genetic Diseases in the 1970s and AIDS in the 1980s

Regina Kenen
Robert Schmidt

A national genetic disease program was established with the enactment of the Health Research and Health Services Amendments of 1976.[1, 2] As of November 1977, Congress had yet to provide full funding for the program. This delay may actually serve a useful purpose by allowing time for educational and research endeavors. Advances in applied human genetics have proceeded at a rapid rate, and integration of the new knowledge and technology into the norms and values of the social system have lagged behind. Couples facing reproductive decisions have an array of new options open to them, some inimical to previously held moral and religious beliefs, some offering hope where there was none before, all raising questions for which satisfactory answers are difficult to obtain.

These new developments in genetics require major educational efforts. There is need to design programs for both the general population and the medical community. For example, physician training in the area of applied human genetics needs updating. Many physicians to whom couples might ordinarily turn for advice do not possess the necessary biological expertise or background in medical humanities.

In its original form, this article appeared under the title "Stigmatization of Carrier Status: Social Implications of Heterozygote Genetic Screening Programs" in the *American Journal of Public Health*, vol. 68, no. 11 (November, 1978), pp. 1116–1119.

In 1974 the National Academy of Sciences conducted a survey of physicians' knowledge and attitudes toward genetic screening. It was found that nearly three-fourths of the group reported that no courses in genetics had been available during their medical training.[3] Another recent survey of members of a professional society of obstetricians and gynecologists in the Pittsburgh area revealed that approximately 20 per cent of these physicians did not know that the gene is the basic unit of inheritance, or that Down's syndrome is the result of a chromosomal aberration and sickle-cell anemia a result of an inherited hemoglobin defect.[4]

Moreover, in the early days of large-scale genetic screening programs, a lack of understanding of the complexities involved resulted in organizing efforts that were premature, poorly designed, and had inadequate client safeguards. Health officials, understandably wanting to bring the benefits of promising new technology to the public as rapidly as possible, frequently did not give adequate consideration to possible negative psychosocial and economic consequences. Thus carriers were sometimes denied employment and life insurance because sickle-cell trait and sickle-cell disease were confused.[5, 6]

However, awareness of some of the excesses of previous genetic screening programs is now widespread. Many of the errors have been considered and corrected, but others have not.[7–10] Fortunately, recent publications indicate that psychosocial issues

145

raised by previous genetic screening and counseling programs are beginning to be investigated.[11–14]

The number of genetic diseases and carrier states that can be detected by screening tests continues to grow. Means of effectively treating or preventing many disorders are also increasing, although at a slower pace. Indications for genetic screening programs are: 1) to provide health services; 2) to carry out research; 3) to provide information on reproduction; and 4) to enumerate, monitor, and survey.[15] This paper will stress the third category, providing information on reproduction to prospective parents.

Knowledge of genetic predisposition for a disease, verification of carrier status, or antenatal diagnosis of a genetic disorder may create feelings of inadequacy or strangeness that are themselves damaging to health. The individual may view himself differently and, if the information is public, so may society. Even though geneticists now estimate that each individual carries four to eight recessive deleterious genes, a carrier label cannot be applied to an individual carrying mutant alleles not yet identified. It is the recently achieved technology and ability to identify carriers of a large number of genetic diseases that changes the definition of the situation.

Past experience suggests that people have difficulty in comprehending the concept of probability and risk and that they may misunderstand genetic information presented to them.[16, 17] The concept that genetic mutation can sometimes be beneficial and may, under certain conditions, offer a selective advantage, is often neglected when heterozygote screening programs are explained. Confusion between the carrier state and the disease state may result in the carrier being stigmatized. Public misinformation may even lead to entire ethnic and racial subgroups being stigmatized, a "courtesy stigma" applied to those affiliated only by common ancestry to the stigmatized individuals.[18] These affronts are being afflicted on a group already suffering from a long history of prejudice and discrimination. An example of recent research with potentially stigmatizing effects is a study of the relationship between sickle-cell trait and intelligence.[19] This type of research, involving use of information gathered from a screening program designed to benefit the individuals agreeing to be tested, adds an additional ethical

consideration to the already heated hereditary vs. environmental I.Q. controversy.[20]

Results from the only prospective study of genetic screening and counseling that has been completed illustrate the unanticipated negative consequences that can result even from a carefully planned and executed program. This study was conducted in Orchemenos, a small farming village in Greece;[21] 23 per cent of the population were sickle-cell carriers, and 1 in 100 babies were born with sickle-cell anemia. In this peasant community, about two-thirds of the marriages were still arranged, and health was a factor traditionally considered in the betrothal negotiations. A team of physicians hoped that by screening the population and counseling the villagers about sickle-cell disease and sickle-cell trait, they could persuade the villagers to include information about their genotypes in the marriage arrangements and thus avoid marriages between two sickle-cell carriers.

Seven years later the researchers returned to see how the villagers used the screening and counseling information provided them. They discovered that, although genotype information was shared in these discussions, possession of sickle-cell trait had become a socially stigmatized status, introducing new anxieties into this rural community. After counseling, the number of carrier-carrier matings was the same as if the marriages had occurred randomly in the population. In this village, the educational effort did not lead to objective and rational decision-making or to the desired change in marriage patterns, but to the creation of a new stigmatized status.

This program was undertaken in a rural, traditional society with a cultural heritage different from that of our urbanized, industrial nation. In this small village everyone knew everyone else—a situation typical of social systems based upon primary relationships. As a result of the mass screening effort, carrier status entered into the stratification system of the village along with their reproductive norms and became an "inferior good" on the marriage market. It should be noted, however, that the Orchemenos experience may not be representative of thalassemia screening or sickle-cell screening in the United States. A stigmatized status may not develop as strongly within the more anonymous context typical of American society today. One recent study reported that over 90 per cent of individuals who were sought out and offered counseling, after it was discovered that relatives had hemophilia or muscular dystrophy, claimed that they were gratified that they had been given the opportunity to use this genetic information in their childbearing decisions.[14]

Follow-up studies being carried out by Kaback and associates on their 1973 Tay-Sachs screening programs in Baltimore and Washington will provide more useful data about carrier stigmatization in the U.S. population.[22] Preliminary data suggest that little stigmatization resulted from this program and that there was no evidence of adverse reactions toward interpersonal relations or reproductive decisions. Yet, despite overall approval of the genetic screening program, about one-half of the carriers detected expressed unease in being told they were heterozygotes. These feelings were assuaged by counseling, but some residual anxiety remained.[23] Another study of a Tay-Sachs screening program undertaken in Montreal, Canada high schools showed similar results.[12]

The Tay-Sachs program is quite different from the Greek sickle-cell screening program in several basic ways. The population being screened for Tay-Sachs trait is urban, highly-educated, and sophisticated; moreover, Tay Sachs disease is more readily diagnosed *in utero,* and selective abortion can be chosen as an option. In contrast even if prenatal diagnosis and selective abortion had been an option for the Greek villagers, it is not clear whether it would have been a viable one. A Greek peasant community tends to be religious, and an additional conflict between advances offered by medicine and religious convictions might have erupted. It would be useful to conduct further social-psychological studies of genetic screening programs in American small towns and rural areas before any generalizations are made.

The Greek experience and the experiences of some American Blacks screened for sickle-cell trait in the early 1960s suggest that modern technology may have introduced a new biological and social label—"carrier"—with yet unknown psychological and social consequences. We do not have any direct, cultural experience with a stigmatized carrier status or any cultural tradition to guide us. The newly identified carriers of mutant alleles are, in a sense, both biological and social pioneers. Previous experiences relating social stigma to illness may be relevant.

For example, tuberculosis was heavily stigmatized at the end of the 19th century. The National Tuberculosis Association expended considerable resources to eradicate the stigmatized image. In fact, Susan Sontag cites tuberculosis, along with syphilis and cancer, to be diseases most often used as metaphors for evil during the past two centuries.[24] Even after Villemin published his treatise on the epidemiology of TB and Koch identified the tuberculin bacillus, it took years for the disease to be unequivocably accepted as being caused by a specific transmissible agent.[25]

Ostracism of the severely physically and mentally handicapped, especially if the defect was thought to be of genetic origin, has also been a prevalent social reaction. Only very recently have more enlightened educational approaches to the handicapped been promulgated, including attempts to counteract the stigmatized label and to integrate these individuals into the normal routine of social life. Previously, the handicapped were treated as a stigmatized minority, isolated from the eyes of the world in sheltered workshops and special schools.[26] Although political and educational efforts have wrought tremendous changes, we still too often refer to "handicapped people" and "defective fetuses," rather than to people who *have* specific handicaps or fetuses *with* specific defects. The first usage robs the individual of his normal identity and implies that he is somehow of less value as a human being. To a lesser extent, will a carrier, one who is phenotypically normal but a carrier of a recessive defective gene, be exposed to social stigmatization of this kind? Will his or her freedom of mate selection be restricted? How will these individuals feel about themselves as marital partners and future parents? Will they suffer from self-stigma and entertain doubts about their own worth?

Fear of procreating a child with a severe birth defect has always existed but, without specific information to the contrary, couples usually push this fear into the background and, at least on a superficial level, assume that their baby will be all right.[27] However, when an individual who plans to parent children in the future finds out that he carries a deleterious gene, his self-image is changed. His previous image of being completely healthy (genotypically as well as phenotypically) has been spoiled. No longer can he take for granted that he will have normal offspring, fulfilling society's expectations. According to Erving Goffman,[28] the typical reaction to a spoiled image is to attempt to keep the "failure" secret and compensate in other areas of life. If the individual cannot sustain the injury to his self and adapt to his loss, he often seeks psychological help. In Goffman's terms, the psychotherapist can act as "society's cooler." Perhaps the genetic counselor also acts as "society's cooler" by presenting carriers of genetic defects with acceptable alternatives to biological parenthood and sustaining and supporting couples if they decide either to take a high risk or withdraw from the social role of parent entirely.

Severity of the deleterious gene and visibility of the carrier status are two important factors to consider in an estimation of potential stigma. The degree of severity implies the degree of failure involved. Of course, if prenatal diagnostic tests and selective abortions or, better yet, cures for the diseases are available, the amount of failure is minimized and the resulting stigma is reduced. Moreover, public disclosure of carrier identity influences the types of defenses, strategies, and consolations available to the individual attempting to minimize his or her loss. Using this framework, let us look at the stigma implications for a few genetic disorders.

Tay-Sachs disease is a recessively inherited disorder most frequently occurring among Jews of Eastern European origin. It is characterized by the onset in infancy of developmental retardation, paralysis, dementia, and blindness, ending in death during early childhood. Yet, a combination of screening for carrier status, amniocentesis, and selective abortion of a defective fetus enables a couple to achieve desired normal biological parenthood, provided the couple at risk monitors each pregnancy. Thus, by following these procedures the couple has neither to relinquish socially approved biological parenthood nor to give birth to a defective child.

Sickle-cell anemia is also a recessive hereditary disorder. It is characterized by a chronic anemia related to destruction of red blood cells and damage to various organs. It occurs in approximately 1 in 800 Blacks in the United States. The disease can range from mild to extremely severe. At present, couples at risk for sickle-cell disease do not have the same options available to them as couples at risk for Tay-Sachs disease. A carrier test for sickle-cell trait exists, but no simple prenatal diagnostic technique is now readily available. The couple can either risk being stigmatized for having a sickle-cell child or stigmatized for giving up biological parenthood. The couple can, of course, adopt a child or use artificial insemination with donor sperm, a technique far from being fully accepted.[29]

Hemophilias A and B are lifelong bleeding disorders inherited through the mother. They are caused by a lack of factors VIII or IX respectively in the clotting system. If the mother is a carrier, each of her male children runs a 50 per cent risk of inheriting the defect. Cases vary from mild to moderate to very severe. Individuals suffering from hemophilia have repeated bleeding episodes that can lead to orthopedic, neurological, and other physical and psychological complications. The development of plasma concentrates and freeze-dried factor concentrates has enabled victims to lead more normal lives. The genetic responsibility for the disease is pinpointed for all to see once a hemophilic son is born, but not necessarily before. Scientists are working on carrier tests and prenatal diagnostic techniques, but at present only sex determination is possible. If male fetuses of carrier mothers are aborted, there is a 50 per cent chance that the fetus is afflicted and a 50 per cent chance that it is normal. Couples deciding to abort all male fetuses may also risk social censure for this decision.

Huntington's disease presents a different problem. This degenerative neurological disease is autosomal dominant and does not appear until middle life. A progressive loss in brain cells produces difficulties in speech, muscular control, and motor coordination, as well as changes in personality and intellectual deterioration. Usually, the onset of the disease occurs after the age when most couples have already borne their children. So far, there is no test to determine whether an individual carries the defect. At present, the disorder can be diagnosed only after symptoms appear. Each child of a parent suffering from Huntington's disease has a 50 per cent chance of inheriting the disease, and thus lives his life in a suspect state. He is neither fully stigmatized nor considered fully normal—the label of defective individual lurks in the background of both those eventually afflicted and those who are not. Marriage, parental, and career plans may be in limbo or in jeopardy.

A screening test for Huntington's disease would clarify the status of these individuals, eliminating the uncertainty and freeing the ones found not to be carrying the lethal gene. For those unlucky enough to be carrying the defect, however, uncertainty may be replaced by self and social stigmatization and limitation of opportunities based on the handicapped status expected to occur 30 or 40 years later. Screening tests provide relief for those found not to carry a suspected deleterious gene, but for those identified as possessing the genetic defect, the new technology presents problems as well as benefits.

Goffman's work suggests the need for investigation into the operation of individual and social coping mechanisms. Our present meager information is primarily derived from clinical reports describing experiences of couples at risk in genetic counseling centers and a few studies carried out in conjunction with Tay-Sachs screening programs.[12, 23] Current data suggest that some individuals have difficulty in coping with the carrier status. As yet, we cannot identify the variables most likely to be associated with feelings of self-doubt and the inadequacies stemming from carrier identification. This knowledge is essential for public education aimed at minimizing self and social stigmatization. It would be useful to understand whether males or females are more likely to feel self-stigma. Being a carrier of a recessive genetic defect may strike hard at the male who is frequently expected to be the stronger marital partner in American society. Yet carrier status for a female may be felt even more deeply, because the woman carries the fetus as well. Will self-stigma become stronger in the future if small family size becomes the accepted norm? If couples only have one or two children, and these for psychosocial reasons,[30–32] is the quality of those fewer offspring likely to be more important than it was when children were considered economic assets and large families were common?

Furthermore, reproductive and family values have been traditionally intertwined with ethical and religious beliefs. Yet, we do not know what part an individual's religion affiliation or degree of commitment plays in his ability to accept his carrier status without denigrating his human worth. Two studies indicate that religious couples accept the birth of a child with a severe defect with fewer guilt feelings than do more secularly oriented parents, the event being accepted as "God's will."[33, 34] Will these religious individuals also be more likely to accept carrier status as God's will, thus alleviating their anxieties and feelings of inadequacy?

These are only a few of the issues that require further study; but even the study of these issues may involve latent consequences. The terrain of psychological and sociological implications is delicate to enter. Public discussion helps clarify issues and furthers dissemination of knowledge; yet discussion of these problems may also inadvertently lead to an increase of the stigmatization we are trying to avoid by making a given status more visible and publicly labeling it as a stigmatized one. What may begin as a feeling of unease or as a sense of diffuse anxiety on the part of the individual can become more focused and upsetting when it is given a name and treated as a social problem.

Therefore, educational efforts specifically designed to prevent the onset of self and social stigma may be warranted as part of the planning phase of national genetic screening programs. A careful, deliberate, and thorough approach allows planners time to evaluate results of the few prospective long-term research investigations already being conducted, time to design comprehensive programs based on previous research and to direct future research toward questions still awaiting answers.

AIDS POSTSCRIPT, JANUARY 1986

Current national efforts to implement an effective service and research program for the acquired immune deficiency syndrome (AIDS) have generated problems analogous to the national sickle-cell disease and genetic disease programs of the 1970s. Although the Department of Health and Human Services is using existing legislative authorities to carry out AIDS related functions in the United States Public Health Service, issues of effective implementation of a unified, coordinated national program that protects the rights of the individual remain.

Negative social consequences resulting from genetic screening programs in the early 1970s added "carrier status" to the list of what Goffman called discreditable stigma—those blemishes of person or character that are not immediately perceivable but, if made public, could be stigmatizing.[18] In the 1970s, mass screening of Blacks for the recessive sickle-cell trait was eventually abandoned, largely because the harm caused by social and economic misuse of the information was greater than the personal and public health benefits.

In the mid 1980s, some public health advocates are once again pushing for extensive screening—this time to identify carriers of antibodies to the AIDS virus, which indicates the presence of past and usually present infection. This public health approach is more understandable in the case of an infectious and almost always fatal disease like AIDS, where the immune system is destroyed, than it was with a genetic disease such as sickle-cell anemia. The mass hysteria regarding AIDS, however, provides a social climate that is not very amenable to protecting the rights and privacy of affected individuals or those falsely labeled. The advent of local and national computerized disease registries makes confidentiality even more difficult to protect than it was in the 1970s, and the rapid number of new cases may increase the likelihood that the public will confuse carrier and disease states. Yet AIDS poses a major public health threat. How can both the public good and the individual be best served?

In December 1985, the Centers for Disease Control reported that more than 15,000 cases of AIDS in the United States had been diagnosed and over 7000 deaths had been attributed to AIDS. Currently, the number of new cases is expected to double every 12 to 14 months. Researchers are investigating promising clues in the development of a vaccine against AIDS and drugs that will cure or ameliorate the disease, but so far no breakthrough has been made.

Thus far, AIDS has been largely confined to minority groups in the United States, groups that have been actively lobbying for the same issues those affected by sickle-cell disease lobbied for in the 1970s.

- Increased funding for research and services
- Effective education and prevention programs, especially for the general public
- Increased support of clinical research, including alternative therapies
- Confidentiality; informed consent; protection of human rights; guarantees against loss of job, life, and health insurance
- A coordinated approach by the agencies of the United States Public Health Service

To name a few.

See Table 1 for analogies between sickle-cell and AIDS screening programs.

The public health community needs to decide whether it can incorporate genetic disease screening program guidelines into suggested AIDS screening programs and, most importantly, what it can learn from the 15-year-old national sickle-cell disease experience to prevent unnecessary psychosocial/legal/ethical problems with this "new" disease.

Early problems with the national sickle-cell dis-

TABLE 1   Acquired immune deficiency syndrome. Analogies to the National Sickle-Cell Disease Program

	SCD	AIDS
CLINICAL		
Existing Therapy	−	−
New Therapy	+/−	+/−
ETHICAL/PSYCHOSOCIAL ISSUES		
Involves Minority Groups	+	+
Confidentiality Issues	+	+
Employment Discrimination	+	+
Insurance Discrimination	+	+
National Blood Supply	+	+
Improper Laboratory Diagnosis	+	+
Procreation Decisions	+	+
Social Morals and Values	+	+
Damage to Self-Esteem	+	+
LAWS		
Federal	+	*
State	+	+
FUNDING		
Local Government	+	+
State Government	+	+
Federal Government	+	+
Private	+	+
PUBLIC POLICY		
Lobbies	+	+
State/Local	+	+
Federal	+	+
EDUCATION		
Public	+/−	+/−
Patient/Client	+	+/−

* Have been proposed. The Center for Disease Control is currently using existing authority for surveillance. The National Institute of Health is using existing authority to fund research.

+/− Varies according to location. No uniform national program.

ease program were many, and they parallel many of those facing the development of a national AIDS program today.[15, 35, 36, 42] They included improper laboratory diagnosis, lack of confidentiality of results, stigmatization of carriers, mandatory screening programs, employment disruption, loss of health and life insurance, and inadequate health care services and counseling programs. In 1976, the National Genetic Disease Program, PL 94–278, emphasizing health education and prevention, was passed.[1] Its passage was, in part, due to intensive community-based concern and efforts to reverse the untoward effects of sickle-cell screening. Yet this bill raised further public policy questions that are still unresolved in 1986.[41]

Current public health measures dealing with the spread of AIDS and the care of AIDS patients vary from locale to locale and are in a state of rapid flux. The same troubling issues that plagued the early sickle-cell disease prevention initiatives are resurfacing and being replayed. We will look at a few of the areas of concern.

A New Phase: Approval of a Blood Screening Test

The development of a blood screening test for a specific defect or disease heats up the controversy between advocates of voluntary, private health measures and those promoting aggressive, public health initiatives. This is what happened when a blood test to detect antibodies to the AIDS virus was approved by the Federal Drug Administration in mid-1985 to help rid the nation's blood supply of AIDS-virus contaminated blood.

The Centers for Disease Control estimate that anywhere between 300,000 and 1 million individuals already carry the AIDS virus.[39] Only about 5 to 10 per cent are expected to be at high risk for developing AIDS. Another 10 to 15 per cent are expected to come down with ARC (AIDS related complex), which is less severe and more chronic. The remaining 75 to 80 per cent are not expected to show any symptoms, though they may be infected for life and may be able to transmit the virus to others. Nobody knows for sure. In the face of uncertainty and the possibility of serious harm, the Public Health Service is disseminating information about the transmission of AIDS and is suggesting "safe" sex practices and a healthy life style. The question is whether extensive screening for carriers of antibodies to the AIDS virus (an indicator of past and probable present infection) should be added to the preventive measures already promulgated.

Many ethical and social considerations are at issue. Mass screening programs have a great potential for infringing on individual rights, particularly when a great deal of medical uncertainty exists; the advantages of the screening approach are not overwhelmingly clear; and an already stigmatized minority group is involved. Breaches of confidentiality, false labeling, and the harm to individuals resulting from just the knowledge that they are carriers are crucial concerns.

Issues of Confidentiality and Misuse of Information
Do employers and insurance companies have the right to demand the results of blood screening tests? Will carrier status be used to discriminate in hiring or promoting employees? The military has begun to test recruits, and some individuals who were diagnosed as having AIDS have been discharged. The authorities claim that the discharges were not related to the disease but to the sexual preference that it revealed.[43]

Isolated cases of blacklisting antibody-positive carriers have already occurred and the American Civil Liberties Union is concerned that these injustices are spreading. For example, in Abilene, Texas, a young man is now living on unemployment insurance as an indirect result of his being a good samaritan and giving blood every eight weeks. He was fired from his job as a cafeteria worker in a medical center because he tested positively on the mandatory test now given to all blood donors. Further medical tests showed no sign of AIDS. Hospital officials state that the employee was fired because he told other employees about his condition. The employee denies this and claims that a supervisor told him the hospital received an anonymous letter threatening to disclose his test results.[44]

Insurance companies want access to the screening information, and some want the right to request the blood test from high-risk individuals before issuing them medical insurance. As of the end of 1985, more than 75 insurance companies had requested this information.[38] California and Wisconsin have passed legislation restricting the insurance companies' use of the screening tests for AIDS antibodies. Wisconsin has already modified its position after the state epidemiologist and insurance commission approved the tests as reliable. At the other end of the spectrum, Colorado has the distinction of being the first state to pass a law requiring mandatory reporting of AIDS-antibody-positive individuals by name and address. Other states are likely to follow.

In September 1985, thousands of parents refused to send their children to public schools in the borough of Queens, New York City, because one seven-year-old child with AIDS was allowed to attend school. This child had already attended school for the two previous years without any health problems for herself or others. Later, physicians reevaluating her medical record decided the child probably didn't have AIDS after all. In a town in New Jersey, the nine-year-old brother of a child suspected of having AIDS was prevented from attending school.

The parents in these cases could not accept evidence that the chance of contracting AIDS through casual contact is negligible and that sex and blood are the only confirmed paths of infection. The fact that the AIDS virus has been found in saliva—even though no cases are known to have been transmitted in this manner—became paramount. All of a sudden, parents voiced great concern about little children's proclivity to bite one another. What if the experts were wrong was the repeated worry.

False Labeling   The blood test gives some false negatives (not identifying individuals who have antibodies against the AIDS virus in their blood) and some false positives (identifying people as having antibodies who really do not). A small percentage of individuals register false negative on the test because of yet unknown reasons or because they have so recently been infected that their systems have not yet generated antibodies to the virus. These people are then given the label of "healthy" when they may not be. On the other hand, those with false positive results may be labeled "diseased" when they are in fact healthy.

For example, out of 8 million blood donations each year, 40,000 will be false positives.[39] Another, more sophisticated and more expensive test is needed to detect those falsely labeled. Most blood banks are adding the names of antibody-positive donors, even if the finding has not been confirmed by a second test, to their lists of individuals to be excluded from donating blood. Although this is a justified precaution from a public health perspective, there are problems for the falsely labeled individuals.

According to the American Red Cross regulations issued July 1, 1985, individuals who test positive on a single test only will not be notified. Their names will be kept in the *local* registry and future blood donations will be discarded. Therefore, such individuals may continue to give regular blood donations not knowing that their blood is not being used.[39] They may also face the possibility that the fact their names are on these lists may be leaked.

Self-Knowledge of Carrier Status   The psychological burden can be extremely traumatic for individuals who receive notification that they tested antibody positive. Their lives are turned upside down. They do not know if they ever will develop a full-blown case of AIDS or ARC. They carry this cloud for five years or longer before they can be reasonably sure they will not succumb. One man in Sydney, Australia, committed suicide after receiving his positive result.

Major restrictions on sexual activities and childbearing are recommended. The risk of giving an unborn child AIDS is assumed to be great, but precisely what that risk is or whether all carriers are at equal risk is yet unknown. In New York City, public health officials plan to promote the antibody test aggressively among women who are considered to be at high risk for contracting AIDS. This will be an attempt to intervene in the transmission of the disease. Women who test positive or whose partners test positive are advised to delay childbearing indefinitely.[37]

Those couples who adhere to the warnings relinquish biological parenthood and must psychologically adapt to that loss; those that take a chance bear the responsibility for playing Russian roulette—no easy choice. Couples who carry the sickle-cell trait face similar choices and have expressed similar feelings of inadequacy and conflict.

The American Red Cross plans to notify donors with confirmed positive-antibody findings and to advise them to seek medical evaluation. Their names will be kept on its confidential *national* registry of individuals whose blood is unacceptable. Test sites will provide counseling or counseling referrals to those receiving the positive notification.

Continuing Controversies

Suggestions have been made for mandatory screening of couples seeking a marriage license, pregnant women, health care workers, foodhandlers, teachers, prostitutes, individuals being admitted to hospitals for non-AIDS related reasons, and those applying for medical insurance. What is the purpose of these testing requirements? Are marriage licenses going to be refused to individuals who test antibody positive? Are pregnant women who test positive going to be pressured to have abortions? Are hospital patients who have been exposed to the AIDS virus going to be placed in separate areas? Are workers who test positive going to be fired or placed in jobs where they have little contact with other employees or the public?

As of now, the value of extensive use of the screening test is questioned. Physicians believe that the test is most helpful to people who have a very small chance of infection; for example, those who have had a blood transfusion between 1980 and 1985 and those who will not alter their lifestyles unless they have firm evidence they are harboring the virus. Doctors disagree as to the value of the procedure for most male homosexuals and drug users in major cities. Most of these individuals are believed to be already infected, and the test is not seen to be of proven value in preventing the spread of the disease within these high-risk groups. These individuals need to take precautionary measures whether or not they test positive.

Furthermore, social morality is at issue. In a Gallup Poll taken in November, 1985,[40] one-third of the respondents said that their disapproval of homosexuals has increased as a result of the AIDS epidemic, and a substantial proportion of those interviewed believe that homosexuals should not be members of the armed forces, doctors, members of the clergy, or school teachers. If the public associates being antibody positive with homosexuality, job and housing discrimination may increase both for homosexuals and for those mislabeled as homosexuals.

The surfacing of latent prejudice toward homosexuality and the public's phobic fear of AIDS may shift the delicate balance between the public good and the protection of individual rights. Effective implementation of a unified, coordinated, and comprehensive national program for dealing with AIDS, based on the lessons learned in the 1970s, is a top public health priority. It is necessary to head off an unhealthy siege mentality under which unwarranted and needless quarantines and isolation measures will be promulgated in the guise of public health necessity.

ACKNOWLEDGMENTS

We thank James E. Bowman, MD, Marc D. Hiller, DrPH, Richard Levinson, PhD, and Godfrey P. Oakley, MD, MPH, for reviewing a draft of this manuscript.

References

1. PL 94–278, 94th Congress, HR 7988, April 22, 1976.

2. Schmidt RM and Curran WJ: A national genetic-disease program: Some issues of implementation. N Engl J Med 295:819–820, 1976.

3. National Research Council. Committee for the study of inborn errors of metabolism. In Genetic Screening Programs, Principles, and Research. National Academy of Sciences, Washington, DC, 1975, pp. 161–162.

4. Naylor EN: Genetic screening and genetic counseling: Knowledge, attitudes, and practices in two groups of family planning professionals. Social Biology, 22:304–314, 1975.

5. Gustafson J: Genetic screening and human values: An analysis. In Ethical, Social and Legal Dimensions of Screening for Human Genetic Disease, Bergsma D, ed. New York: Stratton Intercontinental Medical Book Corp., 1974, pp. 201–224.

6. Powledge T: Genetics screening as a political and social development. In Ethical, Social and Legal Dimensions of Screening for Human Genetic Disease, Bergsman D, ed., New York: Stratton Intercontinental Medical Book Corp., 1974, pp. 25–56.

7. Young WI, Peters J, Houser HB and Jackson EB: Awareness of sickle cell abnormalities. A medical and lay community problem. Ohio State Med J 70:27–30, 1974.

8. Hampton ML, et al.: Sickle cell 'nondisease.' A potentially serious public health problem. Am J Dis Child 128:58–61, 1974.

9. Rutkow IM and Lipton JM: Some negative aspects of state health department policies related to screening for sickle cell anemia. Am J Public Health 74:217–221, 1974.

10. Whitten CF and Fischoff J: Psychosocial effects of sickle cell disease. Arch Intern Med 133:681–689, 1974.

11. Hsia YE, Hirschhorn K, Silverberg R, Godmilow L, eds. Counselling in Genetics, New York: Alan Liss, Inc., 1977.

12. Clow C and Scriver CR: Knowledge about and attitudes toward genetic screening among high school students: The Tay-Sachs experience. Pediatrics 59:86–91, 1977.

13. Headings VE: Alternative models of counseling for genetic disorders. Social Biology 22:297–303, 1975.

14. Lubs HA and de La Cruz F: Genetic Counseling, Grand Haven, MI: Raven Press, 1977.

15. National Research Council. Committee for the study of inborn errors of metabolism. Genetic Screening Programs, Principles and Research. National Academy of Sciences, Washington, DC, 1975.

16. Carter C, Roberts JAF, Evans KA and Berck AR: Genetic clinic, a follow-up. The Lancet 1:281–285, 1971.

17. Leonard C, Chase G and Childs B: Genetic counseling: A consumer's view. N Engl J Med 287:433–439, 1970.

18. Goffman E: Stigma: Notes on the Management of Spoiled Identity. Englewood Cliffs, NJ: Prentice-Hall, 1963.

19. McCormack M, et al.: A comparison of the physical and intellectual development of black children with and without sickle-cell trait. Pediatrics 56:1021–1025, 1975.

20. Block N and Workin G: eds. The IQ Controversy. Westminster, MD: Pantheon Books, 1976.

21. Stamatoyannopoulos G: Problems of screening and counseling in the hemoglobinopathies. In Birth Defects: Proceedings of the Fourth International Conference, Motulsky AG and Ebling J, eds. Excerpta Medica, Vienna, 1974, pp. 268–275.

22. Kaback MM, Becker M and Ruth VM: Sociologic studies in human genetics: I. Compliance factors in a voluntary heterozygote screening program. In Ethical, Social and Legal Dimensions of Screening for Human Genetic Disease, Bergsma D, ed., New York: Stratton Intercontinental Medical Book Corp., 1974, pp. 145–164.

23. Childs B, et al.: Tay-Sachs screening: Social and psychological impact. Am J Human Genetics 28:550–558, 1976.

24. Sontag S: Disease as Political Metaphor. The New York Review of Books: 29–33, Feb. 17, 1978.

25. The Encyclopedia Americana. Tuberculosis. New York: Americana Corp., 27:194, 1974.

26. Scott R: The selection of clients by social welfare agencies: The case of the blind. Social Problems 14:248–257, 1967.

27. Apgar V and Beck J: Is My Baby All Right? New York: Pocket Books, 1974.

28. Goffman E: On cooling the mark out. Psychiatry 15:461–463, 1952.

29. Sorenson J: Some social and psychologic issues in genetic screening. In Ethical, Social and Legal Dimensions of Screening for Human Genetic Disease, Bergsma D, ed. New York: Stratton Intercontinental Medical Book Corp., 1974, pp. 165–184.

30. Hoffman LW and Hoffman ML: The value of children to parents, In Psychological Perspectives on Population, Fawcett JT, ed., New York: Basic Books, Inc., 1973, pp. 19–76.

31. Coombs LC: Preferences about sex of children, In Cross Cultural Comparisons: Data on two Factors in Fertility Behavior, Freedman R and Coombs L, eds., the Population Council, New York, 1974.

32. Westoff C and Rindfuss R: Sex preselection in the United States: Some implications. Science 184:633–636, 1974.

33. Levinson RM: Family Crisis and Adaptation: Coping With a Mentally Retarded Child. Doctoral Dissertation, University of Wisconsin, Madison, 1975.

34. Zuk GH: The religious factor and the role of guilt in parental acceptance of the retarded child. Am J Ment Defic 64:139–147, 1959.

35. Bowman JE: Genetic screening programs and public policy. Proceedings of the Conference on the Health of Black Populations, Athens, Georgia: University of Georgia Press, 1977.

36. Chapman CB, Lemke JE: The Status of the Sickle Cell Program, Fiscal Years 71 through 74: An Analysis of Federal Legislation, Federal Support and Public Reaction. Washington, D.C.: Congressional Research Service, 1973.

37. Eckholm E: City in Shift to Make Blood Test for AIDS Virus More Widely Available: The New York Times: B8, December 23, 1985.

38. Kristof N: More Insurers Screen Applicants for AIDS: The New York Times: D1, D4, December 26, 1985.

39. Levine C and Bayer R: Screening Blood: Public Health and Medical Uncertainty. Hasting Center Report: 8–11, August, 1985.

40. The New York Times: 37% in Poll Say AIDS Altered Their Attitudes to Homosexuals: 41: December 15, 1985.

41. Schmidt, RM and Curran W: A national genetic-disease program: Some issues in implementation: N Engl J Med 295:819–820, 1976.

42. Schmidt, RM: Hemoglobinopathy screening: Approaches to diagnosis, education and counseling: Am J Public Health 64:799–804, 1974.

43. Silverman M and Silverman D: AIDS and the Threat to Public Health: Hasting Center Report: 19–22, August 1985.

44. Ziegler, Lou: Safer Blood—But at What Cost? USA Today: 1–2A, Dec. 12, 1985.

Labeling Theory and Community Care of the Mentally Ill in California: The Relationship of Social Theory and Ideology to Public Policy

Paul R. Benson

During the past 20 years, labeling theory has become one of the most influential and controversial theoretical orientations in American social science to the study of deviant behavior. The employment of the perspective has provoked debate in a number of areas (see Gove 1975a), but the most disputed application of labeling theory has probably been to mental illness. The polemic interchanges between labeling theory's proponents and its antagonists regarding this application (Scheff 1975; Gove 1975b; Chauncey 1975; among others) illustrate, I believe, a fundamental clash between two divergent sets of belief regarding the nature of mental disorder: the interactional and the medical models of mental illness (Siegler and Osmond 1974; Begelman 1971). Considering the profound differences between these competing models, it is unlikely that a synthesis of the perspectives can be achieved[1] (see, for example, the comments of Kitsuse and Schur in Gove 1975a).

Rather than adding to the present debate in this area by attempting to demonstrate one model of mental illness to be "more correct" than the other, I will take a different tack in this paper. I will examine, in some detail, one piece of mental health policy, at least in part generated from one of these two opposing conceptualizations—in this case, the interactional or labeling model of mental disorder. I will not focus on traditional evaluative criteria in an assessment of labeling theory. Rather, I will discuss the use of the perspective within the public policy

Reprinted by permission of the Society for Applied Anthropology from *Human Organization*, vol. 39 (Summer, 1980), pp. 134–141.

arena, that is, its employment in the conceptualization, development, and implementation of mental health policy programs.

To date, a rich literature has accumulated concerning public policy implications associated with a medical model of mental illness (Szasz 1960; Goffman 1961; Scheff 1963, 1966; Leifer 1969; Perrucci 1974; Schrag 1978). However, few researchers have directed attention to policy implications of labeling theory in this area. One exception is Back (1975:139–40), who has detailed the *potential* mental health policy implications of labeling theory in the following manner:

> If taken to its logical conclusion, labeling theory would lead to radical changes in mental health policy. Instead of providing more facilities, especially for inpatients, policy would have to be directed toward protecting "residual deviates" from being caught in a bureaucratic network in which they may be stigmatized and changed but from which they rarely benefit. Thus acceptance of this theory would imply a radical change in policy, including the closing, or at least reorganization, of mental hospitals, and either an educational program to improve tolerance of deviance, or designing institutions to protect helpless labeled-individuals from the nefarious influences of the mental health establishment. Merely improving established institutions—or using additional funds to provide more mental health facilities— would only compound current mistakes.

Back correctly alerts us here to the potential consequences of an applied labeling approach to mental disorder and its treatment. This "translation" of theory into policy, however, has already taken place in the state of California where, since 1968, a radically decentralized community mental health program has closed all but a handful of state mental hospitals and released thousands of former psychiatric patients into the community.

An analysis of the California community mental health program, I believe, offers an excellent opportunity to observe labeling theory "in action," so to speak, and to evaluate its usefulness in terms of its application to the development of public policy. This analysis does not, however, suggest a unilinear

causal relationship between labeling theory and California's community mental health program. Many who advocated the deinstitutionalization of mental health services in the state during the late 1960s and early 1970s did not express their views in terms of the labeling perspective. Arguments based on labeling theory (as well as on associated antipsychiatric models of mental illness) were one of a number of factors influencing mental health politics in California at the time.[2]

The effect of labeling theory on contemporary California mental health treatment policy has been profound. Weiss (1975, 1977), in this regard, has suggested two major (although largely unacknowledged) uses of social science theory and research in the public policy arena. The first is the "sensitization" of political decision makers to certain problems and methods for dealing with them. The second covert use of social science in the policy process, according to Weiss, is as "political ammunition," employed by political partisans to legitimate or discredit policy proposals and programs. Labeling theory, I suggest, served both of these implicit policy functions in the case of community mental health in California during the late 1960s and early 1970s. Initially, the perspective served to focus state decision makers on mental health (specifically, the issue of involuntary civil commitment) as an area for legislative reform. Later in the policy process, the labeling perspective provided policymakers with a coherent intellectual and ideological rationale for their actions.

Due to the pervasive relationship between these two developments, labeling theory significantly influenced both the scope and the content of the California mental health program. I believe that this affinity, unfortunately, led to a number of major problems in the implementation of the California policy. These problems are at least partly due to the incorporation into policy of several problematic features of the labeling perspective; in particular, the failure to adequately consider the consequences of unlabeled deviant behavior. Placed in this framework, this paper may be viewed as a case study in the interrelationship of social theory, social ideology, and public policy, as well as an examination of the responsibility of social scientists in the application of their work to the "real world" of political decision making and policy development.

LABELING THEORY AND THE CONSPIRATORIAL MODEL OF MENTAL ILLNESS

The general thrust of the labeling position is, by this time, a fairly familiar one to most social scientists; thus, my description of the perspective will be brief.[3] In essence, labeling theory shifts major theoretical attention in the study of deviance from a question of etiology to one of how persons come to be *defined* by others as deviant and in need of social control. From the labeling viewpoint, variables characterizing the interactional milieu of the defined deviant assume critical importance, although initial acts of unlabeled rule-breaking behavior receive little attention. Actual deviant behavior is assumed by most proponents of the perspective to be relatively inconsequential; it is the labeling process which generates social deviance.

Scheff's concept of mental illness (1966) is one of labeling theory's most important contributions to the study of deviant behavior. Briefly, Scheff posits the roots of the mental illness label to lie in the continued violation of commonly held, but implicit, social norms which he terms "residual rules." Once the residual rule-breaker becomes labeled by others as "being mentally ill," and becomes involved with social control agents, such as the police, the courts, and mental health professionals, the deviant is basically assured of hospitalization and formalization of the mentally ill role. Continued treatment, rather than benefiting the patient, serves instead to finalize the deviant role through a process of institutionalization.

To fully understand the ideological underpinnings of Scheff's theory, it should be viewed as part of a more comprehensive orientation toward mental illness and its treatment. This orientation has been referred to by various authors as the "sociological" (Leifer 1969), "communal" (Perrucci 1974) or "conspiratorial" (Siegler and Osmond 1974) model of mental illness. Numbered among the proponents of this model are Szasz, Sarbin, Laing, Leifer, and (in some of his writings, e.g. *Asylums*) Goffman. Within the conspiratorial model it is assumed that:

> . . . *the person labeled as mad is not different than the rest of us* [*who are not so labeled*], *but*

> *for some poorly understood reason . . . members of his society choose to call attention to some of his acts, label them as deviant, and move against him in a concerted fashion.* [*Siegler and Osmond 1974:65–66*]

Or as Perrucci (1974:17) has noted: "[Within the conspiratorial model] persons called mentally ill are not seen as patients, but as *victims*" (emphasis in original).

The basic theoretical and ideological thrust of Scheff and the other conspiratorial theorists is the same: each places primary emphasis on interactional processes in the genesis of mental disorder. In their opinion, before labeling, "mental illness" is a relatively inconsequential disruptive and maladaptive form of personal behavior. They perceive the defined mentally ill deviant as the passive victim of an arbitrary labeling process, the mental health profession as a coercive agency of social control, and psychiatric treatment as, at best, of little or no benefit to patients (and, at worst, actively harmful to them). Finally, as Siegler and Osmond (1974:69) have noted: "Szasz, Lain, Goffman, Scheff, and others using the conspiratorial model have stated or implied that the elimination of the category, 'mental illness,' would end the suffering of those so labeled." As we shall see, these ideological tenets have significant public policy implications.

LABELING THEORY AND THE DEVELOPMENT OF COMMUNITY MENTAL HEALTH IN CALIFORNIA

Though the movement toward decentralization of California mental health services dates from the late 1950s, the documented association between labeling theory and mental health policy in the state begins in 1965.[4] During that year, the California legislature enacted a large-scale experimental community treatment program in the area of mental retardation (California Assembly Subcommittee 1965a). This program marked the first major legislative victory of the then newly created Subcommittee on Mental Health Services of the California State Interim Committee on Ways and Means and its chairperson, Assemblyman Jerome R. Waldie.[5]

Encouraged by its initial success in the mental

retardation field, Waldie and the subcommittee were anxious to turn their attention to the area of mental health as well. At this time, a staff assistant to the subcommittee with ties to the California academic community arranged for Arthur Bolton, Waldie's chief assistant, to read a research report by a student of Erving Goffman's (then at the University of California at Berkeley). The student's report dealt with the workings of a state civil commitment court she had observed.[6] Its findings were unsettling: the average length of the hearings observed was a brisk 4.1 minutes, with involuntary hospitalization recommended in nearly all cases. In addition, the author of the report noted that often commitment cases were heard without the presence of legal counsel on the part of the alleged mentally ill defendant.

Spurred on by this early report, the subcommittee proceeded to gather additional evidence regarding the civil commitment process in the state. As Bardach (1972:102) summarizes:

> During the next few months Bolton and Waldie obtained two more pieces of graduate research, one by a law student . . . and the other by a student of Thomas Scheff at UC-Santa Barbara. The latter documented the perfunctory nature of the prehearing examination in the psychiatric observation ward of one county hospital [see Note 7]. In this particular unit the research reported the average psychiatric interview lasted four or five minutes.

Reviewing this material, Waldie, Bolton, and the subcommittee concluded that they had found their issue and they systematically began to push for the abolition of civil commitment in the state and the general reform of the California mental health treatment system.[8]

As part of this process, during late 1965 and early 1966 the subcommittee held preliminary public hearings in Los Angeles and San Francisco. A number of groups were represented at these hearings and speakers included psychiatrists, public defenders, social workers, hospital administrators, and social scientists. Included among the speakers at the Los Angeles hearing was Thomas Scheff. Scheff's testimony dealt primarily with his research on civil commitment in Wisconsin (Scheff 1963, 1964), as well as on his recommendations for changes in the California mental health law. In addition, he noted:

> It is my judgment from a scientific point of view [the notion that mental illness is a disease] is a dubious proposition for most of the cases that we are concerned with. . . . We're dealing in the mental hospital system largely with other kinds of problems—non-conformers, various kinds of psychological problems, economic problems, sometimes problems of physical disease, welfare problems. I think that in the long run it will be shown that trying to treat these problems under the classification of mental illness and disease is a mistaken one. [California Assembly Subcommittee 1965b:40–41]

Scheff later noted that his testimony "greatly impressed" subcommittee members. His opinion, I believe, is substantiated by the fact that his advice on the development of the LPS Act and other mental health reforms was solicited by the assembly subcommittee staff throughout 1966 and 1967. Indeed, Scheff's influence on the work of the subcommittee was so pervasive that Bolton related to Scheff at the time that his book, *Being Mentally Ill* (1966), "was their bible" (Scheff 1979—personal communication).

In June of 1966, the assembly subcommittee contracted with a research firm, Social Psychiatric Associates of San Francisco, to carry out a number of studies on the civil commitment process in the state. The director of the firm was Dr. Dorothy Miller. It was Miller's paper on the "county lunacy hearings" (written while she was a graduate student at Berkeley) that had initially drawn Bolton and Waldie's attention to civil commitment as a potential area for reform a year and a half earlier. Miller's description of Social Psychiatric Associates was that of "a group of researchers . . . engaged in a series of social surveys on the community careers of persons *labeled as deviant*" (cited in Bardach 1972:107, emphasis in original).[9] The Miller group, grounded largely in the labeling model, played a significant role in the production of a highly influential background report written by Bolton and the subcommittee staff regarding the problem of civil commitment and mental hospitalization in the state. The report, entitled *The Dilemma of Mental Commitments in California,* was released in late 1966—less than a year before the passage of the LPS Act.

The 200-page document, liberally sprinkled with

references to and quotations by labeling and conspiratorial theorists,[10] questioned the basic wisdom of state mental hospital care for the mentally disturbed and proposed broad changes in the organization of mental health treatment in the state. The influence of labeling theory on the report is clear. Early in the document, "mental illness" is defined as ". . . a non-scientific, generalized, popular label used to explain or describe a wide range of behavior which is considered "peculiar" or "sick" or "objectionable" (California Assembly Subcommittee 1966:9). The report continues:

> It is also evident that when a person's behavior is labeled as "mental illness," those who do the labeling are guided by their own conceptions of what is normal and abnormal. Madness, like beauty, may exist in the eye of the beholder. [Ibid.: 11]

The recommendations of the subcommittee report were wide-ranging. They included: the repeal of existing state commitment laws; the limitation of involuntary psychiatric hospitalization to a maximum of 17 days; the conversion of California state hospitals to short-term, voluntary "open-hospitals"; and the creation within each county of community mental health crisis units. The report concluded its recommendations by noting: "When these steps are taken, the state hospitals as we know them, will no longer exist" (ibid.:105).

The LPS Act, passed by the California legislature and signed into law by Governor Reagan in August of 1967, incorporated many of the recommendations of the subcommittee report. Prior state commitment laws were repealed and replaced by a set of statues which greatly increased the difficulty of initiating involuntary treatment. Concurrently with the enactment of LPS in 1968, the California legislature mandated the creation of community mental health programs for all counties in the state with a population of 100,000 or more (before that, such programs were voluntary on the part of each county). In addition, the legislature increased the state's share of mental health costs to 90% of the total (up from a previous state–county funding formula of 50–50% and 75–75%). The joint impact of these related pieces of mental health legislation was to discourage use of state hospitals by the counties, while at the same time encouraging (through legislative fiat and financial incentives) the creation of community-care facilities and programs. Major responsibility for the care of California's mentally ill shifted from the state to the local counties.

During 1969, the Reagan administration began to close mental hospitals for the mentally ill. By 1973, three state institutions had been completely shut down and mentally ill patients removed from several others (mentally retarded remain in these latter facilities). In 1973, the California Department of Mental Hygiene announced its intention of closing all state hospitals for the mentally ill by 1978 and all state hospitals for the retarded by 1981. While this plan has been temporarily shelved by the current administration of Governor Brown, the deinstitutionalization of mental health services in the state has continued largely unabated.[11]

THE IMPACT OF DEINSTITUTIONALIZATION

Although there have been many ramifications of the decentralization of California's mental health program (see ENKI 1972; Segal and Aviram 1978), the most obvious and dramatic effect of the policy has been the rapid depopulation of the state's mental institutions. In the first two years following the enactment of the LPS Act, the mentally ill patient population of the California state hospital system declined by one-third—from 18,831 in 1968 to 12,671 in 1970 (see Table 1). From 1970 to 1975, the patient population again declined dramatically—this time by nearly one-half—to a low of 6,458.

As the patient population of the California state hospitals has dropped, an increasing proportion of state mental health funds has shifted from the hospitals to community services. This trend is clearly shown in Table 2, which depicts state funding for the mentally ill for selected years between FY 1958 and 1978. During this 20-year period, two-thirds of California's total state mental health budget was shifted to community-care services. In FY 1958, for example, only 1.1% of the state mental health budget went to local programs. By FY 1968, 10 years later, community mental health funding had increased to 22.4% of the state mental health budget. In FY 1978, this figure had risen to 69.9%. With the ascendancy of community mental health in California, what have

TABLE 1   Year end mentally ill patient population, California State Hospital System (fiscal years 1961 through 1976)

FISCAL YEAR	YEAR END PATIENT POPULATION
1960–61	36,851
1961–62	36,048
1962–63	35,743
1963–64	34,955
1964–65	32,622
1965–66	30,193
1966–67	26,557
1967–68	21,966
1968–69	18,831
1969–70	16,116
1970–71	12,671
1971–72	10,814
1972–73	8,179
1973–74	7,011
1974–75	6,689
1975–76	6,468

Source: California State Department of Health (1977).

been the consequences of the policy for the mentally ill, especially the severely and chronically disturbed former residents of the state's mental institutions?

Following Kirk and Therrein (1975), in the following discussion I will place primary emphasis on three major aspects of the California community-care program and its impact on the mentally ill: (1) the *rehabilitation* of the mentally ill within a community context; (2) their *reintegration* back into the community; and (3) the *quality and continuity of care* provided by community-based mental health services in the state.

Rehabilitation

One major ideological tenet which buttressed the deinstitutionalization movement in California (and elsewhere) was the belief that mental hospitalization hurt the patient more than it helped, and that treatment within the patient's own community—close to family, friends, and job—would facilitate rapid recovery and rehabilitation. However, a large percentage of the patients released from California state hospitals during the early 1970s had nowhere to go. They had neither family nor friends who desired their return, nor the financial or social resources necessary to maintain themselves in the community in an autonomous fashion (Lamb and Goertzel 1971; Place and Weiner 1974). Many had lost all personal identification with the outside world. The hospital was their "home"; the community was an alien environment. In sum, many released mental patients were unable to exist outside the hospital without considerable support (Segal 1975). One major attempt to mitigate this problem was the development of community-based "sheltered-care" facilities for the California mentally ill during the early 1970s.

According to Segal and Aviram (1978), by 1977 there were approximately 1,115 sheltered-care facilities in California serving 12,400 mentally disordered individuals between the ages of 18 and 65. These facilities vary a great deal in terms of size and quality. They include halfway houses, small "family-care" homes, larger "board and care" homes, and "skilled nursing facilities" or nursing homes. Let us examine these two latter sheltered-care facilities somewhat more closely.

The board and care (B & C) homes are the most common form of sheltered-care facility employed in

TABLE 2   California state mental health budget (selected fiscal years)

FISCAL YEAR	TOTAL BUDGET	LOCAL PROGRAMS	STATE HOSPITAL	STATE HOSPITAL
1957–58	$ 69,324,545	$ 786,000	$ 68,538,545	98.9%
1962–63	97,306,939	3,225,000	94,081,939	96.6
1967–68	135,888,281	23,901,030	111,987,251	78.6
1972–73	198,913,087	124,537,980	74,375,107	37.4
1977–78	337,893,792	229,761,737	101,572,966	30.1

Source: Teknekron, Incorporated. Improving California's Mental Health System: A Framework for Public Contributions. Report prepared for the California Assembly Permanent Subcommittee on Mental Health and Departmental Disabilities, September 1977. Berkeley: Teknekron, Inc., Health and Human Sciences Division.

California. They care for a full 82% of the state sheltered-care population and comprise 72% of California's sheltered-care facilities (Segal and Aviram
1978). B & C homes are privately owned and operated
boarding houses which specifically serve the community-based mentally ill. They are profit-making enterprises and are generally operated by nonlicensed
and untrained personnel. Federal disability (Supplemental Security Income) funding is, in most instances, the sole means of support enjoyed by B & C
home residents. Very little or no rehabilitative activities are provided in the vast majority of these facilities (Wolpert 1974; Segal and Aviram 1978). Evidence indicates that the level of care provided by
many of these boarding houses is similar to that
provided in the "back-wards" of the traditional state
hospital. As Wolpert, Dear, and Crawford (1974)
have commented:

> While there is little or no evidence to suggest
> that the residents [of these boarding homes] are
> mistreated or exploited by the operators, there
> is ample evidence of inadequate community facil-
> ities for their further rehabilitation, recreation,
> or other support systems. At least half of the
> residents are not employable and their daily rou-
> tine largely involves confinement to their homes
> watching television . . . [cited in Bachrach
> 1976:7]

Or as Lamb and Goertzel (1971:31) state:

> We feel it is only an illusion that patients who
> are placed in boarding and family-care homes
> are "in the community." These facilities are in
> most respects like small, long-term state hospital
> wards isolated from the community.

The skilled nursing facility (SNF) is a high-
security, long-term convalescent home serving the
chronically and severely disturbed mental patient
who cannot be maintained in a less restrictive form
of sheltered care. These facilities, again privately
owned, profit-making businesses,[12] are characteristically plagued by chronic staff shortages (particularly
in terms of trained physicians and nursing personnel) and low operating budgets (Community of Communities 1973; American Justice Institute 1974). A
position paper regarding SNF's by the Greater [San

Francisco] Bay Area Committee on Continuing Care
(1976:3), an umbrella association of northern California mental health professionals, for example, has
noted:

> Unfortunately, most of the "skilled nursing facili-
> ties" currently in operation appear to be inferior
> to the level of care required by the patients placed
> there. It is [California] state policy that skilled
> nursing facilities ". . . should present an atmo-
> sphere which is psychologically conducive to re-
> covery. . . . Regular daily exercise and recre-
> ation should be an integral part of the milieu
> program . . . [and] in any facility the treatment
> staff is of prime importance in aiding patient
> recovery." In many SNF's known to the represen-
> tatives of this committee, such standards do not
> prevail.

Later in the same position paper, the committee continues:

> [C]riticism . . . about SNF's regarding flagrant
> examples of poor patient care, inadequate, filthy
> living conditions, physical, financial, and sexual
> exploitation of patients by other patients and/
> or by staff, lack of activity, and poor medical
> and psychiatric care, can be cited by us with
> reference to the SNF's where our patients are
> housed. [Ibid.]

As in B & C homes, rehabilitative activities are,
for the most part, nonexistent in SNF's, due to a
paucity of personnel and funds. California SNF's
and B & C homes, in addition, rely heavily on the
use of antipsychotic medication to manage their residents (see Segal and Aviram 1978: 232–51).[13] Although these drugs have been shown to produce serious and long-term side effects in some individuals
(American College of Neuropsychopharmacology
1973), in many instances they appear to be the only
treatment method in use (Crane 1974; Benson 1978).

Reintegration

The reintegration of the mentally ill into the community, for the most part, has not occurred in California
with deinstitutionalization. As Aviram and Segal
(1973) have pointed out, numerous exclusionary tactics (zoning ordinances, fire regulations, etc.) have
been developed by California communities in order

to segregate the community-based mentally ill from their nondisturbed neighbors. This has led, in some instances, to the virtual "ghettoization" of the mentally disordered within deteriorated, transitional urban centers. In the city of San Jose, for example, nearly two thousand former state hospital patients reside in sheltered-care facilities concentrated within a 20-square-block area of the central city.[14] Arrests and jailing of the mentally ill have increased in the state (California State Senate Select Committee 1975). In addition, studies of public support for community care in the state indicate a continued public attitude of fear, hostility, and intolerance toward the mentally ill. Breithaupt (1975), for example, in one series of surveys taken in the San Jose area found that nearly one-half (47%) of those questioned opposed the idea of community care for the mentally ill, while over 70% expressed support for the reopening of a nearby state mental hospital to the mentally disturbed.

Quality and Continuity of Care

As noted above, many former California mental patients were not self-supporting after their discharge into the community and were in need of a wide array of services. Unfortunately, for the most part, these services have not been adequate to meet the needs of the community-based mentally ill. Most California communities were unprepared to accept or adequately care for the influx of former state hospital patients that accompanied the deinstitutionalization of mental health services in the state. Often, patients were released into the community with little or no aftercare planning.[15] As a result, it has been estimated that only 10% of all state hospital patients released into the community in California during the five-year period following the enactment of the LPS Act (1968 to 1973) had any contact whatsoever with their local community mental health clinics (Weiner, Place, and Ahmed 1974). Furthermore, as Weiner and his associates (1974:18) have noted:

> [I]n many areas [of California] not large enough to support adequate mental health programs, there are no facilities for either chronically or acutely disordered patients. . . . [P]rograms in these areas too often consist of putting the potential client on a bus for the next county.

Thus, many of California's chronically mentally ill, either by choice or design, end up in large urban centers (such as Los Angeles, San Francisco, Fresno, and San Jose) that have the facilities and services necessary to support them.

One last point deserves comment. While the state hospital system provided a unitary agency for the care of the mentally ill patient, community care in California has generated a fragmented system of services, scattered among a host of public and private agencies. This fragmentation of services, as Kirk and Therrein (1975) have pointed out, often leaves the mentally ill client unaware of where to turn for assistance. In addition, ex-mental patients are among the most undesirable clients of helping agencies, and their undesirability often prevents them from obtaining necessary services (Bord 1971; Allen 1974; Kirk and Therrein 1975). Thus, while the state hospital (at least in theory) was responsible for the care and treatment of the "whole patient," the community-based mentally ill person's needs are provided for by an array of often poorly coordinated organizations. In some cases, it appears the needs of these people are not adequately provided for by any of these groups.

In summary, then, available evidence casts severe doubt on the adequacy of community mental health care in California. Whether the problems of the program are due simply to a too-rapid shift from an institutional to decentralized system of care or, instead, to a more profound defect (such as an inadequate or imprecise conceptualization of the policy itself) is unclear. The second conclusion, I believe, should not be dismissed.

CONCLUSION: SOCIAL THEORY, IDEOLOGY, AND POLICY

In this paper I have attempted to assess the merit of a labeling approach to mental illness through an examination of the perspective's application in terms of public policy, i.e., community mental health policy in the state of California. In this regard, I gave special consideration to the deinstitutionalization of mental health services in that state, the closing of several state mental hospitals, and the release of former psychiatric patients into the community. The relationship between social theory and public policy is an elusive association to demonstrate empirically. For this reason, I presented, in some detail, illustrations of direct, as well as indirect, influence by labeling theorists and researchers on contemporary California community mental health policy. I also assessed the consequences of that policy. It is clear that California's decentralized community mental health program has failed to live up to the original expectations of many who formulated and supported the policy. In many respects, community mental health in California has not worked. The question remaining is "Why?"

A partial explanation, I believe, may lie in the association that developed between the labeling model of mental illness and California mental health policy during the late 1960s and early 1970s. A cause-effect relationship between theory and practice, however, is not suggested—labeling theory did not "cause" community mental health in California. Rather, I suggest that a type of Weberian "elective affinity" (Howe 1978; Marx, Rieker, and Ellison 1974) existed between the two—an affinity illustrated by their mutual antipsychiatric orientation, their common emphasis on the sociogenic character of mental disorder, and also by their shared belief that psychic distress, in many cases, need not be defined as constituting "mental illness" at all. Labeling theory's influence on California community mental health policy, I claim, stems from this elective affinity.

In my opinion, the major analytic flaw of the labeling approach to mental illness is its failure to take the consequences of unlabeled psychotic behavior explicitly into account within its theoretical framework. It fails to recognize that serious mental illness does exist irrespective of labeling. Instead of recognizing the problematic nature of unlabeled deviance (going on to relate the initial rule-breaking behavior to processes of labeling and societal reaction), labeling theorists have, for the most part, ignored them. Furthermore, by neglecting the potential positive factors associated with mental hospitalization (Linn 1968; Braginsky, Ring, and Ring 1969; Siegler and Osmond 1974), and the potential deleterious effects of community care (Brown et al. 1966; Grad and Sainsbury 1966; Grad 1968; Davis et al. 1974; Arnhoff 1975), the perspective generated an ideological thrust uncritically endorsing community treatment for *all* mentally ill. However, as Mechanic (1969) has correctly observed:

From the point of view of public policy, we should recognize that the construction and modification of effective environments for mental patient care is not exclusively a community or *hospital venture. . . . [I]n condemning bad institutions we need not abandon the institutional idea entirely since some persons probably function best in them.*

Social science theory and research are being increasingly consulted in the formulation and implementation of public policy, both on the state and national level. The use of social science by political decision makers, however, has its pitfalls as well as its promises. Perhaps the greatest potential problem of the use of social science in public policy is that policy initiation and development are not usually the primary objectives of the social scientific enterprise. Social science theory, in particular, is often constructed with quite another point in mind than its practical policy implications. The primary purpose of theory within any scientific discipline is to further scientific progress in that discipline. This means, especially within the social sciences, that theoretical formulations are not always constructed by the scientists to serve as a fully accurate reflection of empirical reality. Scheff (1974:445) has, for example, noted that his labeling theory of mental illness (with which this paper has been so concerned) was actually meant to be used as a "sensitizing-theory"— used to "jostle the imagination, to create a crisis of consciousness that will lead to new visions of reality." According to Scheff, contrary to formal deductive theory, ". . . a sensitizing-theory may be *ambiguous, ideologically-biased,* and *not literally true,* and still be useful and even necessary for scientific progress" (emphasis added). This being the case, it is not surprising that labeling theory encountered major problems when applied to practical policy issues.

Social science theory and research have two principal, although often contradictory, aims. The first is scientific advancement. The second is the application of social scientific knowledge and judgment to the "external world"—often through policy research, program evaluation, and the like. Both are integral aspects of the social scientific enterprise. They are, however, quite different, often involving contrary methods of theory construction and research. As such, they should remain distinct from one another, in the minds of both the policymaker and the social scientist. To do otherwise, I believe, is to invite the problematic consequences put forth in this paper.

POSTSCRIPT, MARCH 1986

The preceding article was written during the late 1970s and focuses primarily on deinstitutionalization in the state of California. The shift to community care for the mentally ill has, however, been a nationwide movement. In this postscript, I will present an updated overview of deinstitutionalization and community care as they have unfolded in the United States through the mid-1980s.

It is unquestionable that deinstitutionalization succeeded in terms of one of its primary goals: the depopulation of the nation's state mental hospitals. In 1955, the resident population of U.S. state and county mental hospitals was 559,000. By 1980, the number of patients housed in these institutions had dropped to 138,000—a reduction of more than 75% (Brown 1985). There is, however, considerable evidence suggesting that deinstitutionalization has *not* achieved a second major aim: the provision of adequate care for the tens of thousands of mentally ill individuals now residing in the community.

Where Have the Mentally Ill Gone?

Recent studies by the National Institute of Mental Health (NIMH) estimate that 1.7 to 2.4 million Americans suffer from a chronic mental illness (Goldman, Gattozzi, and Taube 1981). Of this total, 900,000 are institutionalized, 83% in community nursing homes. It has been well documented that much of the national decline in the state mental hospital patient population during the 1970s was due to the transinstitutionalization of the elderly mentally ill to nursing homes (Kramer 1977). Currently, 58% of the patients residing in U.S. nursing homes are chronically mentally ill (Shadish and Bootzin 1981). The large numbers of chronically mentally ill in these facilities, along with the poor quality of care these facilities often provide (Stotsky and Stotsky 1983), have prompted some to refer to nursing homes as "the new back wards in the community" (Schmidt et al. 1977).

Estimates of the number of noninstitutionalized chronically mentally ill total approximately 800,000 (Goldman 1984). Living conditions, service utilization, and general quality of life among these individuals vary greatly. Many community-based mentally ill (estimates range from one-third to two-thirds) reside—at least periodically—with their families (Minkoff 1978; Goldman 1982). Whereas most families welcome their mentally ill relatives into the home, research has also documented the often severe psychological, social, and economic burdens that family members must bear caring for a disordered loved one (Creer and Wing 1974; Hatfield 1984).

Large numbers of mentally ill also reside in a variety of boarding homes, often located in large urban centers (Lamb 1979). In many states, a good number of these facilities are unlicensed and are staffed by untrained personnel. Social, employment, or rehabilitative programs in these facilities are rare. Van Putten and Spar (1979) have described the typical resident of the psychiatric boarding home as "a chronic schizophrenic between the ages of 16 and 70 . . . [who] spends . . . the day in virtual solitude, either watching TV or wandering aimlessly around the neighborhood" (p. 461). In many large U.S. cities, as well, chronically mentally ill individuals inhabit single-room occupancy "welfare hotels" or "SROs." In New York City, for example, estimates of the citywide mentally ill SRO population range from 10,000 to 20,000 (Baxter and Hopper 1980).

Finally, some mentally ill in the community become homeless persons, a fact that has received considerable recent professional and media attention (Lamb 1984; Newsweek 1986). Although the actual number of homeless mentally ill is unknown, estimates have suggested that one-third to one-half of the approximately 2.5 million homeless persons in the United States today are chronically mentally ill (Baxter and Hopper 1984). Although the causes of homelessness among the mentally ill are myriad, the lack of adequate, low-cost housing for this group is certainly a major contributing factor. Without available community housing and ready access to public mental institutions, many of the chronically mentally ill have nowhere to live but the streets.

The Dilemmas of Deinstitutionalization

There are many reasons why community care has largely failed to provide adequately for the needs of the mentally ill. Three will be briefly mentioned: (1) inadequate funding for community services, (2) lack of coordination among agencies dealing with the mentally ill, and (3) naivete among early proponents of community care concerning the inherent difficulties of treating severe and chronic mental disability.

In many states, the programmatic emphasis upon deinstitutionalization was never matched by an adequate budget for community mental health programs. Although individual states varied in their fiscal enthusiasm for community care, many state governments perceived deinstitutionalization largely as an opportunity to cut costs and shift much of the economic burden for the care of the mentally ill from the state to the federal level through the utilization of Medicare, Medicaid, and Supplemental Security Income programs initiated by the federal government during the 1960s and 1970s (Rose 1979). Furthermore, even where money was adequately provided for state mental health services, the dollars often did not follow the patients into the community but instead remained tied to state hospital programs that were treating only a fraction of their former patient populations.

A lack of coordination between agencies and service providers for the deinstitutionalized mentally ill has also reduced the quality of their care in the community (U.S. General Accounting Office 1978). Prior to deinstitutionalization, services for the mentally ill were provided under one roof—the state mental hospital. In the community, however, the mentally ill must contend with a complicated bureaucratic maze of agencies, regulations, and programs. The mentally ill require a broad array of specialized services to function satisfactorily in the community, including housing, income support, medical follow-up, psychosocial rehabilitation, crisis management, vocational training, and leisure and social activities. As a result of the lack of coordination among these many service providers, clients are underserved or "fall through the cracks" of the system. One promising approach to this problem has been the Community Support Program initiated by NIMH in 1978 (Turner and TenHoor 1978). One of the major thrusts of the Community Support Program has been to provide state and local governments with funding and expertise to assist them in developing comprehensive and integrated mental health, rehabilita- tion, and support services for the chronically mentally ill in the community. Between 1978 and 1984, NIMH committed over $42 million to Community Support Program activities (Love 1984). However, given the massive scope of the problem, the program has not been adequately funded and has, since its inception, faced an uncertain future (for each of the past four years, for example, Congressional intervention has been necessary to rescue the program from being eliminated by the Reagan administration).

A third factor contributing to the problems of deinstitutionalization was the naivete and excessive optimism of many early proponents of the policy. Advocates of deinstitutionalization often expressed the hope that patients would be able to live normal lives and blend into the mainstream of society if treated outside the mental hospital. However, the experience of the past several decades has shown that mental illness is not simply an artifact of inadequate hospital treatment that will disappear if institutionalization is avoided. Many social disabilities once thought to be associated only with long-term hospitalization (the so-called "institutional neuroses") have now been noted among a new generation of young chronically mentally ill whose treatment has involved only brief hospitalization and community care (Pepper et al. 1981; Estroff 1981). It is now clear that mental illness is not a mythical entity but a serious clinical condition that can cause immeasurable suffering to the mentally ill and those close to them, regardless of where treatment is received.

Should Community Care Be Abandoned?

No one clearly knows how many chronically mentally ill are "doing well" in the community and how many are "doing poorly" (Braun et al. 1981). By a number of conventionally employed indices of "success," however, deinstitutionalization has clearly failed: only about 10 to 30% of former mental patients become employed (even temporarily) and between 35 and 50% are rehospitalized within one year of release (Anthony, Cohen, and Vitalo 1978). This high rate of recidivism has been dubbed the "revolving door" syndrome. As noted previously, many early proponents of deinstitutionalization hoped that the mentally ill in the community could be "normalized" and reintegrated back into society. I believe this is too much to expect from any current treatment program, hospital or community based. We simply do not know enough about mental illness.

Nevertheless, in my view, community care of the mentally ill should not be abandoned. Given adequate resources, we should certainly be able to create programs that can vastly improve the quality of life of the community-based mentally ill. More and better quality housing must be provided—"satellite housing," where the mentally ill live in small groups of two to five, without live-in staff but with some professional supervision, is one innovative option (Lamb 1981). More psychosocial rehabilitation centers, such as the Fountain House in New York and the Friendship Club in New Orleans, must be developed where the mentally ill can meet, socialize, and learn new social and employment skills (Beard, Probst, and Malamud 1982). More patient self-help groups, such as GROW, must be encouraged (Rappaport et al. 1985), as well as family support organizations, such as the National Alliance for the Mentally Ill. We as a society must learn to live with the mentally ill in our communities without stigmatization and undue fear. And the majority of the elderly prefer life in the community to an institutional existence (Estroff 1981; Segal and Aviram 1978; Lehman, Reed, and Possidente 1982).

This is not to say that state mental hospitals will no longer be necessary. There is considerable evidence on the positive side concerning the present level of performance of these hospitals. Those still residing in mental hospitals, whether public or private, face a good staff-to-patient ratio of 1.5 to 1, and as one observer puts it, "as hospitals have reduced their censuses, they have been able to direct an increased share of their resources to meet needs of these long-term patients" (Greenblatt and Norman 1983). We must, of course, remain aware of the past insufficiencies of many of these hospitals to make sure that those conditions will never reoccur.

Notes

1. The debate between the supporters of the medical and the interactional models of mental illness may be profitably viewed as a clash between two opposing "paradigms" in the Kuhnian sense. Paradigms may be incomparable in that they address different problems, embody different standards and even definitions of sci-

ence. Proponents of each paradigm inhabit opposing worlds of discourse and often tend to "talk past" each other in discussion. As Kuhn (1962:148) has observed: "The proponents of competing paradigms are always at least slightly at cross-purposes." Paradigm debates thus cannot be understood in terms of the categories of rational argument and they can seldom be resolved through a scientific "meeting of the minds." One paradigm must fail to make logical or cognitive sense in terms of the other, owing to a fundamental failure of translation, and so, of communication. (See Kuhn 1962 and Scheffler 1967.)

2. Other important influences included, among others, a desire on the part of the state to reduce its financial and administrative burden in the mental health area, extensive lobbying by civil libertarians to end involuntary mental commitment in the state, and a wish by individual California counties to increase their share of the state mental health budget. In addition, these influences need to be placed in the historical context of a steady national decline in mental hospital population—a decline powered largely by the introduction of antipsychotic medication in the 1950s, as well as by the initiation of federal mental health and public assistance programs for released mental patients in the 1960s.

3. For a more detailed discussion of labeling theory, see, for example, Schur 1971 and Scheff 1966.

4. Much of the material discussed in this section is drawn from the work of Bardach (1972).

5. In May of 1966, Waldie was elected to the U.S. Congress and was replaced by Assemblyman Nicholas Petris as subcommittee chairperson.

6. Later published as "County Lunacy Hearings: Some Observations of Commitments to a State Hospital" (Miller and Schwartz 1966).

7. Kreplin (1966).

8. Waldie and the subcommittee's general plan was that the end of the involuntary commitment process in the state would lead to other major changes in California's overall mental health program. As Valarie Bradley (1972), a staffperson for the subcommittee during the period the LPS Act was developed, has noted:

If the commitment system was abolished . . . a chain-reaction would start, resulting in fewer involuntary placements, shorter periods of hospitalization, diversion of patients and dollars to a variety of community services, development of new attitudes and procedures among treatment personnel and most importantly, a change in public attitudes toward mental disorders and how to deal with them. [p. 184]

9. For an example of Miller's work, see her 1966 article.

10. Of the 62 general references cited in the subcommittee report, 15, or nearly one-fourth, are by individuals associated with either the labeling or conspiratorial model of mental illness.

11. Under Brown, the deinstitutionalization of mental health services in California has continued. In 1976, for example, a law was signed by the governor mandating community mental health care for mentally ill offenders. It is interesting to note in this regard that Brown himself appears to be sympathetic toward the conspiratorial model of mental disorder. In an interview published in February of 1978, Brown was quoted as stating: "I've had some doubts about the role of psychiatry and their approach to mental illness. I've had a lifelong interest in the field. . . . I'm aware of Thomas Szasz—I've read everything he's written" (Lewis 1979).

12. Many SNF's and other sheltered-care facilities are owned by large medical-care corporations. One major corporation, Beverly Enterprises of Pasadena, California, for example, was formed in 1964 with a total of 3 SNF's. As of 1977, the corporation operated 150 such facilities nationwide. The firm's revenues rose from $66.6 million in 1976 to $81.3 million in 1977 (Traska 1978).

13. Segal and Aviram in their 1976 survey of the mentally ill in California's sheltered-care facilities found that 76% of their respondents were taking antipsychotic medication at the time. Sixty-one percent were found to be taking two or more psychotropic drugs daily and 10% were taking four or more of these medicines daily (Segal and Aviram 1978).

14. In 1973 a local San Jose television station, for example, ran the following as part of an editorial regarding community mental health care:

If you are a citizen of San Jose and have not visited the areas between Santa Clara and Williams Streets [the sheltered-care area] you should do so, but only in a locked car and never alone. . . . We have been told that there are 15,000 residents of half-way houses in San Jose, many of them within blocks of San Jose State University. A co-ed walking home alone at night is taking her life in her hands. [Cited in testimony, California State Senate Select Committee on the Proposed Phaseout of State Hospital Services, July 16, 1975. Agnews State Hospital, San Jose, California (Transcript, p. 279)]

15. Interview with Ruth Baird, MSW, Director, Continuing Care Services, Santa Clara County (California) Department of Health, Mental Health Division, August 1977.

References Cited

ALLEN, P.
1974 A Consumer's View of the California Mental Health Care System. Psychiatric Quarterly 48:1–13.

AMERICAN COLLEGE OF NEUROPSYCHOPHARMACOLOGY
1973 Neurologic Syndromes Associated With Antipsychotic Drug Use. Archives of General Psychiatry 29:463–67.

AMERICAN JUSTICE INSTITUTE
1974 Santa Clara County Mental Health Aftercare Evaluation: First Year Final Report. Sacramento, California.

ANTHONY, W. A., M. R. COHEN, and R. VITALO
1978 The Measurement of Rehabilitation Outcome. Schizophrenia Bulletin 4:365–383.

ARNHOFF, F. N.
1975 Social Consequences of Policy Toward Mental Illness. Science 188:1277–81.

AVIRAM, U., and S. P. SEGAL
1973 Exclusion of the Mentally Ill: Reflections on an Old Problem in a New Context. Archives of General Psychiatry 29:126–31.

BACHRACII, L. L.
1976 Deinstitutionalization: An Analytical and Sociological Perspective. DHEW Publication No. (ADM) 76–351. Washington, D.C.: U.S. Government Printing Office.

BACK, K. W.
1975 Policy Enthusiasms for Untested Theories and the Role of Quantitative Evidence: Labeling Theory and Mental Illness. In Social Policy and Sociology. N. J. Demarath III, O. Larson, and K. P. Schuessler, eds. New York: Academic Press, pp. 135–48.

BARDACH, E.
1972 The Skill Factor in Politics: Repealing the Mental Commitment Laws in California. Berkeley: University of California Press.

1977 The Implementation Game: What Happens After a Bill Becomes a Law. Cambridge, Massachusetts: MIT Press.

BAXTER, E., and K. HOPPER
1980 Pathologies of Place and Disorders of Mind. Health/PAC Bulletin 11:1–22.

1984 Troubled on the Streets: The Mentally Disabled Homeless Poor. In The Chronic Mental Patient: Five Years Later. J. A. Talbott, ed. Orlando, Florida: Grune and Stratton, pp. 49–62.

BEARD, J. H., R. N. PROBST, and T. J. MALAMUD
1982 The Fountain House Model of Psychosocial Reha-

bilitation. Psychosocial Rehabilitation Journal 5: 47–53.

BEGELMAN, D. A.
1971 Misnaming Metaphors, the Medical Model, and Some Muddles. Psychiatry 34:38–58.

BENSON, P. R.
1978 Psychiatric Drugs and the Deinstitutionalization of the Mentally Ill. Unpublished paper presented at the annual meetings of the Society for the Study of Social Problems, San Francisco.

BORD, R. J.
1971 Rejection of the Mentally Ill: Continualities and Further Developments. Social Problems 18:496–509.

BRADLEY, VALARIE J.
1972 California Moves Rapidly to Community Centered Mental Health Programs under 1967–68 Legislation. California Journal, July:184.

BRAUN, P., G. KOCHANSKY, R. SHAPIRO, et al.
1981 Overview: Deinstitutionalization of Psychiatric Patients; A Critical Review of Outcome. American Journal of Psychiatry 138:736–749.

BROWN, G. T., et al.
1966 Schizophrenia and Social Care. London: Oxford University Press.

BROWN, P.
1985 The Transfer of Care: Psychiatric Deinstitutionalization and Its Aftermath. London: Routledge and Kegan Paul.

CALIFORNIA STATE ASSEMBLY SUBCOMMITTEE ON MENTAL HEALTH
1965a A Redefinition of State Responsibility for California's Mentally Retarded. Sacramento, California.
1965b Edited Transcript of Hearing of the Subcommittee on Mental Health, December 20, 1965, Los Angeles, California. Sacramento, California.
1966 The Dilemma of Mental Commitments in California. Sacramento, California.

CALIFORNIA STATE SENATE SELECT COMMITTEE ON THE PROPOSED PHASEOUT OF STATE HOSPITAL SERVICES
1975 Final Report of Senate Select Committee. Sacramento, California.

CHAUNCEY, R.
1975 Comment on the Labeling Theory of Mental Illness. American Sociological Review 40:247–51.

COMMUNITY OF COMMUNITIES
1973 Report on 'L' Facilities in Santa Clara County. San Jose, California: Community of Communities.

CRANE, G. E.
1974 Two Decades of Psychopharmacology and Commu-

nity Mental Health: Old and New Problems of the Schizophrenic Patient. Transactions of the New York Academy of Sciences 36:644–56.

CREER, C. and J. WING
1974 Schizophrenia in the Home. London: Institute of Psychiatry.

DAVIS, A., et al.
1974 Schizophrenics in the New Custodial Community. Dayton: Ohio State University Press.

ENKI CORPORATION
1972 A Study of California's New Mental Health Law (1969–1971). Chatsworth, California: ENKI Corporation.

ESTROFF, S. E.
1981 Making It Crazy: An Ethnography of Psychiatric Clients in an American Community. Berkeley: University of California Press.

GOFFMAN, E.
1961 Asylums: Essays on the Social Situation of Mental Patients and Other Inmates. Garden City, New York: Doubleday.

GOLDMAN, H. H.
1982 Mental Illness and Family Burden: A Public Health Perspective. Hospital and Community Psychiatry 33:557–559.
1984 Epidemiology. In The Chronic Mental Patient: Five Years Later. J. A. Talbott, ed. Orlando, Florida: Grune and Stratton, pp. 15–32.

GOLDMAN, H. H., A. GATTOZZI, and C. A. TAUBE
1981 Defining and Counting the Chronically Mentally Ill. Hospital and Community Psychiatry 32:21–27.

GOVE, W. R.
1975b The Labeling Theory of Mental Illness: A Reply to Scheff. American Sociological Review 40:242–47.

GOVE, W. R., ed.
1975a The Labeling of Deviance: Evaluating a Perspective: New York: Wiley.

GRAD, J.
1968 A Two Year Follow-up. In Community Mental Health: An International Perspective, R. H. Williamson and L. D. Ozarian, eds. San Francisco: Jossey-Bass, pp. 429–54.

GRAD, J., and P. SAINSBURY
1966 Evaluating the Community Psychiatric Services in Chicester: Results. Milbank Memorial Fund Quarterly 44:242–77.

GREATER BAY AREA COMMITTEE ON CONTINUING CARE
1976 Position Paper: Skilled Nursing Facilities. San Francisco. Mimeographed.

GREENBLATT, N., and M. NORMAN
1983 Deinstitutionalization: Health Consequences for the Mentally Ill. Annual Review of Public Health 11:131–54.

HATFIELD, A. B.
1984 The Family. *In* The Chronic Mental Patient: Five Years Later. J. A. Talbott, ed. Orlando, Florida: Grune and Stratton, pp. 307–324.

HOWE, R. H.
1978 Max Weber's Elective Affinities: Sociology Within the Bounds of Pure Reason. American Journal of Sociology 84:366–85.

KIRK, S. A., and M. E. THERREIN
1975 Community Mental Health Myths and the Fate of Former Mental Patients. Psychiatry 38:207–17.

KRAMER, M.
1977 Psychiatric Services and the Changing Scene, 1950–1985. DHEW Publications no. (ADM) 77–433. Washington, D.C.: Government Printing Office.

KUHN, THOMAS
1962 The Structure of Scientific Revolutions. Chicago: University of Chicago Press.

KREPLIN, KARL W.
1966 Mental Illness Commitment: A Study of the Decision-Making Process. M.A. thesis, University of California at Santa Barbara.

LAMB, H. R.
1979 The New Asylum in the Community. Archives of General Psychiatry 36:129–134.
1981 What Did We Really Expect from Deinstitutionalization? Hospital and Community Psychiatry 32:105–109.

LAMB, H. R. (ed.)
1984 The Homeless Mentally Ill. Washington, D.C.: American Psychiatric Association.

LAMB, R. H., and V. GOERTZEL
1971 Discharged Mental Patients: Are They Really in the Community? Archives of General Psychiatry 24:29–34.

LEHMAN, A. F., S. K. REED, and S. M. POSSIDENTE
1982 Priorities for Long-Term Care: Comments from Board and Care Residents. Psychiatric Quarterly 54:181–189.

LEIFER, R.
1969 In the Name of Mental Health. New York: Science House.

LEWIS, ANTHONY
1979 A Brown Study III. New York Times, February 13:A–21.

LINN, L.
1968 The Mental Hospital from the Patient Perspective. Psychiatry 31:213–33.

LOVE, ROBERT E.
1984 The Community Support Program: Strategy for Reform? *In* The Chronic Mental Patient: Five Years Later. J. A. Talbott, ed. Orlando, Florida: Grune and Stratton, pp. 195–214.

MARX, J. H., P. P. RIEKER, and D. ELLISON
1974 The Sociology of Community Mental Health: Historical and Methodological Perspectives. *In* Sociological Perspectives on Community Mental Health. P. Roman and H. Trice, eds. Philadelphia: F. A. Davis, pp. 9–40.

MECHANIC, D.
1969 Mental Health and Social Policy, Englewood Cliffs, New Jersey: Prentice-Hall.

MILLER, DOROTHY
1966 Worlds that Fail: Part I. Retrospective Analysis of Mental Patients' Careers. Research Monograph #6. Sacramento: California Department of Mental Hygiene.

MILLER, DOROTHY, and MICHAEL SCHWARTZ
1966 County Lunacy Hearings: Some observations of Commitments to a State Hospital. Social Problems 14:26–35.

MINKOFF, K.
1978 A Map of Chronic Mental Patients. *In* The Chronic Mental Patient. J. A. Talbott, ed. Washington, D.C.: American Psychiatric Association, pp. 11–37.

NEWSWEEK
1986 Abandoned. Newsweek (January 6, 1986): 14–19.

PEPPER, B., M. KIRSCHER, and H. RYGLEWIEZ
1981 The Young Adult Chronic Patient: Overview of a Population. Hospital and Community Psychiatry 32:475–78.

PERRUCCI, R.
1974 Circle of Madness. Englewood Cliffs, New Jersey: Prentice-Hall.

PLACE, D. M., and S. WEINER
1974 Re-entering the Community: A Pilot Study of Mentally Ill Patients Discharged from Napa State Hospital. Unpublished manuscript. Stanford Research Institute, Menlo Park, California.

RAPPAPORT, J., E. SEIDMAN, P. A. TORO, et al.
1985 Collaborative Research with a Mutual Help Organization. Social Policy 15:12–24.

ROSE, S. M.
1979 Deciphering Deinstitutionalization: Complexities in Policy and Program Analysis. Milbank Memorial Fund Quarterly 57:429–60.

SCHEFF, T. J.

1963 Decision Rules, Types of Error, and Their Consequences in Medical Diagnosis. Behavioral Science 8:97–107.

1964 The Societal Reaction to Deviance: Ascriptive Elements in the Psychiatric Screening of Mental Patients in a Midwestern State. Social Problems 11:403–13.

1966 Being Mentally Ill: A Sociological Theory. Chicago: Aldine.

1974 The Labeling Theory of Mental Illness. American Sociological Review 39:444–52.

1975 Reply to Chauncey and Gove, American Sociological Review 40:252–57.

SCHEFFLER, ISRAEL

1967 Science and Subjectivity. Indianapolis: Bobbs-Merrill.

SCHMIDT, W., A. M. REINHARDT, R. L. KANE, et al.

1977 The Mentally Ill in Nursing Homes: New Back Wards in the Community. Archives of General Psychiatry 34:687–91.

SCHRAG, P.

1978 Mind Control. New York: Pantheon.

SCHUR, EDWIN M.

1971 Labeling Deviant Behavior: Its Sociological Implications. New York: Harper and Row.

SEGAL, S. P.

1975 Transition from Mental Hospital to Community: Issues in Providing a Continuing Sheltered-Care Environment. Paper presented at the National Conference on Social Welfare, San Francisco. Mimeographed.

SEGAL, S. P., and U. AVIRAM

1978 The Mentally Ill in Community-Based Sheltered-Care. New York: Wiley-Interscience.

SHADISH, W. R., and R. R. BOOTZIN

1981 Nursing Homes and Chronic Mental Patients. Schizophrenia Bulletin 7:488–498.

SIEGLER, M., and H. OSMOND

1974 Models of Madness, Models of Medicine. New York: Macmillan.

STOTSKY, B. A., and E. S. STOTSKY

1983 Nursing Homes: Improving a Flawed Community Facility. Hospital and Community Psychiatry 34:238–242.

SZASZ, T. S.

1960 The Myth of Mental Illness. American Psychologist 15:113–18.

TRASKA, MARCIA R.

1978 Nursing Home Survey: Proprietary Chains Operated 20% More Beds During 1977. Modern Health Care, June: 38–42.

TURNER, J., and W. TENHOOR

1978 The NIMH Community Support Program: Pilot Approach to a Needed Social Reform. Schizophrenia Bulletin 4:319–348.

U.S. GENERAL ACCOUNTING OFFICE

1978 Returning the Mentally Disabled to the Community: Government Needs to Do More. Washington, D.C.: GAO.

VAN PUTTEN, T., and J. E. SPAR

1981 The Board and Care Home: Does It Deserve a Bad Press? Hospital and Community Psychiatry 32:488–501.

WEINER, S., D. M. PLACE, and P. I. AHMED

1974 A Report on the Closing of a State Hospital. Administration in Mental Health (Summer): 13–20.

WEISS, C. H.

1975 Improving the Linkage Between Social Research and Public Policy. *In* Knowledge and Policy: The Uncertain Connection. L. E. Lynn, ed. Pp. 23–81. Washington, D.C.: The National Research Council.

1977 Research for Policy's Sake: The Enlightenment Function of Social Science. Policy Analysis 3:531–45.

WOLPERT, J.

1974 The Relocation of Released Mental Hospital Patients into Residential Communities. Unpublished manuscript. School of Architecture and Urban Planning, Princeton University.

WOLPERT, J., M. DEAR, AND R. CRAWFORD

1974 Mental Health Satellite Facilities in the Community. Paper presented at the National Institute of Mental Health Center for Studies in Metropolitan Problems Seminar Series, Rockville, Maryland.

The Patient–Practitioner Relationship

The doctor–patient relationship was one of the earliest issues of interest to medical sociologists when the field was getting on its feet in American colleges and universities during the 1950s and 1960s. During that time, Samuel Bloom's book *The Doctor and His Patient* was often required reading in courses in medical sociology, and Parsons' notion of the sick role was a key concept to be discussed. The perspective used was that of an asymmetrical relationship in which the doctor was completely dominant. Parsons' sick role has often been criticized for its perceived limitations in this regard.

Sociologists are still fascinated with the relationship between doctor and patient, but some portion of the current interest is devoted to speculation about the possible erosion of the relative power of the physician. For a number of reasons related to factors associated with both the changing character of consumers and the manner in which the practice of medicine is changing, it is felt that a subtle realignment might be taking place. At the same time, the literature includes more and more articles on the possible effects on the doctor–patient relationships of so many more women coming into medicine.

It is notable that, overwhelmingly, the focus of medical sociologists has been on the doctor–patient relationship to the virtual exclusion of the consideration of relationships between patients and any other health professionals. Thus, little has been done within sociology on the nurse–patient relationship without also relating it to the nurse–doctor and/or doctor–patient relationship.

The first article in this chapter is Thomas S. Szasz and Marc H. Hollender's classic analysis of three types of doctor–patient relationships, which range from the doctor-dominant one to one emphasizing mutual participation. The authors note that the different types of relationships are relevant to different medical situations. The typology put forth by Szasz and Hollender is clearly normative in nature since it deals with what the doctor–patient relationship *should* be in each of three particular sets of circumstances. The second article in this chapter shows that real life is somewhat more complicated and that while circumstances would seem to call for the guidance–cooperation mode, the active–passive mode seems to be more in evidence. Here, Marcia Millman looks at the relationship that coronary care patients have with their surgeons and with additional significant others at Lakeside Hospital (which is a fictitious hospital that represents a composite of three hospitals—all nonprofit, teaching hospitals associated with prestigious medical schools—studied by Millman over a two-year period). According to Millman, the prime consideration of both the medical professionals and patients is to avoid allowing threatening aspects of the situation to impact on the patient, and she describes the ways in which each side attempts to "neutralize" potential threats.

It will be recalled that in the second of the two articles introducing the field of medical sociology in Chapter 1, Renée Fox announced her enthusiasm for a research agenda that would include analyses of the impact of women physicians. In the next article in Chapter 5, Carol S. Weisman and Martha Ann Teitelbaum discuss some of the implications, for patient care, of the increasing presence of women in medicine. Following this article, Irving Kenneth Zola briefly discusses, simply and in a straightforward manner, subtle aspects of the patient–physician relationship through which the physician exerts control. He also introduces the concept of "compliance." Zola's feeling is that much of the reason for the patient's complying or not complying with the doctor's orders can be traced to the doctor. On the other hand, Peter Conrad speculates in the following article that the noncompliance of epileptics in ignoring doctors' orders concerning the proper use of medications may derive from forces outside the doctor–patient relationship. In his conclusion, Conrad suggests that his discussion may have applicability to other cases of chronic illness in which patients must manage medications over the long-term.

In the final article in Chapter 5, Howard D. Schwartz and Ian S. Biederman provide an overview of sociological thinking on the roles played by patients in servicing their own health needs as well as in securing the services of health care professionals. The wide-ranging discussion presents sociological perspectives on self-care (it can be seen that the material on self-medication is an extension of Conrad's discussion in the previous article), lay referral, self-help groups, and "consumerism." As regards the last issue, Schwartz and Biederman critically evaluate the contention that there now exists in the United States a broad-based and activist consumer movement aimed at gaining more power for patients in their relationships with health-care providers.

The Basic Models of the Doctor–Patient Relationship

Thomas S. Szasz
Marc H. Hollender

When a person leaves the culture in which he was born and raised and migrates to another, he usually experiences his new social setting as something strange—and in some ways threatening—and he is stimulated to master it by conscious efforts at understanding. To some extent every immigrant to the United States reacts in this manner to the American scene. Similarly, the American tourist in Europe or South America "scrutinizes" the social setting which is taken for granted by the natives. To scrutinize—and criticize— the pattern of other peoples' lives is obviously both common and easy. It also happens, however, that people exposed to cross cultural experiences turn their attention to the very customs which formed the social matrix of their lives in the past. Lastly, to study the "customs" which shape and govern one's day-to-day life is most difficult of all. (Ref.1).

In many ways the psychoanalyst is like a person who has migrated from one culture to another. To him the relationship between physician and patient—which is like a custom that is taken for granted in medical practice and which he himself so treated in his early history—has become an object of study. While the precise nature and extent of the influence which psychoanalysis and so-called dynamic psychiatry have had on modern medicine are debatable, it seems to us that the most decisive effect has been that of making physicians explicitly aware of the possible significance of their relationship to patients.

The question naturally arises as to "What is a doctor–patient relationship?" It is our aim to discuss this question and to show that certain philosophical preconceptions associated with the notions of "disease," "treatment," and "cure" have a profound bearing on both the theory and the practice of medicine.

WHAT IS A HUMAN RELATIONSHIP?

The concept of a relationship is a novel one in medicine. Traditionally, physicians have been concerned with "things," for example, anatomical structures, lesions, bacteria, and the like. In modern times the scope has been broadened to include the concept of "function." The phenomenon of a human relationship is often viewed as though it were a "thing" or a "function." It is, in fact, neither. Rather it is an abstraction, appropriate for the description and handling of certain observational facts. Moreover, it is an abstraction which presupposes concepts of both structure and function.

The foregoing comments may be clarified by concrete illustrations. Psychiatrists often suggest to their medical colleagues that the physician's relationship with his patient per se helps the latter. This creates the impression (whether so intended or not) that the relationship is a thing, which works not unlike the way that vitamins do in a case of vitamin deficiency. Another idea is that the doctor–patient relationship depends mainly on what the physician does (or thinks or feels). Then it is viewed not unlike a function.

When we consider a relationship in which there is joint participation of the two persons involved, "relationship" refers to neither a structure nor a function (such as the "personality" of the physician or patient). It is, rather, an abstraction embodying the activities of two interacting systems (persons). (Ref. 5).

Reprinted from the *Archives in Internal Medicine,* vol. 97 (1956), pp. 585–592. Copyright © 1956 by the American Medical Association.

THREE BASIC MODELS OF THE DOCTOR–PATIENT RELATIONSHIP

The three basic models of the doctor–patient relationship (see Table 1), which we will describe, embrace modes of interaction ubiquitous in human relationships and in no way specific for the contact between physician and patient. The specificity of the medical situation probably derives from a combination of these modes of interaction with certain technical procedures and social settings.

1. The Model of Activity–Passivity

Historically, this is the oldest conceptual model. Psychologically, it is not an interaction, because it is based on the effect of one person on another in such a way and under such circumstances that the person acted upon is unable to contribute actively, or is considered to be inanimate. This frame of reference (in which the physician does something to the patient) underlies the application of some of the outstanding advances of modern medicine (e.g., anesthesia and surgery, antibiotics, etc.). The physician is active; the patient, passive. This orientation has originated in—and is entirely appropriate for the treatment of emergencies (e.g., for the patient who is severely injured, bleeding, delirious, or in coma). "Treatment" takes place irrespective of the patient's contribution and regardless of the outcome. There is a similarity here between the patient and a helpless infant, on the one hand, and between the physician and a parent, on the other. It may be recalled that psychoanalysis, too, evolved from a procedure (hypnosis) which was based on this model. Various physical measures to which psychotics are subjected today are another example of the activity–passivity frame of reference.

2. The Model of Guidance–Cooperation

This model underlies much of medical practice. It is employed in situations which are less desperate than those previously mentioned (e.g., acute infections). Although the patient is ill, he is conscious and has feelings and aspirations of his own. Since he suffers from pain, anxiety, and other distressing symptoms, he seeks help and is ready and willing to "cooperate." When he turns to a physician, he places the latter (even if only in some limited ways) in a position of power. This is due not only to a "transference reaction" (i.e., his regarding the physician as he did his father when he was a child) but also to the fact that the physician possesses knowledge of his bodily processes which he does not have. In some ways it may seem that this, like the first model, is an active–passive phenomenon. Actually, this is more apparent than real. Both persons are "active" in that they contribute to the relationship and what ensues from it. The main difference between the two participants pertains to power, and to its actual or potential use. The more powerful of the two (parent, physician, employer, etc.) will speak of guidance or leadership and will expect cooperation of the other member of the pair (child, patient, employee, etc.). The patient is expected to "look up to" and to "obey" his doctor. Moreover, he is neither to

TABLE 1   Three basic models of the physician-patient relationship

MODEL	PHYSICIAN'S ROLE	PATIENT'S ROLE	CLINICAL APPLICATION OF MODEL	PROTOTYPE OF MODEL
1. Activity–passivity	Does something to patient	Recipient (unable to respond or inert)	Anesthesia, acute trauma, coma, delirium, etc.	Parent–infant
2. Guidance–cooperation	Tells patient what to do	Cooperator (obeys)	Acute infectious processes, etc.	Parent–child (adolescent)
3. Mutual participation	Helps patient to help himself	Participant in "partnership" (uses expert help)	Most chronic illnesses, psychoanalysis, etc.	Adult–adult

question nor to argue or disagree with the orders he receives. This model has its prototype in the relationship of the parent and his (adolescent) child. Often, threats and other undisguised weapons of force are employed, even though presumably these are for the patient's "own good." It should be added that the possibility of the exploitations of the situation—as in any relationship between persons of unequal power—for the sole benefit of the physician, albeit under the guise of altruism, is ever present.

3. The Model of Mutual Participation

Philosophically, this model is predicated on the postulate that equality among human beings is desirable. It is fundamental to the social structure of democracy and has played a crucial role in occidental civilization for more than two hundred years. Psychologically, mutuality rests on complex processes of identification—which facilitate conceiving of others in terms of oneself—together with maintaining and tolerating the discrete individuality of the observer and the observed. It is crucial to this type of interaction that the participants (1) have approximately equal power, (2) be mutually interdependent (i.e., need each other), and (3) engage in activity that will be in some ways satisfying to both.

This model is favored by patients who, for various reasons, want to take care of themselves (at least in part). This may be an overcompensatory attempt at mastering anxieties associated with helplessness and passivity. It may also be "realistic" and necessary, as, for example, in the management of most chronic illnesses (e.g., diabetes mellitus, chronic heart disease, etc.). Here the patient's own experiences provide reliable and important clues for therapy. Moreover, the treatment program itself is principally carried out by the patient to help himself.

In an evolutionary sense, the pattern of mutual participation is more highly developed than the other two models of the doctor–patient relationship. It requires a more complex psychological and social organization on the part of both participants. Accordingly, it is rarely appropriate for children or for those persons who are mentally deficient, very poorly educated, or profoundly immature. On the other hand, the greater the intellectual, educational, and general experiential similarity between physician and patient, the more appropriate and necessary this model of therapy becomes.

THE BASIC MODELS AND THE PSYCHOLOGY OF THE PHYSICIAN

Consideration of why physicians seek one or another type of relationship with patients (or seek patients who fit into a particular relationship) would carry us beyond the scope of this essay. Yet, it must be emphasized that as long as this subject is approached with the sentimental viewpoint that a physician is simply motivated by a wish to help others (not that we deny this wish), no scientific study of the subject can be undertaken. Scientific investigation is possible only if value judgement is subrogated, at least temporarily, to a candid scrutiny of the physician's actual behavior with his patients.

The activity–passivity model places the physician in absolute control of the situation. In this way it gratifies needs for mastery and contributes to feelings of superiority. (Ref. 6 and 7.) At the same time it requires that the physician disidentify with the patient as a person.

Somewhat similar is the guidance–cooperation model. The disidentification with the patient, however, is less complete. The physician, like the parent of a growing child, could be said to see in the patient a human being potentially (but not yet) like himself (or like he wishes to be). In addition to the gratifications already mentioned, this relationship provides an opportunity to recreate and to gratify the "Pygmalion Complex." Thus, the physician can mold others into his own image, as God is said to have created man (or he may mold them into his own image of what they should be like, as in Shaw's "Pygmalion"). This type of relationship is of importance in education, as the transmission of more or less stable cultural values (and of language itself) shows. It requires that the physician be convinced he is "right" in his notion of what is "best" for the patient. He will then try to induce the patient to accept his aims as the patient's own.

The model of mutual participation, as suggested earlier, is essentially foreign to medicine. This relationship, characterized by a high degree of empathy, has elements often associated with the notions of friendship and partnership and the imparting of expert advice. The physician may be said to help the patient to help himself. The physician's gratification cannot stem from power or from the control over someone else. His satisfactions are derived from more abstract kinds of mastery, which are as yet poorly understood.

It is evident that in each of the categories mentioned the satisfactions of physician and patient complement each other. This makes for stability in a paired system. Such stability, however, must be temporary, since the physician strives to alter the patient's state. The comatose patient, for example, either will recover to a more healthy, conscious condition or he will die. If he improves, the doctor–patient relationship must change. It is at this point that the physician's inner (usually unacknowledged) needs are most likely to interfere with what is "best" for the patient. At this juncture, the physician either changes his "attitude" (not a consciously or deliberately assumed role) to complement the patient's emergent needs or he foists upon the patient the same role of helpless passivity from which he (allegedly) tried to rescue him in the first place. Here we touch on a subject rich in psychological and sociological complexities. The process of change the physician must undergo to have a mutually constructive experience with the patient is similar to a very familiar process: namely, the need for the parent to behave ever differently toward his growing child.

WHAT IS "GOOD MEDICINE"?

Let us now consider the problem of "good medicine" from the viewpoint of human relationships. The function of sciences is not to tell us what is good or bad but rather to help us understand how things work. "Good" and "bad" are personal judgments, usually decided on the basis of whether or not the object under consideration satisfies us. In viewing the doctor–patient relationship we cannot conclude, however, that anything which satisfies—irrespective of other considerations—is "good." Further complications arise when the method is questioned by which we ascertain whether or not a particular need has been satisfied. Do we take the patient's word for it? Or do we place ourselves into the traditional parental role of "knowing what is best" for our patients (children)?

The shortcomings and dangers inherent in these and in other attempts to clarify some of the most basic aspects of our daily life are too well known to require documentation. It is this very complexity of the situation which has led, as is the rule in scientific work, to an essentially arbitrary simplification of the structure of our field of observation. (We omit any discussion of the physician's technical skill, training, equipment, etc. These factors, of course, are of importance, and we do not minimize them. The problem of what is "good medicine" can be considered from a number of viewpoints [e.g., technical skill, economic considerations, social roles, human relationships, etc.]. Our scope in this essay is limited to but one—sometimes quite unimportant—aspect of the contact between physician and patient.)

Let us present an example. A patient consults a physician because of pain and other symptoms resulting from a duodenal ulcer. Both physician and patient assume that the latter would be better off without these discomforts. The situation now may be structured as follows: healing of the ulcer is "good," whereas its persistence is "bad." What we wish to emphasize is the fact that physician and patient agree (explicitly or otherwise) as to what is good and bad. Without such agreement it is meaningless to speak of a therapeutic relationship.

In other words, the notions of "normal," "abnormal," "symptom," "disease," and the like are social conventions. These definitions often are set by the medical world and are usually tacitly accepted by others. The fact that there is agreement renders it difficult to perceive their changing (and relativistic) character. A brief example will clarify this statement. Some years ago—and among the uneducated even today—fever was regarded as something "bad" ("abnormal," a "symptom") to be combated. The current scientific opinion is that it is the organism's response to certain types of influences (e.g., infection) and that within limits the manifestation itself should not be "treated."

The issue of agreement is of interest because it has direct bearing on the three models of the doctor–patient relationship. In the first two models "agreement" between physician and patient is taken for granted. The comatose patient obviously can not disagree. According to the second model, the patient does not possess the knowledge to dispute the physician's word. The third category differs in that the physician does not profess to know exactly what is best for the patient. The search for this becomes

TABLE 2   Analysis of the concepts of "disease," "treatment," and "therapeutic result"

DOCTOR–PATIENT RELATIONSHIP	THE MEANING OF "TREATMENT"	THE "THERAPEUTIC RESULT"
1. Activity–passivity	Whatever the physician does; the actual operations (procedures) which he employs	Alteration in the structure and/or function of the patient's body (or behavior, as determined by the physician's judgment); the patient's judgment does not enter into the evaluation of results; e.g., T & A is "successful" irrespective of how patient feels afterward
2. Guidance–cooperation	Whatever the physician does; similar to the above	Similar to the above, albeit patient's judgment is no longer completely irrelevant; success of therapy is still the physician's private decision; if patient agrees, he is a good patient, but if he disagrees he is bad or "uncooperative"
3. Mutual participation	An abstraction of one aspect of the relationship, embodying the activities of both participants; "treatment" cannot be said to take place unless both participants orient themselves to the task ahead	Much more poorly defined than in the previous models; evaluation of the result will depend on both the physician's and the patient's judgments and is further complicated by the fact that these may change in the very process of treatment

the essence of the therapeutic interaction. The patient's own experiences furnish indispensable information for eventual agreement, under otherwise favorable circumstances, as to what "health" might be for him.

The characteristics of the different types of doctor–patient relationships are summarized in Table 2. In this connection, some comments will be made on a subject which essentially is philosophical but which continues to plague many medical discussions; namely, the problem of comparing the efficacy of different therapeutic measures. Such comparisons are implicitly based on the following conceptual scheme: We postulate disease "A," from which many patients suffer. Therapies "B," "C," and "D" are given to groups of patients suffering with disease "A," and the results are compared. It is usually overlooked that, for the results to be meaningful, significant conceptual similarities must exist between the operations which are compared. The three categories of the doctor–patient relationship are concretely useful in delineating areas within which meaningful comparisons can be made. Comparisons between therapies belonging to different categories are philosophically (and logically) meaningless and lead to fruitless controversy.

To illustrate this thesis let us consider some examples. A typical comparison, with which we can begin, is that of the various agents used in the treatment of lobar pneumonia: type-specific antisera, sulfonamides, and penicillin. Each superseded the other, as the increased efficacy of the newer preparations was demonstrated. This sort of comparison is meaningful because there is agreement as to what is being treated and as to what constitutes a "successful" result. There should be no need to belabor this point. What is important is that this conceptual model of therapeutic comparisons is constantly used in situations in which it does not apply; that is, in situations in which there is clearcut disagreement as to what constitutes "cure." In this connection, the problem of peptic ulcer will exemplify a group of illnesses in which several therapeutic approaches are possible.

THE NOTIONS OF DISEASE AND HEALTH	IN MEDICINE (ILLUSTRATIVE EXAMPLES)	IN PSYCHIATRY (ILLUSTRATIVE EXAMPLES)
The presence or absence of some unwanted structure or function The actual state of affairs / The same state without the disability	1. Treatment of the unconscious patient; for example, the patient in diabetic coma; cerebral hemorrhage; shock due to acute injury; etc. 2. Major surgical operation under general anesthesia	1. Hypnosis 2. Convulsive treatments (electroshock, insulin, etc.) 3. Surgical treatments (lobotomy, etc.)
The presence or absence of "signs" and "symptoms"; the physician's particular concept of "Disease" (e.g., infection) / "Health" (usually no disease; e.g., no infection)	Most of general medicine and the postoperative care of surgical patients (e.g., prescription of drugs, "advice" to smoke less, etc.)	1. "Suggestion," counseling, therapy based on "advice," etc. 2. Some modifications of psychoanalytic therapy 3. So-called psychotherapy "combined" with physical therapies (e.g., electric shock)
The notions of disease and health lose most of their relevance in this context; the notions of more-or-less successful (for certain purposes) modes of behavior, adaptation, or integration take the place of the earlier, more categorical concepts	The treatment of patients with certain chronic diseases or structural defects; for example, the management of diabetes mellitus or of myasthenia gravis; "rehabilitation" of patients with orthopedic defects, such as learning the use of prostheses, etc.	1. Psychoanalysis 2. Some modifications of psychoanalytic therapy

This question is often posed: Is surgical, medical or psychiatric treatment the "best" for peptic ulcer? Such a question is roughly comparable to asking, "Is an automobile or an airplane better?"—without specifying for what. See Reference 8. Unless we specify conditions, goals, and the "price" we are willing to pay (in the largest sense of the word), the question is meaningless. In the case of peptic ulcer, it is immediately apparent that each therapeutic approach implies a different conception of "disease" and correspondingly divergent notions of "cure." At the risk of slight overstatement, it can be said that according to the surgical viewpoint the disease is the "lesion," treatment aims at its eradication (by surgical means), and cure consists of its persistent absence (nonrecurrence). If a patient undergoes a vagotomy and all evidence of the lesion disappears, he is considered cured even if he develops another (apparently unrelated) illness six months later. It should be emphasized that no criticism of this frame of reference is intended. The foregoing (surgical) approach is entirely appropriate, and accusations of "narrow-ness" are no more (nor less) justified than they would be against any other specialized branch of knowledge.

To continue our analysis of therapeutic comparisons, let us consider the same patient (with peptic ulcer) in the hands of an internist. This specialist might have a somewhat different idea of what is wrong with him than did the surgeon. He might regard peptic ulcer as an essentially chronic disease (perhaps due to heredity and other "predispositions"), with which the patient probably will have to live as comfortably as possible for years. This point is emphasized to demonstrate that the surgeon and the internist do not treat the "same disease." How then can the two methods of treatment and their results be compared? The most that can be hoped for is to be able to determine to what extent each method is appropriate and successful within its own frame of reference.

If we take our hypothetical patient to a psychoanalyst, the situation is even more radically different. This specialist will state that he is not treating the "ulcer" and might even go so far as to say that he is not treating the patient for his ulcer. The psychoanalyst (or psychiatrist) has his own ideas about what constitutes "disease," "treatment," and "cure." (Ref. 9 and 10.)

CONCLUSIONS

Comments have been made on some factors which provide satisfactions to both patient and physician in various therapeutic relationships. In conclusion, we call attention to two important considerations regarding the complementary situations described.

First, it might be thought that one of the three basic models of the doctor–patient relationship is in some fundamental (perhaps ethical) way "better" than another. In particular, it might be considered that it is better to identify with the patient than to treat him like a helplessly sick person. We have tried to avoid such an inference. In our opinion, each of the three types of therapeutic relationship is entirely appropriate under certain circumstances and each is inappropriate under others.

Secondly, we will comment on the therapeutic relationship as a situation (more or less fixed in time) and as a process (leading to change in one or both participants). Most of our previous comments have dealt with the relationship as a situation. It is, however, also a process in that the patient may change not only in terms of his symptoms but also in the way he wishes to relate to his doctor. A typical example is the patient with diabetes mellitus who, when first seen, is in a coma. At this time, the relationship must be based on the activity–passivity model. Later, he has to be educated (guided) at the level of cooperation. Finally, ideally, he is treated as a full-fledged partner in the management of his own health (mutual participation). Confronted by a problem of this type, the physician is called upon to change through a corresponding spectrum of attitudes. If he cannot make these changes, he may interfere with the patient's progress and may promote an arrest at some intermediate stage in the evolution toward relative self-management. The other possibility in this situation is that both physician and patient will become dissatisfied with each other. This outcome, however unfortunate, is probably the commonest one. Most

of us can probably verify it firsthand in the roles of both physician and patient (Ref. 11).

At such juncture, the physician usually feels that the patient is "uncooperative" and "difficult," whereas the patient regards the physician as "unsympathetic" and lacking in understanding of his personally unique needs. Both are correct. Both are confronted by the wish to induce changes in the other. As we well know, this is no easy task. The dilemma is usually resolved when the patient seeks another physician, one who is more attuned to his (new) needs. Conversely, the physician will "seek" a new patient, usually one who will benefit from the physician's (old) needs and corresponding attitudes. And so life goes on.

The pattern described accounts for the familiar fact that patients often choose physicians not solely, or even primarily, on the basis of technical skill. Considerable weight is given to the type of human relationship which they foster. Some patients prefer to be "unconscious" (figuratively speaking), irrespective of what ails them. Others go to the other extreme. The majority probably falls somewhere between these two polar opposites. Physicians, motivated by similar personal "conflict" form a complementary series. Thus, there is an interlocking integration of the sick and his healer.

SUMMARY

The introduction of the construct of "human relationship" represents an addition to the repertoire of fundamental medical concepts.

Three basic models of the doctor–patient relationship are described with examples. The models are (a) Activity–passivity. The comatose patient is completely helpless. The physician must take over and do something to him. (b) Guidance–cooperation. The patient with an acute infectious process seeks help and is ready and willing to cooperate. He turns to the physician for guidance. (c) Mutual participation. The patient with a chronic disease is aided to help himself.

The physician's own inner needs (and satisfactions) form a complementary series with those of the patient.

The general problem usually referred to with the question "what is good medicine?" is briefly considered. Different types of doctor–patient relationships imply different concepts of "disease," "treatment," and "cure." This is of importance in comparing diverse therapeutic methods. Meaningful comparisons can be made only if interventions are based on the same frame of reference.

It has been emphasized that different types of doctor–patient relationships are necessary and appropriate for various circumstances. Problems in human contact between physician and patient often arise if in the course of treatment changes require an alteration in the pattern of the doctor–patient relationship. This may lead to a dissolution of the relationship.

References

1. Ruesch, J., and Bateson, G.: Communication: The Social Matrix of Psychiatry, New York, W. W. Norton & Company, Inc., 1951.
2. Dewey, J., and Bentley, A. F.: Knowing and the Known, Boston, Beacon Press, 1949.
3. Russell, B.: Power: A New Social Analysis, New York, W. W. Norton & Company, Inc., 1938.
4. Szasz, T. S.: Entropy, Organization, and the Problem of the Economy of Human Relationships, Internat. J. Psychoanal. 36:289, 1955.
5. Dubos, R. J.: Second Thoughts on the Germ Theory, Scient. Am. 192:31, 1955.
6. Jones, E.: The God Complex, in Jones E.: Essays in Applied Psychoanalysis, London, Hogarth Press, 1951, Vol. 2, p. 244.
7. Marmor, J.: The Feeling of Superiority: An Occupational Hazard in the Practice of Psychotherapy, Am. J. Psychiat. 110:370, 1953.
8. Rapoport, A.: Operational Philosophy, New York, Harper & Brothers, 1954.
9. Zilboorg, G.: A History of Medical Psychology, New York, W. W. Norton & Company, Inc., 1941.
10. Bowman, K. M., and Rose, M.: Do Our Medical Colleagues Know What to Expect from Psychotherapy? Am. J. Psychiat. 111:401, 1954.
11. Pinner, M., and Miller, B. F., Editors: When Doctors Are Patients, New York, W. W. Norton & Company, Inc., 1952.

The Enactment of Trust: The Case of Cardiac Patients

Marcia Millman

Just as medical mistakes are systematically neutralized (covered up, ignored, made little of, or justified) by doctors who work together, so does patient anger and mistrust go through a similar process of redefinition. There is collusion in every aspect of hospital routine to ignore patient mistrust and to undermine and cool out patient anger, for the direct expression of these feelings (like the open recognition of mistakes) is highly disruptive to the comfort, schedule and convenience of the medical staff. Patients and their families usually offer no resistance to this carefully engineered neutralization of doubt and anger. Since they feel they have little choice or control over their medical treatment or over what is going to happen to them in the hospital, they prefer, like the medical staff, to avoid acknowledging their doubts in the hope that the less mistrust expressed, the less will be experienced. Indeed, they fear (often with good reason) that unless they are uncritical and undemanding, they run the risk of receiving worse treatment from angry physicians and nurses.

The "backrooms" of medicine, then, refer not only to the places and events that are off-limits to patients, but also to the thoughts and subjects of conversation that are avoided, and the emotional expressions that are not allowed in the doctor–patient or even patient-family relationships. And though these expressions are carefully held in check, they often threaten to break through the social conventions and disrupt the situation. The most upsetting ones have to do with indications of mistrust.

The patient's experience is one familiar to other situations: in many relationships and associations (with friends, spouses, work partners) an individual frequently finds that he must act as if he fully trusted, and felt trusted by, the other individual, for the relationship would be disrupted and mutual action become impossible if the actual mistrust were fully and openly acknowledged. Feelings of trust and mistrust are not simply states of mind that an individual is allowed to experience according to his own preference or temperament, for the expression of mistrust is much too disruptive to social encounters to be allowed such free latitude. Like behavior, feelings are shaped by social conventions and etiquette, and the expression of anger and mistrust comes under such strict social regulation that people are often forced to publicly display trust and confidence when they privately feel most doubtful and apprehensive.

Considering the magnitude of what is at stake, patients are exceedingly successful in masking whatever doubts about their doctors they may have acknowledged to themselves. Still, expressions of mistrust inevitably slip through, or are carefully phrased in indirect or unserious manners, and these expressions must be neutralized in order to prevent them from upsetting and dominating the interaction.

The situation of patients undergoing open heart surgery provides a dramatic illustration of the social neutralization of doubt and mistrust that can be found in ordinary conversations among doctors, patients and families. Although the interaction is orchestrated primarily by the physicians, it is enacted by all of the parties involved, each for their own different reasons.

It is not surprising that patients would wish to ignore their own mistrust. There are times in life when a sense of safety is maximized by ignoring danger in the environment. Sometimes openly showing what one has noticed may subject the observer to further risk (as in the case of the sleeper who

This article originally appeared as Chapter 9, "The Enactment of Trust: Cardiac Surgeons and Patients," in *The Unkindest Cut* by Marcia Millman, pp. 179–198. Reprinted by permission of William Morrow and Company. Copyright © 1976 by Marcia Millman.

awakens to discover a burglar). Sometimes admitting to knowledge may force the individual into public stands or actions that he or she would prefer to avoid (as in the case of the individual who discovers a spouse's extramarital affairs). Finally, as the stock character of the rejected lover always discovers, people are most foolishly trusting and recklessly blind to signs of danger when they want something badly. All of these considerations enter into the situation of surgical patients.

Most of the patients undergoing heart surgery are under the impression (correct or not) that there is little or no choice about their operations. By and large, their surgeons tell them that they have a choice of either refusing surgery and living only a short time (a few months, a few years) with considerable discomfort, or alternatively, of taking a relatively "small" risk in undergoing heart surgery. Since surgical consent forms are designed to protect the doctor and hospital from lawsuit rather than to insure that the patient has full information, the dangers of the operation are made to appear as small as possible. For example, mortality rates that are quoted may reflect the likelihood of death in the operating room but exclude the expectable proportions of surgery-related deaths in the weeks following the operation. Under the circumstances, very few patients refuse to undergo the surgery since the alternative appears so unattractive. Frequently, since they see no choice they would just as well ignore their doubts and misgivings. Like the sleeper who hears strange noises in the house, they figure they are more likely to come through the situation successfully if they ignore suspicious clues and sleep through the experience. Patients are encouraged in this avoidance by hospital staff members who communicate the notion that the "good" patient is the one who asks the fewest questions.

Friends and family members, for their part, feel that it is their special duty to cheer up the patient and help him or her to adjust to the operation and post-surgical "discomforts." With a strained but determined tone of optimism, daily visitors exhort the patient to "listen to the doctor for your own good" and join the hospital staff in discounting or making light of the patient's worries, thereby leaving little room and no social validation for the expression of the patient's anger and mistrust.

Doctors and staff members have the most to gain from the outward display of patient trust and the cloaking of suspicion or doubts. Paying attention to direct or indirect signs of nervousness and mistrust requires a great deal of doctor time and energy, and may make the doctor more vulnerable to uneasy feelings should the surgery go badly. Furthermore, by neutralizing signs of patient mistrust, the surgeon can sustain a more pleasant and amiable atmosphere in his patient contacts.

A display of "trust" by a patient for his surgeon is not, then, an automatic response that wells out of the individual's innermost feelings. Trust, rather, is a dramatic effect produced by the constant, unremitting efforts of everybody concerned to head off, ignore, and if necessary, neutralize the expression of disturbing thoughts. These efforts are expended in several strategic lines of action: they are built, first of all, into the background setting and etiquette of patient-staff contacts and the careful censorship of information that works to prevent the recognition and expression of mistrust. Should this fail, there is a second line of defense: an assortment of expressive techniques for minimizing or neutralizing patient mistrust once it has broken through the social barriers and been experienced or displayed.

An "atmosphere" of safety and trust is introduced by the outward manners of the staff and doctors: physicians present themselves and their surgical proposals with an air of confidence and certainty, and doctors and staff make up a "united front" in support of the procedure being recommended and of one another's expertise. They refrain from showing any doubts or disagreements about the treatment to the patient, and praise one another to the patient (whatever their private assessments may be). Nurses likewise routinely assure the patient that the surgeon is "one of the best" and that patients come from "all over the country" to have this particular surgeon and be in this particular hospital. Then, if a patient should entertain a doubt about a particular doctor, the suspicion is undermined by the belief that if the hospital is so good, so must be each of the doctors. Friends and family members also typically join the staff in singing the praises of the hospital and discounting patient concerns. For example, when one patient expressed doubts to her husband about agreeing to heart surgery, the husband teased her: "Come on, don't make such a fuss about it. These guys do it every day. It's nothing for them."

The first and most obvious technique for insuring "trust" is to keep the patient from hearing any disturbing information once it is known that he will probably consider or undergo surgery. Tales of success and of dramatic improvement following surgery are recounted to the patient. Reassuring visits to the patient might even be paid by members of the Mended Hearts Society, a national club composed of former heart surgery patients who give living testimony to the benefits of the operation. The enthusiastic attitude of these visitors toward surgery is insured by the organization's requirement that they go through a training certification process in order to gain permission to pay visits to prospective surgical patients. In their training they are explicitly instructed to "forget any unpleasant incidents" they may remember about their own surgery while paying visits as members of Mended Hearts. Those who cannot be completely counted upon to censor unpleasant information are told that they are not yet ready to make visits, for their "hearts are still mending."

Family members will usually hide their own doubts from the patient, but occasionally a patient will have to screen himself from a nervous relative. For example, several male patients undergoing cardiac surgery left instructions that their wives were to stay away from the hospital and even refrain from telephoning them in the final days before the operation. After surgery, they allowed their wives only a limited number of visits to the hospital. These men complained that their wives "made them nervous," almost to the point of making it impossible for them to undergo the operation. One such patient reported that a year earlier his wife had made him so apprehensive that he cancelled the operation just a few hours before it was scheduled to take place. Since that time he had suffered an additional heart attack and felt that he now had to submit to the operation. Fearing that a visit from his wife would create the same change of mind in the last moments, he had forbidden his wife to communicate with him in any way. Similarly, many patients dread the thought of seeing their spouses or children just before they are to be taken to the operating room. They fear that at the last moment their relatives will be unable to disguise their anxiety, and that the obviousness of their worry will force them, the patients, to finally experience the full depth of their own doubts and concerns.

Despite everyone's efforts to screen out alarming information, various disturbing elements invariably intrude on the patient's attentions and disrupt the "trust" that has been so carefully developed. Disturbances to "trust" come from many sources: unexpected complications or bad experiences in the hospital, disappointing behavior on the part of the doctors, alarming information from the environment, signs that the doctor or family members are not saying all they know. All of these upsetting intrusions challenge the outward appearance of trust and safety which everyone has gone to such care to produce, and the patient will often have to "neutralize" these signals in order to reinstate his own confidence and faith in his surgical care.

For example, patients who are waiting to undergo heart surgery are often placed in the alarming situation of wondering why another patient has failed to return to the ward even days after an operation. Since all the heart surgery patients in one hospital, both preoperative and postoperative, were kept together on one floor (except for the first twenty-four hours after surgery, which were spent in the Intensive Care Unit), when a patient failed to return to the ward within a few days after surgery there was good reason for the other patients to believe that the patient had either suffered serious complications that kept him in the Intensive Care Unit or, still worse, had died. Since cardiac surgery patients on the ward generally kept careful observations about each other's progress and passed news among themselves about all the cases, it was quite a feat for them to ignore the disappearance of a patient after surgery. Those still awaiting their operations were especially hard-pressed to account for these failures to return. At these times, there was remarkably little inquiry into the absence. If the subject was broached at all, the patients typically reassured one another that the missing patient must have been sent to another floor, even though they had been clearly informed that all cardiac surgery patients were kept in the same ward.

Such a response illustrates a common neutralizing technique of "redefining" the alarming cues in order to give them less upsetting meanings. An interesting example of this process occurred one day when the patients on the cardiac surgery ward heard on the television news that a young, well-known singer had died in heart surgery. Few patients made mention of the event, and those who did agreed that the singer must have been *very* sick (sicker than they were) not to have survived the operation.

Sometimes alarming information about the carelessness of the hospital staff will press itself upon a patient's attention. At about ten o'clock one night a patient who was recovering from heart surgery was exercising by walking up and down the corridor of the hospital wing designated for the special intensive monitoring of post-surgical patients. There were several lights shining over patient doors, indicating that these patients had called for a nurse, but not a single nurse was to be found at the desk or on the floor. Through an opening in the door to the nurses' lounge the patient observed that all of the nurses were crowded into the lounge, enjoying a farewell party for one of the nurses who was leaving the hospital. Disturbed that all of the nurses were seemingly out of range of patient call signals, the patient "redefined" the alarming sign by commenting that the nurses must have had a "lightboard" in their lounge so they could know when a patient was in need.

In addition to "redefining" the situation, another common technique of neutralizing the feelings and expression of mistrust involves the use of humor. It has often been observed that humor is used to express thoughts that cannot be stated directly. When patients make "jokes" about their anger or mistrust, they manage to give some small recognition to their doubts and criticisms, yet simultaneously keep them carefully in check by presenting these concerns as "not really serious."

Sometimes joking may be combined with redefining the situation. One patient who had undergone coronary artery bypass surgery was upset that he had not yet met his surgeon. Before his surgery took place he had consoled himself over not meeting the surgeon with the thought that he *had* met and liked his cardiologist. He explained that even though he had not met the surgeon, as long as the cardiologist was "on the team" (though he had been told the cardiologist would not be in the operating room) he had confidence in the surgery. After the operation he admitted that he was still disappointed when

the surgeon failed to come by but he felt that he could not directly express his disappointment or request a visit. He decided, instead, to make "a little joke" to his cardiologist in the hope that the underlying meaning would be understood and communicated to the surgeon. When he next saw his cardiologist he remarked, "Well, I sure will be embarrassed when I go back to Omaha and everyone asks me how I liked my surgeon and I'll have to say I never met him." The cardiologist expressed surprise that the surgeon had never stopped by and suggested that some unusual circumstance must have interfered with his customary preoperative visit. The patient's strategy was unsuccessful and, in fact, the surgeon never did visit the patient. By the last day of his hospital stay the patient was so disappointed not to have met the surgeon that he redefined events in order to make them less disturbing: he announced that he now believed that one of the young doctors who made daily rounds in the early morning hours was not just another resident but actually his surgeon who had been visiting him every day. Indeed, although the morning visitor in question was actually just another resident, there was some ironic truth in the patient's self-delusion, for the resident had done a much greater part of the operation than had "his surgeon," who was in the operating room during only a small portion of the total surgery.

It is impossible to think about the question of trust and mistrust without considering the extent to which patients "monitor" the environment for danger and observe what is going on around them. Most doctors act as if they assume that patients are thoroughly trusting and that they do not hear, see, think about or notice anything which is not directly addressed to them. From the doctor's point of view, the advantage of making this assumption is that they can conveniently talk in front of patients while making rounds without having to include the patient in their remarks or concern themselves with what the patient might have heard and understood from their conversation. Usually the patients will cooperate with the doctor's treatment of them as insensate by "pretending" not to listen to conversations which do not include them. Thus, while doctors on rounds discuss a patient's case as if the patient were "not present" (for example, by speaking about the patient in the third person even as they touch the patient's body), the patient will often politely remain silent or even cast his eyes upward toward the ceiling or away from the doctors in order to indicate that he is not eavesdropping on a conversation he has not been invited to join. But even when a patient indicates that he has heard what has been said, doctors will frequently persist in their treatment of the patient as an unobservant figure.

For example, one day the thoracic team was making rounds and stopped by the bed of a patient who had been returned to the operating room for repeat operations twice after her original mitral valve replacement surgery. She had required the two subsequent operations because she suffered from excessive post-surgical bleeding which had to be stopped. Since these two reoperations had occurred within a twenty-four-hour period after the original surgery, it was unclear whether the patient remembered any of these complications. Standing around the bed, the chief asked the resident how long it had been since her operation. The resident cryptically answered, "Three weeks since her third op." The chief replied, "Let's try to do it all in one step next time, shall we, gentlemen?" (meaning the residents should be more careful in suturing together the heart). As they turned to leave, the patient, who until now had been listening quietly, asked, "What did you say?" The chief paused and smiled and kept walking out the door. The patient repeated the question to the intern who was trailing behind and still close to her bed. The intern smiled and answered, "He said you're doing very well."

Occasionally one of the senior cardiac surgeons at Lakeside would ignore the customary professional courtesy of hiding mistakes from the patient, and would criticize subordinate staff members for mistakes directly in front of patients. By treating the symbolic social membrane that divided doctors from patients as an actual physical barrier he assumed that since the argument did not include the patient, the patient would not hear the dispute. One day, while examining a patient's surgical wound (which had been purposely left open to allow for drainage after an infection had developed), this surgeon was annoyed to find that the nurses had been using small-sized sponges (bandages) on the open wound. Calling them around the patient's bed, he yelled that they were to use only *large* sponges since the small ones could easily get lost in the gaping wound. After dis-

missing the nurses, he swiftly departed, while the patient was left to silently worry about still one more danger in a postoperative course that had already been filled with serious complications. The patient could not even give voice to his new alarm, since he was attached to a respirator inserted into his throat, making speech impossible. Indeed, such conversations seem to be held most often in front of intubated patients, perhaps precisely because they are unable to speak. For just as blind persons with normal hearing are often shouted at as if they were also deaf, so are patients, unable to speak because they are intubated, often treated by doctors as if they are also blind and deaf.

Indeed, patients are so thoroughly expected to be nonobservant that the rare occasions in which they indicate their watchfulness often seem comical and incongruous. For example, when patients have been given local rather than general anesthesia for an operation, their serious remarks about the operation or their attempts to take part in doctors' conversations as the surgery is underway often bring the staff to laughter.

The humor emerges partly from the fact that the patient's remarks are sober yet "unscientific," but these situations have a comic aspect primarily because there is something incongruously funny about a patient speaking up and making mistrustful observations as the surgery is actually proceeding. Here the patient becomes both a passive object and an active subject at one and the same moment, and the juxtaposition is so extreme as to be humorous.

Thus one surgical team could not restrain from laughing as the patient sagely observed, "I guess you can't smoke in the operating room because you keep a lot of ozone in here." The anesthesiologist, with tears of laughter in his eyes, mockingly agreed, "Oh yes, sir, we always keep the operating room *filled* with ozone." Another surgical team broke into knowing smiles as one alarmed surgical patient (who had been given spinal anesthesia to block sensation in his right leg) kept moaning and insisting that the doctors had made a mistake and were operating on the wrong leg.

Still another example of the unexpectedness and incongruity of patient watchfulness is the following. On the evening before surgery, an anesthesiologist and his intern-assistant paid a visit to a patient in order to make a final check on the patient's condition and to inquire about allergies and explain what would happen the next day. While examining the patient, the anesthesiologist asked about various body scars that indicated previous surgery. When he was done with his questions he asked the patient, "Now is there anything that you would like to ask me?" The patient, treating the doctor's invitation literally, replied, "Yes, what's that growth you have over your lip? Is that a mole, or a wart, or what?" The physician was mildly stunned to have the roles reversed and asked, "What?" The patient repeated his question. Glancing to the intern to smile at how "inappropriate" this question was, the anesthesiologist answered, "Oh, this? It's just a polyp. I've had it all my life and it's completely harmless, although there are a few surgeons who would like to get their hands on it." The patient continued, "Well, you should have it removed." The doctor smiled carefully, "Well, if you have no questions [implying that the patient's question was not a "real" one], I'll be going." As they walked out, the two doctors could be seen shaking their heads.

An interesting exception to the usual lack of appreciation by surgeons of the patient's observing capacities involved the case of a patient who was himself a physician. Immediately following cardiac surgery, the anesthesiologist and cardiologist noticed that the physician–patient had a very rapid heartbeat, which was hard to explain in view of his general condition. When they asked the patient to move his arms and legs and there was no response, they suspected that the patient was still paralyzed from the muscle relaxant that had been used as part of the anesthesia. After some speculation about the possible alternative explanations for the rapid beat, they decided that since the patient was a physician and knowledgeable about the operation and its risks, his rapid heartbeat might have been the result of anxiety from mistaking his temporary paralysis caused by the anesthesia for permanent paralysis due to damage done to the brain during surgery (and being paralyzed he would be unable to speak and communicate his concern). One of the doctors told the other of a case reported in a medical journal of a physician–patient who had erroneously made this same interpretation about his paralysis following surgery, and who had suffered a cardiac arrest (which later proved to be fatal) from the unnecessary anxiety. The two doctors in this case therefore decided to administer

a drug that would sedate the doctor–patient enough to make him unconcerned if indeed he were suffering from this worry. What is significant about this case is the fact that it is only when the surgical patient is himself a doctor that the physicians are likely to speculate about what the patient might be thinking about his inability to move. Obviously, even a non-physician might be alarmed to find himself paralyzed following surgery and unable to speak to learn the reason why, but this possibility was never raised with the other patients, who were presumed not to be worrying about their conditions.

When patients are treated and expected to act as if they are not observant about their condition or treatment, the assumption has many implications. For the patient it creates a further restriction on the legitimacy of expressing doubts or objections about his or her medical care. For the doctor, it is the first protection against having to pay attention to complaints or disappointments. For, if attempts to screen out alarming information and the patients' efforts to ignore, redefine or joke about their concerns are not sufficient to inhibit the recognition and expression of mistrust, then the neutralization process will arrive at its final phase: the doctor's techniques for making as little as possible out of the patient's expressed concerns. Clearly, the doctor's first strategy for neutralizing mistrust or resistance is simply to ignore it.

Treating the patient as if he weren't present and aware is only the most dramatic form of ignoring patient alarm. By routinely making bedside visits short and hurried, the doctor not only protects his time but also makes it practically impossible for the patient to introduce a serious discussion of worries, objections and concerns. Instead, the patient's alarm may only be voiced in more general and indirect questions which the doctor is free to interpret in terms of their most limited and technical meanings.

For example, one man of forty-two who suffered from severe coronary artery disease was told that his condition was very grave and that he would need to have several bypass grafts inserted into his coronary arteries. What he was not told was that his condition was so poor that he did not actually stand a very good chance of surviving the operation. His surgeon would be using a device called an intra-aortic-balloon-pump to support his circulation during the operation (a form of mechanical assistance sometimes used in the poorest-risk cases). Instead of indicating how poor were his chances (40 percent) of surviving the operation, the surgeon told the patient that the usual mortality risk of the surgery was not large but that since his case was more difficult and risky than many they would have to use an intra-aortic-balloon-pump to compensate for his poor condition. The patient, who was not fully convinced that he wanted the operation, asked, "Will the balloon mean my risk of dying is greater?" The patient was obviously referring to his total chances, with the help of the balloon, of surviving the operation compared to the average survival expectancy. The surgeon, however, chose to interpret the question literally. He answered, "No, the balloon will improve your chances." The doctor thereby allowed the patient (who did, in fact, die in surgery) to draw a falsely optimistic inference.

Just as the doctor may interpret and answer patient questions in such ways as to minimize the opportunities for patient resistance, so do doctors frequently "redefine" patient remarks in ways that neutralize the implicit mistrust being conveyed. The following incident, involving a postoperative patient, illustrates how doctors may selectively interpret a patient's remarks in order to ignore mistrust.

On the day he was to be discharged from the hospital following cardiac surgery a patient remarked to the surgical residents (who had come by on rounds and were about to leave), "It's all right for me to drive my car now, isn't it?" A resident answered, "No, you shouldn't drive for at least three weeks. You might get into a situation where you couldn't move quickly enough to turn the wheel or respond to something." The patient, apparently upset that this advice would not have been automatically offered had he not asked, replied with irritation: "Well, it's a good thing I asked, isn't it?" The resident, slightly annoyed, repeated once again the reason for not driving. The patient repeated twice more that it was a good thing he had asked. After they left the room the residents offered the explanation that by his remarks the patient meant that he was sorry he asked if he could drive, since in the residents' view he wanted to get away with taking a vacation while on sick leave from work. By not responding to the more obvious interpretation that the patient was angry and upset with *them* for not having advised him on postoperative restrictions, the resi-

dents avoided having to deal with an unpleasant situation.

Finally, a doctor may "redefine" and thereby neutralize expressions of a patient's alarm or doubts about surgery or hospital care by discounting them as "normal" and "expectable." Just as the last-minute doubts of prospective brides and grooms are cheerfully dismissed by friends and relatives as natural, unserious and even amusing, so is the doubting patient assured that his thoughts and feelings are due to "natural nervousness" rather than to any real fault with the medical staff. In fact, cardiac surgery patients are often warned that they may at times feel suspicious of their care, or fear that a staff member is going to hurt them, but that if they have these experiences they should remember that these are "normal" feelings which follow surgery and that they will eventually disappear. On the nurse's checklist of preoperative duties, such an "explanation of normal feelings" to the patient is often included along with other routine duties such as preoperative shaving and preparation. This advance warning to the patient is probably reassuring at times. Still, the custom illustrates just how systematically the neutralization of mistrust is built into patient care.

In addition to leaving little time for and ignoring or redefining signs of patient mistrust, doctors frequently neutralize these expressions by making jokes about them and treating them as unserious. For example, when a patient directly indicated mistrust for her doctor and his recommendation for surgery, the physician tried to neutralize the situation by joking that he would find the patient a surgeon "who needed the money." By making such a joke the doctor implicitly acknowledged that he knew what the patient really thought of him, yet simultaneously dismissed her opinion as laughable and unserious.

Finally, doctors and staff members often neutralize patients' expressions of watchfulness or mistrust by treating them as "inappropriate behavior." By labeling a patient's alarm as inappropriate doctors not only dismiss the expression of mistrust but may in extreme cases also disqualify the patient from the ranks of persons whose remarks must be taken into account. In most cases the patient is treated in ways that will inhibit any further expressions along these lines.

For example, following cardiac surgery one patient grew accustomed to the regular, even sounds emanating from his cardiac monitor, and these sounds reassured him that his heart was functioning well. When the sounds of his heartbeat suddenly became highly irregular one evening, he became alarmed and rang for the nurse, stating that he felt something was wrong with his heart because the sounds had changed. The nurse briskly replied: "That monitor is none of your business. It's my business, so why don't you just leave it to me."

When staff members respond to indications of mistrust as "inappropriate" they usually apply a wide range of "punishments" to the patient, ranging from gentle rebuke to more extreme measures. An example of the milder response involved a young male patient who was very well liked by the residents and interns. Upon entering his room on rounds one morning, the house officers came upon this patient as he was reading reprints from medical journals about his own particular disease. One of the residents grabbed the reprints from the patient's hands and demanded, "Where did you get these?" "From my brother," replied the patient. The resident continued, "Who's your brother?" The patient smiled and answered, "John." The resident then lectured the patient about how it was "dangerous" for non-medical people to read medical journals because they couldn't understand what they were reading and might reach the wrong conclusions about their illness. After the resident left with the reprints the intern added, "You know, you could have asked us if you had any questions."

From the patient's point of view, the wish to read medical journals (like the tendency to ask questions) might have actually reflected not mistrust of the doctors but rather curiosity and a desire to know more about his illness. Such an interest is often interpreted and treated by doctors, however, as a sign of deficient trust, which is "inappropriate." In making this interpretation they reverse their usual tendency to *underestimate* the patient's mistrust.

When patients attend to what they are supposed to ignore, critical assessments are likely to be made about their characters and personalities. For example, one patient had been kept awake night after night by the sounds of laughter and flirtation between the nurse and orderly who worked on the night shift. The patient had asked her roommate if she would mind if they kept the door to their room closed at night, in order to shut out the noise from the corridor, but her roommate felt she could not sleep with the door closed, since she felt "shut-in." As the laughter one night grew louder and louder, the patient, at three A.M., finally got out of bed, walked to the desk, and asked the nurse and orderly to keep their voices down. That night, the nurse recorded in the patient's chart that the patient "appeared to be nervous and anxious, complained of inability to sleep, and was out of bed walking the corridors." No mention was made of why the patient had been unable to sleep.

Sometimes a complaint or expression of mistrust will be interpreted by doctors as so "inappropriate" as to justify regarding the patient as mentally disturbed. By labeling a patient "crazy," doctors ultimately have the power to dismiss any criticism voiced by a patient. One patient who had been described by the staff as "uncooperative" and a "management problem" kept a diary in which he logged the comings and goings of the staff, and the number of minutes it took for nurses to respond to patient calls. The patient kept the diary unobtrusively in the night table by his bed, but each time he was sent to the x-ray department, the residents would remove the diary from the drawer and laugh together as they read aloud selected excerpts. The entries in the diary were cited by the residents as evidence that the patient was "paranoid." Although the diary seemed peculiar to the residents, it made perfect sense from the patient's point of view. The patient had earlier in the week had the unfortunate experience of spending much of one night with a patient-roommate whose death had gone unnoticed until breakfast time the following morning, an oversight that the patient attributed to the laziness of the nurses. He had subsequently taken to recording nurse arrival times in order to demonstrate his argument that the hospital nursing care was poor.

The doctor's behavior is usually more sympathetic when patient expressions of mistrust are masked or ambiguous enough to be handled by indirect responses such as joking or redefining the situation. A patient who is more direct in expressing his dissatisfaction is more likely to receive a sharper reply to his expression of doubts or misgivings. The same may be said about patient requests for reassurance from doctors (which may themselves be taken as signs of mistrust). When the requests for reassurance are made indirectly, the doctor's responses will probably be generous. For example, when one preoperative patient wished her surgeon "good luck" in her operation, the doctor responded to the implicit fear in her communication by reassuring her, saying, "We're going to do the best we can for you, and everything is working in your favor. When you wake up, the respirator will be breathing for you, so you won't have to worry about a thing."

On the other hand, when another patient made a more direct demand for reassurance from her surgeon on the night before surgery, asking, "Doctor, will I be all right?" the surgeon curtly replied, "Madam, we don't guarantee our work." And when another preoperative patient shook her head worriedly and remarked: "I hope God is with you tomorrow," the surgeon replied with irritation, "Madam, God has nothing to do with this."

Perhaps with direct requests for reassurance patients call too much attention to the fact that they are entrusting their lives to the doctor, and implicitly charge the doctor with full responsibility for the outcome. Many doctors report feeling uneasy when a patient says, "You're the boss, Doc, whatever you want to do, go ahead." For while the doctor wants full control, he doesn't wish to have the full responsibility dumped in his lap. It is at such moments that physicians often protest (by refusing to "guarantee" the work) that the patient is the one, after all, who "decided" on the operation and must take responsibility for the outcome.

Finally, it must be added that instead of neutralizing indications of patient mistrust, doctors occasionally directly acknowledge and "discuss" the mistrust with the patient. Sometimes these direct confrontations will be made in the hope of arriving at a better relationship with the patient. But more often they are used to threaten the patient with withdrawal from the case, and the result is usually to make the patient less openly critical of the doctor. As one surgeon explained, "Whenever a patient asks me if I mind bringing in a consultant for a second opinion, I say to myself, 'This patient is trouble—this is the kind of patient who is looking for a malpractice suit,' and I tell the patient that if he doesn't fully trust me, he's perfectly welcome to go home and find himself another doctor."

Such a threat of withdrawal is one of the most powerful and effective tactics a doctor can employ to stop or control expressions of patient complaints or mistrust. Most patients, when threatened with physician abandonment at a time when they are extremely vulnerable and helpless, will grimly swallow their concerns and apologize to the doctor, requesting forgiveness for having behaved badly. Frightened by the doctor's anger when they are dependent and see little choice, patients usually figure that the doctor must be retained at all cost. Indeed, many patients fear that if a doctor is angry with them, or dislikes them, he is likely to do a worse job on them, especially in surgery.

This broadly enforced enactment of "trust" has enormous consequences for patient care. By having his thoughts and feelings of doubt and criticism subjected to this complicated neutralization process, the patient becomes easy to control from the staff's point of view. The patient, meanwhile, comes to rely less and less upon his own judgment and observational capacities, since these receive no social validation and may even bring sharp rebuke. And while he may earn some small amount of comfort in being able to ignore frightening information, the patient also loses whatever small amount of autonomy he held in the situation. The ultimate result is to grant complete license to the physician and the staff, a license which is already virtually free from any professional regulation.

In daily life individuals normally monitor their surroundings for signs of danger, since survival ordinarily depends upon continuous watchfulness. The fact that most individuals unhesitatingly entrust their bodies and lives to doctors about whom they know nothing is a remarkable testimony to the power of social conventions and etiquette. For it demonstrates that even our most supposedly spontaneous responses, those involving trust and mistrust, are ultimately felt, not according to "authentic inner" experiences, but rather according to frameworks of social reality and behavioral proprieties that are created and sustained by organizations and institutions.

Physician Gender and the Physician–Patient Relationship: Recent Evidence and Relevant Questions

Carol S. Weisman
Martha Ann Teitelbaum

This paper reviews recent evidence and relevant questions regarding the potential effects of physician gender on the physician–patient relationship. Despite widespread interest in sex differences in health care utilization and illness behavior [1, 2] and recent criticism of the content and process of health care for women [3–5], little research has addressed the impact of physician gender on the physician–patient interaction and its outcomes. The lack of research in the area of physician gender is partly because few women, until recently, have entered those medical specialities most responsible for adult health care—namely, family and general practice, internal medicine and obstetrics–gynecology [6–8]. In addition, few health care settings are likely to be willing to randomly assign patients to male and female physicians for purposes of analyzing effects of physician gender on the process or outcomes of care. Nevertheless, the patient care issues raised by questions of the effects of physician gender are important ones to be considered, particularly as more women enter the practice of medicine and more consumers have the opportunity to be treated by female physicians.

We would like to emphasize that the current state of research in this area is such that no definitive statement can be made that physician gender has any discernible effects on the quality of physician–patient interactions or on the nature of patient outcomes. Such effects may exist, but no research tradition has addressed the question in a systematic way and only one brief review of studies in this area was found [9]. This paper will discuss the theoretical rationale for expecting gender effects and then present recent research that provides suggestive evidence on some aspects of the question.

THEORETICAL RATIONALE

This paper takes the view that if physician gender were to affect the quality of care, this would be likely to occur through subtle effects on the physician–patient relationship. In the most general sense, the nature and outcomes of physician–patient interactions are determined by the physician's attitudes and role expectations, by the patient's attitudes and role expectations and by the nature of the situation (e.g. clinical setting) in which the interaction takes place [10]. Thus although our present purpose is to discuss the potential effects of physician gender on the relationship, it will be necessary to view these effects within the context of the situation and to consider the impact of physician gender on the patient's expectations and behavior. This discussion will therefore consider patient's responses to physicians of different genders as well as the behavior of physicians of different genders.

Reprinted from *Social Science and Medicine,* vol. 20 (1985), pp. 1119–1127.

The success of physician–patient relationships in general has been studied with respect to various outcomes, including patient satisfaction, patient compliance with regimens and appointment schedules and (less frequently) patient health status. Dimensions of the physician–patient relationship that have been found to influence these outcomes include: *communication of information* between physician and patient (i.e. symptom reporting by patients, effective questioning and answering by both parties and communication of information and instructions by the physician); the *affective tone* of the relationship (i.e. empathy, trust, rapport); and the *negotiative quality* of the relationship (i.e. participation by the patient in decision making and conflict resolution when physician and patient have conflicting goals or expectations) [11–14]. These dimensions may be interrelated, in that effective communication of information and stronger rapport may enhance the negotiation process, thus improving outcomes [15, 16].

We reason that physician gender potentially affects these key dimensions of the physician–patient relationship and thus might affect the outcomes of care as well. Physician gender might operate through several mechanisms. First, *physician sex differences* in personality, attitudes or interpersonal skills might affect their interactions with patients. Early sex-role socialization is highly resistant to change and is reinforced through numerous social control mechanisms [17]; it is therefore unlikely that professional socialization processes would completely counteract sex-role differences among physicians. To the extent that female physicians have been socialized to the traditional female sex-role, they could be more nurturant and expressive and have stronger interpersonal orientations than male physicians. By the same reasoning, male physicians could be more reserved and less empathetic than female physicians.

On the other hand, female physicians have broken sex-role stereotypes to some extent by becoming physicians. As a consequence, they might be less likely than male physicians to hold traditional attitudes about sex roles and to impose traditional views on their patients' behavior. Thus the female physician might be inclined to involve the female patient in decision making to a greater extent than a male physician would, since the female physician is less likely to assume that women are passive and dependent; she might also exert more effort to direct or elicit information from male patients, since she is less likely to assume that men are inherently independent and reticent. The overall impact of physician gender on the physician–patient relationship therefore is hypothesized to be more effective communication, greater affect and improved negotiative quality when the physician is female.

It should also be noted that a considerable literature has attempted to explain the often observed sex difference in illness behavior and utilization of health services, in which women are found to receive more services than men. Nathanson has presented some alternative explanations for this phenomenon, including the argument that sex-role socialization may result in women being more expressive and feeling more comfortable disclosing symptoms [18]. Gove argues that traditional sex roles result in women actually experiencing greater morbidity than men, since women's roles are less fixed and more stressful [2]. To date, it is not known to what extent physician gender may be implicated in this phenomenon. Most male and female patients are treated by male physicians, who may impose traditional views of sex roles on their patients—e.g. may assume that women do not hold 'fixed roles' and therefore have more time to utilize health services; or that men are more robust and have less time to indulge in the sick role. Male physicians' attitudes and behaviors might reinforce symptom reporting or health care utilization in women and discourage the same in men. We are not suggesting here that male physicians account for these observed sex differences among patients, but rather that the hypothesis has not been subjected to empirical test [19].

The second way that physician gender might affect the physician–patient relationship is by altering the expectations that *patients* bring to the encounter. Sex-role socialization could result in patients bringing traditional role expectations or stereotypes to the encounter and responding to physicians based on these expectations. Patients might expect female physicians to be empathetic and nurturant, and male physicians to be less demonstrative and more directive. In addition, owing to the historical fact that until recently the vast majority of physicians were men, patients may identify the male physician with the norm of 'affective neutrality'—i.e. professional objectivity to preserve technical judgment [20]. Since there is considerable evidence from patient satisfaction studies that patients desire physicians who display an 'affective quality' in addition to technical competence [11, 21, 22], patients may expect and desire that female physicians will be more expressive or humane. Thus both male and female patients might respond to female physicians with greater self-expression and symptom disclosure, expecting greater affectivity in response. These patient expectations and the physician sex differences hypothesized earlier could be mutually reinforcing during the physician–patient interaction.

Finally, gender might affect the relationship by altering the *status relationship* between physician and patient. Here the relevant issue is not gender or gender role *per se,* but rather the *match* between physician and patient. Gender is a major component of social status, so that same-sex physician–patient dyads are presumed to result in greater 'status congruence' between provider and patient than would occur in opposite-sex dyads [23]. Historically, men have received medical care from same-sex physicians, and women have received care from opposite-sex physicians. Whether and to what extent this might account for sex differences in care received is an open question. Current models of physician–patient interactions support the notion that some degree of negotiation and 'mutual participation' improves outcomes, as compared to the traditional model in which an authoritative physician directs a relatively passive patient [23–25]. Greater status congruence in same-sex physician–patient dyads might be expected to enhance mutual participation by providing a basis for freer communication, including more self-disclosure, as well as more joint decision-making [13]. Thus both female–female and male–male physician–patient dyads would be expected to exhibit more favorable process and outcome attributes than would opposite-sex dyads.

The research literature on effects of physician gender is sparse and does not fit neatly into the framework just presented. To examine empirical support for the proposition that physician gender affects the physician–patient relationship through any of the mechanisms discussed, we must draw together evidence from a diverse set of studies many of which were not conceived or designed to investigate gender effects specifically and most of which varied either physician gender or patient gender,

but not both. With these limitations in mind, we discuss literature from the last decade in three categories pertinent to the topics just presented: (1) studies of sex differences in physicians' attitudes and sex biases; (2) studies of patients' perceptions of male and female physicians; and (3) studies of same-sex vs opposite-sex physician–patient interactions.

PHYSICIANS' ATTITUDES AND SEX BIASES

This section reviews studies of physicians' attitudes and perceptions that are potentially relevant to their treatment of male and female patients. As noted previously, if male and female physicians have been socialized differently or if physicians perceive male and female patients to be different, the physician–patient relationship may be affected. Studies pertinent to this topic are of several types. A number of studies have investigated sex differences in the general attitudes and career orientations of medical students and physicians and several have explored physicians' attitudes toward women's issues specifically. Other studies have investigated physicians' sex biases.

As regards studies of physicians' *general* attitudes and orientations, research has documented that female medical students and physicians are more highly oriented toward interpersonal relationships and affectivity in medical practice, while men are more reserved and science-oriented [26–28]. Recent studies have shown that female medical students are more likely than men to be 'helping-oriented' and to prefer assertive and communicative patients [28] and to value more egalitarian physician–patient relationships involving more information exchange and questioning by the patient [30]. These typical 'female' orientations are presumed by some to be compatible with the needs and expectations of the typical patient, who tends to value these qualities in a physician [9].

A few studies have looked at sex differences in physicians' attitudes toward *women's issues* specifically, since these are presumed to be related to how physicians interact with female patients as well as with female colleagues. Heins *et al.* [31] surveyed 182 practicing physicians in Detroit about their gender role sensitivity (i.e. rejection of sexual bias and traditional sex roles) as well as other attitudes. The sample reflected the universe of practicing physicians in Detroit in terms of age distribution (the men were, on average, older than the women) and specialty distribution. The study reveals that female physicians have greater gender role sensitivity than male physicians, even when age and specialty area are controlled. Women in this study were in general more liberal and egalitarian than the men.

Leichner and Harper [32] report that female practicing physicians in Manitoba, Canada, are more feminist in their views of women than are male physicians, with psychiatrists being more feminist than family practitioners, surgeons and obstetrician–gynecologists. Leserman [29] found that female medical students in North Carolina are more sensitive than males to issues concerning discrimination against female physicians and female patients and that some of these attitudinal sex differences become *more* pronounced, rather than less, over the course of medical socialization. Margolis *et al.* [33] found that female residents in obstetrics–gynecology surveyed as part of a national sample of U.S. residents in the specialty held more liberal views than their male counterparts on such issues as availability of abortion and contraceptive services and sharing medical practice with non-physician providers. These and other authors speculated that such differences may mean that female physicians would be more sensitive providers in dealing with female patients.

Another set of research studies focuses on the question of physicians' sex biases with respect to patients. In 1973, Lennane and Lennane [34] observed that physicians' tendencies to attribute psychogenic causes to a number of women's complaints (e.g. dysmenorrhea, nausea of pregnancy, labor pains), despite evidence of organic causes, was evidence of a sex bias in medical practice. There have been several attempts to demonstrate empirically that such a sex bias occurs in medical practice, but studies are inconclusive. Broverman *et al.* [35] found that providers of mental health services (i.e. psychologists, psychiatrists and social workers in clinical practice) hold stereotypes of male and female patients which characterize men as more inherently 'healthy' than women. In their study, male and female providers held consistent stereotypes, so the argument could not be made that female providers would be less likely to stereotype their female pa-

tients. Similarly, Bernstein and Kane [36] used a self-administered questionnaire and vignettes to study 225 male and 28 female family physicians, asking for diagnosis and attribution of psychological or organic origins to common complaints in male and female patients. No difference was found between male and female doctors, but male and female patients were judged differently by the physicians. Although in the vignettes both male and female patients had the same presenting complaints, men's illnesses were viewed as either psychosomatic or organic in origin depending on the information given, while women's complaints were more likely to be viewed as psychosomatic regardless of the information given. The authors caution that the lack of influence of physician gender is not conclusive because of the small number of female physicians in the study.

Still other studies attempt to infer physicians' attitudes and sex biases from observations of their treatment-related behaviors, without measuring physicians' attitudes directly. Typically, these studies look at volume of services or prescriptions delivered to male and female patients, with some attempt to control for severity of condition, and interpret sex differences in services received as evidence of physician sex bias. A major problem with these studies, from the point of view of this discussion, is that physician gender is not controlled; in most studies to date, physician gender has been unspecified but may be presumed to be overwhelmingly male. For example, Milliren [37] found that among the institutionalized elderly, women receive more major tranquilizers than men, even controlling for the women's higher anxiety levels. Cooperstock [38] concluded that women's higher use of psychotropic drugs cannot be accounted for by the stresses and social roles of women, but may be due to the behavior of physicians and the drug industry in promoting these drugs.

Verbrugge and Steiner [39] used the 1975 National Ambulatory Medical Care Survey to study services delivered in response to selected complaints (fatigue, headache, vertigo/dizziness, chest pain and back pain). A number of significant sex differences in services, prescriptions and return appointments were found, with women receiving more services than men, even after controlling for age, seriousness of problem, diagnosis, prior visit status and reasons for visit. Physician sex bias was suggested as one possible explanation for these findings.

Other data from the 1977 National Ambulatory Medical Care Survey suggest that the physician's sex might affect volume of services delivered. It was found that male psychiatrists prescribed drugs in 33% of their patients' visits, compared to 17% for female psychiatrists. Among the visits to male psychiatrists, 37% of those made by female patients involved drug prescriptions, compared to 28% of the visits made by male patients [40]. The visits to female psychiatrists were not examined by sex of patient.

Studies that do identify sex differences in volume of care delivered to patients, after introducing appropriate control variables, present a major problem in interpretation, however. Is the sex that receives the higher volume of services receiving better quality care, or is it the victim of unnecessary care imposed by physicians as a result of sex stereotyping or other considerations? 'More care' delivered to men may be interpreted as evidence that physicians take men's complaints more seriously or value men's return to healthy functioning more; this is the interpretation offered by Armitage *et al.* in one study that found men receiving more services than women for comparable complaints [41]. 'More care' delivered to women may be interpreted as overuse of tests or treatments on a population perceived as complaining, as dependent or as easily intimidated by the provider. These types of factors are considered by Verbrugge and Steiner. Thus the interpretation of findings of sex differences in volume of services received is problematic without measures of physician gender and sex-role orientations.

In sum, the evidence for physician sex differences in attitudes and sex biases is mixed. On the one hand, there is consistent evidence that male and female physicians at various stages in their careers (medical school, residency and practice) hold different attitudes toward practice and toward women's issues, with women physicians more strongly oriented to the interpersonal aspects of health care and more sensitive to female patients and women's health care issues. However, the translation of these attitudes into sex differences in behaviors toward patients has not yet been observed in the research literature. Vignette and simulation studies have provided some evidence that male and female *patients* are perceived differently, but to date there is no evidence that male and female *physicians* differ in their perceptions of male and female patients. Studies of actual services delivered present evidence of differences in quantity of services received by male and female patients, but again these differences are not linked consistently with gender of the physician.

PATIENT PERCEPTIONS OF MALE AND FEMALE PHYSICIANS

Having considered physicians' perceptions of male and female patients, we now turn to patients' perceptions of male and female physicians. Patients' perceptions of (including preferences for and satisfaction with) male and female physicians are relevant because they may reflect different sets of expectations which patients bring to encounters with male and female physicians. The previous section showed that male and female physicians express different attitudes and orientations regarding the interpersonal aspects of medical care, with women more interested in and oriented toward these aspects of care. As previously noted, studies of patient satisfaction with care received (regardless of sex of the physician) show that a major dimension of patient satisfaction corresponds to this interpersonal aspect of medical care; this dimension is variously labeled 'humaneness,' 'affective quality' or 'personal interest' and is contrasted with dimensions having to do with the physician's technical competence or administrative expertise. If the interpersonal dimension is indeed a major factor determining patients' satisfaction with medical care, and if women physicians are perceived by patients as more likely to excel at this dimension of care, then patients would be expected to prefer female to male physicians, to bring these expectations to the physician–patient encounter and to be more satisfied with care received from a female physician.

What is the evidence that patients perceive female physicians differently than male physicians? In a study of how male and female physicians are perceived, Shapiro *et al.* [42] administered the Bem Sex-Role Inventory to male and female private and clinic patients, medical students and physicians and asked them to describe the typical male or female physician. The women respondents in all three groups tended to view female physicians' behavior toward patients as 'androgynous'—i.e. having both instrumental (technical) and expressive (interpersonal) qualities—while male physicians were viewed by all respondent groups as either low on both dimensions or as only instrumental. The study therefore demonstrated that male and female physicians are perceived as behaving differently toward patients, but it did not address the relationship between these perceptions and either preferences for male or female physicians or patient satisfaction with care received.

There have been several studies of patients' preferences for male or female physicians, with 'preference' operationalized in a variety of ways. Using data from a large 1977 American Medical Association survey of office-based physicians, Langwell investigated potential patient preference for male or female physicians by analyzing the demand for physicians' services as reflected in fees charged for office visits, the number of days a patient must wait for an appointment for a routine office visit and hours spent per week in providing patient care in the office [43]. Using these indicators, the study found no evidence of consumer discrimination against female physicians; indeed, the study found a higher demand for women doctors, with patients (male and female patients are not distinguished) paying more and waiting more days for an appointment with female doctors.

Patient preference for male or female physicians has also been operationalized as potential patients stated preferences for types of providers. Engleman surveyed 500 male and female outpatients at New York City general medical clinics about their attitudes toward male and female physicians [44]. While a majority of both men and women (84% of men and 75% of women) stated a preference for a male doctor as their regular physician, three times as many women (17%) as men (6%) preferred a female doctor. Women subjects stated a preference for a female obstetrician–gynecologist more often than they stated a preference for a female doctor in any other specialty. Having previously consulted a female physician was found to increase the preference for a female physician and to increase subjects' ratings of the competence of female physicians.

Haar *et al.* surveyed 409 female patients of both male and female physicians (gynecologists, internists and psychotherapists) about their attitudes and practices regarding gynecologists and gynecological examinations [45]. The authors found that 34% of all the women stated a preference for a female gynecologist (19.3% stated that they would not prefer a woman gynecologist, and the remainder reported 'no difference' or 'no opinion'). However, 59% of the women who were patients of female physicians preferred a female gynecologist. Preference for a female gynecologist was also found to be associated with subjects' perceptions that pelvic examinations are difficult for them or that their current gynecologist does not understand women's psychological or sexual problems. Patients of psychotherapists were more likely than patients of other specialists to state a preference for a female gynecologist. It is possible to infer from the Engleman and Haar studies that either prior *experience* with a female physician or special problems for which the female physician is perceived by the patient as a more *credible* provider, perhaps due to her inherent expertise as a woman in treating sensitive or female conditions, increases the preference for a female physician.

Other research supporting this 'credibility' argument are recent studies of adolescents in family planning clinics. Philliber and Jones [46] found a greater same-sex than cross-sex provider preference among female adolescent patients seeking family planning services. When asked how important it was to them to have a counselor or examiner of the same sex, ethnicity and age as the patient, patients reported that gender was most important, especially in terms of the examiner. The JWK International Corporation [47] reported similar findings. Fear of the pelvic exam among teenagers has been suggested as one reason why teenage women prefer a female examiner [48].

As regards actual patient behavior in selecting male or female physicians, there is little evidence that patients actively choose physicians on the basis of sex. One recent study in the San Diego Family Practice Department of the Kaiser-Permanente Medical Care Program, a health maintenance organization, investigated members' choice of primary physicians by sex of member and sex of physician [49]. Based on data on visits by 50,018 patients (57% of whom were women) over a 6-month period, it was found that female patients were 1.49 times as likely as males to select a female physician, and male patients were 1.14 times as likely as females to select a male physician. Consequently, the female physicians' panels consisted of 66% female patients, whereas male physicians' panels consisted of 54% female patients. These findings support the conclusion that there is a tendency for patients in this practice setting to select a family physician of their own sex.

Another recent study focuses on the element of choice. Ross *et al.* [50] found that physician status characteristics (including sex) were related to patient satisfaction only in situations where patients were assigned to physicians (i.e. in large prepaid group practices) and not in situations where patients chose their own physicians (i.e. in small fee-for-service practices). When patients were assigned to physicians, they were found to be less satisfied with physicians whose characteristics were non-normative; thus, clients in prepaid groups were less satisfied with older physicians, female physicians and physicians from lower status and Catholic backgrounds. The length of time the patient has been going to the physician modified the impact of some physician characteristics on satisfaction. This study therefore suggests that both choice and length of exposure are important factors in patients' responses to female physicians.

Finally, it should be noted that few studies of patient satisfaction (the above mentioned study is an exception) consider the sex of the physician as an explanatory variable. This may be due to the small number of female physicians available for study until recently and/or to the sensitivity of this question to physicians. Furthermore, the difficulty of interpreting findings of differences in satisfaction associated with physician sex is illustrated by a recent investigation by Comstock *et al.* [51]. These authors studied 150 patients of 15 internal medicine residents (only 4 of whom were women) and found that female patients seeing female doctors were more satisfied with their doctors than were male patients with female doctors *or* male or female patients with male doctors. The authors argue that the greater satisfaction of females with female doctors was in spite of the fact that a trained observer of the physician–patient interactions detected no differences between male and female doctors in caring skills behavior when treating female patients. The findings could be due to women's different *expectations* of female

physicians, rather than to any actual differences in the encounters. No controls for previous experience with a female physician or credibility were included in the study.

To summarize, studies of patient perceptions of male and female providers suggest several tentative conclusions. First, since there is evidence that patients in the aggregate tend to attribute somewhat different traits to male and female physicians and that patient preference for female physicians is increased by previous experience with a female physician, it may be expected that patients' perceptions of female physicians will become more favorable as more patients are exposed to the growing numbers of women practicing medicine. Second, there is evidence that female patients, particularly those previously exposed to female doctors, prefer female doctors, in situations where a female doctor is perceived as a more credible provider (e.g. in family planning services, obstetrics–gynecology or psychotherapy). Third, satisfaction with care received by a doctor may be a function, at least in part, of the patient's ability to act on his or her preferences and select a physician of the preferred gender. These contingencies—experience, credibility and choice—seem to be key variables modifying the impact of physician gender on patients' perceptions of providers.

SAME-SEX vs OPPOSITE-SEX PHYSICIAN–PATIENT INTERACTIONS

To date, there have been very few studies of physician–patient interactions that attempt to compare the patient care process or its outcomes for same-sex vs opposite-sex physician–patient dyads. While some investigators (e.g. Ross *et al.* [50]) have addressed the general question of the effects of physician–patient status congruence, the question of matched or unmatched gender as a component of this congruence has not been studied systematically. Research in which some gender effect may be discussed (either because patient sex has been varied, or because physician sex has been varied, if not both) has consisted primarily of studies of the physician–patient interaction process rather than studies of patient outcomes. Variables pertaining to the care process that have received attention include: length of time spent in the interaction, symptom disclosure by patients, degree of information exchange between physician and patient and degree of empathy expressed by the physician.

There is considerable evidence, to begin with, that female physicians see fewer patients than male physicians per unit of time, thus spending more time on each patient visit and, presumably, more time in direct interaction with each patient. (It should be noted that the question of whether more time per patient equates with higher quality care has not been answered.) For example, Langwell reports, using 1978 AMA data, that in all specialty areas, female physicians see fewer patients per office hour than do male physicians [43]. Interestingly, the greatest differential on this variable between male and female physicians occurs in obstetrics–gynecology, in which nearly all patients are female: male obstetrician–gynecologists saw an average of 3 patients per office hour, compared to an average of 1.73 patients seen by females in the specialty.

Data from The National Ambulatory Medical Care Survey, covering office visits in the United States made by ambulatory patients to office-based physicians, show similar findings [40]. On average, female physicians spend more time in face-to-face contact with each patient than do male physicians. According to 1980–1981 data from this survey, female obstetrician–gynecologists had an average of 49 patient visits per week, with visits averaging 17.1 minutes; this compares with 69.5 visits per week to male obstetrician–gynecologists, with visits averaging 13.8 minutes [52]. In addition, female physicians spend more time, on average, in direct contact with their *female* patients than with their male patients. One possible explanation for the overall difference between male and female physicians in duration of visits is that male physicians may have more office staff to whom they can delegate portions of the patient encounter.

Another possible explanation is that the incentive structures in male and female physicians' practices differ: men are more likely than women to work in private, fee-for-service practices (as opposed to salaried positions), in which income is dependent upon number of patients seen [53]. Alternative hypotheses are that female physicians spend more time per patient because they are more attuned to the interpersonal aspects of health care (as suggested

earlier) or because they are able to establish better rapport with patients, particularly with female patients. Duration of the physician–patient interaction may either *reflect* stronger rapport, since more discussion and information-exchange occurs, or it may *produce* stronger rapport by providing the patient with more attention and more opportunity for discussion.

As previously mentioned, the reporting of symptoms by patients is presumed to be enhanced by stronger rapport and is considered to be a key component of provider–patient communication, affecting both the 'negotiative quality' of the interaction and outcomes of care [15]. An important finding in this area is that the social status of the provider can influence symptom reporting. In epidemiologic field studies of psychiatric disorders, women have been found consistently to report more symptoms than men [54, 55], and this sex difference generally has been interpreted as representing a true sex difference in symptoms rather than response bias [2, 56, 57]. However, other things being equal, status congruence between the physician and patient may influence both the reporting of symptoms by patients and the physician's interpretation of and response to information provided by patients. For example, there is evidence that less social distance between interviewer and respondent increases rapport and may enhance reporting behavior [58]. Riessman [59] reports that in a population-based study in New York City, women respondents tended to report more symptoms of functional psychological disorder than did men and also to report more symptoms when the interviewer was a psychiatrist who did *not* identify himself as a physician (as compared to interviewers who *did* identify themselves as physicians). Male respondents reported more symptoms to higher status interviewers (i.e. those perceived as physicians). (All physician interviewers in the study were male.) The findings suggest that higher status interviewers may 'threaten' female respondents and reduce their reporting.

The sex of the medical interviewer is also an indicator of the interviewer's social status and therefore may affect symptom reporting by patients. Several studies suggest that provider sex *per se* does not affect patients' symptom disclosure, but that the *match* between provider sex and patient sex is the key factor [60, 61]. In a study of subjects' willingness to disclose physical and emotional symptoms to hypothetical family practice physicians, Young found that male and female respondents were more willing to disclose symptoms to a physician of the same sex than to a physician of the opposite sex, especially when disclosing symptoms of a personal nature. It is important to note that these findings are consistent with the status congruence view noted earlier, rather than with the view that female physicians in general would be perceived by patients as more nurturing or sensitive, thus encouraging more symptom disclosure. If the latter were the case, then men as well as women would report more symptoms to female physicians than to male physicians, a finding not supported by the above mentioned studies.

However, one study provides some tentative evidence that male physicians may discourage communication and information exchange with female patients. In a study of 336 taped interactions between male internists and their male and female patients, Wallen et al. [62] observed the information-seeking behavior of patients and the responses of the physicians to males' and females' requests for information. They found, first, that physicians were more likely to attribute psychological causes to the illnesses of female patients than to those of men and to report being more pessimistic about the prognoses for their female patients as compared to their male patients. Further, the researchers found that whereas women asked more questions than men, physicians tended to give shorter answers to women's questions and to give less technical answers to women than their questions were judged to require. The authors interpreted these findings as indicating a tendency for physicians to withhold medical information from women in order to maintain the traditional male–female power relationship.

Another variable examined in the literature is the degree of empathy expressed by physicians during the encounter. In an observational study of residents in obstetrics–gynecology, Scully found that female residents tended to be more empathetic than males in dealing with conditions that are uniquely female and that they themselves have experienced (e.g. dysmenorrhea, labor pains); the author argues that stronger physician–patient bonds are formed in same-sex dyads as a result of empathy [63]. In a recent study of 39 female victims of rape, Bassuk and Apsler [64] found no differences in male and

female therapists' affective responses to victims or treatment of victims; however, female therapists rated victims as having more distress and functional impairment than did male therapists, perhaps as a result of their greater empathy with victims. In this particular study, empathy did not appear to affect the treatment process. However, in a study of 40 mothers' initial infant visit with 11 pediatric residents and nurse-practitioners, Wasserman et al. [65] found that increased empathy from the clinician was associated with higher satisfaction with the visit and a reduction in concern among the mothers. Female physicians provided significantly more empathy than did male physicians (4.3 episodes per visit as compared to 1.9 episodes of empathy per visit). Left unanswered in all of these studies is the question of whether female physicians are generally more empathetic than males, or whether they are more empathetic only in the treatment of female patients.

Studies of outcomes of the care process that examine effects of same-sex vs opposite-sex physician–patient dyads are extremely rare, and no conclusions can be drawn from the available literature. Seiden [66] reports that therapist gender is often considered when assigning patients in mental health clinics, and she presents some evidence of improved patient outcomes in psychotherapy or counseling situations in which the therapist and the client are of the same sex. Biener [67] studied counseling of clients in a drug treatment program and found that female clients were more likely to appear for a screening appointment if they had been interviewed first by a female counselor rather than by a male counselor. For male clients, the sex of the counselor made no difference in subsequent appointment-keeping. The implicit assumption here is that better communication between provider and client in female dyads could result in better client outcomes because of increased rapport between the interviewer and client.

To summarize, there is tentative research evidence that same-sex physician–patient dyads may result in greater opportunities for rapport (perhaps due to increased amounts of time spent in the encounter), in greater symptom disclosure and exchange of information, and in greater empathy expressed by the physician. While this suggests that women's symptom reporting, already found to be greater than men's, might be increased further through treatment by same-sex physicians, it is possible that the communication process surrounding the symptom reporting and the climate of rapport that might be established in same-sex dyads will be better suited to sorting out 'true' symptoms and negotiating treatment based on these symptoms.

CONCLUSIONS

Due to the limitations of the literature to date, we cannot draw definitive conclusions about the effects of physician gender on the physician–patient relationship or its outcomes. However, the research supports the plausibility of the potential mechanisms, discussed earlier in this paper, through which physician gender might exert an impact. We have presented evidence that male and female physicians hold somewhat different attitudes toward medical practice and women's issues, that patients hold different expectations of male and female physicians and that same-sex physician–patient interactions may be characterized by more effective communication and stronger rapport than opposite-sex dyads. Further research will be needed to test the specific hypotheses suggested at the beginning of this paper.

Some of these hypotheses anticipate more favorable outcomes when care is provided by a female physician, as compared to a male physician, regardless of the sex of the patient, and other hypotheses anticipate more favorable outcomes when care occurs in a same-sex dyad as opposed to an opposite-sex dyad. To test these hypotheses, one approach would be to use study designs in which both physician gender and patient gender are varied. The following dyads could be studied, for example, in analyzing physician–patient relationships in treatment of comparable conditions within the same specialty area (e.g. general or family practice, internal medicine):

		PATIENT GENDER	
		Male	*Female*
	Male	Male–Male Dyad	Male–Female Dyad
PHYSICIAN GENDER			
	Female	Female–Male Dyad	Female–Female Dyad

Given a balanced design, studies incorporating these comparisons would permit two-way analysis of variance as a means of independently assessing the effects of physician and patient gender. The presence of an interaction effect would reflect effects of same-sex dyads as compared to opposite-sex dyads. A further design feature that would strengthen such studies is random assignment of male and female patients to male and female physicians at an initial visit; random assignment would reduce the likelihood of a selection effect if patients chose their physicians partly on the basis of sex. Random assignment is likely to be feasible only in certain types of settings, for example, in health maintenance organizations or clinic settings employing a relatively large number of physicians delivering primary health care to adults. Potential modifiers to consider in these designs might include patients' prior experience with a female or male physician and patients' expectations regarding male and female physicians.

Care should also be taken in future studies to control for physician age in order to account for period effects that might confound findings of studies comparing older male physicians with younger female physicians. Since the availability of female physicians in older cohorts is limited, studies of physician gender effects will probably have to focus on younger physicians, who were socialized in the same 'eras' [26]. If the relationship of age, or years in practice, to gender effects is to be studied, then it would appear most appropriate to define a recent cohort of male and female physicians trained during the same period and follow that cohort prospectively.

Finally, research findings to date suggest that it may not be fruitful to seek general or global effects of physician gender on the physician–patient relationship or its outcomes, but rather to focus on identifying specific *conditions* under which physician gender will have an important effect. It is unlikely, for example, that women treating women and men treating men would reduce the aggregate sex difference in health service utilization, affect the overall quality of medical care, or be feasible in any case. However, it is likely that same-sex dyads might produce better relationships and outcomes under the following conditions: (1) when patients *prefer* to be treated by a physician of their own sex, because of their expectations regarding treatment by a same-sex physician; (2) when *sex-specific conditions* are being treated (e.g. in obstetrics–gynecology for women, in treatment of genitourinary conditions in men); (3) when conditions of a highly *personal or sensitive nature* are being treated, such that sex or sexuality are highly salient in the situation (e.g. in psychotherapy, in family planning, in treatment of sexual dysfunction); or (4) when a *longterm relationship* between physician and patient is required, involving negotiation over outcomes, motivating the patient over a period of time, and/or modifying the patient's lifestyle (e.g. in the treatment of such chronic conditions as hypertension or diabetes). Under these conditions, gender congruence may be a key factor promoting communication of information, establishing a climate of rapport and facilitating negotiation. Future research should attempt to identify the specific conditions under which physician gender effects are salient.

References

1. Nathanson C. Sex, illness and medical care: a review of data, theory and method. *Soc. Sci. Med.* **11,** 13, 1977.
2. Gove W. R. Gender differences in mental and physical illness: the effects of fixed roles and nurturant roles. *Soc. Sci. Med.* **19,** 77, 1984.
3. Ruzek S. *The Women's Health Movement.* Praeger, New York, 1979.
4. Corea G. *The Hidden Malpractice: How American Medicine Treats Women as Patients and Professionals.* William-Morrow, New York, 1977.
5. Ehrenreich B. Gender and objectivity in medicine. *Int. J. Hlth Serv.* **4,** 617, 1974.
6. Leeson J. and Gray J. *Women and Medicine.* Tavistock, London, 1978.
7. Weisman C. S., Levine D. M., Steinwachs D. and Chase G. A. Male and female physician career patterns: specialty choices and graduate training. *J. med. Educ.* **55,** 813, 1980.
8. Burkons D. M. and Willson J. R. Is the obstetrician–gynecologist a specialist or primary physician to women? *Am. J. Obstet. Gynec.* **121,** 808, 1975.
9. Gray J. The effect of the doctor's sex on the doctor–patient relationship. *Jl R. Coll. gen. Pract.* **32,** 167, 1982.
10. Bloom S. W. and Wilson R. N. Patient–practitioner relationships. In *Handbook of Medical Sociology* (Edited by Freeman H. E., Levine S. and Reeder L. G.), p. 275. Prentice-Hall, Englewood Cliffs, NJ, 1979.
11. Wasserman R. C. and Inui T. S. Systematic analysis of clinician–patient interactions: a critique of recent approaches with suggestions for future research. *Med. Care* **21,** 279, 1983.
12. Ben-Sira Z. The function of the professional's affective behavior in client satisfaction: a revised approach to social interaction theory. *J. Hlth soc. Behav.* **17,** 3, 1976.
13. DiMatteo M. R. and DiNicola D. D. *Achieving Patient Compliance: The Psychology of the Medical Practitioner's Role.* Pergamon Press, New York, 1982.
14. Garrity T. F. Medical compliance and the clinician–patient relationship: a review. *Soc. Sci. Med.* **15E,** 215, 1981.
15. Anderson W. T. and Helm D. T. The physician–patient encounter: a process of reality negotiation. In *Patients, Physicians, and Illness* (Edited by Jaco E. G.), p. 259. The Free Press, New York, 1979.
16. Lazare A., Eisenthal S., Frank A. and Stoeckle J. Studies on a negotiated approach to patienthood. In *The Doctor–Patient Relationship in the Changing Health Scene* (Edited by Gallagher E. B.), p. 119. DHEW Pub. No. (NIH) 78–183, Washington, DC, 1978.
17. Scanzoni J. H. *Sex Roles, Life Styles, and Childbearing.* The Free Press, New York, 1975.
18. Nathanson C. A. Illness and the feminine role: a theoretical view. *Soc. Sci. Med.* **9,** 1, 1975.
19. Nathanson C. A. Women and health: the social dimensions of biomedical data. In *Women in the Middle Years: Current Knowledge and Directions for Research and Policy* (Edited by Giele J. A.), p. 37. Wiley, New York, 1982.
20. Parsons T. *The Social System.* The Free Press, Glencoe, NY, 1951.
21. Ware J. E. and Snyder M. K. Dimensions of patient attitudes regarding doctors and medical care services. *Med. Care* **13,** 669, 1975.
22. Segall A. and Burnett M. Patient evaluation of physician role performance. *Soc. Sci. Med.* **14A,** 269, 1980.
23. Friedson E. *Profession of Medicine: A Study of the Sociology of Applied Knowledge.* Dodd, Mead, New York, 1970.
24. Szasz T. S. and Hollender M. H. A contribution to the philosophy of medicine: the basic models of the doctor–patient relationship. *Am. med. Ass. Archs intern. Med.* **97,** 585, 1956.
25. Stewart M. A. What is a successful doctor–patient interview? A study of interactions and outcomes. *Soc. Sci. Med.* **19,** 167, 1984.
26. Funkenstein D. H. *Medical Students, Medical Schools and Society During Five Eras: Factors Affecting the Career Choices of Physicians 1958–1976.* Ballinger, Cambridge, MA, 1978.

27. Cartwright L. K. Personality differences in male and female medical students. *Psychol. Med.* **3**, 213, 1972.

28. Cartwright L. K. Personality changes in a sample of women physicians. *J. med. Educ.* **52**, 467, 1977.

29. Bean G. and Kidder L. H. Helping and achieving: compatible or competing goals for men and women in medical school? *Soc. Sci. Med.* **16**, 1377, 1982.

30. Leserman J. *Men and Women in Medical School: How They Change and How They Compare.* Praeger, New York, 1981.

31. Heins M., Hendrick J., Martindale L., Smock S., Stein M. and Jacobs J. Attitudes of women and men physicians. *Am. J. publ. Hlth* **69**, 1132, 1979.

32. Leichner P. and Harper D. Sex role ideology among physicians. *Can. med. Ass. J.* **127**, 380, 1982.

33. Margolis A. J., Greenwood S. and Heilbron D. Survey of men and women residents entering United States obstetrics and gynecology programs in 1981. *Am. J. Obstet. Gynec.* **146**, 541, 1983.

34. Lennane J. K. and Lennane R. Alleged psychogenic disorders in women—a possible manifestation of sexual prejudice. *New Engl. J. Med.* **288**, 288, 1973.

35. Broverman I. K., Broverman D. M., Clarkson R., Rosenkrantz P. and Vogel S. Sex-role stereotypes and clinical judgments of mental health. *J. consult. clin. Psychol.* **34**, 1, 1970.

36. Bernstein B. and Kane R. Physicians' attitudes toward female patients. *Med. Care* **19**, 600, 1981.

37. Milliren J. W. Some contingencies affecting the utilization of tranquilizers in long-term care of the elderly. *J. Hlth soc. Behav.* **18**, 206, 1977.

38. Cooperstock R. Sex differences in psychotropic drug use. *Soc. Sci. Med.* **12**, 179, 1978.

39. Verbrugge L. M. and Steiner R. P. Physician treatment of men and women patients: sex bias or appropriate care? *Med. Care* **19**, 609, 1981.

40. Cypress B. K. *Characteristics of Visits to Female and Male Physicians.* Vital and Health Statistics: Series 13, No. 49. U.S. Department of Health and Human Services, Hyattsville, MD, 1980.

41. Armitage K. J., Schneiderman L. J., Bass R. A. Response of physicians to medical complaints in men and women. *J. Am. med. Ass.* **241**, 2186, 1979.

42. Shapiro J., McGrath E. and Anderson R. C. Patients', medical students', and physicians' perceptions of male and female physicians. *Percept. Motor Skills* **56**, 179, 1983.

43. Langwell K. M. Factors affecting the incomes of men and women physicians: further explorations. *J. Hum. Resour.* **17**, 261, 1982.

44. Engleman E. G. Attitudes toward women physicians: a study of 500 clinic patients. *West. J. Med.* **120**, 95, 1974.

45. Haar E., Halitsky V. and Stricker G. Factors related to the preference for a female gynecologist. *Med. Care* **13**, 782, 1975.

46. Philliber S. G. and Jones J. Staffing a contraceptive service for adolescents: the importance of sex, race, and age. *Publ. Hlth Rep.* **97**, 165, 1982.

47. JWK International Corporation. *Patterns of Utilization of Contraceptive Services for Teenagers.* Executive Summary, Contract No. 240–77–0155, submitted to the Office for Family Planning, Bureau of Community Health Services, Health Services Administration, Amandale, VA, 1979.

48. Zabin L. S. and Clark S. D. Why the delay: a study of teenage family planning clinic patients. *Fam. Plan. Persp.* **13**, 205, 1981.

49. Kelly J. M. Sex preference in patient selection of a family physician. *J. Fam. Pract.* **11**, 427, 1980.

50. Ross C. E., Mirowsky J. and Duff R. S. Physician status characteristics and client satisfaction in two types of medical practice. *J. Hlth soc. Behav.* **23**, 317, 1982.

51. Comstock L. M., Hooper E. M., Goodwin J. M. and Goodwin J. S. Physician behaviors that correlate with patient satisfaction. *J. med. Educ.* **57**, 105, 1982.

52. Cypress B. K. *Patterns of Ambulatory Care in Obstetrics and Gynecology.* Vital and Health Statistics: Series 13, No. 76. U.S. Department of Health and Human Services, Hyattsville, MD, 1984.

53. Bobula J. D. Work patterns, practice characteristics, and incomes of male and female physicians. *J. med. Educ.* **55**, 826, 1980.

54. Tueting P., Koslow S. H. and Hirschfeld R. M. A. *Special Report on Depression Research.* National Institute of Mental Health Science Reports, U.S. Department of Health and Human Services, Rockville, MD, 1981.

55. Clancy K. and Gove W. Sex differences in mental illness: an analysis of response bias in self-reports. *Am. J. Sociol.* **80**, 205, 1974.

56. Weissman M. M. and Klerman G. L. Sex differences and the epidemiology of depression. *Archs gen. Psychiat.* **34**, 98, 1977.

57. Carmen E. H., Russo N. F. and Miller J. B. Inequality and women's mental health: an overview. *Am. J. Psychiat.* **138**, 1319, 1981.

58. Dohrenwend B. S., Colombotos J. and Dohrenwend B. P. Social distance and interviewer effects. In *Research Methods in Health Care* (Edited by McKinlay J. B.), p. 267. Milbank Memorial Fund, New York, 1973.

59. Riessman C. K. Interviewer effects in psychiatric epidemiology: a study of medical and lay interviews and their impact on reported symptoms. *Am. J. publ. Hlth* **69,** 485, 1979.

60. Highlen P. and Gillis S. Effects of situational factors, sex and attitude on affective self-disclosure and anxiety. *J. Counsult. Psychol.* **25,** 270, 1978.

61. Young J. W. Symptom disclosure to male and female physicians: effects of sex, physical attractiveness, and symptom type. *J. Behav. Med.* **2,** 159, 1979.

62. Wallen J., Waitzkin H. and Stoeckle J. D. Physician stereotypes about female health and illness: a study of patient's sex and the informative process during medical interviews. *Women Hlth* **4,** 135, 1979.

63. Scully D. *Men Who Control Women's Health: The Mis-education of Obstetrician-Gynecologists,* Houghton Mifflin, Boston, 1980.

64. Bassuk E. and Apsler R. Are there sex biases in rape counseling? *Am. J. Psychiat.* **140,** 305, 1983.

65. Wasserman R. C., Inui T. S., Barriatua R. D., Carter W. B. and Lippincott P. Pediatric clinicians' support for parents makes a difference. An outcome-based analysis of clinician-parent interaction. *Pediatrics.* In press.

66. Sieden A. M. Overview: research on the psychology of women—II. Women in families, work, and psychotherapy. *Am. J. Psychiat.* **133,** 1111, 1976.

67. Biener L. *On the Need for Women Therapists: The Effect of Sex of Interviewer on the Entry of Women Into a Polydrug Treatment Program.* Wellesley College, Center for Research on Women, Wellesley, MA, 1979.

Structural Constraints in the Doctor–Patient Relationship: The Case of Non-compliance

Irving Kenneth Zola

. . . Too many investigations define non-compliance as almost entirely a patient issue. As such both research and programs emphasize what patient characteristics can be changed (cf. Becker and Maiman 1975 for general review). Study after study (such as Davis 1966) notes that physicians overwhelmingly attribute non-compliance to the patient's uncooperative personality or specifically blame the patient's inability to understand physicians' recommendations. In fact, the individual physician seems extraor-

dinarily well-defended against closely examining the problems of non-compliance. Not only do doctors generally underestimate the rates of non-compliance in their practices but they are also inaccurate in identifying non-compliant individuals (Balint et al. 1970, Barsky and Gillum 1974, Davis 1966). Thus, while almost all clinicians agree that there *is* a problem, it seems to be someone else's.

The truth is, of course, closer to home. General studies of learning indicate the important role played by the transmitter of information. This role may not even be a conscious one. Several reports have noted that experimenter attitudes have even influenced the results of animal research (Freeman 1967). Surely, if the attitudes of an experimenter can affect the behavior of his rats, it is not too much to expect that the beliefs of prescribing physicians about their patients, their problems and their treatment must similarly influence the actions of those very patients.

My general contention is that there are certain structural barriers in the ordinary treatment situation which specifically impede communication. In short, the doctor-patient consult, as presently constituted, is an ill-suited one for learning to take place.

At the most general level, it is important to bear in mind that the doctor-patient encounter is perhaps the most anxiety-laden of all lay-expert consultations. Rarely does someone go for a reaffirmation of a good state. At best, they are told that they are indeed in good health and thus a previous worry should be dismissed (Zola 1972). More likely they learn that a particular problem is not as serious as they feared. Moreover, given all the untreated medical complaints uncovered by epidemiological surveys, seeking a doctor's help is a relatively infrequent response to symptoms (Zola 1966, 1973). The visit to a doctor is likely approached with considerable caution. Delay is the statistical norm. Fear and anxiety the psychological ones. And while some anxiety has been found to be conducive to learning, the amount in the traditional doctor-patient encounter is surely excessive!

It is also not without significance that recall of the timing, if not the frequency, of doctor visitation is found to be notoriously inaccurate. In the large majority of instances the visit may well have been an experience to be finished as quickly as possible. And the most common way to deal with unpleasant events is to suppress them. In such a situation is it any surprise that a patient is likely to forget much that happened, including their physician's instructions?

But I can be more specific. At present I would contend that in the visiting of a physician, a negative context for answering and asking questions has been created—the result of both a witting and unwitting process of intimidation.

The negative context begins early. It starts with place. I am old enough to remember when the most frequent location of seeing a doctor was in my home. Whatever the 'good medical' reasons for the shift of almost all visits to hospitals, clinics, or the doctor's office (Gibson and Kramer 1965), it has resulted in a tremendous loss of the patient's power and security

at a time when he or she is most vulnerable. The visit is no longer on one's home territory. Everything is now unfamiliar. There are now no social and physical supports, no easy way to relax, no private space to move around in or escape to. Moreover, while most examining rooms are physically closed to other patients and staff, they are often so audibly open that complaints and medical advice are easily overheard (Clute 1963, Stoeckle 1978). And little effort is made in medical settings to change this. If anything, the physical set-up emphasizes rather than reduces social distance between patient and the doctor, and heightens the strangeness of the encounter. Thrust amid suffering strangers one is assaulted by medical signs, equipment, uniforms and sterility. Let me be mundane. When I was a child, my mother, to make the situation more relaxed, would offer the doctor a cup of coffee or tea. Is there any remotely analogous experience to defuse or make more 'familiar' our current visits?

From place we can go to physical position. Whether it be horizontal, or in some awkward placement on one's back or stomach, with legs splayed or cramped, or even in front of a desk, the patient is placed in a series of passive, dependent, and often humiliating positions. These are positions where embarrassment and anger are at war with the desire to take in what the doctor is saying. In this battle learning is clearly the loser.

The standard gathering of essential information also brings in its wake a series of problems (cf. Waitzkin and Stoeckle 1972 for a general review). It often starts with the taking of the medical history. It's bad enough that I don't know all my family's medical diseases or of what my grandparents, whom I never knew, died, but I begin to feel positively stupid when at the mature age of forty-four I do not know whether as an infant I had the measles or chicken pox. I may do a little better with more recent conditions but the feeling sinks again when it comes to medications I've taken that have given me trouble. "Those little red pills" seems an insufficient answer and the recording physician's dubious look does not help much. It's with difficulty that I recall that prescription drugs have only been labelled within the last fifteen years. By this point in the interview when I am asked questions about the specific timing and location of my varying symptoms, I begin to answer with a specificity born more of desperation than accuracy. Any vagueness I report is responded to as related to my faulty memory than the very reality of the symptoms I am experiencing. The scenario may be different in detail from patient to patient. In short, being confronted with a situation in which we already feel stupid not only sets a tone for the rest of the encounter but makes it very difficult, if not impossible, to ask the physician simple questions or admit that you do not understand certain things—no matter how much the physician may later encourage one to do so.

Another impediment to communication is the quantity of information to be transmitted in the doctor-patient encounter. Regardless of the potentially upsetting nature of the advice, there is quite simply the problem of *data-overload*. The patient is asked to remember too much, with too few tools, in too short a time. In most other teaching situations, the learner is encouraged to find ways of remembering (like taking notes). But the traditional position of the patient—without the 'set' or the implements—negates this possibility. Giving patients a printed sheet of instructions, as done occasionally in pediatric practice, is not the complete answer, but it is a start.

Next, there is the method of communication. For here is a situation where the physician attempts to distill, in several minutes, the knowledge and experience accumulated in decades. I have spent much of my professional life at medical schools and teaching hospitals but have yet to see much explicit attention given to this problem. As is the case with college teaching, the degree is regarded as sufficient guarantee of the ability to communicate what was learned. But the task is not so simple. In fact, what few self-evident truths there are, are soon forgotten. Experientially, we know that different subject matters, like mathematics in contrast with literature, must be taught and learned in different ways. By analogy, the same is true for a medical regimen, some things can be told, some demonstrated, some only experienced, some written out, some stated a single time, some repeated with variations. This in itself may lead to the further realization that the teaching cannot be done all at once or by the same person.

On a rather mundane level, there is the matter of language which both in tone and content often patronizes and thus further intimidates, and even confuses the patient. First there is the manner of address. Whether it be to bridge the lack of familiarity, physically or socially, or truly to establish authority and keep distance, the use of first names and diminutives seems to have lost its endearing charm. I will admit that it took the women's movement and a certain amount of personal aging to make me realize how awkward it felt to be addressed by a physician ten years my junior as 'Irv' while I could only call him by his attached label, 'Dr. Smith'. But the ultimate ludicrousness was brought home by a colleague during a recent hospitalization. When visiting her I witnessed the following interaction:

> *Looking down only at the chart and not at the patient in the bed, the physician said jocularly, "Well Anne, how are you today?"*
>
> *"Lousy, Robert how are you?"*
>
> *Taken aback, he responded, "My name is Dr. Johnson, I only called you Anne to make you feel comfortable."*
>
> *"Well," my friend responded, "My name is Dr. Greene, I only called you Robert to make you feel more comfortable."*

While I'm not recommending the above dialogue as a general mode of response, it did seem ludicrous to have my fellow colleague, herself a Ph.D. and several years older than the M.D., addressed in such a manner. Few potential patients would, however, be in such control as to handle the situation as did my colleague. Given that the average time of doctor-patient interaction is so short (one estimate is that the average visit is about five minutes with initial visits ranging to thirty, Waitzkin and Stoeckle 1972) address itself sets a tone. Thus the use of the diminutive and false familiarity further increases the already existing gap between the helping provider and the anxious patient, making the latter feel even more child-like, dependent, and intimidated.

A second aspect of tone that is worth reexamining is that most common and important of the doctor's tools—reassurance. That even this cannot be given without thought was illustrated in a recent study of pediatric practice (Pessen 1978). Confronted continually by what are often referred to as 'overanxious' mothers, doctors often responded straightforwardly with, "There, there. You needn't have worried. Michael is fine." In general I've begun to realize that the admonition, 'not to worry' is perhaps the most overworked and useless advice in the English language (Janis 1958). But here in Pediatric consultation, it had a more dysfunctional effect. It was a truly double-edged sword. While, on the one hand, it did communicate to the mother that her child's condition was not medically serious, it also contained an implicit 'put down' of the mother's concern. It made her feel foolish for being bothered by something that turned out to be 'nothing'. As Pessen revealed, one of the lessons the mother learned was thus a negative one—to be more cautious in consulting a doctor, lest she look foolish. The mother, however, did not learn *what* to be cautious about, but rather in general to think twice about her next visit.

My guess is that in this situation, should the pediatrician try to correct the mother's perspective, she simply cannot take it in. Already feeling foolish for having bothered the doctor, the mother is not in a good position to learn anything—the information the pediatrician is trying to transmit just feels like a further scolding. What should have been communicated were *two* separate and distinct messages. First, the physician should state that the child's condition was not medically serious, i.e., nothing to worry about, then the pediatrician should probably tell her that s/he understood and appreciated her concern, i.e., given her newness as a mother and the inarticulateness of infants, a baby's signs and symptoms are naturally puzzling and disturbing. At this time, truly reassured as to both her being a good mother and the lack of medical seriousness of her child's illness, the mother can then 'hear' the pediatrician's instructions about medically appropriate 'worrisome' signs and symptoms.

My final comment on communications concerns the very words used. The technical jargon confronting a patient might be bad enough but the major confusion is the different meanings assigned to the same word by doctor and patient. I heard recently of a survey where, of all the patients who were told to take diuretics for fluid retention, over half believed that the drugs helped retain fluid and were, therefore, used to treat nocturia. They altered their use accordingly.

In many instances the process is equally insidious. For when heard by the patients, the dictionary meaning of the instructions is absolutely clear. The confusion sets in only after the consultation, when the patient is at home and must operationalize the instructions. Let me illustrate with several routine incidents.

1. "Take this drug four times a day." Since this means taking it every six hours must I wake up in the middle of the night? What if I forget? Should I take two when I remember?
2. "Keep your leg elevated most of the day." How high is elevated? Is it important that it be above my waist or below? How long is 'most'? What about when I sleep?
3. "Take frequent baths." Are they supposed to be hot, cold or warm? Should I soak for a while? Is four times a day frequent? Does it matter when? Should I use some special soap?
4. "Only use this pill if you can't stand the pain." What does "can't stand" mean? How long should I wait? Is it bad to take it? If I do, am I a weak person?
5. "Come back if there are any complications." What is a complication? Must it be unbearable? What if my fingers feel a little numb? Which feelings are related to my problem and which to my treatment? Is it my fault if there are complications?

All of the issues in this paper I have delineated become even more complicated when the health professional is treating a person with chronic disease. When that person is also poor and a woman they are triply cursed (Emerson 1970, Boston Women's Health Book Collective, Cartwright 1964, Kosa and Zola, 1976). Everything becomes more complex—both in the telling and the hearing. Accordingly, the instructions and teaching, like the disorder itself, is a long-term event. Thus, the patient will, in the course of their disorder, inevitably have more questions, more troubles, and more doubts. They must not be 'guilted' for things that are just starting to bother them now. This should be regarded as the expected and natural course of events and communicated thusly to the patient.

Finally, we come to what the reality of treating a person with a chronic disease means for the provider of care. Particularly for physicians, this is a frustrating task, one for which their training in acute care has left them largely unprepared. Most of the diseases affecting us today cannot be cured, only abated. Death cannot be defeated, only postponed.

And these are realities that both doctor and patient must deal with, not deny. Nor will the medical world's previous defense against dealing with their own as well as their patients' frustration be any longer possible. The objectification of the patient as a disease state and the distance this produced will no longer be tolerated. The appendicitis in Room 104 or the rheumatoid arthritis down the hall will not stand for it. There is at long last in this country a consumer health movement. In its wake come many demands: a demystification of expertise, a right to know everything about one's body, and a sharing of power in any decision affecting one's life. Thus health personnel are forced to look at their patients as people and in many cases people who are quite different from themselves in gender, in class, race, ethnicity and some of whom they may simply not like. There is no easy answer to these new found feelings but they are there and must be dealt with.

While I have been detailed in my criticism of the present structure of the doctor-patient relationship, I am by no means pessimistic that it will remain so. As I just mentioned, there is a growing patient movement which will make them continually more assertive of their rights. It is, however, necessary that the medical world react not merely from a defensive posture. It can and should realize that an altering of a position of dominance, while initially experienced as loss, will in the long-run give us more freedom. (This is a lesson the women's movement is trying to teach men—that their 'liberation' will indeed help men in their own struggles to be free.)

Being mundane, a change in communication patterns with our patients can only improve our basic task. There is already research showing that the more information we share the greater is the likelihood of patient medical compliance (Davis 1968; Francis et al. 1969; Williams et al. 1967; Korsch et al. 1968). I believe that this sharing, including the sharing of uncertainty, will also decrease the psychological burden that physicians carry—a burden that I think is reflected in the alarmingly high rates of suicide, emotional breakdown, drug and alcohol addiction among health-care workers. A demystification of the doctor and his power, an opening up of communication, including angry communication between doctors and their patients, may also help stem the growing tide of malpractice suits. Part of the latter is, I believe, a response to dashed expectations.

When there is no place to vent dissatisfaction within a system (i.e. the standard doctor-patient consult) the only recourse is to go outside (i.e. to seek redress in the legal system).

I am essentially arguing for more open communication between the doctor and the patient. As I have delineated in this paper, part of the barrier to such communication lies both in the unjustified assumptions about patient behavior held by the health provider as well as a series of socio-psycho-physical elements which currently structure the ordinary medical consult. Hopefully, my description of these misconceptions and these barriers has been sufficiently concrete to show how they can be dismantled. . . .

There are many elements of the clinical encounter itself which can and should be changed. While many changes are fairly explicit in my listing of barriers to communication let me deal with some that may not be. The patient's position within the consult must be strengthened. Some, as I have mentioned, must take place outside our purview but others we can at least encourage. We must look more explicitly at the encounter as a didactic one and thus analyze how learning can best take place. At least one suggestion is a more explicit separation in time if not space between the examination and the information that the patients must have to know about their diagnosis, their prognosis, and their care. Where, for whatever reason, there can be no substantial separation, then at least let us give the patient a chance to absorb what s/he has been through— some way of gathering themselves together before we proceed. In a workshop I am currently running, we are teaching patients 'relaxation exercises' so that they can 'center' themselves before (a) they receive more information and/or (b) they start asking questions.

A second element is a recreation in certain ways of the patient's territory. It may be impossible to shift the place of most medical encounters back to the home, though particularly in long-term care an occasional home-visit seems appropriate to keep health providers in touch with the reality of their suggestions. What we can do, however, is encourage a trend that is already beginning, what the self-help movement calls the presence of an advocate. To the degree that certain medical conditions as well as regimens involve patients' families and 'significant others' we should take this into consideration when we explain the implications of a particular diagnosis and its treatment. Without taking responsibility away from the patient we can encourage and allow the presence of others during all phases of the medical encounter. We have I think 'overprivatized' the medical interview to the detriment of all concerned.

This concludes my remarks on this contribution of health researchers and providers to the communication barriers in the doctor-patient relationship. In reference to non-compliance I am contending that part of what patients are responding to when they do not cooperate is not the medical treatment but how they are treated, not how they regard their required medical regimen but how they themselves are regarded. Unless we fully recognize this phenomenon, we will live out the warning of Walt Kelly's immortal Pogo, "We have met the enemy, and they are us!"

Hopefully, I have taken a step in this paper to reverse this process. It is time to reexamine many of the traditional assumptions of what it takes to heal and to help. I am naive enough to believe that knowledge and awareness are powerful tools. While acknowledging the dilemmas in the doctor-patient relationship will not be sufficient to make the problem of non-compliance disappear, it will at least change the context of discussion. The participants in deciding what is best must be patients as well as doctors. We must remember that giving up power is NOT the same as abdicating responsibility. There must be less talk of persuasion and more of negotiation. And when we do so, a change in philosophy will be reflected in a change in language. We will no longer speak of 'medication compliance' but rather of 'therapeutic alliance'.

References

BALINT, M., J. HUNT, D. JOYCE, M. MARINKER, and J. WOODCOCK
1970 Treatment or Diagnosis—A Study of Repeat Prescriptions in General Practice. London: Tavistock Publications.

BARSKY, A. and R. GILLUM
1974 The Diagnosis and Management of Patient Non-Compliance. Journal of the American Medical Association 228:1563–1567.

BECKER, M. H. and L.A. MAIMAN
1975 Sociobehavioral Determinants of Compliance with Health and Medical Care Recommendation. Medical Care 13:10–24.

Boston Women's Health Book Collective
1976 Our Bodies Ourselves. New York: Simon and Schuster.

CARTWRIGHT, A.
1964 Human Relations and Hospital Care. London: Routledge and Kegan Paul.

CLUTE, K. F.
1963 The General Practitioner—A Study of Medical Education and Practice in Ontario and Nova Scotia. Toronto: University of Toronto Press.

DAVIS, M. S.
1966 Variations in Patients' Compliance with Doctors' Orders. Journal of Medical Education 41:1037–1048.
1968 Variations in Patients' Compliance with Doctors' Advice: An Empirical Analysis of Patterns of Communication. American Journal of Public Health 58:274–288.

EMERSON, J. P.
1970 Behavior in Private Places: Sustaining Definitions of Reality in Gynecological Examinations. In Recent Sociology, J. P. Dreitzel, ed. pp. 74–97. London: MacMillan Co.

FRANCIS, V., B. M. KORSCH, and M. J. MORRIS
1969 Gaps in Doctor-Patient Communication: Patients' Response to Medical Advice. New England Journal of Medicine 280:535–540.

FREEMAN, N.
1967 The Social Nature of Psychological Research. New York: Basic Books.

GIBSON, C. D. and B. M. KRAMER
1965 Site of Care in Medical Practice. Medical Care, 3:14–17.

JANIS, I.
1958 Psychological Stress-Psychoanalytic and Behavioral Studies of Surgical Patients. New York: John Wiley & Sons.

KORSCH, B. M., E. K. GOZZI, and V. FRANCIS
1969 Gaps in Doctor Patient Communication: Doctor-Patient Interaction and Patient Satisfaction. Pediatrics 42:855–871.

KOSA, JOHN and IRVING KENNETH ZOLA, eds.
1975 Poverty and Health: A Sociological Analysis (rev. edition). Cambridge: Harvard University Press.

PESSEN, B.
  1978 Learning to be a Mother: The Influence of the Medi-
       cal Profession. Ph.D. dissertation, Department of
       Sociology, Brandeis University.

STOECKLE, J.
  1978 Encounters of Patients and Doctors—A Book of
       Readings with Commentary. Unpublished Manu-
       script.

WAITZKIN, H. and J. STOECKLE
  1972 Communication of Information about Illness. *In*
       Advances in Psychomatic Medicine, Vol. 8, Z. Li-
       powski, ed. pp. 180–215. Basel: Karger.

WILLIAMS, T. F., et al.
  1967 The Clinical Picture of Diabetes Control Studied
       in Four Settings. American Journal of Public
       Health 57:441–451.

ZOLA, I. K.
  1966 Culture and Symptoms—An Analysis of Patients'
       Presenting Complaints. American Sociological Re-
       view 31:615–630.

  1972 Studying the Decision to See a Doctor: Review,
       Critique, Corrective. *In* Advances in Psychomatic
       Medicine, Vol. 8, Z. Lipowski, ed. pp. 216–236. Ba-
       sel: Karger.

  1973 Pathways to the Doctor—From Person to Patient.
       Social Science and Medicine 7:677–684.

The Meaning of Medications: Another Look at Compliance

Peter Conrad

Compliance with medical regimens, especially drug regimens, has become a topic of central interest for both medical and social scientific research. By compliance we mean "the extent to which a person's behavior (in terms of taking medications, following diets, or executing lifestyle changes) coincides with medical or health advice" [1]. It is noncompliance that has engendered the most concern and attention. Most theories locate the sources of noncompliance in the doctor patient interaction, patient knowledge or beliefs about treatment and, to a lesser extent, the nature of the regimen or illness.

This paper offers an alternative perspective on noncompliance with drug regimens, one situated in the patient's experience of illness. Most studies of noncompliance assume the centrality of patient–practitioner interaction for compliance. Using data from a study of the experience of epilepsy, I argue that from a patient-centered perspective the meanings of medication in people's everyday lives are more salient than doctor–patient interaction for understanding why people alter their prescribed medical regimens. The issue is more one of self-regulation than compliance. After reviewing briefly various perspectives on compliance and presenting a synopsis of our method and sample, I develop the concept of medication practice to aid in understanding patient's experiences with medication regimens. This perspective enables us to analyze 'noncompliance' among our sample of people with epilepsy in a different light than the usual medically-centered approach allows.

Reprinted from *Social Science and Medicine*, vol. 20 (1985), pp. 29–37.

PERSPECTIVES ON COMPLIANCE

Most studies show that at least one-third of patients are noncompliant with drug regimens; i.e. they do not take medications as prescribed or take them in correct doses or sequences [2–4]. A recent review of methodologically rigorous studies suggests that compliance rates with medications over a large period tend to converge at approx. 50% [5].

Literally hundreds of studies have been conducted on compliance. Extensive summaries and compilations of this burgeoning literature are available [1, 6, 7]. In this section I will note some of the more general findings and briefly summarize the major explanatory perspectives. Studies have found, for example, that noncompliance tends to be higher under certain conditions: when medical regimens are more complex [8]; with asymptomatic or psychiatric disorders [9]; when treatment period lasts for longer periods of time [5]; and when there are several troublesome drug side effects [4]. Interestingly, there seems to be little consistent relationship between noncompliance and such factors as social class, age, sex, education and marital status [8].

Two dominant social scientific perspectives have emerged that attempt to explain variations in compliance and noncompliance. One locates the source of the problem in doctor–patient interaction or communication while the other postulates that patients' health beliefs are central to understanding noncompliant behavior. These perspectives each are multicausal and in some ways are compatible.

There have been a series of diverse studies suggesting that noncompliance is a result of some problem in doctor–patient interaction (see [10]). Researchers have found higher compliance rates are associated with physicians giving explicit and appropriate instructions, more and clearer information, and more and better feedback [2, 10]. Other researchers note that noncompliance is higher when patients' expectations are not met or their physicians are not behaving in a friendly manner [12, 13]. Hulka *et al.* [3], Davis [2] and others suggest that the physician and his or her style of communicating may affect patient compliance. In short, these studies find the source of noncompliance in doctor–patient communication and suggest that compliance rates can be im-

proved by making some changes in clinician–patient interaction.

The importance of patient beliefs for compliant behavior is highlighted by the 'health-belief model.' The health-belief model is a social psychological perspective first developed to explain preventative health behavior. It has been adapted by Becker [14–16] to explain compliance. This perspective is a "value-expecting model in which behavior is controlled by rational decisions taken in the light of a set of subjective probabilities" [17]. The health-belief model suggests that patients are more likely to comply with doctors' orders when they feel susceptibility to illness, believe the illness to have potential serious consequences for health or daily functioning, and do not anticipate major obstacles, such as side effects or cost. Becker [15] found general support for a relationship between compliance and patients' beliefs about susceptibility, severity, benefits and costs.

Both perspectives have accumulated some supporting evidence, but make certain problematic assumptions about the nature and source of compliant behavior. The whole notion of 'compliance' suggests a medically-centered orientation; how and why people follow or deviate from doctors' orders. It is a concept developed from the doctor's perspective and conceived to solve the provider defined problem of 'noncompliance.' The assumption is the doctor gives the orders; patients are expected to comply. It is based on a consensual model of doctor–patient relations, aligning with Parsons' [18] perspective, where noncompliance is deemed a form of deviance in need of explanation. Compliance/noncompliance studies generally assume a moral stance that not following medical regimens is deviant. While this perspective is reasonable from the physician's viewpoint, when social scientists adopt this perspective they implicitly reinforce the medically-centered perspective.

Some assumptions of each perspective are also problematic. The doctor–patient interaction perspective points to flaws in doctor–patient communication as the source of noncompliance. It is assumed that the doctor is very significant for compliance and the research proceeds from there. Although the health belief model takes the patient's perspective into account, it assumes that patients act from a rational calculus based on health-related beliefs. This perspective assumes that health-related beliefs are the most significant aspects of subjective experience and that compliance is a rational decision based on these beliefs. In an attempt to create a succinct and straight-forward model, it ignores other aspects of experience that may affect how illness and treatment are managed.

There is an alternative, less-developed perspective that is rarely mentioned in studies of compliance. This patient-centered perspective sees patients as active agents in their treatment rather than as "passive and obedient recipients of medical instructions" [19]. Stimson [19] argues that to understand noncompliance it is important to account for several factors that are often ignored in compliance studies. Patients have their own ideas about taking medication—which only in part come from doctors—that affect their use of medications. People evaluate both doctors's actions and the prescribed drugs in comparison to what they themselves know about illness and medication. In a study of arthritis patients Arluke [20] found that patients evaluate also the therapeutic efficacy of drugs against the achievement of specific outcomes. Medicines are judged ineffective when a salient outcome is not achieved, usually in terms of the patient's expected time frames. The patient's decision to stop taking medications is a rational-empirical method of testing their views of drug efficacy. Another study found some patients augmented or diminished their treatment regimens as an attempt to assert control on the doctor–patient relationship [21]. Hayes-Bautista [21] notes, "The need to modify treatment arises when it appears the original treatment is somehow not totally appropriate" and contends noncompliance may be a form of patient bargaining with doctors. Others [22] have noted that noncompliance may be the result of particular medical regimens that are not compatible with contexts of people's lives.

These studies suggest that the issue of noncompliance appears very different from a patient-centered perspective than a medically-centered one. Most are critical of traditional compliance studies, although still connecting compliance with doctor–patient interactions [19, 21] or with direct evaluation of the drug itself [19, 20]. Most sufferers of illness, especially chronic illness, spend a small fraction of their lives in the 'patient role' so it is by no means certain that the doctor–patient relationship is the only or even most significant factor in their decisions about drug-taking. A broader perspective suggests

that sufferers of illness need to manage their daily existence of which medical regimens are only a part (cf. [23]). Such a perspective proposes that we examine the meaning of medications as they are manifested in people's everyday lives.

This paper is an attempt to further develop a patient- or sufferer-centered perspective on adhering to medical regimens. We did not set out to study compliance *per se;* rather this paper reflects themes that emerged from our larger study of people's experiences of epilepsy [24]. We examine what prescribed medications mean to the people with epilepsy we interviewed; and how these meanings are reflected in their use.

METHOD AND SAMPLE

The larger research project from which these data are drawn endeavors to present and analyze an 'insider's' view of what it is like to have epilepsy in our society. To accomplish this we interviewed 80 people about their life experiences with epilepsy. Interviews were conducted over a 3-year period and respondents were selected on the basis of availability and willingness to participate. We used a snowball sampling technique, relying on advertisements in local newspapers, invitation letters passed anonymously by common acquaintances, and names obtained from local social agencies, self-help groups and health workers. No pretense to statistical representativeness is intended or sought. Our intention was to develop a sample from which theoretical insight would emerge and a conceptual understanding of epilepsy could be gained (see [25]).

We used an interview guide consisting of 50 open-ended questions and interviewed most of our respondents in their homes. The interviews lasted 1–3 hours and were tape-recorded. The recordings were transcribed and yielded over 2000 single-spaced typed pages of verbatim data.

Our sample ranged in age from 14 to 54 years (average age 28) and included 44 women and 36 men. Most respondents came from a metropolitan area in the midwest; a small number from a major city on the east coast. Our sample could be described as largely lower-middle class in terms of education and income. None of our respondents were or had been institutionalized for epilepsy; none were interviewed in hospitals, clinics of physicians' offices. In short, our sample and study were independent of medical and institutionalized settings. More detail about the method and sample is available elsewhere [24].

EPILEPSY, MEDICATION AND SELF-REGULATION

The common medical response to a diagnosis of epilepsy is to prescribe various medications to control seizures. Given the range of types of epilepsy and the variety of physiological reactions to these medications, patients often see doctors as having a difficult time getting their medication 'right.' There are starts and stops and changes, depending on the degree of seizure control and the drug's side effects. More often than not, patients are stabilized on a medication or combination at a given dosage or regimen. Continuing or altering medications is the primary if not sole medical management strategy for epilepsy.

Medications are important to people with epilepsy. They 'control' seizures. Most take this medication several times daily. It becomes a routine part of their everyday lives. Although all of our respondents were taking or had taken these drugs, their responses to them varied. The effectiveness of these drugs in controlling seizures is a matter of degree. For some, seizures are stopped completely; they take pills regularly and have no seizures. For most, seizure frequency and duration are decreased significantly, although not reduced to zero. For a very few of our respondents, medications seem to have little impact; seizures continue unabated.

Nearly all our respondents said medications have helped them control seizures at one time or another. At the same time, however, many people changed their dose and regimen from those medically prescribed. Some stopped altogether. If medications were seen as so helpful, why were nearly half of our respondents 'noncompliant' with their doctors' orders?

Most people with illnesses, even chronic illnesses such as epilepsy, spend only a tiny fraction of their lives in the 'patient role.' Compliance assumes that the doctor–patient relationship is pivotal for subsequent action, which may not be the case. Consistent with our perspective, we conceptualize the issue as one of developing a *medication practice*. Medication practice offers a patient-centered perspective of how people manage their medications, focusing on the meaning and use of medications. In this light we can see the doctor's medication orders as the 'prescribed medication practice' (e.g. take a 20 mg pill four times a day). Patients interpret the doctor's prescribed regimen and create a medication practice that may vary decidedly from the prescribed practice. Rather than assume the patient will follow prescribed medical rules, this perspective allows us to explore the kinds of practices patients create.* Put another way, it sees patients as active agents rather than passive recipients of doctors' orders.

Although many people failed to conform to their prescribed medication regimen, they did not define this conduct primarily as noncompliance with doctors' orders. The more we examined the data, the clearer it was that from the patient's perspective, doctors had very little impact on people's decisions to alter their medications. It was, rather, much more a question of regulation of control. To examine this more closely we developed criteria for what we could call self-regulation. Many of our respondents occasionally missed taking their medicine, but otherwise were regular in their medication practice. One had to do more than 'miss' medications now and again (even a few times a week) to be deemed self-regulating. A person had to (1) reduce or raise the daily dose of prescribed drugs for several weeks or more or (2) skip or take extra doses regularly under specific circumstances (e.g. when drinking, staying up late or under 'stress') or (3) stop taking the drugs completely for three consecutive days or longer. These criteria are arbitrary, but they allow us to estimate the extent of self-regulation. Using this definition, 34 of our 80 respondents (42%) self-regulated their medication.†

* Two previous studies of epilepsy which examine the patient's perspective provide parallel evidence for the significance of developing such an approach in the study of 'noncompliance' (see [26] and [27].

†Reports in the medical literature indicate that noncompliance with epilepsy regimens is considered a serious problem [28–32]. One study reports that 40% of patients missed the prescribed medication dose often enough to affect their blood-level medication concentrations [33]; an important review article estimates noncompliance with epilepsy drug regimens between 30 and 40%, with a range from 20 to

To understand the meaning and management of medications we need to look at those who follow a prescribed medications practice as well as those who create their own variations. While we note that 42% of our respondents are at variance with medical expectations, this number is more suggestive than definitive. Self-regulators are not a discrete and separate group. About half the self-regulators could be defined as regular in their practice, whatever it might be. They may have stopped for a week once or twice, or take extra medication only under 'stressful' circumstances; otherwise, they are regular in their practice. On the other hand, perhaps a quarter of those following the prescribed medical practice say they have seriously considered changing or stopping their medications. It is likely there is an overlap between self-regulating and medical-regulating groups. While one needs to appreciate and examine the whole range of medication practice, the self-regulators provide a unique resource for analysis. They articulate views that are probably shared in varying degree by all people with epilepsy and provide an unusual insight into the meaning of medication and medication practice. We first describe how people account for following a prescribed medication practice; we then examine explanations offered for altering prescribed regimens and establishing their own practices. A final section outlines how the meaning of medications constructs and reflects the experience of epilepsy.

75% [34]. Another study suggests that noncompliant patients generally had longer duration of the disorder, more complicated regimens and more medication changes [35]. Attempts to increase epilepsy medication compliance include improving doctor–patient communication, incorporating patients more in treatment programs, increasing patient knowledge and simplifying drug regimens. Since noncompliance with anti-convulsant medication regimens is deemed the most frequent reason why patients suffer recurrent seizures [30], some researchers suggest, "If the patient understands the risks of stopping medication, he *will not stop*" [36]. Yet there also have been reports of active noncompliance with epilepsy medications [37]. In sum, epilepsy noncompliance studies are both typical of and reflect upon most other compliance research. In this sense, epilepsy is a good example for developing an alternative approach to understanding how people manage their medications.

A TICKET TO NORMALITY

The availability of effective seizure control medications early in this century is a milestone in the treatment of epilepsy (Phenobarbital was introduced in 1912; Dilantin in 1938). These drugs also literally changed the experience of having epilepsy. To the extent the medications controlled seizures, people with epilepsy suffered fewer convulsive disruptions in their lives and were more able to achieve conventional social roles. To the extent doctors believed medications effective, they developed greater optimism about their ability to treat epileptic patients. To the degree the public recognized epilepsy as a 'treatable' disorder, epileptics were no longer segregated in colonies and less subject to restrictive laws regarding marriage, procreation and work [24]. It is not surprising that people with epilepsy regard medications as a 'ticket' to normality. The drugs did not, speaking strictly, affect anything but seizures. It was the social response to medication that brought about these changes. As one woman said: "I'm glad we've got [the medications] . . . you know, in the past people didn't and they were looked upon as lepers."

For most people with epilepsy, taking medicine becomes one of those routines of everyday life we engage in to avoid unwanted circumstances or improve our health. Respondents compared it to taking vitamins, birth control pills or teeth brushing. It becomes almost habitual, something done regularly with little reflection. One young working man said: "Well, at first I didn't like it, [but] it doesn't bother me anymore. Just like getting up in the morning and brushing your teeth. It's just something you do."

But seizure control medications differ from 'normal pills' like vitamins or contraceptives. They are prescribed for a medical disorder and are seen both by the individual and others, as indicators or evidence of having epilepsy. One young man as a child did not know he had epilepsy "short of taking [his] medication." He said of this connection between epilepsy and medication: "I do, so therefore I have." Medications represent epilepsy: Dilantin or Phenobarbital are quickly recognized by medical people and often by others as epilepsy medications.

Medications can also indicate the degree of one's

disorder. Most of our respondents do not know any others with epilepsy; thus they examine changes in their own epilepsy biographies as grounds for conclusions about their condition. Seizure activity is one such sign; the amount of medications 'necessary' is another. A decrease or increase in seizures is taken to mean that epilepsy is getting better or worse. So it is with medications. While two may be related— especially because the common medical response to more seizures is increased medication—they may also operate independently. If the doctor reduces the dose or strength of medication, or vice versa, the patient may interpret this as a sign of improvement or worsening. Similarly, if a person reduces his or her own dose, being able to 'get along' on this lowered amount of medication is taken as evidence of 'getting better.' Since for a large portion of people with epilepsy seizures are considered to be well-controlled, medications become the only readily available measure of the 'progress' of the disorder.

TAKING MEDICATIONS

We tried to suspend the medical assumptions that people take medications simply because they are prescribed, or because they are supposed to control seizures, to examine our respondents' accounts of what they did and why.

The reason people gave most often for taking medication is *instrumental:* to control seizures, or more generally, to reduce the likelihood of body malfunction. Our respondents often drew a parallel to the reason people with diabetes take insulin. As one woman said, "If it does the trick, I'd rather take them [medications] than not." Or, as a man who would "absolutely not" miss his medications explained, "I don't want to have seizures" (although he continued to have 3 or 4 a month). Those who deal with their medication on instrumental grounds see it simply as a fact of life, as something to be done to avoid body malfunction and social and personal disruption.

While controlling body malfunction is always an underlying reason for taking medications, psychological grounds may be equally compelling. Many people said that medication *reduces worry,* independent of its actually decreasing seizures. These drugs can make people feel secure, so they don't have to

think about the probability of seizures. A 20 year-old woman remarked: "My pills keep me from getting hysterical." A woman who has taken seizure control medication for 15 years describes this 'psychological' function of medication: "I don't know what it does, but I suppose I'm psychologically dependent on it. In other words, if I take my medication, I feel better." Some people actually report 'feeling better'—clearer, more alert and energetic—when they do not take these drugs, but because they begin to worry if they miss, they take them regularly anyhow.

The most important reason for taking medication, however, is to insure 'normality.' People said specifically that they take medications to be more 'normal': The meaning here is normal in the sense of 'leading a normal life.' In the words of a middle-aged public relations executive who said he does not restrict his life because of epilepsy: "Except I always take my medication. I don't know why. I figure if I took them, then I could do anything I wanted to do." People believed taking medicine reduces the risk of having a seizure in the presence of others, which might be embarassing or frightening. As a young woman explained:

> I feel if it's going to help, that's what I want because you know you feel uncomfortable enough anyway that you don't want anything like [a seizure] to happen around other people; so if it's going to help, I'll take it.

This is not to say people with epilepsy like to take medications. Quite the contrary. Many respondents who follow their medically prescribed medication practice openly say they 'hate' taking medications and hope someday to be 'off' the drugs. Part of this distaste is related to the dependence people come to feel. Some used the metaphor of being an addict: "I'm a real drug addict"; "I was an addict before it was fashionable"; "I'm like an alcoholic without a drink; I *have* to have them [pills]"; and "I really don't want to be hooked for the rest of my life." Even while loathing the pills or the 'addiction' people may be quite disciplined about taking these drugs.

The drugs used to control seizures are not, of course, foolproof. Some people continue to have seizures quite regularly while others suffer only occasional episodes. Such limited effectiveness does not necessarily lead these people to reject medication as a strategy. They continue, with frustration, to express "hope" that "they [doctors] will get it [the medication] right." For some, then, medications are but a limited ticket to normality.

SELF-REGULATION: GROUNDS FOR CHANGING MEDICATION PRACTICE

For most people there is not a one-to-one correspondence between taking or missing medications and seizure activity. People who take medications regularly may still have seizures, and some people who discontinue their medications may be seizure-free for months or longer. Medical experts say a patient may well miss a whole day's medication yet still have enough of the drug in the bloodstream to prevent a seizure for this period.

In this section we focus on those who deviate from the prescribed medication practice and variously regulate their own medication. On the whole, members of this subgroup are slightly younger than the rest of the sample (average age 25 vs 32) and somewhat more likely to be female (59–43%), but otherwise are not remarkably different from our respondents who follow the prescribed medication practice. Self-regulation for most of our respondents consists of reducing the dose, stopping for a time, or regularly skipping or taking extra doses of medication depending on various circumstances.

Reducing the dose (including total termination) is the most common form of self-regulation. In this context, two points are worth re-stating. First, doctors typically alter doses of medication in times of increased seizure activity or troublesome drug 'side effects.' It is difficult to strike the optimum level of medication. To people with epilepsy, it seems that doctors engage in a certain amount of trial and error behavior. Second, and more important, medications are defined, both by doctors and patients, as an indicator of the degree of disorder. If seizure activity is not 'controlled' or increases, patients see that doctors respond by raising (or changing) medications. The more medicine prescribed means epilepsy is getting worse; the less means it is getting better. What doctors do does not necessarily explain what patients do, but it may well be an example our respondents use in their own management strategies. The most common rationales for altering a medication practice

are drug related: the medication is perceived as ineffective or the so-called side effects become too troublesome.

The efficacy of a drug is a complex issue. Here our concern is merely with perceived efficacy. When a medication is no longer seen as efficacious it is likely to be stopped. Many people continue to have seizures even when they follow the prescribed medication practice. If medication seemed to make no difference, our respondents were more likely to consider changing their medication practice. One woman who stopped taking medications for a couple of months said, "It seemed like [I had] the same number of seizures without it." Most people who stop taking their medicine altogether eventually resume a medication practice of some sort. A woman college instructor said, "When I was taking Dilantin, I stopped a number of times because it never seemed to *do* anything."

The most common drug-related rationally for reducing dose is troublesome 'side effects.' People with epilepsy attribute a variety of side effects to seizure control medications. One category of effects includes swollen and bleeding gums, oily or yellow skin, pimples, sore throat and a rash. Another category includes slowed mental functioning, drowsiness, slurred speech, dullness, impaired memory, loss of balance and partial impotence.* The first category, which we can call body side effects, were virtually never given as an account for self-regulation. Only those side effects that impaired social skills, those in the second category, were given as reasons for altering doctors' medication orders.

Social side effects impinge on social interaction. People believed they felt and acted differently. A self-regulating woman described how she feels when she takes her medication:

I can feel that I become much more even. I feel like I flatten out a little bit. I don't like that feeling. . . . It's just a feeling of dullness, which I don't like, almost a feeling that you're on the edge of laziness.

If people saw their medication practice as hindering the ability to participate in routine social affairs,

---

* These are reported side effects. They may or may not be drug related, but our respondents attribute them to the medication.

they were likely to change it. Our respondents gave many examples such as a college student who claimed the medication slowed him down and wondered if it were affecting his memory, a young newspaper reporter who reduced his medication because it was putting him to sleep at work; or the social worker who felt she 'sounds smarter' and more articulate when 'off medications.'

Drug side effects, even those that impair social skills, are not sufficient in themselves to explain the level of self-regulation we found. Self-regulation was considerably more than a reaction to annoying and uncomfortable side effects. It was an active and intentional endeavor.

SOCIAL MEANINGS OF REGULATING MEDICATION PRACTICE

Variations in medication practice by and large seem to depend on what medication and self-regulation mean to our respondents. Troublesome relationships with physicians, including the perception that they have provided inadequate medical information [14], may be a foundation on which alternative strategies and practices are built. Our respondents, however, did not cite such grounds for altering their doctors' orders. People vary their medication practice on grounds connected to managing their everyday lives. If we examine the social meanings of medications from our respondents' perspectives, self-regulation turns on four grounds: testing; control of dependence; destigmatization; and practical practice. While individual respondents may cite one or more of these as grounds for altering medication practice, they are probably best understood as strategies common among those who self regulate.

Testing

Once people with epilepsy begin taking seizure-control medications, given there are no special problems and no seizures, doctors were reported to seldom change the medical regimen. People are likely to stay on medications indefinitely. But how can one know that a period without seizures is a result of medication or spontaneous remission of the disorder? How long can one go without medication? How 'bad' is this case of epilepsy? How can one know if epilepsy

is 'getting better' while still taking medication? Usually after a period without or with only a few seizures, many reduced or stopped their medicine altogether to test for themselves whether or not epilepsy was 'still there.'

People can take themselves off medications as an experiment, to see 'if anything will happen.' One woman recalled:

I was having one to two seizures a year on pheno-barb . . . so I decided not to take it and to see what would happen . . . so I stopped it and I watched and it seemed that I had the same amount of seizures with it as without it . . . for three years.

She told her physician, who was skeptical but 'allowed' her this control of her medication practice. A man who had taken medication three times a day for 16 years felt intuitively that he could stop his medications:

Something kept telling me I didn't have to take [medication] anymore, a feeling or somethin'. It took me quite a while to work up the nerve to stop takin' the pills. An one day I said, "One way to find out. . . ."

After suffering what he called drug withdrawal effects, he had no seizures for 6 years. Others test to see how long they can go without medication and seizures.

Testing does not always turn out successfully. A public service agency executive tried twice to stop taking medications when he thought he had 'kicked' epilepsy. After two failures, he concluded that stopping medications "just doesn't work." But others continue to test, hoping for some change in their condition. One middle-aged housewife said:

When I was young I would try not to take it . . . I'd take it for a while and think, "Well, I don't need it anymore," so I would not take it for, deliberately, just to see if I could do without. And then [in a few days] I'd start takin' it again, because I'd start passin' out . . . I will still try that now, when my husband is out of town . . . I just think, maybe I'm still gonna grow out of it or something.

Testing by reducing or stopping medication is only one way to evaluate how one's disorder is progressing. Even respondents who follow the pre-scribed medication regimen often wonder 'just what would happen' if they stopped.

Controlling Dependence

People with epilepsy struggle continually against becoming too dependent on family, friends, doctors or medications. They do, of course, depend on medica-tions for control of seizures. The medications do not necessarily eliminate seizures and many of our re-spondents resented their dependence on them. An-other paradox is that although medications can in-crease self reliance by reducing seizures, taking me-dications can be *experienced* as a threat to self reli-ance. Medications seem almost to become symbolic of the dependence created by having epilepsy.

There is a widespread belief in our society that drugs create dependence and that being on chemical substances is not a good thing. Somehow, whatever the goal is, it is thought to be better if we can get there without drugs. Our respondents reflected these ideas in their comments.

A college junior explained: "I don't like it at all. I don't like chemicals in my body. It's sort of like a dependency only that I have to take it because my body forced me to. . . ." A political organizer who says medications reduce his seizures com-mented: "I've never enjoyed having to depend on anything . . . drugs in particular." A nurse summed up the situation: "The *drugs* were really a kind of dependence." Having to take medication relin-quished some degree of control of one's life. A woman said:

> I don't like to have to take *anything*. It was, like, at one time birth control pills, but I don't like to take anything everyday. *It's just like, y'know, controlling me, or something*.

The feeling of being controlled need not be substanti-ated in fact for people to act upon it. If people *feel* dependent on and controlled by medication, it is not surprising that they seek to avoid these drugs. A high school junior, who once took medicine because he feared having a seizure in the street, commented:

> And I'd always heard medicine helps and I just kept taking it and finally I just got so I didn't depend on the medicine no more. I could just

> fight it off myself and I just stopped taking it in.

After stopping for a month he forgot about his medi-cations completely.

Feelings of dependence are one reason people gave for regulating medicine. For a year, one young social worker took medication when she felt it was necessary; otherwise, she tried not to use it. When we asked her why, she responded, "I regulate my own drug . . . mostly because it's really important for me not to be dependent." She occasionally had seizures and continued to alter her medication to try to 'get it right':

> I started having [seizures] every once in a while. And I thought wow, the bad thing is that I just haven't regulated it right and I just need to up it a little bit and then, you know, if I do it just right, I won't have epilepsy anymore.

This woman and others saw medications as a power-ful resource in their struggle to gain control over epilepsy. Although she no longer thinks she can rid herself of epilepsy, this woman still regulates her medication.

In this context, people with epilepsy manipulate their sense of dependence on medications by chang-ing medication practice. But there is a more subtle level of dependence that encourages such changes. Some reported they regulated their medication in-take in direct response to interventions of others, especially family members. It was as if others *wanted* them to be more dependent by coaxing or reminding them to take their medications regularly. Many re-sponded to this encouraged greater dependence by creating their own medication practice.

A housewife who said she continues regularly to have petit mal seizures and tremors along with an occasional grand mal seizure, remarked:

> Oh, like most things, when someone tells me I have to do something, I basically resent it. . . . If it's my option and I choose to do it, I'll probably do it more often than not. But if you tell me I have to, I'll bend it around and do it my own way, which is basically what I have done.

Regardless of whether one feels dependent on the drug or dependent because of others' interven-tions around drug taking, changing a prescribed medication practice, as well as continuing self-regulation serve as a form of *taking control* of one's epilepsy.

Destigmatization

Epilepsy is a stigmatized illness. Sufferers attempt to control information about the disorder to manage this threat [38]. There are no visible stigmata that make a person with epilepsy obviously different from other people, but a number of aspects of having epilepsy can compromise attempts at information control. The four signs that our respondents most frequently mentioned as threatening information control were seizures in the presence of others, job or insurance applications, lack of a driver's license and taking medications. People may try to avoid seizures in public, lie or hedge on their applications, develop accounts for not having a driver's license, or take their medicine in private in order to minimize the stigma potential of epilepsy.

Medication usually must be taken three or four times daily, so at least one dose must be taken away from home. People attempt to be private about taking their medications and/or develop 'normal' pill accounts ("it's to help my digestion"). One woman's mother told her to take medications regularly, as she would for any other sickness:

> When I was younger it didn't bother me too bad. But as I got older, it would tend to bother me some. Whether it was, y'know, maybe somebody seeing me or somethin', I don't know. But it did.

Most people develop skills to minimize potential stigmatization from taking pills in public.

On occasion, stopping medications is an attempt to vacate the stigmatized status of epileptic. One respondent wrote us a letter describing how she tried to get her mother to accept her by not taking her medications. She wrote:

> This is going to sound real dumb, but I can't help it. My mother never accepted me when I was little because I was "different." I stopped taking my medication in an attempt to be normal and accepted by her. Now that I know I need medication it's like I'm completely giving up trying to be "normal" so mom won't be ashamed of me. I'm going to accept the fact that I'm "differ-

ent" and I don't really care if mom gives a damn or not.

Taking medications in effect acknowledges this 'differentness.'

It is, of course, more difficult to hide the meaning of medications from one's self. Taking medication is a constant reminder of having epilepsy. For some it is as if the medication itself represents the stigma of epilepsy. The young social worker quoted above felt if she could stop taking her medications she would no longer be an epileptic. A young working woman summed up succinctly why avoiding medications would be avoiding stigma: "Well, at least I would not be . . . generalized and classified in a group as being an epileptic."

Practical Practice

Self-regulators spoke often of how they changed the dose or regimen of medication in an effort to reduce the risk of having a seizure, particularly during 'high stress' situations. Several respondents who were students said they take extra medications during exam periods or when they stay up late studying. A law student who had not taken his medicine for 6 months took some before his law school exams: "I think it increases the chances [seizures] won't happen." A woman who often participated in horse shows said she "usually didn't pay attention" to her medication practice but takes extra when she doesn't get the six to eight hours sleep she requires: "I'll wake up and take two capsules instead of one . . . and I'll generally take it like when we're going to horse shows. I'll take it pretty consistently." Such uses of medication are common ways of trying to forestall 'possible trouble.'

People with epilepsy changed their medication practice for practical ends in two other kinds of circumstances. Several reported they took extra medication if they felt a 'tightening' or felt a seizure coming on. Many people also said they did not take medications if they were going to drink alcohol. They believed that medication (especially Phenobarbital) and alcohol do not mix well.

In short, people change their medication practice to suit their perceptions of social environment. Some reduce medication to avoid potential problems from mixing alcohol and drugs. Others reduce it to remain 'clear-headed' and 'alert' during 'important' performances (something of a 'Catch-22' situation). Most, however, adjust their medications practically in an effort to reduce the risk of seizures.

CONCLUSION: ASSERTING CONTROL

Regulating medication represents an attempt to assert some degree of control over a condition that appears at times to be completely beyond control. Loss of control is a significant concern for people with epilepsy. While medical treatment can increase both the sense and the fact of control over epilepsy, and information control can limit stigmatization, the regulation of medications is one way people with epilepsy struggle to gain some personal control over their condition.

Medication practice can be modified on several different grounds. Side effects that make managing everyday social interaction difficult can lead to the reduction or termination of medication. People will change their medication practice, including stopping altogether, in order to 'test' for the existence or 'progress' of the disorder. Medication may be altered to control the perceived level of dependence, either on the drugs themselves or on those who 'push' them to adhere to a particular medication practice. Since the medication can represent the stigma potential of epilepsy, both literally and symbolically, altering medication practice can be a form of destigmatization. And finally, many people modify their medication practice in anticipation of specific social circumstances, usually attempting to reduce the risk of seizures.

It is difficult to judge how generalizable these findings are to other illnesses. Clearly, people develop medication practices whenever they must take medications regularly. This is probably most true for long-term chronic illness where medication becomes a central part of everyday life, such as diabetes, rheumatoid arthritis, hypertension and asthma. The degree and amount of self-regulation may differ among illnesses—likely to be related to symptomatology, effectiveness of medications and potential of stigma—but I suspect most of the meanings of medications described here would be present among sufferers of any illness that people must continually manage.

In sum, we found that a large proportion of the people with epilepsy we interviewed said they themselves regulate their medication. Medically-centered compliance research presents a skewed and even distorted view of how and why patients manage medication. From the perspective of the person with epilepsy, the issue is more clearly one of responding to the meaning of medications in everyday life than 'compliance' with physicians' orders and medical regimens. Framing the problem as self-regulation rather than compliance allows us to see modifying medication practice as a vehicle for asserting some control over epilepsy. One consequence of such a reframing would be to reexamine the value of achieving 'complaint' behavior and to rethink what strategies might be appropriate for achieving greater adherence to prescribed medication regimens.

References

1. Haynes R. B., Taylor D. W. and Sackett D. L. (Eds) *Compliance in Health Care*. Johns Hopkins University Press, Baltimore, 1979.

2. Davis M. Variations in patients compliance with doctor's advice: an empirical analysis of patterns of communication. *Am. J. publ. Hlth* **58**, 272, 1968.

3. Hulka B. S., Kupper L. L., Cassel J. LC. and Babineau R. A. Practice characteristics and quality of primary medical care: the doctor–patient relationship. *Med. Care* **13**, 808–820, 1975.

4. Christenson D. B. Drug-taking compliance: a review and synthesis. *Hlth Serv. Res.* **6**, 171–187, 1978.

5. Sackett D. L. and Snow J. C. The magnitude of compliance and non-compliance. In *Compliance in Health Care* (Edited by Haynes R. B. *et al.*), pp. 11–22. Johns Hopkins University Press, Baltimore, 1979.

6. Sackett D. L. and Haynes R. B. (Eds) *Compliance With Therapeutic Regimens*. Johns Hopkins University Press, Baltimore, 1976.

7. DiMatteo M. R. and DiNicola D. D. *Achieving Patient Compliance*. Pergamon Press, New York, 1982.

8. Hingson R., Scotch N. A., Sorenson J. and Swazey J. P. *In Sickness and in Health: Social Dimensions of Medical Care*. C. V. Mosby, St Louis, 1981.

9. Haynes R. B. Determinants of compliance: the disease and the mechanics of treatment. In *Compliance in Health Care* (Edited by Haynes R. B. *et al.*), pp. 49–62. Johns Hopkins University Press, Baltimore, 1979.

10. Garrity T. F. Medical compliance and the clinician–patient relationship: a review. *Soc. Sci. Med.* **15E,** 215–222, 1981.

11. Svarstad B. L. Physician–patient communication and patient conformity with medical advice. In *Growth of Bureaucratic Medicine* (Edited by Mechanic D.), pp. 220–238. Wiley, New York, 1976.

12. Francis V., Korsch B. and Morris M. Gaps in doctor–patient communication: patients' response to medical advice. *New Engl. J. Med.* **280,** 535, 1969.

13. Korsch B., Gozzi E. and Francis V. Gaps in doctor–patient communication I. Doctor–patient interaction and patient satisfaction. *Pediatrics* **42,** 885, 1968.

14. Becker M. H. and Maiman L. A. Sociobehavioral determinants of compliance with health and medical care recommendations. *Med. Care* **13,** 10–24.

15. Becker M. H. Sociobehavioral determinants of compliance. In *Compliance With Therapeutic Regimens* (Edited by Sackett D. L. and Haynes R. B.), pp. 40–50. Johns Hopkins University Press, Baltimore, 1976.

16. Becker M. H., Maiman L. A., Kirscht J. P., Haefner D. L., Drachman R. H. and Taylor D. W. Patient perceptions and compliance: recent studies of the health belief model. In *Compliance in Health Care* (Edited by Haynes R. B. *et al.*), pp. 79–109. Johns Hopkins University Press, Baltimore, 1979.

17. Berkanovic E. The health belief model and voluntary health behavior. Paper presented to Conference on Critical issues in Health Delivery Systems, Chicago, 1977.

18. Parsons T. *The Social System.* Free Press, Glencoe, 1951.

19. Stimson G. V. Obeying doctor's orders: a view from the other side. *Soc. Sci. Med.* **8,** 97–104, 1974.

20. Arluke A. Judging drugs: patients' conceptions of therapeutic efficacy in the treatment of arthritis. *Hum. Org.* **39,** 84–88, 1980.

21. Hayes-Bartista D. E. Modifying the treatment: patient compliance, patient control and medical care. *Soc. Sci. Med.* **10,** 233–238, 1976.

22. Zola I. K. Structural constraints in the doctor–patient relationship: the case of non-compliance. In *The Relevance of Social Science for Medicine* (Edited by Eisenberg L. and Kleinman A.), pp. 241–252. Reidel, Dordrecht, 1981.

23. Strauss A. and Glaser B. *Chronic Illness and the Quality of Life,* pp. 21–32. C. V. Mosby, St Louis, 1975.

24. Schneider J. and Conrad P. *Having Epilepsy: The Experience and Control of Illness.* Temple University Press, Philadelphia, 1983.

25. Glaser B. and Strauss A. *The Discovery of Grounded Theory.* Aldine, Chicago, 1967.

26. West P. The physician and the management of childhood epilepsy. In *Studies in Everyday Medicine* (Edited by Wadsworth M. and Robinson D.), pp. 13–31. Martin Robinson, London, 1976.

27. Trostle J. *et al.* The logic of non-compliance: management of epilepsy from a patient's point of view. *Cult. Med. Psychiat.* **7,** 35–56, 1983.

28. Lund M., Jurgensen R. S. and Kuhl V. Serum diphenyl-hydantoin in ambulant patients with epilepsy. *Epilepsia* **5,** 51–58, 1964.

29. Lund M. Failure to observe dosage instructions in patients with epilepsy. *Acta neurol. scand.* **49,** 295–306, 1975.

30. Reynolds E. H. Drug treatment of epilepsy. *Lancet* **II,** 721–725, 1978.

31. Browne T. R. and Cramer I. A. Antiepileptic drug serum concentration determinations. In *Epilepsy: Diagnosis and Management* (Edited by Browne T. R. and Feldman R. G.). Little, Brown, Boston, 1982.

32. Pryse-Phillips W., Jardine F. and Bursey F. Compliance with drug therapy by epileptic patients. *Epilepsia* **23,** 269–274, 1982.

33. Eisler J. and Mattson R. H. Compliance with anticonvulsant drug therapy. *Epilepsia* **16,** 203, 1975.

34. The Commission for the Control of Epilepsy and its Consequences. The literature on patient compliance and implications for cost-effective patient education programs with epilepsy. In *Plan for Nationwide Action on Epilepsy,* Vol. II, Part 1, pp. 391–415. U.S. Government Printing Office, Washington, DC, 1977.

35. Bryant S. G. and Ereshfsky L. Determinants of compliance in epileptic conditions. *Drug Intel. Clin. Pharmac.* **15,** 572–577, 1981.

36. Norman S. E. and Browne T. K. Seizure disorders. *Am. J. Nurs.* **81,** 893, 1981.

37. Desei B. T., Reily T. L., Porter R. J. and Penry J. K. Active non-compliance as a cause of uncontrolled seizures. *Epilepsia* **19,** 447–452, 1978.

38. Schneider J. and Conrad P. In the closet with illness: epilepsy, stigma potential and information control. *Soc. Probl.* **28,** 32–44, 1980.

Lay Initiatives in the Consumption of Health Care

Howard D. Schwartz
Ian S. Biederman

Sociological interest in the nature and extent of the public's active involvement in the many day-to-day decisions surrounding the health of the individual has had four major foci. These are (1) the existence of a very considerable amount of self-care; (2) the impact of friends, relatives, and similar significant lay others on individuals' decisions about their health, which has been conceptualized most notably in relation to a "lay-referral system"; (3) the operation of a large and growing number of self-help groups; and (4) speculation on the degree to which a so-called "consumerist" orientation—a set of client attitudes demanding a greater sharing of control with health-care providers—can be found among individuals as they interact with these providers.

Self-care refers to decisions and accompanying behaviors where there is little or no contact with the professional medical system in the person's attempt to remedy his or her problem.

The lay-referral system, articulated by Eliot Freidson, refers to a process of decision-making involving steps which may or may not lead to the use of the health-care delivery system.[1] (In some instances, then, lay referral can be tied up with self-care.) Those playing key roles in this network of lay influences include family and friends who may do such things as recommend home remedies or a well-respected physician to visit.

Self-help groups provide mutual support systems for those falling into particular illness categories. One Day at a Time, a group in which terminally ill patients assist one another in coping with life, is one example of such a support group.

Consumerism, as viewed by those who write about it, refers to a growing awareness among consumers of health care of their potential power in their encounters with providers, and their actions in response to this awareness. Those, like Marie Haug, who have written on the subject maintain that changing social conditions, such as a more educated population, have led to a broad-based activist consumer movement. The evidence for this assertion willl be analyzed in the last part of this paper.

SELF-CARE

When we think of health care, paid medical professionals immediately come to mind as those to whom we look for maintenance and restoration of our health. It is an established fact though that most of our decisions, in this regard, involve not the traditional physician–hospital centered system, but our own actions. The notion of self-care, as already mentioned, refers to individually determined health-related actions, where the person perceiving himself or herself to be ill is the decision maker and actor. Self-care has recently been receiving increasing attention, but as DeFreise and Woomert have noted, "The fact of the matter is self-care has always been the predominant way in which most people have dealt with most of their health problems."[2]

The self-care category includes a wide assortment of health-related activities. In *The Hidden Health Care System,* which presents one of the clearest and most comprehensive discussions of self-care, Levin and Idler describe the essential components of the phenomenon.[3] They first note that self-medication seems to be, by far, the most important element in self-care. In support of this contention, they cite data from several countries as well as a study of

This is an original article written for this edition of *Dominant Issues in Medical Sociology.* The authors wish to thank Kenneth Perkins for his technical assistance.

the Food and Drug Administration (FDA) that surveyed the health practices and attitudes of Americans. The FDA, in its conclusions, placed great emphasis on the practice of Americans of "taking something" to either prevent or cure disease. Common medication practices include use of vitamins and nutritional supplements, health foods, weight control medications, medication for both common and serious ailments, aids to stop smoking, and medications for arthritis/rheumatism and cancer. Of course, self-care involves more than taking medication, as Levin and Idler make clear in the following passage:

> Self-medication is certainly the most researched aspect of self-care for minor illness and injury, but the wide range of other such activities deserves mention and further study; first aid for minor injuries, cuts, scrapes, bruises and burns; vaporizers and bed rest for colds and flu; ointments, compresses, and astringents for skin problems; home surgery for blisters and splinters; kisses and Bandaids for imaginary "boo-boos"; massage and hot tub bath for sore muscles; chicken noodle soup and "a nice hot cup of tea" for anything; hot water bottles and heating pads for menstrual cramps; ice packs for swellings; vinegar douches and yogurt for vaginal infections; hydrogen peroxide for ear wax; salt water gargles—the list could go on and on. In addition to these treatments, certain diagnostic and monitoring equipment are increasingly found in home use, such as thermometers, sphygmomanometers (to measure blood pressure), otoscopes, home throat culture and urine-testing kits, and home pregnancy tests.[4]

What is perhaps most interesting about self-care is its sheer magnitude. There is a consensus among researchers that the amount of self-care in the United States far exceeds the care delivered by health-care professionals. Obtaining information from the daily diaries of a sample of over 500 families in upper New York State, Roghmann and Haggerty found that more than 90% of health-related actions taken were based on self-decision.[5] Riessman notes that from 65–85% of all health and medical care is provided by nonprofessional sources, and that probably 85% or more of the care of minor and common illnesses is provided by these sources. Put in another way, Riessman concludes that the ratio of nonprofessional to professional care for all health problems is somewhere around 7 to 1.[6] Similarly, Demers and his colleagues found that only 10 to 20% of the health-care problems of Americans receive professional attention.[7]

The pervasiveness of self-care is as characteristic of other countries as it is of ours. Citizens of industrialized nations with well-developed medical systems treat four out of five illnesses without the help of the medical system.[8] Thus, self-care is a fundamental part of any health-care system regardless of the political or economic nature of the particular society.

Unlike the United States, Great Britain has a system of universal health-care coverage. Yet, a study of that country determined that 63% of all disease/illness interventions involved self-care (another 16% involved not taking any action).[9] The finding of such a high level of nonuse of the National Health Service for health problems seems to bring into question the conventional wisdom that self-care is most commonly a response of those who lack access to professional health resources. In Great Britain the professional health resources are available to the population free of charge and there is still a great deal of self-care.

The enormous amount of self-care existing in the United States and elsewhere points up a significant but somewhat unrecognized function of such care—its role as a first-line of defense against overuse of the established health-care system. As Fry and his colleagues, the authors of the above-cited British study, conclude, "Self-care is an inevitable, important but totally neglected level of care in all systems of health care. . . . Without self-care any system of health care would be swamped."[10]

What factors distinguish between those who engage in self-care and those who do not? Unfortunately, there has not been a great deal of research directed specifically to this question. Nevertheless, there is some agreement about one influence on self-care usage, social class. It seems to be the case that self-care is most likely to be found among those of higher socioeconomic status. Levin and Idler, looking at the available research concerning self-medication, conclude that "the amount of nonprescription medications may be related to socioeconomic status, the more affluent and better educated purchasing more of them."[11] One study they mention, for example, found that families of lower socioeconomic status use less of both over-the-counter and prescribed drugs.

A recently published study provides support for the link between higher social class and greater use of self-care. Using data from the 1984 Illinois Comparative Health Survey Cockerham, et al., found that, in response to a list of symptoms of illness, the lower classes were more likely to view the symptoms as warranting going to the doctor and were also more likely to visit a physician in response to the symptoms.[12] Conversely, the researchers found that the more affluent "perceive the . . . symptoms more selectively and as conditions that they can perhaps deal with themselves."[13] These class differences were related to the existence of a greater sense of control over one's health among the higher classes.

Self-care is also a central element in certain religious groups, including Christian Scientists and Catholic Pentacostals. The latter group and the role of self-care in it has been discussed at some length by Levin and Idler, a discussion from which the following is drawn.[14] Catholic Pentecostalism, also known as Catholic Charismatic Renewal, is a religious movement that began in the United States in 1967 at Duquesne University. Catholic Pentacostals believe that healing is a gift from God that can be gained from prayer-activated "baptism in the Holy Spirit." Healing acquired increased importance for Catholic Pentecostals as a consequence of a 1974 conference held at Notre Dame University. On the first day, the movement's leadership conducted a mass healing service attended by 30,000 people. At that service about seventy physical healings were reported immediately, including cases of blindness, cancer, back problems, deafness, and blood disease. Since then, the movement's magazine *New Covenant* has printed testimonies of healings that occurred at Notre Dame involving cases of coronary heart disease, rheumatoid arthritis, and epilepsy.

The growth of Catholic Pentacostalism has been steady. The International Directory of Charismatic Prayer Groups listed over 1,000 groups in 1973, and by 1980 some 4,500 groups were registered in the United States and Canada. The membership is predominantly middle class and comes largely from university communities.

Catholic Pentecostals desire to expand medical definitions of healing to include spiritual faith, which is relied upon to restore health and which is thought to be as effective as any medical treatment. Unlike some other groups, there is an absence of antagonism between health professionals and leaders of the Pentacostal movement. Catholic Pentecostals say the professional model of health care is incomplete because it ignores faith; but they also recognize the legitimacy of some medical treatment. The movement's literature urges those who have experienced charismatic healing to return to their physicians for confirmation of the healing and to remain on any prescribed medication until the doctor says it is no longer necessary to do so.

There seem to be parallels between the healing aspect of Catholic Pentecostalism and childbirth at home. Both are very old practices undergoing renewed popularity and both have middle-class support. Both attempt to inject a component of self-care into a particular kind of health-care-related experience. In this regard, according to Levin and Idler, each demonstrates "a demand for a certain type of experience, one that is profound and binds very tightly together those who share in it."[15]

In any discussion of self-care, something must be said about the cultural factor and its relationship to self-care, a connection which has been of somewhat greater interest to medical anthropologists than to medical sociologists. EM, a designation which the reader will come across again in the article by Irwin Press in Chapter 11, stands for "explanatory model." An EM refers to the underlying belief system through which one understands the nature of illness, and consequently, defines the appropriate type of care. Self-care modalities, deriving from such cultural belief systems, can vary from the more esoteric, such as placing keys on a chain around the neck for a bloody nose or placing camphor on the chest, with red scarves around the chest, for a sore throat to the more conventional use of honey or tea for a variety of ailments.

There has been within the medical establishment a growing recognition that to be effective with certain groups of patients, health professionals must take into account these culturally-based self-care modalities when they encounter them, for example, in the emergency room setting. Increasingly, major medical journals have included articles on EMs, and how health professionals can incorporate them into the treatment. One of the best known studies appeared in 1971 in the *Journal of the American Medical Association* and dealt with the "Hot–Cold" EM of many Puerto Rican Americans.[16] Based on the Hippocratic theory of four bodily humors (blood, phlegm, black bile, and yellow bile), the EM holds that illnesses classified as cold must be treated with medications and foods classified as hot, while hot illnesses are to be treated with cold substances. (The classification of an illness, medication, or food as hot or cold follows no apparent logic from the point of view of an outsider.) The task of the physician should be to try and blend the hot–cold theory in with the treatment so that the patient will be more likely to comply with the physician's directives and to seek medical care in the future. For example, during menstruation, to make up for the loss of potassium, women will frequently eat bananas or dried fruit. However, within the hot–cold theory, menstruation is a cold bodily state while bananas and dried fruit are considered cold foods. Thus, the Puerto Rican woman will avoid these foods during menstruation. A physician might, however, place potassium in a solution and present it as a "vitamin," which is considered hot and which would make it acceptable from the patient's point of view.

Before leaving the discussion of self-care, mention of two further points seems in order. First, self-care is likely to dramatically increase as the number of chronically ill persons treated at home increases. With the rapid aging of our population, there will be more persons with such degenerative, incurable diseases as diabetes, arthritis, cancer, heart disease, and the like. Allowing those who so desire to remain at home seems to many to be the most humane kind of treatment as well as a way to relieve the enormous demand for nursing-home care that continues to outstrip the supply. And such care can also be effective. For example, research has shown that in cases of stroke, self-care at home which includes both patient and family is as effective for rehabilitation as is care in a hospital.

Second, and this is an elaboration of the last point above, research has also shown that the public has a substantial capacity to learn and employ self-care skills. In this regard, DeFreise and Woomert carried out a study to assess the degree to which laypersons could learn over 250 self-care skills taught through the use of popular instructional textbooks used in self-care courses. Their conclusion was that "the major self-care curricula used in the United States consist of skills the majority of which are significant to health, relatively low in risk when performed by a layperson, and easily taught to persons without professional health backgrounds."[17]

LAY REFERRAL

The previous examination of self-care revealed that the majority of health-care decisions made by individuals regarding their health problems are made without contact with the professional medical community. The present section deals with the process by which "lay" individuals—that is, nonprofessionals—depend on each other in making decisions about whether or not to seek professional help, and if so, what kind of professional expertise to seek.

Sociological interest in the process by which people make their health-care-related decisions has centered around the concept of the lay-referral system. There is nothing particularly unique about the notion of lay referral except that, as with self-care, it is very important but so often ignored in our thinking about how health-care consumers make their decisions.

The term lay-referral system was coined by Eliot Freidson as an outgrowth of his research on subscribers to a prepaid medical plan in the Bronx, New York.[18] The study centered on how the lay and professional social structures influence the ways in which individuals utilize medical care. More specifically, Freidson showed how the lay system is often critical in bringing the prospective patient in contact with the medical system. (Lay influences can just as easily lead individuals away from use of the medical system but Freidson's focus was on how patients select medical care.)

According to Freidson, the lay-referral system is made up of a series of steps, each step likely to include diagnosis, prescription, and referral, involving how the individual deals with his or her illness. Freidson's description of how the process typically operated in the lives of the subjects of his research is as follows:

> . . . *in the Bronx the process of seeking help began with personal, tentative self-diagnosis that implied their own self-administered treatments.*

Upon failure of those first prescriptions, members of the household were consulted. Aid in self-diagnosis was sometimes sought from laymen outside the household—friends, neighbors, relatives, fellow workers, a former nurse, or someone with the same trouble. Indeed, when explorations of diagnoses were drawn out and not stopped early by cessation of symptoms or immediate recourse to a physician, the prospective patient referred himself or was referred through a hierarchy of consultant positions. The hierarchy ran from the intimate and informal confines of the nuclear family through successively less intimate lay consultants until the professional was reached.[19]

A recent study supports Freidson's view of the critical role played by lay referral in the seeking of medical care. Using a national sample, Wolinsky and Steiber directed themselves to the question of how people choose a new physician.[20] Their major finding was that the recommendation of friends or neighbors was, by far, the most frequently cited reason for the choice, and that typically individuals exploit the lay-referral system concerning medical matters before consulting health professionals.

In his pioneering study, Freidson found that, for a variety of reasons, the lay-referral system was more highly developed among the lower classes. Among the reasons was the fact that lower-class individuals feel more removed from medical institutions and, thus, feel the need for group support and counsel in medical matters. Within this context, it is noteworthy that American gypsies have among the most highly developed lay-referral systems. Documentation for this fact comes from several sources including an early article by anthropologist Jeffrey Salloway[21] and a 1985 piece by physician James Thomas which appeared in the *Annals of Internal Medicine*.[22]

A central element of gypsy culture is its adversarial relationship with the larger American society. Gypsies are suspicious of, and often hostile to, non-gypsies whom they collectively refer to by the perjorative term "gaje." Any kind of exploitation of the gaje is permissible, and gypsies are well known for illegal economic activities, such as various types of petty thievery, carried out at the expense of the gaje. Gypsies assiduously retain their separation from outsiders. For example, gypsy children attend grade school irregularly and, thus, are rarely literate and have little extracurricular contact with gaje children.

The gypsies have a rich tradition of self-care through folk medicine. One traditional remedy is johal (ghost vomit), a slime mold of algae used to treat hemorrhage or epilepsy. Although the use of these remedies is less common today, Thomas reports that they have not vanished and he provides an example of one patient who treated an enlarging breast carcinoma (cancerous tumor) for 3 years with garlic compresses before seeking medical help.

At as great a social distance from mainstream middle-class America as most any group in the society, gypsies nonetheless use, as Thomas observes, "remarkable savvy" in their interactions with the health-care system. Gypsies are found to have remarkably accurate knowledge about such things as floor numbers, doctors' names, clinic hours, differences in the quality of care available at various hospitals, which hospitals have teaching hospitals, which have specialties in various departments, and which have long waits in crowded out-patient departments. And, as Thomas notes, the information gypsies have about the best hospitals and physicians is not confined to a local area but covers the entire nation. Thus, they "seek only the biggest physician" (i.e., a doctor with an impressive reputation), and can identify who such a doctor is in a particular specialty.

As Salloway puts it, the questions arises, "How do people who appear to be poor, who lack formal education to the point of widespread illiteracy, and who speak English as a second language come to know so much about a complex . . . medical system?"[23] The answer, according to both Salloway and Thomas, is the social network which we have called the lay-referral system. Speaking of the operation of the lay referral among gypsies, Salloway writes:

It is through this network that they inform one another who is sick, where he is being treated, who is treating him, and how pleased or displeased the patient, the family, and other interested parties are with the care that is being received. It is through this network that the Gypsy community seems to learn of care providers who are receptive to Gypsies, who understand their culture and their needs, and who provide the kind of care they want. They seem to substitute effective social networks and experience for formal education.[24]

The importance of "lay consultations" about health among the elderly has been documented by Furstenberg and Davis.[25] The researchers found discussion of health issues and the sharing of health-related information among members of this group to be so salient as to constitute an important kind of "social currency" used as a medium of exchange in interactions with one another. On the other hand, it was found that those who did not communicate with friends, and/or relatives, and/or acquaintances on health matters were more likely to be elderly men than elderly women. This conclusion is in line with other research which has shown men less predisposed to seek social support in health matters than women. For example, a recent study found that the initial diagnosis of cancer is much more traumatic for women than men. However, women are more able, over time, to cope with the fact of their illness due to their greater use of social support systems.[26]

The importance of the lay-referral system to the elderly can be partially attributed to the link between the incidence of chronic illness and increasing age. As people get older they increasingly share with others of the same age persistent health problems for which modern medicine can provide few, if any, curative remedies. As a result they frequently turn to nonprofessionals for advice based on life experiences with particular chronic illnesses. Arluke has described, for example, how arthritis sufferers often decide on the amount of a prescribed drug to take, the frequency with which to take it, and the point at which to cease taking it by soliciting opinions from fellow arthritis sufferers who have taken the same medication.[27] In addition, they receive information about drugs which have been effective with others but which their doctors may not have not mentioned.

SELF-HELP GROUPS

Another aspect of lay referral is the pervasive self-help movement which has arisen in this country. As a counterpart to the individual-to-individual network described in the preceding section, self-help groups, or mutual aid groups as some have called them, help fill a void in areas of health care in which medical professionals have relatively little interest. As with self-care, what is most striking about these self-help groups is their pervasiveness. It has been estimated that about 500,000 such groups (including health and nonhealth related ones) exist in the United States today.

Although health-related self-help groups can be categorized in various ways, a most commonly used typology distinguishes four such types of groups.[28] First, there are those groups involved in changing behavior related to smoking, overeating, drug abuse, alcoholism, and the like. Examples of behavioral change groups are Smokenders, Weightwatchers, Narcotics Anonymous, and Alcoholics Anonymous— the latter, of course, being perhaps the most well-known of all self-help organizations.

Alcoholics Anonymous (AA) was begun in 1935 by a stockbroker and a physician. Their goal was to help themselves and others to sobriety by creating, in an intimate discussion-group setting, a supportive atmosphere in which members could speak about their problems. The communalism of AA is rooted in the Oxford Group of the 1930s, a religious movement stressing confession-oriented social exchange among its members. As a result, AA has the quality of a quasireligious organization and the process undergone by its members has many similarities to religious spiritual renewal. Three years after its founding, AA published the book *Alcoholics Anonymous* in which the principles of the organization— the 12 "steps" to recovery—were systematically laid out. These 12 steps lead the alcoholic through the process of redefining alcoholism from a vice to a disease.

As mentioned above, many self-help groups serve individuals who have health conditions on which health professionals do not place a high priority. Thus, as Conrad has noted, the existence of AA "serves to free the physician from what is often considered the bothersome responsibility of treating the chronically intoxicated."[29] In this regard, one study of physicians found that the majority of those viewing alcoholism as a disease believed that referring drinkers to AA was the best professional strategy.[30]

Many behavioral change groups share as part of their programs a clearly identifiable process through which the group's ideology is instilled in its new members. This is often achieved through written texts, such as AA's "Big Book." Further, long-time members act as sponsors for a newcomer (a type of lay-referral outreach). This serves a dual purpose of indoctrinating new members while at the same time renewing the commitment of well-established members. In fact, it was found that those AA members who sponsored a newcomer were more likely than nonsponsors to remain in the group.

While behavioral change groups share a number of characteristics in common, there are frequently important differences that distinguish one from another. For example, an important difference between AA and Recovery, which is composed of ex-psychiatric patients, concerns their quite dissimilar ideologies. An underlying principle of AA is the need to accept the fact of having a long-term chronic disease. Recovery, on the other hand, emphasizes that one can overcome one's symptoms by working hard to act healthy. As Antze puts it, where AA stresses a sick role posture, Recovery rests upon a belief in the efficacy of will power to the end of getting well.[31]

A second type of self-help group is composed of those organizations whose goal is rehabilitation. Examples of this genre are Mastectomy, Inc. (for women who have had breasts removed due to cancer), Mended Hearts, and Make Today Count (for terminally ill cancer victims). Rehabilitative self-help groups take up where physicians leave off—at the so-called postacute phase—and concentrate on helping members adjust to their changed life situation. Of these groups, Gartner has written: "Interaction with others who have undergone a similar experience provides a body of special inside knowledge about the stages of recovery and how to function, coping techniques, role models, an emotional outlet, and support and encouragement."[32]

Riessman has offered an insightful examination of "stroke clubs," another example of a rehabilitative group. These clubs cater to a clientele that, at the onset of their rehabilitation, have largely lost the capacity to speak but retain their hearing ability. Left unabated, the consequent frustration could lead to total withdrawal from others. One method used by stroke clubs to avoid this withdrawal is instructing stroke victims to communicate by a code transmitted through finger pressure.[33]

Still another type of self-help group focuses on aspects of prevention, such as the control of hyper-tension. It has become increasingly apparent that such groups can be of enormous benefit to those individuals whose life situations make them particularly vulnerable to stress as, for example, the elderly. In 1983, after decades of decline, the suicide rate of Americans 65 and older began to rise once again due, in part, to what experts referred to as the increasing pressures facing members of that group. In that year, there were 19.2 suicides per 100,000 among people 65 and older, while the rate was 11.2 for young people 15–24. One of the factors impacting heavily on the mental health of senior citizens is the loss of a spouse. While both men and women feel the emotional toll of the death of a spouse, the impact is felt differentially by the sexes. Looking at the considerable research, Gartner has noted that although women comprise the bulk of the widowed—as high as 75%—it is men who appear to suffer more from widowhood. Gartner[34] cites other evidence concerning the relative vulnerability of widowers to stress: a community survey which found widowed males were more depressed than widowed females, a 1983 report of the House of Representative's Select Committee on Aging which concluded that widowers over 75 had the highest alcoholism rate in the country, and a related study, in which researchers at Johns Hopkins discovered that widowed men had a 28% greater mortality than their married counterparts and, moreover, that widowers (in this case the ages ranged between 55 and 65) had a mortality rate 60% higher than that of married men at the same age. Women, on the other hand, according to the last study, were found to be much less affected by the death of a husband.

Self-help groups, thus, can play an important role for those who lose a spouse. Groups like THEOS (They Help Each Other Spiritually), Widowed Persons Service, and Widow to Widow can provide emotional support systems and the possibilities for new relationships. It has been shown that bereavement time is significantly shortened by an individual's participation in these self-help groups.

The last category of self-help groups includes those concerned with primary care. (Of course, primary care is sufficiently broad so as to overlap, at points, with the functions of behavior change, prevention, and rehabilitation.) These groups range from those directed to teaching patients with chronic illness to adjust and exist with such illness to those providing health education to women, and other constituencies.

Perhaps the most highly publicized self-help groups of all are those [primary-care groups] directed to the health problems of women. For some, these groups represent more than just a social service. To them, these groups are a most successful element of a political movement to wrest control of health care from the professional establishment.

Whatever the ultimate impact of these women's groups, they have gained an extraordinary foothold in a relatively short period of time as, among other things, a network of women's health centers, largely staffed by laywomen, have sprung up throughout the United States. The publication in the early 1960s of *Our Bodies, Ourselves,* a text written by non-health professional women who were members of a Boston women's health collective, and the work of Carol Downer, a nonhealth professional women's activist, who, at about the same time, traveled the country demonstrating self-examination techniques to women, were two important elements in the recent historical development of the women's health movement. Frankfort has vividly described a typical Downer session in which women were provided the first inspection of their own reproductive organs through the use of a speculum (a device used to separate the walls of the vagina) with a mirror attached. An excerpt from Frankfort follows:[35]

An old church basement, a long table, a woman, a speculum—and pow! In about five minutes you've just about destroyed the mystique of the doctor.

I saw it happen this week when Carol, a woman from the Los Angeles Self-Help Clinic, slipped off her dungarees and underpants, borrowed somebody's coat and stretched it out on a long table, placed herself on top, and with her legs bent at the knees, inserted a speculum into herself. Once the speculum was in place, her cervix was completely visible and each of the fifty women present took a flashlight and looked inside.

"Which part is the cervix? The tiny slit in the middle?"

"No, that's the os. The cervix is the round, doughnut-shaped part."

"Have you had any children?"

"Yes, six, and two abortions and two miscarriages."

"My God, how old are you?"

"Thirty-eight."

"You know, it's changing. The cervix now looks more protruded and the os has opened slightly."

"Yes, we're very flexible inside."

"How much of this can you see yourself?"

"Come, take a look from here."

Carol placed the dime-store mirror so the women could see from her vantage point. The cervix, as reflected in the mirror, was clear and distinct.

Before actually demonstrating the use of the speculum, Carol had talked about self-examination while Lorraine, another woman from the clinic, showed slides.

"This is what a speculum looks like, the thing the doctor puts inside. Except it doesn't feel cold because it's not made of stainless steel.

"Here's a picture of cancer of the cervix. There's the tumor—that bulbous structure attached to the bottom. It takes about ten years for most tumors to reach that advanced stage. Each year 13,000 women die of tumors of the cervix. And the so-called danger signs we're told to look for are usually associated with late stages. But if each woman had her own speculum and knew how to examine herself, she could note any changes immediately.

"At our self-help clinic, we believe very much in sticking to our own experiences. We don't talk about what we've read in books. For example, one woman said, 'We can have twenty-five orgasms.' 'Well, have you?' I asked. 'No.' Now I'm not saying it's impossible, I'm just saying I haven't personally met a woman who has.

"The same thing applies to health. For instance, doctors have been telling women they have tipped or retroverted uteri. They're at the wrong angle, they say. You know the picture the textbooks have of the so-called normal uterus. Well, now that we've been examining each other, we see that the 'normal' uterus is the least common. The uterus can assume all angles of flection. And they're about as relevant as the shape of a nose. Yet one woman had her uterus removed because of its shape and another

had braces stuck up to force it not to be tipped.

"*But what really gave us the biggest charge was hearing a doctor check an IUD [intrauterine device]. You know, doctors talk in real fancy language. The eleven o'clock position, he says. For that he had to go to medical school and we have to pay $15. Well, if you look at the cervix in this slide at the eleven o'clock position, you can see exactly what the doctor sees: a little string. Generally, you have cervicitis where the string is. We recommend that the string be longer so you can pull it out.*

"*Now in this slide, the woman has monilia, a yeast-like infection. It's the milky white area over the cervix. And if you put a cotton swab to it, it will be cheesy. The smell is not foul, which is one way you can distinguish it from other vaginal infections.*

"*Here is a woman with cervicitis, an inflammation. Most of us have it. Yet many women are cauterized for it by doctors. We say watch it by checking whether it is still there a week later. In most women it goes away. We found that the frequency increased in the summer. At first we said women don't have odors, that's a male myth. But then the warm months came and we found that there was a distinct odor when we examined women.*

"*Here's a cervix of a woman who's had several children. It's slightly protruding. But if we touch it, it will retreat. Once we became tuned in to our uterus, we saw we had great control. What had previously been referred to as gut level, we now call uterus level.*"

"*Do you notice anything different about this cervix?*"

"*Color.*" *(It was very red.)*

"*Any idea why?*"

"*She's pregnant?*"

"*Right. She* was, *that is. By the next day, she wasn't.*"

"*Right on!*"

"*If you look at your cervix every week, you can see when it's softer, when the os opens and the color becomes darker or blotchy or reddish. And then you can know you're pregnant before a test tells you.*"

Regarding gynecological self-help groups, Marieskind has documented a rich history of such lay type organizations which date back to the Egyptian and Sumerian civilizations and which have responded to the "consistent effort to exclude women from anatomical and medical knowledge."[36] The success of these groups in contemporary America in the area of health education has been documented in the literature. Table 1 presents the often cited results of one such study in which scores on a gynecological awareness test were compared for women who frequented clinics staffed by physicians (the tra-

TABLE 1   Correct scores of knowledge measurements of women in three types of medical facilities (percentages)

TEST	TRADITIONAL	PARAMEDIC	SELF-HELP	ALL FACILITIES
Anatomy identification (Clitoris, uterus, vagina, os, Fallopian tube, urethra, ovary, labia, cervix, hymen)	46.2	54.6	72.2	57.7
Definition of gynecological procedures (Breast exam, Pap smear, speculum, pelvic exam, D & C, biopsy)	82.0	85.6	98.0	88.6
Knowledge of appropriate frequency of performing procedures	60.0	67.6	73.2	67.0
Contraceptive Contraindications (Pill, IUD, diaphragm, foam, condom)	22.0	39.2	39.2	33.4

From "Helping Oneself to Health" by Helen I. Marieskind, *Social Policy*, September/October, 1976, p. 65.

ditional means of gaining information), by paramedics, and self-help groups. As can be seen from Table 1, as regards every type of information, women served by the self-help groups were more knowledgeable.

Any mention of primary care self-help groups must take note of the Yale Self-Care Project under the direction of Lowell Levin.[37] This project involves the development of self-care abilities on a communitywide basis. The project is actually four different subprojects carried out at each of four separate health care facilities serving different neighborhoods. An underlying belief of Levin and his associates is that the most effective and appealing self-care education is that which allows the laypersons involved to determine the structure and desired outcomes of the program. Through this type of self-direction laypersons can be "empowered" to gain more control over their health and health care.

CONSUMERISM

Up to now the discussion has centered on health-care seeking behaviors which deemphasize the use of health professionals, and frequently avoid such use altogether. The notion of health-care consumerism as it has been used in the sociological literature refers, in sharp contrast, to a set of attitudes and strategies which bring the public into a challenging, and oftentimes adversarial position, in relation to the health-care establishment.

Marie Haug[38] and John McKinlay[39] are among those who posit the existence of a strong, and ever-growing, consumer movement in the United States. Their arguments are based essentially on the premise that changing conditions in American society are impacting on the relationship between the health professional and the client to make that relationship a far more egalitarian one. First, decreasing respect for physicians is seen to be the end result of the convergence of two factors, the prominence of anti-authoritarian attitudes toward traditional institutions—a legacy of the 1960s—and the increasing "proletarianiziation" of physicians as many of them move from being office-based, fee for service, independent entrepreneurs to being employees on salary in bureaucratic organizations like multinational (i.e., run by a chain) for-profit hospitals and health main-

tenance organizations. (The increasing unionization of doctors is also seen as contributing to the proletarianization of physicians.) The increase in chronic disease is viewed as still another factor moving the patient–practitioner relationship toward one in which the patient takes on greater responsibility for all aspects of his or her treatment. Finally, it is postulated that an increasingly educated population is more and more able to bring relevant health information to bear on their relationships with physicians and other health professionals.

Despite the number of arguments in the literature linking the above conditions to the development of a broad-based consumer movement, such a connection is, at the present time, still highly problematical. While it is true that confidence in traditional institutions has declined, medicine (as well as physicians) still rates highest among all of the major institutions. Although a substantial proportion of Americans display a cynicism toward physicians in general, the vast majority have very favorable attitudes toward their own physicians, a dichotomy which Blendon and Altman have referred to as part of the American public's "schizophrenia" toward the health-care system.[40] For example, one representative study found that while 66% of Americans say they had lost faith in doctors in general, only 15% had lost faith in their own doctor.[41] In another study, 66% said that doctors are too interested in making money, 68% that physician fees are not usually reasonable, and 62% that physicians do not spend enough time with their patients. In contrast to these responses, 72% of the same people said that their own physician is not too interested in making money, 71% that their own physician's fees are usually reasonable, and 77% that he or she spends enough time with them.[42]

A lot has been said and written about the meaning of the rise in malpractice suits against physicians. A view singling out decreasing respect toward physicians on the part of the public as the main cause would be an oversimplification of the issue. As just noted, Americans, for the most part, hold very favorable attitudes toward their own physicians. In addition, ours is an increasingly litigious society in which, for a wide variety of reasons, it has become fashionable and profitable to sue. In such an environment, physicians do not stand alone as defendants in such suits. It is also true that medicine's very success in treating illness may also be a culprit here. Innovations like by-pass surgery and organ transplants have given people access to health who only a few years ago would have had no hope for better health. At the same time, the public's expectations about what medicine can do has risen as have the risks involved in many of the new procedures. As far as the high-risk issue is concerned, it must be noted that malpractice suits are most likely to be directed against physicians in the most high-risk specialties.

Concerning the role of bureaucratic medicine on the status of physicians, Freidson has noted that physicians will still exert a good deal of control in these organizations since it is they who ultimately must attract patients and are, on a day-to-day basis, most responsible for patient care.

There is no question that the development of chronic disease (rather than acute disease) as the major problem facing the health-care system will create great problems for that system which is relatively unprepared to deal with chronic health problems. However, the ramifications of this fact are yet to be known. The effect of the increasing prevalence of chronic disease on public confidence in health care will depend on a number of factors including the capacity of the health-care system to adapt to the changing mix of illness in America. It is impossible to say, at this point, that mass disaffection has occurred among the chronically ill, and that modern medicine will not, in the future, meet many of the challenges presented by chronic illness.

Perhaps most important to a consumer challenge to the established health-care system is the need to decrease the "knowledge gap" between health-care professionals and their clients. While the educational level of Americans has risen to unprecedented heights, it is not clear how this education translates into more knowledge about health care since the need for adequate health education has only been given lip service in our society. At that same time, with medical knowledge growing exponentially, even medical professionals are finding it difficult to keep up with new developments in their specialities.

Further impediments to a narrowing of the knowledge gap are the obstacles that the medical establishment has placed in the path of attempts to provide the public with greater health-care infor-mation. For example, when Ralph Nader attempted to collect comparative information on Washington, D.C., physicians which would be disseminated to the public, a minority of doctors supplied the information. The American Medical Association recently opposed publication of a list of cancer specialists which would be available only to physicians. The fear was that the public would gain access to the list. In that case, physicians not current or expert in cancer treatment who nevertheless treat patients (thought to be a very large percentage of physicians due to the rapidity with which cancer research has generated new treatment) might suffer a loss of patients. It is true that in 1986, in a very significant development, the Department of Health and Human Services did make public information on the mortality rates of hospitals throughout America. However, the publication of this kind of information is rare, particularly as concerns the performances of individual physicians (which was not provided in this instance).

The history of "informed consent" is an excellent illustration of medicine's reluctance to share knowledge with its clientele. Informed consent refers to a legal doctrine that has evolved gradually since the late 1950s through a body of court decisions. In one of the most detailed analyses of the evolution of the doctrine, Katz describes informed consent as a physician's "affirmative duty to acquaint patients with the important risks and plausible alternatives to a proposed procedure."[43]

The concept of informed consent developed out of the case of Salgo versus the Stanford University Board of Trustees in 1957. It first appeared in a judge's opinion which was taken verbatim from an *amicus curiae* (friend of the court) brief, submitted in support of Stanford University, by the American College of Surgeons. There is enormous irony in the fact that the doctrine of informed consent, of which many doctors have been exceedingly critical, had its genesis in the medical community.

To be sure, informed consent can present a real dilemma for physicians in particular instances. In the Salgo versus Stanford case the Court stated, in part, "In discussing the element of risk a certain amount of discretion must be employed consistent with the full disclosure of facts necessary to an informed consent." As Katz has pointed out, achieving both discretion *and* full disclosure is no easy task.

Questions arise as to how much information doctors should withhold in order to avoid further alarming an already fearful patient, and what kinds of information should be disclosed so as not to unduly influence a patient's consent.

The difficulties of reconciling discretion and disclosure aside, it is true that organized medicine has consistently opposed informed consent and that, in clinical situations, physicians have paid little attention to it. Informed consent often amounts to nothing more than a mechanical and perfunctory rendering of the facts to the patient in a presentation dotted with technical jargon. Katz concludes that "the law of informed consent is substantially mythic and fairytale like as far as advancing patient's rights to self-decisionmaking is concerned."[44] Similarly, the recent report of the President's Commission for the Study of Ethical Problems in Medicine and Biomedical and Behavioral Research concluded that, in general, "physician/patient communication in practice bore little relation to informed consent as envisioned by law," and that despite the doctrine's "substantial foundations in law, it is essentially an ethical imperative."[45] A Louis Harris poll found that 79% of patients, and 55% of physicians believe that the informed consent document primarily protects the physician against a lawsuit.[46]

Much like the doctrine of informed consent, the more inclusive Patient's Bill of Rights, which includes an informed consent right within it, does little to change the relationship between patient and professional. Passed by the American Hospital Association in 1973, the Patient's Bill of Rights reads as follows.

PATIENT'S BILL OF RIGHTS

The American Hospital Association presents a Patient's Bill of Rights with the expectation that observance of these rights will contribute to more effective patient care and greater satisfaction for the patient, his physician, and the hospital organization. Further, the Association presents these rights in the expectation that they will be supported by the hospital on behalf of its patients, as an integral part of the healing process. It is recognized that a personal relationship between the physician and the patient is essential for the provision of proper medical care. The traditional physician–patient relationship takes on a new dimension when care is rendered within an organizational structure. Legal precedent has established that the institution itself also has a responsibility to the patient. It is in recognition of these factors that these rights are affirmed.

1. The patient has the right to considerate and respectful care.

2. The patient has the right to obtain from his physician complete current information concerning his diagnosis, treatment, and prognosis in terms the patient can be reasonably expected to understand. When it is not medically advisable to give such information to the patient, the information should be made available to an appropriate person in his behalf. He has the right to know by name, the physician responsible for coordinating his care.

3. The patient has the right to receive from his physician information necessary to give informed consent prior to the start of any procedure and/or treatment. Except in emergencies, such information for informed consent, should include but not necessarily be limited to the specific procedure and/or treatment, the medically significant risks involved, and the probable duration of incapacitation. Where medically significant alternatives for care or treatment exist, or when the patient requests information concerning medical alternatives, the patient has the right to such information. The patient also has the right to know the name of the person responsible for the procedures and/or treatment.

4. The patient has the right to refuse treatment to the extent permitted by law, and to be informed of the medical consequences of his action.

5. The patient has the right to every consideration of his privacy concerning his own medical care program. Case discussion, consultation, examination, and treatment are confidential and should be conducted discreetly. Those not directly involved in his care must have the permission of the patient to be present.

6. The patient has the right to expect that all communications and records pertaining to his care should be treated as confidential.

7. The patient has the right to expect that within its capacity a hospital must make reasonable response to the request of a patient for services. The hospital must provide evaluation, service, and/or referral as indicated by the urgency of the case. When medically permissible a patient may be transferred to another facility only after he has received complete information and explanation concerning the needs for and alternatives to such a transfer. The institution to which the patient is to be transferred must first have accepted the patient for transfer.

8. The patient has the right to obtain information as to any relationship of his hospital to other health care and educational institutions insofar as his care is concerned. The patient has the right to obtain information as to the existence of any professional relationships among individuals, by name, who are treating him.

9. The patient has the right to be advised if the hospital proposes to engage in or perform human experimentation affecting his care or treatment. The patient has the right to refuse to participate in such research projects.

10. The patient has the right to expect reasonable continuity of care. He has the right to know in advance what appointment times and physicians are available and where. The patient has the right to expect that the hospital will provide a mechanism whereby he is informed by his physician or a delegate of the physician of the patient's continuing health care requirements following discharge.

11. The patient has the right to examine and receive an explanation of his bill regardless of source of payment.

12. The patient has the right to know what hospital rules and regulations apply to his conduct as a patient.

No catalogue of rights can guarantee for the patient the kind of treatment he has a right to expect. A hospital has many functions to perform, in- *cluding the prevention and treatment of disease, the education of both health professionals and patients, and the conduct of clinical research. All these activities must be conducted with an overriding concern for the patient, and, above all, the recognition of his dignity as a human being. Success in achieving the recognition assures success in the defense of the rights of the patient.*

While an impressive list of protections, the Patient's Bill of Rights is simply a set of guidelines for providers. Many patients are not even aware of its existence, and, in actuality, the document is more a statement of existing problem areas than it is a mechanism to actually address these problems.

One mechanism which could enhance the likelihood of patients' rights being fulfilled is that of the patient advocate or representative. A very promising idea when first conceived a few decades ago, the idea of someone to act as an advocate for the patient in his or her encounters with health professionals has gained little momentum. The first school to develop a program to train patient representatives, Sarah Lawrence, remains the only school to have such a program. Additionally, patient representatives have gained only moderate acceptance within hospitals and other health settings where they work, and the organizational constraints under which they work have severely limited their capacity to act vigorously on behalf of patients. (In an article in Chapter 3, Marjorie Glassman strongly asserts that social workers should act as patient advocates for the elderly in cases where there is an incorrect diagnosis of senile dementia.)

The foregoing material concerning consumerism should not be taken to mean that there is no evidence of a stronger public stance in the matter of health care nor that a consumerist perspective will not eventually characterize the American consumer of health care. Up to this point, the argument has only been that claims of a broad-based consumer movement generated by such things as anti-authority attitudes and increased education are highly speculative at this time.

There is certainly evidence of important pockets of health consumerism such as among a substantial number of women; among gypsies as we have mentioned; among some of the intellegensia if the Norman Cousins case,[47] in which Cousins developed his own treatment for a serious disease of the connective tissue, is more than an isolated incident; among some younger, more educated Americans if the work of Haug is correct, and among some other groups as well. In addition, Kasteler and her colleagues[48] have discovered a surprising amount of "doctor-shopping" (i.e., changing doctors) among a sample of lower- and upper-class families in Salt Lake City, Utah, as has Norman Cousins in a more informal California survey, the findings of which were presented in *The New England Journal of Medicine*.[49]

What about the future? Any steam gained by consumerism in the future is less likely to stem from the conditions which Haug and others have focused upon than from changes in the way in which health care is paid for and delivered in this country as well as from consequent pressures such changes bring to bear on providers.

In a competitive health-care environment labeled by the phrase "consumer choice" and spawned by the Reagan administration, many employees are now obligated to choose annually during the so-called "open-season" from various health-care plans and options. These choices, as with employees of the Federal government, can be very complicated, involving over 20 different plans and even a greater number of options within the various plans. In addition, consumers are now being asked to act on behalf of insurance companies and to be wiser consumers by getting second opinions, or more, before submitting to a wide range of surgical interventions. Fielding[50] and Freidson[51] have also suggested that health maintenance organizations, the choice of an increasing number of Americans, may provide patients with a better grievance procedure than found in other kinds of health delivery systems.

Greater concern for consumers may be generated as a result of the interests of providers themselves. Hospitals, for example, have entered a new era of hospital "hospitality" due to, among other things, a dramatic decline in patients as a result of the increase in ambulatory care such as same-day surgical centers. Among the benefits are increased attention to the needs of hospitalized patients. The options hospitals now provide husbands and wives in the situation surrounding the birth process derive, in large part, from a decline in the number of children being born and competition from competing facilities such as birthing centers.

SUMMARY

The preponderance of attention which has been paid to the mode of health-care delivery involving the traditional relationship between the doctor and his or her client has resulted in neglect of the substantial role played by the client in response to health-care matters. Such neglect overlooks the fact that for most health problems, individuals do not engage the health-care system but attend to such problems themselves. Lay-referral networks and self-help groups are additional manifestations of the role members of the lay public play in responding to their health needs. Finally, while questions have been raised about the existence of a broad-based health care consumer movement at this time, it has been suggested that recent changes in the health-care delivery system may result in an acceleration of consumerism in the future.

References

1. Freidson, E., *Patients' View of Medical Practice,* New York: Russell Sage Foundation, 1961.

2. DeFreise, G. and Woomert, A., The Policy Implications of Self-Care in the Study of Health and Illness Behavior, *Social Policy,* Fall, 1982, p. 55.

3. Levin, L. S. and Idler, E. L., *The Hidden Health Care System: Mediating Structures and Medicine,* Cambridge, Mass.: Ballinger, 1981.

4. Levin and Idler, *Ibid.,* p. 75.

5. Roghmann, K. J. and Haggerty, R. J., The Diary as a Research Instrument in the Study of Health and Illness Behavior: Experiences with a Random Sample of Young Families, *Medical Care,* 1972, 10, 143–63.

6. Reissman, F. The Self-Help Ethos, *Social Policy,* Summer, 1982, p. 42–45.

7. Demers, R. Y., Altamore, R., Mustin, H., Kleinman, A., and Leonardo, D., An Explanation of the Dimensions of Illness Behavior, *The Journal of Family Practice,* 1980, 11, pp. 1085–1092.

8. Cited in Light, D., Lay Medicine and the Medical Profession: An International Perspective, in Herder, D. and Schuller, A. (eds.), *Die Herausforderung der Rung der Laienmedizin,* Stuttgort: Kholhimmer, 1982, p. 97.

9. Fry J. and the Panel on Health Care, Self Care: Its Place in the Total Health Care System, 1973, unpublished paper.

10. Fry, *Ibid.*, p. 10.

11. Levin and Idler, *op. cit.* p. 75.

12. Cockerham, W. C., Lueschen, G., Kunz, G., and Spaeth, J. L., Social Stratification and Self-Management of Health, *Journal of Health and Social Behavior,* 1986, 27, pp. 1–14.

13. *Ibid.,* p. 7.

14. Levin and Idler, *op cit.*, pp. 137–152.

15. *Ibid.,* p. 152.

16. Harwood, A., The Hot-Cold Theory of Disease: Implications for Treatment of Puerto Rican Patients, *Journal of the American Medical Association,* 1971, 216, pp. 1153–1158.

17. DeFreise, G., and Woomert, A., *op. cit.*, p.

18. Freidson, E. *op. cit.*

19. *Ibid.,* p. 198.

20. Wolinsky, F. D. and Steiber, S. R., Salient Issues in Choosing a New Doctor, *Social Science and Medicine,* 1984, 16, pp. 759–767.

21. Salloway, J. C., Medical Care Utilization Among Urban Gypsies, *Urban Anthropology,* 1973, 2, pp. 113–125.

22. Thomas, J. D., Gypsies and Medical Care, *Annals of Internal Medicine,* 1985, 102, pp. 842–845.

23. Salloway, *op. cit.*, p. 115.

24. *Ibid.* p. 118.

25. Furstenberg, A. L. and Davis, L. J., Lay Consultation of Older People, *Social Science and Medicine,* 1984, 18, pp. 827–837.

26. Men, Women, and Cancer: The Emotional Reaction Differs Between the Sexes, *Washington Post,* Oct. 17, 1984.

27. Arluke, A., Judging Drugs: Patients' Conceptions of Therapeutic Efficacy in the Treatment of Arthritis, *Human Organization,* 1980, 39, pp. 85–87.

28. Gartner, A., A Typology of Women's Self-Help Groups, *Social Policy,* Winter, 1985, pp. 25–30.

29. Conrad, P. and Schneider, J. W., *Deviance and Medicalization: From Badness to Sickness,* St. Louis: C. V. Mosby, 1980, p. 90.

30. Jones, R. W. and Helrich, A. R. Treatment of Alchohism by Physicians in Private Practice: A National Survey. *Quarterly Journal for the Study of Alcoholism,* 1972, 33, pp. 117–131.

31. Antze, P., The Role of Ideologies in Peer Psychotherapy Organizations: Some Theoretical Considerations and Three Case Studies, *Journal of Applied Behavioral Science,* 1976, 12, pp. 323–346.

32. Gartner, A., *Ibid.*, p. 28.

33. Reissman, F., Moody, H. R., and Worthy, E. H., Self Help and the Elderly, *Social Policy,* Spring, 1984, pp. 19–24.

34. Gartner, A., *op. cit.*

35. Frankfort, E., Vaginal Politics, in C. Dreifius, (ed.), *Seizing Our Bodies: The Politics of Women's Health,* New York: Vintage Boosk, 1977, pp. 263–265.

36. Marieskind, H. I., Helping Oneself to Health, *Social Policy,* September/October, 1984, pp. 63–66.

37. A detailed discussion of the Yale study appears in Savo, C., Self-Care and Empowerment: A Case Study, *Social Policy,* Summer, 1983, pp. 19–22.

38. Haug, M. and Lavin B., *Consumerism in Medicine: Challenging Physician Authority,* Beverly Hills: Sage, 1981.

39. McKinlay, J. and Arches, J., Towards the Proletarianization of Physicians, *International Journal of Health Services,* 1985, 15.

40. Blendon, R. J. and Altman, D. E., Public Attitudes About Health-Care Costs, *New England Journal of Medicine,* 1985, 311, pp. 613–616.

41. Jeffe, D. and Jeffe, S. B., Losing Patients with Doctors: Physicians vs. The Public on Health Care Costs, *Public Opinion,* March. 1984, 7, p. 55.

42. Blendon and Altman, *op. cit.*, p. 614.

43. Katz, J., *The Silent World of Doctor and Patient,* New York: Free Press, 1980, p. 60.

44. *Ibid.,* p. 83.

45. President's Commission for the Study of Ethical Problems in Medicine and Biomedical and Behavioral Research, *Summing Up: Final Report on Studies of the Ethical and Legal Problems in Medicine and Biomedical and Behavioral Research,* March, 1983, p. 20.

46. Cited in Abram, M. B., To Curb Medical Suits, *New York Times,* March 31, 1984.

47. Cousins, N., Anatomy of an Illness (As Perceived By The Patient), *New England Journal of Medicine,* 1975, 295, pp. 1458–1463.

48. Kasteler, J. R., Kane, R., Olsen, D., and Thetford, C., Issues Underlying Prevalence of "Doctor-Shopping" Behavior, *Journal of Health and Social Behavior,* 1976, 17, pp. 328–339.

49. Cousins, N., How Patients Appraise Physicians, *New England Journal of Medicine,* 1985, 313, pp. 1422–1424.

50. Fielding, S. L., Organizational Impact on Medicine: The HMO Concept, *Social Science and Medicine,* 1984, 18, pp. 615–620.

51. Freidson, E. The Changing Nature of Professional Control, *Annual Reviews of Sociology,* 1984, 10, pp. 1–24.

PART TWO

The Practitioner

CHAPTER 6 _____

The "Loss of Idealism" Theme

Occupational socialization is a key issue in the sociology of occupations and professions. It involves the way in which an individual learns to play an occupational role. Although sociologists are concerned with the way in which technical skills are acquired, this is only of secondary interest to them. Their main interest is in the process through which the values and attitudes that members of a given occupational group have in common are learned. These predispositions to action determine the manner in which and the patients to which the technical skills are applied. Two of the classic works dealing with the occupational socialization of physicians are Becker's *Boys in White* and Merton's *The Student Physician*. More recently, a surprising number of excellent studies of the socialization of medical residents have come out. These include Scully's *Men Who Control Women's Health,* Light's *Becoming a Psychiatrist,* and Bosk's *Forgive and Remember. Dominant Issues* includes material from the first two of these.

The three themes most commonly found in the literature on the socialization of health professionals are the "loss of idealism"—which is the subject of this chapter—"training for uncertainty" and the learning of the "medical model."

In mid-1983, a report of the prestigious Association of American Medical Colleges criticized medical schools for not training students to be more sensitive to the psychological and social needs of patients. As a result many have called for the development of a somewhat more humanistically-oriented medical school curriculum.

The first section of this chapter includes articles dealing with the loss of idealism of medical residents—doctors-in-training who, following graduation from medical school, embark on a program of training in a specialty area. Terry Mizrahi describes the increasing cynicism of overworked medical residents as a response, in part, to very difficult working conditions. In the second article, Diana Scully reveals how residents in the dual specialty of obstetrics–gynecology manipulate patients to gain more surgical experience.

The second section of this chapter focuses on the lack of idealism among practicing physicians. "The Undesireable Patient" appeared as the lead editorial in a specialized medical journal. Written by a prominent doctor, Solomon Papper, it delineates several categories of patients that doctors are likely to see as undesirable. The article that follows is used as an addendum to Papper's article. Taken from Michael Medved's bestselling book *Hospital,* it presents quotes taken from interviews with health professionals at a medical center. In the concluding article in this chapter, David Sudnow shows how social class and other nonmedical factors can determine who gets treatment and who doesn't—who lives and who dies—in the emergency room setting. (Among those staffing the emergency room are a range of physicians from those with vast experience to residents-in-training.)

References

BECKER, H. S., B. GEER, E. C. HUGHES, and A. L. STRAUSS 1961. *Boys in White: Student Culture in Medical School.* Chicago: University of Chicago Press.

BOSK, C. 1979. *Forgive and Remember: Managing Medical Failure.* Chicago: University of Chicago Press.

LIGHT, D. 1980. *Becoming Psychiatrists: The Professional Transformation of Self.* New York: W. W. Norton.

MERTON, R. K., G. G. READER, and P. L. KENDALL (eds.) 1957. *The Student-Physician: Introductory Studies in the Sociology of Medical Education.* Cambridge, Mass.: Harvard University Press.

SCULLY, D. 1980. *Men Who Control Women's Health: The Miseducation of Obstetrician-Gynecologists.* Boston: Houghton Mifflin.

Coping with Patients: Subcultural Adjustments to the Conditions of Work Among Internists-in-Training

Terry Mizrahi

Internship and residency are important and stressful rites of passage for young physicians. During this part of their training, doctors have full responsibility for the care of patients for the first time. The house staff—as residents and interns are called collectively—usually has a very large case load of patients and is exploited by the hospital as a relatively cheap source of labor. Doctors feel that the medical profession makes the greatest demand on their time and energy during this phase of their career. They devote nearly all their waking hours to the practice of medicine, working at a feverish pace in life-and-death situations under less than optimal conditions.

Many studies of the professional socialization of doctors have viewed internship and residency as a necessary and even desirable system of medical training (Fox, 1959; Merton et al., 1957; Mumford, 1970). The adverse effects of this system on the normal day-to-day relationships between doctors and patients have rarely been examined. Researchers such as Bucher and Stelling (1977) have largely accepted the medical field's own definition of graduate medical education and have concentrated on how novices learn technical skills and become medical professionals.

On the other hand, a growing literature on doctor-patient interaction has revealed considerable dissatisfaction among patients with the provision of medical care (Hulka et al., 1975a, 1975b; Korsch, et al., 1968; Korsch and Negrete, 1972; Wartman et al., 1981). Recent studies also show that stressful aspects of training and unsatisfactory encounters with patients contribute to disillusionment among medical students, interns and residents, and even physicians in private practice (American Medical Association, 1974; Coombs, 1978; Gerber, 1983; Light, 1980; Lipp, 1980; McCue, 1982; Mawardi, 1979; Nadelson and Notman, 1979; Pfifferling, 1983; Preston, 1981; Rosenberg, 1980; Shapiro and Driscoll, 1979; Tokarz et al., 1979; Werner and Korsch, 1979).

In this research, I show how distortions of the doctor-patient relationship and negative reactions to patients develop as subcultural adjustments by interns and residents to their work environment. Sociological accounts of professional training have described the common perspective (Becker et al., 1957) or subculture that emerges as a collective solution to shared problems in work settings. This

Reprinted from *Social Problems*, vol. 32 (December, 1984), pp. 156–165. Copyright © 1984 by The Society for the Study of Social Problems.

approach to adult socialization has been applied to numerous occupational situations, including the training of medical students. In the first part of this paper, I apply and extend this approach to more advanced stages of medical training—internship and residency in internal medicine. Like other work groups, the house staff is faced with distinctive problems that are solved or, at least, made more manageable by subcultural definitions and techniques.

In the second part of the paper, I describe intense emotional reactions by interns and residents that go beyond these more practical, subcultural adaptations to their work environment. House staff members share and express very negative feelings about their work and, especially, about their patients. These emotional responses are also ways of coping with aspects of medical practice that these doctors believe are wrong in a fundamentally moral sense. Since they must do this work, they develop "techniques of neutralization" or shared coping mechanisms in which they display their moral ambivalence through exaggerated expressions of hostility toward patients and, occasionally, toward lower-ranking staff.[1] These findings focus attention on graduate medical training as a source of serious and enduring consequences for doctors' views and treatment of patients.

---

[1] Examination of coping or defense mechanisms (Coelho et al., 1974) among physicians is rare. In their review of the literature, Spitz and Block (1981) were unable to find any studies of the use of denial, disavowal or minimization by normal physicians. Nevertheless, the family physicians in their study were found to employ these techniques in telephone contacts with patients, resulting in distorted diagnoses and treatment plans. Coombs and Goldman (1973) identified several coping mechanisms that are used by medical personnel: humor; escape into work; language alteration; and rationalization. Physical and psychological avoidance of patients have been noted in studies of medical students (Coombs and Powers, 1978; Martin, 1957) and psychiatric residents (Coser, 1967; Light, 1980). The subcultural strategies that were shared among house staff in this study also parallel neutralization techniques (Sykes and Matza, 1957) and other mechanisms that various deviant groups develop to cope with oppressive environments and to rationalize deviant acts (also see Cohen, 1966; Goffman, 1961).

METHOD

In the late 1970s, I was a participant observer in a graduate training program in internal medicine in an urban medical center that I will call the Southern Area Medical School (SAMS) which included 102 interns and residents. I also interviewed a total of 83 randomly selected interns and residents at different stages of their three years in training.[2] Additionally, I spoke with seven family practice interns who each spent a four-month rotation in internal medicine.

I was identified to the house staff as a sociologist, and they were informed about basic aspects and goals of my research. The house staff usually seemed oblivious to my presence as they performed their duties. At times, I helped out or ran a necessary errand. On other occasions, some members of the house staff confided in me about their frustrations or grievances.

THE WORLD OF INTERNS AND RESIDENTS IN INTERNAL MEDICINE

Upon graduation from medical school, specialists in internal medicine spend three years as members of a hospital house staff as interns and residents. This period of their career is also known as graduate medical training. For the first time, they are paid to have major responsibility for patients. In teaching hospitals affiliated with SAMS, staff members assume responsibility for the primary health care for many poor patients by default. As undergraduate medical students, they had assisted the medical staff and had few, if any, patients of their own. Because the teaching institutions were primarily public hospitals, the patients these doctors faced were difficult to treat. They came predominantly from lower-class backgrounds and suffered from socially- and self-induced diseases, many of which were chronic and untreatable. Because of the monthly system of rotations, there were few patients with whom the house staff had ongoing relationships.

Interns and residents are in hospitals to learn as well as to treat. Although one learns through

---

[2] See Mizrahi (forthcoming) for additional information on fieldwork and interview procedures.

treating patients, most patients at SAMS present mundane or untreatable conditions. The house staff spends the great bulk of its time on routine medical care in which there is little to be learned after basic patient management skills have been acquired. This is referred to in the house staff subculture as "scut work." Continued learning comes from the occasional "interesting" case which, more often than not, is appropriated by the attending faculty or sub-speciality fellows for teaching purposes.

Interns and residents are in the middle of a hierarchy, with medical students below and faculty above them. The medical students, because of their status, are protected from assuming responsibility for patient care, since they are presumed to be unqualified to treat patients without close supervision by the house staff. Some routine work can be sloughed off on students as learning experiences. However, the house staff, especially the intern, is effectively at the bottom of the hierarchy in which responsibility is delegated. This means that unwanted patients are "dumped" (their term) on house staff by faculty, other medical services within the medical center, private hospitals that exclude indigent patients, and local private practitioners. Because of the sheer volume of patients referred to them, house staff members are usually overwhelmed with responsibilities. I observed them to be constantly at work—writing on patient charts, filling out forms, ordering laboratory tests, reading voluminous records, preparing for, conducting or following up on a variety of "rounds" (discussions and conferences), performing myriad procedures, transporting patients, etc. As I will show later, time with patients was a minor share of this daily routine.

Interns spend most of their time keeping patient charts and presenting cases to the senior staff. They are immersed in laboratory tests and technical procedures, which generate a voluminous amount of paper work. The house staff calls this "laboratory/technical-based medicine" as opposed to clinical medicine in which the doctor makes a diagnosis primarily by examining and talking to a patient. The house staff likens its role to that of a "sleuth" or detective, who uses the latest technology to make the diagnosis. They give a low priority to developing skills in relating to patients, emphasizing instead the intellectual challenge of their specialty.

When they are not involved in the preparation, implementation or evaluation of diagnostic or therapeutic procedures, the most significant portion of the house staff members' time was spent with the patients' medical records. Indeed, it appeared that as much, if not more, of their actual time and energy each day was devoted to the patients' charts as to any other activity. Hours each day were occupied with requesting, waiting, reading, reviewing, discussing, and writing in medical records.

While careful record-keeping is important, the chart seemed to be the pivotal point of action around which everything else revolved—ultimately, it was the actual embodiment of the patient.[3] Tension in the house staff was visible when they were forced to act or make a decision without a chart being present. To preclude missing anything, the house staff needed to know "everything"—past and present—about the patient, and the chart was the vehicle for becoming so informed. Not only did doctors commonly believe that they could learn more from the chart than from patients, but often that they would learn more accurately. For example:

In the Intensive Care Unit (ICU) Intern Zorez consulted with a surgeon about a patient who had become a surgical emergency . . . When the surgeon asked Zorez about the patient's pulses, he replied, 'Actually, I never checked them, but in the chart it said . . .'

When there was a discrepancy between what appeared on the chart and what was reported by the patient or family, staff members frequently believed the medical record.

A patient was presented by a medical student . . . It was mentioned in her social history that she had a 45 year history of smoking and occa-

---

[3] Mumford (1970) makes a passing reference in a footnote to the possibility that the patient chart may become an end in itself. Freidson (1975:167–182) shows how doctors in practice discount the appropriateness of the chart for evaluation of their performance, while, at the same time, recognize it as the only "objective" assessment of their work. Hence, he characterized it as a tool, weapon, and cover. The doctors Freidson studied saw their work experience and not the chart as the reality. For members of the house staff at SAMS, the political uses of the chart were limited primarily to the informal system of social control—that is, for unofficial assessments of each other's work.

sional drinking. The medical student added emphatically, 'But her chart says she was a heavy user.'

Given the cultural and class barriers between the house staff and the typical patient, and the lack of time to communicate comprehensibly to patients, the chart often became an easier and surer source of information. At times, the chart seemed to replace the patient.

In the settings I observed, then, the main reason for patient contact was to obtain information for medical charts. To accomplish this primary objective while restricting other demands of their heavy case load, the interns and residents collectively developed several strategies: 1) avoiding patients and their families; 2) narrowing the focus of interaction to strictly "medical" concerns; and 3) treating patients as non-persons—even in their presence.

AVOIDING PATIENTS

The actual amount of physical time house staff members spent in direct interaction with patients was (with a few exceptions) brief. The substance of any house staff-patient encounter was directed almost exclusively at acquiring information directly related to the disease. As suggested by the testimony of a family practice intern, staff members gave low priority to direct interaction with patients and their families:

> *The amount of time the [internal medicine] house staff spends with the patient after initial history and physical depends. It may be as little as 5 minutes a day, 3–5 minutes on morning rounds . . . Sometimes if the family can catch you, you may spend more time [answering their questions] if they actually grab you and drag you into the room.*

Another staff member described the strategy of avoidance as follows:

> *If I was really busy I was avoiding patients. I wouldn't avoid those who were critically ill. It would be the patients who were just on 'automatic pilot' where the family would want to know— say—'Would she ever play the violin again?'*

As opposed to patient contact, the house staff wanted as much experience as possible in the use of various technical medical procedures. The house staff sometimes engaged in "shot-gunning"—ordering every possible test to avoid a small chance of error—or "rubber banding"—stretching the diagnostic indications for a procedure for educational rather than patient care purposes. To a great extent, involvement with these technical procedures and tests insulated the house staff from personal involvement with patients.[4] As staff members learned that the policies for obtaining patients' or family members' written permission were quite lenient for certain tests, they limited these personal contacts even further. When they did return to the patient's bedside, it was almost always to collect additional information. These doctors were so intent on doing things *to* patients, that they seemed to have little time or desire to do anything *for* them—such as simply comforting them. As an intern told me before I accompanied him on his rounds:

> *You'll see. You have to spend so much of your time doing these things [he points to the computer] such as entering lab data, scheduling tests, labeling lab data . . . instead of being a doctor. I have no time to think about my patients' problems.*

NARROWING THE FOCUS OF INTERACTION

A second subcultural strategy for managing the demands on house staff is based on the inequality of the doctor-patient relationship. Medically, if not socially, patients occupy an inferior status in this relationship because of their necessary dependence on doctors. Interns and residents quickly learn how to use their dominant status to control and direct interaction with patients. In order to extract all necessary information from patients in the shortest amount of time, house staff members narrow both the scope and substance of interaction to "medically pertinent" topics. As in the following example, doctors view this as an efficient solution to a difficult problem:

[4] Others have labeled these types of coping mechanisms as "escape into work" (Coombs and Goldman, 1973) or "turning to technique" (Light, 1980).

*I used to get frustrated with people because pa-
tients rambled. Now I just don't give them a
chance to ramble. People might be offended because I do that, but on the other hand, it is much
more efficient than to have somebody take a half
hour or 45 minutes of your time and really not
be able to get everything that you want. You need
to be able to get the gist . . . what's important.*

A thorough medical history and physical examination can take as long as two hours. To be "textbook"
correct, the history should include current medical
problems, past medical history, family history, and
social history. House staff members indicated that
they learned how to complete this process in substantially less time without sacrificing thoroughness.
This skill—often considered the essence or art of
internal medicine—is taught by more experienced
colleagues or acquired through observation. However, the pressures to reduce patient contact to a
minimum tended to undermine the breadth and
quality of patient histories. Interns and residents
frequently blamed patients when histories were incomplete or incorrect. I repeatedly heard comments
like the following in formal presentations and informal conversations among staff and supervisors: "The
patient is a poor historian."; "She may not be telling
you the whole story."; "The patient is an unreliable
or unbelievable historian."

The house staff learned that it was acceptable
to take short cuts and omit information if it did
not seem to be directly pertinent to the medical diagnosis. At the same time, they learned that time invested in the doctor-patient relationship went unre-
warded, and might indeed be costly if their mentors
felt more significant activities were being ignored
or postponed. A junior resident summed these expectations up as follows:

*You know I'd love to sit there and hold their
hand for half an hour and more but you also
want to get home sometime before midnight and
you have other things to do. If you don't sit and
talk with the cancer patient for a half hour, in
terms of your job description and what's expected,
nobody will be upset with you. But if you don't
know what the hemoglobin is on that patient
they [the resident and chief of medicine] are going
to be very upset.*

Among the topics that were defined as less "pertinent" medically were social aspects of the patient's
history. The shared belief that social factors were
irrelevant to medical treatment generally deepened
and hardened as house staff progressed through their
training. As one doctor put it:

*The amount of time spent on social factors de-
pends on the situation. Sometimes I probably
did a lot and sometimes I probably did little
. . . If it affects them either going home or coming
back and was medically appropriate, I dealt with
it. Otherwise, I didn't get into it. I don't feel
that I have the time or the energy or really the
desire to get into their personal lives.*

In this vein, several house staff referred to the former
T.V. series, *Marcus Welby, M.D.,* to highlight the
discrepancy between the public's image of medical
practice and their own expectations about doctor-
patient interaction. For example:

*I guess I could use the excuse that I don't have
the time to do that [deal with social factors] . . .
It would be nice to* bullshit *with your patients
for an hour or so and get a feel for their social
situation . . . It may affect the complaints they
present with . . . If I was Marcus Welby and
saw one patient per week, maybe I would be more
concerned. I doubt it though, because it's really
not appealing to me. If I really wanted to do it,
I would have majored in social work or psychiatry. What appeals to me is treatment of sick people
by diagnosing their diseases and giving medications. I like good hard facts and physical findings—things I can deal with on a tangible basis—
not some intangible nebulous feeling of what
their social situation is.*

I observed a number of means by which the
more experienced house staff members and supervisors taught new interns and medical students to
focus on "medically-relevant" aspects of cases. Whenever anything defined as non-essential was presented by the novices, the more experienced members gestured to them to "get to the point" or exhorted
them to "give only the pertinent facts." Sometimes
house officers would snap their fingers impatiently.
At other times they fell asleep, yawned, and otherwise communicated boredom and restlessness.

From their own experiences, several of the house staff and all of the family practice informants corroborated how they narrowed the focus of their interest in patients. One family practice intern summed up this process:

> We were taught that the social history is supposed to be anything that pertains to patient's life outside the hospital . . . But the only thing that ever gets asked is smoking and drinking habits. I think a lot of people start out with the attitude, 'These factors are important, but I don't have the time'. . . As your training goes on, you ignore them more and more; eventually there comes a time when those things don't even enter your consciousness anymore—you become more and more narrow in your approach . . . A lot of it is not intentional . . . It's what's rewarded.

Little in the organization or culture of medical training contradicts this narrow and detached view of the doctor-patient relationship. Hence, house staff members oriented themselves to subculturally approved and rewarded instrumental ends. Obtain "just the (medical) facts" was not merely a slogan, but it represented a normative guideline for encounters between patients and house staff.

THE PATIENT AS "NON-PERSON"

Goffman (1959:151) described the role of being neither audience nor actor as the status of "non-person." He pointed out that it is a discrepant role and that the classic non-person is the servant. Treating patients as absent when they are physically present denies the existence of the human subject. In spite of considerable evidence of the importance of involving patients as active participants in the treatment process (Howard and Strauss, 1975; Sorenson, 1974), house staff members denied this possibility by treating most patients as subjectless objects. I observed such techniques of "objectification" in both collegial conversations and interaction with patients.

These techniques are not only based on the conceptual orientation of medical science—i.e., the separation of the patient from the disease—but they are grounded in the structure and interactional processes of graduate medical training, such as doctors' practices on rounds (Mumford, 1970; Roberts, 1977).

During rounds a visit was often made to the bedside of new patients by house staff. While conducting a brief physical exam and interview, staff members talked about patients—often in their presence—in the third person. They used medical terminology which was incomprehensible to most patients and often looked past them, avoiding eye contact. Patients and, especially, family members were frequently treated as if they were invisible.

> There was much discussion on rounds about what kinds of procedures to do on a Black male middle-aged patient. Intern Old was in a quandary about how to treat his 'UTI' (Urinary Tract Infection). All this time the patient was trying to eat. Intern Cory said something about the patient's hand. The patient looked up and said, 'I sprained it.' Everyone looked surprised as the patient clearly understood what was being discussed although he had been ignored.

Even when patients or family members tried to interject themselves into a conversation for social or medical purposes, they rarely received a full response. Sometimes they were teased or occasionally given a curt or patronizing answer:

> The room of an 80 year old patient was entered. She immediately said she was feeling worse. Junior Resident Cape joked with her. She commented, 'I didn't sleep well last night because I've been worried about what's going to happen.' No one spoke directly to her. Instead Cape asked the medical student to present her case to the assembled physicians. Someone mentioned the patient's blood gases by the patient's bed. The patient asked what those were. The medical student responded they were to measure oxygen. The patient persisted: 'Is that good or bad?' The medical student smiled and said, 'Oh you're doing fine,' and continued talking to his senior colleagues.

By ignoring or dismissing patients as social participants, this strategy presumably focuses activity during rounds on the process of teaching and learning. However, it conveys the passivity of the patient role—both to novices on the staff and to patients. Some instances of objectification unintentionally frightened or even hurt patients, as in the following example:

Ms. Gim was visited by the team. While they talked to her she had to tell the house officers several times that her hand hurt terribly and asked them not to touch it. Both the Chief Resident and the Junior Resident touched it several times [without explaining to her or anyone why it may have been necessary to ignore her wishes]. They were preoccupied with the discussion of symptoms and the physical exam. This seemed to prevent them from actually hearing the patient who tried to talk.

Much of the doctor's time spent away from patients was occupied in discussions with peers and superiors (and occasionally with students) on a specific patient's medical status or on general aspects of the diagnosis or treatment of a patient's disease. During these informal conferences, the patient was often discussed as a thing. This type of objectification during collegial interaction was continually used and encouraged by faculty as well as by senior residents. Comments like the following are typical: "The stroke is over there."; "Look at the nice little fits."; "Look at those 'sicklers' [people with sickle cell anemia]."

In the novice internist's interactions with attending faculty and other house staff members, such uses of objectification impressed upon them that the all-important goal in internal medicine is to understand and detect disease—not to understand the patient as a person.[5] Everyday conversations I heard reflected this view of the patient as object:

The Junior Resident was observed commenting loudly, 'You can see some great 'Pathology' coming in the Emergency Room and then there are the patients!' which led to laughter and more joking among his peers.

THE EMOTIONAL ENVIRONMENT

The strategies of patient avoidance, focused interaction, and objectification allowed house staff members to manage their demanding case load by restricting the range and depth of their personal involvement with patients. However, I also observed numerous instances in which interns and residents reacted with exaggerated expressions of aggression and hostility toward patients and their families, and even toward coworkers. These negative reactions—like strategies for keeping patients at a distance—reflected subcultural solutions to the emotional strains and moral dilemmas imposed upon staff members by their work environment.

Much of the language used by the house staff to describe patients went well beyond the affectively bland process of objectification. The use of pejorative slang terms and sarcastic black humor is virtually universal in the U.S. house staff culture and was abundantly in evidence in the settings I observed.[6] Direct, verbal abuse of patients was infrequent; but when interns and residents were in the protected company of their peers, they spoke disparagingly of patients and deprecated their diseases. This was especially likely to occur on those services where there were fewer faculty or less administrative supervision—the emergency rooms, certain V.A. hospital rotations, and the outpatient clinics. Most of the patients in these services came in with common medical complaints, or else they had serious medical problems that were seen as self-inflicted (e.g., alcoholism). These patients were viewed as system abusers or as staff abusers, and staff members often referred to this in justifying their ridicule of them:

Everyone has jokes about the VA. The typical 'vet' is an alcoholic. One doctor once told me that God created veterans as the closest experimental model to man. That's not nice but at the same time, it relieves a lot of tension . . . You don't know why you're helping this person because they are making no contribution to society—and yet you're working your ass off to save

---

[5] Roberts (1977) presents a functional explanation for physician behavior which focuses on the case instead of the person. By describing the symptoms (e.g., "the 'burn' is doing fine"), she asserts that the doctors are probably transmitting a much more precisely coded message than by using names.

[6] Spontaneous references to the popular satirical novel on internship, *The House of God* (Shem, 1978), abounded in interviews and in my field observations. It portrays a bizarre, "Catch-22" world of medicine in which destructive behavior toward patients was endemic. Interns and residents occasionally cited examples from this novel while describing their own experiences or reactions toward patients.

that person. It leaves you with a dichotomy in your feelings toward that patient.

A number of researchers similarly interpret black humor among medical staff as a tension-relieving mechanism that prevents more serious expressions of hostility or mistreatment of patients (e.g., Coombs and Powers, 1978; Coser, 1959; Fox, 1959; Robinson, 1977). However, my interviews and observations revealed some less benign consequences of negativity toward patients.

Some of the house staff members acknowledged that demeaning remarks and slang were probably overheard by outsiders, including patients and their families:

> *It's the way the doctor keeps his sanity . . . calling people 'trolls,' 'gomers,' 'SHPOS' (Subhuman pieces of shit), etc. Guess it's sort of sick humor and I probably use it too much. We use it too much.* People say it in the elevators and use it in the streets and places where they shouldn't . . .

I observed some instances where patients were characterized in abusive terms in their presence during heated exchanges between staff members:

> *In the Emergency Room, Senior Resident Fable was still complaining to his peers that his interns were slow. He saw Intern Kots taking a history from a male patient and said in an annoyed tone, 'You don't need the whole medical history, just find out what's wrong now'. . . Later, Fable questioned Intern Kots, 'Why the work-up?' Fable said to him in a voice loud enough to be heard anywhere in the Emergency Room, 'Let's get the turkey out of here. Let's get those other winos out of here now.' He told both interns to their faces, 'You're all slow as shit! Let's get moving.'*

As suggested by this incident, many house staff members stated that they tended to give less thorough treatment to patients who were labeled derogatorily. Some informants admitted to making mistakes because of their attitudes toward these patients—e.g., by delaying tests or sending them out of the emergency room prematurely. Regardless of whether patients are physically harmed or neglected as a result of black humor or demeaning labels, these reactions make patients the object of derision and create a

dehumanizing climate similar to that observed among rehabilitation workers (Wiseman, 1970), police, and other "street-level bureaucrats" (Lipsky, 1969) who perceive themselves as working in a hostile environment.

House staff members' reactions to death provided some of the most striking illustrations of distortion of the doctor-patient relationship within this work environment. As shown by the following two examples, interns and residents frequently referred to death as a "relief"—as one less patient for whom they were responsible (cf. Coombs and Goldman, 1973; Glaser and Strauss, 1964):

> *At that point [when a patient dies], you're just interested in your own survival. Sometimes it's hard to relate to people who die, and it's a relief when they die, not only because they're so sick and what you put them through is often worse than death but the fact that you don't have to do that any more. It saves time and energy, so you think in terms of the overall benefit.*

> *[When my first patient died] it was terrible. Now if they die, it's usually, you know, it's almost a relief. Especially if the patient has 101 problems and, you know, should die. Best for him, best for the family, that he should die.*

Death became a subject of black humor when house staff members and, occasionally, their supervisors joked about ways to get rid of patients by acts of omission or commission:

> *Junior Resident Jover came by and talked to Cape about a patient who last night was in the DTs [delirium tremens]. Cape said, 'Apparently, the Haldol [a drug] didn't work.' Jover responded, 'I don't like Haldol. I prefer to give Valium until he's sedated and stops breathing, then he'll go into arrest and the ICU [Intensive Care Unit] will have to take him and I'll get rid of him.' Cape smiled. They looked at the observer as if to acknowledge their humorous intentions.*

The line between black humor and more serious discussions of responsibility for a patient's death was sometimes hazy. Deliberations took place daily about who was to live or die, and more specifically, about how "aggressive" house staff members should be in their efforts to sustain patients' lives. The moral dilemma that lay just beneath the surface of these discussions was conveyed in the comment of a family practice intern:

> It's my feeling that the decision about whether a patient should be a 'code' or a 'no-code' (resuscitation or not) should never be left in the hands of the intern because there's always a sub-conscious realization that if the patient is a 'code' you're going to have to be the one to code it.
> Also if the patient is a code, it means they'll be alive that much longer for you to take care of.
> In other words, the intern really has the motivation for letting someone die, and that can't help but influence you subconsciously in your decision.

House staff members constantly complained to each other about the amount of work they had to do with terminally ill patients, especially elderly individuals who lingered near death for days. Some characterized death as the ultimate process that lessened their patient load.

Nonetheless, house staff members often defined the death of a patient as a failure, even if it was viewed as inevitable. Most of them felt compelled to keep patients alive at all costs. The sense of failure that surrounded a patient death not only stemmed from the demands of medical ethics but also from a concern with professional and administrative repercussions. A patient death—even when all agreed that nothing could have been done to avoid it—potentially reflected upon the competency of staff members. Too many deaths, regardless of the reason, resulted in lengthy inquiries and explanations which they wished to avoid. As a consequence, the house staff frequently tried to transfer a patient to another service before death occurred. This often entailed dogged negotiation with other doctors or medical services. One typical attempt at negotiation (which failed) involved a patient who died in the Intensive Care Unit:

> Attending Physician Paul discussed with Senior Resident Leeds the problem of trying to get the patient upstairs [off their service] before 'disaster' came. Senior resident Mora reported, 'The patient was here to 'rule out' chest pain, and then

> the nurses tried to get him back to [the private hospital] but were hampered.

Thus, patient deaths confronted house staff members with a stressful mixture of moral and professional conflicts. Their efforts to cope collectively with these dilemmas through avoidance, rationalization, and expressions of apathy or antipathy toward dying patients seriously affect their views and performance of their professional role.

CONCLUSION

The current system of graduate medical education subjects interns and residents to long hours of extremely demanding work in poor facilities. This, combined with the increasing technical development of medicine, requires that interns and residents develop ways of lightening their major burden—their patient load. The avoidance of contact with patients seems on the surface to contradict the very reason for becoming a doctor. However, given the structure of this work setting, limitation of involvement with patients emerges as the most efficient and subculturally legitimate solution to the practical and emotional demands placed upon the house staff. While the strategies and rationalizations that interns and residents learn allow them to cope with the frustrations of work with unrewarding patients, these subcultural adjustments also gradually alter their view of their professional role. Techniques that doctors acquire as interns for managing their case load evolve into a detached and distant orientation to the doctor-patient relationship.

The subcultural strategies examined here are in some ways similar to defense mechanisms (Mechanic, 1974), in that they represent short run means of managing or avoiding immediate frustrations rather than more fundamental solutions to these problems. They do not appear to allow many novice internists to resolve the dissonance between their medical ideals and the harsh reality of their experiences as house staff members. Not all staff members were "successfully" desensitized to the emotional demands of their patients; some remained ambivalent about the doctor-patient relationship. Others became disillusioned with medicine, and a few terminated their residency with cynicism and apathy toward patients.

The question of whether these physicians-in-training regain their humanity if not their idealism in their permanent career settings is important. However, for thousands of patients across the U.S., the teaching hospital is their "here and now," and they are receiving care from novice internists undergoing a highly stressful experience. The treatment of future patients is not relevant to those currently under the collective care of the house staff who view this as the worst year of their lives. As I have shown, the subcultural strategies and negative reactions that develop as these doctors attempt to cope with their work adversely affect the quantity and quality of care that patients receive. Several of my informants told me that none of the patients in this system received optimal treatment. This is a troubling moral dilemma for many of these young doctors. From a broader perspective, it is a serious problem in the training of medical professionals and the delivery of health care in the U.S.

References

AMERICAN MEDICAL ASSOCIATION
1974 Helping the Impaired Physician. Chicago: American Medical Association.

BECKER, HOWARD S., BLANCHE GEER, EVERETT C. HUGHES and ANSELM L. STRAUSS
1957 Boys in White. Chicago: University of Chicago Press.

BUCHER, RUE, and JOAN STELLING
1977 Becoming Professional. Beverly Hills, CA: Sage.

COELHO, GEORGE V., DAVID A. HAMBURG and JOHN E. ADAMS (eds.)
1974 Coping and Adaptation. New York: Basic Books.

COHEN, ALBERT K.
1966 Deviance and Control. Englewood Cliffs, NJ: Prentice-Hall.

COOMBS, ROBERT H.
1978 Mastering Medicine. New York: Free Press.

COOMBS, ROBERT H., and LAWRENCE J. GOLDMAN
1973 "Maintenance and discontinuity of coping mechanisms in an intensive care unit." Social Problems 20 (April):342–355.

COOMBS, ROBERT H., and P. S. POWERS
1978 "Socialization for death: The physician's role." Urban Life 4(January):250–271.

COSER, ROSE LAUB
1959 "Some social functions of laughter." Human Relations 12(May):171–82.
1967 "Evasiveness as a response to structural ambivalence." Social Science and Medicine 1(June):203–218.

FOX, RENEE
1959 Experiment Perilous. Glencoe, IL: Free Press.

FREIDSON, ELIOT
1975 Doctoring Together. New York: Elsevier Books.

GERBER, LANE A.
1983 Married to Their Careers: Career and Family Dilemmas in Doctors' Lives. London: Tavistock.

GLASER, BARNEY G., and ANSELM L. STRAUSS
1964 "The social loss of dying patients." American Journal of Nursing 64(June):119–121.

GOFFMAN, ERVING
1959 The Presentation of Self in Everyday Life. New York: Doubleday.
1961 Asylums. New York: Doubleday.

HOWARD, JAN, and ANSELM L. STRAUSS
1975 Humanizing Health Care: The Implication of Technology, Centralization and Self Care. New York: John Wiley.

HULKA, BARBARA, LAWRENCE L. KUPPER, JOHN C. CASSEL and F. MAYO
1975 "Doctor-patient communication and outcomes among diabetic patients." Journal of Community Health 1(Fall):15–22.

HULKA, BARBARA, LAWRENCE L. KUPPER, JOHN C. CASSEL and ROBERT A. BABINEAU
1975 "Practice characteristics and quality primary medical care: The doctor-patient relationship." Medical Care 13(October):808–820.

KORSCH, BARBARA M., ETHEL K. GOZZI and VIDA F. NEGRETE
1968 "Gaps in doctor-patient communication, doctor-patient interaction and patient satisfaction." Pediatrics 42(November):855–871.

KORSCH, BARBARA M., and VIDA F. NEGRETE
1972 "Doctor-patient communication." Scientific American 227(August):66–75.

LIGHT, DONALD
1980 Becoming Psychiatrists: The Professional Transformation of Self. New York: W.W. Norton.

LIPP, MARTIN
1980 The Bitter Pill. New York: Harper and Row.

LIPSKY, MICHAEL
1969 Toward a Theory of Street Level Bureaucracy. Madison, WI: University of Wisconsin Press.

McCUE, JACK D.
1982 "The effects of stress on physicians and their medical practice." New England Journal of Medicine 306(February 25):458–463.

MARTIN, WILLIAM
1957 "Preference for types of patients." Pp. 189–206 in R. K. Merton, G. G. Reader and P. L. Kendall (eds.), The Student Physician. Cambridge, MA: Harvard University Press.

MAWARDI, BETTY HOSMER
1979 "Satisfactions, dissatisfactions, and causes of stress in medical practice." Journal of the American Medical Association 241(April):1483–1486.

MECHANIC, DAVID
1974 "Social structure and personal adaptation: Some neglected dimensions." Pp. 133–144 in C. V. Coelho, D. A. Hamburg and J. E. Adams (eds.), Coping and Adaptation. New York: Basic Books.

MERTON, ROBERT K., GEORGE G. READER, and PATRICIA L. KENDALL (eds.)
1957 The Student Physician. Cambridge, MA: Harvard University Press.

MIZRAHI, TERRY
Forthcoming Getting Rid of Patients: Contradictions In the Training of Internists. (working title) New Brunswick, NJ: Rutgers University Press.

MUMFORD, EMILY
1970 Interns: From Students to Physicians. Cambridge, MA: Harvard University Press.

NADELSON, CAROL C., and MALKAH T. NOTMAN
1979 "Adaptation to stress in physicians." Pp. 201–215 in E. C. Shapiro and L. M. Lowenstein (eds.), Becoming a Physician: Development of Values in Medicine. Cambridge, MA: Ballinger.

PFIFFERLING, JOHN HENRY
1983 "The impaired physician: An overview." Durham, NC: Center for Professional Well-Being.

PRESTON, THOMAS
1981 The Clay Pedestal. Seattle: Madrone Press.

ROBERTS, CECILA M.
1977 Doctor-Patient in the Teaching Hospital: A Tale of Two Life Worlds. Lexington, MA: D.C. Heath.

ROBINSON, VERA M.
1977 Humor and the Health Professions. Thorofare, NJ: Charles B. Slack.

ROSENBERG, PEARL
1980 "Catch-22: The medical model." Pp. 81–92 in E. C. Shapiro and L. M. Lowenstein (eds.), Becoming a Physician: The Development of Values in Medicine. Cambridge, MA: Ballinger.

SHAPIRO, EILEEN C., and SHIRLEY G. DRISCOLL
1979 "Training for commitment." Pp. 187–198 in E. C. Shapiro and L. M. Lowenstein (eds.), Becoming a Physician: Development of Values in Medicine. Cambridge, MA: Ballinger.

SHEM, SAM
1978 The House of God. New York: Richard Marek Press.

SORENSON, JAMES R.
1974 "Bio-medical innovation, uncertainty and doctor-patient interaction." Journal of Health and Social Behavior 15(December):366–380.

SPITZ, LOUIS, and ELLEN BLOCK
1981 "Denial and minimization in telephone contacts with patients." Journal of Family Practice 12(January):93–98.

SYKES, GRESHAM, and DAVID MATZA
1957 "Techniques of neutralization: A theory of delinquency." American Sociological Review 22(October):664–670.

TORKARZ, J. PAT, WILLIAM BREMER and KEN PETERS
1979 Beyond Survival. Chicago: American Medical Association.

WARTMAN, STEVEN A., LAURA L. MORLOCK, FAYE E. MALITZ and ELAINE PALM
1981 "Do prescriptions adversely affect doctor-patient interactions?" American Journal of Public Health 71(December):1358–1361.

WERNER, EDWENNA R., and BARBARA M. KORSCH
1979 "Professionalization during pediatric internship: Attitudes, adaptations and interpersonal skills." Pp. 113–138 in E. C. Shapiro and L. M. Lowenstein (eds.), Becoming a Physician: The Development of Values in Medicine. Cambridge, MA: Ballinger.

WISEMAN, JACQUELINE
1970 Stations of the Lost. Englewood Cliffs, NJ: Prentice-Hall.

Negotiating to Do Surgery

Diana Scully

I have argued that residents emerged from training with different amounts of practice in surgical skills. The amount of experience or practice a resident had in what he defined as important skills was significant in determining not only his actual level of ability, but also his confidence as a surgeon. Simply stated, residents sought the opportunity to gain experience. This chapter will illustrate how this was accomplished within the social context of training and the effect these efforts had on patient care.

Formal policies of hospitals and the medical profession set limits on the kinds of acts in which physicians can engage. In spite of formal rules, most forms of organization tolerate variation within a range of quasi-legitimate behaviors. This is true also of medical training. Residents developed a group perspective in which questionable acts were justified because they were interpreted in terms of their usefulness as learning experiences. To some extent, residents had to negotiate for the opportunity to carry out these acts.

Residents believed that those among them who went through training complying with formal rules gained less experience than residents who intervened on their own behalf and who could negotiate and bargain for access to certain types of work and patients. At Elite and Mass, residents used the term "aggressive" to mean "the ability to intervene successfully on one's own behalf." Aggressive residents, it was believed, were more successful in gaining experience.

> An aggressive resident is one who places himself in a position so that he is able to accomplish and observe and do those things he wants to do, as opposed to a more quiet guy who doesn't make his presence known and who sort of gets lost in the shuffle . . . I think that perhaps I'm more aggressive than some. I know how to get more out of relationships than some do. I'm a finagler; I mean I can always make it a point to come out smelling good . . . I think I can control my environment a little more than some can. (Interview, Elite.)

The object was to control others' actions so that personal goals could be accomplished. To some degree, a resident's ability to control was related to his year of training; senior residents had important advantages that junior residents lacked. However, at every level of training, residents were engaged in a process of negotiation and bargaining that involved attendings, colleagues, and patients. At Elite and Mass, though residents' acts and behavior differed because of differences in the training institutions and programs, the twofold objective was the same. Residents negotiated for a position in which they could optimize the opportunity to do work that was defined by them, at any point, as contributing to their professional development. At the same time, they attempted to decrease or avoid work that they did not perceive as making a similar contribution. It will become apparent that the needs of patients were often secondary to the residents' own needs and that cooperation on the part of the attending staff was often necessary in order for residents to accomplish their goals. . . .

FINDING "MATERIAL"

The single most important resource in training, from the resident's view, is the patient who presents a medical problem that corresponds to the resident's need for experience in a particular skill and who agrees to undergo surgery. The residents at Elite and Mass believed that a prerequisite of successful training was the ability to locate patients and to convince them that surgery was in their best interest.

Reprinted from Men Who Control Women's Health by Diana Scully, pp. 198–199, 219–232 with permission of the Houghton Mifflin Company. Copyright © 1980 by Diana Scully.

At Elite, residents looked for patients primarily in the various clinics administered and staffed by the department. The chief of ward gynecology was expected to spend two afternoons a week in the clinic "looking for material." Some residents went to the extent of arranging their third-year schedules so that their clinic rotation preceded their labor room rotation. This was done so that they could look for potential cases from among the women who would deliver while they were in obstetrics. They were hoping most of all to find candidates for cesarean hysterectomies. One resident explained:

> You have to look for the kind of person in the clinic and if you don't have that rotation beforehand, you have to hope that the person in the clinic is looking for you, because once she gets into the hospital—once she is in labor—it's difficult to talk someone into a hysterectomy. (Interview, Elite.)

Another source of surgical material was the evening family planning clinic. Aggressive residents tried to work as many evenings as possible to enlarge their range of patients seen and increase their probability of locating pathology.

At Mass, the clinic was one of two major sources of cases. Because all three services occupied the same clinic space and all of the residents on each service were looking for their own cases, competition often reached an extreme. For example, if the clinic coordinator happened to assign one service more than its share of postoperative cases, residents complained: someone who just had surgery wasn't a potential surgical case. There was so much competition that some residents felt the clinic was worthless as a source of cases. By the time a patient reached the clinic, she either had a clearly nonsurgical problem or she was postoperative.

> You go to the clinics and everybody tries to get the operating cases, so by the time they reach the gyn clinic, they are usually postoperative. Sometimes they are first visit. They have a reference from another doctor and they come to the clinic. You examine the patient, they need surgery, OK. But most of the time you don't get much from the gyn clinic, so you have to go to other clinics like family planning, like the emergency room. In the family planning clinic, they come for birth control and they have five or six babies and maybe a prolapsed uterus or incontinence, so you take the case. (Interview, Mass.)

Many residents believed that the emergency room was the most fruitful source of cases. At Mass, the emergency room functioned as the main examining and intake area of the hospital, and patients were seen there before referral to a clinic. As a result, a resident who worked in the emergency room had first choice over all the patients who used the hospital. Residents could increase their case load by working in the emergency room during the night shift and on weekends when the regularly scheduled resident was off.

Every resident had to spend three months in the emergency room as part of his second-year rotation. Following this rotation, residents usually returned to one of the gynecology services. The resident faced the dilemma of knowing that when, in two or three months, he would be on the gynecology service, he would be very much in need of cases, but here were the cases passing through his hands while he was in the emergency room. The solution was what the residents called "saving cases," instead of referring them to the resident on call or to the clinics, as the rules stipulated.

> I worked in the emergency room a month ago. I was assigned there but I wasn't in the hospital at the time, so if I sent the patients to the clinic, I would miss them. So you keep the names and telephone numbers and say I will call you. Of course, if it is an emergency, you have to admit the patient. If it is a fibroid uterus, it can wait for a couple of weeks. (Interview, Mass.)

Some residents were unaware of this practice and naïvely sought the most expedient solution for the patient. One second-year resident explained:

> If you have a rotation in gyn before you go to the emergency room, you learn the tricks. If you just go to the emergency room, you just want the patients to be taken care of, and you think when your time comes, you will get your cases and you just look for the betterment of the patient because you don't know that the patient can wait for a week or two without any problem . . . You can just as easily save the patient for yourself.

Say a patient comes in with a fibroid uterus; the patient doesn't need surgery right away, the patient can wait. Most people keep their names and give them a call and tell them to come to the clinic when they know they will be there. But these things you only know after you have had a rotation in gyn. (Interview, Mass.)

Often, because gynecological surgery is elective, and waiting would not imperil the woman's health, residents told patients that the hospital was full and they would be called as soon as there was space. In this way, residents could accumulate a large number of cases. One resident proudly showed me twelve pages of names he had collected in six weeks in the emergency room.

SELLING THE HYSTERECTOMY

After a potential patient was located, she had to be persuaded to have surgery. As one resident put it:

You have to look for your surgical procedures; you have to go after patients. Because no one is crazy enough to come and say, hey, here I am, I want you to operate on me. You have to sometimes convince the patient that she is really sick, if she is, of course, [laugh] and that she is better off with a surgical procedure. (Interview, Elite.)

One important skill residents acquired during their four years' training was that of talking women into agreeing to surgery. Since surgical indications were sometimes questionable, persuasion became an important skill for a resident to have. When there was no indications at all, surgery was not approved. However, when minor pathology was present, indications were sometimes stretched and surgery approved. An attending at Mass announced at a residents' meeting, "Doing cases in residency that aren't indicated because you want to do a few cases while you are still in training is not OK when the indications are way off." (Field Notes, Mass.) In other words, surgery was permissible as long as the indications weren't "way off."

Besides the practice of performing hysterectomy for sterilization, another abused form of gynecological surgery was hysterectomy for small, benign, asymptomatic fibroids, which can disappear without surgical intervention or remain intact without symptom. I asked residents what they would do with nine-to-ten-week-size asymptomatic fibroids and received the following answer from a fourth-year resident:

Uh, most likely I would do the surgery. I will offer the woman, you would probably offer the woman, you would explain the situation. I don't think it would be right to say you have a horrible disease or you have cancer or anything like that, I have to do this surgery.

I would explain to her that she has fibroids that are nine-to-ten-week size, that she isn't going to have a family anymore, she doesn't want a family anymore, that these fibroids may some time in the future grow bigger, may get symptoms, may cause her trouble, she may need surgery at some point in time, and if she would like to have surgery done now, it can be easy surgery, vaginally. As a consequence she won't have any more children, but she won't have any fibroids and she won't have any potential for disease.

[Q. Put like that many people would say yes.]

Right, but is that being dishonest?

[Q. Those fibroids may also disappear by themselves.]

Right, but you are only saying they may do this or they may do that and essentially you let the patient make up her mind. Usually when patients hear they have fibroids and there is some bleeding, there is a sufficient symptomatology. (Interview, Elite.)

A resident at Mass explained it this way: "Well, you stretch a little bit a minor indication but no major indication. For example, a sterilization in those patients over thirty-five with mild pelvic relaxation, you could stretch the indications for a vaginal hysterectomy." (Interview, Mass.)

After spending months in the clinics and emergency room listening to residents talk to women about surgery, I saw a pattern emerge. The residents' tactics, based on high volume, were similar to that of any effective salesperson, regardless of the product; that is, the greater the number of contacts, the greater the probability of making a sale. This type of high-turnover sale was especially suited to the high-volume, quick-turnover conditions in the clinics and emergency room. Like any sophisticated salesperson, a resident could judge within minutes whether a woman was going to buy a hysterectomy. When it appeared that she wasn't, he used another tactic. Many women came to the clinic simply to obtain birth control and were completely unaware that anything was going to be found amiss. Residents believed that women would eventually accept surgery if they were given some time to think it over. Thus, after a resident had completed his pitch and the woman was still reluctant, he would tell her that he would call her in a week and discuss the surgery further. The woman was dismissed and the next prospective case was brought into the examining room. The entire interaction, including physical examination, usually took three to four minutes.

The sales pitch used by residents at both hospitals was remarkably similar; in some cases the very same words were used. The resident opened by moving from a general problem for which a number of solutions, including doing nothing, were possible, to the solution he was going to try to sell, usually a hysterectomy. The more supporting evidence that could be brought to bear on the problem, the more secure the resident was in his pitch. The pitch frequently began when a woman over the age of thirty-five requested birth control or permanent sterilization in the form of a tubal ligation. If, in addition, the resident could locate evidence of some pathology, he would attempt to sell a hysterectomy. Essentially, the resident was substituting a hysterectomy (surgery he wanted to do) for a tubal ligation (surgical scut work). The tactic was similar to the "bait and switch" technique used in sales in which the advertised item is discredited and another, more expensive, product is substituted in its place. For example:

Dr. W. saw a woman with a class III Pap smear. He explained to her that it could be a precancerous condition, in which case surgery was indicated, or an infection, in which case medical treatment was indicated. Then she told him she had eleven children and wanted a tubal ligation but had fibroids so that it couldn't be done. In that case Dr. W. told her it was even more likely that she should have a hysterectomy. (Field Notes, Mass.)

Dr. S. examined the woman and then told her that her uterus had slipped a little and it would be best to take it out. He told her that eventually she would have problems with it. It would press on her bowels and she would be constipated. She was told that it should come out through her vagina and they wouldn't have to cut her stomach. (Field Notes, Mass.)

Dr. Z. told her she had moderate dysplasia and if she thought about having her tubes tied, then she should think about a hysterectomy because that was the only thing that would really cure her. (Field Notes, Mass.)

My observations indicated that clinic women were never advised of the relative dangers or rates of complication of the vaginal hysterectomy versus the tubal ligation. Instead, residents stressed that the vaginal hysterectomy was easier than the abdominal hysterectomy because "you don't have to be cut." Even if this statement were true, the reasoning is dishonest, because the real comparison is between the vaginal hysterectomy and the tubal ligation.

When the pathology involved a fibroid, "the tumor" was presented in such a way that the woman would initially become alarmed. Later, when the resident assured her that fibroids weren't cancerous, the psychological impact had already been made. Many women were frightened into surgery by the word "tumor," which is closely associated with cancer and death in our health-conscious society.

Dr. Z. told her she had a tumor in her stomach and that while it wasn't an emergency, she should have it out as soon as possible. He said, "It is not cancer but there is a possibility of small cancer tumors within it." (Field Notes, Mass.)

After fear and doubt had been planted in a woman's mind, the next step was to discuss the purpose and utility of a uterus. These discussions illustrated the residents' basic disregard for the female reproductive tract, which they saw as functional only for childbearing.

He told the woman that the only function of a womb was to carry a baby, and with a tumor [fibroid] she couldn't get pregnant so she might as well have it out. (Field Notes, Mass.)

He told the woman that a uterus was only needed for babies and that her problem could turn into cancer in five or ten years, and to guard against it, she should have it out now. (Field Notes, Mass.)

Dr. P. told the woman she didn't need her womb, that it was only a cradle for the baby, and if she wasn't going to have children, she didn't need the cradle. (Field Notes, Mass.)

The next step in the pitch was to assure the woman that a hysterectomy would not reduce her femininity, attractiveness, or sex drive.

Dr. S. told the woman that ovaries make you feminine, the vagina would stay, and sex drive would be the same. She just wouldn't have a uterus. (Field Notes, Mass.)

Dr. W. told her that a hysterectomy wouldn't make her any less a woman, that she would still have a sex drive, but she wouldn't have to worry about things anymore. (Field Notes, Mass.)

Finally, the pitch was concluded with a summary of the "advantages" of a hysterectomy and the promise of a simple, quick operation.

Dr. S. explained to her the advantages of a vaginal hysterectomy: no more periods, no fear of cancer, no loss of sex drive, the operation would only take twenty-five minutes, and she would probably have to have it out sooner or later because of the fibroids. (Field Notes, Mass.)

Once the woman agreed to surgery, she lost whatever power she previously had had—the power of refusal. The situation changed from one of negotiation to complete control by the resident. The patient was expected to trust the knowledge and wisdom of her doctor. She was not consulted on the form her surgery would take nor was it expected that she was capable of understanding medical-surgical mysteries. The resident, influenced by his own need for practice, decided what operation he would do. Women were not aware that there was a choice.

You might have a borderline, say ten-to-twelve-week-size uterus, and rather than doing it from above [abdominally] you can do it from below [vaginally] and do a little bit more difficult vagi-

nal hysterectomy but hopefully not increase the morbidity for the patient. You have an older woman who has a pessary in with a fourth-degree prolapse, you may want to do a LeFort [sewing the vagina closed] on her. Namely, because it will be good for her condition and otherwise because you have never done a LeFort before. You know, you have that option. [Laugh.] You disagree with me? (Interview, Elite.)

Likewise, women were not consulted on the type of childbirth experience they would have. Residents exercised the option to use forceps until they felt confident of their technique with them.

Once the woman was in the operating room and her abdomen was open, residents tended to want to remove more than just the organ originally bargained for. A healthy appendix or ovaries were sometimes removed.

Occasionally we do an appendectomy, but occasionally you could be in trouble doing an appendectomy at the same time you are doing other surgery. To do an appendectomy when the appendix is well, usually, most of the time it doesn't increase morbidity. It's a preventive measure. (Interview, Elite.)

"Prophylactic" appendectomies became so frequent at Mass that the department ruled they could not be performed without the approval of the head of the gynecology division. Appendectomies performed while tubal ligations were being done were especially censured.

Not all residents used all of these techniques to the same extent. The extent to which they were used, however, was, as we have seen, closely related to the amount of surgery the resident wanted to do and only marginally related to ethical issues. Most of the residents condoned these practices if the surgery was done for training purposes, and, for the most part, many attendings complied. . . . once a resident became satisfied with the amount of surgery he had performed, the patient's interest received more consideration. However, until the resident developed a sense of confidence in his ability to perform a particular surgical technique, his need for practice was a salient influence on patient care.

AVOIDING WORK

In order for the residents to achieve what they regarded as a successful training experience, it was necessary for them not only to secure desirable work but to avoid scut work, work involving skills already mastered. Attending physicians who by reputation did not usually turn cases and patients who possessed characteristics or pathology that residents found not to their liking were also to be avoided.

At Elite and Mass, the most common avoidance technique was dumping. When a resident had a relatively higher status than others, he would dump undesirable work or uncooperative attendings on a more junior resident. Senior residents, because they more often held positions of high status, were better able to dispose of work and attendings than were junior residents.

Another method of avoiding unwanted work was to discourage women from undergoing certain procedures—or at least to refrain from encouraging them. These procedures always involved routine skills the resident believed he had mastered.

> Dr. X. mentioned to me that there was a gravida 14, para 13 in the labor room and she didn't want a tubal ligation. He said many of the women are afraid tubal ligations will affect their sexual functioning and it needs to be explained to them. However, he said, from a resident's point of view, a tubal ligation is a nuisance because there is nothing new to learn from them after you have done a few. So if the woman says no, they don't push it because they don't want to do them anyway. (Field Notes, Elite.)

At Elite, some work was avoided to such an extent that an important medical service was not available to patients. This was the case with abortions. Although numerous first- and second-trimester abortions were performed by attendings on private clients, they were not available to the residents' institutional patients. When questioned about the lack of an abortion service for institutional patients, the hospital staff reported that, for religious and moral reasons, residents could not be required to perform them. On questioning residents, though, I found that with few exceptions all of them planned to offer abortion as a service to their patients in private practice. Either residents didn't have convictions preventing them from performing abortions, or the desire for financial reward was greater than their convictions. It should be noted that first-trimester abortion involves dilation and curettage, which is one of the skills acquired very early because it is used to treat a number of uterine conditions, abortion being one. When I probed further, residents finally told me, "We don't learn anything from abortions. All you do is insert a drug and wait. Residents want to do things they learn from." (Interview, Elite.) Another resident said, "Well you see, this is the whole point. We are residents; we don't get anything out of abortions; we don't learn anything from it. It's a pain in the neck." (Interview, Elite.)

It was also to the resident's advantage to avoid some individual patients. At Elite, "undesirable" patients could be transferred elsewhere, usually Mass, where residents did not have a similar option because the institution was legally bound to treat all who came to its door. Thus, Mass was known at Elite—and elsewhere in the area, I'm sure—as a dumping ground for unwanted patients.

At Elite, residents frequently referred to some women as "Mass patients." The term was used to denote women who presented a trait or a combination of traits residents disliked, including certain pathology, physical features such as obesity, attitudes, and kinds of behavior.

At Elite, patients in the terminal stages of cancer were frequently transferred to another hospital, usually Mass, where, they were told, there were experts to handle their problems. This was accurate, but it was also usually true that part of the motivation was to dispose of dying patients who were going to require a great deal of care. One night, for example, an elderly woman with terminal cancer was brought to the emergency room by her family. The resident on call asked the family to return the next day, when the chief of ward gynecology could examine the patient. The resident on call explained that if he admitted a patient like that to the ward gynecology service without the chief's approval, the chief would hate him every day until the woman died. The next day the woman was transferred to Mass. (Field Notes, Elite.)

Patients who came to the emergency room requiring what was viewed as scut work were also transferred to Mass if possible. One resident explained:

> A considerable number of ladies come in with incomplete abortion or vaginal bleeding. Now if we accepted all those cases, we would do nothing but D & Cs all day and night. A certain percentage of those patients need to be transferred. (Interview, Elite.)

At Elite, where residents had to do most of their own scut work, avoiding patients who required such work was attempted whenever possible. To the residents, a labor room filled with women who were not in active labor but nonetheless required care was such a situation. A woman who came to Elite in the early stage of labor but had not received prenatal care there was told to go to Mass for her delivery. The Elite resident would then contact a Mass resident and explain that their obstetric beds were full, which, of course, Mass residents were unable to check. When the woman was one of Elite's own, she was made an offer she couldn't refuse: she would be told that she could remain in the hospital, in bed with a needle in her arm, prevented from eating, drinking, or smoking, or she could go home and return when her labor was active. Women usually went home.

> Mass residents didn't have the option of transferring patients. Patients, however, could frequently be avoided through stalling. Often this was done when the resident was unsure about treatment and couldn't arrange for a consultation with someone more experienced. Residents on the labor row told me they could evaluate the ability of the resident on the shift before their own by the work that was left undone or decisions unmade when they arrived.

Another method of stalling involved postponing treatment until the resident knew he would be off the particular service. A patient could be given a Band-Aid-type of remedy and asked to return to the clinic at some later date. This method was used in the infertility clinic at Mass.

> Infertility clinic, there aren't any attendings. There is supposed to be but he doesn't come very often. Most of the residents don't like endocrinology because you have to read—they like surgery. So the residents have a two-month rotation in the endocrinology clinic and the patients have been coming for five or six years. They keep coming and the resident knows that in two months he is going to be off the rotation. So the resident tells them to take their temperature and wait for lab results and he gives them an appointment to come back in two months when he is out of the clinic. (Interview, Mass.)

Referral to other clinics within the hospital was another stall tactic. At Elite patients on whom nobody wanted to operate might go through several stalls before finding a chief who would handle their case.

All of these tactics facilitated the residents' personal objective: performing the type of medical task, usually surgical, that would contribute to their skill as surgeons. In a very real sense, residents' training was incomplete until these tactics had been mastered. It is reasonable to suggest, as I did earlier, that the attitudes learned while in training continue to influence the behavior of surgeons in private practice. It is not surprising that surgeons perform unnecessary operations. After all, they are trained to do it.

Equally serious is the lack of concern and the disrespect residents learned to display in dealing with patients. Human beings are entitled to considerate treatment and good health care, but "material" is a commodity that can be manipulated and exploited for personal gain. Even if residents did change when they reached private practice, the women I observed and the poor who must receive health care in institutions like Elite and Mass would continue to be victims.

The Undesirable Patient

Solomon Papper

While the position of being undesirable is an unwelcome eventuality in any interpersonal relationship, for a patient to be regarded by his physician as "undesirable" can be catastrophic. Not only may such a patient sense his situation with uneasiness, but in general he is likely to receive less than the best total care, including emotional, physical, and social aspects. Despite the Oath of Hippocrates and the high aspirations of the profession, biases, attitudes, and circumstances may result unconsciously in certain patients being regarded by the physician as "undesirable." We wish to explore briefly only some examples of undesirability beginning with those founded in the personal individual biases of physicians: especially, but perhaps not exclusively, in the teaching setting.

(i) Some patients may be classified as *Socially Undesirable*. In general, this category is based on apparently irreconcilable differences between the patient and the physician. There is much in the background of many medical students and physicians that makes the *alcoholic* broadly unacceptable. To be aged and sick in a teaching hospital, surrounded by the young staff, may be less than a strong vantage point for excellent care. While not all cultures accept the notion that cleanliness is next to godliness, the physically *dirty* patient is undesirable: and any other lofty qualities he may have will have little opportu-

nity to penetrate the barrier established by the physician. The *uneducated* (often confused with unintelligent) may be patronized and denigrated by the physician who is not necessarily blessed with as much perceptiveness as his patient. The *very poor* may be viewed as undesirable unrelated to their inability to pay. Even when the physician has genuine concern for the economically disadvantaged he may, because of his own background, unwittingly regard the extremely poor as "different," with a flavor of "inferiority" included in the difference. We shall not mention further the generally recognized biases that can lead to a patient's undesirability—race, religion, region or country of origin.

(ii) *Attitudinal Undesirability* results from other types of personal bias. One of the most common examples is the *ungrateful* patient, and sometimes a physician thinks that a patient should be very grateful indeed. The failure to deify, or at least pedestalize, the physician can provoke remarkably strong negative responses. Then there is the patient who *"wants to know too much"* or who *"thinks he knows so much,"* implying something less than total and absolute faith in the physician. Another example is the patient *"who does know"* a good deal; it is in this framework, at least in part, that the physician as a patient is undesirable and suffers accordingly. Of course, in the teaching setting, it can be a tactical error for the patient, during rounds, *to correct* the student or house officer presentation or to provide the attending physician with historical facts previously unrevealed. There are other examples, but basically

Reprinted from the *Journal of Chronic Diseases*, vol. 22 (1970), pp. 777–779.

the problem here is the patient's lack of knowledge of, or failure to meet, the physician's expectations and needs.

(iii) A patient may be *Undesirable* on *physical* grounds. To some physicians the *absence of physical illness* is sometimes cause for negativism rather than an opportunity to share the patient's sense of relief with his good fortune; he may even be labelled a "crock." In other instances the *presence of physical illness* may be grounds for rejection, especially if the data prove the physician's initial assessment to be in error. Patients may be undesirable because of their *lack of response to good treatment;* it is as if the patient is to blame. The patient with *chronic illness,* and especially with *malignant disease,* not uncommonly becomes undesirable, particularly when he does not respond to treatment and recognizes his deterioration. This occurs more readily where the physician has implied promises he ultimately cannot fulfill. The physician may become anxious, angry with himself, and unwittingly separate himself from the patient, even at a time when the patient has his greatest need. And who in the teaching setting has not observed the undesirable nature of the patient with *an ordinary illness;* "just another stroke," for example.

(iv) *Circumstantial Undesirability* derives from conditions totally apart from the patient and beyond his control. For example, if the patient arrives on the ward "late" (at the end of a long, exhausting day for the physician) and is not desperately ill, he may be resented. This is especially true if, through no fault of his own, the patient has been sitting in the Admitting Room for hours and has no knowledge of a feud between Ward Staff and Admitting Room. We can also all recall the depressing *outpatient clinic* setting that is poorly furnished, overcrowded, inadequately equipped, and staffed with vastly overprogrammed and harassed house officers. In this setting it takes a highly mature, disciplined house officer and a patient skillful in the art of being loved to avoid undesirable status.

(v) Finally, we wish to consider a more recent mechanism for the genesis of undesirability: this might be called *Distraction Undesirability* or *Incidental Undesirability.* In fact, it is simply that the patient does not fit with the interests and orientation of the times. In current jargon, his status as a patient places him outside the mainstream. An example was

provided during the great *research* development beginning with the termination of the second World War. People primarily or exclusively interested in research sometimes found patient care responsibilities sufficiently distracting to make the entire clinical setting undesirable—inevitably including individual patients.

Another form of *Distraction Undesirability* is now coming to the fore. Here we refer to the major and even global *"preventive medicine"* programs. In this context any patient can become undesirable simply because to some people deep concern with the health problems of any given individual is perhaps unconsciously regarded as a digression from the "greater" problem and "higher" calling of the care of millions of people. We have gained the impression that, in some instances, it is almost as if one can love humanity with minimal direct concern for individuals.

In both examples of Distractive Undesirability, the academic community has been in the position of pursuing economic practicality rather than, or in addition to, nobility; at first in the research area and more recently by large-scale preventive medicine programs. While some of our remarks may be misinterpreted, we do regard research and programs in preventive medicine as good and essential ingredients of the teaching setting, even if, in some instances at least, they are examples of good things being done for less than the best reasons.

SUMMATION

Patients can achieve "undesirability" in many ways, including: biases on the part of physicians, being victims of circumstance in a hospital, and being apart from another major and worthy interest.

We recognize that one cannot eliminate bias or background as one excises tumors. On the other hand perhaps it is helpful to acknowledge to ourselves that there are times when we, as individual physicians, participate in patient care in a manner that we really think and feel is not optimal. Honest recognition should stimulate and enhance a sense of self-discipline that minimizes the numbers of patients who become Undesirable.

For the Distractive varieties of Undesirability, we again need acknowledgment as well as perspective. We also need to recognize that, while research and preventive medicine programs are essential even beyond the dollar value to the institution, for that

"moment" in which we assume responsibility for *any individual* patient, surely this must have higher priority than any other consideration.

Addendum: The Patient as the Enemy

Michael Medved

DR. HARRISON O'NEILL, GASTROENTEROLOGIST

I get rid of patients I don't like. It's better for me and it's better for them. I usually react badly to people who have destructive characteristics that are part of my own personality. The ones I dislike the most are the alcoholic people who could get well, but choose not to. Who choose to hang on to their disease, who choose to suffer. And I, in turn, choose not to suffer with them. . . .

DR. MILTON TESSLER, CARDIOLOGIST

One afternoon I was putting a temporary pacemaker in a lady who was about seventy. I had given her a local anesthetic, but of course she was uncomfortable and she kept nagging me to hurry up and finish the procedure. I said, "Look, it's only going to take a couple of minutes," but she kept on complaining. Finally she shouted at me, "Stop this minute! If you don't stop I'm going to sue you for malpractice."

So I looked up at her and said, "Lady, you just

Reprinted from *Hospital* by Michael Medved, pp. 237–241 by permission of Simon & Schuster, Inc. Copyright © 1983 by Michael Medved.

said the magic word!" I called the nurse and I said, "Let's go. Let's take her back." And I started walking away with this procedure half completed. The lady really panicked. She said, "No, wait! I was just kidding! Come on back."

For the rest of the procedure she didn't say a word. But it still bothered me, and it's typical of a common problem. Part of the ego gratification of being a physician is the feeling that you're appreciated by patients. I like being thought of as a good guy, and I get miffed when I'm doing something that's good for the patient and they keep bitching and moaning and telling me it's terrible.

DR. ARNOLD BRODY, DIRECTOR OF MEDICAL ONCOLOGY

I'm a controller. And when a patient bucks my control it pisses me off, because I know better than they do. I listen to what they have to say, but when someone starts giving me a bunch of crap, questioning me every step of the way, I get pissed.

I'll give you an example. There was a gal I'd been taking care of for a year and a half who would come in wide-eyed, dry-mouthed, saying, "What's this? I think I've got something." And I would feel and feel and feel. "Jeez, I can't feel anything." Then she says, "Here it is." And you finally feel some little pinpoint of nothing. Now I could go to another part of her body and feel around long enough and come up with the same thing. Admittedly this gal is terrified. She had breast cancer. She's lost her breast, she's lost her husband. She wasn't good-looking before the mastectomy. Her breasts were the best-looking part of her. And she lost half of that. I mean, there's a whole laundry list of things that explain this woman's behavior. But that behavior is still neurotic and she's still a pain in the ass. Now she's gone to another doctor. She was just somebody that wanted too much from me.

There's a worse kind of patient, even though they don't want anything at all. That's the GOMER, an old decrepit bastard who's just a shell of his former self. Not a person. These poor hulks should be laid to rest somehow and not messed with. Some of the crap that goes on with the young docs and their GOMERs is just sickening. They get these poor people out of the nursing homes and they use 'em as pathology museums. Four or five or six doctors working on these derelicts, sending the fees to Medicare. For the docs it's sort of enjoyable. You don't even have to spend a lot of time talking to them, because there's nothing to talk to.

DR. DAVID ANZAK, OBSTETRICIAN-GYNECOLOGIST

I like patients who are intelligent, responsible people and I hate patients who are irresponsible slobs. The Medi-Cal patients—the people on welfare—are the worst of the bunch. Since the government is paying for it, they just don't care about what's going on. They don't show up for appointments, and they never call to tell you. They don't take their medicine. They call you Saturday night, three in the morning, with a problem that could have been taken care of on Wednesday afternoon.

On top of that they have very unrealistic expectations. People who are well educated are a little more realistic about what a doctor can do. But often the uneducated, welfare-type patients have wild ideas about what medicine can accomplish. They come in thinking that the doctor waves his magic wand and you get cured. They don't understand our limitations and they don't take responsibility for their own health. Half of the problems these people

have could have been avoided by just minimal precautions. Abortions, infections, venereal diseases and all their complications. It's irritating to have to take care of people when they don't make the slightest effort to take care of themselves. . . .

DR. EDWARD FERRARO, MEDICAL ONCOLOGIST

The alcoholic patients are the worst. I used to see quite a few of them when I was just starting out and I worked for this internist in town. I used to go on housecalls. There was this one couple I remember very well. He was a famous jazz musician and he and his wife used to have terrible quarrels at night. He was a drunk and she was a drunk and they used to call in the middle of the night. What they wanted was a referee. They used me, and I felt lousy. I felt obligated to go and I hated it. The whole experience was degrading. That's the trouble with patients who are alcoholics—they tend to drag you down into their world.

JOE RIVERA, EMERGENCY CARE TECHNICIAN

The patients I really hate are the gypsies. There are a whole lot of them in this area, so they come in maybe once a week. And they are just the worst, the absolute worst. Their whole culture is based on lying, stealing, cheating. Anything to survive. In the ER you don't have time to deal with all their problems. I mean, you're talking about people who still believe in obesity, who think it's beautiful. I don't know how often they take baths but they all come in with terrible body odor. And you have to deal with the ignorance of the whole family. If one of 'em comes in you'll have twenty-five in the waiting room, and each one of those twenty-five will get up and ask you what's going on. It drives you nuts.

DR. JACK BUCKMAN, DIRECTOR OF EMERGENCY MEDICINE

All patients are pretty much the same to me, but I don't like the cry-babies and complainers. You have to deal with them like you'd handle an immature child. Sometimes we get a lot of that type in the emergency room—faggots in particular.

It's hard for me to understand them, and what they do to themselves. I mean, talk about a bizarre social aberration! I'm convinced that faggotism is a result of the breakdown and failure of the whole society. You ought to see what these guys do to themselves, all the stuff they shove up their assholes. They perforate their colons, they do all kinds of damage, then they come in here and we have to fix 'em up. The other day we took out a big rubber fist about two feet long, a black latex fist. We've also had table legs, light bulbs, jars of Alka-Seltzer, dildos, pool balls. This is what they do for fun! As far as I'm concerned, that's pretty much on the raggedy end.

But I feel more out-and-out disgust for the rich suburban ladies who come into my emergency room demanding that you instantly make their sore throats better. Whatever they have, they'll demand the maximum amount of attention, and it has to be cured instantly. They should suffer no pain, no inconvenience. They should be able to make their bridge game or whatever else is on their mind. So unrealistic compared to the rest of the world! Who says you have a right to feel healthy every minute of every day? Whoever says it hasn't spent time in the emergency room. Let 'em come sometime and take a look.

Dead on Arrival

David Sudnow

In County Hospital's emergency ward, the most frequent variety of death is what is known as the "DOA" type. Approximately 40 such cases are processed through this division of the hospital each month. The designation "DOA" is somewhat ambiguous insofar as many persons are not physiologically *dead on arrival,* but are nonetheless classified as having been such. A person who dies within several hours after having been brought to the hospital might, if upon arrival he was initially announced by the ambulance driver to be dead, retain such a classification at the time he is so pronounced by the physician.

When an ambulance driver suspects that the

Reprinted from *Transaction/Society,* vol. 5, no. 1 (1967) with permission of Transaction, Inc. Copyright © 1967 by Transaction, Inc.

person he is carrying is dead, he signals the emergency ward with a special siren alarm as he approaches the entrance driveway. As he wheels his stretcher past the clerk's desk, he restates his suspicion with the remark, "possible," a shorthand reference for "possible DOA." (The use of the term *possible* is required by law, which insists, primarily for insurance purposes, that any diagnosis unless made by a certified physician be so qualified.) The clerk records the arrival in a log book and pages a physician, informing him in code of the arrival. Often a page is not needed, as physicians on duty hear the siren alarm, expect the arrival, and wait at the entranceway. The patient is rapidly wheeled to the far end of the ward corridor and into the nearest available foyer or room, supposedly out of sight of other patients and possible onlookers from the waiting room. The physician arrives, makes his examination, and pronounces the patient dead or not. If the patient is dead, a nurse phones the coroner's office, which is legally responsible for the removal and investigation of all DOA cases.

Neither the hospital nor the physician has medical responsibility in such cases. In many instances of clear death, ambulance drivers use the hospital as a depository because it has the advantages of being both closer and less bureaucratically complicated a place than the downtown coroner's office for disposing of a body. Here, the hospital stands as a temporary holding station, rendering the community service of legitimate and free pronouncements of death for any comers. In circumstances of near-death, it functions more traditionally as a medical institution, mobilizing lifesaving procedures for those for whom they are still of potential value, at least as judged by the emergency room's staff of residents and interns. The boundaries between near-death and sure death are not, however, as we shall shortly see, altogether clearly defined.

In nearly all DOA cases the pronouncing physician (commonly that physician who is the first to answer the clerk's page or spot the incoming ambulance) shows in his general demeanor and approach to the task little more than passing interest in the event's possible occurrence and the patient's biographical and medical circumstances. He responds to the clerk's call, conducts his examination, and leaves the room once he has made the necessary official gesture to an attending nurse. (The term "kaput," murmured in differing degrees of audibility depending upon the hour and his state of awakeness, is a frequently employed announcement.) It happened on numerous occasions, especially during the midnight-to-eight shift, that a physician was interrupted during a coffee break to pronounce a DOA and returned to his colleagues in the canteen with, as an account of his absence, some version of "Oh, it was nothing but a DOA."

It is interesting to note that, while the special siren alarm is intended to mobilize quick response on the part of the emergency room staff, it occasionally operates in the opposite fashion. Some emergency room staff came to regard the fact of a DOA as decided in advance; they exhibited a degree of nonchalance in answering the siren or page, taking it that the "possible DOA" most likely is "D." In so doing they in effect gave authorization to the ambulance driver to make such assessments. Given that

time lapse which sometimes occurs between that point at which the doctor knows of the arrival and the time he gets to the patient's side, it is not inconceivable that in several instances patients who might have been revived died during this interim. This is particularly likely in that, apparently, a matter of moments may differentiate the revivable state from the irreversible one.

Two persons in similar physical condition may be differentially designated dead or not. For example, a young child was brought into the emergency room with no registering heartbeat, respirations, or pulse—the standard "signs of death"—and was, through a rather dramatic stimulation procedure involving the coordinated work of a large team of doctors and nurses, revived for a period of eleven hours. On the same evening, shortly after the child's arrival, an elderly person who presented the same physical signs, with—as one physician later stated in conversation—no discernible differences from the child in skin color, warmth, etc., arrived in the emergency room and was almost immediately pronounced dead, with no attempts at stimulation instituted. A nurse remarked, later in the evening: "They (the doctors) would never have done that to the old lady (attempt heart stimulation) even though I've seen it work on them too." During the period when emergency resuscitation equipment was being readied for the child, an intern instituted mouth-to-mouth resuscitation. This same intern was shortly relieved by oxygen machinery, and when the woman arrived, he was the one who pronounced her dead. He reported shortly afterwards that he could never bring himself to put his mouth to "an old lady's like that."

It is therefore important to note that the category DOA is not totally homogeneous with respect to actual physiological condition. The same is generally true of all deaths, the determination of *death* involving, as it does, a critical decision, at least in its earlier stages.

There is currently a movement in progress in some medical and lay circles to undercut the tradiional distinction between "biological" and "clinical" death, and procedures are being developed and their use encouraged for treating any "clinically dead" person as potentially revivable. Should such a movement gain widespread momentum (and it, unlike late 19th-century arguments for life after death, is legitimated by modern medical thinking and technology), it would foreseeably have considerable conse-quence for certain aspects of hospital social struc-ture, requiring perhaps that much more continuous and intensive care be given "dying" and "dead" pa-tients than is presently accorded them, at least at County. (At Cohen Hospital, where the care of the "tentatively dead" is always very intensive, such de-velopments would more likely be encouraged than at County.)

Currently at County there seems to be a rather strong relationship between the age, social back-ground, and the perceived moral character of pa-tients and the amount of effort that is made to at-tempt revival when "clinical death signs" are detected (and, for that matter, the amount of effort given to forestalling their appearance in the first place). As one compares practices in this regard at different hospitals, the general relationship seems to hold; although at the private, wealthier institu-tions like Cohen the overall amount of attention given to "initially dead" patients is greater. At County efforts at revival are admittedly superficial, with the exception of the very young or occasionally wealthier patient who by some accident ends up at County's emergency room. No instances have been witnessed at County where, for example, external heart massage was given a patient whose heart was stethoscopically inaudible, if that patient was over 40 years of age. At Cohen Hospital, on the other hand, heart massage is a normal routine at that point, and more drastic measures, such as the injec-tion of adrenalin directly into the heart, are not un-common. While these practices are undertaken for many patients at Cohen if "tentative death" is discov-ered early (and it typically is because of the attention "dying" patients are given), at County they are re-served for a very special class of cases.

Generally speaking, the older the patient the more likely is his tentative death taken to constitute pronounceable death. Suppose a 20-year old arrives in the emergency room and is presumed to be dead because of the ambulance driver's assessment. Be-fore that patient will be pronounced dead by a physi-cian, extended listening to his heartbeat will occur, occasionally efforts at stimulation will be made, oxy-gen administered, and often stimulative medication given. Less time will elapse between initial detection of an inaudible heartbeat and nonpalpitating pulse and the pronouncement of death if the person is 40 years old, and still less if he is 70. As best as can be detected, there appeared to be no obvious difference between men and women in this regard, nor between white and Negro patients. Very old pa-tients who are initially considered to be dead solely on the basis of the ambulance driver's assessment of that possibility were seen to be put in an empty room to wait several moments before a physician arrived. The driver's announcement of a "possible" places a frame of interpretation around the event, so that the physician expects to find a dead person and attends the person under the general auspices of that expectation. When a young person is brought in as a "possible," the driver tries to convey some more alarming sense to his arrival by turning the siren up very loud and keeping it going after he has already stopped, so that by the time he has actu-ally entered the wing, personnel, expecting "some-thing special," act quickly and accordingly. When it is a younger person that the driver is delivering, his general manner is more frantic. The speed with which he wheels his stretcher in and the degree of excitement in his voice as he describes his charge to the desk clerk are generally more heightened than with the typical elderly DOA. One can observe a direct relationship between the loudness and length of the siren alarm and the considered "social value" of the person being transported.

The older the person, the less thorough is the examination he is given; frequently, elderly people are pronounced dead on the basis of only a stetho-scopic examination of the heart. The younger the person, the more likely will an examination preced-ing an announcement of death entail an inspection of the eyes, attempt to find a pulse, touching of the body for coldness, etc. When a younger person is brought to the hospital and announced by the driver as a "possible" but is nonetheless observed to be breathing slightly, or have an audible heart beat, there is a fast mobilization of effort to stimulate increased breathing and a more rapid heartbeat. If an older person is brought in in a similar condition there will be a rapid mobilization of similar efforts; however, the time which will elapse between that point at which breathing noticeably ceases and the heart audibly stops beating and when the pronounce-ment of death is made will differ according to his age.

One's location in the age structure of the society

is not the only factor that will influence the degree of care he gets when his death is considered possibly to have occurred. At County Hospital a notable additional set of considerations relating to the patient's presumed "moral character" is made to apply.

The smell of alcohol on the breath of a "possible" is nearly always noticed by the examining physician, who announces to his fellow workers that the person is a drunk. This seems to constitute a feature he regards as warranting less than strenuous effort to attempt revival. The alcoholic patient is treated by hospital physicians, not only when the status of his body as alive or dead is at stake, but throughout the whole course of medical treatment, as one for whom the concern to treat can properly operate somewhat weakly. There is a high proportion of alcoholic patients at County, and their treatment very often involves an earlier admission of "terminality" and a consequently more marked suspension of curative treatment than is observed in the treatment of nonalcoholic patients. In one case, the decision whether or not to administer additional blood needed by an alcoholic man bleeding badly from a stomach ulcer was decided negatively, and that decision was announced as based on the fact of his alcoholism. The intern in charge of treating the patient was asked by a nurse, "Should we order more blood for this afternoon?" and the doctor answered, "I can't see any sense in pumping it into him because even if we can stop the bleeding, he'll turn around and start drinking again and next week he'll be back needing more blood." In the DOA circumstance, alcoholic patients have been known to be pronounced dead on the basis of a stethoscopic examination of the heart alone, even though such persons were of such an age that were they not alcoholics they would likely have received much more intensive consideration before being so decided upon. Among other categories of persons whose deaths will be more quickly adjudged, and whose "dying" more readily noticed and used as a rationale for apathetic care, are the suicide victim, the dope addict, the known prostitute, the assailant in a crime of violence, the vagrant, the known wife-beater, and, generally, those persons whose moral characters are considered reproachable.

Within a limited temporal perspective at least, but one which is not necessarily to be regarded as trivial, the likelihood of "dying" and even of being "dead" can be said to be partially a function of one's place in the social structure, and not simply in the sense that the wealthier get better care, or at least not in the usual sense of that fact. If one anticipates having a critical heart attack, he had best keep himself well-dressed and his breath clean if there is a likelihood he will be brought into County as a "possible."

The DOA deaths of famous persons are reportedly attended with considerably prolonged and intensive resuscitation efforts. In President Kennedy's death, for example, the *New York Times* (Nov. 23, 1963) quoted an attending physician as saying:

> *Medically, it was apparent the President was not alive when he was brought in. There was no spontaneous respiration. He had dilated, fixed pupils. It was obviously a lethal head wound. Technically, however, by using vigorous resuscitation, intravenous tubes and all the usual supportive measures, we were able to raise the semblance of a heart beat.*

There are a series of practical consequences of pronouncing a patient dead in the hospital setting. His body may properly be stripped of clothing, jewelry, and the like, wrapped up for discharge, the family notified of the death, and the coroner informed in the case of DOA deaths. In the emergency unit there is a special set of procedures which can be said to be partially definitive of death. DOA cases are very interestingly "used" in many American hospitals. The inflow of dead bodies, or what can properly be taken to be dead bodies, is regarded as a collection of "guinea pigs," in the sense that procedures can be performed upon those bodies for the sake of teaching and research.

In any "teaching hospital" (in the case of County, I use that term in a weak sense; that is, a hospital which employs interns and residents; in other settings a "teaching hospital" may mean systematic, institutionalized instruction) the environment of medical events is regarded not merely as a collection of treatable cases, but as a collection of experience-relevant information. It is a continually enforced way of looking at the cases one treats to regard them under the auspices of a concern for experience with "such cases." That concern can legitimately warrant the institution of a variety of procedures, tests, and inquiries which lie outside and may even on occasion conflict with the strict interests of treatment; they fall within the interests of "learning medicine," gaining experience with such cases, and acquiring technical skills.

A principle for organizing medical care activities in the teaching hospital generally—and perhaps more so in the county hospital, where patients' social value is often not highly regarded—is the relevance of any particular activity to the acquisition of skills of general import. Physicians feel that among the greatest values of such institutions is the ease with which medical attention can be selectively organized to maximize the general benefits to knowledge and technical proficiency which working with a given case expectably affords. The notion of the "interesting case" is, at County, not simply a casual notion but an enforced principle for the allocation of attention. The private physician is in a more committed relation to each and every one of his patients; and while he may regard this or that case as more or less interesting, he ideally cannot legitimate his varying interest in his patients' conditions as a basis for devoting varying amounts of attention to them. (His reward for treating the uninteresting case is, of course, the fee, and physicians are known to give more attention to those of their patients who shall be paying more.)

At County Hospital a case's degree of interest is a crucial fact, and one which is invoked to legitimate the way a physician does and should allocate his attention. In surgery, for instance, I found many examples. If on a given morning in one operating room a "rare" procedure was scheduled and in another a "usual" procedure planned, there would be no special difficulty in getting personnel to witness and partake in the rare procedure, whereas work in the usual case was considered as merely work, regardless of such considerations as the relative fatality rate of each procedure or the patient's physical condition. It is not uncommon to find interns at County who are scrubbed for an appendectomy taking turns going next door to watch a skin graft or chest surgery. At Cohen such house staff interchanging was not permitted. Interns and residents were assigned to a particular surgical suite and required to stay throughout the course of a procedure. On the medical wards, on the basis of general observation, it seems that one could obtain a high order correlation between the amount of time doctors spent discussing and examining patients and the degree of unusualness of their medical problems.

I introduce this general feature to point to the predominant orientation at County to such matters as "getting practice" and the general organizational principle that provides for the propriety of using cases as the basis for this practice. Not only are live patients objects of practice, so are dead ones.

There is a rule in the emergency unit that with every DOA a doctor should attempt to insert an "endo-tracheal" tube down the throat, but only after the patient is pronounced dead. The reason for this rule (on which new interns are instructed as part of their training in emergency medicine) is that the tube is extremely difficult to insert, requires great yet careful force, and, insofar as it may entail great pain, the procedure cannot be "practiced" on live patients. The body must be positioned with the neck at such an angle that the large tube will go down the proper channel. In some circumstances when it is necessary to establish a rapid "airway" (an open breathing canal), the endo-tracheal tube can apparently be an effective substitute for the tracheotomy incision. The DOA's body in its transit from the scene of the death to the morgue constitutes an ideal captive experimental opportunity. The procedure is not done on all deceased patients, the reason apparently being that it is part of the training one receives in the emergency unit and is to be learned there. Nor is it done on all DOA cases, for some doctors, it seems, are uncomfortable in handling a dead body whose charge as a live one they never had, and handling it in the way such a procedure requires. It is important to note that when it is done, it is done most frequently and most intensively with those persons who are regarded as lowly situated in the moral social structure.

No instances were observed where a young child was used as an object for such a practice nor where a well-dressed, middle-aged, middle-class adult was similarly used. On one occasion a woman supposed to have ingested a fatal amount of laundry bleach was brought to the emergency unit, and after she died, several physicians took turns trying to insert an endo-tracheal tube, after which one of them suggested that the stomach be pumped to examine its contents to try to see what effects the bleach had on the gastric secretions. A lavage was set up and the stomach contents removed. A chief resident left the room and gathered together a group of interns with the explanation that they ought to look at this woman because of the apparent results of such ingestion. In effect, the doctors conducted their own autopsy investigation without making any incisions.

On several similar occasions physicians explained that with these kinds of cases they didn't really feel as if they were prying in handling the body, but that they often did in the case of an ordinary death—a "natural death" of a morally proper person. Suicide victims are frequently the objects of curiosity, and while there is a high degree of distaste in working with such patients and their bodies (particularly among the nursing staff; some nurses will not touch a suicide victim's dead body), "practice" by doctors is apparently not as distasteful. A woman was brought into the emergency unit with a self-inflicted gunshot wound which ran from her sternum downward and backward, passing out through a kidney. She had apparently bent over a rifle and pulled the trigger. Upon her "arrival" in the emergency unit she was quite alive and talkative, and though in great pain and very fearful, was able to conduct something of a conversation. She was told that she would need immediate surgery and was taken off to the operating room; following her were a group of physicians, all of whom were interested in seeing the damage done in the path of the bullet. (One doctor said aloud, quite near her stretcher, "I can't get my heart into saving her, so we might as well have some fun out of it.") During the operation the doctors regarded her body much as they do one during autopsy. After the critical damage was repaired and they had reason to feel the woman would survive, they engaged in numerous surgical side ventures, exploring muscular tissue in areas of the back through which the bullet had passed but where no damage had been done that required repair other than the tying off of bleeders and suturing. One of the operating surgeons performed a side operation, incising an area of skin surrounding the entry wound on the chest, to examine, he announced to colleagues, the structure of the tissue through which the bullet passed. He explicitly announced his project to be motivated by curiosity; one of the physicians spoke of the procedure as an "autopsy on a live patient," about which there was a little laughter.

In another case, a man was wounded in the forehead by a bullet, and after the damage was repaired in the wound, which resembled a usual frontal lobotomy, an exploration was made of an area adjacent to the path of the bullet, on the forehead proper, below the hair line. During this exploration the operating surgeon asked a nurse to ask Dr. X to come in, and when Dr. X arrived, the two of them, under the gaze of a large group of interns and nurses, made a further incision, which an intern described to me as unnecessary in the treatment of the man, and which left a noticeable scar down the side of the temple. The purpose of this venture was to explore the structure of that part of the face. This area of the skull, that below the hair line, cannot be examined during an autopsy because of a contract between local morticians and the Department of Pathology to leave those areas of the body which will be viewed free of surgical incisions. The doctors justified the additional incision by pointing to the "fact" that since he would have a "nice scar as it was, a little bit more wouldn't be so serious."

During autopsies themselves, bodies are routinely used to gain experience in surgical techniques, and many incisions, explorations, and the like are conducted that are not essential to the key task of uncovering the "cause" of the death. Frequently specialists-in-training come to autopsies though they have no interest in the patient's death; they await the completion of the legal part of the procedure, at which point the body is turned over to them for practice. Mock surgical procedures are staged on the body, often with co-workers simulating actual conditions, tying off blood vessels which obviously need not be tied, and suturing internally.

When a patient died in the emergency unit, whether or not he had been brought in under the designation DOA, there occasionally occurred various mock surgical procedures on his body. In one case a woman was treated for a chicken bone lodged in her throat. Rapidly after her arrival via ambulance a tracheotomy incision was made in the attempt to establish an unobstructed source of air, but the procedure was not successful and she died as the incision was being made. Several interns were called upon to practice their stitching by closing the wound as they would on a live patient. There was a low peak in the activity of the ward, and a chief surgical resident used the occasion to supervise teaching them various techniques for closing such an incision. In another case the body of a man who died after being crushed by an automobile was employed for instruction and practice in the use of various fracture setting techniques. In still another instance several interns and residents attempted to suture a dead man's dangling finger in place on his mangled hand.

What has been developed here is a "procedural definition of death," a definition based upon the activities which that phenomenon can be said to *consist of*. While in some respects this was a study of "dying" and "death," it might be better summarized as a study of the activities of managing dying and death as meaningful events for hospital staff members. My attention has been exclusively given to the description of staff behavior occurring in the course of doing those things which daily ward routines were felt to require.

It was in the course of these routines—handling bodies, taking demographic information on incoming and outgoing patients, doing diagnosis, prognosis, medical experimentation, and teaching—that certain patients came to be recognized as persons legitimately accorded special treatments—the "dying" and "death" treatments. In the hospital world these treatments—organized to fit institutionalized daily ward routines built up to afford mass treatments on an efficiency basis, to obtain "experience," avoid dirty work, and maximize the possibilities that the intern will manage to get some sleep—give "dying" and "death" their concrete senses for hospital personnel. Whatever else a "dying" or "dead" patient might mean in other contexts, in the hospital I investigated, the sense of such states of affairs was given by the work requirements associated with the patients so described. For a "dying" patient to be on the ward meant that soon there would be a body to be cleansed, wrapped, pronounced dead, and discharged, and a family to be told. These activities and the work requirements they entailed provided the situational frame of interpretation around such states.

At least one question that has not been directly addressed is that which would ask why hospital personnel feel treatments must be organized on a mass basis. Its answer, I believe, is to be found in a historical analysis of the development of the medical ideology toward the nonpaying patient and in the peculiarly impersonal environment of the charity institution I examined. I decided at the outset of my investigation to leave unexplained general matters of ideology about patient care and to proceed from there to learn something about the ways in which existing practices were organized and what

these practices entailed as regarded the occurrence of "dying" and "death."

While hospital personnel managed, on the whole, to sustain a detached regard for the event of death, it occurred, on occasion, that routinely employed procedures and attitudes became altered and upset. The successful daily management of "dying" and "dead" bodies seemed to require that patients have a relatively constant character as social types. So long as the patient whose death was anticipated or had occurred was an elderly, poor, and morally proper person, the occasion of his "dying" and "death" was treated with little notice and in accord with ordinarily enforced routines of "death care." On critical occasions, however—when, for example, a child died or a successful, middle-class person was brought into the emergency unit as a DOA—ordinarily employed procedures of treatment were not instituted, and special measures were felt to be necessary. Nowhere was this disruption clearer than with the deaths of children. Nurses have been known to break down in tears when a child died, and in such cases, particularly, "dying" and "death" temporarily cease to have their firmly grounded, organizationally routinized meanings, activities, and consequences. When an intoxicated or suicidal or "criminal" patient was treated, these persons' moral characters intruded as prevalent considerations in the way in which they were regarded, providing a special frame of interpretation around the way care was organized over and above that which the category "patient" established. In key instances, patients' external attributes operated to alter the institutional routine in significant ways, causing vehemence, disgust, horror, or empathetic dismay, and—particularly in the case of children's deaths—a radical though short-lived movement entirely out of role on the part of staff members. No matter how routinized an institution's methods for handling its daily tasks, those routines remain vulnerable at certain key points. No matter how nonchalantly staff members managed to wrap patients' bodies for discharge to the morgue, taper off in the administration of drugs and care to the "dying," pronounce deaths, and return to other tasks, special circumstances caused these routines to be upset—either made more difficult to carry off, more interestedly attended, or substantially revised.

In regarding these special cases—those persons deemed particularly obnoxious or particularly worthy—perhaps insight may be gained into the requirements for usual, orderly ward activities. On those occasions when a nontypical death caused staff members to step outside their regularly maintained attitudes of indifference and efficiency, one could glimpse a capacity for emotional involvement which ordinary work activities did not provide proper occasions for displaying. The maintenance of appropriate impersonality in the hospital requires an enforced standardization to the types of events and persons which personnel confront. This work of *affect* management is aided by staff-held theories of proper fate, proper deaths, proper persons, and notions regarding the appropriate role of medicine and surgery in prolonging life and delaying death. These theories are invoked on a daily basis to support the patterns of care given the dying, the tentatively dead, and the decidedly dead, but they can be employed only as long as the patient in question can be construed to fit the categories for which the theories are relevant. I made every effort to construct classifications of patients so as to provide for the propriety of treating them in organizationally routine ways, but occasionally there was a case which resisted that classification. The death of a child, a young adult, or the deaths of those persons who were regarded as morally imperfect stirred a noticeably atypical degree of moral sentiment.

This class of atypical deaths, those occurring for atypical persons or in atypical ways, became set off as the specially noteworthy events of hospital life, the cases which staff members recounted for long periods of time and built into stories that were frequently retold when death was made a specific topic of conversation. In selecting certain cases to invest with special meaning, staff members demonstrated that despite their work involvements in matters of life and death and their routinely casual attitude toward such events, death nonetheless was an event which could call forth grief and empathy.

"Dying" and "death" are categories that have very broad currency, being variously used in many settings throughout the society. I have examined only one setting, only one locus of meanings and associated activities. The use of the categories in the hospital is to be regarded as hospital specific, although in other domains their usages may share features in common with those found in the hospital. While clinical death occurs, in American society at least, chiefly within the hospital setting, that setting provides only one of a variety of socially organized worlds within which its meaningful character is provided. What "dying" and "death" procedurally entail among staff physicians within the hospital would seem to share little in common with those activities anticipatorily organized by and consequential for the patient himself and members of his family—those for whom doing autopsies, handling the census of a hospital ward, cleaning up dead bodies, and the rest are not relevant considerations. My restricted interest in death in the hospital requires that the formulation of the notions "dying" and "death" given here be clearly confined in generality to this highly instrumental domain of technical activity.

CHAPTER 7 _____

The "Uncertainty" Theme

Although a good portion of the public is likely to see medicine as a relatively exact science, medical professionals are well aware of its inexact nature. Therefore, one function of training is to make students aware of the uncertainties that surround the practice of medicine. An important consequence of this awareness is an understanding of where medical responsibility lies. Medical practitioners must learn the distinction between errors deriving from the inexact nature of medicine and those resulting from errors in their own judgment.

At the same time, some writers like Donald Light (1979) have begun to focus on the ways in which physicians try to develop certainty in response to uncertainty. Light notes how residents training for a career in psychiatry often focus on technique—like the "beautiful hour" with the patient—rather than on the more elusive goal of cure. Specialization is another way in which physicians limit the degree of uncertainty with which they may be confronted. Moreover, within a specialty there are "schools of thought" to which physicians attach so as not to have to make decisions between competing alternative treatments.

This chapter, like the previous one, is separated into two sections. The first looks at uncertainty during the training period and begins with a classic piece by Renée C. Fox. Fox points out how specific aspects of the medical school curriculum are used to impress upon students the uncertain nature of medicine. The following article, by Deborah B. Leiderman and Jean-Anne Grisso, looks at how the presence of severely chronically ill individuals called "Gomers" (as in "Get out of my emergency room") symbolizes to residents the limitations and uncertainties in medicine. Kathleen Knafl and Gary Burkett then discuss how residents in orthopedic surgery learn medical judgment. They also note the existence of alternative means of treatment for the same surgical problem and describe how residents learn to accept one or another "treatment philosophy" as a way of imposing a degree of certainty on the situation.

The second section looks at how aspects of the socialization process, as regards uncertainty, manifest themselves in the professional lives of physicians, once they are through training and are practicing on their own. It begins with an article by a physician, David Hilfiker, that is a very personal account of how physicians make mistakes. Hilfiker's discussion about the different sources of physician mistakes is reminiscent of Fox's description of the kinds of uncertainties to which the medical students she studied were being exposed. The final article, by John Wennberg and Alan Gittelsohn, concerns their study, which has received a great deal of national attention. Comparing surgery rates in geographical areas within New England, the researchers found large differences that were not explained by differences in the health of the populations of the different areas. Although the number of surgeons in an area influenced the overall rate of surgery, this factor failed to explain why certain surgical procedures were practiced so much more often in one area than in another. An explanation, according to Wennberg and Gittelsohn, lies in the existence of the "surgical signature"—individual preferences that individual surgeons have for particular surgical procedures. The choice of a "surgical signature" by a practicing surgeon may be seen as parallel to, and perhaps a consequence of, the choice of a given "treatment philosophy" by residents-in-training. Although limiting treatment options may be an effective way of limiting physician uncertainty, it may deprive patients of choices that they may not be aware are available to them.

References

LIGHT, D. 1979. Uncertainty and Control in Professional Training. *Journal of Health and Social Behavior* 20, 310–322.

Training for Uncertainty

Renée C. Fox

There are areas of experience where we know
that uncertainty is the certainty.

James B. Conant

Voluminous texts, crammed notebooks, and tightly packed memories of students at Cornell University Medical College attest to the "enormous amount"[1] of established medical knowledge they are expected to learn. It is less commonly recognized that they also learn much about the uncertainties of medicine and how to cope with them. Because training for uncertainty in the preparation of a doctor has been largely overlooked, the following discussion will be focused exclusively on this aspect of medical education, but with full realization that it is counterbalanced by "all the material [students] learn that is as solid and real as a hospital building."

There is of course marked variation among students in the degree to which uncertainty is recognized or acknowledged. Some students, more inclined than others to equate knowing with pages covered and facts memorized, may think they have "really accomplished a lot . . . gained valuable knowledge," and that what they have learned is "firmly embedded and clear in their minds." Other students are more

sensitive to the "vastness of medicine," and more conscious of ignorance and superficiality in the face of all they "should know," and of all the "puzzling questions" they glimpse but cannot answer. Many students fall somewhere between these two extremes, half-aware in the course of diligent learning, that there is much they do not understand, yet not disposed "at this point to stop and lament." Discussion will be limited to the training for uncertainty that seems to apply to the largest number of students, admitting at the outset that inferences from the data must be provisional.

THE KINDS OF UNCERTAINTY THAT THE DOCTOR FACES

In Western society, where disease is presumed to yield to application of scientific method, the doctor is regarded as an expert, a man professionally trained in matters pertaining to sickness and health and able by his medical competence to cure our ills and keep us well. It would be good to think that he has only to make a diagnosis and to apply appropriate treatment for alleviation of ills to follow. But such a Utopian view of the physician is at variance with facts. His knowledge and skill are not always adequate, and there are many times when his most vigorous efforts to understand illness and to rectify its consequences may be of no avail. Despite unprecedented scientific advances, the life of the modern physician is still full of uncertainty.[2]

Two basic types of uncertainty may be recognized. The first results from incomplete or imperfect mastery of available knowledge. No one can have

Reprinted by permission of the publisher from *The Student Physician: Introductory Studies in the Sociology of Medical Education* edited by Robert K. Merton, George C. Reader, and Patricia L. Kendall (eds.), Harvard University Press, Cambridge, Mass., pp. 207–218, 228–241. Copyright © 1957 by the Commonwealth Fund.

at his command all skills and all knowledge of the lore of medicine. The second depends upon limitations in current medical knowledge. There are innumerable questions to which no physician, however well trained, can as yet provide answers. A third source of uncertainty derives from the first two. This consists of difficulty in distinguishing between personal ignorance or ineptitude and the limitations of present medical knowledge. It is inevitable that every doctor must constantly cope with these forms of uncertainty and that grave consequences may result if he is not able to do so. It is for this reason that training for uncertainty in a medical curriculum and in early professional experiences is an important part of becoming a physician.

An effort will be made to identify some experiences as well as some agencies and mechanisms in medical school that prepare students for uncertainty and to designate patterns by which students may gradually come to terms with uncertainty. In the initial inquiry we shall content ourselves with a general view of the sequences through which most students pass, but in a concluding section we shall suggest some variations that might be considered in further investigation of training for uncertainty.

THE PRECLINICAL YEARS

Learning to Acknowledge Uncertainty

The first kind of uncertainty which the student encounters has its source in his role as a student. It derives from the avoidance of "spoon-feeding," a philosophy of the preclinical years at Cornell Medical College (as at many other medical schools).

> You will from the start be given the major responsibility for learning [students are told on the first day that they enter medical school]. Most of your undergraduate courses to date have had fixed and circumscribed limits; your textbooks have been of ponderable dimensions. . . . Not so with your medical college courses. . . . We do not use the comfortable method of spoon-feeding. . . .[3] Limits are not fixed. Each field will be opened up somewhat sketchily. . . . You will begin to paint a picture on a vast canvas but only the center of the picture will be worked in

> any detail. The periphery will gradually blur into the hazy background. And the more you work out the peripheral pattern, the more you will realize the vastness of that which stretches an unknown distance beyond. . . . Another common collegiate goal is to excel in competition with others. . . . [But] because an overly competitive environment can hinder learning, student ratings are never divulged [in this medical school], except to the extent that once a year each student is privately informed as to which quarter of the class he is in.

From the first, the medical school rookie is thus confronted with the challenge of a situation only hazily defined for him. Information is not presented "in neat packets";[4] precise boundaries are not set on the amount of work expected. Under these conditions the uncertainty which the beginning student faces lies in determining how much he ought to know, exactly what he should learn, and how he ought to go about his studies.

This uncertainty, great as it is, is further accentuated for the beginner by the fact that he does not receive grades, and therefore does not have the usual concrete evidence by which to discover whether he is in fact doing well:

> In college, if you decide to work very hard in a course, the usual result is that you do very well in it, and you have the feeling that studying hard leads to good grades. You may tell yourself that you don't give a damn about grades, but nevertheless, they do give you some reassurance when you ask yourself if the work was worth it. . . . In medical school, there is no such relationship. Studying does not always lead to doing well—it is quite easy to study hard, but to study the wrong things and do poorly. And if you should do well, you never know it. . . . In my own case, I honestly think the thing that bothers me most is not the lack of grades, but rather the feeling that even after studying some in a given course, I always end up knowing so little of what I should know about it. . . . Medicine is such an enormous proposition that one cannot help but fall short of what he feels he should get done. . . .

Thus, it would seem that avoidance of spoon-feeding by the preclinical faculty encourages the student to take responsibility in a relatively unstructured situation, perhaps providing him with a foretaste of the ambiguities he may encounter when he assumes responsibility for a patient.

From the latter parts of the comment under review it would appear that the same teaching philosophy also leads to the beginning awareness of a second type of uncertainty: by making the student conscious of how vast medicine is, the absence of spoon-feeding readies him for the fact that even as a mature physician he will not always experience the certainty that comes with knowing "all there is to know" about the medical problems with which he is faced. He begins to realize that no matter how skilled and well-informed he may gradually become, his mastery of all that is known in medicine will never be complete.

It is perhaps during the course of studying Gross Anatomy that the student experiences this type of uncertainty most intensely. Over the centuries this science has gradually traced out what one medical student describes as the "blueprint of the body." As a result of struggle to master a "huge body of facts," he comes to see more clearly that medicine is such an "enormous proposition" he can never hope to command it in a way both encompassing and sure:

> . . . Men have been able to study the body for thousands of years . . . to dissect the cadaver . . . and to work on it with the naked eye. They may not know everything about the biochemistry of the body, or understand it all microscopically . . . but when it comes to the gross anatomy, they know just about all there is to know. . . . This vast sea of information that we have to keep from going out the other ear is overwhelming. . . . There's a sense in which even before I came to medical school I knew that I didn't know anything. But I never realized it before, if you know what I mean—not to the extent that it was actually a gripping part of me. Basically, I guess what I thought before was, sure, I was ignorant now—but I'd be pretty smart after a while. Well, at this point it's evident to me that even after four years, I'll still be ignorant. . . . I'm now in the process of learning how much there is to learn. . . .[5]

As in this case, the student's own sense of personal inadequacy may be further reinforced by the contrast he draws between his knowledge and that which he attributes to his instructors. Believing as he does that "when it comes to the gross anatomy, they know just about all there is to know," he is made increasingly aware of how imperfect his own mastery really is.

There are other courses and situations in preclinical years which acquaint the Cornell student with uncertainties that result, not from his own inadequacies, but from the limitations in the current state of medical knowledge. For example, standing in distinction to the amassed knowledge of a discipline such as Gross Anatomy is a science like Pharmacology, which only in recent years has begun to emerge from a trial-and-error state of experimentation:

> Throughout the history of pharmacology, it would appear that the ultimate goal was to expedite the search for agents with actions on living systems and to provide explanations for these actions, to the practical end of providing drugs which might be used in the treatment of the disease of man. As a result of many searches there now exist such great numbers of drugs that the task of organizing them is a formidable one. The need for the development of generalizations and simplifying assumptions is great. It is to be hoped that laws and theories of drug action will be forthcoming, but the student should at this point appreciate that few of them, as yet, exist.[6]

The tentativeness of Pharmacology as a science, then, advances the student's recognition that not all the gaps in his knowledge indicate deficiencies on his part. In effect, Pharmacology helps teach medical students that because "there are so many voids" in medical knowledge, the practice of medicine is sometimes largely "a matter of conjuring . . . possibilities and probabilities."

> When Charles was over for dinner last week, I remarked at the time that I was coming to the conclusion that medicine was certainly no precise science, but rather, it is simply a matter of probabilities. Even these drugs today, for example, were noted as to their wide range of action. One dose will be too small to elicit a response in one individual; the same dose will be sufficient to get just the right response in another; and in

yet another individual, the same dose will produce hypersensitive toxic results. So, there is nothing exact in this, I guess. It's a matter of conjuring the possibilities and probabilities and then drawing conclusions as to the most likely response and the proper thing to do. And Charles last week agreed that a doctor is just an artist who has learned to derive these probabilities and then prescribe a treatment.

In Pharmacology (and in the other basic medical sciences as well) it is assumed that "laws and theories will be forthcoming" so that the uncertainties which result from limited knowledge in the field will gradually yield to greater certainty. However, the "experimental point of view" pervading much of early teaching at the Cornell Medical College promotes the idea that an irreducible minimum of uncertainty is inherent in medicine, in spite of the promise of further scientific advance. The preclinical instructors presenting this point of view have as a premise the idea that medical knowledge thus far attained must be regarded as no more than tentative, and must be constantly subjected to further inquiry. It is their assumption that few absolutes exist:

If you were having a great deal of trouble finding some simple sort of cell in histology and you asked him about it, Dr. A. always made a point to give you information from the experimental point of view. He would (a) point out that this cell has five different names; (b) point out that this cell might actually be a _____ cell or a ____ cell that has undergone a transformation and that indeed, this cell might be able to change into almost anything; (c) also mention that even though the cell has five names, it may not, in fact, exist in the first place—perhaps it's just an artifact.

Or, take the way the Bacteriology Department pushes the theme of "individual differences"— how one person will contract a disease he's been exposed to, while another one won't. The person may have a chill, or not; the agent may be virulent or not; and that determines whether pneumonia will occur or not. . . . "The occurrence, progression and outcome of a disease is a function of the offense of the microorganism and the defense of the host." That's the formula they keep pounding home. . . .

. . . In the course of the demonstration of drugs affecting respiration, Dr. S. quoted Goodman and Gilman [a pharmacology textbook universally recommended and respected] as to the dramatic effect of one certain drug in respiratory failure. And then, they proceeded to show the falsity of that statement. So pharmacologists are now debunking pharmacologists! Heretofore they simply showed the drugs commonly used by many physicians had no effect. If this keeps up, we will all be first-class skeptics!

This is not to say, a student cautions, that we don't learn "a lot of established facts . . . tried and true things about which there is little or no argument." But in course after course during the preclinical years at Cornell, emphasis is also placed on the provisional nature of much that is assumed to be medically known. The experimental point of view set forth by his teachers makes it more apparent than it might otherwise be that medicine is something less than a powerful, exact science, based on nicely invariant principles. In this way, the student is encouraged to acknowledge uncertainty, and, more than this, to tolerate it. He is made aware, not only that it is possible to act in spite of uncertainties, but that some of his teachers make such uncertainties the basis of their own experimental work.

Up to this point we have reviewed some of the courses and situations in the preclinical years at Cornell which make the beginning student aware of his own inadequacies and others which lead him to recognize limitations in current medical knowledge. The student has other experiences during the early years of medical school which present him with the problem of distinguishing between these two types of uncertainty—that is, there are times when he is unsure where his limitations leave off and the limitations of medical science begin. The difficulty is particularly evident in situations where he is called upon to make observations.

Whether he is trying to visualize an anatomical entity, studying gross or microscopic specimens in pathology, utilizing the method of percussion in physical diagnosis, or taking a personal history in psychiatry, the preclinical student is being asked to glean whatever information he can from the processes of looking, feeling, and listening.[7] In all these situations, students are often expected to see before they know how to look or what to look for. For, the ability to "see what you ought to see," "feel what you ought to feel," and "hear what you ought to hear," students assure us, is premised upon "a knowledge of what you're supposed to observe," an ordered method for making these observations, and a great deal of practice in medical ways of perceiving. ("We see only what we look for. We look for only what we know," the famous Goethe axiom goes.)

Nowhere does this kind of uncertainty become more salient for medical students during their preclinical years than in Physical Diagnosis:

> Physical Diagnosis is the one course I don't feel quite right about. I still have a great deal of difficulty making observations, and I usually don't feel certain about them. . . . Dick and I had a forty-year-old woman as our patient this morning. Though I thought we were doing better than usual at the time, we nevertheless missed several important things—a murmur and an enlarged spleen. . . .

"This sort of thing happens often in a course like Physical Diagnosis," the same student continues, and "it raises a question that gives me quite a bit of concern—Why do I have . . . difficulty making observations?"

There are at least two reasons for which a student may "miss" an important clinical sign, or feel uncertain about its presence or absence. On the one hand, his oversight or doubt may be largely attributable to lack of knowledge or skill on his part:

> One of the problems now is that we don't know the primary clinical signs of various disease processes. . . . For example, today we suspected subacute bacterial endocarditis, but we didn't know that the spleen is usually enlarged, and as a result, we didn't feel as hard as we should have. . . .

On the other hand, missing a spleen, for example, or "not being sure you hear a murmur" is sometimes more the "fault of the field" (as one student puts it) than "your own fault." That is, given the limitations in current medical knowledge and technique, the enlargement of a spleen may be too slight, the sound of a murmur too subtle, for "even the experts to agree upon it."

The uncertainty for a student, then, lies in trying to determine how much of his own "trouble . . . hearing, feeling or seeing is personal," and how much of it "has to do with factors outside of himself." (Or, as another student phrases the problem: "How do you make the distinction between yourself and objectivity?")

Generically, the student's uncertainty in this respect is no different from that to which every responsible, self-critical doctor is often subject. But because he has not yet developed the discrimination and judgment of a skilled diagnostician, a student is usually less sure than a mature physician about where to draw the line between his own limitations and those of medical science. When in doubt, a student seems more likely than an experienced practitioner to question and "blame" himself.

His course in Gross Anatomy, it has been suggested, gives a Cornell student some awareness of his own inadequacies; Pharmacology emphasizes the limitations of current medical knowledge; and his training in observation, particularly in Physical Diagnosis, confronts him with the problem of distinguishing between his own limitations and those in the field of medicine. But in his second year his participation in autopsies simultaneously exposes the student to all these uncertainties. The autopsy both epitomizes and summarizes various other experiences which together make up the preclinical student's training for uncertainty.

Before witnessing their first autopsy, second-year students may, on occasion, sound rather complacent about the questions which death poses. For example, speculating on the causes of death, one group of sophomores decided to their satisfaction that the cessation of life could be explained in simple physiological terms and that, armed with this knowledge, the doctor stands a good chance of "winning the fight" against death:

> We found that one very important matter could be traced back to one of two basic actions. The important matter—death. The two basic actions—the heart and respiration. For death is caused, finally, by the stopping of one of these two actions. As long as they both continue, there is life. . . . It's all a fight to keep the heart beating, the lungs breathing, and, in man, a third factor—the brain unharmed. . . . With all the multitude of actions and reactions which are

found in this medical business, it seems strange and satisfying to find something that can really be narrowed down. . . .

But the conviction that death "can really be narrowed down" is not long-lasting. Only a short time later, commenting on an autopsy he had just witnessed, one of these same students referred to death with "disquietude" as something you "can't pinpoint" or easily prevent.

One of the chief consequences of the student's participation in an autopsy is that it heightens his awareness of the uncertainties that result from limited medical knowledge and of the implications these uncertainties have for the practicing doctor. This is effected in a number of ways. To begin with, the experience of being "on call" for an autopsy ("waiting around for someone to die") makes a student more conscious of the fact that, even when death is expected, it is seldom wholly predictable:

In groups of threes, we all watch at least one autopsy—and my group is the third one in line. The first group went in for theirs this morning; this means that ours may come any time now. You can't be sure when, though, so you have to stay pretty close to home where you can be reached. . . .

In other words, although ultimate death is certain, medical science is still not far enough advanced so that the physicians can state with assurance exactly when an individual will die.

Of even greater importance, perhaps, in impressing the student with the limitations of current medical knowledge is the fact that, although the pathologist may be able to provide a satisfactory explanation of the patient's death, the student usually finds these "causes of death" less "dramatic" and specific than he expected them to be:

While our case was unusual, it was a bit of a letdown to me, for there was nothing dramatic to be pointed to as the cause of death. The clinician reported that the patient had lost 1,000 cc. of blood from internal bleeding in the G.I. tract. . . . Well, we saw no gaping hole there. There was no one place you could pinpoint and say: "This is where the hemorrhage took place." . . . Rather, it was a culmination of a condition relating to various factors. I suppose most causes of

death are this way. But still . . . (though I'm not really sure why it should be) . . . it was somewhat disquieting to me.

A third limitation of the field is implied in lack of control over death. For example, the student observes that "the various doctors connected with the case being autopsied . . . wander in while the procedure is going on." This serves to remind him that the " body on the autopsy table" belongs to a patient whose death no physician was able to prevent.

It is not only the limits of the field which are impressed upon the student during his participation in an autopsy. This experience also serves to make him aware of the personal limitations of even the most skilled practitioners. For instance, an autopsy gives a student an opportunity to observe that "the doctors aren't always sure what caused the patient's death"; rather, as one student puts it, "they come . . . to find out what was really wrong." Furthermore, the student may be present at an autopsy in which the pathologist's findings make it apparent that the physician was mistaken in his diagnosis (when, for example, the pathologist "doesn't find any of the things in the doctors' diagnoses"). From experiences such as these the student learns that, not only he, but also his instructors have only an imperfect mastery of all there is to know in medicine.

These varied aspects of the autopsy, in other words, give it central significance in the student's training for uncertainty.

Training for Uncertainty in the Comprehensive Care and Teaching Program

The sense of sureness expressed by students about to complete their third year at Cornell is, in some respects, premature. At any rate, the fourth-year student's perspective on the uncertainties of medicine is usually different from that of a junior:

Experience makes you less sure of yourself, [a senior explains]. What you realize is that even when you've been out of medical school twenty years, there'll be many times when you won't be able to make a diagnosis or cure a patient. . . . Instead of looking for the day, then, when all the knowledge you need will be in your posses-

sion, you learn that such a day will never come. . . .

A fourth-year student who faces up to uncertainty in this way has departed considerably from his third-year self. Part of this change seems attributable to experiences in the Comprehensive Care and Teaching Program.[8] A central feature of the Program is the extensive responsibility for patients who are defined as *his* patients, and he is expected to deal with all the problems that each case presents.[9] Stemming from this degree of responsibility are varied situations and experiences which make the fourth-year student more aware of the uncertainties of medicine.[10]

One important way in which students exercise the broad responsibility offered them is by following their patients over a period of months. This gives them more insight into the prevalence of uncertainties in the practice of medicine. What began as the "classical case" of Mrs. B., for example, illustrates the fact:

My new patient arrived first . . . Mrs. B., a 32-year-old housewife and mother of two children, who had a sudden onset of typical thyroid symptoms complete with the physical findings to go with them. . . . I ordered several diagnostic tests for her and advised her to return in a week. . . .

In this initial contact, the student-physician considered Mrs. B.'s case "typical," and the tests which he ordered were presumably intended merely to confirm the diagnosis. There is no indication that he anticipated special difficulty in handling Mrs. B.'s problems.

On the second visit the student and the attending physician who was supervising him agreed that Mrs. B.'s case was clear-cut, and that surgery would be appropriate. But they did not reckon with the response of the patient to that proposal:

By the time I got to my second revisit, Mrs. B., my toxic thyroid case, she had been waiting some time. . . . She gave me the story of continuation of her previous symptoms with shaking even more apparent at present. Of the tests ordered, only the BMR came back, but this was conclusive, being 59 percent above normal. I informed her that all her problems were related to these findings, and after discussing her with Dr. D. told

her that hospitalization and surgery were her best chance for a permanent cure. At this she broke down in tears, and after composing herself, made many arguments against surgery. . . . Dr. D. and I quickly agreed that I should treat her with propylthiouracil on an ambulatory basis until she has quieted down. This is an unnatural response to hospitalization and surgery, and I'll be interested in seeing if she becomes more logical with the quiescence of her toxic symptoms. . . .

The patient's fear of an operation forced the student and the attending physician to adopt a plan of therapy which they believed was less effective than the one they originally set forth.

On a later visit the full complexity of Mrs. B.'s case became more apparent:

I went in to see Mrs. B. and found that the threat of her husband's quitting his job was related to hysterical crying most of the day. She admitted that her reaction wasn't wholly because of her disease state, but that she had been easily unnerved prior to this. I assured her that although this might be so, her thyroid was making it much worse, and that we would shortly be rid of part of it. . . . She mentioned that a lump on her daughter's wrist was bothering her, and I suggested that she bring her in on the next visit. . . . We discussed surgery at her initiation, and arrived at the same conclusion as before: my insisting that surgery was the best solution to her problem, and her insisting that she, her husband and friends all agree that if a cure is possible without surgery, that it is to be embarked on. . . .

Mrs. B.'s emotional response to the diagnosis and recommendations made by the student-physician, her eagerness to accept the antisurgical opinions of her family and friends, her anxiety over her husband's job and her daughter's health all proved relevant to the appraisal and management of her case. With each visit it became more apparent to the student-physician that Mrs. B.'s problems were psychological as well as physical, and this realization evoked new questions. Was Mrs. B.'s long-standing nervousness wholly attributable to her disease state? Would it be possible to "ever get this woman over some of her anxious moments," and thus ready her for a needed operation? "I'm not too certain about any of these things," Mrs. B.'s student-physician reported at the end of his third visit with her. But had he seen her only once, this student would not have had any reason to alter his original impression that the case of Mrs. B. was diagnostically and therapeutically "clear-cut."

The continuous nature of his contact with patients in the Program, then, alerts a student to some of the clinical uncertainties that lie beyond first medical judgments and the appearance of things. Furthermore, it confronts him with the problem of managing a long-term doctor-patient relationship in the face of these uncertainties. For example:

I saw Mr. T. again and gave him the sad news— no ulcer demonstrated. What could this be if it wasn't an ulcer? I tried my best to put him off so that I wouldn't be obligated to further diagnostic procedures which would be useless and expensive. I did my best to convince him that it sounded like nothing but ulcer, and that we planned to treat it as such because not all ulcers are demonstrated by x-ray. This wasn't good enough. . . .

Mrs. J. puts up a pretty good front, but I think she worries a good deal about her problem. And today she asked me what she had. I was kind of up a tree. . . . I told her that what she had was somewhat different in that it didn't respond to the usual therapy—but that we had many other weapons and she shouldn't be concerned. . . .

With every revisit, the need for a solution may grow more intense in both the patient and the student-physician. Mr. T., for example, becomes harder to convince or reassure. Mrs. J. shows evidence of worrying a great deal and begins to press her doctor for an explanation of her problem. And the student, feeling responsible for the welfare of this man and woman (defined by the Program as *his* patients), is likely to feel frustrated and disappointed by his inability to resolve these cases.

These frustrations may be all the more provoking because the student has not been completely prepared for them by his earlier experiences. His relatively brief and circumscribed contact with patients in the third year had led him to assume that a good doctor ought to be able to arrive at a "definitive

diagnosis" and to evolve a successful plan of treatment for most of the cases with which he deals. But the broad and continuous experience provided by the Program teaches a student that cases like those of Mr. T. and Mrs. J. are more widespread than he had supposed them to be.

Not only do his continuing relationship with patients and the growing magnitude of his responsibility for them increase a student's awareness of the uncertain aspects of the cases with which he deals; they often lead to his being deeply affected by these uncertainties. Because he is working with patients in a sustained way, a student is more susceptible to positive and negative countertransference than he was before entering the Program. As time goes on, he may become attached to some patients and alienated from others. Furthermore, the relatively large degree of responsibility assigned to him by the Program makes a student feel more accountable for what happens to patients than he formerly did. As a result, the uncertainties that a student experiences in the Program "make an emotional impact on [him]," so that he is sometimes inclined to react subjectively to the uncertain features of cases he cannot bring to a satisfactory conclusion. Usually these reactions involve the placing of "blame," either on himself or on his patient:

I blame myself, not Mrs. H. [her student-physician declares]. I can't get her to reduce, and I don't know what I'm doing wrong. I have remained pleasant and sympathetic, but have applied strong urging and have registered disappointment (not wrath) at her failure to cooperate. . . . The reason I find her so difficult is that I feel if someone else were handling her, he could get the pounds off her. . . .

Mrs. C. has caused me quite a bit of consternation [another student asserts]. Though we have taken adequate physical measures to ascertain that her difficulty is on an emotional basis, she's still showing bodily overconcern. . . . She complains of pains in her legs; that her arms are too weak; that she's tired; that she feels pressure in her abdomen. . . . And then, these gripes about her husband. I can understand them in a way—because he's the type of man who comes home from work, picks up the paper, looks at TV for a while, and then goes to bed without saying a word.

. . . But she makes no effort to do anything about the situation. . . . She just sits there and tells me, "That's the way he is. . . ." Another thing about this woman is, in all instances she will discontinue whatever treatment you prescribe and proceed on her own conception. . . .

The "failure" is his, the first student claims; it's the "fault" of the patient and her environment, says the second.

As the cases of Mrs. H. and Mrs. C. suggest, a student is particularly apt to respond in one or the other of these affectual ways when the uncertainty he faces concerns either the social and psychological aspects of a patient's illness, or his own management of the doctor-patient relationship. Partly because psychiatry and the social sciences are in a more embryonic state of development than the disciplines from which medicine derives its understanding of the human body, the student encounters uncertainty more frequently in trying to handle the emotional and environmental components of his patient's disorder than in trying to cope with problems that are largely physical in nature. The classification of psychological disturbances thus far evolved, for example, is not precise enough to permit a high degree of diagnostic exactitude. The relationship between social factors and illness is only beginning to be systematically explored. And most of the available methods for treating sociopsychological difficulties are still grossly empirical, their relative merits and demerits a focus of present-day medical controversy, interest, and concern.

Intellectually, a student is aware of these things before he enters the Comprehensive Care Program; but he has not yet fully learned to acknowledge the uncertainties and limitations in this realm, or to proceed comfortably within the framework of such a realization. This is partly because, prior to his semester in the Program, a student has had little opportunity to take active responsibility for the "personal problems" of his patients. In the third year, for example, as we have seen, a student's work centers primarily on physical diagnosis. The only personal therapy he has occasion to administer to his patients is a simple and limited form of reassurance, which, on the whole, he judges to be effective. His success in this respect he deems "understandable" for he is inclined to feel that the so-called art-of-

medicine skills are based not so much on trained experience as they are on personal qualities. Such an attitude is reflected, for example, in the way that a number of third-year students look upon their psychiatry instructors:

There is a general feeling of great respect for most of the psychiatry people we have come in contact with [one student tells us]. We are impressed to note that the psychiatrist almost always suggests the honest, straightforward, direct approach to things . . . and most of us feel these people make sense. . . .

Yet "the regard we have for psychiatrists is not the same as the respect we have for surgeons," this student goes on to say. In the case of surgery, "it's a matter of respecting skill," in the case of psychiatry, "respecting common sense."

This distinction is one that students carry with them into the Program. It helps explain the observed tendency of many students in Comprehensive Care to reproach themselves when they are unable to formulate the "human aspects of a patient's case" or to decide upon an effective way of dealing with those aspects. ("I can't get Mrs. H. to reduce . . . and I don't know what I'm doing wrong.") For a student who tends to regard problems like "getting the patient to lose weight" as more contingent on personal attributes than on learned skill, the case of Mrs. H. may seem to represent a personal failure on his part.

The more common tendency of a student to blame the patient under such circumstances is a different manifestation of the same emotional involvement. In the face of medical uncertainties that may impede his attempts to be decisive about the sociopsychological dimensions of the cases he handles, a student often projects his own sense of inadequacy upon the patient. In Comprehensive Care, for example, students frequently apply the epithet "crock" to "patients who do not have an organic lesion" or whose behavior appears to be "psychoneurotic." "The central feature in all these patients we call 'crocks' is that they threaten our ability as doctors," one student points out. This is both because such patients do not respond to the diagnostic and therapeutic efforts of the student-physician in the way he would like ("You don't get a foothold anywhere and do something to give them better adjustment. . . ."), and because the student is emotionally "more vulnerable when thinking about the human aspects of a case, rather than just the strict medical problems involved."

> *Whether you're conscious of it or not, a lot of the things disturbed patients talk to you about are the kinds of things you're likely to react to very strongly in a positive or negative way. . . . I mean, it's all very well to say you're not judging these people, for instance. But you can get annoyed as heck with some of them, or lose your sympathy even though you know they're psychoneurotic. . . .*

To sum up: the fourth-year student is repeatedly impressed by the diagnostic and therapeutic uncertainties he encounters in dealing with patients during his semester in Comprehensive Care. Some of these uncertainties, he realizes, result from his own lack of medical knowledge and some from the limitations of medicine itself. In this respect, they are no different from those he has met at earlier points in his training. However, the physician-like responsibilities ascribed to him by the Program, along with the continuing and holistic nature of his relationship to patients, magnify the problem of uncertainty for the student, and make it harder for him to deal with it in a dispassionate way. In turn, the student's emotional involvement increases the difficulty he has in distinguishing between those uncertainties that grow out of his personal ignorance and those that stem from the current limitations of medical science. It is particularly when he feels unsure about how to classify the ulcer-like symptoms of a Mr. T., or what to do about the obesity of a Mrs. H., that a student "doesn't know whether [his] uncertainty is a reflection of his lack of knowledge and technique or whether such cases would be perplexing" even to more experienced physicians. As we have seen, a student is at first more apt to blame himself, or by projection, the patient, than he is to attribute his uncertainty to gaps in medical science.

Coming to Terms with Uncertainty in Comprehensive Care

The student's increased awareness of uncertainties in medicine is of course not the chief by-product of his term in Comprehensive Care. The same experi-ences which lead to such awareness also enlarge his skills in the realms of diagnosis and patient management. From the absence of expected findings in a case like that presented by Mr. T., for example, he learns how to appraise conflicting evidence in arriving at a diagnosis. From the complex problems of Mrs. B. he learns something of the connection between emotional stress and physical illness and gains some experience in dealing with patients who are under such stress. When he leaves the Program the student, therefore, has considerably more confidence about his ability to cope with these problems than he did six months before.

Moreover, the fourth-year student finds ways of adjusting to his remaining uncertainties. The organization of the Comprehensive Care Program and some of its precepts help the student to recognize that he shares part of his uncertainty with fellow classmates and instructors. This enables him to meet his uncertainty with greater confidence and equipoise.[11]

In contrast to the many small groups into which the class is divided during the third year, half of the senior class is enrolled in Comprehensive Care at one time, spending a continuous six months together in the Program. This arrangement facilitates that kind of interchange between students which from the earliest days of medical school provided them with mutual aid and the supportive knowledge that "others feel the way [they] do."

> *In the process of a routine physical, I performed a pelvic and rectal, and the glove specimen of the stool was strongly guaiac positive! And I didn't quite know what to do. The patient lives in upstate New York and can come to the city only when her husband drives in once a month. A decent GI workup would require her spending four full days at the Hospital. To further complicate matters, I wasn't sure of the significance of the positive test. I had rinsed my glove between pelvic and rectal, but the possibility of a positive test from blood in the vagina remains. . . . In the course of describing this experience at lunch . . . one of my classmates suggested that it was a crime to let her out of the building without a GI series, Ba, enema, and proctoscopy. He felt that even if subsequent stool examinations are negative, such a workup is obligatory. . . . This*

is the sort of decision I would prefer to force on someone else. I would feel foolish if such a workup showed nothing and subsequent stools were negative, but I'd feel worse if she showed up with an inoperable cancer a few months hence. . . . The lunch table of four was evenly divided on the question of what one should do if such a circumstance arose in general practice. . . . This problem is a real threat to the young physician. . . .

Although uncertainties such as these are "threatening," the student can perhaps find some reassurance in the fact that his classmates experience the same difficulties in deciding on appropriate action.

The opportunity to work as coequal with the attending physicians of Comprehensive Care also gives the student a chance to see that, at times, expert doctors are no more facile than he in making a diagnosis or deciding upon a course of treatment:

My second case was a three-year old girl with a swollen, red, warm left hand, which seemed to itch more than it hurt. No signs of infected wound—only history of a possible insect bite. I felt this was a contact dermatitis. The pediatrician felt it was obvious cellulitis, but insisted we call in a surgeon to confirm him. The surgeon leaned toward my diagnosis—and we called in a dermatologist who felt this was definitely infection—which was very amusing. . . .

Finally, the experimental milieu of the Program also furthers the student's realization that neither his classmates nor his instructors have sure and easy answers to some of the questions he finds puzzling. Because one of the primary aims of the Program is self-critically to develop a more comprehensive type of medical care, students and staff are continuously engaged in a process of inquiry. Conjoined by a living experiment, they openly express their feelings of doubt and uncertainty, and systematically try to resolve them. In one of the weekly Comprehensive Care conferences, for example, we can see this process taking place. A fourth-year student is presenting the history of the Gonzales family, whom he serves as general physician:

The Gonzales family is a Puerto Rican family that has been in this country for sixteen months.

It consists of eight members: Mr. Gonzales, a 38-year-old unskilled laborer; Mrs. Gonzales, his 25-year-old uneducated wife; and their six children. . . . They live in a three-room, unheated apartment on 60th Street. From the outset of our contact with this family, it was obvious that there were a number of interrelated sociological, economic, and medical problems, all of which could not be treated at the same time. We have tried to proceed in the most logical manner, but often our efforts have had to be side-tracked by the appearance of new problems. First, there was the real possibility of the family breaking up under the existing stresses. This immediate crisis passed. Then, there was the problem of tuberculosis with the diagnosis of Anna's active case, the question of Mrs. Gonzales' status, and the necessity of evaluating other members of the family. Coincidental with this investigation was the series of upper respiratory infections, otitis medias, episodes of gastro-enteritis and pyelitis, Carlo's seizure disorder, and finally, Mr. Gonzales' admission to the Hospital. Many of the family are known to be anemic, so following our satisfaction that none of the other children had tuberculosis, it was agreed that the known parasitic infections should be next attacked. . . . It seems certain that poor nutrition is another contributing factor to the anemias, and we have taken steps along this line as well. . . . One of the family's food difficulties has been the inability to shop properly. Previous to our contact with them, they purchased all of their groceries from a store uptown where Spanish was spoken, and high prices asked. On our advice, Mr. Gonzales now does most of his shopping at the A & P. . . . The situation has been in a constant state of flux since we first came in contact with the family, and shows every evidence of continuing in the same state. . . . All our efforts still leave many of the major problems of the family unsolved. . . . We will welcome any suggestions and opinions you may have. . . .

A series of student comments followed upon this presentation, gradually crystallizing around one of the major ideas of the Program. ("There is consensus that adequate care must include preventive, emotional, environmental, and familial aspects if it is to offer the most that modern knowledge can supply in the management of those who are ill."[12] But it has not yet been determined how inclusive "adequate care" can and should be):

> I was thinking as I sat there listening to the Gonzales case . . . is it or isn't it part of the doctor's job to be concerned with such things as where his patients buy their food?
>
> Theoretically, I guess it's part of the doctor's job. . . . But from my own point of view, I'm afraid that if I had a family like this, all I'd want to do is throw up my hands completely. . . .
>
> As far as the question of whether or not the doctor is obligated to look into such matters as the food people buy is concerned, I'd say yes . . . so long as those things pertain to medical illness. And in this particular family, it's especially important because they're all anemic. . . . But as for the social problems of this Puerto Rican family, they're beyond the scope of an everyday doctor to crack, in my opinion. . . .
>
> What we have here is a group of Americans coming from highly sordid conditions to live in highly sordid conditions. . . . Well, I think it's part of our responsibility to do something about this problem. . . .
>
> We had another case in a session on Thursday that bears on this. This is an Irish woman who's tied down with arthritis and who has a number of problems in addition. Among them is the fact that she lives in a one-room flat—dirty and with no heat. Well, the question arose as to whether it's the doctor's responsibility to get her another apartment and encourage her to move . . . or whether it's beyond the scope of the physician's work. . . .

The variety of opinion voiced in the course of such a conference provides a student with intimations that not only his classmates, but his instructors and physicians in general, are as perplexed as he is by questions about such matters as the boundaries of the doctor's professional task and the unsolved problems of patients like the Gonzales family. In the words of a faculty member who spoke up at the end of this conference:

> These questions don't only concern students . . . They concern doctors as well. . . . There just aren't many "ground rules" in this area. . . .

CONCLUSION

This paper reviews some experiences which acquaint the medical student with the different types of uncertainty he will encounter later as a practicing physician, and some of the ways in which he learns to deal with these uncertainties.

Because this is a preliminary description of what, it turns out, are rather complex processes, we have not organized the analysis around several basic distinctions that could be made. But it seems appropriate to introduce these now so that lines of a more systematic analysis can begin to emerge.

One basic type of uncertainty distinguished at the outset is that deriving from limitations in the current state of medical knowledge. Clearly, the different medical sciences vary in this respect. It has been indicated, for example, that limitations in a field like Pharmacology are now considerably greater than they are in, say, Anatomy. There are comparable differences among the clinical sciences. There would probably be general agreement that gaps in psychiatric knowledge are considerably greater than those in the field of Obstetrics and Gynecology. Such distinctions would provide a focus for further and more rigorous study of training for uncertainty. The different fields would be arranged according to the degree of uncertainty which characterizes them in order to see whether this ranking is paralleled by what the student learns from his different courses about the uncertainties of medicine. Are students made most aware of uncertainties when they are exposed to fields in which these uncertainties are greatest? More important, perhaps, is the question whether those fields in which limitations of knowledge are particularly prominent offer more or fewer means of coming to terms with uncertainty.

The second type of uncertainty, resulting from imperfect mastery of what is currently known in the various fields of medicine, was not analyzed in terms of its variability. We chose rather to concentrate on the "typical" or "model" student at different phases of his medical school career. But, obviously, there are significant individual differences, and these could provide a second focus in a more systematic study of training for uncertainty. Students vary in the level of skill which they achieve at any particular stage of their training. For example, those who find it easy to memorize details may have an advantage over their classmates in the study of Anatomy; those whose manual dexterity is highly developed may not experience the same degree of personal inadequacy as the less adroit students when they begin to carry out surgical procedures; extroverted students may find it easier to get along with patients than introverted classmates. These variations in aptitudes, skill, and knowledge may lead to individual differences in the extent to which students experience the uncertainties which derive from limitations of skill and knowledge. Students probably differ in awareness of their own limitations and in response to these limitations. Some may be more sensitive than others to their real or imagined lack of skill. Some may be more able than others to tolerate the uncertainties of which they are aware. As we have seen, distinctions such as these would have to be considered in a more precise investigation of training for uncertainty. Are relatively skilled students less likely than relatively unskilled students to become aware of those uncertainties that derive from limits on medical knowledge? Are students especially sensitive to the uncertainties which confront them better able than less sensitive classmates to cope with such uncertainties? Or, to raise a somewhat different sort of problem, do students with a low level of tolerance for such uncertainty perform less effectively in their medical studies than students who are able to accommodate themselves to uncertainty? The level of tolerance might also affect the choice of a career: for example, do students who find it difficult to accept the uncertainties which they encounter elect to go into fields of medicine in which there is less likelihood of meeting these uncertainties?

A third distinction involves the experiences through which the student becomes acquainted with the uncertainties of medicine. Some of them are directly comparable with those which a mature physician would encounter. For example, when he meets the tentative and experimental point of view of pharmacologists or when inconsistent findings make a definitive diagnosis problematic, the student is faced with exactly the same sort of unsurenesses met by a practicing physician. But other experiences seem to derive their elements of uncertainty from the teaching philosophies or curricular organization of the medical school. For instance, the uncertainties which a student experiences as a result of the avoidance of spoon feeding by the basic science faculty at Cornell or the atomistic division of his class in the third year are by-products of particular conditions in the medical school, although they may have their analogues in actual practice. This distinction would consequently have to be incorporated into a more detailed analysis of training for uncertainty. Which type of experience is more conducive to recognition of the uncertainties in medicine? Which is more easily handled by students? In view of the wide range of experiences in medical school which have a bearing on training for uncertainty, what is the relative balance between those experiences which are inherent in the role of physician and those which inhere in the role of student?

This concluding section is clearly not a summary of what has gone before. Instead, we have chosen this opportunity to make explicit some of the variables and distinctions which were only implicit in earlier pages in order to indicate further problems for the more systematic qualitative analysis of a process like training for uncertainty.

	PERCENTAGE OF EACH CLASS			
PROBLEM OF "UNCERTAINTIES"	FIRST YEAR	SECOND YEAR	THIRD YEAR	FOURTH YEAR
Quite sure I can deal with this	10	11	21	25
Fairly sure I can deal with this	52	61	60	72
Not sure I can deal with this	38	28	19	3
No. of students	(82)	(82)	(85)	(85)

Notes

1. Unless otherwise indicated, all the quoted phrases and passages in this paper are drawn from the diaries that eleven Cornell students at various points along the medical school continuum have kept for us over the course of the past three years; from interviews with these student diarists and some of their classmates; and from close-to-verbatim student dialogue recorded by the sociologist who carried out day-by-day observations in some of the medical school situations cited in this paper.

2. It is not only the doctor, of course, who must deal with the problem of uncertainty. To some extent this problem presents itself in all forms of responsible human action. The business executive or the parent, for example, has no assurance that his decisions will have the desired results. But the doctor is particularly subject to this problem for his decisions are likely to have profound and directly observable consequences for his patients.

3. This particular sentence was taken from the "Address of Welcome to the Class of 1957" delivered by Dr. Lawrence W. Hanlon. Everything else in the paragraph quoted above is extracted from "Some Steps in the Maturation of the Medical Student," a speech delivered by Dr. Robert F. Pitts at Opening Day Exercises, September 1952.

4. Pitts, *ibid.*

5. Such a felt sense that there will always be more to learn in medicine that he can possibly make his own, is the beginning of the medical student's acceptance of limitation. It might also be said that this same realization is often one of the attitudinal first signs of a later decision on the part of a student to enter a specialized medical field. This is of some relevance to the discussion of specialization by Patricia L. Kendall and Hanan C. Selvin, "Tendencies toward Specialization in Medical Training."

6. Joseph A. Wells, "Historical Background and General Principles of Drug Action" in: Victor A. Drill, ed., *Phar-macology in Medicine* (New York: McGraw-Hill Book Company, 1945), p. 6.

7. The physician is called upon to use his sense of smell and of taste on occasion, too, but not as frequently as those of sight, touch, and hearing.

8. Though the fourth year at Cornell is made up of three terms, we will discuss only the Medicine semester (Comprehensive Care) in this paper. The qualitative data (diaries, interviews, and observations) are not sufficient to do justice to the Surgery and Obstetrics-Gynecology terms that also form part of the fourth year.

9. For a more detailed description of the Comprehensive Care and Teaching Program and the kinds of experiences which students have in it, see: George G. Reader, "The Cornell Comprehensive Care and Teaching Program," and Margaret Olencki, "Range of Patient Contacts in the Comprehensive Care and Teaching Program."

10. The types of uncertainties a student encounters in the Comprehensive Care and Teaching Program seem to be like those he has dealt with recurrently since his days as a freshman. However, it is no longer so easily possible to distinguish which fourth-year experiences are salient for which types of uncertainty. Rather, in the situations in which the fourth-year student finds himself all types of uncertainty seem to converge and to be intertwined. For this reason we have found it necessary here to modify the pattern set in earlier sections of this paper, and we talk now largely in terms of undifferentiated uncertainties.

11. An indication of the marked increase in confidence is contained in a simple statistical result. In May 1955, all four classes at Cornell were asked how capable they felt about dealing with a number of problems encountered by practicing physicians. One of these problems concerned "the uncertainties of diagnosis and therapy that one meets in practice." The class-by-class distribution of replies on this item is shown in the Table.

12. From a report of the Comprehensive Care and Teaching Program to the Commonwealth Fund, March 30, 1954.

The Gomer Phenomenon

Deborah B. Leiderman
Jean-Anne Grisso

INTRODUCTION—THE CULTURE OF MEDICINE

Medical training and practice comprise both a cognitive world of facts and theories and a social world of relationships, symbols, values and specialized language. Informal labels of patients are part of the distinctive language that characterizes the medical subculture. It is a language not intended for the ears of patients, constituting a form of doctor-doctor, rather than doctor-patient communication. It belongs to what Goffman (1959) has termed "backstage behavior." Despite the widespread use of informal language by physicians and heightened societal interest in medical culture, the private medical language and informal labeling of patients by doctors has received scant attention from sociologists and physicians interested in the social aspects of medical practice. Scholarship has focused on professional socialization (Becker et al., 1961; Bucher and Stelling, 1977; Fox, 1957; Light, 1980; Mumford, 1970), management of time (Zerubavel, 1979), error (Bosk, 1979), and decision-making (Bosk, 1980), rather than physicians' perceptions of patients.

Elaborate descriptive terminology or extensive folklore and humor surrounding a particular theme frequently point to an aspect of culture that involves particular stress or conflict. Among the many terms used by young house physicians to describe patients are "gork," "crock," and "gomer." Gomer, one of the most commonly used terms has achieved recognition and lay usage through popularization in the novel, *The House of God* (Shem, 1978). In this fictionalized account of a medical internship at a large teaching hospital, gomers appear as patients whose illnesses frustrate the housestaff's every effort to ameliorate their condition. It is the purpose of this paper,

Reprinted from the *Journal of Health and Social Behavior*, vol. 26 (1985), pp. 222–231.

through analysis of the characteristics and physician perceptions of a group of patients labelled gomers, to attain some insight into the social system of medicine and its values and conflicts.

Given the nature of the house officers' role—the routine confrontation with suffering and death—one can understand why a private culture and language arise and flourish. As Fox has detailed, the work of physicians and nurses demands that they constantly confront "some of the most basic and the most transcendent aspects of the human condition" (Fox, 1979:12). In caring for patients, health professionals are obliged to violate strong cultural taboos against examining, penetrating, and handling the substances of other human bodies. Among the mechanisms physicians adopt for coping with the successful aspects of their work are the development of a scientific, unemotional style and the elaboration of "gallows" humor (Fox and Lief, 1963; Fox, 1979; see Coser, 1959, for a discussion of the function of humor in social groups, using the case of patients on a hospital ward). As Fox (1979) has observed, gallows humor is most florid in situations of extreme stress; in the medical setting, this brand of humor is often a reaction to stress-arousing medical uncertainty and inability to halt the approach of death. The special language and humor serve to maintain group solidarity among house officers and permit aspiring young professionals to express emotion in a ritualized fashion. The medical argot and in-group humor is, for the most part, hidden from public view by the outward adherence of physicians to their formal role-prescriptions of neutrality and detachment.

"GOMER": ORIGINS AND DEFINITIONS OF THE TERM

On the basis of a survey of physicians and nurses throughout the United States about the meaning and use of "gomer," George and Dundes (1978) conclude that the term originated in the late 1950s and was used in Veterans Administration Hospitals, large county hospitals, and university teaching hospitals. Its etymology has been variously traced to the television figure Gomer Pyle and to an old English word meaning fool. George and Dundes' physician informants suggested that it was an acronym for "Grand Old Man of the Emergency Room" (west coast) or "Get Out of My Emergency Room" (east coast).

On the basis of their survey, George and Dundes defined gomers in terms of the management problems they presented for doctors—poor hygiene, incontinence, habitual malingering, and a tendency to pull out intravenous lines. The profile of their typical gomer is an older man, debilitated, and in many cases, a chronic alcoholic on public assistance. He has a history of multiple hospitalizations and prefers life inside the hospital to life outside.

In their discussion, George and Dundes emphasize the human predicament of hospital staff and their need to give vent to their frustration through such mechanisms as "gomer assessment scales." They see young house officers' encounters with the gomer as a severe test of their capacity for role-prescribed compassion.

PURPOSE OF THE STUDY

For health professionals, the phenomenon of informal labeling of patients, especially the use of "gomer," is both interesting and troubling in that physicians are departing from the "ideal" norms and values of respect for the patient and professional role prescriptions. It raises several questions: Who are gomers? How do they differ from other patients? What function does the ascription serve? What occurs in the interaction between particular patients and young physicians-in-training that leads physicians to depart, at least in language, from the "ideal" value of respect for the patient and from the prescribed attitude of sympathetic but detached concern? Another legitimate question is: does labelling affect the care the patient receives? That question will have to await future investigations as it was not within the scope of our study to address it nor do we wish

to imply that any particular impact occurred. The intensity and energy invested in gomer lore suggest that we are dealing with a situation of particular stress and conflict, and that gomerism is not an isolated phenomenon but is, rather, related in a larger way to modern medicine.

STUDY PROCEDURE

To reach an understanding of the meaning of gomerism, an analysis was undertaken of the hospital records of "gomer" patients and of the attitudes and perceptions of the housestaff treating them. A pilot project involving review of charts of four patients identified by medical residents at University Hospital as gomers was conducted to identify the salient variables. This review, combined with our experience with the private medical language at University Hospital, suggested the following variables as important: the patient's social and occupational background, mental status, nature of the illness, diagnostic and/or therapeutic dilemmas posed, number of medical complications, and length of hospital stay. Two other factors that emerged from the preliminary study as potentially important were: behavior management problems posed by the patient and staff frustration with the patient's medical problem.

The final data base used included the patient's age, race, education, occupation, admission and discharge dates, admitting diagnosis, discharge diagnosis, social background, problems identified during hospitalization, consultations obtained, and number and nature of complications. In addition, the hospital course was summarized from the progress notes of physicians and nurses. All comments about patient behavior, indications of diagnostic or therapeutic disputes, and comments conveying staff responses to the patient were extracted.

Several demographic variables, such as age, sex, and social background, were taken directly from the patient's chart. Other variables, such as mental status decline and presence of a therapeutic or diagnostic dilemma, required a more complex judgment. For these variables, each case was rated independently by the two authors. In the rare instances of disagreement, a consensus determination was attained. The variables requiring observer rating and their definitions are listed in the Appendix.

Data were collected on two dates, in December 1979 and January 1980. All the junior residents in internal medicine supervising inpatient services at University Hospital were asked at a regular morning report for the names of gomer patients on their service. There was no discussion of the project and no definition of the term was offered. The residents simply listed the names. Eleven names were listed in December and eleven in January. One named appeared on both lists. Two charts could not be located. One chart, the subject of legal proceedings, also proved unobtainable. The final "gomer" sample thus comprised eighteen of the original twenty-one patients identified in the residents' lists.

A control sample of eighteen general medical patients was selected from the same hospital. For each gomer, one control patient matched by age, sex, and date of admission to a medical service was selected at random from computerized hospital admission records. The charts of the control patients were then reviewed in the manner described above and the same variables were rated.

The final step consisted of interviews with house physicians to learn how they used the term "gomer." Group interviews were conducted informally on regular work rounds with the medical teams each consisting of two interns and one resident.

WHO ARE GOMERS?

Analysis of the chart material compared the gomer to the control patients along three dimensions: patient background characteristics, events occurring during hospitalization, and outcome and disposition.

The gomers were in many ways a more heterogeneous group than George and Dundes' study suggests. They were both male (11) and female (7), black (8) and white (10), and their educational and socioeconomic backgrounds varied considerably. A doctor and a lawyer were among the gomers, as were retired laborers. Their ages ranged from 52 to 91 (see Table 1). The mean age was 69 years compared to the University Hospital medical patient mean age of 54 years (twelve month cumulative data for 1979). They were admitted to the hospital by both private attending physicians and the ward physician team. The shortest hospitalization was four days, the longest nine months. The medical diagnoses ranged from biopsy-confirmed cancer and end-stage renal disease to psychosomatic blackouts and drug-resistant pulmonary tuberculosis.

Neither occupational background nor race distinguished gomers from the control patients. However, at the time of hospital admission, gomer patients had diminished levels of activity and diminished ability to function in adult social roles relative to nongomer patients. Furthermore, one-half of the gomer patients suffered some degree of impairment in mental functioning on admission, compared to less than one-quarter of the control group.

The number of problems the two groups of patients presented to physicians was comparable; however, the patterns of their hospital stays contrasted dramatically. Gomer patients remained in the hospital longer than other patients, had more consultations for diagnosis and therapy, and posed more diag-

TABLE 1   Ascriptive characteristics of gomers (N = 18), controls (N = 18), and all University Hospital medical patients

		GOMER	CONTROL	ALL UNIVERSITY HOSPITAL MEDICAL PATIENTS
Sex	Male	11 (61%)	11 (61%)	55%
	Female	7 (39%)	7 (39%)	45%
Race	White	10 (56%)	11 (61%)	56%
	Black	8 (44%)	7 (39%)	43%
Age	Mean (range)	69 (52–91 yrs.)	69 (51–93 yrs.)	54 yrs.

nostic and therapeutic dilemmas for the physicians who cared for them.

The gomer patients presented more difficult medical and behavior management problems for their physicians. For example, twice as many gomers as nongomers suffered serious medical complications during hospitalization and more than two-thirds of the gomers suffered a deterioration in mental status, becoming, at least temporarily, disoriented and confused; only two nongomer patients became disoriented. Not surprisingly, then, house officers consulted the neurology service more frequently for assistance with their gomer patients than with their control patients. Many of the gomer patients became combative and required physical restraints or tranquilizing medication. Few gomer patients recovered fully, and three-quarters had some mental impairment at discharge, in contrast to the controls, who tended to be mentally intact and able to resume their adult roles at discharge.

Except for low social functioning score at the time of hospital admission for which a missing data problem existed, there was a significant difference ($p < .05$, chi-square) between gomers and controls on the following variables: prolonged hospital stay, greater number of specialist consultations, presence of a diagnostic dilemma, presence of a therapeutic dilemma, mental status decline during hospitalization, neurology consultation, behavior management problem, and nursing home placement at discharge.

In Table 2, gomers are compared with controls on a number of important variables dealing with the delivery of hospital services. Chi-square analysis reveals significant differences ($p < .05$) on a number

of these with three exceptions—impaired mental health status on admission, medical complications, and the presence of a psychiatric consultation. Gomers were significantly different (t-test of difference between the means) with regard to the mean number of consultations required during hospitalization (4.5 vs. 1.8) and the mean length of hospital stay in days (69.8 for gomers vs. 9.4 for controls). It is important to note that the mean length of stay for all University Hospital medical patients was 9.9, similar to the controls. . . .

The importance of psychiatric distress or disorders as a factor underlying the label *gomer* was apparent for several gomer patients whose complaints were diagnosed as psychosomatic. Two gomer patients had psychiatric disorders as the major discharge diagnosis, and in several others, major psychiatric problems complicated their medical illnesses; no psychiatric disorders were recorded for the control patients. Housestaff consulted the psychiatry service to aid in diagnosis and treatment of five of the eighteen gomers, but only one of the controls.

The dramatic contrast between gomer and control patients emerges most clearly from analysis of the whole pattern of hospitalization. (See Table 2.) Control patients tended to be admitted for specific diagnostic or therapeutic interventions, while gomers' admissions were characterized by an ambiguity of definition that was frustrating to housestaff. Seven of eighteen control patients were admitted specifically for diagnostic or therapeutic procedures that were performed without incident. The procedures, including hemodialysis, endoscopy, colonoscopy, bronchoscopy, and cardiac catheterization, were all

TABLE 2 Chi-square comparison of gomers (N = 18) and controls (N = 18) for nine hospital course events

HOSPITAL COURSE EVENTS	GOMERS	CONTROLS	p
Admission Mental Status Impaired	9	4	<.10
Discharge Mental Status Impaired	15	4	<.0004
Mental Status Decline	13	2	<.0007
Diagnostic Dilemma	6	0	<.025
Therapeutic Dilemma	12	3	<.007
Management Problem	9	2	<.03
Medical Complications	10	5	<.17
Neurology Consultation	12	1	<.0005
Psychiatry Consultation	5	1	<.15

elective, and the patients were discharged immediately.

The diagnostic or procedure focus of many of the control admissions did not indicate that the control patients were less seriously ill than the gomers. For example, among the control patients, two diagnostic procedures confirmed cancer and two revealed severe heart disease. That the presence of life-threatening illness did not differentiate the two groups is further supported by the finding that the number of resuscitations and transfers to the intensive care unit were comparable for the two groups (three in each).

The hospitalizations of the control patients appear as organized sequences of events, which provided definitive diagnoses, and a predictable, if not always happy, outcome. In contrast, the admitting problems of the gomers were much harder to define, the course of treatment much less predictable, and the outcome much less satisfactory. Their troublesome illnesses appeared to defy medical categories and procedures. None of the gomers was admitted for a single diagnostic procedure and only one for a single therapeutic procedure. This one therapeutic procedure, a knee replacement, resulted in multiple complications and deterioration in the patient's quality of life and functioning.

Gomers also differed from other patients in the outcome of the hospitalization. Consistent with their mental and functional impairment, nearly one-half of the gomer patients (8) were discharged to nursing homes, as compared to only two control patients (by chi-square, $p < .05$). Because of delays in obtaining nursing home beds, gomer patients frequently were hospitalized long after the resolution of their acute problems. Housestaff progress notes became less frequent and less descriptive, eventually consisting of such perfunctory comments as, "Stable. Awaiting nursing home placement." The average length of hospital stay for the eight gomer patients placed in nursing homes was 132 days as compared to 27 days for the other ten gomers. The prolonged wait for nursing home beds accounts for much of the difference in length of hospitalization between gomer and control patients, and also, we think for much of the housestaff's frustration with their gomer patients.

The gomer patients all lived to be discharged from the hospital; four of the control patients died. Significantly, in three of these four cases, the presence of terminal metastatic cancer was clearly documented and the physicians made the decision to abjure heroic interventions and make the patient comfortable. No resuscitations of these patients were attempted; they were allowed to die without aggressive therapy. Indeed, when asked on work rounds about the defining characteristics of gomers, house physicians did not include the outcome of hospitalization. Rather, their responses emphasized their frustration with the ongoing medical and behavioral management difficulties posed by gomer patients. Several house physicians emphasized the lack of gratification these patients provide; one even described them as "hurting interns." Over and over again, interns and residents defined a gomer as a patient for whom conventional medical practices are ineffective or even harmful, as "someone who, when we help him, gets worse, when we leave him alone, gets better." The perception of the management of these patients as "not right" intensified as the number of diagnostic and therapeutic procedures perceived to be futile, or even deleterious, increased.

Gomerism is defined not by the patients' physical illnesses—which do not clearly distinguish them from other patients—but rather by the patterns and events of their hospitalization and the social outcomes of their illnesses.

CASE STUDIES

Descriptions of the demographic characteristics, medical illnesses, and hospitalization courses of the gomer patients in the aggregate does not adequately capture the human complexity of the gomer, his or her illness and his or her hospital experience. Nor do general descriptions convey the frustration, fears, and compassion of the hospital staff who care for gomer patients. The following profiles of five gomer patients are included to give concrete illustration to the composite profile presented above.

Case #1: Mrs. C.

Mrs. C. was a sixty-year-old white woman, brought to the hospital emergency room after being found comatose at home. Her admitting diagnosis was hypothermia (life-threatening state of sub-normal body temperature). She was described as unresponsive and as having all the signs of "long-term self neglect."

Her arthritic bodily deformities were so severe that advanced radiologic studies were mechanically impossible to perform. She had severe bedsores extending to the bone and was covered with excrement. No cause for her hypothermia could be identified. The patient lived with her son, who carried a diagnosis of schizophrenia. He reported that his mother had been lying on the floor for several days prior to hospitalization. During his mother's hospitalization, the son, a regular visitor, became acutely psychotic. He roamed the hospital's wards seeking out his mother's doctors. After several suicide attempts, he too was hospitalized.

Housestaff notes over several months indicated little progress for Mrs. C. Continuous diarrhea aggravated her bedsores. Warm-water tank therapy for her arthritis was impeded by incontinence. Other complications of her hospitalization included a fractured arm, gastrointestinal hemorrhage, and intermittent fevers attributed to reinfection of her ulcers. Initial treatment with anti-depressants improved her mental status but she subsequently developed the side-effect of urinary retention. Her behavior toward hospital staff was described as hostile and aggressive. She repeatedly asked, "Why are they keeping me half-alive?" The consulting psychiatrist diagnosed a chronic dementia and recommended nursing home placement, but the patient and her son refused to consider it.

Mrs. C. and her son, unable to care for themselves and socially destitute, with no family or institution to care for them, are tragic figures. The enormous management problems the patient and her suicidal son presented to the housestaff, in combination with the extremely slow rate of the patient's clinical improvement, were sources of stress and frustration. The patient's own articulation of the misery of her hospital existence starkly emphasized for the housestaff the futility of endless heroic interventions in the face of refractory illness and the patient's loss of dignity and will to life.

Case #2: Mr. L.

Mr. L., a fifty-seven-year-old man, was a successful businessman prior to the onset of his debilitating neurological symptoms which left him unable to meet his daily responsibilities. He epitomized a subtype of gomer: the patient with a *debilitating chronic ill-*

ness who posed a difficult diagnostic and therapeutic problem. On admission to the hospital, he was described as a demented and pathetic recluse with gait ataxia (unsteadiness). Although his condition was labeled idiopathic (of unknown etiology) by the attending physicians, the housestaff privately attributed his neurological illness to alcoholism. His hospital admission was prompted by complaints of blackouts, which had not been observed by his family. The standard battery of diagnostic tests for syncope was performed, although the same battery had been unrevealing at another hospital. Again, no cause was identified. Mr. L. did, however, develop complications from the tests. A severe scalp infection at the site of an electroencephalography lead resulted in worsening of his previously well-controlled diabetes. He became confused and incontinent and, after being "found on the floor" several times, was restrained in bed. The intern and the attending physician disagreed over management of the patient's diabetes. The house officer argued that, given the limited value of prolonged hospitalization, the patient's wish to return home should be honored.

The case of Mr. L. embodies several value conflicts endemic to modern medical practice. The gomer label derived from housestaff frustration with an evolving situation of increasingly inappropriate care, in this instance, a patient subjected to prolonged hospitalization and repeated tests, despite evidence strongly suggesting that little could be done. Not only did hospitalization fail to help the patient, but, indeed, it had the opposite effect—intensifying illness and psychological distress. The uncertainty aroused by symptoms that resist definition and placement in a recognizable disease category was intensified by the lack of consensus among team physicians about what might reasonably be done. This case exemplifies the potential conflict between the physician's desire for diagnostic certainty and the traditional medical ethic which places the patient's welfare above all other considerations.

Case #3: Mr. F.

Mr. F. presented a different set of frustrations for the housestaff. In no way did this fifty-two-year-old white man resemble the ill-kept, malingering gomer described by George and Dundes. Nor was he a senile, social reject with multiple, chronic problems. He was a successful office manager until fifteen months before admission, when his complaints commenced. After two hospitalizations, thousands of dollars spent on laboratory tests, and exploratory surgery in a community hospital had all proved unrevealing and no therapy ameliorated his symptoms, he was referred to University Hospital for further evaluation.

At the time of admission, he was unable to work. He complained of headaches, shortness of breath, staggering, pains in his arms and hands, fatigue, light-headedness. He told nurses that he was anxious and often hyperventilated, and worried that his doctors would say his symptoms were "all in his head." Past medical records were obtained and reviewed; consultants in cardiology, otolaryngology, and neurology were brought in.

The cardiologist felt the patient's symptoms were non-cardiac in origin; the consultant neurologist suggested that "part of the trouble is functional." The admitting physician, a specialist in pulmonary medicine, had agreed that if all studies were negative, a psychiatric consultation would be requested. When all the studies failed to define an underlying organic pathology, the patient was referred back to his local physician without the recommended psychiatric evaluation. The discharge diagnosis was: "Dizziness, probably functional, followup with local M.D."

Mr. F.'s multiple somatic complaints presented both diagnostic and therapeutic dilemmas. Furthermore, the failure to diagnose organic pathology aroused uncertainty in the hospital staff. A patient like Mr. F. forces doctors to confront the limits of medical science and to question their own professional expertise. Psychosomatic illness such as Mr. F.'s is particularly problematic for physicians ill-prepared by technologically-oriented medicine to manage problems in which the pathologic mechanism or lesion cannot be identified. Mr. F. was perhaps the antithesis of the prototype control patient, who presented a readily identified symptom constellation defined by a diagnostic procedure and amenable to appropriate therapy.

Case #4: Dr. D.

A particularly poignant patient was an eighty-three-year-old single woman who received a medical degree from the university whose hospital ER she was now compelled to enter in the much reduced circumstances of a frail elderly patient with vague somatic complaints. A consultant psychiatry resident diagnosed an organic brain syndrome. The admitting medical resident's diagnosis, however, perhaps reflecting a combination of experience and cynicism, read: "Social complaints—nursing home placement." Dr. D.'s private attending physician described her on the second hospital day as "more confused than ever, no longer able to take care of herself."

Dr. D. presented an unending management problem in the hospital. A sympathetic resident, whose physical examination Dr. D. refused, noted: "She is a very proud woman who is distressed at her failing memory." Repeatedly, progress notes describe her as agitated, and refusing medication. Nursing notes document at least three falls, two of which involved head lacerations requiring sutures.

Dr. D.'s impaired mental status and her social isolation made discharge planning difficult. Because she had no relative to take responsibility for her, a legal guardian had to be appointed before nursing home placement could be arranged. The legal proceedings that culminated in the appointment of a fellow church member as her guardian spanned five weeks.

Dr. D. was one of several patients who had no illness requiring acute hospital care, but were housed in University Hospital for months awaiting the availability of a nursing home bed because they had nowhere else to go.

Despite the major management difficulties which Dr. D. presented and the lack of medical interest which her disease provided for the housestaff, the physician and nursing notes convey enormous empathy for this woman. Nursing notes repeatedly state: "She is off floor with R.N. to snack bar, . . . off floor with extern for coke . . ." The residents' empathic notes suggest respect for this fiercely independent, pioneering woman. They also suggest a degree of identification with this elderly physician patient whose condition underscores the harsh reality that physicians themselves are in no way protected from the universal human experiences of illness, suffering, aging and death.

Case #5: Mrs. J.

An unanticipated and haunting category of gomer specified by house physicians was the "iatrogenic gomer," that is, a patient whose gomer characteristics were acquired as a consequence of hospitalization.

Mrs. J. was an eighty-two-year-old black woman, a retired domestic worker who at the time of admission lived independently, cared for herself and did volunteer work in her church. On admission to the hospital—the first hospitalization of her life—to the orthopedics service for an elective total knee replacement, she was described as mentally intact, a "lovely patient." Her only complaint was the pain of her degenerative joint disease. After a routine medical consultation, Mrs. J. was declared fit for surgery. Postoperatively she developed a urinary tract infection secondary to an indwelling catheter and was treated with antibiotics, as a consequence of which she developed acute renal failure, with the attendant complications of vomiting, bleeding, and anemia. Hemodialysis was complicated by bleeding at the catheter site severe enough to require transfusions. Her surgical wound broke down and she was returned to the operating room. She became febrile and confused. Bedsores developed while she was in traction. Her kidney failure and consequent anorexia and nausea resulted in malnutrition and impaired healing of her incision. Mrs. J.'s hospital stay lasted five months, and a previously aging, but independent and cognitively intact woman was discharged to a nursing home. Housestaff feelings about Mrs. J. were revealed in the sardonic billing of her as an "iatrogenic gomer," in repeated references in her chart to "this unfortunate woman," and in the housestaff's reiteration of the maxim, "Patients over seventy years old are to be revered, not admitted to the hospital."

DISCUSSION

The gomer image that emerges from this study is not a simple stereotype. Gomer is neither a class-linked nor race-linked pejorative term, nor is the term applied merely to malingering, self-destructive patients. Several characteristics did, however, distinguish gomers from other medical patients. As a category, gomers were patients whose illnesses and management posed special frustrations for resident physicians. Gomers suffered irreversible mental deterioration; their illnesses were complex and intract-

able; they were unable to resume normal adult social roles; and they had no place to go upon discharge.

Gomers have a symbolic significance for house officers out of proportion to their numbers and even out of proportion to the efforts they require. The process of labeling gomers both identifies a problem and provides a kind of resolution. Gomers may be seen as an index of medicine's insoluble problems—the diagnostic dilemmas, the gradual deterioration in mental function, the chronic disabling problems that lead neither to death nor cure but to the new twentieth century institution, the nursing home.

The inconsistencies in the system—the gap between the myth of omnipotence of technologic medicine and the realities of gomer patients on the wards—become starkly visible to young physicians in the early stages of professional socialization. Although the recourse to informal labeling of patients may be construed as a breakdown in defenses—the perfectly defended and socialized physician would not need such outlets—it may also be viewed as one mode of coping with the enormous physical and emotional demands placed on housestaff.

On another level, gomerism signals major points of stress in the system, situations that involve peculiarly modern social and medical dilemmas as well as universal existential problems. Modern high-technology, interventionist medicine not only makes possible, but frequently appears to dictate, intervention in patients whose illnesses were merely passively observed by doctors only decades ago. Yet in some patients (cf. our cases Mr. F. and Mrs. J.), medical intervention is to no avail, or even harmful.

The gomer patient, who deteriorates in the hospital, whose illness is unlikely to be significantly improved by medical treatment, who has no concerned family to place him in a meaningful social network and confer personhood (Crane, 1975) as opposed to mere patienthood upon him, confronts resident physicians with two profound threats to their ideals of themselves as physicians. The lingering presence on acute medical wards of patients for whom modern medicine can provide no therapy, or frequently even diagnosis, challenges physicians' ideals about the powers of medicine. The gomer patient forces the young physician to confront uncertainty—that which arises from the limits and gaps in the present state of medical knowledge and perhaps that arising from doubts about his own competence as well (Fox, 1957 and 1979; Light, 1979). Which failure does the gomer represent—the system's or the individual doctor's? Why do the gomer's problems not yield to the aggressive meliorism that is the hallmark and pride of modern medicine? Gomers defy the expectations of both physicians and laymen in an age of seemingly miraculous advances in medical technology.

It is significant that the use of a private internal language is largely confined to physicians in residency training, that is, to idealistic and ambitious young persons in a transitional phase in their careers. Tales abound of severe censure of housestaff by older attending physicians at various university hospitals for the use of epithets like gomer. Senior physicians tend not to use terms like gomer perhaps because they are protected from the frustration, helplessness, and uncertainty that these patients generate. Such physicians are not "front-line," that is, they are not required to care for the difficult hospitalized patients in the intensive, minute-to-minute way required of housestaff. More important, their experience has tempered and made more realistic their expectations of medicine and of themselves. They presumably have learned to tolerate uncertainty, to accept the limits of medicine. While the professional values of attending physicians have been shaped by their earlier experiences in caring for chronically ill patients who do not improve, young residents who have been socialized in the meliorist culture of technologic medicine find their conceptions of medicine and physicianhood challenged by their ward encounters with gomers.

Another difference between senior physicians and house staff is that the latter are formally still at the learning stage. Despite the fact that housestaff often have heavy amounts of responsibility for patient care, they are neophytes, and, indeed, look to patients as sources of learning. From patients they expect to derive much of the knowledge they will need to function on their own, without supervision. House staff are compelled by the nature of their position as trainees to judge patients in terms of their learning value. The so-called "interesting case" epitomizes the desirable patient from an educational vantage point. Gomers are rarely, if ever, interesting cases.

Elderly people are deposited, with increasing frequency, in the hands of a medical profession increasingly concerned with science and its applications. At the same time that society tries to impose limits on the power and jurisdictions of professionals in general and physicians in particular, it expects modern medicine and scientific physicians to provide solutions for many human woes which are really social and existential in nature (Knowles, 1977). That it may be utterly unreasonable to expect a medical solution to the problems of aging and social isolation does not relieve the pressure upon young physicians to use science to heal the patient.

In an era in which the goal of medical care has become cure even though only a few decades ago relief and comfort were acceptable ideals for physician and patient alike, it is little wonder that patients with refractory problems are particularly troubling to housestaff. For overworked, young physicians, the seemingly inexorable decline of patients whose humanness, in their often confused and combative states, may be difficult to perceive represents failure which underscores the impotence of modern medicine. Gomer image and lore captures the universal human fears of illness, intellectual decline, loss of autonomy, and aging as well as the doctor's frustration that modern medicine which promises to do so much, too often fails to deliver on its promise.

In conclusion, gomerism is a phenomenon arising out of the interaction of physicians in training with patients who present complex chronic, medical, psychological, and social problems in the setting of the acute care technologically-oriented hospital. It remains for future research to determine more precisely which characteristics of the patient and the setting lead to the application of the gomer label; and to determine whether this application affects the care and treatment of patients.

APPENDIX

Definitions of Variables Requiring Observer-Rating

1. Admission Mental Status—A rating of intact or impaired was derived from the neurologic section of the admitting resident's history and physical examination.
2. Discharge Mental Status—A rating of intact

or impaired was derived from the discharge note. If mental status was omitted from the discharge summary, a rating was derived from the final hospital day's progress note.

3. Mental Status Decline—This was defined as any deterioration, temporary or permanent, from admission mental status, occurring at any point during the hospitalization. For example, a patient admitted confused who subsequently lapsed into coma was considered to have had a mental status decline even if he returned to baseline mental state prior to discharge.

4. Social Functioning at Admission—Patients were defined as functionally active if they were employed or, if retired, were able to perform volunteer work or housework. Patients were considered to be inactive if illness rendered them unable to perform their customary roles and activities.

5. Occupational Status—Three categories, professional/managerial, skilled labor, and unskilled labor were used. Housewives were categorized as skilled if no other occupation was specified.

6. Diagnostic Dilemma—Cases were coded for the presence of a dilemma if physician progress notes explicitly described the illness as a diagnostic problem or if overt or covert disagreement among team doctors or consultants was evident.

7. Therapeutic Dilemma—Judged present if initial therapeutic interventions were unsuccessful and at least two consultations were obtained for advice regarding therapy.

8. Behavior Management Problem—Judged present if both housestaff and nursing notes documented at least one event in which physical restraints or tranquilizing drugs were used to restrain the patient.

9. Medical Complications—Complications were considered present when major new medical problems developed during the hospitalization, e.g. infection following urinary tract catheterization or post-operatively. This category was coded conservatively, and mental status deterioration after diagnostic or therapeutic procedures was specifically excluded to retain independence of the two variables.

References

BECKER, HOWARD S., BLANCHE GEER, EVERETT C. HUGHES, and ANSELM STRAUSS.
1961 Boys in White: Student Culture in Medical School. Chicago: University of Chicago Press.

BOSK, CHARLES L.
1979 Forgive and Remember: Managing Medical Failure. Chicago: University of Chicago Press.
1980 "Occupational rituals in patient management." New England Journal of Medicine 303:71–76.

BUCHER, RUE, and JOAN G. STELLING.
1977 Becoming Professional. Beverly Hills, CA: Sage Publications.

COSER, ROSE LAUB
1959 "Some social functions of laughter: A study of humor in a hospital setting." Human Relations 12:171–182.

CRANE, DIANA
1975 The Sanctity of Social Life: Physicians' Treatment of Critically Ill Patients. New York: Russell Sage Foundation.

FOX, RENÉE C.
1957 "Training for uncertainty." Pp. 207–241 in Robert K. Merton, George G. Reader, Patricia L. Kendall (eds.), The Student-Physician: Introductory Studies in the Sociology of Medical Education. Cambridge: Harvard University Press.
1979 "The Human Condition of Health Professionals." Lecture delivered at the University of New Hampshire; November 19, 1979.

FOX, RENÉE C., and HAROLD I. LIEF
1963 "Training for detached concern in medical students." Pp. 12–35 in Harold Lief, Victor F. Lief, and Nina R. Lief (eds.), The Psychological Basis of Medical Practice. New York: Harper and Row.

GEORGE, VICTORIA, and ALAN DUNDES
1978 "The gomer: A figure of American hospital folk speech," Journal of American Folklore 91:568–581.

GOFFMAN, ERVING
1959 The Presentation of Self in Everyday Life. Garden City, NY: Doubleday.

KNOWLES, JOHN H.
1977 "Introduction," in Doing Better and Feeling Worse: Health in the United States. Proceedings of the American Academy of Arts and Sciences 106:1–8.

LIGHT, DONALD, JR.
1979 "Uncertainty and control in professional training." Journal of Health and Social Behavior 20:310–322.

1980 Becoming Psychiatrists: The Professional Transformation of Self. New York: Norton.

MUMFORD, EMILY
1970 Interns; From Students to Physicians. Cambridge:
Harvard U. Press.

SHEM, SAMUEL
1978 The House of God. New York: Dell.

ZERUBAVEL, EVIATAR
1979 Patterns of Time in Hospital Life. Chicago: U. of
Chicago Press.

Professional Socialization in a Surgical Specialty: Acquiring Medical Judgment

Kathleen Knafl
Gary Burkett

The ability to exercise sound judgment is a highly valued component of the physician's professional skill system. The physician's image of medical work suggests that the practice of medicine is more complex than the routine application of abstract therapeutic principles to specific cases. It is believed to require, in addition, a large degree of an ability to make successful decisions in the face of ambiguous circumstances. In previous work [1] we have described the factors which tend to minimize the amount of routine, and maximize the necessity for the exercise of judgment in medical practice. In this paper we concentrate on the process through which the skill is acquired in the postgraduate phase of medical education.

Any contemporary discussion of the place of judgment in the practice of medicine needs to take cognizance of the fact that important political issues are involved [2]. A variety of current legislative proposals related to the delivery of medical care, includ-

ing various schemes for regulating payment for physician services, are bringing the issue of the importance of judgment in medical practice to the fore. The notion that the work of an occupation demands skills which are not easily codified nor easily learned is an important part of the ideology of, not only the medical profession, but any profession or occupation seeking to maximize its own autonomy. It is in the self-interest of any occupation to claim that its work involves capacities which are beyond the understanding of any lay person and hence beyond evaluation by an individual from outside the ranks of the occupation itself. Within medicine the element of individual judgment is sometimes held to be so important and so elusive that evaluation of one physician by other physicians, as well as by outsiders, is precluded. The future of proposals for various types of regulation of medical practice hinges, in part, on the degree to which medicine is able to convincingly substantiate its claim that much of its work involves making judgments which are beyond evaluation.

Phrased most concisely the most cogent question

Reprinted from Social Science and Medicine, vol. 9 (1975), pp. 397–404.

seems to be, "Is the emphasis on judgment in the ideology of medicine a consequence of self-serving professional interests?" To answer that question would seem to require a thorough examination of the nature of medical work so as to describe the actual degree of complexity and ambiguity involved. Such an approach has been taken by Freidson [3] who finds the emphasis on the necessity for judgment unwarranted by the nature of the actual medical work. David Mechanic, another long-time observer of the medical care scene, has recently repeated the position that the practice of medicine is characterized by qualities which necessitate the exercise of judgment.

> *Even though there are particular medical procedures for which there is wide agreement on the proper course to follow, much activity in the health field and the management of many of the most common diseases are characterized by considerable imprecision and disagreement [4].*

In a previous work we contended that:

> *To the extent that the practice of medicine consists of the application of techniques which must be selected from a body of conflicting opinion to patients whose individual attributes are seen as presenting unique problems by practitioners who possess special abilities and who value the evidence of their own experience, the exercise of judgment will be required [5].*

The actual extent to which medical work is, and must be, such a complex and ambiguous matter is open to question. What is clear is that the surgical residents who were the subjects of this study strongly believe that the ability to exercise judgment is a fundamental prerequisite for medical practice. By the time individuals have reached the specialty or residency phase of training they are fairly well along in the process of professional socialization. Lay conceptions of medicine have long since been replaced by the medical subculture of the professional. An important aspect of this subculture is the comparatively greater value placed on clinical as opposed to academic learning and knowledge [6,7]. Individual experience can, and often does, take precedence over findings reported in scientific journals. The residents we studied were engaged in accumulating such a store of clinical experience for themselves.

In this paper we concentrate on the process through which these residents go about pursuing and acquiring this highly valued skill. After discussing the mechanisms through which judgment is learned, we will describe those strategies employed by the residents to maximize their learning. Our purpose is to demonstrate the ways in which medical judgment, like scientific knowledge and technical skills, is a component of medical practice which is cultivated in medical training.

METHODOLOGY

Data for this paper were gathered as part of an ongoing study of professional socialization. The study subjects were all 20 residents of a 4-yr state university training program in orthopedic surgery. Data were collected over a 9-month interval during which time we observed the residents in a variety of settings. The residents were equally divided, five apiece in each year of the training program and systematically rotated through four different hospitals at 10-week intervals. These hospitals were varied in nature and included a university hospital, a public county hospital, a Veterans Administration facility and a private community hospital. The bulk of our observations were carried out at the university and Veterans Administration hospitals. Within these settings we observed in a variety of contexts, with particular care being taken to cover the entire range of the residents' professional activities. We had ample opportunity to observe and often informally interview residents on the hospital wards, in various outpatients clinics, during surgery and at their weekly academic conferences.

Immediately following a field observation, we dictated our field notes for later transcription. Transcripts were double checked for accuracy, coded and transferred to sort cards in order to facilitate a systematic analysis of the data. Field observations were supplemented with intensive interviews, which were processed in a similar manner.

There is a good deal of equality in the program's official division of labor. Residents in each year of the program spend roughly the same amount of time in surgery and in seeing clinic patients. Neither the residents nor the more formal structure of the training program specify a sharp distinction in the division of labor by year of the residency. The pervading belief is that one learns orthopedics by doing it and a 1st-yr resident is expected to become immediately involved in both the clinical and academic aspects of the program. This does not mean that no differences exist in the capabilities and responsibilities of 1st- and 4th-yr residents. However, it is in the area of orthopedic judgment that the residents acknowledge important differences between the junior and senior residents.

Although our original interest had been to investigate the acquisition of technical surgical ability, our initial field encounters pointed us in other directions. From the onset, the residents stressed to us and to each other that the development of sound orthopedic judgment is more important than the mastery of specific technical skills. Our own emphasis on the issue is thus firmly grounded in our data.

LEARNING JUDGMENT IN ORTHOPEDICS: DECISION MAKING

It is important to emphasize again that trainees enter the residency already convinced of the importance of judgment in the practice of medicine. In a study of the prior socialization of incoming trainees of several professional training programs, Bucher and her associates emphasize that "It is not enough to focus solely on the events of the training period because these events are experienced by persons who already have a perspective toward the situation" [8]. Trainees entering the specific program studied had all completed 4 yrs of medical school and an additional year of internship. Several had completed a year of general surgical training prior to entering orthopedics and about half had served in a medical capacity in the armed services. In short, the residents studied were not newcomers to the medical subculture which stresses the necessity of clinical experience. Such experience and the knowledge it brings is viewed as a crucial buttress to theoretical knowledge when making decisions in the face of uncertain circumstances. As such, it is a key component of judgment. Residents entered the program fully aware of the uncertain circumstances surrounding much of the decision making that goes on in medicine. A 1st-yr resident expressed the situation to a group of medical students saying that "medicine isn't black or white; it's all shades of grey."

The trainees' awareness of the often ambiguous nature of medical decision making is further confirmed and strengthened upon entering the residency program where they immediately find themselves in situations where decisions are being made. Here they can hear for themselves that the residents ahead of them in the program believe orthopedics to be one of the most ambiguous of specialties. The predominance of this belief came as an initial surprise to the investigators who had selected orthopedic surgery for the study on the grounds that it seemed to be one of the most clearly defined medical specialties.

> I (field worker) say, "I've been surprised that everything doesn't seem as clear-cut as I thought it was in the beginning." He (the resident) sort of picks this up saying, "That's for sure. I thought everything was going to be fairly clear-cut, but it just isn't that way."

Thus, while the relative ambiguity of the practice of orthopedics may come as a surprise to a few of the incoming residents, the understanding that specific cases will not always "follow the book" is well within their frame of reference. It is something with which they have had ample experience within their previous training.

Having already been exposed to a professional culture in which medical judgment is given high value, the residents quickly become involved in the process of decision making. When asked how one developed judgment, one resident summed up the process simply saying, "You do a case and you see what happens." In short, orthopedic judgment is seen as developing in a continual process of deciding how a specific case is to be treated and evaluating the outcome of that treatment, with the growing store of such evaluations contributing to the quality of one's judgment in subsequent decisions. The residents view the process as being a simple one:

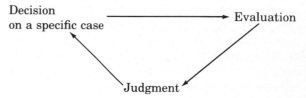

Medical judgment is formed in orthopedics during 4 yrs of continually more active involvement in the decision making and subsequent evaluative processes of patient treatment.

Beginning with his 1st day as a new resident the new trainee is confronted with situations in which he must learn to integrate and apply the raw materials of orthopedic decision making. Two prime ingredients of decision making are clinical experience and the orthopedic literature. The interplay of practical and theoretical knowledge in determining diagnosis and treatment is readily observable during grand rounds, where second, third and fourth year residents present cases of special interest to a gathering of orthopedic residents and attending physicians. An interesting case is one involving singularly difficult diagnostic and/or treatment problems; a case in which greater than usual input and judgment are needed in order to reach a decision. The following passages from notes taken during grand rounds illustrate the interplay of these two factors in determining treatment:

> After the residents finished presenting the case to the audience, one of the attendings asked, "What about doing a cup arthroplasty on him?" Morrison replied, "There's some literature to back it up but it's my experience that 'cups' just aren't that successful on young people."

Clinical and theoretical knowledge are not necessarily compatible, as the following selection from our field notes shows:

> The second case is presented by Dr. Lee, a 4th-yr resident. He shows slides of a 13-month-old girl whose one leg is shorter than the other. The reason for presenting the case is to discuss whether or not the leg should be surgically lengthened. In presenting the case, Dr. Lee quotes from a source in favor of such a procedure. Dr. Eddy, an attending physician, interrupts with, "I know that's what he says, but that's not the way we do it here." Another one of the attending men adds, "That's the way some of us do it!"

Presentation of cases during grand rounds is one of the few responsibilities of the residency in which the 1st-yr residents are not expected to participate. Presumably their knowledge and their clinical experience in orthopedics are too scant to allow them to make meaningful contributions to grand rounds. The following excerpt from our field notes reflects this:

> I asked Mitchell if the residents generally talked much at these conferences. He said, "not usually, not unless they are called on . . . (pause). Oh, they might if there was something they really wanted to bring up. Certainly no one of my status (1st yr) would ever say anything."

First-year residents do, however, show a great deal of interest in the kinds of information used in resolving highly ambiguous cases as well as the manner in which such evidence is assessed and applied.

A similar process of integrating diverse types of information in making decisions takes place on the wards and in the clinics. Here too, the process is most readily observed when the case in question is particularly difficult. The following incident is an example of decision making as it routinely occurs in the daily round of activities:

> Stevens and Giles look at the X-ray of the man's foot and Stevens says, "Well, technically it doesn't meet the criteria for (cites a specific procedure), but clinically I think it's indicated, since he's had repeated sprains." Kramer, the attending, walks in and Stevens repeats what he's just said. Kramer seems to disagree, saying how it's been his experience that what Stevens wants to do just doesn't work in practice. He suggests a more conservative treatment of injecting the foot with cortisone. After a bit more discussion, Stevens agrees with this and prepares the injection.

During the 4th yr of an orthopedic surgery residency the trainee has many opportunities to integrate and apply his continually growing knowledge of orthopedic theory and practice. Thus, not only is he learning new kinds of relevant information, but more importantly, he is continually required to bring this information to bear when making a decision.

If such learning is to occur, residents must have access to situations in which decisions are made. The occasions at which the majority of decisions are made are such that decision-making inputs usually take place in a group setting, providing ample opportunity for junior residents to begin learning judgment. The following incident taken from our field notes is an example of a typical discussion concerning patient treatment:

> *The case was of a man who had previously had his hip fused. He was currently in the hospital because of a fractured femur on the same leg. The fact that his hip joint no longer bent was making treatment of the femur more difficult. The attending was leading the discussion with the residents asking such questions as, "Give me three good reasons why not to do. . . ." He would then name specific procedures which were rather methodically discussed in terms of reasons to and not to do them. All four residents present were making suggestions concerning the treatment of the case. Generally, somebody would say, "What about doing. . . ." and name a specific technique or form of traction. Everyone else would point out the specific pitfalls of the suggested technique—sometimes including the person making the suggestion.*

While junior residents are thus able to enter into discussions regarding various treatment options and while their opinions are solicited and given consideration, the actual responsibility for decision making lies with the senior residents, with varying degrees of involvement by the attending physicians. The more junior residents are thus able to concentrate on developing decision making skills without having to assume full responsibilities for outcomes. In contrast, the situation of the 4th-yr resident who is responsible for all the cases on his service comes closer to approximating the position of the practicing specialist.

The group context of decision making is similarly essential to the residents' learning to recognize and evaluate unique qualities of the patient which are relevant to the choice of a treatment regimen. The importance of being sensitive to the individual patient's characteristics and needs was described to one of the investigators by a 4th-yr resident. He said:

> *Some people think orthopedics is the most impersonal specialty, but this really isn't true at all. You really have to work with the patient—work through the decision with him about what kind of surgery is best, whether or not to do surgery and when is the best time to do it. There has to be a lot of cooperation with the patient in orthopedics.*

At times unique patient characteristics can actually compete with the more technical principles practitioners must consider in reaching a decision in a specific case. In such circumstances collective input regarding the final decision is likely as in the following incident where all the residents and two of the attendings assigned to the rotation were present:

> *The X-rays are of a woman in her early thirties who has an infected hip. The question is whether or not to do a hip disarticulation, i.e. an amputation, or to pursue a more conservative form of treatment. Adams (senior resident) indicates that he wants to get Dr. Simons' (attending) opinion. After the X-rays have been presented, Dr. Bowen (attending) notes that there is no guarantee that disarticulation is going to help. In response Adams says, "I agree with you completely, but this lady has just seen the third decade of her life fly by in a cast. Are we going to tell her that's the way she is going to spend the fourth decade, too? She is psychologically prepared for the operation. She came back expecting it!" Dr. Simons says, "The problem with a disarticulation is that it's a poor prosthesis and there's a huge wound with much greater risk of infection." Shaking his head, Hancock says to me, "The residents wanted to do surgery on that one. The woman has been in pain, she's had pus, and been infected for eight years now. I mean, at what point do you start having a little empathy for the patient? You wonder how long you can keep up with the so-called conservative treatment."*

It is apparent from the last speaker's remarks that the residents, as a group, had already considered the case and felt that their decision to do an extensive surgical procedure required the attendings' corroboration. In weighing the same information the attendings settled on a very different course of treatment. The actual discussion was much more extensive than the above excerpt with the residents and attendings considering the pros and cons of the alternative treatments. In so doing, they referred to theoretical knowledge and clinical experience as well as the patient's unique situation. It is clear that there were differences of opinion over the course of treatment based on technical considerations vs. considerations related to the patient's psychological state and history. This interchange exemplifies the way in which various kinds of relevant information are brought to bear on a case in the decision-making process and the group context in which these decisions are often made.

Such patient characteristics as emotional state or number of previous surgeries may influence the decision with regard to a course of treatment, and the discussion of these characteristics provides a context for developing judgment. The decisions are a result of a group process involving both junior and senior residents and often attending physicians. In these situations various kinds of knowledge or information are recognized as pertinent and subsequently taken into account when deciding on a course of action. As the following discussion between a 4th-yr resident and a 1st-yr resident demonstrates, a central function of the residency is to provide the prospective orthopedic surgeon with adequate time and opportunity to cultivate the judgment needed to make successful decisions:

> They begin discussing two different kinds of hip surgeries. Mitchell (1st-yr resident) says, "I'll tell you, George (4th-yr resident), I don't know enough to tell you which one of some of these procedures to do." George replied, "This is the thing about being a resident. It is time to decide what you are going to do in the real practice."

In short, the residency is viewed as a learning experience, a situation which should provide, among other things, the information and experiences necessary to equip one to arrive at sound medical decisions.

Central to the concept of judgment, however, is the notion that there is often no such thing as the right decision in treating a case. Very often there seems to be a variety of alternatives, each of which may be considered plausible. The choice between these alternatives may be made on the basis of clusters of values or "treatment philosophies" held by the physician. These philosophies provide a general orientation or perspective which serves as a guide in decision making, limiting the number of treatment options which are given serious consideration. In orthopedics, such philosophies center around whether or not one takes a conservative or liberal stance with regard to doing surgery. These orienta-

tions stem from the fact that often the same case can be treated satisfactorily either through surgery or by a more conservative approach involving medications, traction, or braces, etc. As indicated in the following excerpt from our field notes, individual practitioners may become strongly committed to one of these general treatment perspectives:

> A rather lively discussion by the attendings followed Chilton's presentation at grand rounds. The issue was whether or not to do surgery on the man's arm, which was deformed. The problem being that while surgery might improve the appearance it could further limit the function. Dr. Eddy (attending) spoke first, strongly recommending surgery on the basis that "it is a grotesque deformity and a good job would entail no further loss of function." The second private attending said in effect that it would be impossible to do surgery without loss of function. After he had finished speaking, the residents clapped. Finally, Bowen (attending) briefly said that he thought the surgery could be done. Mitchell (resident) said to me, "as you can see there are conservative and liberal philosophies in regard to doing surgery. Obviously Dr. Eddy is very liberal."

Our notes and interviews indicate that taking on one of these philosophies as one's own is something that occurs at least partially during the course of one's residency. Moreover, what appears to be the genesis for such philosophies is apparent in the residents' attitudes toward specific procedures. For example, the 1st-yr residents in the following excerpt speak of "believing in" or "not believing in" specific procedures:

> I (field worker) ask him to explain exactly what the bone graft entails and he says, "Well, I'm not really sure I believe in them. I mean I'm not sure I understand the philosophy behind them." Becker says. "It's an interesting procedure. Not everyone would pin a femur. A lot of people don't see any point in pinning a femur. Keeler (4th-yr resident) believes in this and I believe in it, too, now. I think it's the way to do it."

While narrower in scope than the previously discussed treatment philosophies, these emergent beliefs similarly serve as guides to decision making on specific cases. In other words, if judgment involves the ability to arrive at decisions, which prove more successful, in the face of ambiguous circumstances, the development of general perspectives can make the exercise of judgment less problematic. Such perspectives limit the number of options, and, thus, the uncertainty of making a decision in a specific case.

LEARNING JUDGMENT IN ORTHOPEDICS: EVALUATION

Involvement in decision making prior to treatment is not the only mechanism through which residents learn to develop judgment. As was previously stated, one resident said that judgment is developed by "doing a case and seeing what happens." "Seeing what happens" or evaluating the consequences of the treatment is a more diverse process than decision making, which is virtually always a group process. While in particularly difficult cases, the evaluation of a treatment procedure may be a group phenomenon, more often it is a spontaneous, individual occurrence. The following incidents from our field notes provide typical examples:

> Giles calls for a patient who comes into the examining room, his arm in a sling. Giles removes the sling and asks the man to take off his shirt. He then begins examining the man's shoulder. As he does so he gets a big smile on his face and says, "Beautiful, just beautiful."

> I followed Mitchell on rounds. He begins to unwrap the man's foot and says to me, "Look at that, he's really doing well, see how well it's healing. Only one spot that's a little bit moist. We were able to save almost the entire ball of the foot. That will make it easier for walking." I ask, "Did you do this case?" Mitchell replies, "Yes, I did."

Criteria for evaluation of treatment are more readily available in orthopedic surgery than in many other specialties such as internal medicine or psychiatry. X-rays, various range-of-motion tests and other aids and measurement techniques make it possible to measure improvement with a great deal of precision. As one resident expressed it:

> See, the thing is with orthopedics, if you choose to do surgery on a patient and you put a nail in their fractured hip, you take an X-ray in the recovery room and it shows an excellent alignment and excellent position, and you have then, depending on the type of hip fracture you fixed, anywhere from a 98 percent chance of an excellent result for trochanteric fracture to maybe only 75 percent for a femoral neck fracture, but still, you're going to be feeling by the X-ray if it's good, then you've done your job well. You have a feeling of accomplishment.

Patients and their X-rays often provide relatively unambiguous indicators of success or failure as residents consider specific cases with regard to an improvement in function and/or appearance. Such evaluations may be taken into account in the making of subsequent decisions as the residents indicate in the following example:

> The next patient is an old man with diabetes who has had all the toes on one foot removed. Chilton has the nurse remove the dressing. The foot has turned black for about 2 in. up from the stump. I confirm my diagnosis of gangrene with one of the medical students making rounds with us. Adams turns to Chilton and says, "Look at that, a total failure." We walk down the hall where Adams stops and says to the group, "Rather than keep slicing him up like a piece of salami, we'll go in and take off enough this time." One of the students asks, "Why didn't you take off more last time?" Adams answered, "We had promised the man only to take the toes. . . . This often happens in a case like this. You think you have enough and then a few days later the patient's temperature spikes and you know you're in trouble. You learn to be less conservative in what you take off."

In especially difficult or controversial cases evaluation may become both formalized and collective. In the following instance a case has been presented during grand rounds for the purpose of evaluation. In discussing the case later in the week with two of the residents the investigator asked if the case had been presented to determine whether or not surgery should have been done. One of the residents responded saying, "Yeah, that's more or less right.

Their attendings over there made them do it. The residents thought the patient would have healed just as well in bed." While residents would often share with one another the results of particular cases, we observed very few instances where the actual evaluation of an outcome was the kind of group process so often viewed in decision making. The situation was nicely summed up for us by one of the residents who noted that "the thing with orthopedics is that everything you do is so visible. It's really pretty obvious to everyone when something goes wrong."

While it may be that it is "pretty obvious to everyone when something goes wrong" this does not imply that we observed much group discussion in regard to mistakes. Hughes [9] has pointed out that:

> In some occupations it is assumed that anyone on the inside will know by subtle gestures when his colleagues believe that a mistake has been made. Full membership in the colleague-group is not attained until these gestures and their meaning is known. When they are known, there need not be conscious and overt discussion of certain errors even within the colleague group. And when some incident makes an alleged failure or mistake a matter of public discussion, it is perhaps the feeling that outsiders will never understand the full content of risk and contingency that makes colleagues so tight-lipped.

On a few occasions the field worker was distinctly made to feel like an outsider in situations where the residents and attendings observed cases where something had gone wrong. On one occasion during morning rounds a resident placed an X-ray of a patient, on whom he had performed surgery on the previous day, on the viewer for the attending physician to observe. The attending examined the X-ray with a solemn expression and in a suddenly hushed voice said to the resident, "What happened?" The resident's reply and the brief discussion which followed were inaudible to the field worker but the attending kept nodding his head without changing his expression and with his eyes directed downward. The attending said a few final words to the resident and we moved on to the next patient. Whatever was said between the resident and the attending, it was clear that the attending felt that the explanation was a reasonable one.

The contrast between the open and elaborate discussions which often preceded decisions in regard to treatment and the more isolated and brief evaluations which followed treatment is interesting. The tendency of professionals to focus on the process of professional work rather than the consequences has also been noted by Hughes [10]:

> One of the differences between lay and professional thinking is that to the laymen the technique of the occupation should be pure instrument, pure means to an end, while to the people who practice it, every occupation tends to become an art.

The residents in orthopedics were not indifferent toward the consequences of their work: many of them indicated in interviews that the immediacy and visibility of the results in orthopedic surgery were major factors in their decision to enter that specialty. The process of doing the work, however, was decidedly more interesting to them than the consequence of the work. Consequences of treatment were more taken for granted and while the evaluation of methods of treatment was important for forming judgment on the part of the resident individually, it was not collectively emphasized in the residency program.

The process of decision-making prior to treatment was highly institutionalized in the residency program. Grand rounds every Saturday, visiting rounds every morning and many other formal events of the residency program centered around the gathering of information and the making of decisions with regard to the treatment of specific cases. There was no such institutionalization of subsequent evaluative processes. The evaluation of results tended to be a much more highly individual matter. The setting of the residency program thus may have tended to promote what Freidson has called:

> norms or attitudes that encourage a very special, limited sense of responsibility. In brief, they encourage in the practitioner an emphasis on personal rather than general or communal responsibility, which in turn leads to only limited attempts to assure adequate performance. [11].

SUMMARY AND CONCLUSIONS

Residents in orthopedic surgery de-emphasize the importance of perfecting technical skills. They emphasize, instead, the importance of developing medical judgment; a more elusive ability requiring both understanding and experience in the theoretical and clinical aspects of the specialty. Judgment is developed in a continual process of decision making and evaluation in regard to treatment of specific cases.

Residents entering the program are already well indoctrinated with the belief that the practice of medicine, orthopedic surgery in particular, is fraught with ambiguities which can only be dealt with through the exercise of individual judgment. While clear descriptions of therapeutic procedures can be read in textbooks and while surgical skill can be developed through practice, clinical judgment depends to a great degree on individual values, preferences, and experiences. If the consequence of surgical practice is skill, the additional consequence of developing judgment is confidence. As one senior resident put it, "I now feel confident that I can handle the problems that an orthopedic surgeon would typically see."

The development of confidence in one's judgment is partly the result of having previously handled decision-making situations successfully. A second important component of confidence-building consists of the opinions significant others (attending physicians in particular) express toward the resident. One resident described a situation where an attending:

had enough confidence in me to let me go ahead and do the procedure without him being present. And that really made the biggest difference during this year. Because after that, I felt well, if he's got enough confidence in me to let me do that, then maybe he knows something about me that I don't. . . . If I'm in the operating room and something happens, I feel I can handle it, you know, I think I've got the judgment to handle it. . . . I think that in order to gather the responsibility and the maturity in judgment that you need when you finish, you've got to be put in a situation where you have to make the decisions. . . . And it's a nice feeling to know that someone's got the confidence in you to let you make the decisions.

With such importance placed on developing sound judgment and with the importance attached to attendings' evaluations, it is no surprise that residents develop strategies for maximizing attendings' evaluations of their own judgment and ability. These strategies might be seen as "secondary adjustment," following Goffman's definition of secondary adjustment as ". . . any habitual arrangement by which a member of an organization employs unauthorized means, or obtains unauthorized ends, or both, thus getting around the organization's assumption as to what he should do and get and hence what he should be" [12]. Trainees develop strategies for maximizing the various attendings' evaluation of their orthopedic abilities. For example, rather elaborate secondary adjustments have evolved around residents' performances at grand rounds.

Ostensibly, the purpose of grand rounds is to present particularly difficult or interesting cases to a gathering of attendings in order to benefit from their broader range of knowledge and greater accumulation of clinical experience. In practice, however, residents try to carefully select cases with which the attendings will have little familiarity as the following field note demonstrates:

As we walk out of the clinic together we run into Rosen who is on his way in. Rosen says to Adams, "Hey, guess what I've got to present on Saturday, a case of pseudo sarcomita faciada." Adams laughs, shakes his head and continues down the hall. I ask, "Is that particularly good to present, or what?" Rosen answers. "The attending men won't know a thing about it. I bet none of them have ever heard of it. I've only been able to find 12 articles."

Residents view grand rounds as a game, at which one succeeds by performing in such a way that the attendings are favorably impressed. Moreover, at least certain attendings are quite aware of what is really going on but find the game enjoyable:

He (an attending) pauses for a moment and then adds, changing the subject, "You know something that would really be good for you to study is the kinds of games that the residents play." I say, "You mean like Saturday rounds? It's been my impression that residentmanship more or less reaches its height at Saturday rounds as if their real purpose was for the residents to impress the attending men." Woods responds, "Yes, that's why it's such great fun. That's why the attendings show up. If you'll excuse the expression, another purpose of rounds is to "pimp" the attendings. Have you noticed how they don't give the diagnosis."

In the end, grand rounds is as closely related to demonstrating that one is well along in acquiring medical judgment as it is to actually developing such judgment. Thus, although the attendings assume that the residents will devote themselves to mastering orthopedic skills and knowledge, the trainees also engage a large part of their energies in developing and implementing strategies for enhancing the attendings' opinions of them. Since the attendings' opinions are, in turn, important for the residents' developing confidence in their own judgment, the gamesmanship of the residency is an important component of professional socialization.

Rue Bucher has suggested that role playing, in learning a professional role, "May entail considerable reality or have a playing-at quality. The roles may be central to professional identity, or peripheral, secondary roles" [13]. She suggests that these kinds of variations in the quality of role-playing may be related to the intensity with which one identifies with a professional role. In this sense the roles played by the residents in our study with regard to the exercise of judgment in making decisions can be seen as entailing a considerable degree of the reality of professional work. They include a great deal of actual responsibility for the care of patients in contrast with the roles of medical students who "play-at" being professionals while having little real responsibility. They can be seen as roles which are central to professional identity, as is evidenced by the degree of consensus with which the residents define the capacity to exercise judgment as the fundamental skill of a good orthopedic surgeon.

The medical subculture places great value on individual judgment. The training program we studied operates in such a way as to both reinforce the value placed on this skill and to provide opportunities for the residents to develop it. People in this program often used the phrase, "the way we do it here" to indicate that there may be institutional variations in the ways in which "good judgment" and "bad judgment" are defined. Further investigations of the role of judgment in decision making and the acquisition of judgment in professional socialization might include systematic comparisons with other training programs. Such a comparison could enable the researcher to assess the relative emphasis given to various kinds of information used in reaching decisions. In addition, it might contribute to a more thorough understanding of the development of distinctive judgment philosophies and professional identities.

In addition, further questions need to be raised regarding the adequacy of present methods for developing decision-making abilities in medical education. It is clear, for example, that the fundamental importance attached to personal clinical experience in the exercise of judgment may lead physicians to reject established scientific opinion in favor of personal preferences. Since the individual clinical experience of physicians is subject to many kinds of bias, one might question the appropriateness of assigning such a high value to personal experience in medical decision making. We have described the place of judgment in the subculture of this residency program and the development of judgment in the professional socialization experiences of these residents as an initial step toward further critical research and analysis of these issues.

References

1. Burkett G. L. and Knafl K. A. Judgment and decision-making in a medical specialty. *Sociology of Work and Occupations: an International Journal* 1, 82, 1974.

2. We are indebted to Rachel Jahn-Hut for helping us to see this point more clearly.

3. Freidson E. *Profession of Medicine.* Dodd Mead & Company, 1970.

4. Mechanic D. *Public Expectations and Health Care: Essays in the Changing Organization of Health Services,* p. 2. Wiley-Interscience, New York, 1972.

5. Burkett G. L. and Knafl K. *op. cit.,* p. 108.

6. Becker H. S. *et al. Boys in White: Student Culture in Medical School.* University of Chicago Press, Chicago, 1961.

7. Miller S. J. *Prescription for Leadership: Training for the Medical Elite.* Aldine, Chicago, 1970.

8. Bucher R. *et al.* Differential prior socialization: a comparison of four professional training programs. *Soc. Forces.* 48, 222, 1969.

9. Hughes E. C. *The Sociological Eye: Selected papers,* p. 300. Aldine, Chicago, 1971.

10. *Ibid.,* p. 321.

11. Freidson E. *op. cit.* p. 164.
12. Goffman E. *Asylums: Essays on the Social Situations of Mental Patients and Other Inmates,* p. 189. Doubleday, Garden City, New York, 1961.

13. Bucher R. The psychiatry residency and professional socialization. *J. Hlth Soc. Behav.* 6, 205, 1965.

Epilogue: The Uncertainty in the Practice of Medicine

Making Medical Mistakes

David Hilfiker

A warm July morning. I finish my rounds at our small county hospital around nine o'clock and walk across the parking lot to the clinic. I am a primary-care practitioner, a family doctor; my partners and I work together in a small office building. After greeting the receptionist, I look through the list of my day's appointments and notice that Barb Daily will be in for her first prenatal examination. "Wonderful," I think, recalling the joy of helping her deliver her first child two years ago. Barb and her husband, Russ, had been friends of mine before Heather was born, but we grew much closer with the shared experience of her birth. In a rural family practice such as mine, much of every workday is taken up with disease; I look forward to the prenatal visit with Barb, to the continuing relationship with her over the next months, to the prospect of birth.

At her appointment that afternoon, Barb seems to be in good health, with all the signs and symptoms of pregnancy: slight nausea, some soreness in her breasts, a little weight gain. But when the nurse tests Barb's urine to determine if she is pregnant, the result is negative. The test measures the level of a hormone that is produced by a woman and shows up in her urine when she is pregnant. But occasionally it fails to detect the low levels of the hormone during early pregnancy. I reassure Barb that she is fine and schedule another test for the following week.

Barb leaves a urine sample at the clinic a week later, but the test is negative again. I am troubled. Perhaps she isn't pregnant. Her missed menstrual period and her other symptoms could be a result of a minor hormonal imbalance. Maybe the embryo has died within the uterus and a miscarriage is soon to take place. I could find out by ordering an ultrasound examination. This procedure would give me a "picture" of the uterus and of the embryo. But Barb would have to go to Duluth, 110 miles from our village in northern Minnesota, for the examination. The procedure is also expensive. I know the Dailys well enough to know they have a modest income. Besides, by waiting a few weeks, I should be able to find out for sure without the ultrasound: Either the urine test will be positive or Barb will have a miscarriage. I call her and tell her about the negative test result, about the possibility of a miscarriage, and about the necessity of seeing me again if she misses her next menstrual period.

I work in a summer resort area, and it is, as usual, a hectic summer; I think no more about Barb's troubling state until a month later, when she returns to my office. Nothing has changed: still no menstrual period, still no miscarriage. She is confused and upset. "I feel so pregnant," she tells me. I am bothered, too. Her uterus, upon examination, is slightly enlarged, as it was on the previous visit. But it hasn't grown any larger. Her urine test remains negative. I can think of several possible explanations for her condition, including a hormonal imbalance or even a tumor. But the most likely explanation is that she is carrying a dead embryo. I decide it is time to break the bad news to her.

"I think you have what doctors call a 'missed abortion,'" I tell her. "You were probably pregnant, but the baby appears to have died some weeks ago, before your first examination. Unfortunately, you didn't have a miscarriage to get rid of the dead tissue from the baby and the placenta. If a miscarriage doesn't occur within a few weeks, I'd recommend a re-examination, another pregnancy test, and, if nothing shows up, a dilation and curettage procedure to clean out the uterus."

Barb is disappointed; there are tears. She is college educated, and she understands the scientific and technical aspects of her situation; but that doesn't alleviate the sorrow. We talk at some length and make an appointment for two weeks later.

When Barb returns, Russ is with her. Still no menstrual period; still no miscarriage; still another negative pregnancy test, the fourth. I explain to them what has happened. The dead embryo must be removed or there could be serious complications. Barb could become sterile. The conversation is emotionally difficult for all three of us. We schedule the dilation and curettage for later in the week.

Friday morning, Barb is wheeled into the operating room of the sixteen-bed county hospital. Barb, the nurses, and I all know one another—small-town life. The atmosphere is warm and relaxed; we chat before the operation. After Barb is anesthetized, I examine her pelvis again. Her muscles are now completely relaxed, and it is possible to perform a more reliable examination. Her uterus feels bigger than it did two days previously; it is perhaps the size of a small grapefruit. But since all the pregnancy tests were negative and I'm so sure of the diagnosis, I ignore the information from my fingertips and begin the operation.

Dilation and curettage, or D & C, is a relatively simple surgical procedure performed thousands of times each day in this country. First, the cervix is stretched by pushing smooth metal rods of increasing diameter in and out of it. After about five minutes of this, the cervix has expanded enough so that a curette can be inserted through it into the uterus. The curette is another metal rod, at the end of which is an oval ring about an inch at its widest diameter. It is used to scrape the walls of the uterus. The operation is done completely by feel after the cervix has been stretched, since it is still too narrow to see through.

Things do not go easily this morning. There is considerably more blood than usual, and it is only with great difficulty that I am able to extract anything. What should take ten or fifteen minutes stretches out into a half-hour. The body parts I remove are much larger than I expected, considering when the embryo died. They are not bits of decomposing tissue. These are parts of a body that was recently alive!

I do my best to suppress my rising panic and try to complete the procedure. Working blindly, I am unable to evacuate the uterus completely; I can feel more parts inside but cannot remove them. Finally I stop, telling myself that the uterus will expel the rest within a few days.

Russ is waiting outside the operating room. I tell him that Barb is fine but that there were some problems with the operation. Since I don't completely understand what happened, I can't be very helpful in answering his questions. I promise to return to the hospital later in the day after Barb has awakened from the anesthesia.

In between seeing other patients that morning I place several almost frantic phone calls, trying to piece together what happened. Despite reassurances from a pathologist that it is "impossible" for a pregnant woman to have four consecutive negative pregnancy tests, the realization is growing that I have aborted Barb's living child. I won't know for sure until the pathologist has examined the fetal parts and determined the baby's age and the cause of death. In a daze, I walk over to the hospital and tell Russ and Barb as much as I know for sure without letting them know all I suspect. I tell them that more tissue may be expelled. I can't face my own suspicions.

Two days later, on Sunday morning, I receive a tearful call from Barb. She has just passed some recognizable body parts; what is she to do? She tells me that the bleeding has stopped and that she now feels better. The abortion I began on Friday is apparently over. I set up an appointment to meet with her and Russ to review the entire situation.

The pathologist's report confirms my worst fears: I aborted a living fetus. It was about eleven weeks old. I can find no one who can explain why Barb had four negative pregnancy tests. My meeting with Barb and Russ later in the week is one of the hardest things I have ever been through. I describe in some detail what I did and what my rationale had been. Nothing can obscure the hard reality: I killed their baby.

Politely, almost meekly, Russ asks whether the ultrasound examination would have shown that Barb was carrying a live baby. It almost seems that he is trying to protect my feelings, trying to absolve me of some of the responsibility. "Yes," I answer, "if I had ordered the ultrasound, we would have known the baby was alive." I cannot explain why I didn't recommend it.

Mistakes are an inevitable part of everyone's life. They happen; they hurt—ourselves and others. They demonstrate our fallibility. Shown our mistakes and forgiven them, we can grow, perhaps in some small way become better people. Mistakes, understood this way, are a process, a way we connect with one another and with our deepest selves.

But mistakes seem different for doctors. This has to do with the very nature of our work. A mistake in the intensive care unit, in the emergency room, in the surgery suite, or at the sickbed is different from a mistake on the dock or at the typewriter. A doctor's miscalculation or oversight can prolong an illness, or cause a permanent disability, or kill a patient. Few other mistakes are more costly.

Developments in modern medicine have pro-

vided doctors with more knowledge of the human body, more accurate methods of diagnosis, more sophisticated technology to help in examining and monitoring the sick. All of that means more power to intervene in the disease process. But modern medicine—with its invasive tests and potentially lethal drugs—has also given doctors the power to do more harm.

Yet precisely because of its technological wonders and near-miraculous drugs, modern medicine has created for the physician an expectation of perfection. The technology seems so exact that error becomes almost unthinkable. We are not prepared for our mistakes and we don't know how to cope with them when they occur.

Doctors are not alone in harboring expectations of perfection. Patients expect doctors to be perfect, too. Perhaps patients have to consider their doctors less prone to error than other people: How else can a sick or injured person, already afraid, come to trust the doctor? Further, modern medicine has taken much of the treatment of illness out of the realm of common sense; a patient must trust a physician to make decisions that he, the patient, only vaguely understands. But the degree of perfection expected by patients is no doubt also a result of what we doctors have come to believe about ourselves, or, better, have tried to convince ourselves about ourselves.

This perfection is a grand illusion, of course, a game of mirrors that everyone plays. Doctors hide their mistakes from patients, from other doctors, even from themselves. Open discussion of mistakes is banished from the consultation room, from the operating room, from physicians' meetings. Mistakes become gossip, and are spoken of openly only in court.

Unable to admit our mistakes, we physicians are cut off from healing. We cannot ask for forgiveness, and we get none. We are thwarted, stunted; we do not grow.

During the days, and weeks, and months after I aborted Barb's baby, my guilt and anger grew. I did discuss what had happened with my partners, with the pathologist, with obstetric specialists. Some of my mistakes were obvious: I had relied too heavily on one test; I had not been skillful in determining the size of the uterus by pelvic examination; I should have ordered the ultrasound before proceeding to the D & C. There was no way I could justify what

I had done. To make matters worse, there were complications following the D & C, and Barb was unable to become pregnant again for two years.

Although I was as honest with the Dailys as I could be, and although I told them everything they wanted to know, I never shared with them my own agony. I felt they had enough sorrow without having to bear my burden as well. I decided it was my responsibility to deal with my guilt alone. I never asked for their forgiveness.

When I began at the age of thirty to practice medicine, I was certainly not prepared for the reality of my mistakes or my emotional responses to them. Like many other physicians, I had entered medical school out of a deep desire to serve people and to relieve suffering. I chose to practice in a remote rural area because it desperately needed physicians, because it seemed to offer the opportunity to establish a practice with the kind of personal care I wanted to provide, and because it seemed to be a good place for me and my family to live.

Along with three other doctors also committed to personal medical care, I practiced for seven years in that small Minnesota town. Marja and I raised our family, entered into the life of our community, and tried to live out our dreams. Finally, however, I could no longer tolerate the stresses, and I chose to leave. Dealing with my mistakes was among the stresses.

Doctors' mistakes come in a variety of packages and stem from a variety of causes. For primary-care practitioners, who see every kind of problem, from cold sores to cancer, the mistakes are often simply a result of not knowing enough. One evening during my years in Minnesota a local boy was brought into the emergency room after a drunken driver had knocked him off his bicycle. I examined him right away. Aside from swelling and bruising of the left leg and foot, he seemed fine. An X-ray showed what appeared to be a dislocation of the foot from the ankle. I consulted by telephone with an orthopedic specialist in Duluth, and we decided that I could operate on the boy. As was my usual practice, I offered the patient and his mother a choice: I could do the operation or they could travel to Duluth to see the specialist. My pride was hurt when she decided to take her son to Duluth.

My feelings changed considerably when the specialist called the next morning to thank me for the referral. He reported that the boy had actually suffered an unusual muscle injury, a posterior compartment syndrome, which had twisted his foot and caused it to appear to be dislocated. I had never even heard of such a syndrome, much less seen or treated it. The boy had required immediate surgery to save the muscles of his lower leg. Had his mother not decided to take him to Duluth, he would have been permanently disabled. . . .

Many situations do not lend themselves to a simple determination of whether a mistake has been made. Seriously ill, hospitalized patients, for instance, require of doctors almost continuous decision-making. Although in most cases no single mistake is obvious, there always seem to be things that could have been done differently or better: administering more of this medication, starting that treatment a little sooner . . . The fact is that when a patient dies, the physician is left wondering whether the care he provided was adequate. There is no way to be certain, for it is impossible to determine what would have happened if things had been done differently. In the end, the physician has to suppress the guilt and move on to the next patient.

Maiya Martinen first came to see me halfway through her pregnancy. I did not know her or her husband well, but I knew that they were solid, hard working people. This was to be their first child. When I examined Maiya, it seemed to me that the fetus was unusually small, and I was uncertain about her due date. I sent her to Duluth for an ultrasound examination and an evaluation by an obstetrician. The obstetrician thought the baby would be small, but he thought it could be safely delivered in the local hospital.

Maiya's labor was quite uneventful, except it took her longer than usual to push the baby through to delivery. Her baby boy was born blue and floppy, but he responded well to routine newborn resuscitation measures. Fifteen minutes after birth, however, he had a short seizure. We checked his blood-sugar level and found it to be low, a common cause of seizures in small babies who take longer than usual to emerge from the birth canal. We immediately administered intravenous glucose, and baby Marko seemed to improve. He and his mother were discharged from the hospital several days later.

It was about two months later, a few days after

I had given him his first set of immunizations, that Marko began having short spells. Not long after that he started to have full-blown seizures. Once again the Martinens made the trip to Duluth, and Marko was hospitalized for three days of tests. No cause for the seizures was found, and he was placed on medication. Marko continued to have seizures, however. When he returned for his second set of immunizations, it was clear to me that he was not doing well.

The remainder of Marko's short life was a tribute to the faith and courage of his parents. He was severely retarded, and the seizures became harder and harder to control. Maiya eventually went east for a few months so Marko could be treated at the National Institutes of Health. But nothing seemed to help, and Maiya and her baby returned home. Marko had to be admitted frequently to the local hospital in order to control his seizures. At two o'clock one morning I was called to the hospital; the baby had had a respiratory arrest. Despite our efforts, Marko died, ending a year and a half struggle with life.

No cause for Marko's condition was ever determined. Did something happen during the birth that briefly cut off oxygen to his brain? Should Maiya have delivered at the high-risk obstetric center in Duluth, where sophisticated fetal monitoring is available? Should I have sent Marko to the neonatal intensive care unit in Duluth immediately after his first seizure in the delivery room? I subsequently learned that children who have seizures should not routinely be immunized. Would it have made any difference if I had never given Marko the shots? There were many such questions in my mind and, I am sure, in the minds of the Martinens. There

was no way to know the answers, no way for me to handle the guilt I experienced, perhaps irrationally, whenever I saw Maiya.

The emotional consequences of mistakes are difficult enough to handle. But soon after I started practicing I realized I had to face another anxiety as well: It is not only in the emergency room, the operating room, the intensive care unit, or the delivery room that I can blunder into tragedy. Medicine is not an exact science; errors are always possible, even in the midst of the humdrum routine of daily care. Was that baby I just sent home with a diagnosis of mild viral fever actually in the early stages of serious meningitis? Will that nine-year-old with stomach cramps whose mother I just lectured about psychosomatic illness end up in the hospital tomorrow with a ruptured appendix? Did that Vietnamese refugee have a problem I didn't understand because of the language barrier? A doctor has to confront the possibility of a mistake with every patient visit.

My initial response to the mistakes I did make was to question my competence. Perhaps I just didn't have the necessary intelligence, judgment, and discipline to be a physician. But was I really incompetent? My University of Minnesota Medical School class had voted me one of the two "best clinicians." My diploma from the National Board of Medical Examiners showed scores well above average. I knew that the townspeople considered me a good physician; I knew that my partners, with whom I worked daily, and the consultants to whom I referred patients considered me a good physician, too. When I looked at it objectively, my competence was not the issue. I would have to learn to live with my mistakes. . . .

The Effect of Practice Style on Rates of Surgery: The Role of the "Surgical Signature"

John Wennberg
Alan Gittelsohn

There is a city in Maine where the surgical procedure of hysterectomy (removal of the uterus) was done so frequently in the past decade that if the rate persists, 70 percent of the women there will have had the operation by the time they reach the age of 75. In a city less than 20 miles away the rate of hysterectomy is so much lower that if it persists, only 25 percent of the women will have lost their uterus by age 75. What could account for the disparity? It seems unlikely that there would be any large difference in the general health of the populations of the two neighboring cities, and after looking into the matter we have found none. The populations are similar in economic status. Differences in the number of physicians, the supply of hospital beds and coverage by medical-insurance plans cannot explain the difference in the rate of surgery. Instead the most important factor in determining the rate of hysterectomy seems to be the style of medical practice of the physicians in the two cities. In one city surgeons appear to be enthusiastic about hysterectomy; in the other they appear to be skeptical of its value.

We have examined the rate of surgery and other forms of medical treatment in 193 small areas in the six states of New England. The overall rate of surgery varies more than twofold among the areas. The total rate in a given area is correlated strongly with the number of surgeons there and with the number of hospital beds per capita; these are factors

This article originally appeared under the title "Variations in Medical Care among Small Areas" in *Scientific American*, April 1, 1982, pp. 120–134. Copyright © 1982 by Scientific American, Inc. All rights reserved.

that themselves vary substantially. The amount spent per capita on treatment in hospitals is also quite different from one area to the next. The rates of three of the most common surgical procedures (hysterectomy, prostatectomy and tonsillectomy) vary even more dramatically: the highest rate is six times the lowest one. Even in communities with the same overall rate of surgery the rates of individual procedures can differ greatly. Hysterectomy, prostatectomy and tonsillectomy cause much controversy among physicians. In the absence of general agreement on their value for individual patients the style of practice of the individual physician appears to take precedence.

The substantial variation from area to area in the consumption of medical care and in its per capita cost is sustained by the policies of hospital boards and administrators, regulatory agencies and providers of medical insurance. The policies seldom take into account the existing level of health care in a community; a common result is an increase in medical services in areas that already have high rates of consumption. When such inequities develop, the people receiving the greater number of medical and surgical procedures do not necessarily benefit, particularly when the procedures entail substantial risk.

The 193 areas employed in our work cover the states of Connecticut, Maine, Massachusetts, New Hampshire, Rhode Island and Vermont. Our aim in constructing the areas was to specify the population that attends one local hospital. Except in cases of disorders requiring elaborate treatment (such as cardiac surgery) people are generally treated at a nearby hospital. The attitude of the physicians at that hospital therefore has a strong influence on the rate of a given procedure in the surrounding area.

The analysis of medical care in small geographic areas has been made possible by the establishment of computer-encoded records of hospital admissions in specific regions. In Maine, Rhode Island and Vermont there are registries that include information on each patient admitted to a hospital. The registry lists the patient's age, sex, place of residence, diagnoses, surgical procedures, dates of admission and discharge and health on discharge. For Connecticut, Massachusetts and New Hampshire our data on hospital admissions come from studies in which only the hospital and the patient's place of residence are recorded. The expansion of health-insurance coverage, particularly the passage of the Federal Medicare Act in 1966, has yielded additional information about the medical care of specific populations.

To construct the geographic areas we extracted from the records each patient's residence and the community in which treatment was received. In the records we utilized, the residence of the patient is recorded in the form of his Zip Code, minor civil division (township, for example) or census tract. For each of these small units of residence we determined the community in which residents are most likely to be hospitalized. All townships, census tracts and so on whose residents were most likely to go to a particular community to be treated were combined to form a hospital area.

The 193 hospital areas defined in this way generally have populations of between 10,000 and 200,000, which is large enough for them to have stable rates of medical procedures. In almost all the areas the majority of hospital treatment is provided by facilities within the area.

By counting the surgical procedures done on the population of a hospital area in a given period, the per capita rate of surgery can be calculated. Similar methods give the rate of other kinds of medical treatment. Insurance-reimbursement rates can be calculated by totaling the reimbursements received by residents and dividing by the number of residents who are members of an insurance program. The number of hospital beds per capita is also readily determined.

Although the hospital areas can be employed in a variety of analyses, much of our work has concerned rates of surgery because the information on surgical procedures in regional record-keeping systems has been shown to be more reliable than that for other forms of treatment or for diagnosis.

After adjusting for differences in age among populations we have calculated the rates of hospital admission for surgical procedures in the 11 most populous hospital areas in each of three states: Maine, Rhode Island and Vermont. Procedures done on residents of a hospital area are counted toward the area's total whether the operation took place within the area or outside it. Among the hospital areas in each state the overall rate of surgery varies by a factor of about two.

The variation in the rates of certain common procedures are more dramatic than the variation in the total. The highest hysterectomy rate in the 33 areas (some 90 procedures per 10,000 women per year in 1975) is about four times the lowest rate. The highest rate of prostatectomy is also about four times the lowest rate. For tonsillectomy the highest rate (about 60 procedures per 10,000 people per year) is six times the lowest rate. In many cases the difference between the extreme rates for a procedure and the average rate for all the areas is statistically significant, indicating that the difference is unlikely to be a result of chance variation.

Because of the wide range of rates residents of different areas face very different probabilities of having surgery. In one area of Vermont the tonsillectomy rate from 1969 through 1971 was such that if it had persisted, 60 percent of all children would have had their tonsils removed by age 20. In a second Vermont area the rate was such that only 8 percent would have had their tonsils removed by age 20. In the area with fewer tonsillectomies, however, the prostatectomy rate was such that 59 percent of all men would have had their prostate gland removed by age 80. In a neighboring area only 35 percent would have had a prostatectomy by age 80.

It is important to note that such large disparities in the rate of surgery are not observed for all common surgical procedures. The rates of cholecystectomy (surgical removal of the gallbladder) and appendectomy, for example, vary by a ratio of less than three to one. In few cases is the difference between the rate for an individual area and the average rate statistically significant. The rate of herniorrhaphy (surgical repair of hernia) varies even less, and most of the variation seems attributable to chance.

The ratio of hospital beds to population and the average cost of being hospitalized also vary greatly among New England communities. In the 11 most populous hospital areas in Vermont the highest ratio of hospital beds to population is 6.8 beds per 1,000 people; the lowest is 3.7. In Connecticut the highest ratio is more than four per 1,000; the lowest is less than two. (The ratios have been adjusted to compensate for residents treated outside their hospital areas.) The Federal Health Planning Program has specified four beds per 1,000 people as its standard for health-care planning; the ratios in New England thus range from well below the standard to well above it. Furthermore, the difference between small areas is so great that the number of beds per capita in a state or a county (a measure often used in health planning) is not a reliable indicator of conditions in each community.

The average reimbursement per area resident by agencies that provide medical insurance is another highly variable quantity. In Boston, the area of Massachusetts with the highest rate of Medicare reimbursement, an average of $640 was paid to each person enrolled in the program in 1975. Across the Charles River in Cambridge the amount was $540. In Manchester, N.H., less than 50 miles away, it was $176.

The amount spent per capita on all treatment in hospitals is also quite inconsistent. In 1975, $324 was spent per capita in Boston; in Providence, $225 was spent. In New Haven, on the other hand, per capita expenditure was $153; in Hanover, N.H., it was $120. In all these areas the majority of admissions are to major teaching hospitals. The services provided in the hospitals are probably similar; one would not expect such a disparity in the amount spent on treatment.

Our work has shown that residents of some areas receive much more medical treatment than others and spend more on that care. Why? One might assume that such differences are caused by better health in some communities, but this does not appear to be the case. Surveys we made in selected hospital areas show that differences in the health of residents and in the other factors that affect the demand for medical care account for only a small amount of the difference in the consumption of services.

Ronald M. Andersen and Lu Ann Aday of the University of Chicago have listed certain characteristics that influence whether or not an individual will seek medical treatment. The most important factors are those that affect the person's health or the perception of health. A variety of studies, however, have found that "enabling factors" such as income, health-insurance coverage and education can also have a strong effect. In addition "predisposing factors" such as skepticism or faith in medicine appear to play a role. In the course of our work we have tried to determine how much of the observed difference in medical care could be explained by such characteristics. With Floyd J. Fowler, Jr., of the University of Massachusetts at Boston we interviewed residents of six Vermont hospital areas. The residents were chosen to provide a representative sample of the local populations.

The total surgery rate and the amount spent per capita on hospital treatment differed as much as twofold in the six areas; rates of some surgical procedures varied even more. The interviews, however, showed that the residents differed little in the factors affecting the consumption of medical services. The average numbers of episodes of acute and chronic illness in each area were similar, as were the proportion of people with an income below the poverty level, the proportion with various kinds of health insurance and the proportion with access to a physician. Indeed, approximately equal proportions of the people in the areas visit a physician each year, as would be expected in populations of similar wealth and health. The large differences in surgical rates and the amount spent on hospital care must therefore be traced to factors that come into play after patients have contact with physicians.

What is it that takes effect after the patient sees a physician to increase the patient's chance of being hospitalized or of having surgery or a diagnostic procedure? The crucial factor appears to be the system of medical care in the community. Although health and other demographic factors do not differ much among the six areas, the number of hospital beds and the number of physicians in proportion to the population vary widely. Moreover, the supply of hospital facilities and the types of physicians who practice in the area are closely correlated with overall consumption rates. Where there are many hospital beds per capita and many physicians whose specialty or style of practice requires frequent hospitalization, there is more treatment in hospitals and greater expenditure per capita for hospital care. In hospital areas where there are many general surgeons the surgery rate is high. The surgery rate and the rate of hospitalization are also high in communities where a large proportion of the general practitioners do surgery. In areas where there are many internists many diagnostic tests are given.

That the overall rate of surgery is influenced by the ratio of surgeons to population has been known for some time. In 1970 John P. Bunker of the Stanford University School of Medicine found that the total surgery rate in the U.S. was about twice that in Britain, where there are fewer surgeons per capita. In 1973 a study supported by the American College of Surgeons showed an analogous relation in regions of the U.S.

The total rate of surgery and the likelihood of being admitted to a hospital for treatment thus depend on the supply of physicians and hospital beds in the area. The wide variations in the rates of individual procedures, however, are not caused by differences in the supply of resources alone. Our work suggests that such variations are due to differences in the style of medical practice of local physicians. We examined the total surgery rate and the rate of individual procedures in the five most populous hospital areas in Maine. In three of the areas the total rate is close to the average for the state, in one area the rate is above average and in one it is below average. In each area, however, a different surgical procedure is the commonest one; all the commonest procedures are among those whose rates vary widely. For example, hysterectomy is the commonest procedure in one of the areas but the least common in another, although the two areas have the same overall rate of surgery.

In each of the five areas of Maine the rates of common surgical procedures constitute a "surgical signature" that tends to be consistent over many years, unless physicians leave the area or enter it. In each signature the rates of some procedures exceed the state average; those of other procedures fall below the average. Nora Lou Roos, Leslie L. Roos and their colleagues of the University of Manitoba Faculty of Medicine reached similar conclusions after analyzing variations in small areas in Manitoba.

Figure 1 presents the surgical signatures, as they relate to five common surgical procedures, for each of five of the most populous hospital areas in Maine. The rates are expressed in relation to the state average.

Figure 1 clearly shows the existence of the surgical signature. For example, while areas 2 and 3 have the same total rate of surgery, the surgical signatures are quite different. In area 2 hysterectomy is the commonest procedure; in area 3 it is the least common.

We have accounted for the factors that might influence the rates of surgical procedures, including the health of residents, the supply of hospital beds and the number of physicians. Even taken together, these factors cannot explain all the variation in rates of individual procedures. The strongest remaining hypothesis is that the judgments and preferences of physicians give rise to the surgical signature.

Some of the most persuasive evidence that the style of practice adopted by physicians has a strong influence on surgery rates comes from studies in which physicians are told of geographic variations in the rates. The studies also show that physicians' attitudes can be changed. In the 1950's Paul Lembke of the University of Rochester employed information similar to ours to calculate per capita rates of surgery in communities near Rochester, N.Y. He also persuaded physicians there to undertake an audit of surgical procedures. Soon afterward the rates were reduced in some areas where they had been high. We followed a similar course in Vermont, except that no formal audit was made. Information on the rate of tonsillectomy in each hospital area was given to the Vermont Medical Society. In the area with the highest rate physicians established the requirement that a second opinion be obtained before a tonsillectomy was done. As a result the probability that a child living in the area would have a tonsillectomy before age 20 declined from 60 percent to less than 10 percent. It had been suggested that if tonsillectomy became much less common at the local hospital, the people of the area would go to other nearby hospitals to obtain the surgery for their children. This did not happen, implying that demand by residents

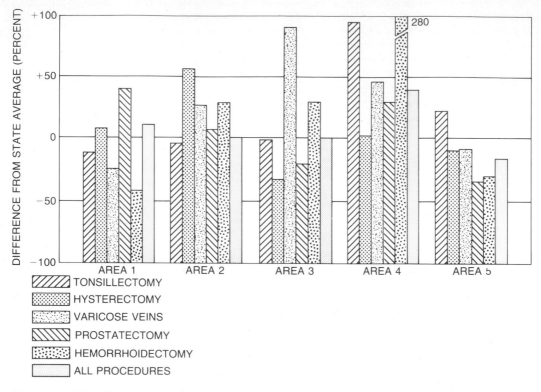

Figure 1 The "Surgical Signature": Variations in Area Rates of Surgery for Five Common Procedures

for the procedure had not been a major factor in maintaining the high tonsillectomy rate.

How can the decisions made by physicians vary so widely from one community to another a few miles away? It seems that the procedures whose rates vary the most are the ones whose risks and benefits are least well established in the medical profession. In some instances the value of the procedure itself has been questioned; in others the criteria for selecting patients for the operation are not definitive. Tonsillectomy, for example, was once done almost routinely for minor inflammation but is now usually reserved for more serious cases. Some practitioners, however, retain the older attitude. In the case of hysterectomy there is general agreement on its necessity in uterine cancer. The operation is most often done, however, for a variety of less threatening conditions; the appropriateness of the procedure in these circumstances has been widely questioned.

In contrast, the procedures whose rates vary little are those that provoke little disagreement. Inguinal hernia, for example, is easily recognized; the treatment of choice is surgical repair. Only where the simultaneous presence of other conditions makes surgery dangerous is any other therapy employed, at least in the U.S. Consequently the rate of surgical repair of hernia is relatively constant in the hospital areas.

The uncertainty of the medical profession about the controversial procedures can be great indeed. Ira M. Rutkow and George D. Zuidema of the Johns Hopkins University School of Hygiene and Public Health and one of us (Gittelsohn) recently surveyed a group of randomly selected surgical specialists. Each surgeon was given a set of fabricated case histories and asked whether he would recommend a particular surgical procedure for them. There was a marked divergence of opinion. For the three fictitious cases related to hysterectomy 25 percent of the surgeons thought none of the cases warranted surgery; 5 percent thought all three did. The remaining 70 percent recommended surgery in one case or two cases. Similar inconsistencies appeared for breast surgery, varicose-vein surgery, tonsillectomy, gallbladder removal, cataract surgery and prostatectomy.

Earlier studies had also demonstrated extreme conflicts of opinion. In 1934 workers from the American Child Health Association chose 1,000 school-children to be examined by physicians, who were to determine whether or not they should have their tonsils removed. Six hundred children had already had the procedure and were removed from the sample. The remaining 400 were examined by school physicians, who recommended that 45 percent have a tonsillectomy. Those that remained after the first round of examinations were examined by another group of physicians who recommended that 46 percent of them have their tonsils out. A third examination by still another group of physicians led to 44 percent of the remainder having tonsillectomy recommended. After three successive rounds only 65 of the original 1,000 children had not had tonsillectomy recommended for them.

For many common illnesses well-designed clinical studies to test alternative forms of therapy have not been done. For this reason there is conflicting information on whether a particular procedure will improve a patient's health or the quality of his life. Many diagnostic and therapeutic techniques are adopted or discarded on the basis of fashion or a physician's personal experience rather than on more reliable grounds.

. . .

In the absence of authoritative standards differences among physicians in perceptions of illness and preferences for treatment appear to be the cause of much variation in rates of surgery and other kinds of treatment.

The savings in lives and money that would result from making rates of medical care correspond to the health needs and preferences of informed consumers might be considerable. How could this be achieved? If physicians in an area where rates are high are made aware of that fact, rates may fall, eliminating some unnecessary surgery. Reliable studies of the effects of various kinds of treatment might lead to a consensus on their value and could provide consumers with more information on which to base their decisions. If regulatory agencies consider the level of health care in the community, some of the tendencies toward excess may be restrained. If premiums for medical insurance reflect the amount of treatment per capita in a given area, subsidization could be reduced.

The most important factor, however, may be the emergence of an informed consumer of medical services. When patients are aware that different forms of treatment are available, they can demand information on risks and benefits and make their own preferences known. If they know that rates of surgery are high at the local hospital, they may choose another. If they realize that a particular operation is a controversial one, they may seek the opinion of a second and even a third physician. Informed patients may therefore be the most important factor in making rates of treatment reflect health needs and eliminating unnecessary medicine.

Suggested Readings

COSTS, RISKS AND BENEFITS OF SURGERY. Edited by John P. Bunker, Benjamin A. Barnes and Frederick Mosteller. Oxford University Press, 1977.

A SMALL AREA APPROACH TO THE ANALYSIS OF HEALTH SYSTEM PERFORMANCE. John E. Wennberg and Alan M. Gittelsohn. Department of Health and Human Services. U.S. Government Printing Office, 1980.

THE NEED FOR ASSESSING THE OUTCOME OF COMMON MEDICAL PRACTICES. John E. Wennberg, John P. Bunker and Benjamin Barnes in *Annual Review of Public Health*, Vol. 1, pages 277–295; 1980.

CHAPTER 8 _____

The "Medical Model" Theme

Medicine's dominant perspective, the one that is taught to medical students to the virtual exclusion of others, is the "biomedical model," sometimes simply called the "medical model." The medical model derives much of its motivating force from the work of nineteenth-century scientists who discovered that certain diseases were associated with the presence of bacteria. As a consequence, much of medicine is devoted to isolating specific bacteriological, physiological, and biochemical causes of physical and emotional illness.

A major criticism of the medical model, and a very valid one, is that it fails to take into account the role of social causation in the development and treatment of illness. The article by Marjorie Glassman in an earlier chapter of this book supports the need to expand the medical model. In looking at how senile dementia is frequently misdiagnosed in the elderly, she observes that physicians frequently neglect to explore the individual's social environment before making such a diagnosis. The call is for a more holistic view of health and illness. The differences between a more limited medical view and a holistic one are represented clearly in the table on page 319.

Two other consequences of the medical model have also been targets of criticism. The first is its failure to emphasize the prevention of disease. The second is its tendency to redefine normal biological conditions as medical problems (e.g., those related to the reproductive function of women).

The two articles in this chapter deal with the limitations of the medical

Comparison of holistic and biomedical concepts of health and disease

	HOLISTIC CONCEPTS	BIOMEDICAL CONCEPTS
Health:	A sense of well-being is the essential feature of the healthy individual. The precondition for health is the integration of the physiological, psychological, and spiritual dimensions of the individual.	Health is the absence of disease. It can be evaluated in relation to physical and physiological function within the normal range. Social, psychological, and spiritual dimensions are rarely considered as essential areas for intervention for a somatic problem. The preconditions for health are reasonably sanitary conditions, moderate exercise, and good eating and sleeping habits.
Disease:	Disease is caused by more factors than a simple pathogenic agent. It should be viewed as an indicator of disharmony between the individual and his/her environment or a disintegration of the essential dimensions of the individual.	Disease can be thought of as "Deviations from the norm of measurable biological (somatic) variables."** It is commonly caused by a specific pathogenic agent, such as a chemical irritant or bacteria, and can be identified by distinctive symptoms. In essence, complex disease phenomena are ultimately derived from one or a few primary events such as contact with a pathogenic agent.
Healing:	Healing must entail a reintegration of basic dimensions. The central factors in the process of successful healing are the intimacy of the patient-practitioner relationship, the quality of the spiritual experience, and the developing ability of the patient to deal with the problem independently.	The necessary prerequisite for healing is an attitude of cooperation with the physician. Disease can be "conquered" either by self-limitation of the pathogen or by a specific therapy. Steps in the healing process itself are congruent with our economic tradition. Prerequisites for cure are often presented to the patient as a set of consumable products (drugs, operations, days in the hospital, etc.).
Role of the Practitioner:	The primary function of the practitioner is to teach the patient how to manage his/her illness and how to achieve and maintain a healthier state.	The physician possesses the necessary specialized technical knowledge and skill to cure the disease. His/her role is to develop the correct therapeutic measures to attack and conquer the disease.
Role of the Patient:	The individual patient is essentially responsible for the outcome of an illness episode. The patient must engage in activities such as physical exercise, stress management, and nutritional awareness, which help maintain health as well as promote healing.*	The patient must cooperate with the physician and comply with instructions.

* Donald B. Ardell, *High Level Wellness* (Emmaus, Pa.: Rodale Press, 1977).
** George L. Engel, "The Need for a New Medical Model: A Challenge for Biomedicine," *Science* 196: 4286 (April 8, 1977), 130.

model in relation to childbirth. The first is the story of a medical student who found out, early in her medical school career, that she was pregnant. Perri Klass found that medical school defined pregnancy as "a very dangerous condition." As a result, much attention was paid to medical intervention and little was paid to such things as nutrition and the emotional aspects of being pregnant. In the second article, Barbara Katz Rothman describes how nurse—midwives abandon some important elements of the medical model after they have been practicing awhile.

Bearing a Child in Medical School

Perri Klass

One day last year, I sat with my classmates in our reproductive medicine course in Amphitheater E at the Harvard Medical School, listening to a lecture on the disorders of pregnancy. The professor discussed ectopic pregnancy, toxemia, spontaneous abortion and major birth defects. I was eight months pregnant. I sat there, rubbing my belly, telling my baby: "Don't worry, you're O.K., you're healthy." I sat there wishing that this course would tell us more about normal pregnancy, that after memorizing all the possible disasters, we would be allowed to conclude that pregnancy itself is not a state of disease. But I think most of us, including me, came away from the course with a sense that pregnancy is a deeply dangerous medical condition, that one walks a fine line, avoiding one serious problem after another, to reach the statistically unlikely outcome of a healthy baby and a healthy mother.

I learned I was pregnant the afternoon of my anatomy exam. I had spent the morning taking first a written exam and then a practical, centered on 15 thoroughly dissected cadavers, each ornamented with little paper tags indicating structures to be identified.

My classmates and I were not looking very good—our hair unwashed, our faces pale from too much studying and too little sleep. Two more exams and our first year of medical school would be over. We all knew exactly what we had to do next: go home and study for tomorrow's exam. I could picture my genetics notes lying on my desk, liberally highlighted with pink marker. But before I went home, I had a pregnancy test.

My period was exactly one day late, hardly worth noticing—but the month before, for the first time, I had been trying to get pregnant.

Four hours later, I called for the test results. "It's positive," the woman at the lab told me.

With all the confidence of a first-year medical student, I asked: "Positive, what does that mean?"

"It means you're pregnant," she said. "Congratulations."

Somewhat later that afternoon, I settled down to make final review notes for my genetics exam. *Down's syndrome,* I copied carefully onto a clean sheet of paper *the most common autosomal trisomy disorder, one per 700 live births.* I began to feel a little queasy. Over the next 24 hours, I was supposed to memorize the biological basis, symptoms, diagnosis and treatment of a long list of genetic disorders. Almost every one was something that could conceivably already be wrong with the embryo growing inside me. I couldn't even think about it; I would have to pass the exam on what I remembered from the lectures.

Over the following months, as I went through my pregnancy and my second year of medical school, I became more and more aware of two aspects of my life influencing each other, and even sometimes seeming to oppose each other. As a medical student, I was spending my time studying everything that can go wrong with the human body. As a pregnant woman, I became suddenly passionately interested in healthy physiological processes, in my own, normal, pregnancy and the growth of my baby. And yet pregnancy put me under the care of the medical profession—my own future profession—and I found myself rebelling as a mother and "patient" against the attitudes the profession conveyed, particularly that pregnancy was somehow a perilous, if not pathological state.

My pregnancy and the decisions I had to make about my own health care changed forever my feelings about the science of medicine and its view of emergency and intervention. My pregnancy became for me almost a rebellion against this view, a chance to do something healthy and normal with my body, something that would be a joyous event, a complex event but not necessarily a medical event.

Medical school lasts four years, followed by an internship and residency program—three years for medicine and five to seven for surgery—and then maybe a two-year fellowship for those pursuing a specialty.

"The fellowship years can be a good time to have a baby," advised one physician. She was just finishing a fellowship in primary care. "Not internship or residency, God knows—that's when your marriage breaks up since you're working 80 hours a week and you're so miserable all the time."

I was 25 years old. After college, I hadn't gone straight to medical school, but had spent two years doing graduate work in biology and one living abroad. I would probably reach the fellowship stage by around 33. It seemed a long time to wait.

The more I thought about it, the more it seemed that there was no time in the next seven or so years when it would be as feasible to have a baby as the present. As a medical student, I had a flexibility that I would not really have further on, a freedom to take a couple of months off or even a year if I decided I needed it, and without unduly disrupting the progress of my career. Larry Wolff, the baby's father, was also 25 and was finishing his doctoral dissertation on Polish–Vatican relations in the late 18th century for a Ph.D. from Stanford. He was also teaching at Harvard, which allowed him a great deal of flexibility. Both our lives frequently had a slightly

frantic quality, but we didn't foresee a less complicated, less frantic future.

I decided against taking a leave of absence right away. Instead, Larry and I started the juggling games that, no doubt, will be a major feature of the years ahead; I took extra courses so I might manage a comparatively light schedule the following spring and stay with the baby two days a week while Larry worked at home the other three. Perfect timing was, of course, of the essence; happily, we'd managed to conceive the baby so it would be born between the time I took my exams in December 1983 and the time I started my hospital course work the following March.

There was one other factor in my decision to have a baby when I did. All through my first year of medical school, in embryology, in genetics, even in public health, lecturers kept emphasizing that the ideal time to have a baby is in the mid-20's—safest for the mother, safest for the baby. "Do you think they're trying to tell us something?" grumbled one of my classmates after a particularly pointed lecture. "Like, why are we wasting these precious childbearing years in school? It almost makes you feel guilty about waiting to have children."

Ironically, I knew no one else my age who was having a baby. The women in my childbirth class were all in their mid-30's. "Having a baby is a very 1980's thing to do," said a friend who is a 27-year-old corporate lawyer in New York. "The only thing is, you and Larry are much too young." In medical school one day, when I was several months along, a lecturer mentioned the problem of teen-age pregnancy, and half the class turned to look at me.

In theory, medical education teaches first about normal anatomy and normal physiology, and then it builds upon this foundation by teaching the processes of pathology and disease. In practice, everyone—students and teachers alike—is eager to get to the material with "clinical relevance," and the whole thrust of the teaching is toward using examples of disease to elucidate normal body functions; specifically, what happens when such functions fail. For example, we understand sugar metabolism partially because of studies on diabetics, who can't metabolize sugar normally. "An experiment of nature" is the phrase often used.

Although we learned a great deal about disease,

we did not, in our first year of medical school, learn much about the nitty-gritty of medical practice. As I began to wonder more about what was happening inside me and about what childbirth would be like, I tried to read my embryology textbook but, again, the pictures of various abnormal fetuses upset me. Instead, I read some books written for pregnant women, not medical students.

Suzanne Arms's "Immaculate Deception: A New Look at Childbirth in America," for instance, was a passionate attack on American childbirth which argues that many routine hospital practices are psychologically damaging and medically hazardous. In particular, the author protested the "traditional birth," a euphemism for giving birth while lying down, a position that is less effective and more dangerous than many others, but convenient for the doctor. An intravenous line is often attached to the arm or an electronic fetal heart monitor strapped to the belly. "Traditional" almost always means a routine episiotomy, a surgical incision to allow the baby's head to emerge without tearing the mother.

Whose "traditions" are these, incorporating interventions designed for problem births into each and every birth? They are traditions developed and perpetuated by doctors trained to define a normal birth as a "negative" event—one with the fortuitous absence of complications. I did not want that kind of traditional birth. I found myself nervously reviewing my own risk factors: I was the perfect age to be having a baby, I had no diabetes or heart disease, I had "a completely negative family history"—none of my close relatives have suffered from obstetrical problems or birth defects. I actually expected to discover some horrendous, lurking source of danger. I reassured myself that I would accept intervention if things went wrong; I just resented the idea that it might be routine.

I decided I would have to shop for a doctor. By this time, I had begun to wonder whether I wanted to have the baby in a hospital at all; when I was a graduate student in California, I knew several people, all biologists like me, who had given birth at home. In the Netherlands, home birth is the norm, and infant mortality rates there have consistently been lower than in the United States.

In our reproductive medicine course last fall, the issue of home birth came up exactly once, in a "case" for discussion. "B B is a 25-year-old married graduate student," the case began. B B, who showed no unusual symptoms and had no relevant past medical problems, had a completely normal pregnancy. When the pregnancy reached full term, the summary concluded, "No factors have been identified to suggest increased risk." Then, the first question: Do you think she should choose to deliver at home?

The doctor leading our discussion section read the question aloud and waited. "No," chorused the class.

"Why not?" asked the doctor.

"Well, there's always the chance of a complication," said one of the students.

B B went two and a half weeks past her due date, began to show signs of fetal distress and was ultimately delivered by Caesarean section after the failure of induced labor. Clearly, B B's case was supposed to teach us something. It was hard for me to read the case without getting the impression that all of B B's problems were a kind of divine retribution for even considering a home birth.

When Larry and I looked into a home birth, we found other problems. For one thing, although it is much cheaper than a hospital birth, my insurance would pay only for the latter. For another, I was frankly not sure I had the moral strength to go ahead with a home birth in a situation in which I would meet with nothing but disapproval from the people around me. As a woman who had given birth at home told me, "You have to accept that if anything goes wrong—even if it's something that would have gone wrong in a hospital, even if it's something like a birth defect—if you have the baby at home, everyone will blame you."

We eventually decided on a hospital birth with a doctor whose inclination was clearly against intervention except when absolutely necessary. In our interview with him, he volunteered the Caesarean and episiotomy figures for his practice. He also regarded the issue of what kind of birth we wanted as an appropriate subject for our first meeting. "A low-tech birth?" he said, sounding amused. "You're at Harvard Medical School and you want a low-tech birth?"

Our doctor suggested we inspect several hospitals at which he performed deliveries. We toured a large teaching hospital where I would probably spend part of the next two years. The labor and delivery floor is usually busy, often with five or six women in labor at one time, and residents and interns and medical students all trying to get the "clinical experience" that is the real stuff of medical training. Inevitably, in such a busy place, some regimentation develops. And perhaps also inevitably, with so many people eager to get their hands on patients, the regimentation may be biased in the direction of more procedures, more interventions. The nurse leading the tour told us exactly what would happen to us, and, if we questioned a procedure, referred us to our doctors in a tone of surprised disapproval.

We chose another hospital, a smaller one near our home. The nurse who took us around referred decisions to us as well as to our doctor and suggested we send a "wish list" to the hospital a few weeks before our due date, specifying any particular requests we had for the birth.

At the beginning of my eighth month, we went to the hospital for the first meeting of a childbirth class. I had great hopes for this class; I was tired of feeling like the only pregnant person in the world. My medical school classmates had continued to be extremely kind and considerate, but as I moved around the school I was beginning to feel like a lone hippopotamus in a gaggle of geese. I wanted some other people with whom Larry and I could go over the questions we discussed endlessly with each other: How do we know when it's time to leave for the hospital? What is labor going to feel like? What can we do to make it go more easily?

At the first meeting it became clear that the class's major purpose was to prepare people to be good patients. It was like that first hospital tour. The teacher exposed us to various procedures so that we would cooperate properly when they were performed on us. Asked whether a given procedure was absolutely necessary, she said that it was up to her doctor.

I found a childbirth class that met at a local day-care center; we sat on cushions on the floor, surrounded by toys and children's work. Many members of the class were fairly hostile toward the medical profession; once again I was greeted with the odd remark: "A medical student and you think you want a natural birth? Don't you get thrown out of school for that?" This class was, if anything, designed to teach people how to be "bad patients." The teacher

explained the pros and cons of the various interventions, and we discussed under what circumstances we might or might not accept them.

The childbirth classes not only prepared me well for labor, but also provided that feeling of community I wanted. Yet they also left me feeling pulled between two poles, especially when I went to medical school during the day to discuss deliveries going wrong in one catastrophic way after another ("C-section, C-section!" our class would chorus when the teacher asked what we would do next) and to childbirth class in the evening to discuss ways to circumvent unwanted medical procedures. As a medical student, I knew I was being trained to rely heavily on technology, to assume that the risk of acting is almost always preferable to the risk of not acting. I consciously had to fight these attitudes when I thought about giving birth.

In our reproductive medicine course, the emphasis was on the abnormal, the pathological. The only thing said about nutrition, for example, was in passing—nobody knows how much weight a pregnant woman should gain, but "about 24 pounds" is considered good. In contrast, the other women in my childbirth class and I were very concerned with what we ate; we were always exchanging suggestions about how to get through those interminable four glasses of milk a day. We learned nothing in medical school about exercise, though exercise books and classes aimed at pregnant women have proliferated.

Will we, as doctors, be able to give valid advice about diet and exercise during pregnancy?

We learned nothing about any of the problems encountered in a normal pregnancy. All we learned about morning sickness was that it could be controlled with a drug, a drug some women were reluctant to take because some studies had linked it to birth defects. (The drug, Bendectin, which had been on the market 27 years, was withdrawn last year.) We learned nothing about the emotional aspects of pregnancy, nothing about helping women prepare for labor and delivery. In other words, none of my medical-school classmates would have been capable of answering even the most basic questions about pregnancy asked by the people in my childbirth class. The important issues for future doctors simply did not overlap with the important issues for future parents.

I mentioned this to my doctor, explaining that

I was tormented by fears of every possible abnormality. "Yes," he said, "normal birth is not honored enough in the curriculum. Most of us doctors are going around looking for pathology and feeling good about ourselves when we find it because that's what we were trained to do. We aren't trained to find joy in a normal pregnancy."

I tried to find joy in my own pregnancy. I am sure that the terrors that sometimes visited me in the middle of the night were no more intense than those which visit most expectant mothers. (Will the labor go well? Will the baby be O.K.?) But I probably had more specific fears than many, as I lay awake wondering about atrial septal heart defects or placenta previa and hemorrhage. And perhaps I did worry more than I might once have, because my faith in the normal had been weakened. In my dark moments, I, too, had begun to see healthy development as less than probable, as the highly unlikely avoidance of a million abnormalities.

I knew that many of my classmates were worrying with me; I cannot count the number of times I was asked whether I had had amniocentesis, the procedure by which fluid is drawn from the amniotic sac and tested for chromosomal abnormalities, particularly Down's syndrome. When I pointed out that we had been taught that amniocentesis is not generally recommended for women under the age of 35, my classmates tended to look worried and mutter something about being *sure*.

The height of the ridiculous came when a young man in class asked me: "Have you had all those genetic tests? Like for sickle-cell anemia?"

I looked at him. He is white. I am white. "I'm not in the risk group for sickle-cell," I said gently.

"Yeah, I know," he said, "but if there's even a one in a zillion chance . . ."

My class in medical school was absorbing the idea that when it comes to tests, technology and interventions, more is better. No one in reproductive medicine ever talked about the negative aspects of intervention, and the one time a student asked about the "appropriateness" of fetal monitoring, the question was cut off with a remark that there was no time to discuss issues of "appropriateness." There was also no time to discuss techniques for attending women in labor—except as they related to labor emergencies.

We were also absorbing the attitude, here as in other courses, that most decisions were absolutely out of the reach of nonphysicians. The risks of catastrophe were so constant—how could we let patients take chances like this with their lives? Dangers that could be controlled by pregnant women—cigarettes, alcohol and drug use—were de-emphasized. Instead, we were taught to think in terms of medical emergencies. Gradually, pregnancy itself began to sound like a medical emergency, a situation in which the pregnant woman, referred to as "the patient," must be carefully guided to a safe delivery, almost in spite of herself. As we spent more and more time absorbing the vocabulary of medicine, we became less inclined to think about communicating our knowledge to those lacking the vocabulary.

Some aspects of having a baby while in medical school were very positive. My courses in anatomy, physiology and embryology deepened my awe of the miracle going on inside me. When I looked ahead to the birth, I thought of what we learned about the incredible changeover taking place during the first minutes of life, the details involved in the switch to breathing air, changes in circulation. I appreciated pregnancy in a way I never could have before.

Another wonderful thing about having a baby in medical school was the support and attention I got from my classmates. Perhaps because having a baby seemed a long way off to many of them, there was some tendency to regard mine as a "class baby." My classmates held a baby shower for Larry and me, and presented us with a fabulous assortment of items for infants. At the end of the shower, I lay back on the couch with five medical students feeling my abdomen, finding the baby's bottom, the baby's foot.

I want to believe that I will be a better doctor because I have combined medical school with this experience of having to choose and control medical care for myself. I want to believe that the classmates who were feeling my abdomen, all people I like very much, will also be good doctors. I want to believe that we will take away the important factual knowledge from our courses, but without absorbing all the attitudes that come with it. I also want to believe that obstetrical medicine will change, but I do not really believe that it will change from within.

And so, in the end, I find myself hoping most of all that expectant parents and others will continue to pressure the medical profession to change, to relinquish some of its control over childbirth, to take a more fair-minded attitude toward the risks of intervention versus the risks of nonintervention, to provide more options and more information and, above all, to stop regarding pregnancy and childbirth as exclusively "medical" events.

Our son, Benjamin Orlando, was born on Jan. 28. Naturally, I would like to be able to say that all our planning and preparing was rewarded with a perfectly smooth labor and delivery. But, of course, biology doesn't work that way. The experience did provide me with a rather ironic new wrinkle on the whole idea of interventions. Most of the labor was quite ordinary. "You're demonstrating a perfect Friedman labor curve," the doctor said to me at one point. "You must have been studying!"

At the end, however, I had great difficulty pushing the baby out. After the pushing stage had gone on for quite a while, I was absolutely exhausted, though the baby was fine. There were no signs of fetal distress, and the head was descending steadily. Still, the pushing had gone on much longer than is usual, and I was aware that two doctors and a number of nurses were now in the birthing room.

Suddenly, I heard one of the doctors say something about forceps. At that moment, I found an extra ounce of strength and pushed my baby out.

As I lay back with my son wriggling on my stomach, the birthing room was suddenly transformed into the most beautiful place on earth. I heard one of the nurses say to another, "You see this all the time with these birthing-room-natural-childbirth mothers—you just mention forceps and they get those babies born."

Midwives in Transition: The Structure of a Clinical Revolution

Barbara Katz Rothman

There has been considerable interest in the United States in recent years in the medical management of the reproductive processes in healthy women. Much of this interest represents a growing recognition by many mothers that hospital births impose structures upon the birth process unrelated to and in many cases disruptive of the process itself.

This paper contends that changing the setting of birth from hospital to home alters the timing of the birth process, a result of the social redefinition of birth. Through an analysis of the medical literature on birth, I compare the social construction of timetables for childbirth—how long normal labor and birth takes—by hospital and home-birth practitioners. I argue that, like all knowledge, this knowledge is socially determined and socially constructed, influenced both by ideology and social setting.

This paper is based on interviews I conducted in 1978 with one subgroup of the home-birth movement: nurse-midwives certified by the State of New York to attend births. I located 12 nurse-midwives in the New York metropolitan area who were attending births in homes and at an out-of-hospital birth center. Nurse-midwives in the United States are trained in medical institutions one to two years beyond nursing training and obtain their formative experience in hospitals. They differ from lay midwives, who receive their training outside of medical institutions and hospitals. Once nurse-midwives are qualified, most of them continue to practice in hospitals. I use the term *nurse-midwives* throughout this paper to distinguish them from lay midwives. I discuss those parts of the interviews with these nurse-midwives which focus on their reconceptualization of birth timetables as they moved from hospital to home settings.

This sample was selected for two reasons: first, because of the position that nurse-midwives hold in relation to mothers compared with that held by physicians; while physicians in hospital settings control the birth process, nurse-midwives in home settings permit the birth process to transpire under the mother's control. Second, because nurse-midwives have been both formally trained within the medical model and extensively exposed to the home–birth model, data gathered in monitoring their adjustment to and reaction to the home–birth model provide a cross-contextual source for comparing the two birth settings.

Observation of the reactions of nurse-midwives to the home–birth setting demonstrates the degree to which their medical training was based on social convention rather than biological constants. The

Reprinted from *Social Problems*, vol 30 (February, 1983), pp. 262–270. Copyright © 1983 by The Society for the Study of Social Problems.

nurse-midwives did not embrace their non-medical childbirth work as ideological enthusiasts; rather, they were drawn into it, often against what they perceived as their better medical judgment. The nurse-midwives were firmly grounded in the medical model. Their ideas of what a home birth should and would be like, when they first began doing them, were based on their extensive experience with hospital births. While they believed that home birth would provide a more pleasant, caring, and warm environment than that ordinarily found in hospital birth, they did not expect it to challenge medical knowledge. And at first, home births did not. What the nurse-midwives saw in the home setting was screened through their expectations based on the hospital setting. The medical model was only challenged with repeated exposures to the anomalies of the home–birth experience.

The nurse-midwives' transition from one model to another is comparable to scientists' switch from one paradigm to another—a "scientific revolution," in Kuhn's (1970) words. Clinical models, like paradigms, are not discarded lightly by those who have invested time in learning and following them. The nurse-midwives were frequently not prepared for the anomalies in the timetable that they encountered at home. These involved unexpected divergences from times for birthing stages as "scheduled" by hospitals. Breaking these timetable norms without the expected ensuing "complications" provided the nurse-midwives attending home births with anomalies in the medical model. With repeated exposure to such anomalies, the nurse-midwives began to challenge the basis of medical knowledge regarding childbirth.

The medical approach divides the birth process into socially structured stages. Each of these stages is supposed to last a specific period of time. Roth (1963) notes that medical timetables structure physical processes and events, creating sanctioned definitions and medical controls. Miller (1977) has shown how medicine uses timetables to construct its own version of pregnancy. Similarly, medical timetables construct medical births: challenging those timetables challenges the medical model itself.

There are four parts of the birth process subject to medical timetables: (1) term (the end of pregnancy); (2) the first stage of labor; (3) delivery; and (4) expulsion of the placenta. I describe the hospital and home–birth approaches to these four parts and how each part's timetable issues arise. Then I consider the function of these timetables for doctors, hospitals, and the medical model.

(1) TERM: THE END OF PREGNANCY

The Hospital Approach

In the medical model, a full-term pregnancy is 40 weeks long, though there is a two-week allowance made on either side for "normal" births. Any baby born earlier than 38 weeks is "premature;" after 42 weeks, "postmature." Prematurity does not produce any major conceptual anomalies between the two models. If a woman attempting home birth goes into labor much before the beginning of the 38th week, the nurse-midwives send her to a hospital because they, like physicians, perceive prematurity as abnormal, although they may not agree with the subsequent medical management of prematurity. In fact, few of the nurse-midwives' clients enter labor prematurely.

Post-maturity however, has become an issue for the nurse-midwives. The medical treatment for postmaturity is to induce labor, either by rupturing the membranes which contain the fetus, or by administering hormones to start labor contraction, or both. Rindfuss (1977) has shown that physicians often induce labor without any "medical" justification for mothers' and doctors' convenience.

Induced labor is more difficult for the mother and the baby. Contractions are longer, more frequent, and more intense. The more intense contractions reduce the baby's oxygen supply. The mother may require medication to cope with the more difficult labor, thus further increasing the risk of injury to the baby. In addition, once the induced labor (induction) is attempted, doctors will go on to delivery shortly thereafter, by Cesarian section if necessary.

The Home–Birth Approach

These techniques for inducing labor are conceptualized as "interventionist" and "risky" within the home–birth movement. The home–birth clients of the nurse-midwives do not want to face hospitalization and inductions, and are therefore motivated to ask for more time and, if that is not an option, to seek "safe" and "natural" techniques for starting labor. Some nurse-midwives suggest nipple stimulation, sexual relations, or even castor oil and enemas as means of stimulating uterine contractions. As I interviewed the 12 nurse-midwives about their techniques it was unclear whether their concern was avoiding postmaturity *per se* or avoiding medical treatment for postmaturity.

The nurse-midwives said that the recurring problem of postmaturity has led some home–birth practitioners to re-evaluate the length of pregnancy. Home–birth advocates point out that the medical determination of the length of pregnancy is based on observations of women in medical care. These home–birth advocates argue that women have been systematically malnourished by medically ordered weight-gain limitations. They attribute the high level of premature births experienced by teenage women to malnourishment resulting from overtaxing of their energy reserves by growth, as well as fetal, needs. The advocates believe that very well nourished women are capable of maintaining a pregnancy longer than are poorly nourished or borderline women. Thus, the phenomenon of so many healthy women going past term is reconceptualized in this developing model as an indication of even greater health, rather than a pathological condition of "postmaturity."

The first few times a nurse-midwife sees a woman going past term she accepts the medical definition of the situation as pathological. As the problem is seen repeatedly in women who manifest no signs of pathology, and who go on to have healthy babies, the conceptualization of the situation as pathological is shaken. Nurse-midwives who have completed the transition from the medical to home–birth model, reject the medical definition and reconceptualize what they see from "postmature" to "fully mature."

(2) THE FIRST STAGE OF LABOR

The Hospital Approach

Childbirth, in the medical model, consists of three "stages" that occur after term. (In this paper I consider term as the first part of the birth process, occurring at the end of pregnancy.) In the first stage of childbirth, the cervix (the opening of the uterus into the vagina) dilates to its fullest to allow for the passage of the baby. In the second stage, the baby moves out of the open cervix, through the vagina, and is born. The third stage is the expulsion of the placenta. The second example of a point at which anomalies arise is in "going into labor," or entering the first stage.

The medical model of labor is best represented by "Friedman's Curve" (Friedman, 1959). To develop this curve, Friedman observed labors and computed averages for each "phase" of labor. He defined a *latent phase* as beginning with the onset of labor, taken as the onset of regular uterine contractions, to the beginnings of an *active phase,* when cervical dilation is most rapid. The onset of regular contractions can only be determined retroactively. *Williams Obstetrics* (Hellman and Pritchard, 1971), the classic obstetric text, says that the first stage of labor (which contains the two "phases") "begins with the first true labor pains and ends with the complete dilation of the cervix" (1971:351). "True labor pains" are distinguished from "false labor pains" by what happens next:

> The only way to distinguish between false and true labor pains, however, is to ascertain their effect on the cervix. The labor pains in the course of a few hours produce a demonstrable degree of effacement (thinning of the cervix) and some dilation of the cervix, whereas the effect of false labor pains on the cervix is minimal (1971:387).

The concept of "false" labor serves as a buffer for the medical model of "true" labor. Labors which display an unusually long "latent phase," or labors which simply stop, can be diagnosed as "false labors" and thus not affect the conceptualization of true labor. Friedman (1959:97) says:

> The latent phase may occasionally be found to be greater than the limit noted, and yet the remaining portion of the labor, the active phase of dilatation, may evolve completely normally. These unusual cases may be explained on the basis of the difficulty of determining the onset of labor. The transition from some forms of false labor into the latent phase of true labor may be completely undetectable and unnoticed. This may indeed be an explanation for the quite wide variation seen among patients of the actual duration of the latent phase.

In creating his model, Friedman obtained average values for each phase of labor, both for women with first pregnancies and for women with previous births. Then he computed the statistical limits and equated statistical normality with physiological normality:

> It is clear that cases where the phase-durations fall outside of these (statistical) limits are probably abnormal in some way. . . . We can see now how, with very little effort, we have been able to define average labor and to describe, with proper degree of certainty, the limits of normal (1959:97).

Once the equation is made between statistical abnormality and physiological abnormality, the door is opened for medical intervention. Thus, statistically abnormal labors are medically treated. The medical treatments are the same as those for induction of labor: rupture of membranes, hormones, and Cesarian section.

"Doing something" is the cornerstone of medical management. Every labor which takes "too long" and which cannot be stimulated by hormones or by breaking the membranes will go on to the next level of medical management, the Cesarian section. Breaking the membranes is an interesting induction technique in this regard: physicians believe that if too many hours pass after the membranes have been ruptured, naturally or artifically, a Cesarian section is necessary in order to prevent infection. Since physicians within the hospital always go on from one intervention to the next, there is no place for feedback; that is, one does not get to see what happens when a woman stays in first stage for a long time without her membranes being ruptured.

Hospital labors are shorter than home–birth labors. A study by Mehl (1977) of 1,046 matched, planned home and hospital births found that the average length of first-stage labor for first births was 14.5 hours in the home and 10.4 hours in the hospital. *Williams Obstetrics* reports the average length of labor for first births was 12.5 hours in 1948 (Hellman and Pritchard, 1971:396). For subsequent births, Mehl found first-stage labor took an average of 7.7 hours in the home and 6.6 hours in the hospital. Hellman and Pritchard reported 7.3 hours for the same stage. Because 1948 hospital births are comparable to contemporary home births, and because contemporary hospital births are shorter, it is probable that there has been an increase in "interventionist obstetrics," as home–birth advocates claim. These data are summarized in Table 1.

The Home–Birth Approach

Home–birth advocates see each labor as unique. While statistical norms may be interesting, they are of no value in managing a particular labor. When the nurse-midwives have a woman at home, or in the out-of-hospital birth-center, both the nurse-midwife and the woman giving birth want to complete birth without disruption. Rather than using arbitrary time limits, nurse-midwives look for progress, defined as continual change in the direction of birth-

TABLE 1 Labor timetables for the first and second stages of birth, for first and subsequent births

BIRTH	LENGTH OF FIRST STAGE OF LABOR (HOURS)		
	HOME 1970s	HOSPITAL 1948	HOSPITAL 1970s
First	14.5	12.5	10.4
Subsequent	7.7/8.5[a]	7.3[b]	6.6/5.9[a]
	LENGTH OF SECOND STAGE OF LABOR (MINUTES)		
First	94.7	80	63.9
Subsequent	48.7/21.7[a]	30[b]	19/15.9[a]

Note:

a. Second births and third births.

b. Second and all subsequent births.

ing. A more medically-oriented nurse-midwife expressed her ambivalence this way:

> They don't have to look like a Friedman graph walking around, but I think they should make some kind of reasonable progress (Personal interview).

Unable to specify times for "reasonable" progress, she nonetheless emphasized the word "reasonable," distinguishing it from "unreasonable" waiting.

A nurse-midwife with more home–birth experience expressed more concern for the laboring woman's subjective experience:

> There is no absolute limit—it would depend on what part of the labor was the longest and how she was handling that. Was she tired? Could she handle that? (Personal interview).

A labor at home can be long but "light," uncomfortable but not painful. A woman at home may spend those long hours going for a walk, napping, listening to music, even gardening or going to a movie. This light labor can go for quite some time. Another nurse-midwife described how she dealt with a long labor:

> Even though she was slow, she kept moving. I have learned to discriminate now, and if it's long I let them do it at home on their own and I try and listen carefully and when I get there it's toward the end of labor. This girl was going all Saturday and all Sunday, so that's 48 hours worth of labor. It wasn't forceful labor, but she was uncomfortable for two days. So if I'd have gone and stayed there the first time, I'd have been there a whole long time, then when you get there you have to do something (Personal interview).

(3) DELIVERY: PUSHING TIME LIMITS

The Hospital Approach

The medical literature defines the second stage of labor, the delivery, as the period from the complete dilatation of the cervix to the birth of the fetus. Hellman and Pritchard (1971) found this second stage took an average of 80 minutes for first births and 30 minutes for all subsequent births in 1948. Mehl (1977) found home births took an average of 94.7 minutes for first births and, for second and third births, 48.7 to 21.7 minutes. Contemporary medical procedures shorten the second stage in the hospital to 63.9 minutes for first births and 19 to 15.9 minutes for second and third births (Mehl, 1977).

The modern medical management of labor and delivery hastens the delivery process, primarily by the use of forceps and fundal pressure (pressing on the top of the uterus through the abdomen) to pull or push a fetus out. Friedman (1959) found the second stage of birth took an average of 54 minutes for first births and 18 minutes for all subsequent births. He defined the "limits of normal" as 2.5 hours for first births and 48 minutes for subsequent births. Contemporary hospitals usually apply even stricter limits, and allow a maximum of two hours for first births and one hour for second births. Time limits vary somewhat within U.S. hospitals, but physicians and nurse-midwives in training usually do not get to see a three-hour second stage, much less anything longer. "Prolonged" second stages are medically managed to effect immediate delivery.

Mehl (1977) found low forceps were 54 times more common and mid-forceps 21 times more common for prolonged second-stage and/or protracted descent in the hospital than in planned home births. This does not include the elective use of forceps (without "medical" indication), a procedure which was used in none of the home births and 10 percent of the hospital births (four percent low forceps and six percent mid-forceps). Any birth which began at home but was hospitalized for any reason, including protracted descent or prolonged second stage (10 percent of the sample), was included in Mehl's home–birth statistics.

The Home–Birth Approach

Nurse-midwives and their out-of-hospital clients were even more highly motivated to avoid hospitalization for prolonged delivery than for prolonged labor. There is a sense of having come so far, through the most difficult and trying part. Once a mother is fully dilated she may be so close to birth that moving her could result in giving birth on the way to the hospital. Contrary to the popular image, the mother is usually working hard but not in pain during the delivery, and as tired as she may be, is quite reluctant to leave home.

Compare the situation at home with what the nurse-midwives saw in their training. In a hospital birth the mother is moved to a delivery table at or near the end of cervical dilation. She is usually strapped into leg stirrups and heavily draped. The physician is scrubbed and gowned. The anesthetist is at the ready. The pediatric staff is in the room. It is difficult to imagine that situation continuing for three, four, or more hours. The position of the mother alone makes that impossible. In the medical model, second stage begins with complete cervical dilation. Cervical dilation is an "objective" measure, determined by the birth attendant. By defining the end of the first stage, the birth attendant controls the time of formal entry into second stage. One of the ways nurse-midwives quickly learn to "buy time" for their clients is in measuring cervical dilation:

If she's honestly fully dilated I do count it as second stage. If she has a rim of cervix left, I don't count it because I don't think it's fair. A lot of what I do is to look good on paper (Personal interview).

Looking good on paper is a serious concern. Nurse-midwives expressed their concern about legal liability if they allow the second stage to go on for more than the one- or two-hour hospital limit, and then want to hospitalize the woman. One told of allowing a woman to stay at home in second stage for three hours and then hospitalizing her for lack of progress. The mother, in her confusion and exhaustion, told the hospital staff that she had been in second stage for five hours. The nurse-midwife risked losing the support of the physician who had agreed to provide emergency and other medical services at that hospital. Even when a nurse-midwife's experiences cause her to question the medical model, the constraints under which she works may thus prevent her from acting on new knowledge. Nurse-midwives talked about the problems of charting second stage:

If I'm doing it for my own use I start counting when the woman begins to push, and push in a directed manner, really bearing down. I have to lie sometimes. I mean I'm prepared to lie if we ever have to go to the hospital because there might be an hour or so between full dilation and when she begins pushing and I don't see—

as long as the heart tones are fine and there is some progress being made—but like I don't think—you'd be very careful to take them to the hospital after five hours of pushing—they [hospital staff] would go crazy (Personal interview).

All my second stages, I write them down under two hours: by hospital standards two hours is the upper limit of normal, but I don't have two-hour second stages except that one girl that I happened to examine her. If I had not examined her, I probably would not have had more than an hour and a half written down because it was only an hour and a half that she was voluntarily pushing herself (Personal interview).

Not looking for what you do not want to find is a technique used by many of the nurse-midwives early in their transition away from the medical model. They are careful about examining a woman who might be fully dilated for fear of starting up the clock they work under:

I try to hold off on checking if she doesn't have the urge to push, but if she has the urge to push, then I have to go in and check (Personal interview).

With more home–birth experience, the nurse-midwives reconceptualized the second stage itself. Rather than starting with full dilatation, the "objective" measure, they measured the second stage by the subjective measure of the woman's urge to push. Most women begin to feel a definite urge to push, and begin bearing down, at just about the time of full dilatation. But not all women have this experience. For some, labor contractions ease after they are fully dilated. These are the "second-stage arrests" which medicine treats by the use of forceps or Cesarian section. Some nurse-midwives reconceptualized this from "second-stage arrest" to a naturally occurring rest period at the end of labor, after becoming fully dilated, but before second stage. In the medical model, once labor starts it cannot stop and start again and still be "normal." If it stops, that calls for medical intervention. But a nurse-midwife can reconceptualize "the hour or so between full dilation and when she starts pushing" as other than second stage. This is more than just buying time for clients: this is developing an alternative set of definitions, reconceptualizing the birth process.

Nurse-midwives who did not know each other and who did not work together came to the same conclusions about the inaccuracy of the medical model:

> My second stage measurement is when they show signs of being in second stage. That'd be the pushing or the rectum bulging or stuff like that. . . . I usually have short second stages [laughter]. Y'know, if you let nature do it, there's not a hassle (Personal interview).

> I would not, and this is really a fine point, encourage a mother to start pushing just because she felt fully dilated to me. I think I tend to wait till the mother gets a natural urge to push. . . . the baby's been in there for nine months (Personal interview).

It may be that buying time is the first concern. In looking for ways to avoid starting the clock, nurse-midwives first realize that they can simply not examine the mother. They then have the experience of "not looking" for an hour, and seeing the mother stir herself out of a rest and begin to have a strong urge to push. The first few times that hour provokes anxiety in the nurse-midwives. Most of the nurse-midwives told of their nervousness in breaking time-table norms. The experience of breaking timetable norms and having a successful outcome challenges the medical model; it is a radicalizing experience. This opportunity for feedback does not often exist in the hospital setting, where medicine's stringent control minimizes anomalies. A woman who has an "arrested" second stage will usually not be permitted to sleep, and therefore the diagnosis remains unchallenged. Forceps and/or hormonal stimulants are introduced. The resulting birth injuries are seen as inevitable, as if without the forceps the baby would never have gotten out alive.

(4) EXPULSION OF THE PLACENTA

The Hospital Approach

Third stage is the period between the delivery of the baby and the expulsion of the placenta. In hospitals, third stage takes five minutes or less (Hellman and Pritchard, 1971; Mehl, 1977). A combination of massage and pressure on the uterus and gentle pulling on the cord are used routinely. Hellman and Pritchard (1971:417) instruct that if the placenta has not separated within about five minutes after birth it should be removed manually. In Mehl's (1977) data, the average length of the third stage for home births was 20 minutes.

The Home–Birth Approach

For the nurse-midwives, the third stage timetable was occasionally a source of problems. Sometimes the placenta does not slip out, even in the somewhat longer time period that many nurse-midwives have learned to accept. Their usual techniques—the mother pulling the baby to suckle, squatting, walking—may not have shown immediate results:

> I don't feel so bad if there's no bleeding. Difficult if it doesn't come, and it's even trickier when there's no hemmorhage because if there's a hemmorhage then there's a definite action you can take; but when it's retained and it isn't coming it's a real question—is it just a bell-shaped curve and that kind of thing—in the hospital if it isn't coming right away you just go in and pull it out (Personal interview).

> I talked with my grandmother—she's still alive, she's 90, she did plenty of deliveries—and she says that if the placenta doesn't come out you just let the mother walk around for a day and have her breastfeed and it'll fall out. And I believe her. Here I would have an hour because I am concerned about what appears on the chart (Personal interview).

> If there was no bleeding, and she was doing fine, I think several hours, you know, or more could elapse, no problem (Personal interview).

WHY THE RUSH? THE FUNCTIONS OF TIMETABLES

The Hospital Approach

There are both medical and institutional reasons for speeding up the birth. The medical reasons are: (1) A prolonged third stage is believed to cause excessive bleeding. (2) The second stage is kept short in order to spare the mother and the baby, because birth is conceptualized as traumatic for both. (3) The anesthetics which are routinely used create conditions encouraging, if not requiring, the use of forceps. The position of the woman also contributes to the use of forceps because the baby must be pushed upwards.

There are several institutional reasons for speeding up birth. Rosengren and DeVault (1963) discussed the importance of timing and tempo in the hospital management of birth. Tempo relates to the number of deliveries in a given period of time. The tempo of individual births is matched to the space and staffing limitations of the institution. If there are too many births, the anesthetist will slow them down. An unusually prolonged delivery will also upset the hospital's tempo, and there is even competition to maintain optimal tempo. One resident said, "Our [the residents'] average length of delivery is about 50 minutes, and the pros' [the private doctors'] is about 40 minutes" (1963:282). That presumably includes delivery of baby and placenta, and probably any surgical repair as well. Rosengren and DeVault further note:

> This "correct tempo" becomes a matter of status competition, and a measure of professional adeptness. The use of forceps is also a means by which the tempo is maintained in the delivery room, and they are so often used that the procedure is regarded as normal (1963:282).

Rosengren and DeVault, with no out-of-hospital births as a basis for comparison, apparently did not perceive the management of the third stage as serving institutional needs. Once the baby is quickly and efficiently removed, one certainly does not wait 20 minutes or more for the spontaneous expulsion of the placenta.

Hospitals so routinize the various obstetrical interventions that alternative conceptualizations are unthinkable. A woman attached to an intravenous or a machine used to monitor the condition of the fetus cannot very well be told to go out for a walk or to a movie if her contractions are slow and not forceful. A woman strapped to a delivery table cannot take a nap if she does not feel ready to push. She cannot even get up and move around to find a better position for pushing. Once the institutional forces begin, the process is constructed in a manner appropriate to the institutional model. Once a laboring woman is hospitalized, she will have a medically constructed birth.

Therefore, not only the specific rules, but also the overall perspective of the hospital as an institution, operate to proscribe hospital–birth attendants' reconceptualization of birth. Practitioners may "lose even the ability to think of alternatives or to take known alternatives seriously because the routine is so solidly established and embedded in perceived consensus" (Holtzner, 1968:96).

The Home–Birth Approach

In home births the institutional supports and the motivations for maintaining hospital tempo are not present; birth attendants do not move from one laboring woman to the next. Births do not have to be meshed to form an overriding institutional tempo. Functioning without institutional demands or institutional supports, nurse-midwives are presented with situations which are anomalies in the medical model, such as labors stopping and starting, the second stage not following immediately after the first, and a woman taking four hours to push out a baby without any problems—and feeling good about it. Without obstetrical interventions, medically defined "pathologies" may be seen to right themselves, and so the very conceptualization of pathology and normality is challenged.

In home or out-of-hospital births, the routine and perceived consensus is taken away. Each of the nurse-midwives I interviewed stressed the individuality of each out-of-hospital birth, saying that each birth was so much "a part of each mother and family." They described tightly-knit extended-kin situations, devoutly religious births, party-like births, intimate and sexual births—an infinite variety. The variety of social contexts seemed to overshadow the physiological constants. That is not to say that constraints are absent, but that at home the constraints are very different than they are within hospitals. At home, the mother as patient must coexist or take second place to the mother as mother, wife, daughter, sister, friend, or lover.

SUMMARY AND CONCLUSIONS

The hospital setting structures the ideology and the practice of hospital-trained nurse-midwives. Home birth, by contrast, provides an ultimately radicalizing experience, in that it challenges the taken-for-granted assumptions of the hospital experience. Timetables provide structure for the hospital experience: structures—statistical constructions, models, or attempts at routinization or standardization—are not necessarily bad in and of themselves. Medical timetables, however, have termed pathological whatever does not conform to statistical norms, which are themselves based on biased samples and distorted by structural restraints imposed in the interests of efficiency. Thus, the range of normal variation does not permeate the model.

One final conclusion to be drawn from this research is a reaffirmation that knowledge, including medical knowledge, is socially situated. Medical reality is a socially constructed reality, and the content of medical knowledge is as legitimate an area of research for medical sociology as are doctor–patient relations, illness behavior, and the other more generally studied areas.

References

FRIEDMAN, EMMANUEL
  1959 "Graphic analysis of labor." Bulletin of the American College of Nurse-Midwifery 4(3):94–105.
HELLMAN, LOUIS, and JACK PRITCHARD (EDS.)
  1971 Williams Obstetrics. 14th edition. New York: Appleton-Century-Croft.
HOLTZNER, BUKART
  1968 Reality Construction in Society. Cambridge, MA: Schenkmann.
KUHN, THOMAS S.
  1970 The Structure of Scientific Revolutions. Chicago: University of Chicago Press.
MEHL, LEWIS
  1977 "Research on childbirth alternatives: What can it tell us about hospital practices?" Pp. 171–208 in David Stewart and Lee Stewart (eds.), Twenty-First Century Obstetrics Now. Chapel Hill, N.C.: National Association of Parents and Professionals for Safe Alternatives in Childbirth.
MILLER, RITA SEIDEN
  1977 "The social construction and reconstruction of physiological events: Acquiring the pregnant identity." Pp. 87–145 in Norman K. Denzin (ed.), Studies in Symbolic Interaction. Greenwich, CT: JAI Press.
RINDFUSS, RONALD R.
  1977 "Convenience and the occurrence of births: Induction of labor in the United States and Canada." Paper presented at the 72nd annual meeting of the American Sociological Association, Chicago, August.
ROSENGREN, WILLIAM R., and SPENCER DEVAULT
  1963 "The sociology of time and space in an obstetric hospital." Pp. 284–285 in Eliot Friedson (ed.), The Hospital in Modern Society. New York: Free Press.
ROTH, JULIUS
  1963 Timetables: Structuring the Passage of Time in Hospital Treatment and Other Careers. Indianapolis: Bobbs Merrill.
ROTHMAN, BARBARA KATZ
  1982 In Labor: Women and Power in the Birthplace. New York: Norton.

_____

CHAPTER 9

The Relationships Among Practitioners

The relationships among health professionals is largely determined by a well-defined stratification system that is dominated by the physician. The issue of professional authority and how it resides in this system will be dealt with explicitly in several articles that come later in the book. Here we are concerned with the doctor–nurse relationship and relationships among doctors.

A substantial amount has been written about the doctor–nurse relationship. Traditionally, the nurse has been characterized as being highly subordinated to the control of the physician and in the role of doctor's assistant rather than professional colleague. Probably the best known description of that role and its subtleties has been written by Leonard I. Stein and is included in the readings in this chapter. In recent years, the nursing profession has become more assertive in pursuit of its goal of greater professional recognition. The sources and consequences of this assertiveness for nursing as a whole is discussed in an article in Part Four.

In the oft-cited article that opens this chapter, Leonard I. Stein analyzes the "doctor–nurse" game. Stein explains how nurses learn to show initiative and make recommendations to a physician in a manner that appears deferential to the physician. The remaining articles look at relationships among physicians. More specifically, they are concerned with the ability of the medical profession to police and exert control over the performance of its members. The first of these is from Marcia Millman's *The Unkindest Cut* and is the second piece from that book to be found in *Dominant Issues*. It describes the Medical Mortality Review, which is a meeting in which suspected physician mistakes that may be linked to the death of a patient are investigated. Millman describes how, in various ways, the consideration of medical errors remains superficial so as to protect the doctors whose performance is under review. It is also true, according to Millman, that only ambiguous cases are selected for review in the first place. The short excerpt from Donald L. Light derives from his research on psychiatric residents. It is treated as an addendum to the Medical Mortality Review discussion, and it shows that Millman's conclusions are generalizable to the case of the Suicide Review, in which psychiatrists review cases where patients have committed suicide while under a psychiatrist's care.

The selection by Eliot Freidson comes from *Doctoring Together*. It is, along with Millman's *The Unkindest Cut,* one of the few books to study firsthand the relationships among physicians. It is not surprising that little research of this kind has been done since obtaining this kind of data from physicians is understandably difficult. In *Doctoring Together,* Freidson presents the conclusions from a study of a large medical group of over 50 doctors serving approximately 25,000 patients on a prepaid basis. He and his colleagues interviewed the physicians and observed them in their daily interactions with each other. In the selection included in this chapter, Freidson analyzes the reasons why physicians in group practice have little control over one another. Central to this lack of control is the fact that information about the performance of one's colleagues is not easily obtained. These conclusions are particularly significant because there had been speculation that a positive by-product of doctors increasingly working in prepaid group practices, as opposed to working alone, would be the greater opportunity for critical scrutiny of each other's performance. According to Freidson, this has not turned out to be the case.

The Doctor-Nurse Game

Leonard I. Stein

The relationship between the doctor and the nurse is a very special one. There are few professions where the degree of mutual respect and cooperation between co-workers is as intense as that between the doctor and nurse. Superficially, the stereotype of this relationship has been dramatized in many novels and television serials. When, however, it is observed carefully in an interactional framework, the relationship takes on a new dimension and has a special quality which fits a game model. The underlying attitudes which demand that this game be played are unfortunate. These attitudes create serious obstacles in the path of meaningful communications between physicians and non-medical professional groups.

The physician traditionally and appropriately has total responsibility for making the decisions regarding the management of his patients' treatment. To guide his decisions he considers data gleaned from several sources. He acquires a complete medical history, performs a thorough physical examination, interprets laboratory findings, and at times, obtains recommendations from physician-consultants. Another important factor in his decision making is the recommendations he receives from the nurse. The interaction between doctor and nurse through which these recommendations are communicated and received is unique and interesting.

THE GAME

One rarely hears a nurse say, "Doctor, I would recommend that you order a retention enema for Mrs. Brown." A physician, upon hearing a recommendation of that nature, would gape in amazement at the effrontery of the nurse. The nurse, upon hearing

Reprinted from the *Archives of General Psychiatry*, vol. 16 (1967), pp. 699–703. Copyright © 1967 by the American Medical Association.

the statement, would look over her shoulder to see who said it, hardly believing the words actually came from her own mouth. Nevertheless, if one observes closely, nurses make recommendations of more import every hour and physicians willingly and respectfully consider them. If the nurse is to make a suggestion without appearing insolent and the doctor is to seriously consider that suggestion, their interaction must not violate the rules of the game.

Object of the Game

The object of the game is as follows: the nurse is to be bold, have initiative, and be responsible for making significant recommendations, while at the same time she must appear passive. This must be done in such a manner so as to make her recommendations appear to be initiated by the physician.

Both participants must be acutely sensitive to each other's nonverbal and cryptic verbal communications. A slight lowering of the head, a minor shifting of position in the chair, or a seemingly nonrelevant comment concerning an event which occurred eight months ago must be interpreted as a powerful message. The game requires the nimbleness of a high wire acrobat, and if either participant slips, the game can be shattered; the penalties for frequent failure are apt to be severe.

Rules of the Game

The cardinal rule of the game is that open disagreement between the players must be avoided at all costs. Thus, the nurse must communicate her recommendations without appearing to be making a recommendation statement. The physician, in requesting a recommendation from a nurse, must do so without appearing to be asking for it. Utilization of this technique keeps anyone from committing themselves to a position before a sub-rosa agreement on that position has already been established. In that way open disagreement is avoided. The greater the significance of the recommendation, the more subtly the game must be played.

To convey a subtle example of the game with all its nuances would require the talents of a literary artist. Lacking these talents, let me give you the following example, which is unsubtle but happens frequently. The medical resident on hospital call is awakened by telephone at 1:00 A.M., because a patient on a ward, not his own, has not been able to fall asleep. Dr. Jones answers the telephone and the dialogue goes like this:

> This is Dr. Jones.
> (*An open and direct communication.*)
> Dr. Jones, this is Miss Smith on 2W—Mrs. Brown, who learned today of her father's death, is unable to fall asleep.
> (*This message has two levels. Openly, it describes a set of circumstances: a woman who is unable to sleep and who that morning received word of her father's death. Less openly, but just as directly, it is a diagnostic and recommendation statement; i.e., Mrs. Brown is unable to sleep because of her grief, and she should be given a sedative. Dr. Jones, accepting the diagnostic statement and replying to the recommendation statement, answers.*)
> What sleeping medication has been helpful to Mrs. Brown in the past?
> (*Dr. Jones, not knowing the patient, is asking for a recommendation from the nurse, who does know the patient, about what sleeping medication should be prescribed. Note, however, his question does not appear to be asking her for a recommendation. Miss Smith replies.*)
> Pentobarbital mg 100 was quite effective night before last.
> (*A disguised recommendation statement. Dr. Jones replies with a note of authority in his voice.*)
> Pentobarbital mg 100 before bedtime as needed for sleep; got it?
> (*Miss Smith ends the conversation with the tone of a grateful supplicant.*) Yes, I have, and thank you very much doctor.

The above is an example of a successfully played doctor–nurse game. The nurse made appropriate recommendations which were accepted by the physician and were helpful to the patient. The game was successful because the cardinal rule was not violated.

The nurse was able to make her recommendation without appearing to, and the physician was able to ask for recommendations without conspicuously asking for them.

The Scoring System

Inherent in any game are penalties and rewards for the players. In game theory, the doctor–nurse game fits the non-zero-sum-game model. It is not like chess, where the players compete with each other and whatever one player loses the other wins. Rather, it is the kind of game in which the rewards and punishments are shared by both players. If they play the game successfully they both win rewards, and if they are unskilled and the game is played badly, they both suffer the penalty.

The most obvious reward from the well-played game is a doctor–nurse team that operates efficiently. The physician is able to utilize the nurse as a valuable consultant, and the nurse gains self-esteem and professional satisfaction from her job. The less obvious rewards are not less important. A successful game creates a doctor–nurse alliance; through this alliance the physician gains the respect and admiration of the nursing service. He can be confident that his nursing staff will smooth the path for getting his work done. His charts will be organized and waiting for him when he arrives, the ruffled feathers of patients and relatives will have been smoothed down, his pet routines will be happily followed, and he will be helped in a thousand and one other ways.

The doctor–nurse alliance sheds its light on the nurse as well. She gains a reputation for being a "damn good nurse." She is respected by everyone and appropriately enjoys her position. When physicians discuss the nursing staff it would not be unusual for her name to be mentioned with respect and admiration. Their esteem for a good nurse is no less than their esteem for a good doctor.

The penalties for a game failure, on the other hand, can be severe. The physician who is an unskilled gamesman and fails to recognize the nurses' subtle recommendation messages is tolerated as a "clod." If, however, he interprets these messages as insolence and strongly indicates he does not wish to tolerate suggestions from nurses, he creates a rocky path for his travels. The old truism "If the nurse is your ally you've got it made, and if she has it in for you, be prepared for misery" takes on life-sized proportions. He receives three times as many phone calls after midnight as his colleagues. Nurses will not accept his telephone orders, because "telephone orders are against the rules." Somehow, this rule gets suspended for the skilled players. Soon he becomes like Joe Bfstplk in the "Li'l Abner" comic strip. No matter where he goes, a black cloud constantly hovers over his head.

The unskilled gamesman-nurse also pays heavily. The nurse who does not view her role as that of consultant, and therefore does not attempt to communicate recommendations, is perceived as a dullard and is mercifully allowed to fade into the woodwork.

The nurse who does see herself as a consultant but refuses to follow the rules of the game in making her recommendations has hell to pay. The outspoken nurse is labeled a "bitch" by the surgeon. The psychiatrist describes her as unconsciously suffering from penis envy, and her behavior is the acting out of her hostility towards men. Loosely translated, the psychiatrist is saying she is a bitch. The employment of the unbright, outspoken nurse is soon terminated. The outspoken, bright nurse whose recommendations are worthwhile remains employed. She is, however, constantly reminded in a hundred ways that she is not loved.

GENESIS OF THE GAME

To understand how the game evolved, we must comprehend the nature of the doctors' and nurses' training which shaped the attitudes necessary for the game.

Medical Student Training

The medical student in his freshman year studies as if possessed. In the anatomy class he learns every groove and prominence on the bones of the skeleton as if life depended on it. As a matter of fact, he literally believes just that. He not infrequently says, "I've got to learn it exactly; a life may depend on me knowing that." A consequence of this attitude, which is carefully nurtured throughout medical school, is the development of a phobia: the overdetermined fear of making a mistake. The development

of this fear is quite understandable. The burden the physician must carry is at times almost unbearable. He feels responsible in a very personal way for the lives of his patients. When a man dies leaving young children and a widow, the doctor carries some of her grief and despair inside himself; and when a child dies, some of him dies too. He sees himself as a warrior against death and disease. When he loses a battle, through no fault of his own, he nevertheless feels pangs of guilt, and he relentlessly searches himself to see if there might have been a way to alter the outcome. For the physician a mistake leading to a serious consequence is intolerable, and any mistake reminds him of his vulnerability. There is little wonder that he becomes phobic. The classical way in which phobias are managed is to avoid the source of the fear. Since it is impossible to avoid making some mistakes in an active practice of medicine, a substitute defensive maneuver is employed. The physician develops the belief that he is omnipotent and omniscient and therefore incapable of making mistakes. This belief allows the phobic physician to actively engage in his practice rather than avoid it. The fear of committing an error in a critical field like medicine is unavoidable and appropriately realistic. The physician, however, must learn to live with the fear rather than handle it defensively through a posture of omnipotence. This defense markedly interferes with his interpersonal professional relationships.

Physicians, of course, deny feelings of omnipotence. The evidence, however, renders their denials to whispers in the wind. The slightest mistake inflicts a large narcissistic wound. Depending on his underlying personality structure, the physician may be obsessed for days about it, quickly rationalize it away, or deny it. The guilt produced is unusually exaggerated, and the incident is handled defensively. The ways in which physicians enhance and support each other's defenses when an error is made could be the topic of another paper. The feeling of omnipotence becomes generalized to other areas of his life. A report of the Federal Aviation Agency (FAA), as quoted in *Time* (August 5, 1966), states that in 1964 and 1965, physicians had a fatal-accident rate four times as high as the average for all other private pilots. Major causes of the high death rate were risk-taking attitudes and judgments. Almost all of the accidents occurred on pleasure trips and were therefore not necessary risks to get to a patient needing emergency care. The trouble, suggested an FAA official, is that too many doctors fly with "the feeling that they are omnipotent." Thus, the extremes to which the physician may go in preserving his self-concept of omnipotence may threaten his own life. This overdetermined preservation of omnipotence is indicative of its brittleness and its underlying foundation of fear of failure.

The physician finds himself trapped in a paradox. He fervently wants to give his patient the best possible medical care, and being open to the nurses' recommendations helps him accomplish this. On the other hand, accepting advice from nonphysicians is highly threatening to his omnipotence. The solution for the paradox is to receive sub-rosa recommendations and make them appear to be initiated by himself. In short, he must learn to play the doctor–nurse game.

Some physicians never learn to play the game. Most learn in their internship, and a perceptive few learn during their clerkships in medical school. Medical students frequently complain that the nursing staff treats them as if they had just completed a junior Red Cross first-aid class instead of two years of intensive medical training. Interviewing nurses in a training hospital sheds considerable light on this phenomenon. In their words they said:

> *A few students just seem to be with it, they are able to understand what you are trying to tell them and they are a pleasure to work with; most, however, pretend to know everything and refuse to listen to anything we have to say and I guess we do give them a rough time.*

In essence, they are saying that those students who quickly learn the game are rewarded, and those that do not are punished.

Most physicians learn to play the game after they have weathered a few experiences like the one described below. On the first day of his internship, the physician and nurse were making rounds. They stopped at the bed of a fifty-two-year-old woman who, after complimenting the young doctor on his appearance, complained to him of her problem with constipation. After several minutes of listening to her detailed description of peculiar diets, family home remedies, and special exercises that have helped her constipation in the past, the nurse politely interrupted the patient. She told her the doctor would take care of the problem and that he had to move on because there were other patients waiting to see him. The young doctor gave the nurse a stern look, turned toward the patient, and kindly told her he would order an enema for her that very afternoon. As they left the bedside, the nurse told him the patient has had a normal bowel movement every day for the past week and that in the twenty-three days the patient has been in the hospital she has never once passed up an opportunity to complain of her constipation. She quickly added that *if* the doctor wanted to order an enema, the patient would certainly receive one. After hearing this report the intern's mouth fell open, and the wheels began turning in his head. He remembered the nurse's comment to the patient that "the doctor had to move on," and it occurred to him that perhaps she was really giving him a message. This experience and a few more like it, and the young doctor learns to listen for the subtle recommendations the nurses make.

Nursing Student Training

Unlike the medical student who usually learns to play the game after he finishes medical school, the nursing student begins to learn it early in her training. Throughout her education she is trained to play the doctor–nurse game.

Student nurses are taught how to relate to physicians. They are told he has infinitely more knowledge than they, and thus he should be shown the utmost respect. In addition, it was not many years ago when nurses were instructed to stand whenever a physician entered a room. When he would come in for a conference, the nurse was expected to offer him her chair, and when both entered a room the nurse would open the door for him and allow him to enter first. Although these practices are no longer rigidly adhered to, the premise upon which they were based is still promulgated. One nurse described that premise as, "He's God almighty and your job is to wait on him."

To inculcate subservience and inhibit deviancy, nursing schools, for the most part, are tightly run, disciplined institutions. Certainly, there is great variation among nursing schools, and there is little question that the trend is toward giving students more autonomy. However, in too many schools this trend has not gone far enough, and the climate remains restrictive. The student's schedule is firmly controlled, and there is very little free time. Classroom hours, study hours, mealtime, and bedtime with lights out are rigidly enforced. In some schools meaningless chores are assigned, such as cleaning bedsprings with cotton applicators. The relationship between student and instructor continues this military flavor. Often their relationship is more like that between recruit and drill sergeant than between student and teacher. Open dialogue is inhibited by attitudes of strict black and white with few, if any, shades of gray. Straying from the rigidly outlined path is sure to result in disciplinary action.

The inevitable result of these practices is to instill in the student nurse a fear of independent action. This inhibition of independent action is most marked when relating to physicians. One of the students' greatest fears is making a blunder while assisting a physician and being publicly ridiculed by him. This is really more a reflection of the nature of their training than the prevalence of abusive physicians. The fear of being humiliated for a blunder while assisting in a procedure is generalized to the fear of humiliation for making any independent act in relating to a physician, especially the act of making a direct recommendation. Every nurse interviewed felt that making a suggestion to a physician was equivalent to insulting and belittling him. It was tantamount to questioning his medical knowledge and insinuating he did not know his business. In light of her image of the physician as an omniscient and punitive figure, the questioning of his knowledge would be unthinkable.

The student, however, is also given messages quite contrary to the ones described above. She is continually told that she is an invaluable aid to the physician in the treatment of the patient. She is told that she must help him in every way possible and that she is imbued with a strong sense of responsibility for the care of her patient. Thus she, like the physician, is caught in a paradox. The first set of messages implies that the physician is omniscient and that any recommendation she might make would be insulting to him and leave her open to ridicule. The second set of messages implies that she is an important aspect to him, has much to contribute, and is duty-bound to make those contributions. Thus, when her good sense tells her a recommendation would be helpful to him, she is not allowed to communicate it directly, nor is she allowed not to communicate it. The way out of the bind is to use the doctor-nurse game and communicate the recommendation without appearing to do so.

Medical Mortality Review: A Cordial Affair

Marcia Millman

A mortality and morbidity conference for doctors bears some resemblance to a wedding or a funeral for members of a family. In all these ceremonies there is some feeling among those who attend that tact and restraint must be exercised if everyone is to leave on friendly terms. But steering a mortality meeting along on a pleasant and even course is occasionally difficult, for as in weddings and funerals, the very nature of the event often prompts participants to come dangerously close to saying to one another those upsetting things that are usually left unsaid.

Mortality meetings are regularly scheduled conferences at Lakeside Hospital; they are held in a large auditorium to accommodate the entire medical staff (private attending physicians, house officers, and teaching staff). Their avowed purpose is to review, in fine detail, those medical cases that ended in an in-hospital patient death, and in which there is some question of error, failure, or general mismanagement on the part of the physicians involved. One of the implicit if unspoken concerns that always underlies the review is the question of whether the patient's death might have been avoided had the medical judgment been more sound for what is usually involved in these cases is a question of misdiagnosis or of appropriate medical action taken too late.

In consideration of the delicacy of the occasion, the meetings are restricted to the medical staff of the hospital. Even the surgical staff is generally not invited. The surgical service has its own mortality meetings, and a surgeon would be considered meddlesome for attending a medical mortality conference simply out of curiosity. Only those surgeons who were directly involved in a particular case under

Reprinted from *The Unkindest Cut* by Marcia Millman, pp. 96–109 by permission of William Morrow and Company. Copyright © 1976 by Marcia Millman.

consideration will be asked to attend a medical mortality meeting. Families are *not* informed that their deceased relative's case has been chosen for review. Although the meetings may be considerably embarrassing for the doctors involved, the Medical Mortality Conference is, at least on the surface, treated as an *educational,* rather than a punitive, affair. At Lakeside, the conferences are not investigations or formal hearings held to consider the competence of particular doctors, although they are often presented this way on television medical dramas. There are no formal sanctions applied to doctors at the end of these conferences. Rather, Mortality Review Conferences are "educational" sessions organized around reviewing particular cases rather than individual doctors, even though the cases are selected because there is disagreement over the appropriate treatment and often a question of physician error involved.

The Mortality Review Conference has a special quality of high tension, and the meetings are better attended than are those of the other regular teaching conferences. At Lakeside Hospital, the Chief of Medicine stands on the stage and presides over the Mortality Review Conference as a master of ceremonies. As the case is reviewed in chronological order, starting with the time of the patient admission to the hospital, and proceeding to the autopsy report, the chief calls on the various doctors who were involved in the case, asks them to step to the front of the auditorium, and instructs them to recall and explain what they did and what they thought at each moment in time. He counsels them not to jump ahead of the chronological order, nor to divulge information gained at a later time, in order not to spoil the final diagnosis for the members of the audience. As one after another of the staff testifies about how they were led to the same mistaken diagnosis, a convincing case for the justifiability of the error is implicitly presented and the responsibility for the mistake is spread so that no one doctor is made to look guilty of a mistake that anyone else wouldn't have made, and in fact, didn't make. As in a good detective story, the case is reconstructed to show that there was evidence for suspecting an outcome different from the one that turns out to be the true circumstance. Responsibility for the error is also neutralized by making much of unusual or misleading features of the case, or showing how the patient was himself to blame, because of uncooperative or neurotic behavior. Furthermore, by reviewing the case in fine detail the doctors restore their images as careful, methodical practitioners and thereby neutralize the actual sloppiness and carelessness made obvious by the mistake. The doctors' discomfort is further minimized by treating the review as an educational occasion rather than an investigatory event.

In order to appreciate the special atmosphere and significance of the Mortality Review, it is important to understand that doctors who work together ordinarily live by a gentlemen's agreement to overlook each other's mistakes. The aim is not merely to hide errors and incompetence from the patients and the public, but also to avoid interfering in one another's work and to avoid acknowledgment of the injury that has been done to patients. Such a conspiracy to look the other way regarding the failures of one's colleagues is not always recognized by the doctors for what it is, for blindness to injury done to patients and a convincing set of justifications and excuses for medical mistakes are carefully built into their training and professional etiquette. Most doctors are therefore capable of comfortably viewing themselves as altruistic and highly responsible practitioners all the while they engage in collective rationalizations for ignoring and condoning each other's errors and incompetence.

Still, there are special occasions in the hospital routine, such as the Mortality Meeting, when doctors are gathered together to examine the sorts of unpleasant facts they would otherwise ignore. At these times a great deal of effort is expended to make the embarrassing facts seem less damaging. For if such medical incompetence or error were fully and publicly (among themselves) acknowledged, physician-colleagues might feel forced to take measures against one another, and this is one of the things they least like to do.

As the Chief of Medicine at Lakeside explained, "Eighty percent of the mistakes made around here are ignored or swept under the rug. I can only pick *certain* cases for mortality review—it's got to be a cordial affair."

Perhaps that description of the selection procedures for mortality review accounts for the curious fact that at Lakeside, most of the medical situations presented at these conferences conveniently seem to involve an illness that would have ended in the patient's death in any case, even if the correct diagnosis had been made immediately. There is a strange absence of cases reviewed in these meetings in which the patient would clearly have lived had it not been for the medical mismanagement. By selecting only those cases in which the physician's error was not fateful in an ultimate sense the discussion of mistakes largely becomes an academic affair.

Practicality rather than sentiment is the key to the tact and reserve with which doctors respond to each other's errors. A doctor's reluctance to criticize a colleague's mistakes to his face at a large meeting is not motivated out of respect or affection. Indeed, many doctors are willing, in small groups, to say that another physician (not present) is a menace or a terrible doctor. And even at the mortality review conferences, those doctors who are not involved in a case may occasionally sit back and enjoy the gentle roasting of a disliked work associate. The reluctance to point out and criticize another doctor's mistakes at an official meeting comes rather out of a fear of reprisal and a recognition of common interests. For each doctor knows that he has made some more or less terrible mistake in his career, and that he is likely to make others—mistakes, moreover, which will be obvious to his colleagues. That is why, in matters of peer regulation, doctors observe the Golden Rule.

So it is that mortality meetings are built upon a simultaneous admission and cover-up of mistakes. For although the avowed purpose of these meetings is to review mistakes and prevent their recurrence, in actuality the meetings are organized and conducted in ways that absolve the doctors from responsibility and guilt and provide the self-assuring but somewhat false appearance that physicians are monitoring each other and their standards of work. In case after case physician errors are systematically excused and justified, and their consequences made to look unimportant.

Before turning to some actual cases, it should be noted that despite the tact and sensitivity with which doctors treat each other's errors, a mortality meeting is not an entirely comfortable situation. Like a family trying collectively to ignore that the father is having an affair, or that the daughter is a drug addict, the doctors at a mortality meeting are often pushed to extreme displays of courtesy to overlook the worst and find good excuses for regrettable behavior.

CASE NO. 1: JONATHAN THOMAS

Jonathan Thomas was a 34-year-old insurance salesman who had complained of abdominal pain and black stool (indicating gastrointestinal bleeding). His problem was diagnosed as gastric ulcer and he was placed on a regimen of tranquilizers and an ulcer diet. His subsequent complaints were explained as being consistent with an ulcer and a neurotic personality. Ten months later Jonathan Thomas died of cancer spread throughout his abdominal cavity.

This was to be a particularly uncomfortable case for the staff to consider in Mortality Review because of a number of factors. First of all, the patient was a young man with a large family, and this made his life more valuable in the eyes of the doctors. Second, mistakes in diagnosis had been made repeatedly, and important information overlooked more than once. Third, a large number of people had been involved in this case, and while this offered the consolation of spreading out the responsibility, it also pointed out the weaknesses of the hospital consulting system. For if not one of a dozen physicians had caught the obvious errors, it was probably because each of the consultants involved in the case had been too accepting of each other's erroneous assumptions instead of carefully doing the diagnostic jobs they were supposed to be doing.

Notices about the mortality meeting had been distributed days beforehand and signs posted around the hospital. The chief's secretary had made sure that all the doctors involved in the case would be there for the review. As always, the meeting was held in the large theater-like auditorium and members of the staff seated themselves in the rows of seats facing the stage in a steep incline.

The meeting was called to order by the Chief of Medicine, who welcomed everyone and made brief announcements of unrelated matters. Next, an intern described the hospital's mortality profile for the preceding month: he described how many patients had died in the hospital in each major disease category. Finally, the Chief of Medicine, Dr. Tanner, returned to the stage and introduced the Thomas case. As usual, the patient's history was reviewed in chronological order, each doctor being called to the front of the room to recall his thoughts and describe his participation at that moment in time in the case.

The early history was reviewed by Dr. Backman, the specialist in gastrointestinal disorders who had managed the case. Backman was highly respected and well liked by most of the staff, and so there were no undertones of questioning his competence but rather friendly empathy for the usually careful physician who had made an uncharacteristic mistake. From the beginning, Backman explained, he had assumed that the gastrointestinal bleeding indicated by the black stool was caused by a stress-induced gastric ulcer: "What led us down the garden path last October was the fact that he was taking on added responsibility for his family's business. The sudden pain seemed to coincide with that, so we put him on an ulcer regimen and gave him tranquilizers and released him in satisfactory condition. After discharge, a GI series was negative, but epigastric pain reappeared and in April he reported severe upper left quadrant pains which became persistent."

Dr. Jenkins, one of the supervisors of the teaching program, interrupted: "Was this severe upper left quadrant pain different from the epigastric pain? Was it something new?"

Dr. Backman: "He described it as different. He had it at night, and it wasn't relieved with antacids."

Dr. Jenkins: "Well, didn't that make you uncomfortable with the diagnosis of gastric ulcer?"

Dr. Backman: "No, because he had resumed smoking and drinking now, and we suspected alcoholic hepatitis, because of his abnormal liver function test. He reported clay-colored stools and we readmitted him to the hospital. From the start of his admission he was quite agitated and needed more sedation, so we called in Dr. Sheingold [the Chief of Psychiatry]."

Dr. Sheingold had considered saying something about Dr. Backman's description of the patient as "drinking again." In fact, he knew the patient drank very little, only a few beers when he went bowling once a week, and it seemed unfair to imply that the man was drinking enough to justify a diagnosis of alcoholic hepatitis. The trouble, Sheingold felt, was that once the doctors decided to bring a psychiatrist into the case most of them no longer believed anything the patient said. And so it had been easy for the doctors to regard this patient as an alcoholic. Still, Dr. Sheingold had observed that Backman was one of the few doctors in the hospital who thought that psychiatry had anything to offer them in their treatment of medical patients, so he had refrained from objecting to the imputation of alcoholism.

Sheingold was motioned to the stage to report on his participation in the case. He began: "Yes, I was invited to walk down the garden path with the others. I talked with the patient on his fourth day of admission. His father-in-law had just retired and appointed the patient as director of the family insurance business. Mr. Thomas had never liked the business and found it morbid. Indeed, he had complicated feelings about his business exacerbated by a long history of depression. Ten years ago he had been responsible for an automobile accident in which his oldest daughter, then three years old, had died. So I was quite sure along with Dr. Backman that this was gastric ulcer disease, and I wrote that in my notes. I also noted that there was an unlikely chance of pancreatic carcinoma [cancer] because I knew that would be considered at some time, but I was quite sure that it was an ulcer."

Dr. Stevens, one of the department chiefs in medicine, had been upset with the reasoning in this case. As he explained, one of his pet peeves was the stupid use of psychiatry, especially by the GI doctors, and he had noticed that Backman was one of the frequent offenders in this regard because as a GI specialist Backman also considered himself something of an expert in the field of psychiatry. As Stevens described the situation, every time one of the GI doctors heard a patient complaint that couldn't be explained he called in a psychiatrist. Stevens wished they would instead just admit to the patient that they didn't know what was wrong, and explain that they would have to wait or do more tests. Instead, complained Stevens, a psychiatrist came in and spoke to the patient and *always* found a psychiatric complication. "And," concluded Stevens, "what did that tell you? That everyone has problems?"

Dr. Rosen, another internist on the hospital staff, was questioning Backman. "Why weren't the clay-colored stools considered? Didn't you believe him?"

Backman replied: "Well, the clay-colored stools could have been caused by the antacids he was taking, but to be perfectly frank, I didn't know how much credence I could give to his reports. He was quite upset and had gone into a rage about having to pay for the use of the television in his room. I should also add that he was now complaining about leg pain as well. He was re-endoscoped and a liver scan was taken. It showed an enlarged liver without focal abnormalities and the liver function was not impaired. A liver biopsy was normal, which surprised us. We expected to find alcoholic hepatitis. After the biopsy there was hemoptysis (coughing up blood). We were concerned because that had never happened and we thought that bleeding from the liver biopsy might have gone into the lung area. We did a cholangiogram and it was normal, but we noted that he had an elevated alkaphosphotase level. We released him from the hospital once again on a bland diet with tranquilizers, and his discharge diagnosis was peptic ulcer."

Dr. Davis, one of the younger internists, directed more questions to Backman: "Why wasn't a surgical exploration done at this time?"

Backman smiled, shaking his head. "I'm not sure. I guess we weren't smart enough." Davis continued: "Why was no attention paid to the calf pain?" Backman answered: "The reason we ignored his complaints of leg pain was that his roommate in the hospital had thrombophlebitis in the leg. So when Thomas complained of it, it just seemed too coincidental and we figured it was just a hysterical reaction."

Dr. Sheingold was afraid that this case was certainly not going to encourage the doctors in the hospital to turn to the psychiatry department for help. It made him angry that the only situation in which most of the doctors considered psychiatry to be useful was for the management of what they considered a "crazy" patient, and once a patient in the hospital was seen by a psychiatrist the doctors would attribute to the patient all sorts of psychological mechanisms that had nothing to do with the patient's personality (in this case they were imputing "hysterical" behavior to a nonhysterical patient) and they wouldn't even read the notes that Sheingold wrote in the patient's chart about which psychological mechanisms were relevant. Also, since they didn't regard psychiatric illness as real, they always disliked patients with psychiatric symptoms. As Sheingold later explained, all the doctors had disliked this patient when they thought that he suffered only from an ulcer, and they had only decided that he was likable after they realized that he was "really" sick with cancer.

Backman was still explaining why he had released the patient despite abnormal laboratory findings. "Oh, and to finish your question about surgery—his abdominal pains went away after three days, so we didn't consider it any more." He leafed through the pages of the chart and continued. "He was readmitted the following week with a swollen foot, and enlarged liver, extensive thrombophlebitis." Backman nodded to Cohen, the cardiologist who had been consulted at this point. Cohen stood up and briefly spoke from his place in the audience. "I was asked to say whether the problem was due to pulmonary emboli or from hemoptysis to the lung from the liver biopsy. I thought he had pulmonary emboli."

Attention was now directed to the Chief of Surgery, who described his part in the case: "I saw him at this point and I knew something terrible was going on. He was going downhill rapidly. It looked like an abdominal mass. The plan was now to deal with his phlebitis—so here we were in a bind. We had a GI bleeder who had to be anticoagulated for his emboli [a treatment that would increase bleeding], and now he had shortness of breath. The problem in dealing with this patient was that he was dead opposed to surgery. He had been in the life insurance business all his life, and every time we talked about surgery he would say, 'Now my family's gonna be collecting on my policy.' " The surgeon turned to Davis, who had earlier criticized Backman for not calling in a surgeon sooner. "I'll tell you why we didn't do an exploratory laparotomy [surgical investiga-

tion] earlier. He was so frantic and had been sick so long. He had abdominal pain, and calf pain and GI bleeding. He dreaded surgery, and frankly I dreaded going in there. His wife kept yelling at me, asking what was wrong, and when I said I didn't know she called me stupid. I guess maybe we *were* stupid. Anyway that's why we didn't do an exploratory earlier." In the back of the auditorium, some of the medical residents were smiling and mumbling that the reason the Chief had delayed surgery was that he hated to operate. Douglas had a reputation among the younger aggressive doctors in the hospital of being too cautious and slow to act. It was not clear whether Douglas noticed their remarks, and he continued. "So we did a venous clip and when we later did an exploratory we saw that there was cancer all over. The patient died three days later, and I just want to add here that according to the chart he was in severe anguish on the last day of his life, and was not given the painkillers we had prescribed, so we can thank our nurses for making the last day of his life as miserable as possible." The surgeon nodded to the pathologist and the lights were switched off. Color slides of the patient's affected organs were flashed on the screen. Each one showed gross abnormalities from the spread of the cancer. Throughout the auditorium murmurs could be heard at the extensiveness of the cancer, as if to emphasize that with so dramatic and pervasive a disease they as doctors could hardly have been expected to stop such an invasion.

When the lights were turned on the surgeon drew the meeting to a close, explaining how at that very moment the patient's brother was waiting in his office; the brother had come to show him an article about a so-called wonder drug, which was illegal, for curing cancer. Douglas added that he had given the brother an appointment so that the man could yell at him for having refused to try this illegal drug. Several doctors in the audience laughed and shook their heads sympathetically, breaking into small groups as they moved into the adjoining room for coffee and doughnuts.

The Thomas case, described above, illustrates how doctors often justify their errors by pointing to misleading or unusual features of the case. By demonstrating that they had good reason (though later shown to be mistaken) for doing what they did, they may avoid censure and discomfort, and save face before their colleagues. Physical symptoms inconsistent with the final diagnosis are the misleading cues which provide the most comforting and persuasive type of excuse for making the wrong diagnosis. However, when physical justifications are unavailable, doctors often resort to psychological and social evidence as the factors which misguided them and justified their behavior. In these cases, the nonphysical evidence is represented as being so convincing as to justify overlooking even physical evidence which should have alerted doctors to the correct diagnosis. In the Thomas case, for example, the doctors overlooked clear symptoms of organic disorder (such as the elevated alkaphosphotase level) because they were so convinced that the patient was neurotic and that his complaints and symptoms could be explained psychologically.

In other cases where physical findings are overlooked, or erroneously discounted, the physician will often excuse his embarrassing error by blaming the patient. If the patient can be "discredited" as crazy, alcoholic, obnoxious, uncooperative, or otherwise difficult or undeserving, then the responsibility for the medical error can be shifted away from the doctor to the patient's own doing. The following case illustrates this process.

CASE NO. 2: ALICE McDONALD

Mrs. McDonald was a 50-year-old woman who died in the Emergency Room of a perforated duodenal ulcer which the staff failed to diagnose, despite her complaints of severe abdominal pain.

The case was introduced in the meeting by the intern who had seen her in the Emergency Room. He opened the discussion by describing her as "An obese, alcoholic woman of Irish extraction who was very uncooperative and used very abusive language," thereby fixing her in the minds of the physicians in the audience as the type of patient who is difficult to treat.

In explaining why they had not paid much attention to her complaints of abdominal pain, the doctors involved in the case made much of her appearance of being "mentally disconnected." Asked to be more specific about her mental state, both the intern and the medical doctor covering the Emergency Room

that night stated that they remembered noting the smell of alcohol on her breath, and therefore felt they could dismiss her complaints as the ravings of a drunken woman.

Toward the end of the meeting someone in the audience offhandedly asked what the alcohol level in the blood had been at the time of the incident. Now the Chief of Medicine sheepishly admitted a fact that had been previously left unmentioned: although much had been made of this woman's drunkenness, the fact was that the alcohol level in the blood had been zero at the time of her examination.

This embarrassing fact was passed over quickly. No longer able to use her drunkenness as an excuse for their failure to take her complaints seriously, the doctors now turned more exclusively to emphasizing her angry, "disconnected" and uncooperative behavior toward them as the factor responsible for the poor treatment she received.

The power of the doctor's self-justification is highlighted in this case. For even after implicitly acknowledging that drunkenness was falsely attributed to the patient, the doctors continued to blame this woman's death on her own anger and abusive language, and ignored the possibility that such behavior was appropriate for a woman dying in great pain while the doctors around her treated her complaints as the fabrications of a hysterical alcoholic.

The case also illustrates how doctors may overlook important physical findings (which should indicate a serious illness) if they have already discounted the complaints by viewing the patient as a certain kind of neurotic individual. For a "neurotic" individual is viewed by doctors as an unreliable reporter, and once characterized this way, a patient's remarks are likely to be ignored. Indeed, these patients are commonly known among many doctors as "crocks" or "turkeys" and are considered undeserving of serious attention.

It is a complicated problem, for certainly doctors will occasionally meet with an anxious patient who will refuse to believe that he is in good health. But serious errors are often made as a result of characterizing patients as "crocks" for doctors are usually not in a position to correctly guess who is really sick and who isn't, from behavior alone. Furthermore, doctors appear to assign the label "crock" quite often on grounds of personal or prejudiced responses. They are more likely, for example, to dismiss a patient as neurotic and not really sick if the patient seems angry, mistrustful, or disrespectful to the doctor.

The label "crock" also seems to be applied erroneously more often to women.

Addendum: Suicide Review

Donald L. Light

Some months after a patient of the hospital or a recently discharged patient has committed suicide, a "suicide review" conference is held by a medical committee. It is an important part of professional management of ethics and crises. Its official purpose is to investigate whether professional mistakes were made and to prevent them from happening again. Daniel Forman was reviewed in December. My field notes of that review follow.

The presentation was very long, detailed and dull. It seemed designed to show that, from the patient's history, suicide was inevitable.

Two patterns emerged in the history. First, that he went quickly into a rage. . . . Second, the pattern of people rejecting him, especially psychiatrists. Not straight rejection, but passing him on.

Then he came here, and in less than a week he went from ward restrictions to group privileges to hospital privileges, to night care so he could work.

Mr. Forman was described as "brilliant" and other such adjectives, so much that finally the reviewing psychiatrist interrupted, "We've got to save the dumb ones too." Everyone laughed sheepishly under their breath.

Reprinted from "Psychiatry and Suicide" from the *American Journal of Sociology,* vol. 77, no. 5 (March, 1972), pp. 833–835.

In the discussion, the senior reviewing psychiatrist analyzed the case. (1) We were the next ones to brush him off. The reviewer made it sound pretty bad; then he added that he was not condemning the staff. "Heaven knows, I've made so many mistakes. . . ."

But the lesson of the day he gave was that what makes a man a professional is that he does not react to a situation as a layman does. If you faint at blood, you go out of surgery. Here, you have always to say, "Am I reacting the way everyone else did? Do I fit the pattern?" To do this, he said, you have to withdraw from being a human and see through professional eyes your humanness.

For the reviewing psychiatrist, this is the most important lesson. . . . (2) No one took the previous suicide attempts seriously. Most psychiatrists who had treated Forman previously thought they were merely manipulations.

"Why did they see the attempts this way?" asked the psychiatrist. "Because the patient used a common technique of deprecating his actions. 'I'm nothing, don't take this stuff seriously.' And you don't; then he kills himself."

Again, the lesson is that a patient is a prism through which you see his life, and as a professional, you learn to correct for distortion.

In the discussion, another member of the Review Board said that had Mr. Forman been kept in the hospital, he would have regressed, so it was not clear that the wrong thing had been done. Then several people in the room and finally the main speaker agreed that Forman would have committed suicide anyway. . . .

Later, the chief said that last year's Suicide Review Board found two common patterns. . . . The second was the person who convinces the doctor that his work or something is the only important part of his life. So the doctor lets him go out to do it, and he kills himself. . . .

The following analysis extracts from this case those features found in all suicide reviews. To understand the suicide review in its stated capacity leaves one disappointed and confused. Officially, the reviewer told the staff that they were rank amateurs who had killed a man by not being professional in their relations with him. Moreover, the mistake was one found to be a pattern in suicide reviews of previous years. The degree of malpractice implied is considerable. Yet everyone left feeling relaxed and fulfilled. All the doctors said that this was a very fine conference. They mainly chatted afterward about the *reviewer* and his performance. The reviewer squarely placed the fault but then excused it very kindly and said everyone is fallible. His main theme—that the service kicked the patient out of the hospital—was disputed, blunting the finger of blame. Finally, the reviewer and audience concluded that the patient would have killed himself anyway, making the rest of the conference academic. But a lesson remained on how to be a professional. The reviewing psychiatrist explored another basic issue: how human is a professional? A professional does not react to crises as do laymen; yet he, too, is fallible.

It is difficult to sustain belief in the manifest function of suicide review—to determine what was done wrong and to learn from it. Not only does the audience respond to other features of the review, but the lessons drawn are not communicated in any serious manner. Psychiatrists generally do not know what patterns previous reviews have found, and what is learned is only communicated to those present on one ward.

Like other acts of reintegration, the suicide review is a ritual designed to reaffirm the profession's worth after a deviant act has cast doubt upon it (Erikson 1966, chap. 1.). Beside suicide, many prob-lems in psychiatric work raise doubts of competence. Accounting professionally for decisions on these problems is a latent function of regular case reviews. Like many of the informal acts which begin when a problem such as suicide occurs, the review must strike a precarious balance between the individual and the profession. It may protect the practitioner in question from blame, but only at the risk of jeop-ardizing the general standards and cohesion of the profession. If, on the other hand, it judges the individ-ual member to be wanting, the profession may reinte-grate itself, but at the cost of embarrassment and admission of lax self-regulation. Thus it serves the organized function mentioned at the beginning of the paper, to spread and allocate losses. Perr (1965) put it well when he said he felt he needed a jury of peers to say he was not guilty.

The suicide review attains a proper balance by diminishing the significance of the suicide and then by effectively removing it as an issue. Its main fea-tures support this inference and follow many rituals of judgment and contrition. The presentation is very long (about 45 minutes) and often succeeds in making one bored with hearing about suicide. The review takes place long enough after the event (four months is average) so that strong feelings on the ward have been talked out, but not so long that the event is forgotten. In the presentation, much evidence points to the inevitability of suicide, much more so than presentations made by the same therapist about the same patient at conferences while he was living. The senior reviewing psychiatrist "explains" the sui-cide and talks about what can be done to become better professionals.

Often, the analysis of the case and the criticism are based on thin evidence, but the collage of bits into some whole is what impresses the audience. As in other aspects of psychiatry, storytelling is im-portant. At the end of the review, the main feeling is one of being impressed by the reviewer, a reaffir-mation of how fine psychiatry is; for in its darkest hour, a clear lesson can be drawn by a model of the profession (the reviewer), implying that, had the best men in psychiatry been handling the case, it would not have happened. In sum, the review of a suicide is temporarily harsh, then uplifting because of the display of psychiatric wisdom which has arisen from an act of ultimate failure.

References

ERIKSON, KAI
1966 *Wayward Puritans.* New York: Wiley.

PERR, HERBERT
1968 "Suicide and the Doctor-Patient Relationship." *American Journal of Psychoanalysis* 28(2): 177–88.

Colleague Relationships among Physicians

Eliot Freidson

Proponents of collective forms of medical practice tend to accept without serious question the assumption that merely by virtue of doctoring together under one roof, having the same patients, doctors will attain a higher quality of medical performance than would be the case if each practiced alone in his individual office. Group practice is thought to facilitate the social control of work by making performance more visible to others and therefore more responsive to critical evaluation. However, not all may be visible, and all that may be visible need not be attended to. The practicing physicians themselves did not consider all the information available to be reliable enough to use as a basis for secure evaluation. Only firsthand experience with the work and talk of the individual would do. When such information was lacking, evaluation could be only tentative and informal, a question of mere opinion and so not a basis for controlling others. Of critical importance for the development of inclinations to exercise social control, therefore, was the extent to which mutual firsthand experience with the work and talk of colleagues was distributed throughout the group, for without it, social control could not take place on a truly collective, or group, basis. *Assumptions about effective social control taking place among colleagues are based solely on faith if they do not rest on detailed, empirical data on how various kinds of information about performance are selected and patterned by various kinds of work arrangements and by the workers' own willingness to display their performance and to communicate their knowledge of others' performance to their colleagues.*

Such issues are almost impossible to address except by reference to an abstract and hypothetical rather than an empirical criterion of completeness. That is, we must assume the possibility of a perfectly complete distribution of information about performance in order to assess what exists as a deviation from such perfection. It was, of course, in reality impossible for all physicians to observe all the performance of all others. But by considering complete information as a possibility, one can better identify the degree and substance of the selectivity of the process which did exist in reality. Thus, we can ask about deviation from universal distribution by asking after the pattern of selectivity to be found in the distribution of information about performance.

Since there were different situations in which information was displayed and perceived, I shall begin my analysis in this chapter by exploring the patterning of exchanges of firsthand information about performance in purposive, consultative interaction and then move on to less formal modes of interaction. I shall point to the selective patterning of particular kinds of interaction which thereby limited direct contact between some kinds of physicians and, where possible, I shall point to the selection of the information conveyed in such interaction, thereby restricting the material available for evaluation. Finally, focusing on performance itself, I shall show evidence that some kinds of information about performance were withheld from other physicians by the performer and by those who learned about it.

FORMAL CONSULTATION

A critical source of information about performance stems from the formal act of referring a patient to a colleague for consultation. As long as a physician himself treats a patient and keeps the patient from seeing other physicians, his colleagues may not observe, let alone evaluate, his performance. Referrals, of course, and the interaction between referrer and consultant around a case, do more than only organize the care of the patient. They also make some facet of the performance of each physician visible to the other and therefore make it possible for each to evaluate the other on the basis of firsthand experience. Formal consultation is thus a basic mode of distributing firsthand information in medical practice in general.[1] In the medical group, however, routine referrals to consultants, particularly in periods of work pressure, tended to minimize interaction, limiting it to a written referral slip and a brief note on the patient's chart. Much of the communication tended to be very perfunctory. Thus, for our purposes it is necessary to distinguish among various kinds of consultation in the medical group. One informant contrasted several:

> If one of the doctors wanted me to see a case other than routine, he'd generally call me about it. Another kind of contact is quite by accident. I'll see a man in the hall, and I'll talk to him about a case or he'll talk to me. But we haven't actually gone looking for each other. The third

> way of informing each other is through the charts. In other words, the consultation is through the routine channels, and I haven't spoken to the doctor about it and I get what information I can from the chart. I get a little bit less from chance meetings in the hall because we are usually going some place and we don't have that much time for talking. And then I get certainly least from the charts. (#39—CONSULTANT)

Let us begin with an examination of the formal referral and consultation, which is usually a two-person relationship joined together by the patient who is seen by both and about whom they confer. Such referrals not only facilitate the care of the patient and the exchange of technical information but also convey, each to each, information about the conscientiousness, judgment, knowledge, and skill of the physicians involved. Prepaid group practice is said to facilitate referral and so to facilitate the display of physician performance to colleagues. However, in the medical group, while referral was very common, the information conveyed about the referred case was often perfunctory, if not inadequate, so that insofar as most referrals were routine, they could *not* be seen to serve as important sources of firsthand information about performance. It was in the exceptional referral—in the more complex case— in which consultation was accompanied by discussion and sufficient interaction was likely to take place for referrer and consultant each to feel he had gained some reliable notion of the capabilities of the other. Nonroutine referrals and consultations between primary practitioners and consultants thus formed one important source of direct experience with colleagues in the medical group, but *they composed a distinct minority of all referrals.*

Furthermore, referral did not make information about the performance of each practitioner available to *all* others. The division of labor was such that pediatricians and internists worked as parallel services, rarely referring to each other and thus rarely having an opportunity to consult each other and so gain firsthand experience with one another's performance. Therefore, while most consultants were likely to have had some firsthand experience with the performance of all pediatricians and internists, and all pediatricians and internists were likely to have had some firsthand experience with most consultants, many if not most consultants were unlikely to have gained much firsthand experience with the performance of those in other specialties, and many if not most pediatricians were unlikely to have gained much firsthand experience with the performance of internists, and vice versa.

Apart from referral and consultation between specialties, there was consultation between colleagues *within* specialties. The possibility for extensive consultation within a single specialty is said to be another of the distinct advantages of prepaid group practice. However, even though no economic competition discouraged sharing cases—as is said to be the case in solo, entrepreneurial practice—among the physicians in the medical group, professional pride did seem to interfere with consultation. The person who had been given the special status of consultant for those in his own specialty described with accuracy the attitude toward him which his colleagues expressed to us in the course of our interviews with them.

> *There probably isn't enough consultation in medicine. Originally the administration hoped that I could have some administrative position in relation to, let's say, hospitalized patients, where I would have to see each one that was hospitalized and oversee the patient. There were some that didn't necessarily have the type of workup that in retrospect he should have got, but there was tremendous objection from most of the family doctors to that. They felt their toes were being stepped on. They're internists and they feel they know how to work up a patient, and they didn't want to have a boss in that sense. So it was left, when they feel they need a consultant, they would call me. (#20—PRIMARY PRACTITIONER)*

In general, my impression was that *within* every specialty it was rare that a consultation took place in which a formal referral of a patient was made. Such a referral was problematic because of the tendency of each physician to feel that his colleagues in the same specialty were no more competent than he and therefore that referral was unnecessary. Only outsiders might serve such a function.

> *In general I don't consider the other men in the service as being any more knowledgeable than I am. So when I run into a real problem I want an outside consultation. (#44—CONSULTANT)*

The major exception to this rule occurred when there were legal or patient-management problems. In such cases, the senior person, or the chief of service, was consulted because of the greater weight his recorded opinion might have and because of some sense that, due to protocol, it was the senior person who "should" receive such referrals. Thus, the potential for formal consultation within specialties at the medical group did not seem to be fully or extensively utilized, each specialist working more or less by himself without much sharing of patients with other specialists except in the parallel, noninteractive sharing that occurred through rotated night and weekend emergency service. And, interestingly enough, the latter were precisely those duties that the physicians of the medical group sought to drop by hiring others from outside the medical group to replace themselves.

In general, it seems fair to say that circumstances in which two practitioners both directly examined the same patient and discussed the issues involved in the case with the deliberate end of arriving at some joint decision on its management formed a rather small proportion of the total universe of everyday work situations in the medical group. By far the bulk of such consultations occurred between specialties rather than within specialties, and they did not occur between every specialty and every other specialty. Thus, *formal consultation,* which had the greatest potential for making available extensive and direct information about the performance of colleagues, *was distributed very unevenly throughout the medical group, and in those segments where it did occur, routinization more often than not led to the minimization of such information.*

INFORMAL CONSULTATION

Apart from communication between colleagues about a patient each had seen, there was a less formal and less easily defined form of communication—consultation without referral.[2] In such a circumstance, the consultant did not usually see the patient. This kind of consultation differed from that in which referral took place in that the problem involved was not one defined as requiring examination or treatment of the patient by the consultant. The person seeking advice assumed that he was competent enough to keep the case but that he nonetheless needed supplementary judgment and information. He knew enough about the case and the issues involved to be able to describe it accurately and completely enough for another to understand the problem, and he wanted the other to give advice about the problem which could be used by the advice-seeker. The consultant might have had some specialized knowledge or experience that the advice-seeker lacked, but it was of such a nature that it could be transmitted verbally to the advice-seeker and then used without the consultant's help.

Such consultation without referral tended to be rather informal: one measure of this informality is the frequent absence of mention of the consultation on the official medical record. Sometimes such a consultation entailed deliberately seeking out a person to gain his advice on a particular problem that could not wait.

> *I had a recent experience of a girl with what looked like a strep infection but with atypical symptoms and a disturbing throat culture, which indicated a possibility of infectious mononucleosis. About this time I called up #29 and described this to him because of the question involved. I had to make a decision that day, and he advised me that he has seen several cases like this that were infectious mononucleosis. As it turns out the tests came back a few days later and they all confirmed the diagnosis. Now in this case you didn't have to send the patient to him, he was just very helpful to talk to on the phone. (#21—PRIMARY PRACTITIONER)*

And, for those questions that could wait, there was the possibility of storing them up so as to be able to ask a particular specialist when one happened to see him.

> *If I have something that's bothering me and I never happen to be in when #27 is around, and I happen to spot him and I could remember what I want to ask him, I will. You know, nail him along the way. #51 the same way. This I could say I do more of. If I'm really up a tree, then, you know, I put in a call. But if it is something so-so, well, I would say about every three or four months, if it is quiet and #27 is in and not too busy, and if I'm just discussing something spe-*

cific, I'll stand around and just talk to him for a while and usually while I'm talking to him, all the things I've been wanting to ask him for the past few months will come to mind and then I get them off my chest and that takes care of it for a while. The meeting just happens. You see him crossing the street or getting out of a car. You see him wandering around in the middle of the hall. And I'll chase after him. (#15—PRIMARY PRACTITIONER)

And there were spur-of-the-moment occasions when a colleague was present and available and when the discussion might be quite casual. Casual or not, all these types of advice seeking were relatively purposive, dealing with particular problems, and seeking advice about them from a given individual. On occasion, however, advice-seeking situations were purely sociable rather than consultative in that an interesting case was made available to another's inspection because of its sheer intellectual value. Interesting cases were treated virtually as gifts between equals, however, and so they depended upon reciprocity for their continued presentation.

> *When it comes to a very complicated case, very often it is not so much calling somebody in for consultation as to say, "Look what I have, how interesting it is." I did call #20 in to look at my cases a few years ago until I decided it was one-sided and I dropped it more and more. I called him in not because I couldn't handle it but because this was a very interesting case, and he was very pleased. He said, "That's very interesting, thank you very much." But he didn't call me in, so after a while I dropped it. (#10—PRIMARY PRACTITIONER)*

Functional considerations of who was useful to consult, formal considerations of who had to be consulted pro forma, intellectual considerations of who would enjoy seeing the case, and social considerations of who was owed a look at a case or was likely to reciprocate when he had the chance constituted some of the complex considerations involved in the process of displaying and receiving information bearing on medical performance in the informal consultations that did not form part of the formal medical record but composed a great part of the working physicians' experience with and consciousness of their colleagues in the medical group. In the case of formal consultation on general technical problems that anyone was competent to discuss, individuals' choices tended to be those whom they felt were approachable and easy to talk to. Their choices could have been but need not have been a matter of personal friendship and could have been but need not have been a matter of seniority and rank. On one service the senior person may have been avoided, while on another the senior person may have been used most often because face was lost less by asking a senior for advice than by asking a peer or a junior. But for minor problems one was more likely to use people with whom one was both friendly and equal. Quite naturally, specialized problems were taken up with those who had themselves devoted more attention than usual to these problems or who were interested in them.

Obviously, because of its very nature, informal consultation was not initiated by all possible parties with all possible others. Indeed, since it was not official or recorded, there was less need for it to follow formal specialty and rank criteria. And since it was, nonetheless, a concession of need for advice or information, a concession with which the physicians were not entirely comfortable in spite of their protestations (Blau 1955:108–109; Goss 1963:178–179), the tendency was to use more particularistic criteria for initiating it than might have been used for initiating formal referrals. Thus, *the patterning of this mode of exchanging information was less narrow, less determinate than that of the formal mode.* And it was considerably more subject to the accident of friendship, of meeting someone in the hall on a particular day, of having hours on the same day as someone else, and of having adjacent offices.

CASUAL SHOPTALK

In reviewing the material on consultation, I have devoted myself largely to advice seeking, which tended to be initiated by one person for a limited, functional purpose. Advice seeking, however, is a comparatively formal mode of interaction even when it takes place informally, without referral. Some of what might be called "consultation" was not so much advice seeking as it was sociable discussion among fellow workers, or casual shoptalk. Such discussion

might have contained within it the request for and granting of advice or information, but it would probably not have taken place between the two people involved if they had not happened to come together when they did. It was often embedded in social, nonfunctional talk. Much corridor or luncheon-table interaction was of this nature, almost always informal and involving more than two people. Unlike an ordinary consultation, which was more the intentional seeking of advice from one by another and which took place as a two-person exchange from which others were excluded, these informal conversations were unplanned and, even if they were two-person exchanges, occurred in the company of other colleagues who listened and sometimes commented on what they heard. In such conversations, the participants displayed their knowledge and acumen to more colleagues than just the one being consulted or consulting them.

The first thing to observe about such casual shoptalk was that a rather limited number of the physicians in the medical group participated in it extensively. It was rare to see one of the part-time consultants sitting at the luncheon table where one found, almost daily, a cadre of full-time primary practitioners. Furthermore, more internists than pediatricians stayed to eat at the luncheon table, as did more male practitioners than females. Apart from the composition of the luncheon groups, however, the mere fact of colleagues meeting and sitting together at a table in the cafeteria led to the exchange of talk beyond the social boundaries of friendship and the functional boundaries of the normal division of labor. Pediatricians chatted with internists, and members of the same specialty chatted with one another. Their exchanges were characterized as small talk or chitchat, but they both educated one another by their comments and tested one another by their questions in ways that spilled over the functional borders of formal consultation.

Such talk was not considered so important as to be defined as consultation, and it included as much, if not more, politics, family, vacations, and hobbies as medicine, but it did include medicine and the practical problems of medical work. The going fees for private patients were discussed on more than one occasion (and such discussion led some individuals to raise their fees). Many problems of practice in the group were discussed, frequently in a jocular, facetious tone but one that nonetheless was instructive.

> About the tricks of the trade, we talk about that. We talk about that more in a joking manner than anything else. We complain about the work load and some of the things we do to try to save time, like not allow a patient to even sit down. (#7—PRIMARY PRACTITIONER)

Such conversation allowed the individuals participating in it to gain some perspective on their difficulties with patients by normalizing them—at the very least gaining catharsis and, even better, comfort and support from complaining publicly (cf. Blau 1955:89–91).

> I think we discussed questions of whether we did the right thing by a patient with our colleagues to protect ourselves, but we discuss always to justify ourselves. In other words, did I make that housecall, should I have made that housecall? And then you want support. . . . So the tendency is when you have gotten angry with a patient, when you've been a little terse, a little fast, if you have been a little discourteous, the tendency is to discuss this with somebody else, more or less to get support. (#12—PRIMARY PRACTITIONER)

In addition to having interviews with the physicians in which we asked them to discuss and classify their varied contacts with colleagues, we took notes on much of the shoptalk that we observed at formal medical-group meetings (usually before the proceedings or just after they had ended), in hallways, and at the cafeteria luncheon tables. It is of course impossible to be precise about the relative distribution of topics in the universe of such exchanges, but my own impression was that talk about medical work composed a small amount of the total. More important was the impression that, in most of the medical shoptalk, the rule of etiquette dominated interaction and restrained what was said in the discussions. That is to say, disagreement with an individual might have been expressed to his face, but only neutrally, as another opinion rather than as a contradiction reflecting on his judgment.

Difficulties in managing patients were almost always responded to supportively in the presence of the person discussing them. And in the case of a mistake that an individual admitted to while seeking support, the tendency was to normalize it by declaring or implying that it was something that could and did happen to anyone, as the following field notes illustrate.

> At the luncheon table, #7 and #3, joined by #6. Before #6 came, the talk was of gasoline and automobiles. #6 came up looking harassed, as usual, and said, "Jesus, what a day! I just finished up. Twelve people this morning and every one of them with pathology. In one case I was going to skip a pelvic and get her out, but I did it and there it was." There was some commiseration, and he continued, "You know, #17 just had a complaint, and is he mad. It was one of those patients he's sat and listened to for years about nothing, and just today he got a letter from her telling him he missed a sacroiliac. She was in [another] hospital and wanted him to pay the bill. And he looked in her chart, and he couldn't find a mention of any symptoms like that. I told him he ought to be grateful because [practicing] here [in the medical group] he could find out what happened to his patients. In private practice he would never find out." Expostulations—"Jesus," "goddamned patients"—were followed by #6 stating that "those damned things were real easy to miss because you send them off to the orthopedist. You should be able to pick it up." #3 said, "But you can do a myelogram," and #6 said, "A good examination or a neurological exam should do it. I missed a lot of those. [Turning to #7] How many of those have you missed, #7?" #7 was noncommittal but left the impression that he had missed some. "How about you, #3?" #3 said, "None, to my knowledge," then hesitated and said, "But I haven't been here long enough to tell. But I think I've diagnosed them more often than they've been really found."

An unusual case, such as that of a 35-year-old woman, very active, with a complaint about her shoulder turning out to have a very serious heart condition, was displayed verbally with great pride by the responsible physician who had "caught it," while a physician who had lost a patient publicly rehearsed self-defenses while colleagues sympathized.

At lunch #4 told a story of a patient who came in complaining of chest pains. He did several cardiograms on him with no results, but the patient finally came in again and had a real infarct. He was hospitalized for two weeks, during which time there were no more symptoms, no cardiogram variations. He was put on anticoagulants and sent home. Two weeks later, another physician on duty got a call that he has chest pains again. He lived two blocks away from the medical group, but by the time the physician got there he was dead. #4 said, "And what could I do? When I discharged him I told him not to worry, that since he'd been walking around so long with it it must be slight. I had to work to get him and his family to prevent putting him in mothballs. I told him not to really exert himself, but otherwise live normally." #10 said something not entirely audible about the inadequacy of anticoagulants, the others making no more than sympathetic noises, and conversation briefly touched on experimental work in the hospital relevant to the issue of coagulation and an article someone read about research on heart disease in zoo animals before shifting entirely back to the original topic of work coverage problems.

CONSTRAINTS ON INFORMATION AND DISPLAY

In all of the contexts I have attempted to describe, information about cases and their management was exchanged between colleagues. The information certainly facilitated medical care and on occasion contributed to the education of at least one of the participants in the exchange. Participation in consultation and conversation, however, besides being an exchange of information also constituted a display to colleagues of one's knowledge, skill, and judgment, a display that constituted the firsthand or direct experience with colleague performance which the physician considered to be the authoritative ground for his evaluation of another. I have already suggested some of the obvious ways in which participation in such interaction was patterned—since not all physicians interacted with all others, not all could

get the direct experience with others which would allow them to feel that they had grounds for consequential evaluation. Thus, many felt that they must either suspend judgment about a colleague or else use other grounds for evaluation. What I wish to suggest now, however, is that *in addition to there being constraints on who could be in interaction with others so as to exchange such firsthand information, there were constraints on the information that was exchanged, producing systematic omissions in what was displayed and evaluated.*

It should not be forgotten that the essential issue being explored here is that of the prerequisites for social control. I have been asking how the physicians in the medical group could discover poor performance on the basis of the information conveyed in their interactions. I have been focusing on the distribution and substance of firsthand experience with colleagues because it was a prerequisite for the development of a sufficiently secure foundation for evaluation to incline the physicians to undertake the deliberate exercise of social control over a colleague. What I have pointed out about the distribution of consultation and shoptalk should come as no surprise. It is obvious, as I found, that universal distribution was impossible and that distribution had to be limited and patterned by a variety of factors— by the division of labor, seniority, friendship, and the like.

It is just as obvious that the substance of the information being distributed would have been controlled so far as possible by the people involved and at risk. There is no reason to expect physicians to be much more open with colleagues about those of their inadequacies of which they are aware than we would expect any other human beings to be. Assuming that the physicians did attempt to control the information they conveyed in interaction, therefore, in some of our questioning we focused on the information they conveyed about the kind of performance that the lay person would call a "mistake." That is, the physicians were asked whether or not and in what context they talked to others about mistakes—whether, in other words, they displayed mistakes in the course of consultation and discussion with their colleagues or whether they attempted to conceal them.

The essence of their answers was related to their

largely implicit criteria for distinguishing types of mistakes. One, for example, claimed that he did not feel he had to hide his mistakes but did not discuss them generally.

I think I have enough security to feel not anxious to hide my mistakes. A doctor makes mistakes, and I feel I try as hard as humanly possible to avoid them and I feel when one comes up that never in my career I felt I must hide it. But of course I don't go around talking about it generally. (#1—PRIMARY PRACTITIONER)

Clearly, while there was some talk about mistakes, it was selective in character. We have already seen evidence that the physicians did tell colleagues who were by no means their close friends and confidants about things they had overlooked and about occasions on which they had made mistakes in their diagnosis and treatment. But did they talk to others about everything?

What seemed to be important in discriminating between mistakes that were displayed and those that were not was the extent to which the mistake could be normalized. When a mistake is normalized it does not function as a reflection on the essential competence of the person involved. The field note on "missing a sacroiliac," several pages back, illustrated rather well how normalization and facesaving occurred in public. . . . *Mistakes that tended to be discussed with others were mistakes that were normalizable.* The physician reported in the field note to have missed a sacroiliac reported missing still another condition without claiming any reluctance to mention it. The same physician, however, protected another colleague from disclosure that he had missed a thyroid, as we shall see below.

Not all physicians seemed to feel that they would mention their mistakes to others, but the problem was what they meant by "mistake." One who claimed in an interview that "doctors generally aren't likely to discuss the fact that they might not have paid attention to some symptom" (#24—PRIMARY PRACTITIONER) and who claimed that he would not discuss it nonetheless himself spoke more than once in his interviews of having missed an acute glaucoma. What is more important, our field observations show that his miss was apparently well known to many of his colleagues, since it was mentioned in public

and they identified him as the person. The context in which he discussed his mistake and in which it was mentioned by others suggested that it served as a symbolic example of a typical and acceptable contingency of medical work. More than one physician had his own personal miss or normal mistake to discuss in interviews and refer to in public. Such mistakes *were* talked about in general.

All mistakes were not normal, however, and the deviant mistake was that one that physicians seemed more inclined to hide.

I'd discuss with others the kind of mistake that others would make. I wouldn't want to discuss one [I made] that was absolutely stupid. You know, something that shows that you're stupid, a fumbler, or a mistake where I just didn't know some basic information. I wouldn't want to discuss this—to broadcast it that I was stupid. I would discuss things with people who I felt would excuse me for making the mistake. (#9—PRIMARY PRACTITIONER)

Deviant mistakes would be discussed only with close friends who could be trusted to be sympathetic and supportive because of their special relationship to the deviant, not because of a mere colleague relationship. They would not be made known to mere colleagues. Indeed, it is likely that, insofar as possible, deviant mistakes would be systematically purged from the information conveyed in consultation and discussion between colleagues. Perhaps this was why one physician described how part of his method of evaluating his colleagues lay in being sensitive to gaps in their discussion, to strategic vaguenesses.

Finally, it seems useful to point out that the entire collegium of the medical group did not have the same concept of deviant mistakes. Each specialty seemed to have its own special normal mistakes, based on its conception of the ordinary contingencies of its specialized work. These conceptions were not necessarily shared by the members of other specialties, which meant that some of what, for members of one specialty, were normal mistakes, mistakes that members might freely concede and discuss among themselves, ran the risk of seeming to be deviant mistakes in the eyes of colleagues outside that specialty. There was a tendency, therefore, for consultants to conceal what they themselves regarded as normal mistakes from the physicians who referred to them.

> *I would talk about my mistakes to personal friends, but not necessarily with referring physicians. The referring physician is so narrow-minded that he would take this error of judgment—well, some of them unfortunately idealize the man they are referring to. They foolishly think he is perfect or near perfect and all that sort of nonsense. . . . You've got to keep them in the dark. But we did discuss these things freely among surgeons. (#41—CONSULTANT)*

It seems accurate to say that, quite apart from being selective in their distribution across the entire collegium, informal discussion and consultation in the medical group were highly selective and defensive in their content. Some of what a layman would call mistakes or errors in performance were freely conveyed in such interaction, but they were accepted in a comparatively uncritical, supportive manner rather than being criticized as reflections on the competence of the physician committing them. In cases in which a physician felt that colleagues—in the same or in a different specialty—would not agree to normalize his mistake, however, he would try to prevent its becoming known to them. If it concerned him so much that he felt obliged to discuss it, he would restrict his confession and discussion to colleagues who were especially close friends—to confidants who could be trusted to keep their knowledge secret. Thus, *unusually critical information about performance was, insofar as possible, withheld from the conversations and informal consultations that constituted a good portion of the firsthand experience with each other which was the physicians' most authoritative source of information about the quality of care their colleagues gave.*

The only source of relatively complete firsthand experience with colleagues which could be affected only minimally by the way its participants chose to display themselves was formal consultation with referral. In that situation, referrer and consultant each could examine both the patient and the medical record independently of the other doctor and could evaluate the other independently of the way he displayed himself. The distribution of formal consultation, however, was as we have seen limited by the nature of the division of labor and by the compara-

tively large number of physicians in each of the major specialty services. And communication was detailed only in nonroutine cases. Thus, in the normal course of events it would take a rather long time for direct, nonroutine consultation to take place among a large proportion of the physicians of the medical group, a long time for each to feel that he had had direct, firsthand experience with many others in circumstances in which performance was directly assessable rather than merely inferable from the display of talk, talk that was potentially dangerous to reputation. The distribution of such experience would not be likely to sustain an effectively organized process of social control.

RESTRICTIONS ON SHARING FIRSTHAND INFORMATION

It would seem that the only way by which such firsthand information about performance as could be obtained from formal consultation could have been quickly and extensively conveyed through the collegium lay in its transmission by its receivers to those who had had no immediate occasion to obtain it themselves. Only by such communication could the patterned bias of consultation be rectified and the slow pace at which information was normally accumulated be speeded up. But by and large this did not occur in the medical group. The rules of etiquette effectively prevented the transmission of such information, though some did get through. Most reported discussion of the unethical or incompetent behavior of others was with colleagues who were close friends, and even there the particular physician involved was not always named. The norm of protecting one's colleagues was firmly adhered to.

Many secrets about physician performance were kept rather well in the medical group. During our study we learned of individuals who seemed to have acted outrageously to patients, falsified their administrative service records, accepted money from patients, and had been dangerously neglectful. We learned that they were, on occasion, encouraged to resign from the medical group, but not all did so. In our investigation of the circulation of information about performance, however, after as much careful probing as we could do without ourselves providing the information to the physicians, we found that far more than a simple majority of the group physicians seemed to know nothing about most of the behavior we learned about. What was perhaps even more revealing was that most physicians did not seem to know of even serious cases of repeated poor performance which occurred in their own specialties, let alone in others. Obviously there were serious barriers to the transmission of information about critical areas of physician performance. Those physicians who discovered poor performance were not inclined to mention it to others.

This disinclination to share with colleagues firsthand information bearing on poor performance was explained by reference to the self-conceptions underlying the rules of etiquette—the view the physicians had of themselves and their work.

> *Well, you talk about mistakes. Maybe that's what interests you. I saw this young girl with a CA of the thyroid yesterday, probably a CA. I'm going to operate next week. I went over the chart very carefully to see that she's been treated, and I couldn't believe that this thing had blossomed, as the chart said, just in the past few weeks. She wasn't sent to me by her regular family doctor but by a subspecialist consultant. After I had seen her he came in and said, "Well, what are you going to do?" I said, "I'll take care of it. . . ." So I said, "Tell me, do you think this has all come up just these last few weeks? She has been under treatment for years. Don't you think that was there to begin with and it should have been noticed and observed?" He said, "Look, the less said about it the better. The man who sent her to me feels horrible about it. He realizes now he missed something and he said, 'Forget it. Don't say anything about it.' He really feels badly about it, you see. . . ." All right, he knows. What more can you do? After a man knows and he realizes, you are not going to go in and twist a knife in his back. He really in my opinion made a very serious error there. This is the first time I've had anything to do with this man. I mean, every once in a while in my opinion one of the medical men in the group makes a mistake, and, as you say, I don't know what's done about it. I don't know what you can do about it. I talk about*

> *it to him, but. . . . I don't go around telling other people. I don't think that's good. (#47—CONSULTANT)*

The physicians collected their firsthand experience with others as their positions in the division of labor permitted, but they did not communicate much of its substance or their evaluation of it to others unless, as we shall see, special conditions held. Under normal circumstances, the tendency was for each physician to accumulate and store his own experience, without sharing anything critical with others. Thus, in the group practice, which provided extraordinary *potential* for collecting and sharing information bearing on performance and for controlling the quality of performance collectively, *much of the patterning of both information and control remained in fact dyadic, almost as it would be had there been no group practice at all.*

Notes

1. For a recent study of referral patterns in a suburban area, see Shortell, n.d.; for a study in West Germany, see Hummel *et al.*, 1970.
2. For useful parallel observations on consultation in a nonmedical setting, see Blau 1955; in a medical setting, see Goss 1959:79–105.

References

BLAU, PETER
  1955 *The Dynamics of Bureaucracy.* Chicago: University of Chicago Press.

GOSS, MARY E. W.
  1959 *Physicians in bureaucracy: a case study of professional pressures on organizational roles.* Unpublished Ph.D. dissertation, Columbia University.
  1963 Patterns of bureaucracy among hospital staff physicians. In Eliot Freidson (ed.), *The Hospital in Modern Society.* New York: Free Press, pp. 176–179.

HUMMEL, HANS J. *et al.*
  1970 The referring of patients as a component of the medical interaction system *Soc. Sci. Med.* **3** (April): 597–607.

PART THREE

The Organization

CHAPTER 10

The Social Organization of the Hospital

There is great variation in the kinds of hospitals that dot the American landscape, and they can be differentiated on a number of dimensions. There are for-profit hospitals that are run both by individuals and by large corporations. The rise of the corporation in the hospital business has been very important, with Hospital Corporation of America and Humana being two of the biggest players. The largest percentage of hospital beds in this country are found in voluntary hospitals, which are nonprofit and are run by boards of directors. The distinction between profit and nonprofit should not obscure the fact that the nonprofits are also interested in making money, although, of course, they are not under pressure from investors who expect a nice dividend at the end of the year. The amount that revenues exceed costs is called "surplus" rather than profit by the nonprofit hospitals. Local and state hospitals, veteran's hospitals, and federal research hospitals are supported by government funds and are run by government employees.

Most of America's hospitals are of the general type, but there are also a wide variety of specialized hospitals that focus on particular medical problems, like Sloan-Kettering in New York City, which is widely known as a leading cancer hospital.

One aspect of hospital care in America has come under intense scrutiny in recent years. There is concern that the for-profit hospitals will ignore poor people and will increasingly place the economic burden of treating them on other hospitals. Recent research has documented the "dumping" of poor patients to public hospitals, and many of these hospitals may not be able to take the financial strain. This would mean that the poor would be without the services of precisely those hospitals that have treated a disproportionate number of them. Arnold Relman, the editor of the *New England Journal of Medicine,* and others have been outspoken critics of hospitals denying the poor access to their emergency rooms, sometimes with dire consequences.

There has also been a dramatic change in the way in which hospitals are being paid for the treatment they provide for the elderly under Medicare. Under new guidelines, hospitals get paid set fees for providing particular treatments according to a set of disease categories called *diagnostic related groups* (DRGs). This system of payment may become the wave of the future, and it will likely place new limits on the great amount of discretion in decision making that physicians have always enjoyed.

This chapter looks at various aspects of the general hospital, a category into which 87 percent of all hospitals in the United States fall.

When the first edition of *Dominant Issues in Medical Sociology* appeared a decade ago, the typical relationship between doctor and hospital was related to a "dual-authority" system. In this system, the hospital administrator had more formal authority than the physician, but the latter actually had more say-so over daily operations within the hospital. Things are changing, however. In the first article, Simone Poirier-Bures and Allen L. Bures examine changes in the doctor–hospital relationship in a changing health-care environment. The rise of for-profit hospitals, the implementation of DRGs, and other factors are looked at as they relate to "an old partnership reconsidered." In the next article, Shizuko Fagerhaugh and her colleagues present a general and wide-ranging exploration of the implications of high technology for various groups within the hospital. This is followed by another discussion of high technology, by the same group of authors, with a more specific focus, the intensive care nursery. This piece provides a detailed description of the many aspects of the social order of this hospital unit.

Next, Emily Mumford describes the development of the hospital emergency room (ER) in America. One important point she makes is that while the ER is still believed be a place for the treatment of medical emergencies, it is frequently used as a resource for those who have relatively routine problems but who may not have a regular physician. In the following article, Marsha Hurst and Pamela Summey look at the "two-class" system of hospital care as it relates to the use of cesarean sections in childbirth.

Lastly, Irwin Press looks at some of the sociological reasons why people sue over their hospital care. His central theme is that whether or not a patient sues is as much or more a result of how he or she feels about the socioemotional aspects of the medical care as it is an objective decision concerning the actual quality of the medical care. This very much parallels sociological arguments about the increase of malpractice at the societal level. These arguments hold, in part, that the increasing impersonality in the doctor–patient relationship due to specialization, the growth of cities, and other things is an important factor in the wave of malpractice suits that now engulfs the country.

Doctor–Hospital Relations: An Old Partnership Reconsidered

Simone Poirier-Bures
Allen L. Bures

Over thirty years have passed since Smith published his seminal article on the dual-authority system that characterized most doctor–hospital relationships.[1] Since then, particularly in the last ten years, changes have occurred that have undermined the old system and may, in fact, render it obsolete. At the very least, these changes are forcing a readjustment in doctor–hospital relations. What those key changes are, how they are affecting traditional relationships, and what future relationships between doctors and hospitals may look like is the subject of this paper.

DUAL AUTHORITY

As recently as ten to fifteen years ago, most hospitals were voluntary (run by boards and funded by revenues) or public (run by localities and funded by public money). These were nonprofit hospitals, and in 1970 they comprised 87 percent of the 5859 nonfederal hospitals.[2] The remaining 13 percent were for-profit hospitals, most of which were individually owned. There was little competition among hospitals then, and hospitals existed in an environment of strong community and philanthropic support. Fees charged by hospitals did not directly correspond to the actual cost of services rendered. Rather, they were adjusted to include the support of equipment, empty beds, emergency rooms, and the care of indigent patients.

This is an original article written for this edition of *Dominant Issues in Medical Sociology*. The authors wish to acknowledge the many contributions of Dr. Howard D. Schwartz to the development of this paper.

Under those conditions, the dual system of authority flourished. Doctors enjoyed a unique relationship with hospitals: they were outside the normal lines of authority that existed for hospital personnel, yet they exercised authority at all levels of the organization. They served on the board and on committees and gave orders to nurses and other hospital employees, yet they were responsible only to their patients, their profession, and themselves. The stereotypical picture that Wilson provided in 1959 was, to a certain extent, still true:

> The high tide of the doctor-dominated hospital, perhaps extending from 1900–1950 . . . , is preserved in the figure of the great doctor making his ward rounds to the bowing of nurses, the scraping of students, and the worshipful gaze of patients. But this picture . . . is . . . simply an exaggerated telling of the truth that the doctor was not only the central figure in the hospital but a towering one.[3]

The doctors' authority was "functional," deriving from their profession and the prestige attached to it, rather than "scalar," deriving from a position within the hierarchy. Organizational theorists have long recognized the existence of two kinds of authority: "formal" (power assigned through a job description) and "informal" (power exercised in day-to-day operations). In hospitals, the administration had "formal" authority, but the real power lay in the "informal" (functional) authority of the doctors.

The dual-authority system reflected the conflict of values that has long been inherent in the hospital structure. This conflict arises from the different orientations of administrators and doctors. Hospitals, like other organizations, require fiscal solvency for survival. Administrators, therefore, have legitimate monetary concerns. Doctors' concerns, however, have traditionally centered on service and the rendering of the best possible care—whatever the cost.

Under the dual-authority system, clashes between "money" and "service" were usually resolved in favor of service—doctors held the edge of power. As a result, hospitals were seen as doctors' cooperatives, run by and for the doctors.[4] The administration existed solely to provide facilities and supplies for the doctors' use.

TIPPING THE SCALES

All that is changing, however. Healthier life styles, the increasing cost of health care, competition among hospitals, and the emergence of new health care delivery systems, like health maintenance organizations (HMOs), are all altering the health care scene. But two factors in particular are profoundly affecting the traditional doctor–hospital relationship. They are the DRGs (diagnosis related groups) with their emphasis on cost containment and the increasing corporatization of hospitals.

DRGs

DRGs are categories into which patients with similar diagnoses are placed. For example, all patients with extensive burns are placed in DRG 457. As such, they are expected to require similar treatment at similar costs. There are 468 DRGs, developed by the Health Care Financing Administration.[5]

In March 1983, Congress adopted the DRGs for use as a guide for Medicare payments to hospitals. This was the beginning of a whole new way of reimbursing hospitals for their services—the prospective payment system. Prior to this time, payments were retrospective, that is, after the fact. Hospitals presented the government with bills for services already rendered to Medicare patients, and the government paid the full amount or a reasonable percentage. With the DRG system, the government designates *in advance* (prospectively) the fee it is willing to pay for each DRG category. The fee is based on a formula that includes average costs for a certain type of care and the nature and location of the hospital. Unlike the old system of artificial costs, DRG

fees are closer to the actual cost of the services rendered.

The idea behind the DRGs was to control the spiraling costs of Medicare. Medicare costs had been increasing at a rate of 17 percent per year since 1970, and hospitals had no incentive to contain those costs. On the contrary, there was always the temptation to enhance revenues by providing more services for a patient—do more, receive more money. The DRG, prospective-payment system, then, was intended to give hospitals the needed incentive for containing costs. It forces them to operate on a fixed budget. If the hospitals can provide the care for less than the prospective fee, they are ahead of the game; if actual costs run higher than the designated amount, the hospitals have to absorb the losses.

There is a good deal at stake here. Currently, Medicare accounts for 40 percent of all hospital revenues.[6] At the present time, hospitals that have a good mix of patients can still recoup losses incurred on Medicare patients in the same way they have traditionally done so for indigent patients: through cost shifting. They can pass on the costs to privately insured patients and other (non-Medicare) payers. However, it is generally believed that the DRGs will eventually become the basis for determining fees for everyone, not just Medicare patients.[7] In fact, New Jersey has been using such a system since 1980. There, DRG fees are set by both the federal and the state government and are applicable to everyone using hospital services.[8]

The DRGs, even in affecting only Medicare, have forced the hospitals to become much more cost conscious. The result of this has been an increase in the "money versus service" conflict that has traditionally existed between hospital administrators and doctors. Whereas administrators need to keep down the cost of patient care, the doctor is the one who actually determines that care. Traditionally, if a doctor wanted to run ten tests on a Medicare patient, ten tests were run. Under the DRG system, the doctor can still order ten tests, but the hospital may only be reimbursed for four. This puts the doctor in a conflict situation, possibly involving a division of loyalties. He or she is caught between the pressure of the administration to contain costs and his or her own professional responsibility to provide the best possible care for the patient. If the doctor ignores costs altogether, the hospital that gives him or her privileges may no longer be able to maintain high-quality facilities. At worst, it may eventually fold. Yet if the doctor gives in to the pressure of containing costs, the health and well-being of the patient may be compromised.

The "money versus service" conflict, however, is not easily resolved. The following case, presented and discussed in a Hastings Center Case Report, illustrates how complex that conflict has become under the DRGs.

The Doctor, the Hospital, and the DRGs[9]

Lakeview hospital in central New Jersey has been reimbursed on the basis of "diagnosis related groups," or DRGs, since May 1980. The hospital's director, Jared Lapin, M.D., acts as a liaison between the hospital's managers and the medical staff. In addition, Dr. Lapin and Ellen O'Connor, director of finance, periodically review the performance of individual physicians from a financial viewpoint.

At a recent meeting, Dr. Lapin and Ms. O'Connor analyzed a lengthy computer report that matched, for each physician, the revenue the hospital received with the costs incurred for treating patients in each of the DRGs in one month. While studying the fifteen DRGs under Major Diagnostic Category number 24 (Pregnancy, Childbirth, and the Puerperium), they noticed that Dr. Daniel Weiner admitted seventeen patients who were later determined to be in DRG 373 (vaginal delivery without complicating diagnosis) but only two in DRG 371 (cesarian section, without complication and/or comorbidity). Yet for the other three obstetricians on staff, fifty-eight came under DRG 373 and nineteen under 371. Across all deliveries, the costs of treating Dr. Weiner's patients exceeded the revenue received from the DRG rates. But the total cost incurred in providing care to the other obstetricians' patients was considerably below revenue and hence the hospital was able to earn a "profit."

The computer report also revealed that the reimbursement rate the hospital received for routine

deliveries fell just short of covering all the incurred expenses, whereas the rate paid for cesarian sections was substantially greater than the actual cost to the hospital. The reason for Dr. Weiner's comparatively poor overall "financial performance," Dr. Lapin and Ms. O'Connor concluded, was that he performed many fewer cesarians than did his colleagues.

Dr. Weiner explained that he did not agree with his colleagues that once a woman had a cesarian delivery, all subsequent deliveries must be cesarian; he felt that most of these women could have normal deliveries. He cited a number of recent studies that found no differences in outcomes (in terms of health risks to both mother and child) associated with the different delivery modes. Dr. Lapin countered that the tradition of performing repeat cesarians was strong and that more time and research were needed before large numbers of physicians changed their practices. He noted too that, if a complication were to arise, the attending physician would likely be faced with a malpractice suit.

Finally, he pointed out to Dr. Weiner that the hospital was losing money on almost every patient he treated. "Dan," he said, "it's in all our interests to look out for the financial health of the hospital. And since it is unclear which of the two approaches benefits the patients more, I urge you to reconsider the way you handle these cases."

Was it ethical for Dr. Lapin to approach Dr. Weiner if there was no indication he was delivering poor quality care? How should financial considerations, both those related to the hospital and to society at large, be weighed against physician judgment? What if Dr. Weiner could convincingly demonstrate that his patients were actually at less risk than those of his colleagues?

Three health care professionals were invited to comment on this case.[10] Each presents a different perspective. The first maintained that Dr. Lapin, representing the interests of the hospital, was right to inform Dr. Weiner of the cost factor. He pointed out that costs (usually to the patient) have always been a consideration in the doctor's decision about treatment, along with other concerns like patient preference. Because the cost factor now includes costs to the hospital or costs to third party payers as well, these too should be considered in the doctor's decision making. This commentator, however, was quick to note that the ultimate decision of treatment should still remain with the doctor.

The second commentator felt that Dr. Weiner should be allowed to continue his practice without pressure from the administration to change. In his opinion, a well-run hospital should be able to provide quality care under a well-constructed DRG system and still survive. A creative administrator, he noted, would find ways to cut costs without compromising the well-being of patients.

The third commentator found the very idea that a doctor might be encouraged to perform more cesarians (which subject the mother to needless stress) in order to preserve the financial health of the hospital "outrageous." Her solution was to correct the DRGs' faulty calculation system, making the reimbursed costs more commensurate with the real ones.

The range of approaches in these commentaries shows that there are no easy solutions. But all three commentators recognized that cost constraints are now a given—doctors will have to live with them. No longer will doctors have the freedom to offer the best possible care "whatever the cost."

In teaching hospitals, the DRGs may aggravate the conflict already existing between attending doctors (private practitioners who admit patients) and house staff (interns and residents who are getting post-doctoral training in a hospital setting). This conflict is summarized by Millman as follows:

> *whereas the private physicians felt that every patient (provided the bills could be paid) should get the maximum amount of health care, including liberal requirements for hospitalization and the benefit of every diagnostic test and treatment that was relevant, the residents and interns felt that certain categories of patients did not deserve hospitalization and "scarce" medical resources.*[11]

If the allocation of resources was a source of conflict in the past, the DRGs, which restrict the amount of care that will be paid for, are likely to worsen this conflict.

Corporatization

In the past ten to fifteen years, individual hospital autonomy has changed dramatically. Thirty-three percent of community hospitals now belong to a multihospital system (a corporation that owns or runs two or more hospitals), and it is estimated that by 1990, 60 percent of all hospitals will be members of systems.[12] This trend for hospitals to become part of corporations (known as "corporatization") has also had a major impact on the relationship between doctors and hospitals.

The for-profit hospitals, in particular, are becoming huge conglomerates. Five companies that did not exist prior to 1968 now own or manage most of the for-profit hospitals in the U.S.[13] Though the proportion of nonprofit to for-profit hospitals has not changed significantly (as in 1970, approximately one out of seven nonfederally owned hospitals is still privately owned[14]), the share of hospital beds has. Moreover, the share of hospital beds owned by for-profit systems is growing at a higher rate than that of the nonprofits: 4.8 percent as opposed to 3.5 percent per year.[15] On the whole, the for-profit systems are larger than the nonprofit systems: they average twenty-three hospitals per system, whereas nonprofit systems average seven hospitals each.[16]

In some ways the distinction between the for-profits and the nonprofits is a spurious one. Both generate "revenues in excess of expenditures"; the nonprofits, however, call these funds "surpluses" rather than "profits." Both use their excess funds to upgrade and expand facilities, attract a higher-quality staff, and handle charity cases. The difference is that the for-profits distribute some of the excess funds to shareholders and pay corporate taxes. Both the for-profits and the nonprofits, however, share a common goal: both must earn a profit/surplus.

The identity of the nonprofits is becoming further obscured as some are becoming holding companies for profit-making businesses. Both the for-profits and nonprofits alike have begun to acquire other enterprises; some are related, such as nursing homes, ambulatory care centers, and health promotion programs; others are unrelated, such as hotels and shopping centers.[17] In short, comparing the traditional community hospital to to-day's corporate, multihospital system is, as Bradford Gray puts it, "like comparing agri-business to the family farm."[18]

An important result of the emergence of the multihospital system has been to shift the locus of decision making more and more from the individual hospital to a separate corporate office. Under the old dual-authority system that existed in most freestanding hospitals, doctors influenced decision making at all levels of the organization. However, when a hospital becomes part of a multihospital system, decision making becomes more complex and more removed. Decisions need to be made with a view to the whole corporation, not just for the good of an individual hospital.

Moreover, with corporatization has come the professional manager. According to Quintana et al., "increased government control of costs and construction, the development of new technology, decreasing resources, increasing competition, and the resulting uncertainty all increase the need for better and professionally trained managers."[19] Yet with the coming of professional managers, doctors often feel that their participation in the decision-making process has diminished. The following passage illustrates how one doctor perceives the changes brought about by a professional manager. The hospital described is part of a large, nonprofit, multihospital system.

One Doctor's Experience[20]

Sister Helen had run the hospital somewhat like a Catholic grade school. She was everywhere. You could pick up a phone, describe a problem with anything from a dirty elevator floor to inadequate staffing during dinner hour in the Emergency Department and have action immediately.

Sister played favorites. She could be sarcastic, even cruel in her anger, but she was personally involved in health care. Her perspective was that of a concerned lay person and she demanded the hospital's service satisfy the patient. When you came in the morning, Sister was already there; when you left at night, she was still there. Doctors and nurses entering the building had to pass by her always open door.

We had expected changes after Mr. Harris's arrival. The frayed brown rug, battered desk, and worn conference table, covered with oil cloth, departed. There came dark paneling on the wall and thick green carpet under the imposing work

station. The door remained open, but the office was empty.

About the time we discovered David was not really "our administrator," but a manager assigned from the . . . (corporate headquarters), strange things happened. The hallway and offices were redesigned. David vanished into a room with no openings to the outside. Even the doorway was plastered over and covered with wallpaper.

Access now is through three secretaries and an assistant administrator. ("Ask Steve, I'm just the conceptualizer.") Memos flow. Strangers in dark, three piece suits with leather attache cases prowl the halls. After thirty years, just short of retirement, Ruth has been cashiered as O.R. supervisor in order to "take control" of that area from the surgeons. In my latest fantasy, I find the administrator, hidden like the Wizard of Oz in his castle, and strangle his memo pad.

With a little effort I can see fiscal benefits from our new association. The . . . Corporation has extended credit so we may build a new facility. They have bought out the pesky private hospital down the hill. But, they will control our Board of Directors; guide us to services which are profitable and meet their ethical standards (no abortions or sterilizations); and, as they have done with the pending construction's contracts, cast aside local firms and people who seem not absolutely cost effective.

As Shortell points out, where once doctors affected the organizational structures of hospitals more than they were affected by it, the opposite is now true: "Physicians are now more affected by the organizational structures of hospitals than the reverse."[21] Doctors are still exercising a good deal of power in individual hospitals, however, and are in fact becoming involved in a wider range of decisions than ever before. Where once doctors involved themselves mostly in decisions involving patient care, "the distinction between 'clinical' and 'administrative' decision making is becoming obscured."[22] As a result, Shortell sees the hospital–doctor relationship moving away from the dual-authority system, where the doctor was dominant, to one of "shared authority," which involves a more equal distribution of power.

Doctors as Employees: Proletarianization

The corporatization of hospitals is affecting doctor–hospital relations in another important way. More and more, the trend is for hospitals to hire doctors as salaried employees. Hospitals have always had some salaried doctors on their staffs, but the dominant model was an autonomous practitioner who brought his or her patients to the hospital and was given privileges there. Private practitioners depended on hospitals to provide them facilities, and hospitals depended on private practitioners to provide them with patients. Under the old system, it was a seller's market for doctors—there were fewer of them and they were able to choose the hospitals with which they preferred to establish relations.

In the last few years, all that has changed. There are now more doctors than ever before, and setting up a private practice has become harder and more expensive because of increased competition and the climbing cost of malpractice insurance. Moreover, many doctors are attracted by the regular hours that come with being a salaried employee.[23] As a result, increasing numbers of young doctors are choosing to become salaried employees of hospitals rather than private practitioners.[24]

This trend, coupled with the fact that corporatization has made hospitals increasingly bureaucratic, has led some to claim that the professional status of doctors is eroding: doctors are moving away from the special "functional" status they once enjoyed and are being absorbed into the "scalar" system as mere employees. One esoteric group even goes so far as to say that doctors will eventually become part of the proletariat, a new type of industrial worker, subject to the same kinds of managerial control as any other worker.[25] Table 1 illustrates some of the factors McKinlay and Arches cite to support this argument.[26]

It is true that the corporatization of hospitals has altered the traditional doctor–hospital relationship. But the theories of Eliot Freidson argue that the professional status of doctors is not eroding.[27] He points out that although professionalism implies a certain measure of control over one's work, being an employee rather than being self-employed does not necessarily mean a loss of that control. Rather, when a professional becomes an employee, the control shifts more to the profession as a corporate body.

TABLE 1 Some general differences between bureaucratically-based and small-scale fee-for-service physicians in control over selected occupational perogatives

KEY PEROGATIVES OF AN OCCUPATIONAL GROUP	PHYSICIANS IN SMALL-SCALE FEE-FOR-SERVICE PRACTICE IN THE PAST	PHYSICIANS IN BUREAUCRATIC PRACTICE THEORY
Autonomy over the terms and content of work	Work typically more generalized and controlled by the individual practitioner him- or herself	Work typically segmentalized and directed by administrators in accordance with organizational contingencies
Object of labor	Patients usually regarded as the physician's "own patients"	Patients are technically clients or members of the organization who physicians must usually share with other specialists
Tools of labor	Equipment typically owned by the practitioner and any employees are hired by the practitioner him- or herself	Technology typically owned by the employing organization and operated by other bureaucratic employees
Means of labor	The physical plant is typically owned and operated by the physicians themselves	The physical plant typically owned and operated in the interest of the organization
Remuneration for labor	The hours work, the level of utilization, and the fees charged pretty much determined by the individual practitioner	Regular hours of work at an established salary level; sometimes limitations on "outside practice"

This can be seen in the system of supervision. Unlike the industrial model, where the rank and file are supervised by professional managers, salaried professionals are supervised by colleagues from their profession who have assumed supervisory duties. The relationship, though it may be that of a subordinate to a superordinate, is still collegial.

Even if hospitals hired all of their doctors as salaried employees, it is unlikely that doctors would lose professional control. Powerful accrediting bodies like the JCAH (Joint Commission on the Accreditation of Hospitals) mandate a self-governing medical staff with exclusive power to admit and discharge patients. The bottom line, according to Starr, is that as long as doctors are responsible for bringing in patients, they will always have power.[28]

THE FUTURE

Traditionally, our health care system has been based on a close collaboration between doctors and hospitals. Once, doctors held the edge of power; now, because of the changes we have discussed here, this is no longer the case. Some observers argue that power is now more equally distributed between doctors and administrators. Others feel that the scales have tipped too far and that doctors have lost and will continue to lose power that rightfully belongs to them.

Where is it all going? How will power lines be drawn in hospitals of the future?

Two things are certain. First, doctors will not easily relinquish power over the medical areas that have always been their exclusive domain. In this regard, they have a good deal of popular support from a public that feels that when "money" becomes more important than "service," the health care of the entire nation suffers. Second, changes like the DRGs and corporatization that have disturbed the old balance of power are also here to stay. Clearly, some arrangement must be made that will allow these two competing groups—doctors and hospital administrators—their own appropriate measures of power.

The solution for some doctors is to disassociate themselves completely from hospitals. In fact, some groups of doctors have formed independent ambulatory care centers (centers that offer, on an outpatient basis, services that used to be provided exclusively by hospitals) to compete directly with hospitals. But such centers will never replace hospitals, and hospitals cannot exist without doctors.

Some theorists suggest that hospitals will have to change their internal structures in order to achieve the optimum balance of power between doctors and hospital administrators. Shortell suggests three organizational models that might become dominant in the future.[29] Each assigns a different role to doctors in relation to hospital governance.

Alternative Organizational Models

One model, "the divisional model" has already been adopted by many large teaching hospitals. The hospital is organized around various functional areas, and each division is headed by a doctor–specialist from that division who serves as manager. This doctor–manager controls all the resources needed to provide cost-effective care within the division, so he or she has a good deal of power.

There are several possible ways to structure a hospital according to division. One way, presently in use, is to form divisions according to diseases, such as cancer, gastrointestinal, cardiovascular, and nervous system, with each of these divisions having both a medical and a surgical component. Or the divisions might be broader, perhaps consisting of four as follows: primary care (including family practice, pediatrics, obstetrics), acute medical/surgical (including surgeons and internal medicine), chronic care (including psychiatry and care for the elderly), and specialized services (including services for drug and alcohol abusers).

The divisional model is essentially a matrix design (an organization where there is coordination across departments as well as up and down the formal line), so it tends to foster cooperation and a team spirit among staff members rather than an "us" versus "them" attitude. The use of a matrix design for hospitals was first proposed by Neuhauser in 1972[30]; it provides a good balance of power between doctors and hospitals by enmeshing doctors in the basic power structure of the hospital.

The other two models that Shortell suggests may emerge in the future are more provocative. The most extreme of the two, "the independent-corporate model," would keep the hospital and its doctors at arms length from one other. The medical staff would become a separate legal entity that would negotiate for its services with the hospital. As a group, then, the doctors would be completely autonomous, completely removed from the hospital's hierarchical structure. In some ways, they would function like subcontractors: the hospital contracts with a patient to provide health care; the hospital subcontracts the medical services portion of that care to a group of doctors.

In this arrangement, individual doctors would be free from the control of hospital administrators. This distance from the administration would allow doctors a significant degree of latitude in medical decision making. However, because doctors would be part of a negotiating entity, it would be in their best interests to provide cost-effective, quality care.

The remaining model, "the parallel model," would leave the traditional structure of the hospital intact but would create a separate mechanism for power sharing. Representatives from the administrative, medical, nursing, and other professional areas of the hospital, selected on the basis of expertise, interest, and experience, would serve on a special committee (what Shortell calls a "parallel structure") "to deal with the major strategic issues facing both the hospital and its medical staff."[31] Members would maintain their primary function within the formal organization, but part of their time would be freed to work with the "parallel structure" in long-range planning.

In this model, doctors would have a chance to influence hospital policy that would ultimately affect them. However, they would probably have less power in this arrangement than in the other two models Shortell describes. For one thing, doctors would be only one of several special interest groups vying for influence. Moreover, whether or not doctors will have any real control will depend on how much authority is given to the parallel structure. If anyone outside that group retains veto power, the parallel structure and, consequently, the various groups it represents will have little "real" power.

Of the three models, the first two—the divisional model and the independent-corporate model—have the most potential for achieving the necessary balance of power between doctors and administrators, between medical integrity and fiscal concerns. Ironically, one does this by enmeshing the two groups completely and the other, by separating the two completely.

No one can predict with certainty what future hospital structures will be, just as no one can predict with certainty what doctor–hospital relationships will be. In all likelihood, there will be no single model but rather a number of different arrangements, depending on the location of the hospital and the climate of negotiations between the hospital and its doctors.

"Negotiation" is the key word. MacNaughton predicts there will be both "winners" and "losers." The "winners" will be

> the ones that define and mutually agree upon the appropriate role for each to play; the ones that innovate and discover new methods to respond to the message of the marketplace; the ones that understand that the individual physician's goal and agenda are not always consistent with those of the institution and that some conflict and adverse behavior can redound to the benefit of patients and society in general. . . .[32]

CONCLUSIONS

The hospital–doctor relationship is a cornerstone of our health care system. This relationship has been seriously threatened by a number of factors, the most important of which are the growth in importance of DRGs and the corporatization of hospitals. The mandate of "do all you can" has become "do as much as is necessary and cost effective." The old partnership, then, has reached a turning point.

There is a Chinese symbol for "crisis" that contains the dual meanings of "opportunity" and "danger." The "crisis" that the doctor–hospital relationship is now facing could well be an opportunity in disguise. The result may be a better health care system for us all.

Notes

1. Harvey L. Smith, "Two Lines of Authority: The Hospital's Dilemma," *Modern Health Care,* March 1955.
2. William C. Cockerham, *Medical Sociology,* 3rd ed., (New Jersey: Prentice-Hall, Inc., 1986), p. 205.

3. Robert N. Wilson, "The Physician's Changing Hospital Role," *Human Organization,* 18 (1959).

4. J. E. Harris, "The Internal Organization of Hospitals: Some Economic Implications," *Bell Journal of Economics,* 8 (1978): 467–482.

5. Danielle A. Dolene and Charles J. Dougherty, "DRGs: The Counterrevolution in Financing Health Care," *Hastings Center Report,* June 1985: 19.

6. B. C. Vladeke, "Medicare Hospital Payment by Diagnosis Related Groups," *Annals of Internal Medicine* 100 (1984): 576–91.

7. Marshall B. Kapp, "Legal and Ethical Implications of Health Care Reimbursement by Diagnosis Related Groups," *Law, Medicine & Health Care,* Dec. 1984: 246.

8. For a history and discussion of the New Jersey system, see James A. Morone and Andrew B. Dunham, "The Waning of Professional Dominance: DRGs and the Hospitals," *Health Affairs,* Spring 1984.

9. Jeffrey Wasserman, "The Doctor, the Patient, & the DRG," *The Hastings Center Report,* October 1983: 23.

10. J. Joel May, Daniel H. Schwartz, and Joy Hinson Penticuff.

11. Marcia Millman, *The Unkindest Cut,* (New York: Morrow, 1976), p. 72.

12. Dan Ermann and Jon Gabel, "Multihospital Systems: Issues and Empirical Findings," *Health Affairs* (Spring 1984): 50–64.

13. James Morone, "The Unruly Rise of Medical Capitalism," *Hastings Center Report,* August 1985: 28.

14. Cockerham, p. 205; and Ermann and Gabel, p. 52.

15. Ermann and Gabel, p. 52.

16. Ermann and Gabel, p. 52.

17. Ermann and Gabel, p. 54.

18. Bradford H. Gray (ed.), *The New Health Care for Profit: Doctors and Hospitals in a Competitive Environment* (Washington: National Academy Press, 1983).

19. Jose B. Quintana, W. Jack Duncan, and Howard W. Houser, "Hospital Governance and the Corporate Revolution," *HMC Review* (Summer 1985): 68.

20. Report to the James Picker Foundation, March 1983. Note: The names in the original report have been changed.

21. Stephen M. Shortell, "The Medical Staff of the Future: Replanting the Garden," *Frontiers,* February 1985: 4.

22. Stephen M. Shortell, "Physician Involvement in Hospital Decision Making," In Gray, p. 74.

23. David Wessel, "Rx for Medics," *The Wall Street Journal.* January, 1986.

24. Wessel.

25. John B. McKinlay and Joan Arches, "Towards the Proletarianization of Physicians," *International Journal of Health Service,* 15.2 (1985): 161–193.

26. McKinlay and Arches, p. 174.

27. Eliot Freidson, "The Changing Nature of Professional Control," *Annual Review of Sociology* 10 (1981): 7.

28. Paul Starr, *The Social Transformation of American Medicine,* (New York: Basic Books Inc., 1982).

29. Stephen Shortell, "The Medical Staff . . . ," pp. 21–38.

30. D. Neuhauser, "The Hospital as a Matrix Organization," *Hospital Administration,* 17 (4): 19.

31. Shortell, "Medical Staff . . . ," 32.

32. Donald S. MacNaughton, "A New Partnership: Physicians, Hospitals, and Their Customers," In Duncan Yaggy and Patricia Hodgson (eds.), *Physicians and Hospitals: The Great Partnership at the Crossroads* (Durham: Duke University Press, 1985), p. 151.

The Impact of Technology on Patients, Providers, and Care Patterns: An Overview

Shizuko Fagerhaugh
Anselm Strauss
Barbara Suczek
Carolyn Weiner

In the last several decades, such innovations in medical technology as open heart surgery, renal dialysis, intensive care units, and CAT scanning have been a mixed blessing. On the one hand, these innovations have saved and extended lives and created opportunities for nurses and other health care professionals in various new specialties. On the other, they have led to immense confusion. Nurses and others have engaged in a frenzied search for solutions to deal with the problems which each innovation has brought in its train; yet, lacking a full understanding of the scope and complexity of the links between technology, changing illness patterns, and social, economic, and political forces acting on the health care system, the solutions have all too often contributed to fragmentation, discord, and sometimes doctrinaire debates.

The confusion is related to a complex interaction of: 1) the rapid impact of technology on health organizations and health practices; 2) the change in the character of contemporary illness, from acute to chronic; and 3) the action of economic, social, and political forces on the health care system. This interaction has created continual shifts in health organizations and practice which, in turn, have resulted in much bewilderment and frustration, not only for the public at large, but also for all health professionals. If we examine each of these issues in turn, we may achieve some understanding of the links between technology and health care. And we may begin to understand also why some solutions put forth often act to increase the confusion and fragmentation within the health care system.

THE IMPACT OF TECHNOLOGY: GROWING LIKE TOPSY

A special feature of technological innovations and medical specialization is that the two are parallel and interactive. Medical specialization leads to technological innovation; then, as a given technology is used, physicians and industrial designers collaborate to improve it. As it is refined, it leads to ever more sophisticated specialization and associated work and procedures.

The growth of intensive care units illustrates this progression. The first ICUs to develop were created to care for a variety of very acutely ill patients, including cardiac patients. Then, because cardiac disease is the major killer, large research funds were made available for further refinements of cardiovascular monitors, drug therapies, and diagnostic procedures and separate cardiac care units evolved. Simultaneously, units that specialized in diagnostic cardiac services, such as cardiac catheterization and cardio-pulmonary function testing, were developed for adults and children. Corresponding to these developments, specialists in heart surgery developed sophisticated cardiac technology. In large medical

Reprinted from *Nursing Outlook,* vol. 28, no. 11 (November, 1980), pp. 662–672. Copyright © 1980, American Journal of Nursing Company.

centers, one finds each medical specialty beginning to have its own intensive care units—the neurological ICU, the respiratory ICU, and so on.

A second illustration is provided by the latest specialties to be highly influenced by technology—obstetrics and pediatrics. Fetal monitoring machines were developed to pick up early signs of fetal distress in high-risk laboring mothers. Simultaneously, intensive care nurseries were developed as adult critical care machinery was refined and scaled down in size in order to care for the increased numbers of high-risk infants saved. Pediatrics then began to be differentiated into perinatology and neonatology, and these specialties spawned a cadre of medical subspecialties, such as pediatric cardiology and pediatric neurology.

As medicine and medical services have become specialized, so too have nursing and other professional groups. This has generated complex relationships among a multiplicity of hospital services and departments, and an increase in the numbers of workers, arrayed both horizontally and hierarchically. The increased numbers of specialists and services result in more bureaucratic organization and rules for efficient administration, and a need for new middle administrators to coordinate work both within and among services.[1] Hence, we find within nursing, for example, the emergence of unit managers, nurse coordinators, liaison nurses, and clinical specialists.

The rapid introduction of technologies has resulted in obsolescence in hospital physical plant, space usage, machinery, health professional skills, and indeed in all institutional arrangements. The effort to keep pace with innovation has increased the complexity, not only of clinical services, but also of the ancillary departments. For example, with the increase in the numbers, kinds, and models of machinery and equipment, the purchase of equipment and supplies requires much consultation from a variety of sources; furthermore, once new machines or pieces of equipment are bought, there tend to be new problems in storing and distributing them. Hence, the emergence of the material management and transport engineer.[2] Equipment repair and maintenance have also become more complex, necessitating such new skilled professionals and technicians as the bioengineer, electronic technician, and ultrasound technician. Environmental safety depart-

ments have expanded in response to the many regulations pertaining to technology and have become differentiated into departments of electrosafety, biochemical safety, radiation safety, etc.

Moreover, as new specialized services are added, workers have to be allocated and new skilled personnel integrated in a continually changing division of labor. The new service may involve training old workers with new skills or introducing new workers whose work is ambiguous or totally unfamiliar to the old workers. Interaction problems often result as the new workers try to carve out roles which impinge on the old workers' roles and tasks. It generally takes some time to delineate the total picture of the work for which a department is responsible so that each specialist can work with the others and get the work done. We see this in the numerous articles related to clinical nurse specialists as they attempt to clarify their roles and gain the acceptance of nurses and other health professionals.[3] The division of labor is constantly negotiated and renegotiated as new technology is added.

ADMINISTRATIVE PROBLEMS

Hospital and nursing administration are faced with the awesome task of coordinating and articulating a multitude of special departments and services, coping with regulations and regulatory agencies in order to stay in operation, arbitrating the demands of workers in competing specialized services for equipment and resources, and at the same time attempting to contain costs.[4] In an effort to attain some measure of order and efficiency, computers are being used for more and more tasks; but computers also require specialized skilled workers, the integration of new workers, and extensive inservice education to upgrade the skills of existing employees. Along with this, there is a search for organizational and administrative theories to bring order to the chaos. A variety of theories abound, among them general systems theory, matrix theory, contingency theory, participative decision-making theory, and many others which are intellectually interesting, but may not provide immediate pragmatic answers.[5–8]

The proliferation of specialized services and their attendant problems of articulation and interface, and the confusion over the division of labor, have resulted in a bewildering profusion of task forces, standing committees, and informal meetings to coordinate and articulate work and to spell out the division of labor. Thus, a common administrators' complaint is that the endless meetings prevent them from getting their jobs done. Patients are also affected; as one patient's relative commented, "I've been trying for days to talk to the charge nurse to resolve some problems about my mother's care, but she's always tied up in meetings." The rapidly changing conditions created either by the new technology, new governmental regulations, or new community pressure groups, mean that "management by ad hoc" or "by putting out fires" becomes the frequent, if not indeed the usual mode.

The technological specialization within hospitals has had a ripple effect on related health care services, such as clinics and home care agencies. The high cost of hospital care has meant that more and more services must be offered through ambulatory clinics, which have had to specialize to meet these needs. In the clinics, just as in the hospitals, new personnel are having to be integrated, with all the problems of working out a division of labor and forging a team to get the job done. With more and more chronically ill patients being sustained at home by means of medical technology such as pulmonary and dialysis machines, special treatments, procedures, and drugs, home care agencies are also having to meet the demands for specialized services and are employing pulmonary, cardiovascular, and cancer nursing specialists. Furthermore, work from the hospital, the clinic, and the home health services must be coordinated. This has created still other categories of nurses—the patient discharge coordinator, the cancer or respiratory liaison nurse, and so on.

The fact that life can be sustained and prolonged to a degree not possible two decades ago poses immense moral and ethical problems for workers in these services. These dilemmas have necessitated still another category of specialist, the bioethicist, in large medical centers. The ethical dilemmas, together with the intensity of work and the frustrations of coping with complex bureaucratic organizations, have created a technologically related work hazard, "burnout."[9,10]

Although most of the above observations pertain to large medical centers, the rate of technological migration to smaller hospitals and communities is becoming more and more rapid.[11] The diffusion to smaller hospitals is due to several factors: 1) the increased role of industry in medical technology, and its need to expand the market; 2) the supply of trained personnel from large research and training centers who are seeking opportunities to practice their skills; 3) the fact that hospitals need prestige if they are to compete and attract patients and physicians; and 4) the demand for equity of services and resources distributed to all citizens. The impact of technology on hospital structure and work is similar in both small and large institutions, differing only in rate and intensity.

CHRONIC ILLNESS AND HALFWAY TECHNOLOGY

The great increase in medical technology and all that it has meant for health care delivery are associated, in part, with the changing character of contemporary illnesses. Since the 1940s, industrially developed nations everywhere have manifested the same patterns of illness; the nature of disease, once chiefly infectious and parasitic, has changed, and there has been a rapid increase in chronic illnesses such as cancer, cardiovascular, and chronic respiratory and renal diseases. The prominence of chronic illnesses has called forth contemporary medical responses which rely heavily on twentieth century technology to contain these diseases, including an array of what Thomas (an eminent cancer research physician) calls "halfway technology."[12] By that he means medical intervention applied after the fact, to make up for the incapacitating effects of a disease whose course one is unable to do much about, or to postpone death. The outstanding example of this is the transplanting of organs.

Thomas argues that this level of technology is both highly sophisticated and, at the same time, primitive. The enormous technology involved in caring for heart disease, for example, includes specialized ambulances, diagnostic services, and patient care units with all kinds of electronic gadgets and an array of new skilled health professionals to maintain the machines and patients hooked to the machines. This type of technology is characteristically costly, calls for a continuing expansion of health facilities, and requires more and more highly trained personnel. It continues until there is a genuine understanding of the mechanism involved in disease—which, as Thomas sees it, means that there should be more basic research to answer questions on the mechanism of disease in the various chronic illnesses. Until these questions are answered, he argues—correctly, in our view—we must put up with halfway technology.

This is not to deny that much of the technology has improved care, provided a better life for many patients, and resulted in the discovery of new and valuable scientific and medical knowledge. Yet halfway technology, together with our current patchwork medical and health services, makes chronic care most difficult to manage. Patients enter a cycle that takes them through the hospital, to home, to the clinic or physician's office, back to the hospital in acute episodes, and back again to home. The problem of articulating the care given in the hospital, clinic, and home is immense.

DEPERSONALIZATION AND SOFT TECHNOLOGY

The acceleration of specialization with the subsequent creation of complex bureaucratic health structures has resulted in 1) fragmentation of chronic care with more possibilities of discontinuity of care; 2) further incorporation of new workers and roles to remedy the ill effects of fragmented care and dehumanization; 3) new social and psychological problems for health workers, patients, and their families; 4) generation of a need for "soft technology"—the expertise of psychiatrists and psychiatric nurse specialists—to manage the social and psychological problems; and 5) a reaction against technology in the form of accusations about the depersonalization and dehumanization it brings about.

These effects of specialization arise because multitudes of departments and layers and layers of workers must be coordinated in the chain of tasks to complete a treatment or a diagnostic test. In the course of carrying out the tasks, the patient is often neglected, because each department has its own situations in which work can go awry. Much has been written about the fragmentation of health care and the depersonalizing effects on patients. Health pro-

fessionals are becoming more and more sensitive to these untoward effects and are trying to remedy the situation by adding liaison workers and fashioning new roles such as primary nurse, primary doctor, and patient advocates.[13–15] But given the organizational considerations outlined earlier, remedying the situation is most difficult. Another complication is that the intricate technologies require very specialized knowledge from many experts who may not agree with one another. Moreover, many of the medical interventions are very uncertain, and there is concern about the possibility of iatrogenic disease.

A characteristic of chronic illness is that the patient and the family must bear the major responsibility for management during the nonacute phase of the illness. This may require teaching the patient and the family the intricacies of operating a machine and giving advice on dietary restrictions, medications to take, possible side effects to watch for, and lifestyle changes which the patient and the family may have to make. New community resources and new forms of patient-professional interactions must be created to assist the patient in managing the medical regimen and in living with a disability.

Among the social and psychological problems for the patients and their families, as well as for health professionals, are the stress of living with the constant threat of death, carrying on in the middle of seemingly never-ending responsibilities to monitor and manage the complex regimen, or coping with social isolation and bodily disfigurement. In response to this there has been a proliferation of support groups for patients and their families, self-help groups, death counseling groups, and many others to cope with these problems. Clearly, the hard technology applied to control chronic diseases has generated a need for the seemingly discrepant soft technology—group work and counseling skills of psychiatrists, psychiatric nurses, social workers, psychologists and so on, as well as lay workers. Soft technology is not only necessary for professionals using hard technology in order to help them maintain their composure and equanimity, but also for the receivers of the hard technology, the patients and their kin.

A reaction has set in against current medical institutions and practices, as evidenced by the growth of alternative health care approaches, such as natural birth centers and holistic health centers.

Among others, more and more nurses are being influenced by this social movement. In general, these alternative approaches are peripheral to the traditional medical institutions, but are beginning to be incorporated into them; for instance, there are alternative birth centers which have opened side by side with traditional medical obstetrical departments.

FUNDING FOR RESEARCH: FEAST OR FAMINE

Although chronic illness is our major health problem, we are unable to cope with it adequately, in part because medical and public attention and support have been directed to specific categories of diseases, such as heart disease, stroke, and, in recent years, catastrophic illness. Chronic illness itself as a major and general health issue is only dimly understood, if at all. Our governmental health commissions and institutes, our privately funded disease-oriented associations and institutes, all support a categorical perspective on chronic illness which is encouraged partly by the tremendous specialization in medicine. This is not to deny that categorical disease approaches do stimulate public interest and support major scientific breakthroughs. Nevertheless, the specialties which have hard technology tend to enjoy generous resources at the expense of other specialties dealing with chronic illnesses. Thus, one finds tremendously expensive medical technology associated with some forms of illness, such as end-stage renal disease, and a paucity of financing and technology with others, such as arthritis, even though the latter may be far more common. This situation generates competition between health specialists and health institutions for research funds and resources, which further detracts from resolving, or at least focusing on, the proper application of technology to the management of chronic illness.

POLITICAL, SOCIAL, AND PHILOSOPHICAL FORCES

A number of political, social, and philosophical concerns enter into any discussion of medical technology—the most important one being its high cost.[16] Some blame this on competition among industries for profit, on physicians' avarice, and on hospitals' drive for prestige.[17,18] (Hence the hue and cry against the dangers of the "medical-industrial complex."[19]) Others argue that competition will reduce costs. The search for causes of high medical costs is clearly related to the issue of who should bear the burden of paying them, which in turn raises the question of equity. The demand for equity implies a fair distribution of medical resources, so that comprehensive health care that includes preventive, diagnostic, therapeutic, and rehabilitative services is provided for all citizens. The issue of just how comprehensive this care should be is hotly disputed. Second, the general public, health workers, and industry are all involved in concern about the regulations governing the use of technology. Debates rage about whether there is too much or too little regulation and about what constitutes appropriate evidence for certification of need for hospitals that want a given innovation; reasonable limitation on a researcher's freedom; or tolerable risk.[20] In industry, there are complaints that governmental safety regulations increase costs and that the bureaucratic system is contrary to the spirit of free enterprise, while among researchers, the regulations are felt to be a roadblock to scientific inquiry and medical breakthroughs.[21] The counterposition is that industry is using this argument to cover up the profit motive and to avoid governmental interference. Moral rationales are applied by opposing groups to support each position.

Third, there are moral and ethical concerns associated with the argument that technology is the root of what is perceived as the current dehumanization of medical care.[22] There are bioethical discussions of informed consent, of sustaining life at the expense of enormous social and economic strains for the family and society, of the extent to which genetics should be tampered with, of the right to die, and so on.[23,24] Moral considerations also enter the debate on cost, leading to such questions as: Is the cost of technology worth the benefits to be gained from using it? Who is worthy to receive costly medical care? And perhaps most important of all: Who shall decide?

In our pluralistic society, many individuals and groups within the general public, health professions, and industry take positions on one or more of these concerns. These groups vary in terms of the stakes involved, self-interest, and ideology. Social diagnoses are made from these varying perspectives and the major causes or culprits responsible for the chaotic state of our health care system are identified. The many special interest groups hold widely divergent views about health problems and therefore find it extremely difficult to resolve either the debates or the profound problems that are inextricably linked with medical technology and chronic illness. Meanwhile, medical knowledge and medical technology continue to advance and help to increase the numbers of chronically ill at home, in hospitals, in clinics and nursing homes, and thus infinitely multiply the problems we have addressed. . . .

References

1. Georgopoulos, B. S., and Mann, F. C. The hospital as an organization. In *Hospital Organization and Management,* 2d edition, edited by J. S. Rakich and Kurt Darr. New York, John Wiley & Sons, 1978, pp. 19–27.

2. Housley, C. E. *Hospital Material Management.* Germantown, Md., Aspen Systems Corporation, 1978.

3. The nurse practitioner: preparation and practice. (9 parts) *Nurs. Outlook* 22:89–127, Feb. 1974.

4. Somers, A. R. *Hospital Regulation: the Dilemma of Public Policy.* Princeton, N. J., Industrial Relations Section, Princeton University, 1969.

5. Kast, F. E., and Rosenzweig, J. E. Hospital administration and systems concept. *Hosp. Admin. Q.* 11:17–33, Fall 1966.

6. Neuhauser, Duncan. The hospital as a matrix organization. *Hosp. Admin.* 17:8–25, Fall 1972.

7. Mockler, R. J. Situational theory of management. *Harvard Bus. Rev.* 49:146–148ff, May 1971.

8. Lowin, Aaron. Participative decision making: a model, literature critique, and prescriptions for research. *Organ. Behav. Human Perf.* 3(1):68–106, 1968.

9. Freudenberger, H. J. Staff burnout. *J. Soc. Issues* 30(1):159–165, 1974.

10. Reichle, M. J. Psychological stress in the intensive care unit. *Nurs. Digest* 3:12–15, May-June 1975.

11. Russell, Louise. *Technology in Hospitals: Medical Advances and Their Diffusion.* Washington, D.C., The Brookings Institute, 1979, pp. 41–98.

12. Thomas, L. *The Living Cell.* New York, Bantam Books, 1974, pp. 35–42.

13. Mundinger, M.O.N. Primary nurse—role evolution. *Nurs. Outlook* 21:643–645, Oct. 1973.

14. Sun Valley Forum on National Health. *Primary Care: Where Medicine Fails,* ed. by Spyros Andreopoulos. New York, John Wiley & Sons, 1974.

15. Hamil, E. M. People power. *NLN Publ.* 20–1623:3–8, 1976.

16. Altman, S. H., and Blendon, Robert, Eds. *Medical Technology: the Culprit Behind the Health Care Cost?* Proceedings of 1977 Sun Valley Forum on National Health. (DHEW Publ. No. (PHS) 79–3216) Washington, D.C., U.S. Government Printing Office, 1979.

17. Health Policy Advisory Committee. *The American Health Empire: Power, Profit and Politics.* New York, Random House, 1971.

18. Waitzkin, Ward, and Waterman, Barbara. *The Exploitation of Illness in Capitalist Society.* Indianapolis, Ind., Bobbs-Merrill, 1974.

19. Health Policy Advisory Committee, *op. cit.*

20. Ivancevich, R. E. American Hospital Association perspective: legislative and administrative thrust in national health policy. In *Evolving National Health Policy: Effects on Institutional Providers.* Proceedings of 1977 National Health Forum, ed. by E. G. Jaco. San Antonio, Tex., Trinity University, Center for Professional Development in Health Administration, 1978, pp. 41–54 (mimeographed).

21. The breakdown of U.S. innovation. *Bus. Week* Feb. 16, 1976, pp. 56–60ff.

22. Illich, Ivan. *Medical Nemesis.* New York, Bantam Books, 1977.

23. Mann, K. W. *Deadline for Survival: A Survey of Moral Issues in Science and Medicine.* New York, Seabury Press, 1970.

24. Williams, P. S., ed. *Ethical Issues in Biology and Medicine.* Proceedings of symposium on the Identity and Dignity of Man, held at Boston University, 1969. Cambridge, Mass., Schenkman Publishers, 1973.

The Social Context of High Technology: The Case of the Intensive Care Nursery

Anselm Strauss
Shizuko Fagerhaugh
Barbara Suczek
Carolyn Weiner

We shall discuss the birth trajectory as it flows through labor and delivery and intensive care nursery units. This involves the impact especially of changes in medical technology and medical specialization on these wards and the reverse impact of that work and those kinds of wards on both technology and specialization; it also involves the lives of families and the children saved in the ICNs and the possible influence of the technological changes on the larger health issues. We shall discuss, too, the influence that ideologies and ideological debate (professional and nonprofessional) seem to have had on the premature-infant trajectory, and vice versa.

A CHANGING TECHNOLOGY AND THE BIRTH TRAJECTORY

Labor and delivery wards are moving from what was considered the practice of an "art" (abetted by analgesic intervention) to heightened application of technology ("we are now more clinically definitive"). With the explosion of new knowledge and new medical technology in the last decade, a quasi-fatalistic

This article was taken from Chapter 9, "Macro to Micro and Micro to Macro Impacts: The Intensive Care Units," in *The Social Organization of Medical Care* by Anselm Strauss, et al., pp. 210–227. Reprinted with permission of the University of Chicago Press. Copyright © 1985 by the University of Chicago.

attitude in obstetrics has been replaced by aggressive intervention in order to maximize the possibility of conception and to maintain formerly hopeless pregnancies. At the same time, goaded by a consumer movement that labeled hospital birth as too impersonal and technological and by the competition of a midwife and home-birth movement, hospitals have opened alternative birth centers (called ABCs), which offer none of the usual technology and no drug intervention. The rationale for acceptance of this radical change has been the closeness of emergency backup. To quote one doctor:

> *Avoiding the hospital is not the answer; humanizing the hospital is. . . . The birth process represents the most dangerous day in the life of the newborn. . . . He has the best chance of dying on that day, and we're not only talking about death but about crippling and handicapping. That's the time that that baby ought to be very close to all care possible. (Fox 1979)*

Alternative birth centers in most cases represent a philosophy rather than actually constitute a separate center. ABC rooms within the conventional hospital have been furnished in a homelike decor, complete with plants, stereo, and a double bed to serve for labor, delivery, and rest. Nurses, who are no longer identifiable by uniforms, remain with the mother the entire time, as may fathers, siblings, and others of the mother's choosing.

Well-baby nurseries have also undergone a change, being sparsely populated since babies now spend more time in their mother's rooms. But adjacent to a near-empty nursery, there is a beehive of activity in the highly machined and highly staffed intensive care nursery, where the radical survival techniques are being performed.

Machines have been to a large extent responsible for who goes to the ICN. But before turning to the ICN and its technology we shall briefly discuss continuous fetal monitoring, the simultaneous electronic recording of fetal heart rate and uterine contractions during labor, which developed out of the desire to assess fetal and/or maternal distress more accurately. Used during pregnancy by applying external electrodes or, if necessary, by adding an intravenous administration of oxytocin, this machine has been found to be a useful tool for gauging fetal capability of withstanding the stress of labor, thereby guiding the best timing and mode of delivery. For indicated cases (such as diabetes, hypertensive disease of pregnancy, intrauterine growth retardation, Rh sensitization, previous stillbirth or premature birth, low esterol excretions), a periodic oxytocin challenge test (OCT), or "nonstress test," as it is sometimes called, can be used to determine whether the respiratory function of the placenta is adequate. The goal is to keep the pregnancy going long enough to give the baby the best start, without endangering either mother or baby. This test is often used in conjunction with drugs and/or other techniques, such as ultrasonography.

A high infant mortality rate gave additional impetus for greater acceptance of the continuous fetal monitoring because of an effort to lower that rate. Moreover, current theory held that mental retardation and cerebral palsy were closely tied to oxygen deprivation during the time immediately before and after birth. Smaller family size, coupled with generous resources for frontier medicine, heightened the value placed on saving each baby. Intensive care nurseries, which started out focusing on babies, soon saw the advantage of monitoring the mother, preferably during pregnancy, but at least during labor, and that led to the expansion from baby transport to mother transport.

What started as a useful tool for high-risk labor, however, became routine in many hospitals, now evoking attack. Critics point to a sharp rise in cesarean births (a riskier and costlier procedure than vaginal delivery), which they attribute to panic readings of the fetal monitor. Defendants maintain that the problem is merely one of interpretation and skill:

A lot of patterns we don't know completely, and sometimes it is difficult to interpret—even if there are late decelerations, it doesn't mean the baby is necessarily distressed. In major centers, where we have a lot of experience, monitor information can be put together with fetal blood samples, but smaller hospitals may not do that.

Participants in a national conference held in the late 1970s on antenatal diagnosis examined the arguments surrounding the growing routine use of monitors. They concluded that although current data were inadequate, no evidence could be found that electronic fetal monitoring reduces mortality or morbidity in low-risk patients (National Institute of Child Health and Human Development, 1979). Thus, the machine's biography has gone through research, development, and refinement to controversy.

Machinery purchased to aid such high-risk cases, however, takes on a life of its own. As stated above, unknowns abound in labor: a woman can evince optimal pelvic physiological construction and still not progress, just as the opposite can occur; labor can be slow for hours and suddenly speed up, requiring quick and pressured decisions. Not only do staff experiential biographies differ (varying degrees of competence at interpretation can lead to confrontations between nurses and physicians), but variability comes into play. Questioned about the routine use of the fetal monitor on low-risk laboring women, nurses answered that it is easier for themselves, that is, the nurse can leave the room, since presumably *someone* is watching the monitor at the central nurses' station (called the "slave monitor" by one nurse). Additionally, there is the ever present fear of malpractice suits. The machine's printout is part of the record and, to quote one physician, "If you've done the right thing, it will support you in court; if you've done the wrong thing, it will damn you" (Neutra 1979). Malpractice notwithstanding, the tyranny of this machine is that a compulsion has been set up to take all possible precautions against missing the signs of fetal and/or maternal distress: "You get afraid after a couple of bad experiences." The fetal monitor has become an evidence machine, by which staff make accusations of negligence or defend action or inaction. As expressed by a nurse, "The old philosophy was everything is normal until proven otherwise; now it's everything is abnormal until proven otherwise." In teaching hospitals especially, this monitor becomes part of the convincing process. As one resident put it:

Because of studies that have been done, criteria develop, and in order to justify [emphasis added] what you have done, you have to go by these criteria. So even if you hear something with the fetascope and it is not on the monitor strip, somehow it is invalid. I don't know whether this is defensive medicine or a preoccupation with hardware.

As machines are assessed on the units—and this information is converted into improvements by industry—specialization and associated work and procedures become more sophisticated. Technological innovation and medical specialization proceed in a parallel and interactive manner (Fagerhaugh et al. 1980). What were the formerly relative static and low-status specialties of obstetrics and pediatrics are being sliced smaller and smaller to correspond with the technology of controlling the correspondingly smaller slices of the birth trajectory itself. Thus, there emerges both perinatology and neonatology. The first is the specialty defined as pertaining to before, during, and after the time of birth, time designation being arbitrary. Neonatology relates to the period immediately succeeding birth, and continuing, roughly, through the first month of life. Each of these medical specialties has spawned attendant clinical nurse specialists and a growing cadre of pediatric specialties in associated services like cardiology and neurology. Staff nursing, too, has become more specialized, requiring special ABC nurses, experienced nurses to accompany and care for high-risk mothers and babies on transports from outlying hospitals. Entwined with the growth of medical machinery has been the expanded knowledge of biochemistry and microchemistry, through which results can be obtained from an ever smaller amount of blood. In addition to juggling the tasks required of all nurses, the intensive care nurse must be an alchemist, striving to achieve and maintain a delicate balance of body chemistry based on sophisticated readings of blood gas studies and keeping an ear ever attuned to the beeping of the heart and respiratory monitor—a far cry from the nurse who

rotated from labor and delivery to postpartum to the nursery.

Moreover, the drive for regionalization of services, in the interest of cost control and better utilization of skills, has divided hospitals into three classifications for the newborn: primary care (small hospitals with no support services for distressed babies); secondary care (minimal support, like oxygen, intravenous assistance); tertiary care (acute services). A medical dispatch center can direct the transport of at-risk babies to the appropriate hospital. These transports allow information to fan out from the medical center to the outlying districts. Since they are vital to the information flow and to the economic structure and prestige of the receiving hospital, staff are ever mindful of the public relations aspect of their work. Greater skill, knowledge, and experience are seeds for judgments of mismanaged labor and/or delivery out there; being received as the saviors from the big city (sometimes augmented by press coverage) adds nourishment to these seeds. The transport staff must be reminded constantly that an irritated and angry local hospital staff is not likely to remain a source of referrals and that effective teaching under these conditions must be tactfully presented in order to be effective.

TECHNOLOGIZED WORK, IDEOLOGIES, AND THE BIRTH TRAJECTORY

Since delivery allows little or no time for quality-of-life decisions, such decisions move from the delivery room to the intensive care nursery. If the infant has a congenital defect, parents may decide they want no corrective procedures. Staff must then continue maintenance care, knowing the baby will not survive. The prolonged agony of such cases is a tremendous strain on parent and staff, and great effort is made to ease the effect on the infant.

With premature births, the staff watches closely during the first six to eight hours. If the baby is judged to be a 25- to 27-weeker, on 80 percent oxygen with oxygen support going higher and higher, the family is told that the outcome is highly questionable and asked if life-sustaining care should be continued. The following is a composite quote about this situation from one ward: "The response can be everything from the father who says 'Where are the autopsy papers?' to one who says, 'I don't care if he's blind and retarded, save him.' In most instances, the family will say, 'Withdraw support.' If we can't read the family, or if the family says they want the baby to survive, we will go great guns." Decisions must be made in rapid succession on the basis of various assumptions. The base of knowledge is recent, rapidly changing, and largely unpredictive. For example, it has only been since 1977 that knowledge about intercranial bleeding has become more conclusive. Now that a brain scan is part of the routine workup, bleeding has been found in 50 percent of the babies who are less than 1200 grams (usually the babies who have been transported). Occasionally the bleeding is massive or shows that major motor function has been affected. More often the results are ambiguous. In addition, it is not unusual for the baby to be too distressed to be subjected to a scan until considerable time has elapsed. Furthermore, a scan that indicates no bleeding does not rule out oxygen damage.

If the infant needs the aid of a respirator to ventilate, the delicate balancing begins: close monitoring of the respirator pressure to minimize lung damage, insertion of tubes to drain air, insertion of an umbilical line to monitor oxygen level through blood gas tests, anticoagulant drugs to correct clogging in the line, drugs to repress the normal breathing that would compete with the respirator, drugs to aid lung development, transfusions to replace blood taken for tests, periodic brain scans and X-rays, insertion of a line to feed through the jugular vein (hyperalimentation), antibiotics to ward off infection. The succession is totally open-ended, as are the complications—from unanticipated, or anticipated but not fully controllable, contingencies—that can further snowball. Such babies may spend as many as six to nine months in the intensive care nursery, during which time staff members and parents may be asking at any point, "What are we doing?"

Faced with a parent who wants "everything done," staff is often unsure if that parent hears or understands what is meant by "brain damage." During this period there may be vast differences of opinion and judgment among staff, and they attend to different indications of improvement. When a physician focuses on trajectory and says, "She's doing well—she's off the respirator," the nurses may still

be agonizing over biography, to wit: "What is her life going to be?"

In intensive care nurseries which place utmost importance on quality of life, although encouraging family involvement in life-sustaining decisions, the staff know that the family does not have the criteria to make such decisions. And they know their own criteria are weak. What sustains the staff is the understanding that as their knowledge base increases, it becomes possible to decrease the implicated assumptions. A baby who survives precarious months as described above (including a succession of some 40 insertions of chest tubes) and goes home breathing room air, showing no intercranial bleed, with eye problems that are correctable, becomes the rationale—despite ethical questions—for continuing treatment on future babies. Bulletin boards covered with snapshots of successes and a Christmas party for graduates serve this same purpose.

Going back to the topic of labor: identity work here also becomes paramount when there are strongly held ideologies. Many childbearing couples who question the hospital system do so on the instruction of theorists like Frederick Leboyer (1975), Fernand Lamaze (1970), and Robert A. Bradley (1974), who teach that birth is a normal process and that with attention to prenatal preparation and an appropriate atmosphere, parents and child can avoid the stress associated with the conventional hospital delivery (see also Arms 1975). For some of these couples, there are ideological stakes. Having reached this final moment of truth, this long-awaited delivery, they place accentuated and negative symbolic significance on each dimension of hospital intervention: enema, prep, drugs, forceps, episiotomies, silver-nitrate for the infant's eyes. Any of the above, if deemed necessary by the hospital staff, are potential points of contention. Conversely, staff, too, may have ideological stakes in the normal childbirth controversy (they may be critical of doctors who believe in responding to the patient's pleas, "Do something!" with, "We'll take care of it, honey") but may not have a choice in their assignment to specific women in labor. And while some prospective mothers have made a conscious choice regarding the camp in which they wished to be placed—some take a defensive posture ("I'm no pioneer"), while others are enthusiastic believers in the alternative birth center—many are not aware that in selecting a physician they may have placed themselves in one ideological camp or another. Most important, they are not likely to be aware of staff ideological stakes. Frequently, the situation will become clear in retrospect. The analysis of one woman ("I think the nurses lost interest in me when my labor was prolonged and it was necessary to induce; I think the challenge for them was gone") was given additional credence by the expressions of frustration voiced by a nurse:

> The mother is doing well. You close the door and cut off the world. Then there's a fluid stain, or the labor is prolonged, or she needs an analgesic. In comes the anaesthesiologist with the crash cart, a tray, a blood pressure machine, the epidural; we attach the monitor.
> And I feel a failure.

The course of each labor is totally unpredictable. As with ethical issues, the absence of clear-cut answers merely increases the rivalry of ideological positions. For every staff member who feels that drug intervention during labor impedes labor, leads to learning or motor disabilities, or detracts from a normal process, another can be found asserting that despite a reassuring physician, partner, and nurse, a significant number of women are going to remain anxious and are going to need intervention. Furthermore, the tone of many of the books about the Leboyer, Lamaze, and Bradley methods has contributed to public competition and peer pressure. (Nora Ephron, writing of her own experience with Lamaze, reflects perhaps a growing reaction: "The trouble is that it has the capability of being every bit as fanatical and narrow-minded as the system it has replaced" [1978].)

Another ideology that has had popular impact concerns parent attachment, labeled "bonding." This term—based on research spanning the last three decades but accelerated in most recent years—signifies the whole range of nurturing stimulation (stroking, swaddling, cuddling) felt to be necessary for the infant's emotional development. Marshall Klaus, whose research led to guidance on how the hospital can fulfill these needs, even in an acute-care setting, has stressed the "fantastic adaptability" of infants and warned against the danger of assuming that bonding must occur immediately at birth (Klaus 1979). Nevertheless, as with all such theories, popu-

larization brings a certain degree of fanaticism. To quote one nurse recalling a "rough case":

> She was a 35-weeker, who wanted an ABC delivery and bonding, and was so freaked out by ending up in labor and delivery with a baby headed for the intensive care nursery. She had already been worn down, and accepted stirrups, draping. I had to convince her that doing an APGAR on the baby during the first five minutes was more important than bonding. [APGAR is a test done to determine the degree of asphyxiation of a baby at birth.]

Belief in the bonding ideology also complicates the imparting of information to parents of sick infants: "You don't want to scare them, and you don't want to affect their ability to bond, so you tell them enough to be concerned and not enough to divorce their feelings. It's hard to know what they understand."

The ward ideology also figures prominently. An intensive care nursery that believes in bonding, is mindful of quality of life, and encourages parent participation is opening up the possibilities of confrontations with parents. Access to the infant's chart may result in a deteriorating relationship between staff and parent, as the following case illustrates. An unfortunate characterization of the mother noted in the chart by her obstetrician both fed into the composite mother biography that staff was building and antagonized her to the extent that her behavior became increasingly withdrawn. A confrontation finally occurred when staff, fearful that the baby was not getting sufficient nutrition, encouraged supplemental bottle feeding. The mother, imbued with the necessity for breast feeding, which is part of bonding ideology, refused. This had been preceded by her accusations of negligence against a midwife and a premature delivery, which thwarted plans for delivery in the alternative birth center. A downward spiral was created which culminated in a mutually agreed on, but earlier than warranted, discharge of the infant. Staff and parent shared concern for the future biography of the infant. They differed on managing the course of the trajectory. Such confrontations arise when an ideology like bonding remains central for parents but, due to other considerations, recedes from staff focus. The emotional blow of an expected ABC delivery that has turned into the nightmare of a sick baby is apparent, and staff are mindful of this trauma. However, ABC parents are quite often assertive—questioning, and sometimes refusing, procedures.

Such behavior is often understood in retrospect but viewed as hostile when it adds to the strain of work. Staff is being called on to do identity work with the parent, when pure medical-nursing work would be preferred.

For the birth trajectory in general, expansion of perinatal and neonatal knowledge, skills, and technology and the ICN itself have made it possible to save babies who formerly were lost, with a paradoxical consequence. It is possible to move infant biographies farther and farther back, thus saving younger babies, who are more at risk by virtue of their being younger and having a less developed physiology. "We used to get excited at saving a 28-weeker; now it's 26 weeks." "Small" has moved from 1500 grams, to 1200, to 1000. This push back is not infinite; prior to 26 weeks there are no lungs and the eyes are sealed. However, there is some ambiguity even here, since each organism progresses at a different rate. Just when the neonatologists feel they have a partial predictive grasp about these babies, along comes a 25–26 weeker, 600 grams, who defies the odds and goes home in five weeks, gaining weight and breathing room air.

This stretching out of the birth trajectory has so far been continuous, for developments have been rapid and revolutionary. As already mentioned, brain scans have provided a tremendous breakthrough in predicting the infant's future. Another fundamental change has come about through the combined efforts of biochemical research and the development of a new technique, continuous positive airway pressure (CPAP). The discovery that surfactant, a detergentlike substance, is essential for normal lung function has led to the administration of hormones to speed the infant's production of this natural substance. CPAP is the application of continuous airway pressure; tubes through the mouth keep the infant's lungs inflated between breaths and can be used continually until the body begins to produce its own surfactant, and the lungs mature. For babies who are not so small and so sick as to need the aid of a respirator, CPAP has been a tremendous boon in radically decreasing the incidence of respiratory disease syndrome, formerly called hyaline membrane disease and formerly the leading cause of death among newborns.

Those who have been in neonatology for as few as five years describe the field as primitive when they started; one physician compared the pace of those five years to twenty in most specialties. During those years, ventilating techniques on the respirator have been vastly improved, in response to the discovery that a type of blindness that affected premature infants (retrolental fibroplasia) was associated with giving too much oxygen. The balancing fight against eye, lung, and brain damage still requires constant monitoring, which is why blood gases must be taken frequently. Hope is now being placed in the transcutaneous oxygen monitor, a machine that measures oxygen through a small platinum and Teflon sensor which is taped to the infant's skin. The sensor warms a small patch of the skin, causing the underlying capillary blood vessels to fill with blood. A current between electrodes in the sensor rises as the oxygen level goes up and is translated into a digital readout on the machine. Since the expectation that this non-invasive technique would replace the umbilical line or heel sticks has not been realized, reaction to this machine varies. What to the physician is a revolutionizing concept that will ultimately measure other values—carbon dioxide, acid-base balance—and with experience may detect an insult to the body like a pneumothorax before it occurs is still an unproven phenomenon to the nurse who now has an added machine to manipulate while still taking periodic blood gas tests. The machine's sensors have to be moved every two hours to avoid a burn; even so, they leave red circles, which recede in twenty-four hours, to be replaced by new marks. For parents, this is one more thing with which to cope. Yet this machine—its development still emerging and its production bursting in growth—is producing unexpected information. It has illustrated that the oxygen level drops when the infant is stuck with a needle for blood tests and, in a surprising tie-in to bonding theory, that just talking to the infant will cause a drop in acidity level.

Such discoveries are sustaining to staff, as when waterbeds, employed as a method of preventing depressed heads, surprisingly were found to decrease the problem of decelerated heart rate. On the other hand, many procedures remain controversial. For example, the administration of hormones to speed lung development is not used in some hospitals for fear of long-term effects. Some parents and staff are wary of subjecting these infants to a substance whose iatrogenic consequences, like those of DES,[1] may not show up for years. But to those working within this arena there is the constant challenge of new discoveries around the bend, new information that will enlarge the possibilities of saving more infants with hopes of better biographies.

So far the follow-up clinic is not yielding guidelines for continuance or withdrawal of treatment from doubtful cases, as hoped. The clinic's immediate value lies in imparting practical information to help parents. One parent's accidental discovery that running the vacuum cleaner was a substitute for the nursery noise which seemed to be needed for sleep, has been passed on to other parents. A grandfather's report of the irritability induced by the diuretic which both he and his infant granddaughter were taking is integrated with the evaluation of this drug. The liaison nurse, the follow-up nurse, and parents are learning together about the problems of coping with ICN infants and are forming family support groups to help parents while babies are hospitalized.

From the staff's perspective, the importance of follow-up care lies in the application of biographical information to the larger view of the birth trajectory. A $10,000 computer that stores information on all drugs and techniques used for each infant is being used to test hypotheses in the hope that over time the assumptions will be replaced by a firm knowledge base. Unit and hospital stakes are high, and a success rate is important justification for the whole enterprise.

The staff members themselves are being shaped by the extended birth trajectory. When the nursery census is high, the unit is hot and noisy with the beeping of machines. The work requires close attention. There is also a complication: since parents are both giving and not giving their child over to the staff, problems arise because of staff expectations

and assessments of parents—judgments about parental qualifications for taking on this child, this artifact that the staff have sustained and nurtured by their skills and technologies. As hospital discharge approaches, further discordances appear; when parents have not conformed to staff values (frequency of visits, visible signs of bonding), staff will be much concerned over the social conditions of the child's future.

Today's birth-trajectory nurses are young and energetic, becoming bored when their learning begins to level off. They place high demands on themselves—how they should function, how much they should accomplish. Faced with the emotional strain and the intensity of the work on such a unit, these nurses are candidates for that technologically related work hazard, "burn-out" (Freundenberger 1974; see also Reichle 1975). Here, too, as for parents, the benefits and satisfactions of this work are incalculable, and individual, and as it is with parents, the staff response is complex. One obstetrical nurse expressed her mixed feelings regarding transport cases: "It's scary. The women may be sick and are terrified. Delivery of a premature or sick baby is emotionally traumatic. The nursing care is all technological—two ambulance sirens going. I, personally, get a kick out of it. It is exciting, intellectually stimulating to see these strange cases."

The effects of an extended birth trajectory are further evidenced in (1) new and expanded career lines, (2) changed hospitals, and (3) altered individual biographies.

1. New and Expanded Career Lines. As already noted, the explosion in perinatology and neonatology has meant that new specialists have evolved and are involved with the increasingly smaller phases of the birth trajectory. Perinatologists rely during various phases on technical experts in specialties like ultrasonography and amniocentesis, as neonatologists do on specialists in radiology, ophthalmology, cardiology, and neurology. In order to qualify as a regional center, the labor and delivery unit must have a full-time obstetrical anesthesiologist who, as patient load increases, calls for increased staff and equipment. Respiratory therapists are employed to help assess respiratory needs of infants, plan and execute this aspect of care, and upgrade physicians'

[1] DES (diethylstilbestrol) is a synthetic hormone (estrogen) which was used by pregnant women between 1941 and 1971. Problems of cervix and vagina are now being found in many DES daughters and minor genital tract abnormalities in DES sons.

and nurses' knowledge of respiratory function. Physical therapists are needed for babies who have had a prolonged stay in the ICN. These particular specialists help assess the infant's development; they exercise the baby, look at muscle tone, and watch for possible signs of cerebral palsy. Specialists on neonatal medical and nursing staff have evolved: they must be experienced, finely skilled, and attuned to every nuance in the given trajectory phase, since they are dealing with delicate bodies, and reversibility can be quick, unpredictable, and damaging.

Expanded services have led to a splintering of the role of the head nurse. Her new title, nursing care coordinator (NCC), is fitting since the major part of her work has to do with coordinating the many services that feed into the unit (for instance, in the nursery: laundry, X-ray, clinical laboratory, pharmacy, and central services for the massive amount of supplies). New middle-level administrative classifications, such as "staff development nurse," have been created to take over some of the former head nurse tasks, like the hiring and orientation of new nurses and their instruction on new equipment. In the labor and delivery ward a liaison nurse handles the administration of the alternative birth center and family follow-up; a master's-level perinatal clinical nurse specialist serves as resource person for transport and other high-risk patients and spreads new obstetrical knowledge to staff nurses and to outlying feeder hospitals.

The ICN has added a liaison nurse whose work also reflects the outward stretch of the trajectory. Families with babies who have spent long months in the nursery need support after discharge. Often these babies have immature nervous systems and are hyperirritable after months of continuous twenty-four-hour stimulation. Emotional adjustment places a huge strain on families:

> It's the isolation that gets to them. They are feeling trapped; they are afraid that the babies will get sick and be back in the hospital and they get to resent their responsibility. These were often first babies—the parents were active, young, vibrant people. If the babies are on oxygen at home, they can't be taken out of the crib. We do have a transport system, but it weighs 11 pounds.

The liaison nurse and the baby's primary nurse look for ways to make the parents' lives easier and contact continues long after hospital discharge. The liaison nurse also reflects the changed organizational structure brought on by regionalization of services. A large part of her job has to do with furthering the network of in-feeding hospitals and tactfully teaching staff nurses in these hospitals. Hers is a dual goal: to decrease mismanaged deliveries while maintaining good public relations in the service of an expanded referral pattern.

A social worker also assists in the support of families and, in conjunction with the above administrative nurses, in sensing and responding to the staff tension which mounts whenever ethical, quality-of-life issues arise. Because of the close interweaving of staff and family biographies, periodic "stress meetings" are held: one hospital's social worker holds weekly social service rounds, while another employs an ethicist, who holds monthly ethics rounds—an open acknowledgment of the need for identity work. Addition of a behavioral pediatrician to record and study infant behavior with computerized recording of a number of variables like sleeping and waking states, motor activity, color is another example of this felt need.

Further support is given to babies who are judged to require long-term evaluation by providing a follow-up clinic which is offered to all babies who fall within the following categories: those under 1250 grams; those with central nervous system bleeds; those who while on the respirator were given drugs to paralyze the musculoskeletal system; those who were given drugs to speed lung development; those who had cytomegalo virus, a respiratory infection that runs about 30 percent in premature babies; those with any other special conditions indicating a need for follow-up. This service is staffed by a nurse practitioner, a pediatrician, and a psychologist.

2. Changed Hospitals. Since it is no longer economically feasible for every hospital to offer every service, in one of the hospitals that we studied the decision was made to focus on geriatric and newborn services. This was in keeping with two considerations. The hospital had a long tradition of support for family services, which could be continued by extending geriatric care and by encouraging family involvement in newborn care through open access to nursery, inclusion of siblings, rooms for parents when babies are hospitalized. The second consideration was economically realistic: reimbursement from the government is greater for critical care (including intensive care for the newborn) than for other services.

Intensive care nursery charges are high. In this hospital (as of 1978) beds were $472 for the most critical level, $333 for semi-intensive care, and $234 for recovery care. These charges covered physicians' and nurses' costs. The major impact on hospital biography lies in the generation of additional income. Every time a blood gas study was done, which could be as frequently as every 10 to 30 minutes, the charge was $35. Respirators cost $150 a day, a brain scan $300, and an X-ray $75. Then a new machine, the transcutaneous oxygen monitor, cost $50 for 4 hours, plus $25 every time the electrodes were shifted— every two hours. Chest tubes were $150 an insertion; suction catheters and gloves used, approximately $25 a day; hyperalimentation $100. "You can figure a baby on a respirator costs $1000 to $1200 a day, and that doesn't count extra procedures." Nursery charges represented a major part of the budget for X-ray and clinical laboratory services. What is more, the nursery provided enough income to cover other hospital losers: labor and delivery, the alternative birth center, postpartum, well-baby nursery, and pediatrics. The interdependency of these particular services may appear one-directional economically, but the needs are reciprocal. A skilled labor and delivery unit will funnel babies into the ICN through its management of high-risk mothers. In order to obtain residents to serve as house staff in the nursery, a full residency in pediatrics must be offered. Of course, knowing that one is being "carried by Big Brother" financially does not make for felicitous feelings: "We have a lot of pull in the hospital; there's resentment that we get a lot, like expensive equipment, which we do."

Other feelings are generated by this interdependency of services. Accusations of mismanaged deliveries—often not explicitly stated—are most often directed toward outlying hospitals, as already discussed. However, the accusations can be intrahospital as well. Disagreements may arise between obstetrical (perinatal) and pediatric (neonatal) staffs over subjecting a woman with a 24-week fetus to a cesarean birth—the former staff focused on what it will do to the mother, the latter on giving every child every chance. When the nursery census is low, wry comments are made about labor and delivery treating premature pregnancies with drugs and forestalling delivery. Conversely, transported mothers

may be greeted happily by a labor and delivery unit that is experiencing a low census of patients or anticipated with groans by a nursery staff already under stress because of a high census.

3. Altered Individual Biographies.   A third general consequence of the stretched-out birth trajectory lies in the shaping of various implicated individual biographies. These include the infant's biography, through the ICN's technology the infant has been given increased biographical time, but it is, in a sense, gestational time. The finished product is still unfinished—the nursery is, in effect, an institutionalized womb. Parents can get their child back at any time—in any shape. Logically, parents can say, "I don't like what you're doing," but structurally they are fatefully locked in. Nurses who remain in contact with these families are learning that the deep anxiety being experienced by parents, as well as any displeasure over staff management, is often suppressed until the baby has been at home for quite awhile. Parental dependency is felt too keenly to risk disturbing the staff.

For parents of a premature or sick child the birth trajectory is of heightened relevance, forcing a new definition of their own biographies and what has happened to them—a realignment of expectations. The financial strain on them is substantial, sometimes causing bankruptcy. Only the very poor (for example, a four-member family making about $11,000 annually) qualify for state support. The rest incur liability proportionate to income before government funding takes over. Financial and emotional costs are interwoven:

> Some of these families are in turmoil. Their financial status takes a tailspin—they're having to live on a shoestring. One family lived in the country; they had birds and horses, lots of land, a nice home. They moved to be near the medical center. They feel trapped—their MediCal status is judged monthly. Only one of them can work, so they can keep their income down to qualify. MediCal doesn't count baby sitters. They express resentment and ask, "How long is this going to go on?"

Some babies are covered by private insurance, but obviously such coverage is not limitless. It is possible, as happened during our research, for a baby born at 27 weeks to be in the nursery for six months, coming close to a lifetime insurance limit of $250,000. In order to qualify for reinsurance, this particular baby cannot be readmitted to the hospital for two years, which places a tremendous, and probably impossible, burden on the family to keep her well. The resulting financial and psychological stress apparently drives some parents to the marriage counselor and perhaps ultimately leads to divorce. If the child is saved through medical intervention, there may still be months and years of turmoil and travail for the parents of a not altogether physically normal child.

OTHER POSSIBLE LARGE-SCALE CONSEQUENCES

What might be said, in addition, about other possible large-scale effects of the highly technologized ICNs and the extended birth trajectory largely produced by them? We dare to speculate a bit about this, since in fact nobody actually knows. What can be said is that there is increasing media coverage on how babies are saved through all this specialized technology, knowledge, and organization. And, correlatively, there is necessarily a heightening of public awareness, thereby, of the hospital as an increasingly technologized workplace and environment. Besides increasing the public's awareness, the media coverage is surely raising expectations of what can be done about babies, and more generally about illness, in these hospitals. ICUs, as we shall see in the next chapter, are very visible in the media and ICNs are undoubtedly central in their public imagery.

On the negative side, public distrust and antagonism to medical technology—perceived as contributing to depersonalized health care—cannot help but be fed by the experiences of parents who have had difficult and highly destructive relationships with ICN staffs (Stinson and Stinson 1979). Those particular parents are accusing these staffs of being so technologically, research-, and career-oriented that they are ultimately indifferent to parents' feelings and to the larger human implications of what they are doing.

> *What sort of memories or thoughts could we have of Andrew? By the time he was allowed to die, the technology being used to "salvage" him had*

> *produced not so much a human life as a grotesque caricature of a human life, a "person" with a stunted, deteriorating brain and scarcely an undamaged vital organ in his body, who existed only as an extension of a machine. This is the image left to us for the rest of our lives of our son, Andrew.* (Stinson and Stinson 1979, p. 72)

This kind of message cannot fail to have some impact on the public image of medical technology and of the ICNs.

The issue of equity is also raised by these wards and their work. Why should so much money be expended on so few births, rather than being spent on the nation's more pressing health needs (the United States, for instance, has an inordinately high mortality rate, contributed to mainly by our more poverty-stricken populations) or on illnesses that affect larger numbers of people? Questions are raised, too, about what kind of "ICN graduates" are being produced, since some proportion of them will be at least disabled and many will be chronically ill for their entire lifetimes. As one pediatrician said to us: "Somebody had better study that!" His exclamation points implicitly to a paradox, namely, that by saving infants the ICN staffs are contributing, in whatever measure, to the numbers of people who are chronically ill. These children constitute, in our terminology, persons whose trajectories have been very much stretched out. In fact these trajectories would never have begun or would have been quickly over if medical interventions had not been partly successful. If the halfway technology does indeed gradually produce visible evidence of its partial failure to a wider public, then, this will be additional evidence that the work on those wards has consequences far beyond the narrow confines of the wards and hospitals themselves.

References

A substantial portion of this article is based on a fairly extensive study of a labor and delivery ward and an intensive care nursery in a hospital located in a metropolitan area, over a five-month period, and rather less intensive fieldwork and interviewing at a comparable metropolitan hospital. An earlier version of this material, organized in somewhat different terms, appeared as "Trajectories, Biographies, and the Evolving Medical Technology Scene," *Soci-*

ology of Health and Illness 1 (1979): 261–83, with Carolyn Wiener as the senior author.

ARMS, S. 1975. *Immaculate Deception*. Boston: Houghton Mifflin.

BRADLEY, R. A. 1974. *Husband-Coached Childbirth*. Rev. ed. New York: Harper & Row.

EPHRON, N. 1978. *San Francisco Chronicle,* December 4, p. 19.

FOX, H. A. 1979. Comment at conference on Technological Approaches to Obstetrics: Benefits, Risks, Alternatives, San Francisco, California, February 3–4.

FREUNDENBERGER, H. J. 1974. "Staff Burnout." *Journal of Social Issues* 30:159–65.

KLAUS, M. 1979. Comment at conference on Technological Approaches to Obstetrics: Benefits, Risks, Alternatives, San Francisco, California, February 3–4.

LAMAZE, F. 1970. *Painless Childbirth: The Lamaze Method*. Chicago: Contemporary Books.

LEBOYER, F. 1975. *Birth without Violence*. New York: Alfred A. Knopf, 1975.

NATIONAL INSTITUTE OF CHILD HEALTH AND HUMAN DEVELOPMENT. 1979. *Antenatal Diagnosis*. Report of a Consensus Development Conference, March 5–7, 1979. Publication No. NIH 79–1973. Bethesda.

NEUTRA, R. 1979. Comment at conference on Technological Approaches to Obstetrics: Benefits, Risks, Alternatives, San Francisco, California, February 3–4.

REICHLE, M. 1975. "Psychological Stress in the Intensive Care Unit." *Nursing Digest* 3:12–14.

STINSON, R., and STINSON, P. 1979. "On the Death of a Baby." *Atlantic Monthly* 244:64–72.

Emergency Room Service: Social History and Current Directions

Emily Mumford

The emergency room, called ER, is used for a widening variety of problems. Most patients seen in emergency rooms have been able to walk in, in contrast to former times when most patients were carried in or brought by ambulance. Changing perceptions of hospitals, of the right to care, of what medicine should be able to do, and of what constitutes an emergency have affected services. While ER utilization was increasing, trends toward centralization and expansion of hospital services created a demand for more interns and residents. One way to attract residents without conflict or challenge from neighboring private practitioners was by expansion of emergency services.

To see what has happened, we will look first at the history of emergency services in one hospital, which illustrates the social and cultural shifts around medicine and gives us some of the reasons why health providers and the public may have different ideas about what constitutes "misuse" of emergency services. We will look at the factors that contribute to the persistence of an image of emergency room services closer to the reality of the 1940s than to the reality of the 1980s, and examine some of the consequences of this culture lag, as well as some of the realities of how emergency services are used today.

THE HISTORY OF ONE EMERGENCY ROOM

The history of emergency room use reflects changes in patients' definitions about when they have a right to expect help. History can shed light on the causes for some of the tension in modern emergency rooms between a public that seeks one kind of help and physicians trained to provide another kind. A combined Almshouse and Penitentiary, with an infirmary on the second floor, the first building in what was to become the giant Brooklyn Kings County Hospital complex was opened in 1831. According to the superintendent of the poor's third annual report, the facility contained: "150 foreigners, 106 of whom were born in Ireland; 2 lunatics; 1 idiot, and 2 mutes. There were 34 deaths; bound out 11; discharged 199; and absconded 21" (Stiles, 1884, p. 465). The lumping together of patient, prisoner, lunatic, derelict, and foreigner typified the concept of a public hospital in those days. Along with the many curious categories used in the annual report, the superintendents of the poor offered an imperious conclusion: "The official situation we have for some time held in relation to the poor, has enabled us to make some practical observations on the principal causes of pauperism; and we do not hesitate to state the appalling fact that three-fourths under our charge, are directly or indirectly caused by intemperance . . . it is a fact that out of the whole number of 401, we could not trust a man of them with a team . . . or a woman with the keys of the medicine closet" (Stiles, 1884, p. 465). Yet the physician's report appended to this document listed four deaths by cholera, "two of the subjects having been brought in in a collapsed state," and thirty other deaths "from various causes." The statistics suggest that these early patients suffered from more than just "intemperance" and the social inferiority the superintendents used to discredit them.

By 1837, a new building provided facilities exclusively for the sick (Hazelton, 1925). Later a separate Pest House and then a Lunatic Asylum further distinguished types of services and problems (Stiles, 1884). Hospital discharge figures suggest that even in the general hospital, the average length of stay may have been over fifty days in the mid-nineteenth century. Many patients died in the hospital. The fact that patients who were admitted tended to stay over a month made for little traffic between the municipal hospital and the community. Under these conditions, the neighborhood around the hospital complex could ignore it, and people in the various hospital units could function with little local intrusion into the way people in the hospital did their work. Nurses and doctors and their students tended to live on the grounds.

The Introduction of the Ambulance

In the summer of 1869, a portent of the eventual impact of daily community life on large city hospitals came with a dramatic innovation in public service, the ambulance. It was another medical invention that developed out of wartime necessity. . . . Ambulances had been used in the Civil War. The first city ones were a resplendent black, even to the sheets, and they were horsedrawn. By 1873 Brooklyn boasted four ambulances.

These early probes into the community were manned by surgeons who served "without compensation" in exchange for training experience (Stiles, 1884); they provided their own functional equivalent of the modern flashing light and loud siren by calling out to scatter pedestrians (Rideing, 1972). At first emergency services did not interfere unduly with life inside hospitals. For example, in the first full year of Brooklyn's ambulance service, there were only 159 calls (Stiles, 1884). Emergency service at the time was synonymous with hospital admission, and not infrequently followed by death. In Manhattan, Bellevue Hospital's figures for 1870 show that of 26 emergency cases admitted, "one died within two hours; 15 of the 25 which remained were treated by amputation. Of this number 10 recovered and five died. Of the ten treated without amputation, three were fractures of the thigh and all of these died. The other patients recovered" (Starr, 1957, p. 95).

Night Medical Service

Before the turn of the century, much medical care was home care or care provided by a doctor willing to visit the home. Some unions and companies had physicians who advised the family about how to care for the patient. Dispensaries that provided free services were available to the poor. As late as 1897, Sears, Roebuck was still doing a brisk business in medicines, including opium, and *Robb's Family Physician* and other "doctor books" were standard works in many homes (Israel, 1968). Private physicians for the rich lived and worked near enough to arrive by carriage (Shyrock, 1966). The doctor might stay for hours when a patient was seriously ill, and a nurse could be hired to live in. At the turn of the century, the new and fashionable private hospitals were beginning to attract wealthy clients. . . .

But the free city hospitals tended to be a final refuge when a family could no longer cope with the illness, or allow the person to die peacefully at home. Orwell (1950) observed:

> *If you look at almost any literature before the latter part of the nineteenth century, you find that a hospital is popularly regarded as much the same thing as a prison, and an old-fashioned, dungeon-like prison at that. A hospital is a place of filth, torture and death, a sort of ante-chamber to the tomb. No one who was not more or less destitute would have thought of going into such a place for treatment.*

Brooklyn as well as other cities began to open municipally sponsored night medical service in the 1880s (Stiles, 1884). The first annual report of the service concluded: "In one instance at least, a human life has been saved by a physician of the service. For the coming year $600 have been appropriated— a sum which will undoubtedly be sufficient to meet all demands" (Stiles, 1884). The relatively large number of physicians who registered to indicate their willingness to make night calls and the small number of calls suggest the marked difference in physician supply and demand then compared with now. But even more significant, the night service was a step along the way to the concept that society had responsibility for care of the person who felt unable to wait for office hours, but who was neither sufficiently ill nor destitute enough to be "put away" in a hospital.

Innovations such as the ambulance and city-run service to provide doctors at night were forerunners of change in the locus of care from home to hospital. The early ambulance formed the first breach in the social wall between the city hospital and its community. Emergency patients who would otherwise have been treated at home appeared in increasing numbers. The number of ambulance calls in Brooklyn increased more than fifteen times from 1873 to 1884 (Stiles, 1884). By the turn of the century ambulances were electrified, painted white instead of an ominous black, and doing a brisk business.

Public Interest and New Hospitals

The public began to show a lot of interest in what went on behind the walls of its municipal hospitals. More people were brought to the hospital for treatment, and with the introduction of asceptic techniques more people survived a hospital admission. A March 22, 1926, *Brooklyn Times* headline read, "Crowding Ignored at Kings Hospital" (Lyndon, 1926). Municipal hospital affairs increasingly became the topic of newspaper reports as more of the population entered them. The article quoted the State Charities Aid report: "As early as 1892 the wards were reported as congested . . . in a space designed for 10 beds there were *12 beds with 19 patients* in them" (emphasis supplied).

In 1931, on the centennial anniversary of the first Kings County combined almshouse/hospital/ penitentiary, New York's Mayor Jimmy Walker dedicated a new main building. He said he had been "shocked" at the condition of the old buildings and announced that the new facility, the largest institution of its kind, would provide "service, not charity." The commissioner of hospitals boasted, "There will be beds for 1500 patients, each of which will have its own radio" (*Brooklyn Daily Eagle,* July 10, 1931). These new facilities suggested neither the old almshouse nor the pesthouse. An imposing stairway dominated a central entrance foyer with an ornate ceiling of carved and painted wood. The magnificent Columbia Presbyterian and the cathedral-like New York Hospital were other products of this same period. Medical advances, rising expectations, and accelerated use of hospitals soon glutted even these facilities.

The giant new citadels of specialized medicine of the 1920s and 1930s represented an innovation. At once the product and the producer of advance in science and technology, they attracted the most eminent physicians and the bulk of research funds. Many forward-looking or youthful patients who wanted the latest in medicine—and did not suffer their elders' fear of big hospitals—became accustomed to specialty outpatient services (Stevens, 1971). With each class of medical students trained in the teaching centers, specialties gained recruits. From 20 specialists per 100,000 in 1931, the number reached 96.1 by 1969 (Stevens, 1971, p. 181).

The decline in numbers of generalist physicians is often suggested as an explanation for accelerated emergency room use. However, in Great Britain, where general practitioners are more readily available (Cartwright, 1967), trends in "nonemergency use" of the emergency room parallel those here (Bergman and Haggerty, 1962). Increased emergency room use seems to reflect emergent demands that services be provided where and when patients say they are necessary.

At Kings County, as elsewhere, traffic between hospital and community continued to increase. The average length of hospital stay shortened from 26 days in 1923 (Hazelton, 1925) to 15.7 in 1942. At the same time outpatient visits increased, bringing still more patients from community to hospital. In 1942, there were 366,534 outpatient visits to Kings County Hospital (*The New York Times,* February 8, 1942). Once more, pressure from existing patterns of use and demand resulted in a new building. Mayor LaGuardia was the luminary at the cornerstone ceremony in 1940 (*Brooklyn Daily Eagle,* September 23) for a building that doubled outpatient capacity. However, the trends once again would mean that the new facility's vaunted capacity would shortly be exceeded.

Changes in Types of Problems

Medicine had been dramatically effective in reducing the threat of infectious disease and acute conditions, which by then had come to mean hospitalization. Infectious diseases, as compared with chronic diseases, accounted for approximately 46 percent of the deaths in 1900, but for only slightly more than 4 percent in 1953 (Oakes, 1973). With each conquest of acute conditions, and with each new means of postponing death in chronic conditions, the potential population for acute care beds would diminish while the number of people who had learned to turn to the hospital and who now needed ambulatory care for their chronic illnesses would expand.

Nationally, outpatient services opened in in-creasing numbers of hospitals, and outpatient visits to hospitals increased. In 1953 there had been two outpatient visits for every inpatient admission. The trend continued, and by 1972 the ratio reached five outpatient visits to one inpatient admission (Petrich and House, 1973). Hospital administrators began to express concern that for the first time in the history of the country, there might be a surplus of hospital beds (Schwartz, 1971).

Through the 1940s, the admitting entrance to city hospitals was still the emergency door where ambulances brought patients. Treatment areas of the emergency rooms tended to be small because so many patients were moved directly into hospital beds, rather than treated and discharged at the same visit. Now treatment areas have been expanded because most patients do not need admission. From the mid-forties on, through what once was the back door, mounting numbers of patients began to arrive by foot, taxi, subway, and bus for immediate consultation, for referral, for care. Impelled by their own sense of need for help rather than by accident or dire illness, fewer patients required admission. Of the thousands who arrived at emergency services, relatively few were brought by ambulance. Concurrently, the term "emergency visit" came into use, and the Kings County emergency services literally moved to front and center of the 1930s buildings, which had been built for extended inpatient care. Though people still called them emergency rooms, they had spread to incorporate huge areas of waiting rooms, hallways, offices, and treatment areas. Between 1955 and 1970, emergency room visits across the nation increased 312 percent, far outstripping the 50 percent rise in outpatient clinic attendance (Petrich and House, 1973).

Changing Social Expectations

During the 1960s, the concept of medical care as a right for all was reinforced and given new impetus by legislation. Medicare, Medicaid, and the Mental Health Act were only a part of the attempt to meet public demand and realize the idea of social responsibility for the health and well-being of all. Funds were authorized for family health clinics, neighborhood health centers, and mental health centers (Stevens, 1971). The creation of a new hospital position, "patient representative," added strength to the community's emerging perception of its right to services. Millis (1969) comments:

> It was not too many years ago that when one listed the necessities of life, he said "food, clothing and shelter." No sane or rational person would today give you a list of less than six: food, clothing, shelter, education, employment and health care. In a sense, we thereby have doubled within my lifetime the list of those things which we call the necessities of life, the basic necessities of life" (p. 499).

At the same time, medical advances and mass media preoccupation with medical "breakthroughs" stimulated demand for the benefits that medicine, particularly hospital medicine, could provide. Rehabilitation services, ambulatory psychiatric services, obesity clinics, stress-reduction programs, sex clinics, family counseling services—all inconceivable in the context of the old hospital—attracted growing numbers of patients. Relieved of some fear and awe of the hospital, and accustomed to going there, successive generations of community members took more initiative for deciding *when* they needed medical attention and *what conditions* justified immediate or emergency service (Pifer, 1970; Ginzberg, 1969; Donabedian, 1974).

The persistent push for new types of medical service, along with the changing patterns of use, became most evident in the emergency room (Bergman and Haggerty, 1962; Reed and Reader, 1967; Shah and Carr, 1974). From an average of 38 emergency room visits a day in a single hospital in 1942, with about two-thirds of them brought by ambulance (*The New York Times,* February 8, 1942), the number went off the top of any charts that projected demand in ensuing years. In 1970, there were 593 visits a day; the figure was 700 by 1974 (Minimum Socioeconomic and Health Profile, 1974). Only a small fraction of these patients in the 1970s were brought by ambulance, and only a fraction were admitted. With the introduction of walk-in neighborhood clinics, the pressure on emergency room use may abate. But pressures for services "on demand" will probably continue. Each generation apparently has been more ready than its parents to use hospital services (McTaggart, 1971), at first for acute illness and inpatient treatment, eventually for specialized outpatient services and now for much more (Stevens, 1971).

Age Distributions in Emergency Room Populations

The adult emergency room population is younger than might be expected if there were no generational differences related to inclination to use this particular service of the hospital. In Kings County, 42 percent of the adults in one survey were between 20 and 29 years old; 76 percent were 40 and younger. Fewer than 5 percent of the emergency room patients were 65 and older, though in the immediate neighborhood of the hospital more than 11 percent are over 65 (Mumford et al., 1976), and it is the older people who generally have the most illness and who in some studies appear to visit physicians most often.

The relative youth of emergency room visitors has been reported in several surveys (Torrens and Yedvab, 1970), and it is particularly striking at those hospitals which have special pediatric emergency services that are crowded with young parents and their children. Emergency services for many have become the functional equivalent of family practices. Hundreds of children served by the emergency room, with its coordinated outpatient facilities, may be expected to arrive at adulthood accustomed to emergency room visits as the natural way to obtain health care.

The explanations offered for the preponderance of youthful people in emergency rooms usually stop with supply and demand. For example, there is a shortage of physicians available to see young mothers and working people at times when they can afford to see a physician. Some clinic hours span only the working day. Older people have Medicaid and time and therefore can "afford" to see a private physician. But these explanations do not fit the phenomenon of the increasing numbers of emergency room visitors also reported in England as well as changing social definitions. Large metropolitan hospitals have provided each successive generation with different probable consequences of emergency room visits.

The press of patients toward the emergency room has been building up with remarkable force since the days of the first ambulance: it is a trend consistent with generational differences in attitudes toward hospitals and illness and toward rights to services (Kadushin, 1969; Gehrig, 1968; Marston, 1968; Fuchs, 1974). Increasingly the public may feel justified in insisting that it is an emergency if the *patient* thinks it is. At the same time, hospital administrators are aware that emergency services attract patients and that young physicians in training for practice seem to want emergency experience. Expansion of emergency services could thus attract patients and also house staff trainees, who are in short supply. The expansion is not likely to be seen as a threat by local physicians, who do not like to be on call at all hours.

Social Definitions of Emergency

Interview responses from one survey in an emergency room suggest that many people may use emergency room services frequently; 71 percent of the sample said they had been in this emergency room before. One-third had been to the emergency room four or more times (Mumford et al., 1976). In a previous study completed in the late 1960s in the same setting, Mesnikoff and associates (1970) had found that 66 percent of their respondents had made a prior visit to the same emergency room. Bergman and Haggerty in a 1962 survey of visits to a children's hospital medical center emergency service found that 12 percent had made *five* or more visits to the same service. A sizable portion of the population apparently was using the emergency room as a walk-in clinic. One patient asked an interviewer, "What is the best time to come here for a checkup?"

More than one out of every five patients in one sample had traveled for more than 30 minutes to get to one metropolitan emergency room. They said: "I have always come here and I get good results." "I would go to no other." One patient had come in to get a second opinion before following a private physician's advice for surgery. Over one-third of the respondents said they were in the emergency room to see a physician about "an old problem." Consistent with this, the diagnoses entered in the emergency room logbook included such chronic complaints as "impotence," "lower back pain," "rheumatism," "chronic headache," and "hypertension."

Among the innovations in response to the fact that the Kings County emergency room is the only site where medical attention is received by large numbers of an impoverished and largely black population, the medical director of the service, Dr. Karl Adler, instituted a system in the 1970s to remind physicians on duty to check specific conditions in charting. One result: Approximately 40 percent of all adult male patients were identified as suffering from hypertension. Rather than simply decrying the fact that patients had come to the emergency room instead of a clinic, the physicians immediately began hypertensive regimens for these patients, and referrals were made to the hospital's hypertension clinic.

Social and Emotional Trauma

. . . [A] potentially stressful life event, or some social or psychological rather than physical trauma, is often associated with a search for medical help (Mechanic, 1972; Zola, 1973; Stoeckle and Zola, 1964; Roghmann and Haggerty, 1973, 1972). The social traumas of assault, accident, or rape are associated with emergency rooms. But more frequently, the connection between social and emotional trauma and an emergency room visit is less obvious, as in the case of the widow who had been robbed a week earlier and appeared in the emergency room complaining of fits of trembling and inability to sleep.

Patients in one emergency room were asked whether within the past six months they had experienced any one of a brief list of events selected from the Social Readjustment Rating Scale developed by Holmes and Rahe (1967). Questions were added to determine whether patients recently had been robbed or mugged, had their homes broken into, or had suffered a financial setback. For each of these events, for which there were reasonably reliable community baselines, more of the population of emergency room visitors had suffered the experience than would be expected, unless such experiences were in some way associated with a search for help in the emergency room (Mumford et al., 1976).

In one study, the emergency room patient population had an incidence of violence nine times that of a comparable community population. Some people apparently had turned to the emergency room instead of the police after victimization. This excess did not include any patients who came in with physical trauma suffered in the course of such an event. One in ten patients reported having been robbed within the past six months, and one in twelve reported that his or her homes had been broken into within the same brief time period. An abbreviated self-rating scale to measure symptoms of depression, anxiety, and emotional distress was given to a sample of general emergency room patients. More than one-third had higher scores on the "anxious neurotic" scale than did *psychiatric patients* in similar reviews.

The "emergency room," or "trauma room," or "accident room" is still aptly named, but now the label includes social and psychological as well as physical trauma. Acute physical and life-threatening conditions of course are brought into every hospital emergency service, but so are many more conditions that in the 1800s would have been handled at home, that a few decades later would have been taken to a general practitioner, and that still more recently would have been taken to an outpatient clinic (Torrens and Yedvab, 1970).

CULTURAL LAG AND ITS RESULTS

The Contrast Between Reality and Image

The first time they approach the large metropolitan hospital emergency room many people seem to expect something they have seen on TV—a setting of blood and heroic action. After the noticeable preponderance of youthful visitors in the emergency room, the next most visible attribute that signifies change in patterns of use is something that a series of student observers have referred to with disappointment: "But it is so quiet!" The adult emergency service that sees some 700 patients a day in quarters that were built for other purposes, and opened to serve fewer patients, is not quiet. But in terms of the expectations of the uninitiated, it seems "calm" or even "peaceful."

A great deal that is of national as well as personal importance happens in emergency rooms today. The fact that many of the patients can, without risk to health, wait for their turn to be seen does not signify that their need for attention on the day they arrive should be dismissed lightly. One physician recalled his early experience in a large emergency service as a time of blood, excitement, and occasional terror. But, he added, after the blood was washed away, most of the patients could be treated with a few stitches. Many patients in the 1940s

looked sicker as they arrived than they turned out to be (Linn, 1976). In contrast, it may be that many patients today are in much more distress than their initial appearance suggests. Crisis is not at first obvious with a patient presenting a lower backache. A look at some of the factors that contribute to perpetuation of the image of the emergency room as the place filled with trauma victims brings us closer to understanding the phenomenon.

Factors That Perpetuate Old Images

Three forces contribute to the persistence of public images of the emergency room. First, in the recent history of the services they were predominantly places where ambulances brought seriously distressed patients for hospital admission. Second, the selective attention and recall of people who do see the services firsthand today tend to obscure daily routine in favor of the big events. It is newsworthy to see a victim of a violent accident. Doctors and nurses may tend to forget selectively all the "common problems" they see in a day and recall the "exciting and interesting ones," where the situation confirms their professional image of dealing with significant events. The young man who sat silently for two hours before being seen may not seem much to talk about. The most frequent events are the least talked about, and the drama surging beneath the apparently calm exterior of the many people waiting is lost.

Third, problems of professional autonomy are generated in situations where it is the patients rather than the professionals who designate when a case is an "emergency." As long as cases are "life and death," the professional does not "lose face" by letting the patient's problem determine timing and priorities. But when there is no such clear external demand, the professional may be uncomfortable letting the patient rather than the doctor's appointment schedule determine the timing of the exchange.

The public image of the emergency room appears fixed in the past, to the time when larger portions of its patients may have been carried in on stretchers. The term "emergency" in association with medical services implies a condition requiring immediate medically directed intervention, or dire outcome in the absence of medical care. The fiction is kept alive in the minds of young physicians who recall drama and forget routine and in the media, where emergency rooms are packed with heroic action and disastrous conditions—in short, with "drama." The press also ignores the routine, the statistical norm, and indeed most of the daily action.

In the context of history, as well as selective reporting, the first response of medical sociology graduate students assigned to emergency rooms for field observations is disappointment, and it makes sense. However, a second phenomenon in the field notes of these students cannot be dismissed as an example of selective exposure. In the first of the field reports, faculty members noticed that at least one staff member in each of the different emergency rooms had volunteered to the student observers something like, "It is very quiet now; you should have been here last night." Or, "This is not a good time to observe; Wednesday was really something." Since students were reporting different days and different hours and different emergency rooms, we wondered at the remarkable coincidence. This "you-should-have-been-here-Wednesday" comment to a field observer turned out to be a recurrent phenomenon in student field reports in following years.

Obviously there are times when staff and facilities in the emergency room are stretched beyond reasonable limits. There are times when health providers in emergency rooms do perform heroically in the face of catastrophic illness. Yet at the same time, staff members are well aware of changing patterns of use in the service; for example, thirty-three of the forty staff members interviewed in one emergency room estimated that only between 25 and 50 percent of the visits were "emergencies" in the medical sense. Six more estimated that more than three-fourths of the patients who came to emergency rooms could have been treated equally well on a later day in an outpatient clinic (Mumford et al., 1976). The effect of the anxiety generated at times of true emergencies may be so powerful that "emergencies" are selectively recalled. The "big event" comes to stand for work done in the emergency room even by the people who work there.

Many people in certain jobs appear to share the outsider's image of work that rests not on routine nor on how most of the day is filled, but on relatively rare "big moments." Police, firefighters, soldiers, and physicians are not identified by the content of most days—standing about, cleaning equipment, waiting, listening to routine complaints, or tediously tying off vessels and suturing in a four-hour operation. The collective demands of each profession are primarily legitimated—and the espirit of the occupation sustained—by the "big event" image and the collective myths that support its work. . . .

Yet another factor probably contributes to the persistence of the old image of the emergency room, and this is the issue of professional autonomy. Medical practice generally rests on the physicians' control of both time and the visibility of the details of their work. The patient waits for an appointment—except in an emergency. In the hospital, when the physician does evoke "medical emergency" as the ultimate legitimation for overlooking rules and regulations, it is often in a case where the patient's condition is one of total dependency and therefore the physician is still fully in charge.

Generally, with the exception of "medical emergency," the physician's work is insulated by space as well as time, so that outsiders generally cannot watch or control the work. As Hughes (1958) pointed out, protection against visibility characterizes many occupations, and it becomes particularly important where risks are significant. The physician's office, with its closed door, protects the privacy of the physician in his work as well as the privacy of the patient. On large, open wards, a circle of house staff members can serve to insulate the physician at work.

In some emergency rooms originally designed to handle "true emergencies," physicians are provided relatively little privacy. Patients sometimes sit and wait in a small examining room, and a lone physician and nurse may clearly be heard in their examination of a patient behind nearby curtains. Patients, relatives, nurses, and physicians move along corridors and in and out of rooms in close proximity with patients and with more blurring of status distinctions than on hospital wards. The physician in the emergency room has his or her autonomy and control diminished both by the relative absence of physical barriers to visibility and by the elimination of protective time schedules. When patients invoke "emergency" for conditions other than extreme physical distress, those patients gain an element of control over the timing of medical attention without being commensurately dependent.

Interviews with staff in one emergency room to assess work satisfaction suggest that satisfaction is inversely correlated with hospital rank. All the clerks, and 80 percent of the nurses, said they liked the work in the emergency rooms "very much." But only half the physicians were so enthusiastic (Mumford, 1976). In relation to their position in the hospital hierarchy, emergency room nurses and clerks gain in autonomy, and sometimes also in grateful attention from patients. But in relation to their situation on other services and their expectations, physicians do *not* gain status and autonomy. Instead, they lose an element of control. They see many patients whose "emergency" does not fit with the traditional medical definition. For physicians who are convinced that the emergency room should be what it may once have been, the present streams of patients with "garden variety" complaints offer little compensation for diminished autonomy and heightened visibility.

Failure to Accept the New Patterns

The tendency to invoke the statistically infrequent event as the ultimate legitimation for privilege is by no means peculiar to the health occupations. Viewing the dramatic or exceptional event as though it necessarily has special force for justifying social action, and as though it is most significant in explaining cause, is apparently ubiquitous. Primitive groups, in their myths, view cause in a similar way. Until recently, history has read as though big events, big plans, and great men alone determined its course. Change in society that is generated by daily patterns within populations has been comparatively ignored.

Physicians' preoccupation with rarity—in their view of history, their attention, and their planning—interferes with perception of the significance of everyday patterns. This is not at all surprising, but it may have unfortunate consequences. In discussions about the delivery of health care, the impact of daily practices and of patients' behavior, although sometimes acknowledged in words, may be labeled as deviant ("misuse") or simply overlooked in planning. Concentrating on the dramatic builds another open heart unit that sometimes stands idle at the expense of added services in a crowded emergency room. In medical schools, concentration on relatively rare dramatic occasions or diseases leaves little time for the problems that are seen most often.

The term "misuse" of the emergency room suggests a tendency to underestimate the force of daily patterns. Labeling current use as deviant results in services remaining unresponsive to new social realities. Chances to intercede effectively on behalf of health are missed, while large investments go toward trying to get people to go elsewhere. New schemes are designed to encourage people to seek medical care early in pregnancy or at early stages of chronic diseases such as hypertension. But many of these people naturally appear at the medical gateway of the emergency service, where they are treated only for the symptom they present and sent away.

On the patient's side, there may be some potentially productive unanticipated consequences of the new pattern of emergency room use, which has grown without benefit of long-range planning or formal rules. The buzzing setting with no pomp and schedule can be less forbidding, less awesome than other medical settings, a factor that may encourage approaches to medical care within the part of the population that tends to neglect health. Patients in this setting see doctors and nurses who work very hard and often with demonstrable compassion. Such visibility may reduce the chances of distrust and hostility within the patient population where distrust of medicine and authority is reported to be high. Merton (1957), in his discussion of mechanisms that make for articulation of role within role sets, comments on "observability by members of their conflicting demands" (374–377). The small examining room where waiting patients can hear another patient "yell at" a beleaguered resident and nurse may be a factor in contributing order to a seemingly chaotic situation. It also may encourage the next patient to speak up and not to be too docile, or to be more appropriately cooperative.

The Emergency Room as a Front Line of Medicine

The health professionals in the emergency room serve at the front lines of medical care in two ways (Garfield, 1970). The emergency room has become the large open door between medicine and the community, and it is exposed to the full force of the rising expectations, demands, and changing priorities of the lay community on the one hand, and on the other to the sometimes opposing priorities, definitions, and expectations of the medical institution (Levine et al., 1969; Freyman, 1971). Those who serve there may find themselves "holding the fort" with relatively little support from headquarters. The people who serve in the emergency room, like the soldiers at the front line, tend to be given lower rank in the hospital hierarchy than is afforded the command staff.

The emergency room functions as a giant triage station for its community. *Triage* is another medical service delivery innovation that developed out of World War I. Many lives were saved by means of a highly developed system in which a medical corpsman on the battlefield quickly decided to which of three categories a wounded soldier belonged. Soldiers who were only superficially wounded and could wait were one category. Those who were gravely ill and could benefit from treatment were given first aid and sent quickly to the nearest hospital. Those who were dying and without a chance were left for last.

Now the triage function is to provide an immediate brief medical evaluation of all incoming patients to determine the general nature of the problem, the type of service needed, and the appropriate referral (Albin et al., 1975). In many emergency services, nurse clinicians or practitioners perform this service. Because emergency rooms are the only places where some patients are presently accessible for screening and referral, it may be a propitious site for effective intervention on behalf of health. As in the frontline battle situation, decisions about referral as well as treatment can have major consequences. The analogy seems even more appropriate when placed in historical perspective, since both the ambulance and the triage system of emergency medical care were actually battlefield innovations.

From the perspectives of logistics, and of economy, and of probability of impact on health, the busy emergency room of an urban general hospital may be the most promising site to influence health in large communities. There is an "orientation to immediate assistance" (Hankoff et al., 1974) that may be a good match for the needs of many people whose lives tend to bump from crisis to crisis. Denying the force of social patterns among the urban poor when trying to improve their health may be analogous to the colonel's approach in *The Teahouse of the August Moon:* "I'll teach these natives democracy if I have to kill everyone to do it."

What happens in the contemporary emergency room may be crucial for people whose only medical contact is through the emergency room and for people who assume that seeing a doctor there is tantamount to a checkup and a clean bill of health unless a referral is made (Bergman and Haggerty, 1962). This may be the attitude of one patient who said, "It was a long wait, but thank God I didn't have anything seriously wrong with me." Bergman and Haggerty, in their study of a pediatric emergency room, report that many of the families apparently believed that they actually received complete care for all their children's needs at the time of these visits, although the staff was attempting to give care only for the presenting problem.

SUMMARY

Emergency rooms provide examples of cultural lag in which definitions have endured, though times and situations have changed. The social and cultural forces that have brought about new patterns of use of emergency services include medical success in curing infectious disease, with consequent shorter hospital stays and more hopeful attitudes about what happens to people in hospitals, and the administrative wish for expansion without incurring the competitive wrath of local physicians. The social and cultural factors that contribute to the persistence of images of emergency services that are closer to what was true in the 1940s than what is true in the 1980s include the persistence of first impressions, selective recall of the dramatic, and the profession's problem in handling situations where patients, not physicians, determine when attention is given. The social consequences of cultural lag about emergency rooms may include missed opportunities for innovation on behalf of health care among populations that are generally considered underserved and hard to reach. . . .

Suggested Readings

BICE, T., and WHITE, K. (March-April 1969). Factors Related to the Use of Health Services: An International Comparative Study. *Medical Care* 124–133.

ROTH, J. (December 1971). Utilization of the Hospital Emergency Department. *Journal of Health and Social Behavior* (12):312–320.

STOECKLE, J. (September 1963). On Going to See the Doctor: The Contribution of the Patient to the Decision to Seek Medical Aid. *Journal of Chronic Disease* 16:975–985.

VINCENT, C. (March 1963). The Family Health and Illness: Some Neglected Areas. *Annals of the American Academy of Political and Social Science* 345:109–116.

References

ALBIN, S., WASSERTHEIL-SMOLLER, S., JACOBSON, S., and BELL, B. (October 1975). Evaluation of Emergency Room Triage Performed by Nurses. *American Journal of Public Health* 65(10):1063–1068.

BERGMAN, A., and HAGGERTY, R. (July 1962). The Emergency Clinic: A Study of Its Role in a Teaching Hospital. *American Journal of Diseases of Children* 104:68–76.

Brooklyn Daily Eagle (July 10, 1931). Walker Lays Cornerstone of Kings Hospital.

Brooklyn Daily Eagle (September 23, 1940). New Dispensary Begun at Kings County Hospital.

CARTWRIGHT, A. (1967). *Patients and Their Doctors.* London: Routledge and Kegan Paul.

DONABEDIAN, A. (1974). Models for Organizing the Delivery of Personal Health Services and Criteria for Evaluating Them. *Organizational Issues in the Delivery of Health Services: A Selection of Articles from the Milbank Memorial Fund Quarterly,* eds. I. Zola and J. D. McKinlay. New York: Milbank Memorial Fund.

FREYMAN, J. (1971). Of Health Care, Hospitals and SSTs. *The New England Journal of Medicine* 284: 272–273.

FUCHS, V. R. (1974). *Who Shall Live?* New York: Basic Books.

GARFIELD, S. (1970). The Delivery of Medical Care. *Scientific American* 222:15–23.

GEHRIG, L. J. (April 1968). Symposium on Health Services: I. Comprehensive Planning for Health. *Journal of Medical Education* 43(4):464–470.

GINZBERG, E. (May 1969). Facts and Fancies about Medical Care. *American Journal of Public Health* 59(5):785–794.

GUY, W., and BONATO, R. (July 1970). Manual for the ECDEU Assessment Battery (Second Revision). Prepared for the Psychopharmacology Research Branch, National Institute of Mental Health. Chevy Chase, Maryland.

HANKOFF, L., MISCHORR, M., TOMLINSON, K., and JOYCE, S. (1974). A Program of Crisis Intervention in the Emergency Medical Setting. *American Journal of Psychiatry* 131(1):47–50.

HAZELTON, H. (1925). *The Boroughs of Brooklyn and Queens, Counties of Nassau and Suffolk 1609–1924. 3.* New York: Lewis Historical Publishing.

HOLMES, T., and RAHE, R. (1967). The Social Readjustment Rating Scale. *Journal of Psychosomatic Research* 11(2):213–218.

HUGHES, E. C. (1958). *Men and Their Work.* Glencoe, Ill.: The Free Press.

ISRAEL, F., ed. (1968). *1897 Sears Roebuck Catalogue.* New York: Chelsea House Publishers.

KADUSHIN, C. (1969). *Why People Go to Psychiatrists.* New York: Atherton Press.

LEVINE, S., SCOTCH, N., VLASAK, G. (1969). Unravelling Technology and Culture in Public Health. *American Journal of Public Health* 59:237–244.

LINN, L. (1976). Personal Communication to E. Mumford.

LYNDON, G. (March 22, 1926). Crowding Ignored at Kings Hospital. *Brooklyn Times.*

MARSTON, R. (1968). To Meet the Nation's Health Needs. *The New England Journal of Medicine* 279:520–524.

McTAGGART, A. (1971). *The Health Care Dilemma.* Boston: Holbrook Press.

MECHANIC, D. (1972). Social Psychologic Factors Affecting the Presentation of Bodily Complaints. *The New England Journal of Medicine* 286(20): 1132–1139.

MERTON, R. (1957). *Social Theory and Social Structure.* New York: The Free Press.

MESNIKOFF, A., SPITZER, R., and ENDICOTT, J. (1970). Program Evaluation and Planning in a New Community Mental Health Service: Two Years' Experience. *Changing Patterns in Psychiatric Care: An Anthology of Evolving Scientific Psychiatry in Medicine,* ed. T. Rothman. Los Angeles, Calif.: Rush Research Foundation, pp. 70–89.

MILLIS, J. (October 20, 1969). The Future of Medicine. *Journal of the American Medical Association* 210(3):498–501.

Minimum Socioeconomic and Health Profile: Comprehensive Planning District. F, Borough of Brooklyn. (January 1974). New York: Comprehensive Planning Agency for the City of New York.

MUMFORD, E. (1970). *Interns: From Students to Physicians.* Cambridge, Mass.: Harvard University Press.

MUMFORD, E., PARDES, H., and LUSK, L. (1976). *History, Present Age Distributions and Future Prospects of Emergency Rooms.* Unpublished Manuscript. Downstate Medical Center, State University of New York.

The New York Times (February 8, 1942). 68,678 Got Help in Kings Hospital.

OAKES, C. (1973). *The Walking Patient.* Columbia, S.C.: University of South Carolina Press.

ORWELL, G. (1950). *How the Poor Die: Shooting an Elephant and Other Essays. New York: Harcourt, Brace.*

PETRICK, F., and HOUSE, M. (November 1973). Improved Data Generation Needed for Ambulatory Planning. *Hospital Progress* (54, Part 2): 84–86.

PIFER, A. (1970). A New Climate. *Journal of Medical Education* 45:79–87.

REED, J., and READER, G. (1967). Quantitative Survey of New York Emergency Room, 1965. *New York State Journal of Medicine* 67:1335–1342.

RIDEING, W. (1972). Hospital Life in New York. *Medical America in the Nineteenth Century,* ed. G. Brieger. Baltimore, Md.: Johns Hopkins University Press, pp. 242–250.

ROGHMANN, K., and HAGGERTY, R. (1973). Daily Stress, Illness and Use of Health Services in Young Families. *Pediatric Research* 7:520–526.

ROGHMANN, K., and HAGGERTY, R. (1972). Family Stress and the Use of Health Services. *International Journal of Epidemiology* 1(3):279–286.

SCHWARTZ, H. (September 12, 1971). Hospitals: Believe It or Not—There Are Too Many Beds. *The New York Times.*

SHAH, C., and CARR, L. (May 4, 1974). Triage: A Working Solution to Overcrowding in the Emergency Department. *Canadian Medical Association Journal* 110: 1039–1043.

SHYROCK, R. (1966). *Medicine in America.* Baltimore, Md.: Johns Hopkins University Press.

STARR, J. (1957). *Hospital City.* New York: Crown Publishers.

STEVENS, R. (1971). *American Medicine and the Public Interest.* New Haven: Yale University Press.

STILES, H. (1884). *The Political, Professional and Ecclesiastical History and Commercial and Industrial Record of the County of Kings and the City of Brooklyn, New York from 1683 to 1884.* 1. New York: W. W. Munsell and Co., pp. 466–567.

STOECKLE, J., and ZOLA, I. (1964). After Everyone Can Pay for Medical Care: Some Perspectives on Future Treatment and Practice. *Medical Care* 2: 36–41.

TORRENS, P., and YEDVAB, D. (1970). Variations Among Emergency Room Populations: A Comparison of Four Hospitals in New York City. *Medical Care* 8(1):60–74.

ZOLA, I. (1973). Pathways to the Doctor: From Person to Patient. *Social Science and Medicine* 7:677–689.

Childbirth and Social Class: The Case of Cesarean Delivery

Marsha Hurst
Pamela S. Summey

It is well known that in 10 years the cesarean delivery rate in the United States has increased almost 300%, a fact that has elicited much debate and concern among consumers and medical professionals alike. It is less well known that middle and upper class women are at higher risk for cesareans than lower class women: the socioeconomic group of women with the lowest risk of pregnancy complications thus runs the highest risk of medical intervention during labor and delivery. In addition to the medical factors that put a woman at risk of cesarean delivery there are many class-related factors including older age at first childbearing, higher educational attainment, more prenatal care, private obstetrical care and birth at a nonpublic hospital. The purpose of our paper is to analyze how obstetrical care in general, and cesarean delivery in particular, varies according to the socioeconomic status of the woman. Our method is to reexamine historical studies of obstetrical intervention for social class differences, and to reanalyze contemporary data on socioeconomic status and type of birth. Some original data are introduced on hospital delivery in the New York City voluntary system, on one New York voluntary hospital, and on physician variation within one hospital.

BACKGROUND

The time-honored relationship between social class and health status is accepted as a given in the United States. Perhaps more complicated, but not less true

is the relationship between social class and medical care. Concern about medical care for the poor classes has generally been based on the assumption that more is better; yet, even with the increased accessibility to medical care that Medicaid has allowed, social class differences in care persist.

Obstetrical history is full of hints, if not full-blown analyses, of substantial and consistent differences in care for women of different classes. In the nineteenth century, a wide range of obstetrical therapies and practices were available, but a woman's choice was dictated by her social class, and choice of type of practitioner meant choice of type of care. Practitioners believed that different obstetrical practices were suitable for a prostitute, a 'worthy' poor woman, a middle class housewife or an upper class society woman; for the woman, her social standing dictated where she would give birth, who would attend her and what her birth experience would be like [1, 2].

The growth of hospitals and particularly obstetrical facilities in hospitals went a long way toward solidifying this relationship between social class and obstetrical care. The early hospitals were for the worthy poor only who were delivered by obstetricians as charity patients [3]. As the usefulness and practicality of hospital care became apparent, the unworthy poor were included in the hospital's obstetrical clientele, which then permitted the hospitals to become sites for obstetrical teaching and experimentation. Social distance between patient and practitioner enabled doctors to experiment on poor women. In Central Park a statue of J. Marion Sims reminds us of this. Sims perfected the technique of repairing vaginal fistulas by purchasing slave women, and

Reprinted from *Social Science and Medicine*, vol. 18 (1984), pp. 621–631.

housing and feeding them in exchange for practicing fistula repairs on their persons. His fame and fortune enabled him to open the first women's hospital in New York City, and his technique provided relief for a problem shared by thousands of women of all classes [4].

A study of nineteenth century obstetrical services in two Boston hospitals—one a teaching hospital staffed by male residents and serving the lowest and least 'worthy' class of poor women, and the other hospital staffed by women physicians who chose to care for only the 'worthy' poor—has shed interesting light on class differences in care. The records of the two obstetrical units are similar. The only significant exception involves neither medical risk of the patient, nor outcome for mother and baby, but rather rates of medication. The women physicians tended to give their 'worthy poor' patients much more pain-killing medication than did the male physicians their 'unworthy poor' [5].

Maternity care in hospitals has always been divided into two classes. In the 1920s, middle class births started moving into the hospital, and hospitals grew in size to accommodate the two classes of patients. The early part of the century was characterized by the interplay of three forces that we have seen in much more recent history. Consumer movements, such as the 'Twilight Sleep' movement among middle and upper income women, were directed at increasing women's decision-making power in obstetrical care. Active obstetrics was becoming the prevailing method of practice. Both national and local investigations of maternal mortality—which had slowed in its decline despite increases in hospital delivery, prenatal care; and the use of aseptic techniques—decried excessive obstetrical intervention, improperly performed [6].

The New York City Maternal Mortality Study [7] noted that the risk of maternal mortality was 'highly correlated with economic status, race, and nativity', with the highest rates among the poorest groups. Yet the cesarean delivery rate in municipal hospitals was roughly half that of obstetric and voluntary hospitals, making the rate of preventable deaths related to cesarean delivery greater among middle income women. Thus this report vividly pointed out the contradiction that we are examining today: poor women are at the greatest medical risk,

but middle and upper class women receive the most medical intervention. Recent obstetrical history and the current state of obstetrical practice bear this out. For the past decade, maternal and child health has focused its concern on the infant. Infant and perinatal mortality today, as maternal mortality in the past, are closely related to social class in the United States [8, 9]. This was shown by Kessner *et al.* [10] on New York City birth data using maternal education as an indication of socioeconomic status. Others have clearly demonstrated the relationship between socioeconomic status and low birth weight [11, 12], pregnancy loss [13], prematurity [14], morbidity and mortality [15] and 'obstetrical competence' [16].

As in the earlier periods, declining mortality and active obstetrics are often said to be causally related; but perinatal mortality has been declining for a long time and has not responded to dramatic increases in active obstetrics [17]. Furthermore, active obstetrics appears to be concentrated in lower risk populations. Although the Collaborative Perinatal Study [18] looked only at race, not social class, it found higher rates of forceps delivery and induction, and lower rates of spontaneous delivery for whites than blacks; and, in the United States, there is a close correspondence between race and class. Induction in particular caused concern in the mid-1970s as rates in private hospitals rose to 35% [19]. In New York City, Pakter and Nelson [20] found hospital induction rates ranging from a high of 18% in a private service to a low of 0.1% in a general service population. When induction was openly an elective procedure, it was overwhelmingly a private procedure, with 80% of elective inductions in New York City performed on private patients.

In his review of medical care in the United Kingdom, Hart [21] noted an 'inverse care law' between medical care and medical need: "the availability of good medical care tends to vary inversely with the need for it in the population served". Chard and Richards [22], after finding that the highest rates of forceps deliveries and inductions were in the areas with the healthiest populations in Britain, concluded that "an inverse care law operates in obstetrical services". We suggest that a form of the inverse care law applies in obstetrics: the amount of medical care women receive in labour and delivery varies inversely with their actual medical need for that care. The following discussion will explore this 'inverse care law' as it applies to cesarean delivery.

VARIATIONS IN CESAREAN DELIVERY

The national cesarean delivery rate in 1981 was 17.9% [23]. This means that almost one out of every five babies born in the United States is born by cesarean, and the rate continues to rise. There is, however, little evidence to show that doing more cesareans improves infant outcome, and considerable data to show substantial risks to mother and baby. Furthermore, the variation in cesarean rates is enormous, and suggests factors other than medical standards are at issue.

If cesarean deliveries are being done for medical reasons alone, we should see any variation in the rates explained by medical risk, and the highest rates among high-risk women. If instead an inverse care law is in operation, we would find the opposite—more cesareans among low-risk women and variation explained by factors other than medical need.

Currently available data on cesarean delivery show wide variation in rates by many nonmedical as well as medical variables. Many of the nonmedical variables suggest that social class may be strongly related to cesarean delivery rates although this relationship is seldom shown directly. Nonmedical factors related to the increase in cesarean delivery rates include characteristics of the childbearing women (age, parity, education, race, amount of prenatal care) and characteristics of the place of birth (region of the country, hospital type, size and ownership).

Age and cesarean delivery have had a consistent relationship, with higher rates for older women. This should not be interpreted to mean older women have more medical complications that lead to cesareans. In fact, the relationship between age and cesarean delivery is largely accounted for by the higher rates of repeat cesareans among older women. Although some studies have shown that women over 35 are more likely to have primary cesareans than younger women [24], recent national data broken into 5 year age groups indicate that primary cesarean rates do not vary consistently by the age of the mother [25]. Actually, the greatest increases over the past decade have been in young women, particularly those under 20 [26, 27].

Women giving birth to their first child are more likely to have a cesarean delivery than are other women. This combined with the increase in women over 30 of higher socioeconomic status having first births may appear to account for the higher rates of cesareans among these middle and upper income women. In fact, however, in 1980, the cesarean rate for first births was only 1.8% higher than the rate for subsequent births [28].

Education of mother, a variable often thought to be a valid indicator of social class, is related to risk of a cesarean delivery [29]. New York City data for 1976–1977 indicate that women with 'some college' had a 17.5% cesarean delivery rate compared to 14.7% for women without a high school diploma [30]. These data, although flawed because age of mother is not taken into account, point to a social class difference in cesarean delivery.

Women who receive more prenatal care and begin that care early in pregnancy are more likely to have a cesarean delivery than women who receive little or no medical care during their pregnancies [31–33]. This is to be expected given the fact that women with complicated pregnancies should have more prenatal visits. Prenatal care, like other preventive medical services, is less likely to be used by low-income patients [34]. Studies done in New York City and in California show that women with no prenatal care whatsoever, almost all of whom are low-income women, have the lowest cesarean rates. In 1975, Petitti *et al.* [35] found that California women with no prenatal care had a cesarean rate of 6.2% compared to 12.8% for women who had received any prenatal care, regardless of the number of visits. New York City studies have found a similar relationship [36, 37]. Once again, these data suggest the influence of social class on cesarean rates.

Racial data are generally poor with large numbers of patients not classified by race. Whites do show a consistently higher cesarean rate than nonwhites, but the differences are not great and vary somewhat by region [38, 39]. California data show a higher cesarean rate in hospitals with more 'white non-Spanish' patients, which is 'perplexing' given the lower perinatal mortality rates and lesser medical risk of that population [40].

Cesarean delivery rates also vary enormously by geographic location of birth. This becomes immediately clear in looking at crossnational data—the United States and Canadian rates are nearly twice as high as the United Kingdom and are triple that of The Netherlands [41]. In Brazil cesarean rates are the highest of anywhere in the world: one survey shows the rate among private patients to be 75% compared to 25% for indigent patients [42]. Within the United States, regional variations have been noted, the Northeast consistently having the highest proportion of cesarean deliveries (20% in 1981), followed by the South (18.8%), the West (17.1%) and the Northcentral (15.9%) regions respectively [43]. The order of the last three varies somewhat over time. This variation—clearly not explained by the medical risk of patients—is likely to be an indicator of the mix of hospitals, doctors and types of patients in each region.

Hospitals themselves have startlingly different cesarean rates. Fleck [44] has put forth a 'high-risk hospital' hypothesis, showing in his data from various upstate New York hospitals that the risk of cesarean delivery is an intrinsic attribute of a specific hospital affecting all patients somewhat equally regardless of their county of origin. National data indicate that large hospitals have consistently higher rates than smaller hospitals and that teaching hospitals have higher rates than nonteaching hospitals [45, 46], a phenomenon commonly thought to be attributable to referral of complicated cases to larger or teaching hospitals.

Both national and New York City data show that hospital ownership is related to cesarean delivery: proprietary and voluntary hospitals have the highest rates; public or government hospital rates are considerably lower. This relationship has been demonstrated to be consistent over a long period of time in New York City [47]. The most recent national figures available (1981) show proprietaries with a 22% cesarean delivery rate, voluntaries 18.5% and government hospitals 15.4% [48]. Since parity has virtually no impact on cesarean rate, the higher rate of primiparous women delivering in nongovernment hospitals should not account for these differences in hospital rates. Furthermore, government hospitals have a significantly larger proportion of low income, high risk birthing women than do other hospitals, and should thus have higher cesarean rates.

Almost a quarter of a century ago, Erhardt and Gold [49] attributed the underlying hospital variation to social class differences. Knowing that proprietary hospitals had only private patients, municipals had only general service patients and voluntaries had a mixture of the two, they divided voluntary hospitals into their private and general service components for comparison. Rates for general service patients in voluntary hospitals resembled those of patients in municipal hospitals and rates for private patients in voluntaries were found to be similar to

TABLE 1   Cesarean delivery in New York City by type of hospital

YEAR	MUNICIPAL (%)	VOLUNTARY (%)		PROPRIETARY (%)	TOTAL (%)
1954–1955*	3.5	5.7		5.0	5.0
1968–1969†	6.1	7.2		7.3	7.0
1976–1977†	14.0	16.4		15.4	15.7
1980	15.0	20.4		21.3	19.1
		General	Private		
1954–1955*	3.5	4.2	6.3	5.0	5.0
1968–1969†	6.1	6.9	7.8	7.3	7.0
1976–1977†	14.0	14.8	17.4	15.4	15.7
1980	15.0	16.4	22.5	21.3	19.1

* Erhardt C. L. and Gold E. M. Cesarean section in New York City: incidence and mortality during 1954–55. *Obstet. Gynec.* **11** 241–260, 1958.

† Cesarean Childbirth: Report of a Consensus Development Conference. U.S. Department of Health and Human Services, Washington, DC, 1981.

those of patients in proprietary hospitals. In fact, the two parts of the voluntary hospital system more closely resemble their non-voluntary counterparts than they do each other. We have elaborated on their work, by reanalyzing the New York City data presented at the Cesarean Consensus Development Conference and by obtaining and analyzing the 1980 New York City hospital data. These data illustrate quite clearly the strong and persistent relationship of social class and cesarean delivery (Table 1).

Variation by hospital does, of course, still exist, suggesting that Fleck's high-risk hospital hypothesis may apply to particular institutions. Referral patterns, reimbursement practices and hospital location all reflect and reinforce social class differences between hospitals. Even within the voluntary system the average cesarean delivery rate of hospitals in

New York City ranged from 14 to 31% in 1981. Within this range, however, it is clear that the social class differences persist: private cesarean rates are higher at nearly every hospital. Indeed although there is some overlap in the spread of general service and private rates, the predominant rates for each are quite obviously different (Fig. 1). The primary cesarean rates (rates for first time cesarean deliveries) for these voluntary hospitals show a similar pattern with an average primary rate of 13.3% overall— 15.3% in the private sector, 10.9% in the general service group.

EXPLANATION AND DISCUSSION

It is clear from national and local data that obstetrical care, and particularly rates of intrapartum inter-

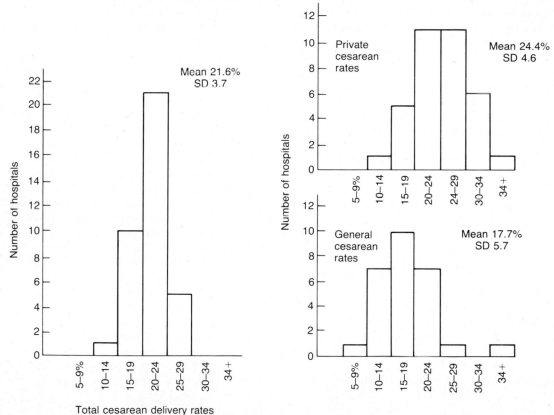

Fig. 1 Cesarean Delivery in New York City Voluntary Hospitals, 1981. Total, Private and General Service Rates.

vention, varies by social class. Both patient and hospital characteristics support the inverse care law when applied, for example, to cesarean delivery. Most data leave it unclear whether type of hospital is the overriding determining characteristic, but our data show that interventions vary by social class even within hospitals. These class differences in care may be less related to patient socioeconomic characteristics than to the two-class structure of medical care in American hospitals [50].

The structure of care for general service obstetrical patients within voluntary hospitals closely resembles that of all obstetrical patients in municipal or most other government hospitals. Pregnant and birthing women are seen by on duty house staff, who may be midwives, residents, or staff physicians. There is rarely continuity of care from one visit to the next, or from one shift rotation to the next during delivery. No fees pass directly from consumer to professional. Most staff are involved in a learning experience and in turn are carrying out an exhausting schedule of care for ob/gyn patients. Private patients see their own physician or group of physicians for prenatal care and delivery. A personal relationship is expected. Consumers are understood to have carefully chosen their birth attendant, and to have certain expectations of care from that professional. In the hospital obstetrical service, general service and private patients are separated. Often they have separate labor and delivery rooms. Almost always they have separate postpartum rooms, and usually on separate floors or wings of the hospital. Given the two structures of care, then, it is reasonable to expect differences in the content of care.

Economic reasons are certainly the most obvious, if not necessarily the most important explanations for the higher rates of cesarean delivery among middle and upper class women. In their exhaustive review of the literature on electronic fetal monitoring [51], Banta and Thacker estimated the added expense of a cesarean over a vaginal delivery to be $2300. Others have estimated that cesarean delivery is 47 percent to 85 percent more expensive [52]. Furthermore, babies delivered by cesarean have higher rates of respiratory distress syndrome which costs between $2700 and $3400 to treat. Increased maternal morbidity resulting from cesarean delivery adds an additional $44 million per year in added bed days alone. Most important a technological arena of birth

featuring expensive pediatric and anesthetic facilities, biochemical and ultrasound facilities, and intensive care units encourages and reinforces a surgical birthing environment. While millions of dollars in cost are added to the obstetrical care system by high rates of cesarean deliveries, the economic incentives to the private care sector alone do not appear to be substantial enough to account for the difference in cesarean rates by social class.

Private physicians, for the most part, add a few hundred dollars to their obstetrical fees for a cesarean delivery. In some areas physicians double their fees for cesareans, and comparisons of these areas with others would be valuable. Since the average gross annual income of an obstetrician is $166,500 [53], including $74,000 of professional expenses, the increment from additional cesarean deliveries is negligible.

Cesarean delivery requires longer hospital stays for the mother and baby at a time when fertility rates are low, particularly among the middle class women who experience higher risk of cesarean delivery. Since most obstetrical services, particularly in larger hospitals, were planned for more fertile times, it could be hypothesized that increased rates of cesarean delivery made up for the loss of bed occupancy that has come with lower fertility rates and shorter stays for both vaginal and cesarean births. According to C. Arden Miller, "These circumstances . . . suggest that Roemer's Law (empty beds tend to become filled) may be operative in the medical market, working to revise the obstetrical practice in order to fill empty beds" [54]. In one large New York City hospital, for example, the number of deliveries steadily declined from 5000 in 1968 to 3000 in 1980, but the increased rate of cesarean deliveries has meant that the number of cesarean births during that period stayed remarkably stable. Nevertheless, in an analysis by the Health Systems Agency of New York City [55] and independent analysis by the authors, it was found that the increased cesarean rate did not go far toward making up for the much more drastic loss of bed days from shorter stays and fewer births. Furthermore, even if higher cesarean delivery rates significantly increased bed occupancy rates, it is not clear why this would provide more of an incentive for cesareans in private than in general service sectors.

Insurance reimbursement policies do not provide any disincentive for doing a cesarean. For most families more costs are reimbursed for cesarean delivery than for vaginal delivery, partly because of the pro-casualty bias of most insurance policies. Williams and Hawes [56] did find lower cesarean delivery rates among HMO hospitals than would be expected given patient characteristics, which argues for the importance of insurance structure in influencing cesarean rates. This finding was also reported recently for maternity patients using the Harvard Community Health Plan and the HMO physicians [57]. A national study, however, found no relationship between type of insurance and cesarean rate [58]. The New Jersey reimbursement experiment might also yield some interesting results since both private and general service deliveries will be reimbursed by diagnosis.

Thus although we feel there are substantial systemic benefits to high cesarean rates in general, we have not found direct evidence that would explain the consistently higher cesarean rates among private patients. The economic argument, however, is critical: for regardless of all else, high cesarean delivery rates among middle class women maintains high risk, and thus high cost obstetrics at a time when consumer pressure is toward lower cost alternatives, and this pressure is reinforced by government concern about hospital costs and health care spending.

The clearest link between higher cesarean rates and private practice in obstetrics is that of the threat of malpractice suit. Although this is very much an economic issue, it is so prevalent, and yet so intangible, that it has become integral to the culture of private obstetrical care. Malpractice suits can be brought directly against a physician by a private patient, but a general service patient is obliged to sue the hospital and it is the hospital that pays if an award is made to the patient. Many doctors leaving residency express some fear at leaving this protective umbrella of the hospital, both because of their increased direct legal responsibility for their performance, and because they will then be required to pay the enormous premium of malpractice insurance themselves. This expense is often the greatest single annual expense of a physician in office practice. Over the last 10 years, the rate paid for this insurance in New York State has increased from $3437 in 1970 to a current high in some counties of nearly $50,000. Fear of malpractice suits was "the most frequent reason for the increase in the Cesarean section rate given by physicians during interviews" conducted by Marieskind [59] for her 1979 DHEW-sponsored report on cesareans. Obstetricians are sued ten times more than the average physician, and their malpractice insurance is generally four times as expensive. Although the number of claims has not substantially increased over the last several years, the average award has tripled, with an estimated average payment for claims in 1981 to be between $100,000 and $150,000. Obstetrical awards making national news have frequently been in the range of one to four million dollars.

Another possible explanation for the social class difference in cesarean deliveries is physician convenience. Private physicians may do cesareans to end long labors in the hospital in order to keep their scheduled office appointments or in order to maximize their evening and weekend leisure time. Staff doctors work regular hospital shifts and thus do not have to cope with the exigencies of private practice in addition to their hospital work. Phillips *et al.* [60] investigated this hypothesis but were unable to show that private physicians were more likely to do cesareans on weekends. Fleck [61], however, found that in certain upstate New York hospitals, cesarean rates were significantly higher on Monday and lower on Sunday. He found that both private and staff physicians exhibited a similar need to sleep rather than perform cesareans at night. Gibbons [62] found that cesarean sections were distributed equally during the day and night on the general service, but that 60% of cesareans were performed during the day on the private service.

Data from one New York City voluntary hospital show that both private and staff physicians are more likely to do cesareans during the daytime hours (Table 2). Looking only at primary cesareans, thus eliminating most of the scheduled cesareans, nearly two-thirds are performed during the day on both services. This may reflect a preference for delivering complicated cases during the day when all hospital facilities are available. When these times are more closely examined, we find that staff physicians are more likely to do cesareans in the afternoon with a peak at about 3:00 P.M.; private physicians do more cesareans in the morning with their peak at 11:00 A.M. These data hold consistently for the 3 year time period examined.

TABLE 2   Primary cesarean deliveries in one voluntary hospital by time of day, 1980

TIME OF DAY	TYPE OF SERVICE	
	SERVICE (%)	PRIVATE (%)
1 A.M.–6 A.M.	17.6	13.2
7 A.M.–12 noon	24.4	35.6
1 P.M.–6 P.M.	35.8	29.6
7 P.M.–midnight	21.9	21.8
Day (7 A.M.–6 P.M.)	60.2	65.2
Night (7 P.M.–6 A.M.)	39.5	35.0
Peak hour (11% of cesareans performed)	3 P.M.	11 A.M.

Differences in daily work patterns between attendings and house staff help explain this finding: private physicians must get to their offices for afternoon scheduled patients; they often begin inducing their patients during the night so that, if induction fails and a cesarean must be performed, it can be done before office hours begin. Furthermore, private physicians have priority for the operating rooms and often schedule cesareans during the desirable morning hours. Staff physicians usually begin inducing patients in the morning, and, if by mid-afternoon labor is not rapidly progressing, they do a cesarean before the 4:00 shift change. It is thought to be inconsiderate for a resident to leave a nonprogressing patient for the next shift to cope with. The responsiveness of even primary cesarean delivery to the schedules of physicians does not in itself explain why private patients have more cesareans. It does indicate to some extent, however, the degree to which physicians treat cesareans as non-emergency surgery, subject to scheduling considerations.

Although the social class difference in cesarean deliveries has persisted over time, the relative risk of cesarean for a private as compared to a general service patient has varied somewhat (Fig. 2). Looking at New York City data, we find a parallel upward trend in cesarean delivery rates for private and general service patients. The difference narrows in the early seventies when the relative risk falls to 1.18. During these years fetal monitors were being tested on general service patients—a factor known to increase cesarean delivery rates [63]. These monitors began to be used widely on private obstetrical patients in the middle to late 1970s at most institutions,

and during this period the relative risk—or private/general service gap—widened again.

Using one voluntary hospital as a case study of this phenomenon (Fig. 3), we see a generally low relative risk private to general service in the early 1970s when only one monitor was available and was used exclusively on general service patients. In fact, one year the general service cesarean rate was higher than the private rate. When a large number of monitors were purchased to be used on all patients in the beginning of 1975, we see the 1975 private cesarean rate jump and the general service rate actually drop. Again, this does not enable us to explain why there are social class differences in the rates. We can conclude, however, that the two services operate as independent structures of care, each responding to its own set of demands and incentives.

Social distance between patient and physician has often been used to explain the social class differences in medical care. Shaw [64] found that identification of doctor with the patient was the most important determinant of the quality of medical care given. Women who most resembled the wives of the male doctors in their social status got "the best treatment and most humanized care. . . . The greater the status differences, the worse the treatment."

Physicians themselves offer this as an explanation of care differences between private and general service patients [65]. One obstetrician interviewed by Summey summed this up:

> *I think the private practitioner becomes less an uninvolved partner or loses some of his objectivity knowing the patient, her family, delivering the other kids, knowing what other social pressures and problems there are. And he may jump to do a cesarean section. A resident who is detached from a clinic patient he's probably never seen before, knowing nothing about her but her name and maybe not even that, may be able to be more objective.*

Many private physicians feel that falling birth rates, increased control over family planning, later timing of births and a wider range of pregnancy diagnostic tools have resulted in an insistence on the part of the private patient and her practitioner for a 'perfect baby.'

> *We probably are doing four or five unnecessary cesarean sections, but I don't want to take that*

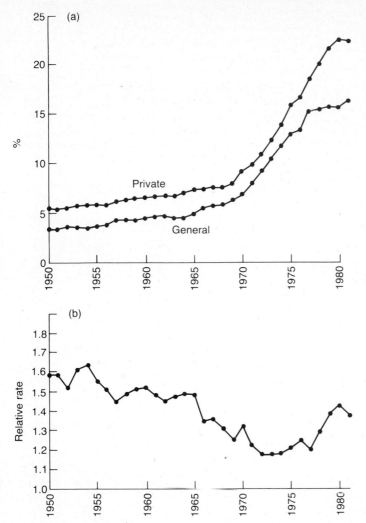

Fig. 2 (a) Percentage of Cesarean Deliveries: Private and General Service. New York City, 1950–1981 (live births). (b) Relative Risk of Cesarean Delivery: Private to General Service. New York City, 1950–1981.

chance. People are only having one or two babies now and they want healthy super human being babies . . . and they don't want any more of these forceps deliveries, these brain damaged children.

Since the 'hazards of the birth canal' are deeply imbedded in obstetrical belief [66], abdominal delivery in case of the slightest chance of risk to the baby, is preferred.

The striking variations both within and between social classes in cesarean delivery rates led us to look at the variation literature for general surgery.

Beginning with Glover's classic 1938 British study of tonsillectomy [67] followed by the Registrar General's study in England in 1954 [68], to the Gittelsohn and Wennberg study in Vermont [69], tonsillectomy rates have been shown to vary widely by geographic region. Wennberg and Gittelsohn [70] found the variation on tonsillectomy and six other procedures related to the number of surgeons practicing in the area:

The wide variations in the rates of individual procedures, however, are not caused by differences in the supply of resources alone. . . . Our

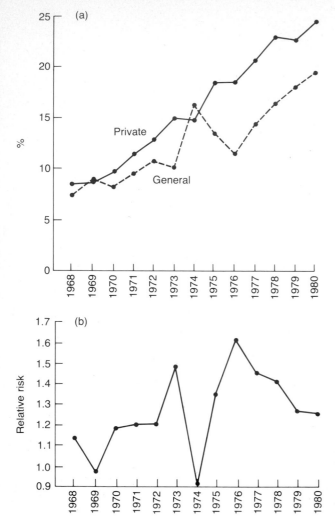

Fig. 3 (a) Percentage of Cesarean Deliveries: Private and General Service. One New York City Voluntary Hospital, 1968–1980. (b) Relative Risk of Cesarean Delivery: Private to General Service. One New York City Voluntary Hospital, 1968–1980.

work suggests that such variations are due to differences in the style of medical practice of local physicians.

Physician variation in obstetrical care has been noted in several studies. Use of induction, forceps, and other interventions has been shown to vary considerably by who does the delivery [71]. Pearson [72] found that doctors with predominantly gynecology practices were most likely to have high cesarean delivery rates. This is consistent with Summey's

finding [73] that physicians with large obstetrical practices tend to have lower cesarean rates. No other information on physician variation is available in the literature to our knowledge.

Just as cesarean delivery is now the 'style' in southern Brazil, we can see changes over time in practice styles of physicians in the United States. Data from one New York teaching hospital indicate the changing nature of preferred style of obstetrical intervention (Fig. 4). In 1968, clearly forceps delivery was the intervention of choice. In 1980, although

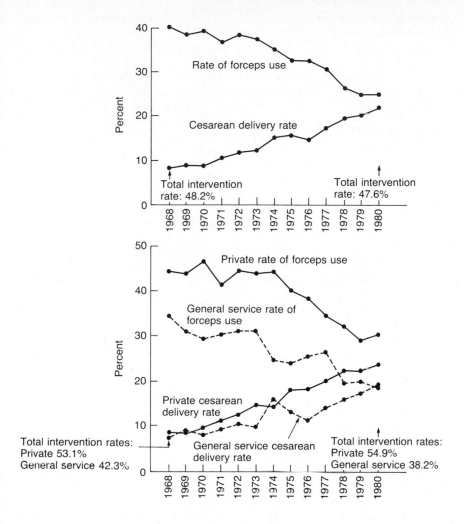

Fig. 4 Forceps Use and Cesarean Delivery Rates in One New York City Voluntary Hospital.

forceps are still used in a large proportion of deliveries, they tend to be low forceps deliveries. In most instances the use of mid or high forceps has been replaced by cesarean delivery which is thought to be safer for the baby than the 'difficult forceps deliveries' of the past. Note that the total proportion of 'interventionist' deliveries does not change—only the preferred intervention changed.

Similarly there seem to be style or fashion preferences among individual physicians at any given time. The 31 busiest New York private obstetricians

practicing at one hospital had cesarean delivery rates for 1980 ranging from 13 to 52%. When the proportion of forceps deliveries was added to the proportion of cesarean deliveries, the total intervention rates ranged from 32 to 93% [74]. In addition, use of forceps and cesarean delivery seemed to vary inversely by practitioner; that is, physicians with lower cesarean rates tended to have high forceps rates, an indication that even physicians who have similar intervention rates may differ in the type of intervention they prefer.

Chalmers and Richards [75] came to a similar conclusion in their examination of variation in obstetrical care:

As in other fields, these international and intranational differences suggest variability in medical fashion rather than in clearly defined need: definitions of need, as perceived by individual obstetric practitioners, vary considerably. Although both the extent to which doctors are responsible for assisting women in childbirth and the way they are paid will influence instrumental delivery rates, the underlying dichotomy between interventionist and conservative practitioners probably plays a more important role.

Given hospital and physician variation in cesarean delivery, we are led to conclude that the medical-ideological beliefs of physicians and the mix of those physicians in a certain setting has an important influence on a patient's risk of cesarean delivery.

CONCLUSION

The 3 to 4-fold increase over the last 10 years in cesarean delivery has occasioned much comment and concern. Given less attention is the fact that population differences in cesarean rates are closely associated with social class characteristics, and appear to follow an inverse care law operative throughout much of obstetrical history: the lower the social class, the higher the medical risk and the lower the intervention rate. Evidence for this in relation to cesarean delivery comes from national, local, and individual hospital data; it can be seen through all measures of socioeconomic status available including size and type of hospital, race and education of the mother, and most important, whether the hospital service used is private or general service.

We feel that the most important factor accounting for the differences in cesarean rates among different social classes is the 'two-class system of care' in obstetrics: private and general service obstetrical patients are part of two almost completely separate environments. Thus, although physician training and prevailing values in practice may be common to physicians in both systems, the financial, personal, practical and professional incentives to practice in

a certain way are quite different in the two structures of care.

The introduction of new technology affects those differences in care, and this is a key to our understanding of the different place of the patient in each system. At these times, an historical pattern prevails: technology is introduced on poorer patients where it is tested, and where physicians learn to use the new methods, devices, or medications; if accepted, it is then passed on to the private sector and becomes the preferred 'modern' style of practice. Once the 'testing' period has passed, and the new technology with its attendant protocols becomes part of the regular training experience, general service intervention rates resulting from the new technology tend to level off or even drop.

The argument about the appropriateness of current intervention rates has been made both ways. On one side are researchers who feel those lower rates for poorer patients indicate poorer care and misallocated resources [76]. On the other hand, one New York City study argues that lower cesarean rates at municipal hospitals is an indication of appropriate caution in obstetrical intervention [77]. According to Kerr [78], "We may have assumed too lightly that more sophisticated management necessarily brings benefits to women, the dangerous argument that more means better".

There is general agreement that the current overall cesarean rate is too high. Minkoff and Schwarz [79], in a lengthy analysis of medical indications for cesarean delivery argue that rates are probably almost ⅓ too high. Even the cautiously worded conclusion of the Consensus Development Conference [80] says birth outcomes can continue to be improved while the cesarean rate increase is halted or reversed. One comparative study of the United States and the United Kingdom clearly argues that a cesarean delivery rate in "excess of 6 percent" would not be "in the best interests of mothers and their babies" [81].

While it is not within the scope of this paper to assess what would be medically appropriate cesarean rates, it does seem clear to us that today's rates are in large measure a result of socioeconomic and not medical factors. Until these socioeconomic factors are acknowledged, sorted out and controlled, there will be no way of delivering safe and appropriate care to birthing women.

References

1. Wertz R. W. and Wertz D. C. *Lying-In: A History of Childbirth in America.* Free Press, New York, 1977.

2. Bogdan J. C. Care or cure? Childbirth practices in nineteenth century America. *Feminist Stud.* **4,** 92, 1978.

3. Rosner D. Health care for the 'truly needy': Nineteenth-century origins of the concept. *Milbank Meml Fund Q. Hlth. Soc.* **60,** 355, 1982.

4. Wertz R. W. and Wertz D. C. *op. cit.*

5. Morantz R. M. and Zschoche S. Professionalism, feminism, and gender roles: a comparative study of nineteenth century medical therapeutics. *J. Am. Hist.* **67,** 568, 1980.

6. Antler J. and Fox D. M. The movement toward a safe maternity: physician accountability in New York City. 1915–1940. *Bull. Hist. Med.* **50,** 569, 1976.

7. New York Academy of Medicine, Committee on Public Health Relations. *Maternal Mortality in New York City: A Study of All Puerperal Deaths, 1930–1932.* The Commonwealth Fund, New York, 1933.

8. Erhardt C. L., Abramson H., Pakter J. and Nelson F. An epidemiologic approach to infant mortality. *Archs Envir. Hlth* **20,** 743, 1970.

9. Brooks C. H. The changing relationship between socioeconomic status and infant mortality: an analysis of state characteristics. *J Hlth Soc. Behav.* **16,** 291, 1975.

10. Kessner D. M. *et al. Infant Death: An Analysis by Maternal Risk and Health Care.* Institute of Medicine. Washington, DC, 1973.

11. Shah F. K. and Abbey H. Effects of some factors on neonatal and postneonatal mortality: analysis by a binary variable and multiple regression method. *Milbank Meml Fund Q.* **49,** 33, 1971.

12. Niswander K. R. and Gordon M. G. *The Women and Their Pregnancies: The Collaborative Perinatal Study of the National Institute of Neurological Diseases and Stroke.* W. B. Saunders, Philadelphia, 1972.

13. Shapiro S., Schlesinger E. R. and Nesbitt R. E. L. *Infant Perinatal, Maternal and Childhood Mortality in the United States.* Harvard University Press, Cambridge, MA, 1968.

14. Garn S. M., Shaw H. A. and McCabe K. D. Effects of socioeconomic status and race on weight-defined and gestational prematurity in the United States. In *The Epidemiology of Prematurity* (Edited by Reed D. M. and Stanley F. J.), p. 127. Urban & Schwarzenberg, Baltimore, 1977.

15. Alberman E. Facts and figures. In *Benefits and Hazards of the New Obstetrics* (Edited by Chard R. and Richards M.), p. 1. J. B. Lippincott, Philadelphia, 1977.

16. Amante D. and Brandt N. The social ecology of obstetrical competence. *Soc. Sci. Med.* **12,** 391, 1978.

17. Dunn P. Obstetric delivery today, for better or worse? *Lancet* **1,** 790, 1976.

18. Niswander K. R. and Gordon M. G. *op. cit.*

19. Anderson S. F. Childbirth as a pathological process: an American perspective. *Am. J. Matern. Child Nurs.* July/August, 240, 1977.

20. Pakter J. and Nelson F. Induction of labor with oxytoxics (elective induction of labor and delivery). Presented at the 103rd Annual Meeting of the American Public Health Association, Miami Beach, FL, 1976.

21. Hart J. T. The inverse care law. *Lancet* **1,** 405, 1971.

22. Chard T. and Richards M. (Eds) Lessons for the Future. In *Benefits and Hazards of the New Obstetrics,* p. 157. J. B. Lippincott, Philadelphia, 1977.

23. Placek P. J., Taffel S. M. and Moien M. Cesarean section rates: United States, 1981. *Am. J. Publ. Hlth* **73,** 861, 1983.

24. Williams R. L. and Chen P. M. Controlling the rise in cesarean section rates by the dissemination of information from vital records. *Am. J. Publ. Hlth* **73,** 863, 1983.

25. Placek P. J., Taffel S. M. and Keppel K. G. Maternal and infant characteristics associated with cesarean section delivery in the United States, 1972 and 1980. *Health, United States: 1983.*

26. Placek P. J. and Taffel S. M. One-sixth of 1980 United States births by cesarean section. *Publ. Hlth. Rep.* **97,** 183, 1982.

27. Petitti D., Olson R. O. and Williams R. L. Cesarean section in California—1960 through 1975. *Am. J. Obstet. Gynec.* **133,** 391, 1979.

28. Placek P. J., Taffel S. M. and Keppel K. G. *op. cit.*

29. Kessner D. M. *et al. op. cit.*

30. Consensus Development Conference Sponsored by the National Institute of Child Health and Human Development. *Cesarean Childbirth.* National Institutes of Health, Bethesda, MD, 1981.

31. Williams R. L. and Hawes W. E. Cesarean section, fetal monitoring and perinatal mortality in California. *Am. J. Publ. Hlth* **69,** 864, 1979.

32. Petitti D., Olson R. O. and Williams R. L. *op. cit.*

33. Consensus Development Conference, *op. cit.*

34. Aday L. A. and Anderson R. *Access to Medical Care.* Health Administration Press, Ann Arbor, MI, 1975.

35. Petitti D., Olson R. O. and Williams R. L. *op. cit.*

36. Erhardt C. L. *et al. op. cit.,* 1970.

37. Albertsen P., Jones E. and Roberts R. Uncomplicated antepartum course as a predictor of uncomplicated labor and delivery. Columbia University College of Physicians and Surgeons, New York, unpublished, 1977.

38. Consensus Development Conference, *op. cit.*

39. Placek P. J. and Taffel S. M. Trends in cesarean section rates for the United States, 1970–78. *Publ. Hlth Rep.* **95,** 540, 1980.

40. Williams R. L. and Hawes W. E. *op. cit.*

41. Consensus Development Conference, *op. cit.*

42. Janowitz B. *et al.* Cesarean section in Brazil. *Soc. Sci. Med.* **16,** 19, 1982.

43. Placek P. J., Taffel S. M. and Moien M. *op. cit.*

44. Fleck A. C., Assistant Commissioner, Division of Child Health, Department of Health, New York State. Letters to Diony Young, 8 and 13 November, 1978.

45. Lowe J. A., Klassen D. F. and Loup R. J. Cesarean sections in U.S. PAS hospitals, time trend in rates, 1967–1974. *PAS Reporter* (Special issue) **14,** 1, 1976.

46. Placek P. J., Taffel S. M. and Moien M. *op. cit.*

47. Erhardt C. L. and Gold E. M. Cesarean section in New York City: incidence and mortality during 1954–55. *Obstet. Gynec.* **11,** 241, 1958.

48. Placek P. J., Taffel S. M. and Moien M. *op. cit.*

49. Erhardt C. L. and Gold E. M. *op. cit.*

50. Krause E. A. *Power and Illness: The Political Sociology of Health and Medical Care.* Elsevier, New York, 1977.

51. Banta H. D. and Thacker S. B. *Costs and Benefits of Electronic Fetal Monitoring: A Review of the Literature.* National Center for Health Services Research, DHEW Publication No. PHS 79–3245, Washington, DC, 1979.

52. Consensus Development Conference, *op. cit.*

53. American Medical Association. *Periodic Survey of Physicians, 1972–1980. Center for Health Services Research and Development,* Monroe, WI, 1981.

54. Miller C. A. What technology breeds: a review of recent U.S. experience with cesarean section. John Sundwall Memorial Lecture, School of Public Health, University of Michigan, Ann Arbor, Michigan, unpublished, 1978.

55. Health Systems Agency of New York City. Summary of maternity and neonatal ICU bed needs, methodologies and recommendation for the city and boroughs. Health Systems Agency of New York, New York, unpublished, 1980.

56. Williams R. L. and Hawes W. E. *op. cit.*

57. Wilner S., Palmer R. H., Mondon R. and Shownbaum S. Differences in obstetric technology utilization and related costs in HMO and fee-for-service settings. Presented at the American Public Health Association, Montreal, Canada, 1982.

58. Cynamon M. J. and Placek P. J. Insurance coverage for prenatal care, hospital stay and physician care: United States, 1964–66 and 1972 National Natality Surveys. Presented at the American Public Health Association, New York, 1979.

59. Marieskind H. I. *An Evaluation of Caesarean Section in the United States.* Report to Office of the Secretary. Department of Health Education and Welfare. Washington, DC, 1979.

60. Phillips R. N., Thornton J. and Gleicher N. Physician bias in cesarean sections. *J. Am. Med. Ass.* **248,** 1082, 1982.

61. Fleck A. C. Letter to Marsha Hurst 20 March, 1980.

62. Gibbons L. K. Analysis of the rise in C-Section in Baltimore. Johns Hopkins University School of Hygiene and Public Health, Baltimore, MD, unpublished doctoral dissertation, 1976.

63. Haverkamp A. D. *et al.* A controlled trial of the differential effects of intrapartum fetal monitoring. *Am. J. Obstet. Gynec.* **134,** 399, 1978.

64. Shaw N. S. *Forced Labor: Maternity Care in the United States.* Pergamon Press, New York, 1974.

65. Summey P. S. Physician variation in the use of technology in childbirth. SUNY Stony Brook, New York, forthcoming doctoral dissertation, 1984.

66. Stone M. L. Presidential Address, The American College of Obstetricians and Gynecologists. 3 April, 1979.

67. Glover J. A. The incidence of tonsillectomy in school children. *Proc. R. Soc. Med.* **31,** 1219, 1938.

68. *Registrar General's Statistical Review of England and Wales, Part I.* Office of the Registrar General, London, 1954.

69. Gittelsohn A. M. and Wennberg J. E. On the incidence of tonsillectomy and other common surgical procedures. In *Costs, Risks and Benefits of Surgery* (Edited by Bunker J. B., Barnes B. A. and Mosteller F.), p. 91. Oxford University Press, New York, 1977.

70. Wennberg J. E. and Gittelsohn A. M. Variations in medical care among small areas. *Scient. Am.* **246,** 120, 1982.

71. Chalmers I. and Richards M. Intervention and causal inference in obstetric practice. In *Benefits and Hazards of the New Obstetrics* (Edited by Chard T. and Richards M.), p. 34. J. B. Lippincott, Philadelphia, 1977.

72. Pearson J. Practice review for the American College of Obstetricians and Gynecologists. ACOG, Chicago, IL, unpublished, 1979.

73. Summey P. S. *op. cit.*

74. *Ibid.*

75. Chalmers I. and Richards M. *op. cit.*

76. Williams R. L. and Hawes W. E. *op. cit.*

77. Norwood C. Cesarean report: a relatively low cesarean rate in an urban population: lessons from the New York City Municipal System. Health and Hospitals Corporation, New York, unpublished, 1981.

78. Kerr M. G. Problems and perspectives in reproductive medicine. University of Edinburgh Inaugural Lecture, No. 61, Edinburgh, unpublished, 1975.

79. Minkoff H. L. and Schwartz R. The rising cesarean section rate: Can it safely be reversed? *Obstet. Gynec.* **56,** 135, 1980.

80. Consensus Development Conference, *op. cit.*

81. Francome D. and Huntingford P. L. Births by cesarean section in the United States of America and in Britain. *J. Biosoc. Sci.* **12,** 353, 1980.

Why People Sue: Sociological Determinants of Malpractice Suits within Hospitals

Irwin Press

The past dozen years have witnessed an astounding rise in costs relating to the prevention and management of medical malpractice claims. Not surprisingly, a crisis of trust has also been building over the same period. Public interest in alternatives to traditional health care has increased as has the plethora of defensive medical procedures in hospitals. In addition, the past decade has seen the rise of such hospital professions as risk management, patient representation, quality assurance, and utilization review. The current high interest in "patient services" and "patient relations" is just that—*current:* a reflection of low priority until gathering crises made such interests relevant.[1]

The cost crisis has led to both reactive and preventive behaviors on the part of hospital personnel. Reactive behaviors are those designed to respond to errors and claims after they occur. Examples are incident investigation, adjustment decisions, and insurance reserve manipulation. Preventive behaviors are designed to head off incidents before they occur, by identifying and reducing sources of clinical error, legal liability, and patient aggravation. Many risk management or quality assurance newsletters include as a regular feature a column listing examples of clinical error (including errors of documentation) which "could have been prevented." Books and articles wholly devoted to examples of clinical error are of particular interest to concerned risk managers.[2] Workshops on informed consent and documentation have drawn packed audiences.

All these books, articles, workshops, and symposia share the assumption that claims can be prevented, or payout minimized, through *mechanical*

This article originally appeared under the title "The Predisposition to File Claims: The Patient's Perspective" in *Law, Medicine and Health Care*, vol. 12, no. 2, 1984, pp. 53–62 and is reprinted with permission. Copyright © 1984, American Society of Law and Medicine, Boston, Massachusetts.

means—that is, via a reduction of medical error or an improvement in documentation. Unfortunately, this assumption has little empirical basis. There is no evidence which indicates that a significant drop in overall clinical error has occurred since the malpractice crisis began, despite the growth of such hospital departments as risk management and quality assurance. Indeed, the increasing rate of litigation has been accompanied by increasing attention to clinical practices and errors. Nor is there evidence suggesting that particular types of error invariably lead to claims, while others do not. Hospital administrators are well aware of the highly idiosyncratic nature of claims and patients' responses to maloccurrences. Similarly, a well-constructed, witnessed and signed consent form may not protect health care providers from suits. In the past two decades, cases such as *Canterbury v. Spence*[3] and *Wilkinson v. Harrington*[4] have demonstrated the courts' growing "material risk" approach—a view that the patient's perception of the exchange of information determines whether consent was informed, and that what is a reasonable disclosure in one instance may not be reasonable in another.[5] Thus, at least in the case of informed consent, a narrow focus upon the mechanical aspects of patient management may not even have a secure legal, let alone empirical, basis.

Given the questionable results thus far produced by an exclusive focus upon the mechanics of harm (whether via an act of medicine or documentation), it would seem that a new approach is required to supplement existing efforts to reduce medical and legal risks. This approach should focus upon patient perception of clinical care and harm.

The opinion that patient perceptions might indeed be relevant to malpractice claim prevention is now being tentatively expressed by some physicians and administrators.[6] The call for greater physician "rapport" with patients, however, does little good if the content and mechanism of establishing rapport are not specified. It is impossible to plan a strategy for overcoming such vague problems as poor "patient relations" or "lack of sensitivity." The goal of this article is to add to the beginning discussion of specifics in patients' perceptions and evaluations.

The cause and continuation of the malpractice crisis cannot result solely from errors by hospitals and physicians, waiting time in emergency rooms, interior decoration, or the legal profession. Rather, patients are perceiving more events and outcomes as negative or claimable. An analysis I made of closed claims at one large inner-city hospital revealed that close to half reflect ambiguous causes or damages: scars from emergency surgery considered unsightly; residual minor impairments from major life-saving treatment; unexpected medical or surgical outcomes when all procedures were routine.[7] These are not clear-cut errors and harm, but were perceived as such by patients or their families. These are formal claims (usually via legal representation), and for every such claim, risk managers usually receive a dozen or more "nuisance complaints" which never get to court, yet which require staff time, legal consultation, and, occasionally, bill write-offs.

Risk managers also have a thick file of serious incidents which never result in claims. Indeed, the number of harmed patients who actually enter a claim appears to be less than 5 percent.[8] This figure appears even smaller when one considers the rate of iatrogenic injury to hospital patients. Some estimate that as many as one-third of all patients may experience an iatrogenic incident.[9] Here, again, it is logical to assume that the operation of patient (or family) perception is a major factor in the genesis of claims. The rather simplistic phrase "Incidents don't sue—patients do" is a fair distillation of the notion that a maloccurrence in itself generates nothing. Rather, incidents (actual or imagined) must be transformed into lawsuits, and this transformation is a socio-emotional process, not a medical or legal one *per se*.[10] The transformation process can begin with either patient or family, and the role of family perceptions of management and interactions cannot be underestimated in the genesis of suits. As Horsley notes: "One thing is certain—if a patient is weighing the question of whether or not to sue, the doctor's indifference to the family in their time of stress can be the deciding factor."[11] "Injury by itself," comments Lander, "does not translate into the intense hostility that a lawsuit expresses. The objective sign must be joined with the subjective state of being angry. . . ."[12] Indeed, "without anger, an act as hostile as a lawsuit, particularly against as well-established an authority figure as a physician, is impossible to contemplate."[13] In short, the incident—the mechanical event itself—is insufficient to explain claims, and thus can only be a partial element in their prevention.

PATIENT PERCEPTION AND CLAIMS: AN INSUFFICIENTLY RESEARCHED AREA

Unfortunately, little research has been directed specifically to the operation of patients' perception and attitudes in the decision to seek a claim. Most data on the motivation to seek a claim are inferential only, and derive largely from studies which were not related to claims but which focused on general "patient satisfaction" or observations of doctor/patient interaction.

In one study, 65 percent of patients experiencing a "bad medical outcome" still expressed satisfaction with the medical care they had received.[14] The authors conclude that patients' evaluations of medical care are influenced primarily by "their assessment of the physician's effort. . . ."[15] A seminal study by Cay and his colleagues suggests that patients evaluate successful outcomes of peptic ulcer surgery more on the basis of psychosocial and interactive factors than upon physical outcome.[16] Segall and Burnett conclude that patients, lacking medical competence themselves, "must rely on the affective dimension of the doctor-patient relationship in evaluating the physician's role performance."[17] Ben-Sira finds that "mechanical" factors, such as waiting time and adequacy of staffing, seem unrelated to patients' reported satisfaction.[18] As Larson and Rootman put it, "satisfaction with medical care is influenced by the degree to which a doctor's *role* performance corresponds to the patient's expectations."[19] Patients' expectations of physicians' roles are based almost wholly upon patient beliefs, attitudes and psychosocial needs—not knowledge of appropriate professional behavioral standards.

Unfortunately, patient attitudes and evaluations of care generally do not receive administrators' attention unless the hospital has a "hot line" or mail-out questionnaire with adequate returns. Questionnaires, however, almost invariably use Likert-scaled items, which produce vague results (such as "nursing staff were *fairly* courteous") useless in pinpointing problems. Questionnaires, furthermore, often fail to contain items about physicians. One study found no correlation between patient satisfaction and staff merit raises, or nurse morale measured on the same services experienced by these patients.[20] Indeed, higher nurse morale was correlated with *lower* patient satisfaction. Researchers here concluded that hospitals and patients evaluate staff performance on very different bases.[21]

Physicians, too, often have little idea of their personal or medical impact upon patients. In observations of physicians' visits with their hospitalized patients, Waitzkin and Stoeckle noted that during an average 20-minute stay, less than one minute was spent by the physician informing the patient about the medical problem or treatment.[22] Patients, following such visits, were quite aware of this, while physicians reported spending 10 to 15 minutes in giving information.[23] Another researcher directly observed that physicians tend to talk more than patients during medical history-taking.[24] For their part, physicians so observed denied having talked more than their patients. Golden and Johnston noted that many physicians are unaware that patients experience "massive amounts of anxiety" during sickness and treatment.[25] Further, physicians tend to be unaware of the part played by their insensitivity to patients' socioemotional needs in patients' noncompliance,[26] and are generally unaware of the extent to which their patients are noncompliant.[27] Indeed, findings of 50 to 60 percent noncompliance are common. This study also found physicians to be unable to judge which of their patients were or would be noncompliant.[28]

While existing research does not directly demonstrate a relationship between the patient's perception of the medical event and the transformation of incidents (again, real or imagined) into claims, there is sufficient suggestion of this connection. Certainly, the very possibility of such a connection demands that we discuss and investigate it seriously. The following sections of this article offer a preliminary discussion of some specific factors which can affect patients' perceptions and their predisposition to claim. These factors most intimately define the patient's sickness and trigger his response to it and to the healing process.

PREDISPOSING AND PRECIPITATING FACTORS

Patients are the final judge of how well they are treated, how well they are healed, and whether they have been harmed in the process. Before entering a claim, patients must first perceive an injury. Such a perception, of course, is never automatic. It depends upon the degree to which the patient is predisposed to view treatment—and incidents—negatively.

Predisposing factors include consciously or subconsciously perceived events, interactions, and phenomena which the patient evaluates negatively, and which affect the patient's perception and evaluation of subsequent treatment and mistreatment. These factors, major or minor, accumulate during the patient's stay in the hospital—the wake-up call for medications at 2 A.M.; the cold lunch because of tests scheduled near noon; the walks in corridors where strangers of both sexes can see the catheter dangling from beneath the short gown and the urine-filled bag clutched in the patient's hand; the physician's quickly passing over the patient's ideas of what his sickness might be. These are all predisposing factors, and essentially condition the patient to expect negative events or to search for them.

Precipitating factors, in contrast, are specific, usually single incidents which trigger a predisposed patient's desire to make a claim. These include the more familiar errors and events that risk managers traditionally emphasize. Frequently, however, the precipitating factor is merely the last in a chain of events perceived negatively (and often unconsciously) by the patient. Predisposing factors are complex, involving subtle interactions between hospital and patient. Each responds to the other on the bases of long-established value systems, and each confronts sickness from its own perspective and with its own agenda.

PATIENT-GENERATED PREDISPOSING FACTORS

As a social scientist working in clinical settings, I have found that consciously or subconsciously, every hospitalized patient asks a multitude of questions about his experience. These questions range from why he is sick, to how his family can manage the complex treatment once he is discharged, to worries about the discomfort of the treatment. Patients ask: Will the physician and staff take my ideas and worries seriously? How emotional will they allow me to be? Will the sickness diminish me in terms of sexual, economic, and other roles? Will anyone con-

sider that I will miss events and obligations because of my sickness and hospitalization? Is there an alternative to this mode of treatment?

It should be noted that the patient also wonders about the housekeeping and hotel functions which figure so prominently in most patient-satisfaction questionnaires. Yet, housekeeping elements are the least important problems confronting the sick patient. It is likely, however, that patients complain heavily about these hostelry phenomena simply because they are intimidated by the health professional staff, dependent upon (and thus afraid to antagonize) them, or embarrassed at demonstrating their fears, inexperience and weakness.[29]

THE MYTH OF MEDICAL PERFECTION

The manner in which the hospital answers or handles these typical concerns contributes to the patient's perception of treatment. The concerns themselves reflect a number of underlying predisposing factors. The most significant of these (and those with broadest impact) are: (1) the general concepts and stereotypes of medicine that patients bring with them to the hospital; and (2) the manner in which the patient's *illness* is managed by the hospital.

The first—general stereotypes—reflects the public image of medicine. Chief among the elements of this image is the "myth of medical perfection." Both hospitals and physicians foster this notion of medical infallibility. Admission of susceptibility to error is viewed by health professionals as terrifying to potential patients—and likely to trigger malpractice suits. From the patient's perspective, medical perfection is desirable (as well as expected) for several rasons. First, one's life may depend upon it. Second, because biomedicine is a monopoly and prevents all competition, it should be perfect. Third, in an era of high technology and mechanical miracle, error becomes intolerable.[30] The "deification" of physicians is probably both a by-product and a cause of the myth of perfection, and stems from their monopoly over health resources. Whatever the reason, deification is an additional source of unreasonably high expectations about performance, which are further fostered by television programming's idealized image of the selfless, warm and sensitive health professional. No hospital, nurse, or physician can meet these constantly and publicly reinforced standards, but the average patient is predisposed to expect them.

ILLNESS VERSUS DISEASE

It is necessary in this analysis to make a convenient distinction between illness and disease.[31] "Disease" is the physical manifestation of sickness, as well as the official medical interpretation and labeling of sickness. "Illness" is the behavioral, emotional, and expressive component of sickness. Since patients' worries, comments, responses, interactions and beliefs about sickness far outnumber the disease components themselves, the bulk of any sickness episode is perceived as illness, not disease, by the patient. All discussions, recollections, comments, and opinions, as well as the medical history, given by the patient constitute illness—perceptions and sensations heavily affected by culture.

Symptoms are largely cultural constructs, from the initial act of identifying sensations as suggestive of sickness, to grouping them as a meaningful syndrome. An aching joint can be interpreted as stiffness resulting from a vigorous tennis game, or as a symptom of sickness such as arthritis. Pain tolerance itself has been shown to be affected by reference group values.[32] Complaining about pain is strongly affected by ethnic definitions of sickness as cues for social cohesion versus social isolation.[33] Different ethnic groups may focus attention upon symptoms in differing body locations as indicators of sickness.[34]

If symptoms have a large cultural component, responses to symptoms are pure culture. Symptoms are almost invariably discussed and evaluated with family and friends.[35] Decisions to self-treat, e.g., with patent medicines, old prescription drugs, or dietary shifts, are pure culture. Most sicknesses (whether seen by physicians or not) are self-limiting, and most never are seen by doctors.[36] Decisions to seek professional care stem as much from symptom-caused social inconvenience, e.g., disruption of everyday life or income or threat to self-image, as from purely physical discomfort. One study concludes that what underlies the final decision to seek medical care is still unknown—but it certainly is not the disease alone.[37] In sum, by the time the patient even sees a physician, his initial *disease* has been sifted through a fine-meshed screen of culture, and converted largely into the *illness* with which he finally presents. This illness is then expressed to the physician as verbal statements about symptoms, feelings and worries. The interaction with the clinical professional thus constitutes yet another cultural element in the evolution of sickness. It is affected by the doctor's and the patient's expectations of one another, social class and ethnic congruence, and other symbolic factors. These factors determine the content and style of the patient's presentation.

While the patient presents with illness, clinical medicine looks exclusively for disease. During research in Bogotá, Colombia, I found that patients of folk healers present with only one-half to two-thirds of the number of symptoms as do patients at the outpatient clinic of the city's major hospital (both groups of patients were identical socially, and many in each group used both healers and physicians regularly).[38] The reason for the difference is that folk healers accept any symptom offered by the patient while clinical physicians accept only those symptoms which fit official biomedical syndromes, or which fit the disease that the physician believes the patient may have. Thus, by presenting with "extra" symptoms, clinical patients in Bogotá increase the possibility that at least one of them will be validated by the physician's attention—thereby giving the patient some proprietary ownership of his own sickness. Patients may thus resent having several symptoms ignored or given cursory attention.

Illness consists of more than symptoms, decisions to seek relief, and presentation strategies. Every individual arrives at the hospital with a full-blown explanation for his sickness. This explanatory model consists of explanations for what the patient has, why he is afflicted and why at this time, and what the treatment should be.[39] The fact that all patients have such explanatory models (EMs) reflects the significant anxiety and threat caused by all episodes of sickness. Such EMs may or may not conform to official orthodox biomedical models, but they enable the patient to understand and attack the unpredictable and threatening. All humans (whether jungle primitives or American urbanites) have a large repertoire of explanatory models. Most self-treat, and most do not seek medical help. Because most sickness episodes are self-limiting, there is usually a return to health, thus reinforcing the EMs employed.

EMs can have multiple origins. In the United States population, explanatory models derive from archaic biomedical beliefs, contemporary mass fads, individual family traditions, ethnic group repertoires, and "common sense."[40] Examples of EMs that I obtained at a major inner-city hospital include: "Hypertension is reflected in tenseness and irritability; so when you feel calm, the pressure is down;" "I think I lost my baby because I started having sex when I was only 14;" and "Diabetes is a sweetness of the blood; eating sour things (lemon, aloe, vinegar) will cure it."

Popular and/or folk EMs are employed for each bout of sickness, and vary by region, rural or urban residence, ethnicity, race, generation, and social class. They affect decisions to seek medical care, interaction and expectations during care, and compliance afterward. It is easy—and misguided—to assume that a white, English-speaking, non-ethnic "standard American" patient will have EMs generally conforming to the biomedical paradigm, and that his response to sickness will be "rational." Unfortunately, there is no such thing as a standard response to sickness and hospitalization. Lower and middle class non-ethnic "WASPs" may differ significantly in EMs and strategies of resort to treatment; the literature on class and response to illness is huge.[41]

Where ethnicity is involved, EMs may vary dramatically from official biomedical concepts and practices. Latin American, African, and Asian peasant and tribal medical traditions are generally humoral in nature, with disease causal concepts linked to maintenance of balance between body, personality, environment, and social context. In such systems, diseases can be caused by such factors as other humans, social and ritual dysjuncture, weather, supernaturals, and purely mechanical means. Here, health and healing are as much social as physical phenomena, and are inseparable from everyday events and places.[42] Where disease is linked to social, religious, and economic life, it threatens a broad spectrum of human concerns and cannot be perceived as being effectively treated if such human concerns are not addressed. The United States has many migrants who still adhere to such variant medical systems or to remnants of them. Elsewhere, I have indicated the broad range of social, economic and psychological functions which ethnic or folk EMs can play, even for urbanites in United States cities.[43]

In conclusion, explanatory models—whether mundane or exotic—are logical and meaningful to the patient, and are invariably mobilized when sickness occurs. EMs form a significant part of the cultural baggage which all patients bring to the clinical setting.

There are additional factors. All humans—particularly adult ones—fill numerous societal and private roles which are generally threatened by sickness. Self-image suffers when sexual, parental, collegial, and other obligations are faced with curtailment. Threats to one's role and image are even greater in the clinical setting, where the already threatened individual is isolated from even the familiar physical trappings of control and competence. The hospital environment provides no potential for the maintenance or the resumption of the obligations, identities, and rewards now undermined by sickness. First-time hospital patients can be severely traumatized by this new experience, thus exacerbating the already significant anxieties created by the disease and its effects on one's role and self-image. Lewis notes:

> For certain medical purposes it might be just as relevant to classify illnesses according to the social attributes of the people affected . . . or by social effects of the illness (stigma, interference with obligations at work, in the home, job performance, chronic or fleeting social inconvenience). Such features as these may correlate better with differences in the behavior of people ill (for instance, delay in seeking advice, readiness to comply with treatment, liability to relapse after discharge) than features that are intrinsic to the kind of disease they suffer from.[44]

Cassell has recently decried modern medicine's inattention to patients' "suffering" (a socio-emotional response to disease, not to be confused with "pain"). People, he comments, "are their roles" and, when sick, "suffer from what they have lost of themselves in relation to the world of objects, events, and relationships. . . . Although medical care can reduce the impact of sickness, inattentive care can increase the disruption caused by illness."[45]

All of these factors—the symptom sensations

and definitions, the attitudes towards health providers, the perceptions of healers and hospitals, the explanatory models, and threats to roles—comprise illness. It is always brought to the hospital along with the disease. Often the elements of illness far outnumber the perceived symptoms of disease. Hospitals and biomedical health care professionals, however, are trained to deal with disease, not illness. Yet, it is the perceived attention to illness that predisposes the patient to a positive or a negative evaluation of his treatment—often long before any maloccurrence.

HOSPITAL VALUES

It is not that patients enter the hospital already predisposed to evaluate its treatment and personnel negatively. Of course, the myth of medical perfection affects pre-hospitalization expectations, but the patient's overall predisposition largely depends upon the manner in which the hospital interacts with his illness. The illness, in short, is the raw material, and the hospital's response can convert this raw material into a negative predisposition. The hospital's response reflects basic clinical predisposing factors, which, no less than the patient's illness, are cultural in nature and reflect values, roles, and legal and economic decisions that are no more scientific, valid or natural than those of the patient. By implication, therefore, they are open to modification.

We can speak of two ways in which hospital predisposing factors are culturally generated: through common medical and clinical values and through the organization of clinical care. Major values include the assumption that only physicians with their specialized training know medicine. Nurses may know a little about medicine, but generally not enough to diagnose, call for tests, or prescribe medications in the physician's absence. The patient, however, knows nothing; in effect, "the customer is always wrong." This value, of course, puts a minimal premium upon eliciting (let alone negotiating with) the patient's explanatory model.[46] It also tends to suppress the provision of information to patients: there is no reason to provide this information if patients do not have the special knowledge to evaluate it properly. While many physicians do ask patients if there is anything they would like to know, patients are often intimidated and incapable of articulating specific queries which can make sense of the strange information just given by the physician. Information-providing often occurs only as part of the mandated informed consent. As such, it is usually one-way, with the providers selecting the agenda.

A corollary value holds that because modern medicine is scientific and true, it works independently of patients' thoughts, desires, and personalities. There are two major consequences of this assumption. One is that patients' anxieties and explanatory models may be considered irrelevant to medical management. The second is that if a patient is noncompliant or insists on his EM, he is considered to be "acting out" and is a potential candidate for a psychiatric consultation. This consequence is reflected in a recent study by Ries and his colleagues, who report that nearly half of all calls by medical staff for psychiatric consultations result from poor interaction and understanding between patients and staff, rather than from patients' problems.[47]

Another basic clinical value leads to the assumption that the patient is able to leave his daily life outside when he enters the hospital. This life is not considered to be the concern of the hospital, nor is it expected to be the patient's. Physicians' sensitivity to the threats made by illness to patients' roles and identities is generally low.[48] History-taking (the basic tool of doctor/patient interaction) is not heavily stressed in medical schools, and doctors frequently talk more than their patients.[49] Interpersonal factors are downplayed in favor of clinical indicators; if the patient has a legitimate address and does not complain, non-medical data are not usually elicited.[50] Where social, economic, familial, and other role problems are expressed, non-medical consultation is frequently sought. By giving these problems to social workers, chaplains, or psychiatrists, clinical medicine is clearly separating disease from illness, and the patient from his social and emotional self.

Another value (which also diminishes the clinical importance of socioeconomic and emotional factors) results in the view of the hospital patient as mainly concerned with diagnosis and treatment of his disease, not with such matters as personal dignity. This leads to such hospital conventions as shared rooms, short gowns, public X-ray areas (which often contain outpatients in street clothes) and other assaults on patients' sensitivities. It is a cornerstone of hospital values that the patient leaves all identity and dignity behind when entering the world of sickness and healing.

The patient must also surrender his autonomy—yet another clinical value. Knowing nothing, and being the legal responsibility of the hospital, he must conform to clinical schedules, treatment modes, and behavioral requirements. Lifelong habits and ego-reinforcing modes of environmental control must be abandoned.

A final value reflects the notion that medical professionals are too busy for "trivia," which usually refers to minor medical problems or irrelevant behavioral manifestations. Here the patient is placed in a double bind. On the one hand, he is expected to know enough about medicine to engage in the self-triage of unimportant symptoms so as to avoid presenting trivia to the physician or, once in the hospital, to avoid requesting nursing care for them. On the other hand, the patient is expected to "have no knowledge and to passively accept what the physician (or hospital) offers."[51] The result for the patient can be confusion and resentment. Knowing neither medicine nor hospital protocol, he must relinquish control over his own sickness and medical management, voicing few questions and worries, or risk being labelled a "crock" which frequently results in slower patient care.

CLINICAL ORGANIZATION

Aside from the values themselves, the ways in which medical care and hospitals are organized significantly affect interactions with patients and their illnesses. One significant organizational aspect concerns the fact that only physicians are licensed to diagnose, test, and treat patients. Patients are aware that nursing and other staff have only limited managerial powers. As a result, when the physician leaves, the patient can easily feel abandoned or have anxiety.

Another organizational aspect is that hospitals are generally geared to deal with sick people, not their healthy retainers. This is reflected in the lack of planned space in sickrooms for families, if not in the visiting policies. The fact that increased room size and more comfortable furnishings will undoubtedly affect hospital revenue is not at issue here, because malpractice claims, successful or not, also affect revenue. Because our medical system generally downplays the effect of symbolic or social phenomena upon either sickness or healing, it tends to view the family as a socially, but not a medically, necessary factor in patient management. Whereas families of young children and the elderly are usually brought into discussions of treatment and post-discharge strategy, the kin of alert, competent adult patients is often neglected. A recent study of emergency room nurses reveals more tolerance for patient emotional outbursts than for emotional demonstrations of family members who accompany them.[52] This is not surprising; the patient, of course, is the sick one. But it reflects a common view that the patient's family is, at best, peripheral to the state of sickness and the process of healing. If the patient's emotionalism is suspect and distracting, his family's demonstrations of anxiety are unacceptable. The above study noted emergency room nurses' tendency to view any emotionalism as more appropriately attended by psychiatric nurses than by themselves.

Underestimation of the effect of family upon patients' attitudes can have serious consequences, with patient compliance and healing directly affected.[53] Equally significant, patients rarely initiate lawsuits without consulting first with significant family members. Where the family as well as the patient have experienced negative interaction with the hospital, the predisposition to claim may be higher.[54]

Another organizational aspect that generates hospitals' predisposing factors concerns the fact that clinical treatment involves only either inpatient or outpatient modes. Although a number of hospitals now offer significant outpatient services and such innovations as same-day surgery, inpatient philosophy is still largely "all or nothing." Procedures for releasing patients temporarily are non-existent or poorly articulated. Patients frequently languish over weekends for tests scheduled on a Monday morning, or are hospitalized for entire days for one or two one-hour diagnostic procedures. It is easy to ignore the fact that patients may be more inconvenienced by the hospitalization than by the sickness itself, once acute symptoms have subsided. Policies which accommodate some patients' needs to be elsewhere for periods during hospitalization might significantly alleviate role stresses that could otherwise lead to a negative predisposition.

The specialized training and skills required of hospital staff necessitate a specialized language for efficient, minimal-error communication. This language also serves, however, to reinforce the hospital staff's higher level of status and competence, and it can confuse and frighten the patient. More important, clinical language is not designed for healer-client interaction, negotiation, or consensus. It is a one-way language that conveys inadequacy along with (and often instead of) information to the patient. Because patients do not know the medical language, it is easy for clinical personnel to fall into the erroneous assumption that patients thus do not have their own terms and concepts for body parts, conditions, or symptoms. Actually, patients are vast repositories of terms for body parts, diseases, causes, and effects.[55]

The increasing dependence of modern hospitals upon complex machinery places them increasingly beyond the comprehension and everyday experience of patients. The machinery depersonalizes and intimidates the patient who has received little or no information. The symbolic effect of clinical procedures upon patients cannot be ignored. For example, fetal heart monitors and IVs are routinely employed in labor rooms around the country. They are used just in case something should happen (e.g., an irregularity in the fetal heart beat or a blood pressure crash). In most cases, there is no incident, yet not to utilize them (and document the use) is to ask for a claim in the event of complications. Thus, they are used for legal as much as medical purposes. Such measures also have the effect of telling the maternity patient that she is sick and dependent and that birth is not a natural process, but one which requires active intervention by specialists and specialized machinery. The procedures imply that she is a dependent. It stands to reason, therefore, that *any* complication is the hospital's fault, not hers.

This raises the general issue of the *claim-generating potential* of patient management modes which have high *dependency-producing impact*. The implications of this extend beyond obstetrics to all clinical patients. It would be useful to investigate the post-discharge claim rates of patients who had varying degrees of invasive and regimented procedures while hospitalized (particularly procedures which kept them bed- or room-ridden), and how patients perceive clinical procedures in the first place. Such routine invasive techniques as IV might be found extremely dependency-producing to an average patient.

Hospitals, unlike families, operate on shifts. This necessarily results in discontinuity of personnel. Patients may feel reluctant or resentful of having to reestablish sick roles and modus vivendi with personnel who at the very least have not seen them for 16 hours. Discontinuity is also significant in teaching hospitals when resident rotations occur.

A different sort of discontinuity is created by staff specialization, which guarantees that the patient will be functionally dismembered, with the parts distributed to a variety of staff members with differing ranks and tasks. This is unquestionably the most depersonalizing aspect of the entire clinical encounter. It could easily outweigh a host of other factors that make patients dislike their clinical experiences. The anxiety created by this lack of continuity in care may have a significant impact upon predisposition to claim. The most obvious effect upon the patient is his suspicion that no single person is wholly "in charge" and his concern that the attending physician is not keeping track of the data generated and procedures delivered by diverse specialists during the clinical stay. Most attending physicians visit patients for only a few minutes per day. That the attending physician may have already perused the charts and spoken with staff in the nursing station is not obvious to the patient, who sees the physician's brief visit as the day's medical highlight. It thus seems that time should be focused on major treatment strategies and prognoses, for physician visits do not usually seem appropriate for minor queries, gripes, or rambling interrogative sessions. The question of who is in charge is easily converted into a question about who is responsible. The lack of a coherent personal relationship with the clinic can result in the most impersonal of quests for remedy—the claim.

A final element is related to both hospital values and organization. The very efficiency of the modern clinic, its mechanical wizardry, and its never-ending stream of minimally to spectacularly sick patients foster an understandably blasé attitude on the part of staff. To staff members, upper chest infections are routine. But to the hard-breathing patient, this new and terrifying problem is life-shattering (not least because it threatens his values and roles). Errors or incidents caused by apparently blasé attendants—as opposed to obviously concerned collaborators in the treatment of a serious and anxiety-provoking condition—are more likely to predispose the patient to claim.

A CONCLUDING COMMENT

These are but some of the factors ostensibly generated within the clinical milieu that predispose patients to file claims. These phenomena appear to operate apart from outright error and incident to affect the patient's evaluation of his clinical experience. These factors, I suggest, involve the interaction of the cultures of both the patient and the clinic. The relationship between this interaction and the predisposition to file claims begs for extensive research. We have enough information at present to look to such research less for actual corroboration than for specific mechanisms and linkages. . . .

References

1. The crisis is still growing. Contrary to the belief that the peak of 1973–75 is past, claims are costing more than ever. St. Paul Fire and Marine Insurance Company (the nation's largest malpractice insurer) estimates that while the actual number of suits may be dropping, cost per exposure is increasing dramatically—up 63 percent between 1976 and 1981. ST. PAUL AND MARINE INSURANCE, PERSPECTIVE SPECIAL #1 (February 1981).

2. *See, e.g.,* N. M. Davis, *et al.,* Medication Errors (George F. Stickley, Publisher, Philadelphia, Penna.) (1981); Furrow, B. R., *Iatrogenesis and Medical Error: The Case for Medical Malpractice,* Law, Medicine & Health Care 9(5): 4–7 (October 1981).

3. Canterbury v. Spence, 464 F.2d 722 (D.C. Cir.), *cert. denied,* 409 U.S. 1064 (1972).

4. Wilkinson v. Harrington (Wilkinson v. Vesey), 243 A.2d 745 (R.I. 1968).

5. Miller, L. J., *Informed Consent, Parts I–IV,* Journal of the American Medical Association 244(15): 2100–03 (November 7, 1980); 244(20): 2347–50 (November

21, 1980); 244(22): 2556–58 (December 5, 1980); 244(23): 2661–62 (December 12, 1980).

6. *See* Vaccarino, J. M., *Malpractice: The Problem in Perspective,* Journal of the American Medical Association 238(3): 861–63 (August 22, 1977); Ladenburger, M., *quoted in* Occurrence 3(6): 4(1983).

7. Press, I., Report to the Department of Risk Management, Jackson Memorial Hospital, Miami, Fla. (1982).

8. St. Paul Fire & Marine Ins. Co., Property and Liability Division Report (1982) (claims per physician were 3.4 percent; hospital claims per exposure were 2.5 percent).

9. Steel, K., *et al., Iatrogenic Illness on a General Medical Service at a University Hospital,* New England Journal of Medicine 304(11): 638–42 (March 12, 1981).

10. Felsteiner, W., Abel, R., Sarat, A., *The Emergence and Transformation of Disputes: Naming, Blaming, Claiming . . . ,* Law and Society Review 15(3 & 4): 631–54 (1980/1981).

11. Horsley, J., *Turning Off the Patient's Family Can Turn On a Lawsuit,* Medical Economics, 56:119, 129 (January 22, 1979).

12. Lander, L., *Why Some People Seek Revenge Against Doctors,* Psychology Today 12(2): 88, 90–91 (July 1978).

13. *Id.* at 91.

14. Woolley, F. R., *et al., Research Note: The Effects of Doctor-Patient Communication on Satisfaction and Outcome of Care,* Social Science and Medicine 12A(2): 123, 127 (March 1978).

15. *Id.*

16. Cay, E. L., *et al., Patients' Assessment of the Result of Surgery for Peptic Ulcer,* Lancet, pp. 29, 30 (January 4, 1975).

17. Segall, A., Burnett, M., *Patient Evaluation of Physician Role Performance,* Social Science and Medicine 14A(4): 269, 277 (July 1980).

18. Ben-Sira, Z., *The Function of the Professional's Affective Behavior in Client Satisfaction: A Revised Approach to Social Interaction Theory,* Journal of Health & Social Behavior 17(1): 3–11 (March 1976).

19. Larson, D., Rootman, I., *Physician Role Performance and Patient Satisfaction,* Social Science and Medicine 10(1): 29 (January 1976) (emphasis added).

20. Taylor, P. W., *et al., Development and Use of a Method of Assessing Patient Perception of Care,* Hospital and Health Services Administration 26:89–99 (Winter 1981).

21. *Id.*

22. Waitzkin, H., Stoeckel, J., *Information Control and the Micropolitics of Health Care: Summary of an Ongo-*

ing Research Project, Social Science and Medicine 10(6): 263, 264 (June 1976).

23. *Id.*

24. Bain, D. J., *Doctor-Patient Communication in General Practice Consultations,* Medical Education 10(2): 125–31 (March 1976).

25. Golden, J., Johnston, G., *Problems of Distortion in Doctor-Patient Communications,* Psychiatry in Medicine 1: 127–49 (1970).

26. Hulka, B., *et al., Communication, Compliance, and Concordance Between Physicians and Patients With Prescribed Medications,* American Journal of Public Health 66(9): 847–53 (September 1976); Sackett, D. L., Snow, J., *The Magnitude and Measurement of Compliance,* in COMPLIANCE IN HEALTH CARE (R. Haynes, *et al.,* eds.) (Johns Hopkins University Press, Baltimore, Md.) (1979).

27. Norell, S. E., *Accuracy of Patient Interviews and Estimates by Clinical Staff in Determining Medication Compliance,* Social Science and Medicine 15E(1):57, 59 (February 1981).

28. *Id.*

29. A study I recently completed in three hospitals in South Bend, Indiana, revealed that hostelry items constitute approximately 45 percent of total complaints, while 25 percent of the patients complained about quality of interaction with physicians and nurses.

30. B. Marks, THE SUING OF AMERICA (Seaview, New York, N.Y.) (1981) at 21.

31. Eisenberg, L., *Disease and Illness: Distinction Between Professional and Popular Ideas of Sickness,* Culture, Medicine, and Psychiatry 1(1): 9–23 (April 1977) at 9.

32. Lambert, W. E., *et al., The Effect of Increased Salience of a Membership Group on Pain Tolerance,* Journal of Personality 38: 350–57 (1960).

33. Zborowski, M., *Cultural Components in Responses to Pain,* Journal of Social Issues 8: 16–30 (1952).

34. Zola, I. K., *Culture and Symptoms: An Analysis of Patients' Presenting Complaints,* American Sociological Review 31(5): 615, 630 (October 1966).

35. *See generally* Suchman, E. A., *Stages of Illness and Medical Care,* Journal of Health and Human Behavior 6(3): 114–28 (Fall 1965); E. Freidson, PATIENTS' VIEWS OF MEDICAL PRACTICE: A STUDY OF SUBSCRIBERS TO A PREPAID MEDICAL PLAN IN THE BRONX (Russell Sage Foundation, New York, N.Y.) (1961).

36. Alpert, J., *et al., A Month of Illness and Health Care Among Low-Income Families,* Public Health Report 82(8): 705, 713 (August 1969); White, K., *et al., The*

Ecology of Medical Care, New England Journal of Medicine 265(18): 885, 890–91 (November 2, 1961).

37. Zola, I. K., *Studying the Decision to See a Doctor,* Advances in Psychosomatic Medicine 8: 216–36 (1972).

38. Press, I., *Urban Illness: Physicians, Curers, and Dual Use in Bogotá,* Journal of Health and Social Behavior 19: 209–18 (1969). *See* Good, M. J., Good, B., *Patient Requests in Primary Care Clinics,* in CLINICALLY APPLIED ANTHROPOLOGY (N. Crisman, T. Maretzky, eds.) (D. Reidel, Dordrecht, Holland) (1982) at 292.

39. A. Kleinman, EXPLANATORY MODELS IN HEALTH CARE RELATIONSHIPS (National Council for International Health: Health of the Family, Washington, D.C.) (1975) at 159–72.

40. *See* Press, I., *Problems in the Definition and Classification of Medical Systems,* Social Science and Medicine 14B(1): 45–57 (February 1980) (discussing the difference between popular and folk medical beliefs and systems). *See also* Weidman, H., *"Falling-Out": A Diagnostic and Treatment Problem Viewed from a Transcultural Perspective,* Social Science and Medicine 13B: 95–112 (1979) (southern black "falling out"); L. Cohn, CULTURE, DISEASE, AND STRESS AMONG LATINO IMMIGRANTS: RIIES SPECIAL STUDY (Research Institute on Immigration and Ethnic Studies, Washington, D.C.) (1979) (hypertension beliefs); Snow, L., *Folk Medical Beliefs and Their Implications for Care of Patients,* Annals of Internal Medicine 84:82–96 (1974) (black American medical concepts); Blumhagen, D., *Hyper-Tension: A Folk Illness with a Medical Name,* Culture, Medicine and Psychiatry 4(3): 197–227 (September 1980) (hypertension beliefs); Helman, C. G., *"Feed a Cold, Starve a Fever"—Folk Models of Infection in an English Suburban Community, and Their Relation to Medical Treatment,* Culture, Medicine and Psychiatry 2(2): 107–37 (June 1978) (non-ethnic beliefs about cold and fever treatment).

41. *See, e.g.,* E. Koos, THE HEALTH OF REGIONVILLE (Columbia University Press, New York, N.Y.) (1954); Hinkle L. E., *et al., An Examination of the Relation Between Symptoms, Disability, and Serious Illness in Two Homogeneous Groups of Men and Women,* American Journal of Public Health 50(9): 1327–36 (September 1960); Rosenblatt, D., Suchman, M., *Blue Collar Attitudes and Information Toward Health and Illness,* in BLUE COLLAR WORLD: STUDIES OF THE AMERICAN WORKER (A. Shostak, W. Gomberg, eds.) (Prentice-Hall, Englewood Cliffs, N.J.) (1964); R. Duff, A. Hollingshead, SICKNESS AND SOCIETY (Harper & Row, New York, N.Y.) (1968); *A Month of Illness and Health Care Among Low-Income Families, supra* note 36; J. Kosa, *et al.,* POVERTY AND HEALTH: A SOCIOLOGICAL ANALYSIS (Har-

vard University Press, Cambridge, Mass.) (1969); Rosenstock, I., Kirscht, J., *Why People Seek Health Care,* in HEALTH PSYCHOLOGY: A HANDBOOK: THEORIES, APPLICATIONS, AND CHALLENGES TO THE HEALTH CARE SYSTEM (G. C. Stone, *et al.,* eds.) (Jossey-Bass, Inc., San Francisco, Calif.) (1979).

42. H. Fabrega, Jr., DISEASE AND SOCIAL BEHAVIOR (MIT Press, Cambridge, Mass.) (1974) at 247–56; Foster, G., *Disease Etiologies in Non-Western Medical Systems,* American Anthropologist 78(4): 773–82 (December 1976).

43. Press, I., *Urban Folk Medicine: A Functional Overview,* American Anthropologist 80(1): 71–84 (March 1978).

44. Lewis, G., *Cultural Influences on Illness Behavior: A Medical Anthropologist Approach,* in THE RELEVANCE OF SOCIAL SCIENCE FOR MEDICINE (L. Eisenberg, A. Kleinman, eds.) (D. Reidel, Dordrecht, Holland) (1981) at 156.

45. Cassell, E. J., *The Nature of Suffering and the Goals of Medicine,* New England Journal of Medicine 306(11): 639, 642 (March 18, 1982).

46. Waitzkin, J., *Medicine, Superstructure, and Micropolitics,* Social Science and Medicine 13A(6): 601–09 (November 1979).

47. Ries, R., *et al., Psychiatric Consultation-Liaison Service: Patients' Requests, Functions,* General Hospital Psychiatry 2(3): 204–212 (September 1980).

48. Cassell, *supra* note 45, at 639.

49. Bain, *supra* note 24.

50. Platt, F., McMath, J., *Clinical Hypocompetence: The Interview,* Annals of Internal Medicine 91(6): 898–902 (December 1979).

51. Twaddle, A., *Sickness and the Sickness Cancer: Some Implications,* in THE RELEVANCE OF SOCIAL SCIENCE FOR MEDICINE, *supra* note 44, at 124. For further discussion of the double bind, see Bloor, M., Horobin, G., *Conflict and Conflict Resolution in Doctor/Patient Interactions,* in SOCIOLOGY OF MEDICAL PRACTICE (C. Cox, A. Mead, eds.) (Collier-MacMillan, London, Eng.) (1975) at 271–84; FRIEDSON, *supra* note 35.

52. Yoder, L., Jones, S., *The Family of the Emergency Room Patient as Seen through the Eyes of the Nurse,* International Journal of Nursing Studies 19: 29–36 (1982).

53. DiMatteo, M., Hays, R., *Social Support and Serious Illness,* in SOCIAL NETWORKS AND SOCIAL SUPPORT (B. Gottlieb, ed.) (Sage Publications, Beverly Hills, Calif.) (1981) at 117–48; Pisarcik, G., *et al., Psychiatric Nurses in the Emergency Room,* American Journal of Nursing 79(7): 1264–66 (July 1979).

54. Horsley, *supra* note 11.

55. *See* Boyle, C. M., *Differences Between Patients' and Doctors' Interpretations of Some Common Medical Terms,* in SOCIOLOGY OF MEDICAL PRACTICE, *supra* note 51, at 299–308.

_____

CHAPTER 11

The Social Organization of Palliative Care

Palliative care refers to the care given to patients who are not curable. It is most commonly associated with the care employed in the service of terminally-ill cancer patients. A relatively new approach to palliative care is the hospice movement, which brings that kind of care to cancer patients and which improves the quality of life in the final phase of one's life. In England, where the hospice movement developed, a great deal of palliative care is given in house—that is, in hospitals designed particularly for the terminally ill. Although such facilities are now found throughout the United States, the emphasis of hospice care in this country is on serving patients at home. Thus, the hospice described by Joan Kron has only a small number of beds, but it is the hospice for the entire state of Connecticut. It is regarded as a backup for the care available in the community.

Nursing homes, which will become even more strategically important as the age of the U.S. population continues to increase, provide a mix of palliative and curative care. The older the nursing home resident, the more likely it is that the mix will emphasize palliative care.

The first article, by Joan Kron, describes the development of the New Haven Hospice—actually the Connecticut Hospice. She looks at its innovative architectural features as well as the priority given to the feelings of the families of patients. When Kron wrote the article, the Connecticut Hospice had not yet opened; it opened its doors on July 7, 1980. Attached to the end of the Kron article is a postscript written by John D. Thompson, a founder of the Connecticut Hospice (and a member of the faculty of the Yale Medical School), and Rosemary Hurzeler, its Executive Director. The second article, by Robert W. Buckingham, III, and his colleagues, presents a discussion of a participant-observation study of the relative merits of standard hospital care versus hospice care for the dying. Because of the great difficulty in gathering data on the lives of the dying and their caretakers, Buckingham played the role of a cancer patient. With an elaborate deception and the aid of physicians, he spent two days in the holding unit, four days on a surgical care ward, and four days on the palliative or hospice care ward of the Royal Victoria Hospital in Montreal. Buckingham's findings support the effectiveness of the hospice system of care for the hopelessly ill.

In the final article in this chapter, J. Neil Henderson introduces us to the notion of "lower participants"—that is, staff at the lower levels of the organizational hierarchy. Marcia Millman (1976) has discussed the questionable care provided by some aides and orderlies on the hospital nightshift. Many articles have been written about the same kind of questionable care by lower-level staff in the nursing home. The most well known, perhaps, is one written by Charles Stannard (1973) concerning the social conditions leading to the abuse of nursing home residents by orderlies and aides. J. Neil Henderson counterbalances these articles by showing how nursing home housekeepers provide an informal and largely unrecognized but very important source of emotional support for patients.

References

STANNARD, C. I. 1973. Old Folks and Dirty Work: The Social Conditions for Patients Abuse in a Nursing Home. *Social Problems* 20: 329–342.
MILLMAN, M. 1976. *The Unkindest Cut*. William Morrow and Company, Inc., Chapter 8.

Designing a Better Place to Die: Structural Characteristics of the Hospice

Joan Kron

I have seen the plans for the New Haven Hospice and I like them. It will change our lives and our deaths—even if we don't live near New Haven.

The hospice movement has arrived from England, and America is ready for it, although most people don't have the vaguest idea what hospices are. But they know why they need them.

Death is on the mind. The Karen Anne Quinlan dilemma and the death-defying efforts of Franco's physicians have sent a number of people I know into panic and therefore into the offices of their physicians with signed Living Wills. (The Euthanasia Educational Council reports that at the height of the Quinlin publicity, requests for the L. W. doubled.)

Granted, some people want every extra dollop of life that medical technology can scrape out of the bowl for them, no matter how severe the physical or emotional suffering. But more and more people I talk to are concerned instead about increasing the *quality* of the last days of life.

Certainly psychiatrist Elisabeth Kübler-Ross, author of the best-seller *On Death and Dying,* has made more people aware of the emotional pain of the terminal patient. Yet anyone who's recently kept a vigil over a critically ill patient knows that in most hospitals very little has changed—the psychological and social needs of the patient, not to mention the family, must still be subordinated to the needs of the institution. This often translates into such travesties as patients dying alone while loved ones are forced to wait out in the hall. And we've heard too often about patients being denied painkillers for fear of addiction.

But awareness precedes change, and change in the care of the dying is on the way. "The old idea of one hospital to satisfy all needs is a thing of the past," says hospital design consultant John Thompson, who has just coauthored a comprehensive design book on the subject, *The Hospital: A Social and Architectural History.*

"We need a *series* of institutions," he says. "We'll always need some health-care factories for efficient, short-term, intensive-care stays, but we'll need others where humanity won't have to overcome the technical apparatus.

"In the terminal situation, the family is as necessary as any other form of care. But we exclude families from intensive-care units. The hospice represents one type of facility where family interaction is possible."

If care of the dying is changing, credit must go to Dr. Cicely Saunders, the dynamic 57-year-old physician who started rewriting the modern deathbed scene (and the days that lead up to it) in 1967 when she opened London's now-renowned St. Christopher's Hospice. Not exactly a traditional hospice (which is a way station for travelers), St. Christopher's is a way station for the dying—a place where people in the final stages of degenerative disease, such as cancer, can go when surgery, chemotherapy, and radiation have failed to cure—a place to go when the doctor says, "There's no more to be done."

"I didn't invent this use of the word *hospice,*" Saunders says, but she has made it synonymous not only with humane care but also with good medical practice.

The six-foot-tall Saunders is a former nurse and medical social worker who went back to school at age 33 to become a physician in order to "look into the problem of pain in the dying patient." A no-nonsense woman, she sees herself as a spokeswoman for the patient, and she resists efforts to romanticize her, a la Florence Nightingale, by joking about her "tarnished halo and feet of clay." But thousands of grateful patients can't be wrong. For them she has taken much of the fear out of the fear of dying.

"People think of St. Christopher's as a place with a little religious music playing in the background," says Saunders, but although it has a very strong religious foundation, she sees it as a cross between a hospital and a patient's own home.

"A kind of convalescent home—no, more like a family . . ." is the way one patient described it in St. Christopher's 1974–75 annual report. Others say: "Not like a hospital—like a big parlour"; "A place where people know what they're doing"; "A kind of annex to a hospital—where you can get better slowly"; and where those who don't get better "have comfort to the end."

At St. Christopher's the unit of care is not just the patient, but also the family; the place of care is the patient's home —where studies show most people would prefer to die —for as long as possible. In fact, St. Christopher's cheery 54-bed inpatient facility is actually a backup unit and patients often go back and forth between the hospice and home. The health care itself is a team effort involving medical, nursing, and social workers, psychiatric and religious workers, and family members. And care doesn't end when the patient dies. Social workers and volunteers follow the family to help them adjust to bereavement. "It's basically very simple, what we do," Saunders says. "It's a family community—a caring place," where nurses are encouraged to sit on a patient's bed, where family members are encouraged to help in the care—give a sponge bath, bring food from home, whatever. Visiting hours there are unlimited except for a day off on Monday—not for the staff's convenience, but because Saunders believes that families need a day off to do the laundry and other personal chores without feeling guilty. And if a patient wants to see a favorite pet, it can visit. So can children, and there's a daycare center on the premises for the children of staff members.

Sounds no different from a good convalescent home, you might say. But it's different in one crucial way. St. Christopher's is known for its expertise in controlling the symptoms of degenerative disease— the nausea, weakness, difficulty in breathing, etc.,

and most important, the pain. Brompton's mixture— a centuries-old formula containing diamorphine (heroin), cocaine, alcohol, syrup, and chloroform water—is used there with excellent results, without psychological addiction and without sacrificing the patient's alertness. The reason for St. Christopher's success in overcoming pain, Saunders believes, is that medication is never administered PRN (*pro re nata,* "as needed"), but before it is needed, to prevent pain and fear of pain, as well as to prevent feelings of dependency in patients who have to ask for relief to get it.

St. Christopher's has no sophisticated resuscitation equipment, explains Saunders, carefully phrasing her answer to this touchy question, "because we do not treat acute remedial patients. We might resuscitate staff or visitors, which we have done on occasion, but mainly we treat irremedial illness. But we certainly do all we can to fulfill a patient's potential for living well until he dies."

As the afflicted flock to Lourdes, so the healthcare professionals flock to St. Christopher's—not for care, but for inspiration. And the dozens I've spoken to have all given it the ultimate accolade. "I often think if I were dying of a terminal illness," said Harvard psychologist William Worden at a recent conference on death and dying, "that I'd like to die at St. Christopher's." So it was inevitable that "the Gospel according to Cicely," as Canadian urologist Balfour Mount fondly refers to it, would beget hospices elsewhere. Mount has recently established a twelve-bed palliative-care unit in Montreal's Royal Victoria Hospital. "The night staff were touched one evening," read its first newsletter, "when two teenage daughters and their friends were softly playing their guitars and singing to their mother as she died, and in those final moments her tense face relaxed, reflecting a new sense of peace and comfort."

Stories like this will multiply, because the United States is on the verge of a hospice proliferation. In New York City, St. Luke's Hospital has a year-old home-care program; there are two hospice-planning groups in California; nurse Joy Ufema set up a hospice service at Harrisburg Hospital; and dozens of committees across the country are studying hospice feasibility. There was even a hospice-planning symposium recently where participants talked of restricting use of the word.

But all eyes are on the New Haven Hospice,

which many people mistakenly think is connected to Yale because it developed out of a Yale study group. New Haven Hospice is unique in that it's the first hospice here to be closely modeled on St. Christopher's. One hundred and seventy cancer patients have already been cared for in Hospice's two-year-old home-care program. Hospice is receiving money from the National Cancer Institute, and many foundations. The program is headed by St. Christopher's alumnae Dr. Sylvia Lack (medical director) and Sister Mary Kaye Dunn (program director). The home-care team is on call 24 hours a day, seven days a week, and because of this program about 50 percent of their patients who have died have been able to die at home and the others have stayed out of hospitals weeks longer than they would have without the team. With Hospice's 26-member staff and 46 essential volunteers already involved in care, planning, financing, research, and evaluation, Hospice will also be the first of the home-grown hospices to build an inpatient facility from scratch. Six acres of land have been purchased in Branford, Connecticut, and plans by Prentice, Chan, & Ohlhausen (who designed the new Henry Street Settlement building and the Roosevelt Island Tramway stations in New York) are almost complete.

"If being humane in the care of the dying is avant-garde, then I guess this is a very avant-garde plan," says Florence Wald, former dean of the Yale School of Nursing and one of the original founders of Hospice, who worked closely with architect Lo-Yi Chan in her role as planning coordinator of the inpatient facility. Wald was the one who first brought Saunders to lecture at Yale in the late sixties.

The Hospice building committee considered a number of well-qualified architects, but one of the many things that impressed them about Chan was that he volunteered to spend time at St. Christopher's if he were to get the assignment.

"What do you want to go for?" Chan's friends asked him. "It'll be so depressing." "I'm going," he replied, "because I know very little about hospices, or for that matter, hospitals." He had never designed one, another plus with the committee. "We didn't want anyone with preconceived ideas," says engineer Henry Wald, Yale's director of health-facilities planning, who wrote the original feasibility study for Hospice as a master's thesis at Columbia, was chair-

man of the Hospice building committee, and who is also Florence Wald's husband.

In December, 1973, as Chan packed for his two-week trip to London, he wondered about whether he should take his favorite red tie. In Canton, China, where the Dartmouth-educated, Harvard-trained architect was born, red means happiness, and it's never worn to funerals. Would the tie be appropriate? Finally, he packed it.

For the first time in Chan's professional career, he took his wife, Millie, along on a business trip. "This was so clearly going to be a situation where emotions would be involved," the 43-year-old Chan recalled recently, "that I thought it was important for us to share it."

"Millie and I walked up to the entrance to St. Christopher's full of anxiety. We didn't know what to expect at St. Christopher's even though we had prepared ourselves by going to thanatology lectures and reading a lot on the subject. But it's all different when you're personally involved. In spite of our fears, the reception St. Christopher's has for families, patients, and visitors is so warm that anxiety is quickly overcome. . . .

"I don't know why I was worried about the tie. It was so cheerful there, full of flowers, children visiting. It wasn't depressing. It was uplifting. I saw people coping and helping each other, and that far overshadowed the fact that some were dying."

Chan came away from St. Christopher's as most visitors do—evangelized. He wanted to create an architecture of healing. "Hospitals are designed to cure," says Lo-Yi Chan, "which means that they are usually designed for staff convenience." But they wanted Hospice to be a therapeutic environment designed from the patient's point of view with an at-home feeling and a place for families.

They got what they wanted. Simply explained, the proposed 44-bed Hospice will consist of two V-shaped patients' wings, each attached at its apex to one long service and administrative spine.

A major theme running through the Hospice design is the concept of transitional spaces—a direct result of Chan's memory of his anxiety at St. Christopher's door. "We need to prepare people more before they see a very sick patient," he says. "Ease them into situations they don't want to confront right away. In Hospice we're building a lot of escape valves in the form of anterooms—devices to let people get in touch with their feelings before they walk into a room. Even a window in a door can be a transitional device."

According to Chan, antianxiety treatment will start outside Hospice. The glass-walled staff dining room and (if the state approves it) the children's day-care-center playground "are to be placed facing the street in order to ease the anxiety of people driving by. They'll see this is not a death house." They'll see patients are mobile and can go outside—all calculated to allay the primitive fear that death is catching and that the dying are weird. (One neighborhood had opposed Hospice's purchase of land near a playground, and, Chan relates, a resident said, "I don't want my children molested by those dying patients.")

"We went in circles about the design of the entrance," Chan recalls. "Our first thought was to have a really familiar entrance, like a standard suburban house with coach lights and a colonial door. But then we realized that it would look false and everyone would realize it. Although we wanted to alleviate anxiety by the use of familiarity, it would be dishonest to do it with stagecraft. We decided it would be better to create an atmosphere that was professional while friendly. And that could be done more with staff than by design."

Now the plan is to use the same entrance for everyone—visitors, inpatients, and home-care patients. That way, the door to the inpatient facility won't have bad connotations for the patient who is transferring in from the home-care program.

"The most critical entrance," says Lo-Yi Chan, "is a patient's first entrance. Some hospitals admit patients arriving by ambulance through a side door. But patients are people, and they should be able to come through the front door like anyone else. Those who are immobilized come in on a litter and have to be transferred to a bed. This transfer is crucial for the family and patient. If it's done well, in a pleasant place, it can fill them with confidence. We thought of doing it out of sight. But it only takes 30 seconds. I timed it. So we decided to make this transfer right in the reception room. Admissions (which are by physician referral) will be by appointment, and it's estimated that there will be no more than two new patients a day so we can have a bed waiting with the patient's name on it."

But for visitors, the entrance to the patient's room is the critical one. "I visited a friend once in the intensive-care unit at Lenox Hill Hospital," recalls Chan. "You walked right into the unit directly from the hall—right into this scene of maybe nine seriously ill patients all lined up. Those are wild spaces." At Hospice each 22-bed patients' wing will be approached through another stopping-off place— a large sky-lit family room with a fireplace and cozy seating groups. "It's a valve," says Chan, "if you're coming to see your aunt and you don't know what condition she's in."

A major problem in the care of the dying anywhere is emotional support for staff members who find the work draining. Staff needs at New Haven Hospice will be dealt with architecturally, by having totally separate staff lounges, dining room, and offices, plus a special innovation: a tiny glass-domed, sound-proof meditation or "screaming room" which will, literally, go through the roof. The carpet-lined retreat will have no furniture except, perhaps, bean bags. And no artificial light, architect Chan says, in order to "cool the psyche. . . . It will be nonobjective and nonfamiliar—like a blank slate."

"Hospice deviates from present hospital trends," says hospital consultant John Thompson, "in its relative unconcern for lack of privacy." Although government regulations generally call for 60 percent single-bedded rooms in all new hospitals, Hospice will have 90 percent four-bedded rooms. "Interaction of staff, patient, and family is the key to Hospice's program, but with private rooms you can't interact," says Thompson. "I believe in four-bedded rooms," says Hospice's home-care medical director Dr. Sylvia Lack, "to create a community of persons—to get peer support from people experiencing the same problems. And families then give support from bed to bed." In order to have wards, though, Hospice has to call them intensive-care units. But ICUs have to have all beds visible from a single point, which was impossible. "It's Catch-22," says Chan. Finally, the government relaxed the last regulation.

Since many people think the sexual needs of the terminal patient are overlooked, Hospice will have four private rooms. Double beds will be available, "even if they're used for nothing more than emotional warmth between a husband and a wife." Private rooms are also necessary for patients who are disruptive, disfigured, or have extremely large families, or perhaps for someone with no family and a lot of personal objects. "I remember a lady at St.

Christopher's," says Dr. Lack, "who brought half her antiques shop with her."

In most hospitals the rooms are distributed in either the double-loaded corridor system (center hall with rooms off it on either side) or the center-core plan (rooms in a circle, corridor in the middle). In both plans, visitors must walk into and out of the patients' rooms through a general-use corridor where the guests invariably are intruding on the privacy of ambulatory patients and in the way of staff.

But Hospice has a unique layout—a double-corridor plan. The rooms will be arranged in a row with corridors on either side. On one side there will be a *private* corridor with bathrooms, supply rooms, doctors' desk, flower-arranging sink, small family conference room, dispensary, etc.; on the other side, a *social* hallway, which will consist of a greenhouse facing the patios—a corridor wide enough for patients' beds, where families and patients can visit and have a change of scene.

The greenhouse windows will be the room windows. Inspired by the fifteenth-century French hospice at Beaune, the Hospice wards will have no walls and no doors, just low partitions. (The partitions will give a *sense* of privacy while permitting the nurses to keep a close watch on patients and giving the patients a sense of community.)

"One characteristic of the terminal patient," says Chan, "is a sense of isolation. We want to go in the opposite direction. There'll be a sense of light, life, and growing things."

"Studies show that patients recover faster in natural light," says Henry Wald. "And skylights accentuate the passage of time," says Chan. "The movement of the sun, shadows, rain, snow—it's all palpable. It gives a patient a point of reference to the outside world. The building won't be insulated from life. It's been established that there are rhythms in day and night, and to deny that is wrong."

Although the interior-design plans aren't complete yet, the concepts are well defined. And trendy supergraphics aren't in the plans. "What's really contemporary in the Hospice design," emphasizes Florence Wald, "is that the design impulse is the humane impulse."

"*Interiors* magazine may not want to photograph it," says Lo-Yi Chan. Rocking chairs and wing chairs will be standard equipment. "We want to do something intensely human, even with the patients' own furniture which they'll be allowed to bring from home.

"We know that some people would rather talk to a dying patient on the phone than come in. We hope that they'll want to come to Hospice, but still there'll be as many phones as we can cram in." And there will be TV outlets—which caused some disagreements. "On the one hand," says Chan, "TV is a separator of people—it makes people zombies. On the other hand, it's what some people want to do, and it can also create shared experiences."

It's estimated that a stay at Hospice, which will probably be covered by Medicaid, etc., will cost $108 a day, as compared to $50 a day in a nursing home and $208 in a general hospital.

Designing for the dying forces an examination of people's attitudes toward death. For instance, how do you handle the newly dead person? And should there be a morgue?

Based on St. Christopher's statistics, two people a day might be discharged to their homes, but there could also be two deaths a day. The decision to have an in-house morgue (or "aftercare facility," as Florence Wald prefers to call it) caused some anguish to New Haven-area undertakers. In England, undertakers don't work on weekends, so St. Christopher's has to have its own facilities for people who die on weekends. But in this country, undertakers work a seven-day week, and the area's funeral people argued that there was no need to spend money on morgue space and refrigeration. It was such an emotional issue that when Chan tried to determine how long it takes for a body to decompose, everyone had a different estimate.

But Florence Wald and the building committee were adamant. "We want to confront death right away," Wald says. "There is a need for a viewing ritual. We want an opportunity for families to view the patient there—to help them accept the reality of death." Recent studies have shown that survivors who don't view the body have difficulty in separating themselves from the dead and can become chronic grievers, making them susceptible to higher morbidity and mortality rates. On the other hand, people who don't want to view will never be forced to. The morgue won't be in the basement, as in most hospitals. It'll be upstairs—physically and symbolically.

The prep room won't have refrigeration, but will

be kept cool to slow natural deterioration, and bodies will be picked up shortly after viewing. Bodies will leave by a back door that is reached through the rear parking lot, where funeral homes will call for them in death-denying station wagons.

Theoretically, there is no room in a hospice for the denial of death. But in practice even some of the most enlightened staff members had trouble. "The subject that tore the hospice-planning group apart," says Chan, "was how to transport the dead from their beds to the morgue." Cover the face? Don't cover the face? Conceal the body? Or move it right past visitors? One group argued that the patient was still a person after death.

"If it's just a body, you throw it in a stainless steel box and forget it. But if it's a person, you compose the face and body and take her down the hall and she's still Mrs. Jones," said Florence Wald. But the other group said that relatives of patients visiting Hospice might not be ready to deal with it. "Suppose the dead body is coming down the hall with a wailing family behind," one member said. "Sometimes you can't compose the face suitably. It can be a shock. Are Americans ready for it? Can anyone handle it?" Clearly, most of the Hospice staff couldn't.

How do other hospitals handle the dead? At New York Hospital there is, surprisingly, no standard procedure. Dr. Eleanor Lambertsen, the director of nursing, says, "It's up to each nurse to decide. One system is to cover the face with a sheet," but it's not Lambertsen's first choice because "it signifies death to other patients and visitors. In general, we try not to upset the other patients." Another technique used in some hospitals is a false-bottom bed—actually a stretcher with a recessed tray in which a body can be concealed. On the surface it looks like an empty bed. And a third technique is to keep the body in an empty room or holding place until you can clear a hall, close all the patients' doors, and move the body. And there are reputable hospitals where it's not unusual for passengers to find themselves in an elevator along with a dead body, a sheet pulled over its face.

In the end, talks with Cicely Saunders resolved the issue. "When a patient dies," Dr. Saunders says, "we pull the curtains around him at the end and say a prayer—unless he's an atheist. We tell the other patients in the bay that he has died, and move the patient in his bed out of the ward into the treat-ment room, do the body prep there, then move him to wherever he will be viewed. We pull the sheet up sometimes, it depends. I don't think a dead patient in a bed should go through where there are other visitors. I feel that would be imposing undue trauma on new patients and family. Of course, the sky won't fall in if someone does see it."

At Hospice, Chan says, they will get around the problem by using one of the two parallel corridors. "We will simply clear one when we are moving a patient's body." But there is no way to avoid passing visitors on the way to the elevator. So Chan calls the space outside the elevator "the intersection of the denial and acceptance of death."

The designing of a hospice is a similar intersection. After all, as Chan says, "What is the job of a patient at Hospice? To be himself or herself. But how do you design for that? Who is he or she? It's hard to find out. So as not to intrude on patients' privacy, I talked to only one client in Hospice's home-care program. That patient was a plumber, and he advised that we have one bathroom for each patient—which was impossible—but after talking to him I moved the bathrooms closer to the patients' beds.

"But one thing I know without asking," says Lo-Yi Chan, who is now doing research in design as a therapeutic tool under a grant from the National Endowment for the Arts: "Pain destroys people and the tasks they have to do. If Hospice can't control pain and suffering, the building is useless. But I think they can guarantee that people won't suffer."

He also thinks that "if Hospice has the wrong staff, you could have the most sensitively designed building and it wouldn't work. But with the right staff it could work in a motel."

So why have a new building? Why not take over an old building, as some people suggested? The venerable Calvary Hospital in the Bronx, everyone reminds you, does an excellent job with terminal-cancer patients. Even Elisabeth Kübler-Ross, chairman of Hospice's National Advisory Council, cautions, "Don't worry about the color of the wallpaper—if you love each other, all the colors will be shiny and beautiful." Can a $3-million building make a difference?

"Yes, of course, a building can help," says Cicely Saunders, who knows from experience, since St. Christopher's was built to her specifications. "We need spaces for patients to look out on trees and for visitors to feel welcome. A good building can make a difference to the backs and feet of the staff and to the patients' spirits. Beauty is very healing. It makes patients see that the creation to which they also belong is good—it can be trusted."

POSTSCRIPT, JULY 1986

The Connecticut Hospice did get built at a cost of 3.5 million dollars; the first specially designed building for terminally-ill patients and their families received its first patient in the summer of 1980. Prior to this opening, the Connecticut Hospice Organization, which runs the facility, had only a home-care program embracing 18 towns and cities in the Greater New Haven Area. This program was the first in the nation. The trouble was that when hospice home-care patients required inpatient services (i.e., needed to be hospitalized), they had to be transferred to acute-care hospitals, which had little expertise in, and were not organized to deal with, terminal illness.

In the first seven years over 7000 patients have been served in the new facility and 7000 families of these patients have been helped through the difficult period of bereavement.

What is perhaps most striking about our hospice program is the high level of use of its services by those to whom the services are relevant. In the Greater New Haven area—which is the area we most directly serve—80 percent of all patients who die of cancer use hospice home-care or inpatient services or both. Although the typical hospice patient is 65 years of age or older, is married, and has some form of cancer, many patients live alone, are younger, and have other terminal diseases.

The patient and family decide with their community physician when hospice care is appropriate. Seven criteria must be met in order for an individual to be eligible to be admitted to the inpatient facility. The most important is that an individual's disease must be terminal—that is, noncurable. Among the other criteria are that the prognosis must indicate that death is likely to occur no more than two to three months hence, and that the patient and his/her physician consent to the admission (this means that the patient's physician agrees to hand over full responsibility for the patient's treatment to the hospice staff).

It is often a painful and difficult process to realize that modern medicine will not offer a cure for a disease, but it is physically and emotionally rewarding to know that a system of hospice care is available that can respond to the physical, spiritual, and emotional problems of dying patients and their families.

The inpatient facility, is a place where love, care, and clinical expertise abound, as symbolized by the carved wooden Tree of Life found on its front door and representing quality of life for as long as life lasts. It is much the way Martin Gehner, Chairman of the Hospice Building Committee, envisioned it back in 1976 in the early planning period. From the moment a patient and his/her family arrive by ambulance, they are made to feel the "family" quality of the facility. They are received warmly by a nurse and a volunteer receptionist who say, "Hello, you are very welcome here." The patient is then brought by stretcher into a four-bed room and is settled comfortably into a hospital bed with a water mattress. There is lots of sunlight and, in addition, a view of the outside patios, where children from our preschool are often seen playing.

The "community of four" (the four-bed room) has been a resounding success, offering a great deal of essential support for patients and families so that individuals are less intimidated by the recognition of what they will eventually face. The physical weakness and changes that occur throughout the long process of terminal illness tend to be very isolating. A four-bed community enables the patient, even one there for but a weekend, to have comforting human interaction without having to reach for it. We have found that, as those who first decided on the four-bed room concept had suspected, it is isolation, not the lack of privacy, that most terminally-ill patients fear the most.

There is no hardware in the hospice facility but rather the technology of skilled human beings giving their talents and devotion to patients and their families. The ratio of nurses to patients is one to three, around the clock, seven days a week. The medically-directed, nurse-coordinated program is enhanced through the efforts of the interdisciplinary team, consisting of physicians, nurses, social workers, pastoral and arts staff, a pharmacist, a chef, a dietician, consultants (psychiatrists and physical therapists), and both professional and lay volunteers. Physicians engage in daily rounds and review pain and symptom management regimens at this time. Seventy-five percent of all medications are Schedule II narcotics (i.e., the potentially most addicting drugs, including morphine). Ninety percent of all medications are administered without injections. (Injections hurt, and hospice care is always directed toward being noninvasive and pain easing.)

Although some patients come to the hospice inpatient facility to be stabilized so that they may return home with comfort, many will not go home and will die within a couple of weeks. (The average stay is between 12 and 16 days). In those weeks, the hospice tries to help patients and families conclude unfinished business, work on personal and family issues, and laugh and cry. One of the ways that the environment of the inpatient facility supports this is through the movement of a patient's bed from one space to another—the spaces include the bedroom, family living room, commons, chapel, and patios. Since most patients are nonambulatory (i.e., confined to bed or chair), this movement creates a sense of control and wellness by not forcing the individual to look at the same scenery or to feel trapped in the same bed in one place. This physical mobility also lets patients and families participate in art happenings and pastoral services and even smell the roses in the garden. (One patient had an art exhibit for friends and families; others have been married, baptized, or confirmed.)

The federal government took a major step in November 1983 by providing financial coverage for hospice patients through the Medicare program (and industry is starting to include hospice coverage in its insurance plans). Yet financial constraints continue to weigh us down. The Tax Equity and Fiscal Responsibility Act, which is the name of the Medicare-hospice legislation, requires that home care constitute 80 percent of the services provided by hospice organizations, thereby limiting the amount of inpatient care that can be provided. Moreover, the act includes severe reimbursement limits or exclusions from reimbursement in relation to such key hospice services as counseling, bereavement, arts, and pastoral care. We are therefore under constant pressure to devise innovative ways to meet these requirements while still keeping true to the high standards of care that make hospice care so unique.

One final point must be made. Hospice is a philosophy of caring. As such, it need not be confined to a particular setting. Hospice can occur anywhere—in the home or within a specialized hospice facility or a hospital. All that is required is that the principles of care that support life for as long as life lasts are upheld.

John D. Thompson
Rosemary Hurzeler

Living with the Dying: The Consequences of Hospice Care for the Patient and the Family

Robert W. Buckingham, III
Sylvia A. Lack
Balfour M. Mount
Lloyd D. MacLean
James T. Collins

How can we best care for our patients who are dying? What do they and their families think about their care? To gain insight into these questions the anthropologic technique of participant observation was used to observe the treatment attitudes and interactions of hospital staff, terminally ill patients and their families, and to compare the effectiveness of two treatment units in meeting the known needs of such patients and their families. Our findings support the view that an acute care hospital does not offer as good a milieu for the dying as a unit specifically designed to meet the known needs of such patients.

BACKGROUND: PARTICIPANT OBSERVATION

The technique of participant observation, which has provided valuable information about the relationships between native patients and their health care providers,[1] has been adapted to the study of modern institutions. Participant observers have assumed roles in prisons[2] and psychiatric wards[3] to study

Reprinted by permission from the *Canadian Medical Association Journal*, vol. 115 (December 18, 1976), pp. 1211–1215.

those subcultures. Participant observation is appropriate when the study requires an examination of complex social relationships or intricate patterns of interaction.

The observer's primary responsibility is to those he studies; when there is a conflict of interest these individuals come first. The anthropologist, for example, must protect their physical, social and psychological welfare and must honour and respect their dignity and privacy. This standard is of particular significance in the present study, in which the observer assumed the identity of a consumer of health services and attempted to represent their attitudes and concerns.

METHOD OF OBSERVATION

The Participant Observer and Preparation for Admission to Hospital

A 31-year-old man, a medical anthropologist (R.W.B.) hereafter referred to as "M," assumed the role of a patient with terminal cancer of the pancreas. A second medical anthropologist acted as his cousin and was his contact during the hospitalization.

To gain admission to the hospital and establish M's assumed identity, certain preparations were required. The medical director, executive director, hospital lawyer and heads of both departments involved (surgery and palliative care service) participated in planning the project to preserve medicolegal standards and to guard against iatrogenic harm that might befall the researcher while in hospital. The palliative care unit physician, having known M previously, was forewarned of his pseudo-patient status but was not advised of the details of the study.

Because of the difficulty of documenting the impact of the palliative care type of medical service, and because of the need to make every effort to evaluate the singularly important pilot project of the palliative care unit, we carefully considered the ethical issues raised by participant observation. We viewed these issues as those of informed consent and of evaluation of medical care and certain persons giving this care (particularly personnel in the palliative care unit). The principal investigator gave his informed consent and the palliative care unit personnel were made aware that the palliative care unit was being evaluated, though the specific form of the evaluative study was not detailed. Furthermore, an ad hoc committee was formed to consider these issues; the view of the committee was that the experiment was acceptable.

In order to impersonate a cancer patient, M prepared himself in a number of ways before entering the hospital. He went on a severe six-month diet and lost 22 pounds from his already spare frame. Exposure to ultraviolet rays made it appear that he had undergone cancer radiation therapy. Puncture marks from intravenous needles on his hands and arms indicated that M had also had chemotherapy cancer treatment. A cooperative surgeon performed minor surgery on him in order to produce "biopsy" scars. This would show that exploratory surgery had been performed. M reviewed medical charts and maintained close contact with patients dying of cancer of the pancreas. He was, thus, able to observe and imitate suitable behavior. A patchy beard and the results of several days of not washing or shaving completed the picture.

Documentation from a major medical centre to substantiate the diagnosis rendered further investigation unnecessary. The following documents, identifying M as the patient, were produced: (a) a university hospital discharge summary detailing investigations, diagnosis and treatment; (b) a summary of radiation therapy; (c) a letter from a collaborating oncologist documenting M's refusal to continue toxic chemotherapy and his terminal state; (d) a pathology slide demonstrating adenocarcinoma in a lymph node compatible with a pancreatic primary site; and (e) selected radiographs from abdominal angiography and retrograde pancreatography.

Admission and Hospitalization

M and his alleged cousin presented themselves at the hospital emergency department, their arrival being preceded by a telephone call from the chief of surgery stating that the patient had been referred to him for assessment of symptoms compatible with bowel obstruction (severe pain and vomiting).

The patient's personal, social, previous medical and family histories were those of the investigator, where possible, to minimize the chance of subsequent inconsistency. After routine radiography and blood tests M was admitted to the emergency holding area and transferred to a general surgical ward the following day. He spent four days on the surgical ward, where oncology and palliative care service consultations were requested. He was then transferred to the palliative care unit, where he spent another four days, subsequently discharging himself to the care of his cousin. He spent a total of nine days in the hospital.

Intrahospital Observation Technique

Apart from simulated pain and nausea and his refusal of a nasogastric tube, M maintained passive behaviour and quiet affect in the hospital. The content of his conversations and his expressed philosophies, likes and dislikes were representative of his personal feelings. M's behaviour included being quiet, ringing for nurses even if he could help himself and showing little verbal initiative.

Throughout his hospitalization M made notes and kept records of quantitative data, with the explanation that he wished to finish writing a book before he died. Nobody took any notice or interest in this activity apart from one nurse on the surgical ward who said she hoped he was not writing about the hospital.

OBSERVATIONS AND DISCUSSION

Impact on Observer

M was surprised to find that he began to experience symptoms: 48 hours after admission he was complaining to his "cousin," "My back really does hurt." M discarded his pajamas to "preserve accurate observations," to "feel better," and to silently protest that he was not sick. Similar behaviour has been noted in other pseudopatients.[3] On the surgical ward he became bored and frustrated with the lack of meaningful social contacts. In spite of his determination to remain passive he found himself exerting stimuli and attempting to engage in conversation. When asked by staff how he was feeling he spoke of his pain and weakness, symptoms he actually experienced much of the time after the first 48 hours.

M was nervous at the thought of being transferred to the palliative care unit, where, with fewer ambulant patients, he thought he might be detected more easily as a pseudopatient, but once on the unit he identified closely with these sick people and became weaker and more exhausted. He was anorexic and routinely refused food. He felt ill. It took all his energy to take a shower. He sat exhausted in a chair. He experienced increasing pain, a constant ache in his left leg together with numbness, and restless nights during which family members of other patients commented sympathetically on his "moaning and groaning." M himself was unaware of this nocturnal behaviour.

Contact with Staff, Patients and Others

Quantitative observations during the project included the frequency and duration of verbal contacts with staff members, other patients, and relatives and friends of other patients (Tables 1 and 2). The number of contacts was almost the same in both the surgical ward and the palliative care unit, yet

TABLE 1 Verbal contact of patient M with staff and other patients and their families in the four-day periods in the surgical ward and palliative care unit

	SURGICAL WARD			PALLIATIVE CARE UNIT			
ITEM	STAFF	PATIENTS AND FAMILIES	TOTAL	STAFF	PATIENTS AND FAMILIES	TOTAL	DIFFERENCE (AND %)
Time spent (min)	164	229	393	512	1354	1866	1473 (374.8)
No. of contacts	30	29	59	27	34	61	2 (3.4)
Mean no. of minutes per contact	5.5	7.9	6.6	19.0	39.8	30.6	24.0 (363.6)

TABLE 2 Mean duration of contacts between staff and patient M

STAFF POSITION	SURGICAL WARD			PALLIATIVE CARE UNIT		
	MIN/D	CONTACTS/D	MIN/CONTACT	MIN/D	CONTACTS/D	MIN/CONTACT
Nurse	8.5	3.5	2.4	45.5	3.5	13.0
Physician[1]	9.5	2.0	4.8	6.3	0.8	8.3
Student nurse[2]	22.8	1.8	13.0	35.0	1.5	23.3
Volunteer[3]	0	0	0	66.3	2.0	16.6

[1] On the surgical ward "Physician" includes attending staff, residents and interns. In the palliative care unit there was only one physician; both he and the admitting surgeon, being aware that the "patient" was not actually ill, may have spent less than the usual amount of time with him.

[2] One student nurse attended M on the surgical ward and continued to visit him following his transfer.

[3] No volunteers were working on the surgical ward during M's stay, whereas volunteers formed an important part of the palliative care team.

the mean duration of contact was substantially longer in the palliative care unit for all categories of personnel as well as for other patients and families who visited M. On the surgical ward only the student nurse, admitting resident and oncology consultant spent more than five minutes in any one contact. In the palliative care unit only three of the professional contacts were less than five minutes in duration.

Physicians' Attitudes to Patients

On the surgical ward, doctors rarely entered the patient's room alone. Ward rounds were typically made by residents traveling in groups of two or three. This practice fostered discussion—both social and medical—between the doctors but completely prevented doctor–patient communication on any but the most superficial level. Many patients appeared intimidated and were reluctant to question a group of young doctors.

Three doctors had a clearly audible and highly critical conversation regarding hospital problems unrelated to patient care. Frequently staff, including doctors, went in and out without any recognition, by word or look, of the people in the room.

This pattern of short, task-oriented contacts between medical staff and patients hampered meaningful communication. Some patients' comments were these:

- "The doctors cover up too much."
- "They don't tell me what's wrong with me."
- "One has to ask if one is to find out."

The patient needs to discuss his anxious and sad feelings but physicians frequently fail to provide this psychological relief.[4] Moreover, the patient needs a sense of continuing self-respect and identity as a person, and only when a doctor can talk about death with the patient will the doctor have a chance of communicating helpfully with his dying patients.[5] Such communication with patients is essential because the patients need to have a sense of control and involvement in decision making.[6] Yet studies by Kübler-Ross[7] and LeShan[8] have shown that doctors avoid their dying patients at a time when the latter are faced with the greatest emotional crisis of their life.

An excellent example of good consultation on the surgical ward was provided by the visiting oncologist. He came alone. He was gentle, compassionate, and honest. He discussed his recommendations but did not press them. He discussed prognosis and questioned whether M was depressed. He promised that if ever he were needed he would be there.

In the palliative care unit the doctors made rounds alone, thus providing the patient with this essential opportunity for communication.

Observations differed on the two types of wards, in part because their functions were different. The goals of a surgical ward are those of any active-treatment hospital ward: investigation, diagnosis, cure and prolongation of life, with the expectation that the patient will return home. In contrast, the palliative care unit is designed to enhance the quality of life remaining to a patient with a terminal disease. A multidisciplinary team attempts to meet not only the medical but also the psychological, interpersonal and spiritual needs of patients and their families.[9]

Other Staff–Patient Relationships

On the surgical ward the threat to personal identity of the patient was accentuated and staff–patient contacts were mostly technical and usually brief (Table 1). The patient had to look up at the staff person who remained standing by the bed. Interviews were rushed and restrictive. Lengthy responses by the patient were tolerated reluctantly and impatience was evidenced if information given was not strictly related to staff concerns.

Minor matters became troublesome on the surgical ward. On the holding ward an orderly had gone out of his way to find saccharin for M's coffee and later he remembered how M liked it. On the surgical ward, however, the request for coffee as desired was repeated daily; sometimes it came, sometimes not. One morning the orderly from the holding ward appeared and for the first time the "right" coffee arrived. Individuals tried to be kind but the system was not set up for it. Food was invariably placed away from the bed and M's bedbound roommates frequently could not touch their food; the full tray would be removed with no comments or questions.

Only the head nurse—a person who radiated concern, efficiency, and quiet authority—and one student nurse took the trouble to explain what their position was in the hospital. No one else came and said "I am an intern" or "I am a resident" or stated what particular interest they had in a given case. Cleaners went in and out as if the patients were not present. They kept their eyes fixed on the floor, looking away immediately if, by chance, an upward glance should catch a patient looking at them.

Patients walked close to the walls, greetings were rare and staff frequently crossed to the other side of the hall, walking by, heads averted. One night on the surgical ward a nurse saw M in the hall and told him to go to bed. At 11 P.M. he was again found in the hall, this time by the head nurse, who said she didn't mind him being here—clearly a special dispensation from a senior person, not a matter of routine. On his second day M was passing the nursing station when he was questioned in a loud voice, "Are you lost? Do you belong to us?" He nodded. "What is your name?" He told her, she checked her list and everything was fine. He belonged there.

M heard laughter for the first time two days after his admission. A student nurse was talking to an elderly man. She took a personal interest in the patients and spoke with openness about herself and the hospital. The only staff groups who initiated conversations were the student nurses and orderlies. Personal requests made to other staff were frequently ignored or forgotten.

Patients, in general, experienced monotony and loneliness on the surgical ward. Typical comments were the following:

- "Nobody talks around here."
- "I'm going stir-crazy. This place is terrible."
- "Reading keeps me from crying and being alone too much."

M's overall impression was that the surgical ward had highly developed skills in acute care. The staff displayed great efficiency in preparing patients for operation and caring for them postoperatively.

On his arrival at the palliative care unit M found some flowers and a card by his bedside saying "Welcome, Mr. M." The initial nursing interview was conducted by a nurse who introduced herself by name, sat down so that her eyes were on a level with M's and proceeded to listen. There was no hurry, her questions flowed from M's previous answers, and there was acceptance of the expression of his concerns. She asked questions such as "What do you like to eat?" and "Is there anything special you like to do?"

In his first few hours on the unit M observed that the professionalism of the staff members was balanced by a notable freedom to express their own personality. This contrasted with the structured role behaviour on the surgical ward, where smiles were rare and personalities hidden. M's notes written in the palliative care unit included many names: "The night nurse R," "Mrs. B," "T.G. (volunteer)" and "Nurse D." In contrast the surgical ward notes identified staff as "another nurse," "the student nurse," "doctors (three)," "orderly," and "young man with black beard."

Kindness and individual attention were a matter of policy and the system facilitated these attributes. M said only once that he liked coffee with milk and saccharin. Thereafter, every morning, no matter who was on duty, coffee with milk and saccharin arrived for breakfast. Every staff member and volunteer seemed to know who each patient was and something about him. Patients in the hall were greeted by name. Patient freedom in activities and mobility was allowed as a matter of policy. Direct orders to patients on the surgical ward were commonplace; they were never given in the palliative care unit. All these details conveyed "a happy spirit" and "an attitude of caring" that was sensed and commented on by patients and their families. This atmosphere was enhanced by touches of the home—flowers in every room, handmade afghans, posters and children's art, a refrigerator used by patients, a community television, and a piano in the lounge.

The range of health disciplines encountered was greater in the palliative care unit. In addition to the nurses and doctors, M and his 22-year-old roommate were visited by clergy, a dietitian, a social worker, and volunteers. Contributions from these persons were significant. The dietitian was much appreciated, she took infinite pains to provide personal preferences such as Eggs Benedict, looking up the recipe and teaching the cook to make it.

Patients were able to cry with staff and conversations of a personal nature occurred. The chief "distancing" maneuver used on the surgical ward to avoid such intimacy was busy concentration on technical skills. Threatening to take the place of the technical skills on the surgical ward was the pain medication regimen in the palliative care unit. A strong arm was brought to bear on patients to take their drugs and sometimes the nurses were extremely forceful. The philosophy of pain control (regular use of analgesics to prevent pain) was repeatedly explained correctly by staff and volunteers. The floor was peaceful. There was no awareness of agony. People died comfortably without intravenous feeding lines or nasogastric tubes. No deaths were observed on the surgical ward.

One thing not observed on either ward was touching of patients by staff except during medical or nursing routines. There was much touching and stroking of patients by family members, however.

Staff–Family Relationships

Relatives suffered from the physician's inaccessibility on the surgical ward. Queries on medication, diet and many other topics were always referred to the doctor and in his absence they were left unanswered. Families would quiz the patients, "What doctors did you see today?" or they complained angrily, "Where the hell are the doctors in this hospital?" When the patient's condition is clearly improving, such ignorance may be bearable. When the condition of a loved one is deteriorating daily, however, much better communication is necessary. In addition, families may need an outlet for grief and help with their own fear, loss, resentment, anger, guilt and other common emotions. They need to begin to plan to fill the role of the dying person in the family.[10]

In the palliative care unit M observed relatives enquiring for the doctor five times. On each occasion the doctor was reached and either came or spoke to the family on the phone. In addition, nurses, volunteers and other staff members were willing and allowed to answer queries.

The visitors' room was a vital space on the surgical ward, where families felt at ease and gathered to give each other support. They sensed that they were in the way at the bedside. In the palliative care unit the television lounge was important but families also spent much time at the bedside participating in the care of the patient. They changed the bed linen, washed and fed the patient, brought the urinal and plumped the pillows frequently. The staff encouraged the family to experience the meaning of death by allowing them to help in the care of

the dying. For one young man this was his first experience with death. He spoke of how he was being brought in touch with himself through helping his dying grandmother. If we deny the family's right to maintain a meaningful relationship with the patient, we may greatly increase the risk of these families suffering a harmful bereavement.[11]

The granddaughter of one patient obtained relief by staying up and watching the sunrise, talking to and comforting M. The night nurse came in three times to attend to M's roommate and there was total acceptance of the presence of the woman by his bedside from 1 to 5 A.M. Later his nurse initiated a conversation with M, affirming the importance of "living life" because "cancer of the pancreas is a fast disease." The policy of open visiting provides flexibility that allows busy families to care for the patient and to be cared for themselves.

Interpatient Family Support

Throughout his hospital stay M noted a little-documented and important phenomenon: patients helping patients and patients' families helping not only their relatives but also other patients and families. On the surgical ward it was a matter of "facing adversity together." This group mechanism has been recognized by the hospice movement[12] but this study emphasized its strength.

Immediately on arrival on the surgical ward an old Swiss man began talking to M with his hands. This bedridden French-speaking man found himself surrounded by English-speaking roommates and staff. By the end of the second day there was a strong sense of unity between the three disparate roommates—a 19-year-old Canadian, a 31-year-old American, and an elderly Swiss. Frequent smiles and knowing glances were exchanged and they all laughed together over the food and service.

Patients were open with each other, freely sharing diagnoses and following each other's progress with concern. During M's stay on the surgical ward a South African man progressed from experiencing symptoms to investigations, diagnosis of cancer, depression, struggling with life-threatening illness, and preparation for radiation therapy. Every step was discussed with other patients. He came by M's room with thanks for his support on his last day.

Interpatient support crossed barriers of social status, age, race, and sex and continued through transfer to other wards. The severity of the illness determined status. The more serious the illness, the more attentive were other patients. The night before one patient was scheduled for operation the floor was hers. Six or seven patients and family members rallied around her, consoling her, all trying to help. This pattern was repeated with other persons, depending on individual needs.

Fellow sufferers tried to soften the professionals' approach to give false hope: "Doctors are 80 percent wrong you know." They comforted each other. When a patient told M not to worry about suffering ("for death is part of life") and not to be afraid ("Be not frightened my friend") and asked "What do you know of dying?," M could only say "Nothing." The patient's reply was wise: "That is why you should not be afraid."

Patients supported each other in many ways. Expression of personal desire was helpful: "I want to sleep at home with my husband again, it is better to die at home with my husband than alone in hospital."

Also helpful were discussions of fear of pain with patients new to the palliative care unit, whose pain medications were being adjusted: expressions of fear such as "I don't mind dying—it's the pain," and questions such as "What kind of life do I have if I have pain?" were met with reassurance by patients who had been in the unit longer, that pain medication would assuredly relieve the pain. Anger was common and real, as reflected in a patient's reaction to being told to be quiet: "Don't tell me to ssh . . . it fucking hurts!"

The palliative care unit facilitated this powerful support system by allowing more patient–family freedom and mobility, with open visiting and encouragement of family participation in the care of the patient. Patients were not as ambulatory on this floor—many stayed in their rooms because of their illness. Interpatient and family contacts were initiated and maintained in many areas, not just the visitors' lounge. Children came in. Families adopted patients other than their own relatives. Flowers, pickled herring, sherry, loving looks and sympathy were freely exchanged between persons who by normal societal standards were strangers. Sorrow and sadness were intermingled with laughter.

SUMMARY AND CONCLUSIONS

The observations made by the anthropologic technique of participant observation are consistent with the view that a greater effort must be made in accomplishing total care of the terminally ill.[9] The findings of the present study are worth enumerating:

1. A powerful support system for patients with terminal disease is the sharing and help provided by other patients.
2. Also of inestimable value is care given by families, a source of support for patients that must be emphasized.
3. Likewise, the interest and care given by student nurses and volunteers is important, particularly in bringing the person out of the patient.
4. The need for the patient as a person to give, and thus to retain his individuality, is largely unrecognized.
5. Certain staff practices that have developed over the years are sources of concern. Most notable are the intimidating traditions of physicians to travel in groups while seeing patients on wards; the lack of eye contact between physician and patient; the referral to patients by the name of a disease rather than of the person; the accentuation of negative aspects of a patient's condition, again in the context of disease, so that hope is negated; the lack of affection given to the complacent patient; and the discontinuity of communication among medical and nursing staff.
6. Hospitals lack areas specifically designed for patients to make important decisions concerning their future and to share their few remaining moments with families.

Although the needs of the dying and of their families are now widely recognized,[13,14] the findings that terminal distress is inadequately controlled in the acute care hospital[15] and that an important factor in relief of distress is personal interest in the terminally ill[16] still need emphasizing. Also stressed are the need for freedom from the fear of abandonment and social isolation[17] and for help for the family, including children, in their adjustment to the impending death.[18] On the other hand, health care professionals appear to be threatened by death and try to avoid proximity to it, even though such an attitude may lead to inappropriate care.[19] Thus it seems that studies of the needs of the dying are still required.

The active treatment wards under study in this hospital, geared as they are to aggressive therapy and prolongation of life, do not offer an optimal environment for the dying. There is a need for comfort, both physical and mental, for others to see them as individuals rather than as hosts for their disease, and for someone to breach the loneliness and help them come to terms with the end. These needs may be better met by a unit specially designed for this purpose. Such a unit, with its higher staff/patient ratio and freedom from busy active treatment schedules, can concentrate on its prime goal of improving the quality of remaining life and focus on the patient as a person.

It is difficult, however, to identify objective parameters and measurable criteria with which to evaluate the care we give to our dying patients and their families. It is in this situation, where there are such limited methods of gathering information, that participant observation can give significant insights into the subcultural behaviour and values of this group and those who care for them.

References and Notes

1. Buckingham RW: The Navajo medicine man as a psychosomatic practitioner of medicine. Paper presented at the Eastern Regional Association of Medical Anthropologists, March 1975

2. Jacobs JW: Participant observation in prison. *Urban Life and Culture* 3: 221, 1974

3. Rosenhan DL: On being sane in insane places. *Science* 176: 250, 1973

4. Parkes CM: Attachment and autonomy at the end of life, in *Support, Innovation and Autonomy,* London, Tavistock, 1973

5. Cramond WA: Psychotherapy of the dying patient. *Br Med J* 3: 389, 1970

6. Kalish RA: The aged and the dying process. *J Soc Issues* 21: 87, 1965

7. Kübler-Ross E: *On Death and Dying.* New York, Macmillan, 1974, pp. 8–11

8. LeShan L, LeShan E: Psychotherapy and the patient with a limited life span. *Psychiatry* 24: 318, 1961

9. Mount BM: The problem of caring for the dying in a general hospital; the palliative care unit as a possible solution. *Can Med Assoc J* 115: 119, 1976

10. Aitken-Swan L: Nursing the late cancer patient at home. *Practitioner* 183: 64, 1959

11. Parkes CM: *Bereavement,* New York, Intl Univs Pr, 1972, pp 83–4

12. Lack SA: In Kron J: Designing a better place to die. *New York Magazine,* no 9, 1976, p 48

13. Saunders CM: The care of the terminal stages of cancer. *Ann R Coll Surg* 41(suppl): 162, 1967

14. Lack SA, Lamberton R: *The Hour of Our Death,* London, Chapman, 1975, pp 19–21

15. Exton-Smith AN: Terminal illness in the aged. *Lancet* 2: 305, 1961

16. Hinton J: *Dying.* Baltimore, Penguin, 1974, p 71

17. Abrams RD: *Not Alone with Cancer: A Guide for Those Who Care—What to Expect, What to Do,* Springfield, Il, CC Thomas, 1974

18. Wessel MA: A death in the family. The impact on the children. *JAMA* 234: 865, 1975

19. Rabin DL, Rabin LH: Consequences of death for physicians, nurses and hospitals, in *The Dying Patient,* Brim OG, Freeman HE, Levine S, *et al.* (eds), New York, Russell Sage, 1970

Nursing Home Housekeepers: Indigenous Agents of Psychosocial Support

J. Neil Henderson

INTRODUCTION

Contemporary American society has experienced leaps in human longevity largely due to remarkable progress in biomedical control of infectious disease and public health. Concomitantly, the nuclear family has become smaller, more mobile, and economically fragile. One outcome is that millions of people survive into old age with incurable chronic, debilitating disease without the resources for self-management. Generated from this social environment is an increasingly common product of the American cultural scene: the nursing home.

Patient care in nursing homes is assumed to be the province of the uniformed members of the nursing staff. However, the results of a 13-month participant-observation research project in a 90-bed proprietary nursing home shows that the housekeeping staff routinely provides patient care in the form of psychosocial support. While the formal administrative job descriptions assign patient care to the nursing staff, an ethnomedical view shows that housekeepers are also caregivers. One primary feature of the social environment which promotes psychosocial caregiving by the housekeepers and reduces it among the nurses is their respective work styles. The nursing staff's brisk, episodic work style contrasts with that of the housekeeping staff, which is deliberate and sustained. The result is a nursing staff that deals with patients' bodily needs and a housekeeping staff that deals with patients' psychosocial needs.

Reprinted by permission of the Society for Applied Anthropology from *Human Organization*, vol. 40, no. 1 (1981), pp. 300–305. (Updated by author, 1986.)

Erving Goffman, in *Asylums* (1961), discusses ways in which patients and staff adjust to the confines of institutional settings. Two general types of adjustments are presented: primary and secondary. By primary adjustments, Goffman (ibid.: 189) means following the official rules of the institution, while "Secondary adjustments represent ways in which the individual stands apart from the role and the self that were taken for granted for him by the institution." Furthermore, Goffman (ibid.: 199) discusses two types of secondary adjustments to institutional settings: disruptive and contained. The nature of the former is obvious. Goffman's secondary contained adjustments are those efforts aimed at negotiating institutional conditions in ways that do not conflict with official goals, and may in fact assist them. It is the secondary contained adjustment that describes the caregiving of the nursing home housekeepers.

This research focuses on the caregiving role of the nursing home housekeeper as a secondary contained adjustment to working in an institutional setting for chronically ill, aged people. The principal operatives due consideration are the nurse's aides, housekeepers, and patients. Nurse's aides are commonly untrained women whose task it is to feed, clothe, shower, shave, change bed linens, and clean incontinence from patients. This is Gubrium's (1975) "bed and body" work, and Freidson's (1970) "domestic service pattern." These tasks, while not highly technical, are still discharged by a uniformed "nurse," who is socially in close proximity to those of the highest certified technical skill level in the nursing home, the licensed nurses. In this sense, the nurse's aides' tasks are instrumental (Parsons 1951). Housekeepers, however, are not uniformed, push mop buckets around, and have no official ties to the nursing staff and its aura of medical authority.

Ethnomedically, the emphathetic facility of the housekeepers' psychosocial support of patients can be seen as expressive tasks (ibid.). This division of labor is predictable, given that instrumental tasks are accorded higher status, and thus professional staff gravitate toward these tasks leaving the lower-status expressive tasks undone or for others. Further, Mechanic (1968:427) suggests that the less interest higher-ranking participants have in some tasks, the more likely it is that lower-ranking participants will be able to dominate such tasks. Since psychosocial care is not provided by the nursing staff, it is available for discharge by lower participants, in this case, the housekeeping staff.

THE AMERICAN NURSING HOME

Elderly people 75 and older, the "old-old" (Neugarten and Hagestad 1976), comprise the fastest growing segment of the American population and face increased risk for serious incapacitating physical or mental declines which require long term care (Besdine 1982). As a result, the American landscape is dotted with an increasing number of nursing homes in both the private and public sector.

While persons over sixty-five that are in the nation's 25,000 nursing homes (Pegels 1981) are about 1.5 million at any one time (U.S. Bureau of the Census 1978), about 25% of the American population at age 65 can expect to live some portion of their later years in a nursing home environment (Kastenbaum and Candy 1973; Vicente, Wiley, and Carrington 1979). Furthermore, the percentage institutionalized varies as a function of age so that the 65–74 age group has 1.2% of its cohort in nursing homes, the 75–84 age group has 5.9% in nursing homes, and the 85 plus group has 23.7% of its group in nursing homes (Johnson and Grant 1985).

The institutional setting most likely encountered by that minority in need of institutional care is a privately-owned, profit-operated business selling various degrees and types of care to the elderly sick. According to Pegels (1981) 77% of all institutions providing care for the aged sick are proprietary in nature. Nonprofit institutions for the aged provide care for 15% of the institutionalized aged, and 8% of the institutionalized aged are in government-funded facilities.

Characteristics of institutionalized aged populations are varied, but even so, certain clusterings of traits are apparent. There are three times as many women as men. Most institutionalized aged people are white and poor and are maintained by public funds. The institutionalized aged population is likely to have a variety of chronic physical impairments including circulatory disorders, arthritis, digestive disorders and mental impairments such as dementia and depression (Johnson and Grant 1985).

Additionally, most institutionalized aged people have no spouse, no close relatives and the majority have no visitors (Johnson and Grant 1985). They stay in the institution almost 2.5 years with only 20% returning home, the remainder dying in the institution or at a hospital. Few can walk unaided, 33% are incontinent and there is an average of more than four drugs taken per person each day (Moss and Halamandaris 1977; Pegels 1981). These people are served by a caregiving staff that is commonly 100% female. Of all staff groups, about 40% are nurse's aides which comprises a work force of 100,000 employees nationally (AOA 1980). Pecan Grove Manor (pseudonym), the site of this research, reflects very accurately the above characteristics.

PECAN GROVE MANOR

This research took place in Pecan Grove Manor (pseudonym), a 90-bed proprietary nursing home in southern Oklahoma. Pecan Grove Manor can be considered fairly representative in that it shares the following attributes with other contemporary American nursing homes; it is a privately owned business; the physical plant is a system of rail-lined corridors covering large distances; the patients are very old (in their 80s) and the female-to-male ratio is 3 : 1; most patients are widowed; most employees are untrained nurse's aides; patients have few visitors and seldom leave the nursing home grounds; and most patients die there or die shortly after transfer to a hospital (see Moss and Halamandaris 1977).

Pecan Grove Manor is situated in a scenic pecan grove near a creek on the edge of a rural town of 2,500 people.[1] The town has three main industries that pay minimum wage to unskilled workers: horse trailer manufacturing, assembly of trousers ("the pants factory"), and Pecan Grove Manor nursing home. The town is bisected by a north/south two-lane highway with one traffic signal near the town square. The local region is economically oriented toward farming and ranching.

The nursing home itself is of gray and white decorative brick with well-manicured grounds. The interior has highly polished tile floors, exposed concrete block painted in pastels, and residential type lobby furniture. Although its first wing was built 17 years ago, Pecan Grove Manor is free of persistent odor.

In this setting, I undertook 13 months of research, modeled on community studies, spanning 1977 and 1978. My involvement in this site ranged from the usual fieldwork tasks to working as a paid nurse's aide.

THE ETHNOMEDICAL PERSPECTIVE

Nursing homes are part of the American health care culture. As such, they are organized along business and medical heirarchical schemes. Status inequities among employees promote the flow of responsibility diffusion from the top down. From the chief administrator to the janitor, everyone knows their status or position within the ranking system. It is often presumed that those ranking high in such systems wield the greatest power and thus control members of lower ranks. However, "lower participants" in organizations can exert a great deal of influence (Hall 1977:227). For example, maintenance personnel in a tobacco farm held considerable power over superiors because they alone could repair the machinery (Crozier 1964), attendants in mental hospitals have made physicians dependent on them (Scheff 1961), nurse's aides in hospitals can punish superiors through their patients (Taylor 1970), and in fact, most people have observed (privately perhaps) that it is the boss's secretary who really runs the show.

In health care organization, the status system generally begins with the physician and moves downward to the untrained orderly or aide. The biomedical view of significant health care personnel views those employees not obviously involved in direct primary care as outside the bounds of the therapeutic agency. The ethnomedical perspective provides a different view of the therapeutic network. The ethnomedical perspective does not presuppose some organizational

delivery framework, but allows for the discovery of the design of the functional therapeutic network regardless of the assigned job titles of the actors. Ethnomedicine can be defined as "those beliefs and practices relating to disease which are the products of indigenous cultural development and are not explicitly derived from the conceptual framework of modern medicine" (Hughes 1968). Consequently, persons in health care settings whose functions appear marginal may emerge as central.

INDIGENOUS THERAPISTS

Indigenous therapists are people whose training and jobs are not psychotherapeutic but who nonetheless possess personality characteristics and job circumstances that allow for the emergence of psychosocially supportive relationships with those whom they contact. Their lack of formal training is no more an obstacle to positive therapeutic outcome than is the presence of formal training with its tenuous diagnostic nosology and therapeutic techniques (Rosenhan 1973; Gross 1978). As in any job requiring intensive personal interaction, factors other than technical expertise influence the psychotherapeutic scene (Torrey 1972). The most effective use of technical psychotherapeutic knowledge may prevail only when these skills serve as an adjunct to pre-existing personal qualities facilitating empathic interactions. Thus, while ". . . training may improve the efficacy of a therapist, it is not necessary for successful psychotherapy to occur" (ibid.:128). Additional support for the subjective demeanor of therapists as a pivotal variable comes from Jerome Frank (cited in Marshall 1980:506) who states that psychotherapeutic benefit is more a product of the abilities of the therapist than of the technical methods used.

Nonprofessionals whose education ranged from high school to graduate school have successfully served as psychotherapists. Evaluation of their efficacy is based on patient self-report of improvement and/or assessments by professionally trained psychotherapists. High efficacy ratings were given to "lesser trained" psychotherapists such as medical students (Heine 1962; Uhlenhuth and Duncan 1968), general college graduates (Yeager, Sowder, and Hardy 1962; Sanders 1967; Beck, Kantor, and Gelineau 1963; Holzberg, Knapp, and Turner 1967), housewives (nonuniversity-trained) (Rioch 1967), bartenders (Dumont 1967), psychiatric aides (Deane 1961) and other "low-level" health care agents (Torrey 1969). To this list can be added the nursing home housekeeper.

NURSING HOME HOUSEKEEPERS AS INDIGENOUS THERAPISTS

The psychosocial support provided patients by the housekeepers is unrecognized by the administrative and nursing staff at Pecan Grove Manor. Texts on nursing home administration likewise exclude maintenance and housekeeping personnel as therapeutic agents, considering their contribution to patient care in vague terms of providing a pleasant environment (Kramer and Kramer 1976; Manard, Woehle, and Heilman 1977; McQuillan 1974; Miller 1969; Rogers 1971). Invisibility of the housekeeper psychosocial support role is due to absence of formal therapeutic scenes and other artifacts and behaviors commonly associated with primary care. Nonetheless, the patients and housekeepers are not only aware of the benefit of their interaction but actively exploit it.

Although nurse's aides constitute the largest number of staff, their potential for giving psychosocial support is attenuated by the short, episodic time spent with patients, accompanied by ritualistic, shallow interactions. The brevity of nurse's aide-patient contact is due to the large number of tasks to do, the number of patients to be cared for, and the time-space inefficiency of corridor architecture. The following is a sample from fieldnotes of nurse's aides activities ((NA) means nurse's aide and (P) patient; all names are pseudonyms).

6:21 A.M.	(NA) Miller and (NA) Foster in (P) White's and (P) Palmer's room. (NA) Foster leaves room. (NA) Foster in and out of (P) Morgan's and (P) Taylor's room.
6:23	(NA) Price in (P) Sprague's and (P) Jones' room. Gives washcloths.
6:24	(NA) Price out. (NA) Price and (NA) Miller in (P) Horne's room.
6:25	(NA) Foster out of (P) White's and (P) Palmer's room saying, "Oh, my

stars. I dread these three," in reference to her next patients.

6:25	(NA) Price and (NA) Miller out of (P) Horne's room. (NA) Foster: "Where is (P) Mrs. Roger?" (NA) Price: "She's home with her son. Don't you remember in report?" (NA) Foster: "No, I didn't hear it." (NA) Foster: "Here's the heavy-weight" in reference to (P) Dunn. (NA) Miller in (P) Cobb's room. (P) Richard's door closed, skipped by, aides don't knock, light showing under door.
6:29	(NA) Miller out of (P) Cobb's room to get help from (NA) Price. Work with (P) Cobb continues. (P) Dunn left on pot.
6:30	(NA) Miller asks (NA) Foster for help getting (P) Dunn into wheelchair. Both aides make comments about effort to lift (P) Dunn.
6:31	(NA) Foster in (P) Polk's room. There have been two aides helping with (P) Cobb on a rotating basis.
6:32	Patient call light comes on in (P) Perkins' and (P) Starn's room. Buzzer not on yet.
6:33	(NA) Foster leaves (P) Polk's room (19 seconds total time to respond to call light).
6:34	(P) Cobb work finishes.

In order to adequately do one's job in an eight-hour shift, brief, efficient interaction, which interrupts engaging interactions, is required.

2:04 P.M.	(NA) Price: "Should we put her, (P) Horne, to bed? Let's do. She's been up since six. (NA) Foster: "OK, (P) Horne." (NA) Price: "Stand up. We're gonna put you to bed. Do you want to go to bed? Come on, hon'. We're gonna be real easy with you. Now see, you're all right. That was real good
2:07	wasn't it?" (3-minute duration)

Such interactions prevent meaningful, time-consuming conversations. Nurse's aides were kind and humane to patients, but still had to conform to job demands. Pecan Grove Manor's registered nurse was explicit:

(Author): What prevents [meaningful conversations between aides and patients] from happening now?

(RN): The number of employees, mainly. All of them [i.e., nursing staff] are needed for basic care, so that the emotional side . . . is kind of left [undone]. . . . it is hard to just sit down and have eye-to-eye contact and really feel close to the patient when you are giving them daily care . . . if [patients] are going to do any talking or visiting, it has got to be done quickly while they have got [the aides], so a lot of things are left out.

On the other hand, the potential for housekeepers to engage in meaningful interaction with patients is naturally enhanced by their job performance demands. While the nurse's aides demonstrate to supervisors their diligence and hard work by quickly flitting from room to room, the housekeepers are in the opposite situation. Demonstration of job fulfillment for housekeepers involves a lengthy stay of about 20 minutes in patient rooms. This indirectly conveys a message of thoroughness of cleaning, and provides a social field for engaging patient-housekeeper interactions. An 80-year-old male patient compares nurse's aides and housekeepers this way:

Well, all the nurse's aides don't have the time [to visit] 'cause [basic care] is more important. Now, Jane [housekeeper, pseudonym], she can come in here and clean that wash basin and talk all at the same time. And the nurse's aide, if I am sick and they come in to give me some attention, why they got their mind on what they are doing . . . they don't know what time that intercom is going to say go to so-and-so room or a certain wing. Jane, she knows that she is going to clean this wing up before going over to that east wing.

A 77-year-old female patient speaks of the housekeeper encounter:

Well, if I am crocheting, well, we will talk about that, or something that she has made. Usually, that's what we talk about—things that we are interested in . . . I enjoy the fellowship with her. She is interesting to talk to. We [i.e., patient and roommate] stay in the room right smart and it is nice to have somebody to talk to.

When comparing nurses' aides and housekeepers she says:

She [i.e., housekeeper] just comes in and cleans up and . . . she's not in a big hurry. And we talk and visit some . . . When [nurse's aides] come in, well, whatever they come to do, why they will talk but they do just what they've got to do and then they just go on.

Other factors that promote the psychosocial support role of the housekeeper include wearing common street clothes like patients and not white nursing uniforms; they are middle-aged, and have previous experience as nurse's aides. Thus, while they have primary care experience, patient-caretaker distinctions diminish and are replaced by adult-adult interactions.

Author: . . . why [do the patients] seem to visit with [the housekeepers] so much?

Housekeeper: I think maybe it's because we're in the rooms longer, and we don't wear white, and [the patients] seem closer to us. You know, we seem closer to 'em because [the patients] will tell things that maybe they won't tell someone else . . . Anita [i.e., the other housekeeper] will probably tell you the same thing. [The patients] tell her things they don't tell the nurses [aides] or even Miss Turner [the R.N.], you know.

Provisions of psychosocial support are invisible cargos. An instance of providing psychosocial support is not showy, does not involve mechanical instrumentation, but revolves about subtle personal demeanor and time to dispense this cathartic cargo.

Housekeeper: . . . [the patients] just feel closer to us because we are really in the wings longer and we have more time to talk to 'em . . . Like little things I say, like . . . maybe they won't like a nurse and you don't run this nurse down, you know, you build her up and then maybe

next time they'll just fall in love with this nurse.
. . . But, it's just little things like that. But it
don't really seem important—not even to the
[nurse's aides], you know. But, to me and to them
it is.

The lack of awareness of the psychotherapeutic
benefit of housekeeper-patient interaction by the
nursing staff is a common theme in conversations
with the housekeepers.

Housekeeper: . . . sometimes, you know, now I
know I never did feel like this, but some of the
aides think the housekeepers are just the housekeepers, you know. But sometimes we understand
the little people more than the nurses do."

Because the other staff groups are unaware of
the multidimensional role of the housekeepers, episodes of significant psychosocial support given to
patients are not only unrecognized, such support is
not promoted.

Housekeeper: . . . like [P] Miss Thompson, for
instance, before she left [for irradiation of a cancer site], she was, you know, just very depressed,
and I came in [the patient's room] and just sat
down on a stool and talked to her a little while
and had her laughing before I went out.

Author: . . . you don't have to do it for your
job?

Housekeeper: No, I don't . . . I just go ahead
and talk to 'em if they're real lonesome. You know,
a lot of [patients] are real, real lonesome, and
if you can just have a little time with 'em . . .
they're just lonely little people and if you can
say a word or two to make them happy or make
'em feel a little better—you have the time—I don't
see anything wrong with it.

Other housekeeper-nurse's aide distinctions operate to alter the patient perception of encounters
with the staff. Being a patient means the surrender
of a large degree of personal autonomy (Taylor 1970).
Nurse's aides can enter patient rooms, inquire about
bowel habits, sleep habits, mood, touch the nude
body and genitals, etc., all as a part of nursing care
regimens. On the other hand, the presence of a
housekeeper in the patient rooms carries no threat
of bodily invasion or other nursing tasks that often
resemble infant care. The subsequent reduction of

role and status inequities enhances the encounter
in the direction of psychosocial independence and
away from institutional dependence.

The housekeepers also function as brokers between the patients and nursing staff. Direct information regarding this part of their patient support repertoire was difficult to collect due to a powerful
administrative dictum that internal problems not
be overblown by gossip and rumor. The result is
an order to not pass along information that could
be troublesome. Therefore, my inquiries were often
met with vague responses regarding specific problems but clear evidence of a broker function.

Author: It sounds like . . . [the housekeepers]
are more reliable ways to get information to [the
licensed nursing staff rather than the nurse's
aides].

Housekeeper: Like, well, [patients] say, "I told
[a nurse's aide] and she told me that she would
see about it, but, you know, I don't believe she
will." And then I have . . . to please them, I
have gone and told Miss Turner [R.N.] things,
you know.

In another response:

Housekeeper: . . . [Patients] don't want to tell
(problems to the nursing staff) theirselves and
they know if they tell me then I will go and tell
[the proper staff members] . . .

In summary, the patients perceive the housekeepers as expected daily visitors who can converse
at length, carry information throughout the nursing
home, and report on local community matters on a
routine basis. Housekeepers, then, not only "keep
house" but also act as a patient resource and a consistent provider of psychosocial support, although outside the standard boundaries of therapeutic agents.
Thus, while nurses tend to the body, housekeepers
tend to the mind.

DISCUSSION

Other nursing home studies (e.g., Gubrium 1975;
Kayser-Jones 1979) have noted that nursing staffs
are unable to provide psychosocial support to patients due to so-called basic care demands and, moreover, fail to see psychosocial support as a primary
nursing task (Henderson 1979). In this study, deliv-

ery of psychosocial support was the province of the housekeepers, who also were used by the patients as liaisons for handling sensitive matters. The ethnomedical view was critically important in the discovery of the housekeeper's role as caregivers. In fact, for the majority of my research project, the unconscious bias of my world view predisposed me to overlook housekeepers as significant functionaries. The ethnomedical perspective, however, not only served as a conceptual model for collecting and organizing data, but eventually undermined this instance of observer bias.

Prominent and more standard forms of nursing home investigation are the periodic government inspection and evaluation surveys. Such inspections assess the quality of psychosocial provisions by reviewing patient activities entered on government forms by nursing home personnel. These activities include arts and crafts, remotivation sessions, religious services, bingo, and other highly visible, easily recorded events. While such rituals are likely beneficial, the additional psychosocial support provided by the housekeepers is overlooked by inspection teams.

The psychosocial support role of the housekeepers at Pecan Grove Manor is the product of several factors in combination: the long-term-care environment, housekeepers' style of work, housekeepers' personal demeanor, and the human need for psychosocial stimulation. Long-term-care environments allow for patients and staff to get to know each other well, develop resource networks based on reciprocal exchange, and learn manipulative strategies for maximizing one's nursing home career experience. The patient-staff experience in acute care hospitals is similar (see Taylor 1970) to that in nursing homes, but to a much lesser degree due to short patient stays.

The work style of the nursing home housekeeper is another critical factor of their psychosocial support role. During an eight-hour shift, nurse's aides may have longer total patient contact times compared to the housekeepers, but their style of interaction is very different. The brisk, episodic discharge of duty by a nurse's aide may produce a sense of medical security in the eyes of families and administration, but for the patients, the slower, sustained visitation by housekeepers produces a sense of humanness and worth.

The personal demeanors of the housekeepers is another significant factor. Without the social skills of communication and empathy, the psychosocial support services would not emerge or would be quite limited.

Last, the common perspective of nursing homes as desolate, resource-meager environments may be unwarranted. For decades, gathering and hunting societies were portrayed by anthropologists as barely existing in an endless morass of desert mirages. However, among the Dobe !Kung, Lee (1968) shows the human capacity for adaptation in a presumed resource-meager environment. Similarly, the nursing home patient shows remarkable adaptation. Thus, nursing homes may have a variety of resources hidden from the common observer. The future is likely to bring the proliferation of proprietary nursing homes as we know them today. Given this projection, applied research should be directed at maximum extraction and enhancement of naturally evolved beneficial behaviors and roles already extant in nursing home communities. Regarding housekeepers, questions for further research should include an assessment of the degree of benefit provided to patients, effects of the sex and age differences of the housekeeper and patient, analysis of housekeeper and patient interactions, and patients' perceptions of the housekeepers. Application of such research findings could be routed through the existing in-service training programs rather than requiring the creation of new jobs with supporting payrolls. Thus, the cost-benefit ratio of the enhancement of existing behavioral systems is seen as economically attractive to proprietary nursing home owners for improving the quality of institutional life.

In summary, Pecan Grove Manor patients have seized upon the housekeepers as a naturally evolved element of their institutional setting for psychosocial support and as a personal resource. The patients have identified and used the housekeeping staff in an unintended, unexpected way. These findings underscore the persistent depth of capacity for human resource identification and use among institutionalized geriatric patients.

Notes

1. The rural setting likely influences the nature of the housekeepers' psychosocial functions at Pecan Grove

Manor. In this community, the friendship and kinship network was localized so that the housekeeping staff knew the family or friends of many of the patients. Also, racial and religious differences were minimal. Although some staff and patients identified themselves as Indian, only one nurse's aide was a native speaker and voted in tribal elections. However, while local demographic factors may shape the specific patterns of psychosocial caregiving, the common institutional work styles of nursing home housekeepers will continue to promote the existence of their psychosocial support role.

References Cited

ADMINISTRATION ON AGING
1980 Human Resources in the Field of Aging: The Nursing Home Industry, Occasional Papers in Gerontology. USDHEW Publication No. (OHDS)80–20093 (Washington, D.C.: H.E.W.).

BECK, J. C., D. KANTOR, and V. A. GELINEAU
1963 Follow-up Study of Chronic Psychotic Patients Treated by College Case-aide Volunteers. American Journal of Psychiatry 120:269–71.

BESDINE, RICHARD
1982 The Data Base of Geriatric Medicine. Pp. 1–14 in John Rowe and Richard Besdine (eds.) Health and Disease in Old Age. Boston: Little, Brown and Company.

DEANE, W. N.
1961 The Culture of the Patient: An Underestimated Dimension in Psychotherapy. International Journal of Social Psychiatry 7:181–86.

DUMONT, M. P.
1967 Tavern Culture: The Sustenance of Homeless Men. American Journal of Orthopsychiatry 37:938–45.

FREIDSON, ELIOT
1970 Profession of Medicine. New York: Dodd, Meade.

GOFFMAN, ERVING
1961 Asylums. New York: Doubleday.

GROSS, MARTIN L.
1978 The Psychological Society. New York: Random House.

HALL, RICHARD H.
1977 Organizations: Structures and Process. Englewood Cliffs, New Jersey: Prentice-Hall.

HEINE, R.
1962 The Student Physician as Psychotherapist. Chicago: University of Chicago Press.

HENDERSON, J. NEIL
1979 Chronic Life: An Anthropological View of an American Nursing Home. Doctoral Dissertation: University of Florida.

HOLZBERG, JULES D., ROBERT H. KNAPP, and JOHN C. TURNER
1967 College Students as Companions to the Mentally-Ill. In Emergent Approaches to Mental Health Problems. Emory L. Cowen, Elmer A. Gardner, and Melvin Zax, eds. Pp. 91–109. New York: Appleton-Century-Crofts.

HUGHES, CHARLES C.
1968 Ethnomedicine. In International Encyclopedia of the Social Sciences. 10:87–93. New York: Free Press/Macmillan.

JOHNSON, COLLEEN L. and LESLIE A. GRANT
1985 The Nursing Home in American Society. Baltimore: Johns Hopkins University Press.

KASTENBAUM, R. S., and S. CANDY
1973 The 4% Fallacy: A Methodological and Empirical Critique of Extended Care Facility Program Statistics. International Journal of Aging and Human Development 4:15–21.

KAYSER-JONES, JEANIE
1979 Care of the Institutionalized Aged in Scotland and the United States: A Comparative Study. Western Journal of Nursing Research 1:190–200.

KRAMER, CHARLES H., and JEANETTE R. KRAMER
1976 Basic Principles of Long-Term Patient Care: Developing a Therapeutic Community. Springfield: Thomas.

LEE, RICHARD B.
1968 What Hunters Do for a Living, or How to Make Out on Scarce Resources. In Man the Hunter. Richard B. Lee and Irven DeVore, eds. Pp. 30–48. Chicago: Aldine.

MANARD, BARBARA, RALPH WOEHLE, and JAMES HEILMAN
1977 Better Homes for the Old. Lexington, Massachusetts: Lexington Books.

MARSHALL, ELIOT
1980 Psychotherapy Works, but for Whom! Science 207:506–8.

MCQUILLAN, FLORENCE L.
1974 Fundamentals of Nursing Home Administration, 2nd ed. Philadelphia: Saunders.

MECHANIC, DAVID
1968 Medical Sociology. New York: The Free Press.

MILLER, DULCY B.
1969 The Extended Care Facility: A Guide to Organization and Operation. New York: McGraw-Hill.

MOSS, FRANK E., and VAL J. HALAMANDARIS
1977 Too Old, Too Sick, Too Bad. Germantown Maryland: Aspen Systems Corporation.

NEUGARTEN, BERNICE C., and GUNHILD HAGESTAD
1976 Age and the Life Course, pp. 35–55 in Robert H. Benstock and Ethel Shanus (eds.), Handbook of Aging and the Social Sciences, New York: Van Nostrand Reinhold.

PARSONS, TALCOTT
1951 The Social System. New York: The Free Press.

PEGELS, C. CARL
1981 Health Care and the Elderly. Rockville, Maryland: Aspen Corporation.

RIOCH, MARGARET J.
1967 Pilot Projects in Training Mental Health Counselors. *In* Emergent Approaches to Mental Health Problems. Emory L. Cowen, Elmer A. Gardner, and Melvin Zax, eds. Pp. 110–27. New York: Appleton-Century-Crofts.

ROGERS, WESLEY W.
1971 General Administration in the Nursing Home. Boston: Cahners Books.

ROSENHAN, D. L.
1973 On Being Sane in Insane Places. Science 179:250–58.

SANDERS, RICHARD
1967 New Manpower for Mental Hospital Service. *In* Emergent Approaches to Mental Health Problems. Emory L. Cowen, Elmer A. Gardner, and Melvin Zax, eds. Pp. 128–43. New York: Appleton-Century-Crofts.

SCHEFF, THOMAS J.
1961 Control Over Policy by Attendants in a Mental Hospital. Journal of Health and Human Behavior 2:93–105.

SUBCOMMITTEE ON LONG-TERM CARE OF THE SPECIAL COMMITTEE ON AGING, U.S. SENATE
1975 Nurses in Nursing Homes: The Heavy Burden (the reliance on untrained and unlicensed personnel). Nursing Home Care in the U.S.: Failures in Public Policy, supporting paper No. 4 Report No. 94–00, 94th Congress, 1st Session.

TAYLOR, CAROL
1970 In Horizontal Orbit: Hospitals and the Cult of Efficiency. New York: Holt, Rinehart, and Winston.

TORREY, E. FULLER
1969 The Case for the Indigenous Therapist. Archives of General Psychiatry 20:365–72.
1972 The Mind Game: Witchdoctors and Psychiatrists. New York: Bantam.

UHLENHUTH, E. H., and D. B. DUNCAN
1968 Subjective Change with Medical Student Therapists: Course of Relief in Psychoneurotic Outpatients. Archives of General Psychiatry 18:428–38.

U.S. BUREAU OF THE CENSUS
1978 Statistical Abstracts of the United States. Washington, D.C.: U.S. Government Printing Office.

VICENTE, LETICIA; JAMES A. WILEY and R. ALLEN CARRINGTON
1979 The Risk of Institutionalization Before Death. The Gerontologist 19:361–67.

PART FOUR

The System

CHAPTER 12

Health and Health Care: Issues in Access and Delivery

The system of health care in the United States stands apart from those of other industrial nations of the world. The point of difference is the absence of a system of universal comprehensive care for its citizens. Instead, the United States has what many have called a "two-class" medical care system, one for the rich and one for the poor. It is, in fact, a "three-class" system, since below the Medicaid poor are those with no coverage at all—the 36 million or so uninsured.

In the mid-1960s, the United States began to move inexorably toward national health insurance with a slow but sure progression of legislation aimed at subsidizing health care for those unable to afford it. Medicare for the elderly, Medicaid for the poor, a federal program to provide kidney dialysis to those who need it, and one to provide hospice care to the terminally ill were all part of that progression. However, with a new administration in Washington, national health insurance has been forgotten, as cost containment, rather than equity, has become the priority.

The programs that were developed have paid dividends—for example, the existence of Medicaid has helped the poor to get a much fairer share of physician care, although where they receive this care is a different story—but gaping holes still exist. As already mentioned, a substantial number of Americans have no insurance; they make too much to qualify for Medicaid but not enough to buy private insurance. Medicaid patients, for their part, are covered, but they do not receive anywhere near the quality of care received by privately-insured patients. One reason for this is the fact that Medicaid reimbursements for services are on the low side. Only one-fourth of the physicians in the United States treat patients covered under Medicaid, and the Medicaid poor are most likely to receive care in clinics, some of which have been called "Medicaid mills," and at understaffed and underfunded public hospitals. The elderly are partially covered under Medicare, but they have to pay a good deal of the cost of care "out-of-pocket." For example, 49 percent of the enormous cost of nursing home care is paid for by the elderly from their own funds. Many become destitute in the process by being forced to "spend down"; that is, they are forced to get rid of most of their financial assets in order to become eligible for Medicaid.

Privately-insured patients do quite well in a system that emphasizes provider competition to the end of quality care at less cost. In particular, health maintenance organizations (HMOs)—prepaid, group health plans—have proven to be good buys for those who have access to them.

The entry of corporately-owned, for-profit hospitals into the competitive marketplace may add a new dimension in satisfying the needs of the wealthy (see the article on the Humana-Louisville hospital in a later chapter). At the same time, they are likely to impact less positively on the satisfaction of the health care needs of the poor.

Alternatives to hospital care that provide care on an "outpatient" basis are an important part of the strategy of keeping costs down. In addition, the elimination of unnecessary use of the system is being encouraged through insurance payments for things like second opinions.

The most pressing problem for the health care delivery system is the increasing proportion of the population made up of the elderly. Not only is the proportion of those 65 and over a concern, but additional concern is being raised over the dramatic growth in the "old-old"—those 85 and over. There is also some concern about a backlash against the elderly. There have been a number of articles of late that are critical of the fact that more of the resources of the nation go to the elderly— primarily because of the costs of health care in the last years of life — than go to the young. Those worried about the elderly getting short shrift in a system that sometimes seems more concerned with cost–benefit analysis than with saving lives look to England and worry more. In that country, where there is explicit rationing of health care—that is, there are clearly defined limits as to how many people can get certain expensive treatments—those over 50 are often rejected for treatments like kidney dialysis simply because they are older and there are not enough machines to go around (although age is not, by itself, supposed to be a factor in determining who lives and who dies).

David Mechanic begins this chapter with a brief but detailed overview of the structure of the U.S. health care delivery system. Howard D. Schwartz then discusses three aspects of the "irrationality" of the U.S. system, where irrationality is defined as a lack of agreement between the provision of services and the needs of the public. The three aspects are the maldistribution of physicians, the duplication of services, and the lack of fit between acute care and chronic illness. Caroline Kaufmann then compares the United States with two countries that do provide universal comprehensive care, Canada and Great Britain. The comparison looks at both structural differences in the provision of health care services and attitudes toward the notion of health care as a right.

The last two pieces in this chapter follow from the Kaufmann article. Karen Davis and Diane Rowland analyze the characteristics of the uninsured. The final piece in this chapter is Thomas Halper's powerful description of the explicit rationing of kidney dialysis in the United Kingdom.

A Brief Anatomy of the American Health Care System

David Mechanic

The purpose of this introduction is to present a short, overall picture of the health care system. It is difficult to describe in brief the dimensions of an industry involving facilities, goods, and services exceeding $400 billion a year. The size, complexity, and diversity is mind-boggling; the system of care is extraordinarily dynamic; and the high stakes intimately involve hundreds of government agencies, professional groups, business interests, consumer organizations, special interest lobbies, employers and unions, public interest groups, and many others. The health industry has been growing rapidly; some estimate it will reach an expenditure level of $2 trillion and 15 per cent of the gross national product by the year 2000.

HEALTH EXPENDITURE PATTERNS AND THE BURDEN OF ILLNESS

The single major component of total health care expenditures is hospital costs, consuming 42 per cent of the total. The second-largest element is physician fees, not already included in hospital budgets, totaling slightly in excess of 19 per cent. Other major components include: nursing home care (approximately 8.5 per cent); drugs and small medical items (almost 7 per cent); dental services (6 per cent); construction of medical facilities (2.5 per cent); and administration of insurance programs (almost 4 per cent). Restricting consideration more narrowly to

personal health expenditures shows that in 1983, 47 per cent of all such expenditures went for hospital care and 22 per cent for physician services. Given the size of the budget, a seemingly small 1 per cent involves expenditures of more than $4 billion.

In 1983, government at all levels accounted for 42 per cent of total health expenditures. The two largest programs, Medicare—a program for persons over 65 and a limited number of others with specific disabilities—and Medicaid—a federal-state matching program for the most impoverished part of the population—accounted for 29 per cent of personal health expenditures. Medicare alone cost $57 billion in 1983, $62½ billion in 1984, and is expected to cost $75 billion in 1985.

The pattern of health expenditures in some measure reflect the burdens of illness and risks of mortality in varying age and other social strata. The elderly and the poor are, of course, at greater risk. In examining the overall profile of mortality, four additional points ought to be considered. First, rates and causes of death vary greatly by sex and age. Women, on average, live more than seven years longer than men, and deaths among children, adolescents, and young adults are relatively low and predominantly due to accidents and self- and other inflicted violence. Second, age-adjusted death rates in the United States have been falling for major diseases with the exception of cancer. The increases in cancer are almost completely explained by smoking patterns. The large drop in age-adjusted mortality from heart disease and strokes in recent years are particularly important gains and account for a significant proportion of the advances in longevity among the American adult and elderly population. Third, while all groups in the population have benefited from downward trends in mortality, the large differentials between males and females and whites and nonwhites persist. Absolute rates have fallen, but the gaps have not significantly closed. Nonwhites and the poor remain at greater risk. Finally, while many biological, environmental, and other factors contribute to the differentials by age and sex, factors associated with behavior clearly have a major role. Cigarette smoking, accidents, excessive drinking, and failure to maintain control over blood pressure together account for massive increments in sickness and mortality.

More than two-thirds of all deaths in the United States are due to heart disease, cancer, and stroke. In excess of 7 per cent of deaths result from accidents, suicide, and homicide. Other major causes include chronic obstructive pulmonary disease (3.3 per cent), pneumonia and influenza (2.7 per cent), diabetes mellitus (1.8 per cent), chronic liver disease and cirrhosis (1.4 per cent), and atherosclerosis (1 per cent). No other single cause accounts for as much as 1 per cent of all deaths.

An alternative way of looking at the burden of sickness patterns is to examine health expenditures in relationship to varying classes of disease. Many diseases causing substantial suffering and disability, and great dependence on the medical care system, do not necessarily result in death. The 10 most costly categories of illness, as measured by expenditures on hospital care, nursing home care, professional services, and drugs, vary from circulatory disease, costing $33 billion in 1980, to endocrine, nutritional, and metabolic diseases, costing almost $8 billion. Intermediate categories, listed in order of importance were: diseases of the digestive system; mental disorders; injuries and poisoning; diseases of the respiratory system; cancer; diseases of the musculoskeletal system and connective tissues; genitourinary disorders; and diseases of the nervous system and sense organs.

The largest costs involve the elderly, who have more chronic and degenerative disorders than younger populations and require more ambulatory, hospital, surgical, and long-term care. These costs accelerate dramatically at the oldest ages and are particularly high in the final year of life. In 1977, per capita health care spending among those 65 and over was 3½ times that of the total population, and the difference has continued to grow since then. In 1978, persons 19 and under had per capita expenditures of $286 while those 65 or older expended

$2,026. Seventy per cent of all Medicare payments were on behalf of 9 per cent of the elderly involving an average payment of over $7,000. Reimbursement for the elderly was high during the last year of life, and particularly in the last 60 days before death. The 5 per cent of Medicare recipients who died in 1978 accounted for 28 per cent of program expenditures, which, on average, was $4,527 during the final year of life.

Most of the population have much of their medical expenses covered to varying degrees by health insurance. More than 90 per cent of the population have third-party insurance, most commonly profit and nonprofit insurance programs associated with the head of household's employment. The elderly are primarily covered by Medicare, and a significant proportion of the poor by Medicaid. It is estimated that in 1985 as many as 35 million people have no private or public insurance coverage. In 1982, nongovernment health insurance programs paid 29 per cent of all health care expenditures while 28 per cent were paid directly by patients. Hospital care and inpatient physician services were predominantly covered by third-party insurance, but coverage is much less comprehensive in the areas of ambulatory care, outpatient diagnostic services, drugs and appliances, preventive care, and dental and other services. Even Medicare, a program perceived as relatively comprehensive, pays only for 44 per cent of total health care costs of the elderly.[1] Out-of-pocket payments by the elderly have increased in recent years, and this population now pays a larger proportion of their total income for medical care then they did prior to the enactment of the program. Per capita out-of-pocket expenditures for the elderly are estimated to rise from $1,683 in 1985 to $2,395 by 1990. They receive, of course, much more medical care than before.

It is commonly noted that the number of poor aged has declined over time, making this age group comparable in economic status to other age categories in the population. While many elderly people have avoided poverty in large part due to social security and other public programs, a disproportionate number of aged persons live close to the poverty line and could become impoverished with cutbacks in federal programs. Moreover, the elderly group is heterogeneous. While some are affluent, many are poor. Some analysts speak of the "two faces" of aging, emphasizing that significant segments of the aged are greatly disadvantaged and face special burdens when sick. In 1981, for example, while elderly persons on average paid 13 per cent of their incomes for out-of-pocket health expenditures, the black elderly paid 23 per cent and black elderly women 27 per cent of their incomes for such out-of-pocket costs. Also, because of the inadequacy of long-term care coverage and complex eligibility criteria for Medicaid coverage, an elderly person may be required to become impoverished before the spouse can receive needed subsidy for essential long-term care. These areas continue to be important challenges for future policy formulation.

I now turn to a description of the basic components of the system: physicians, nurses, and other health care personnel; the organization of primary medical care and first contact facilities; innovative system approaches such as HMOs (health maintenance organizations); the hospital sector and related institutional facilities; tertiary care and the sophisticated teaching hospitals; and research and development in health and health care.

HEALTH WORKERS

Physicians dominate the health sector although they constitute only a small minority of the many millions of health workers. At the beginning of the century there were two health workers per physician, but the present number is more like 15 to 1.[2] There are approximately one-half million physicians in the United States, a ratio of more than 1 for every 500 patients. This reflects an increase from 1.4 physicians per 1,000 patients in 1950 to 2.2 in 1985. The increasing supply reflects the substantial expansion of medical education between 1960 and 1980. In 1960–1961, American medical schools graduated somewhat less than 7,000 doctors. In recent years, they have been graduating between 16,650 and 17,400. As a consequence, we anticipate an excess future supply. The Graduate Medical Education National Advisory Committee (GMENAC), established to advise the secretary of the Department of Health and Human Services, anticipated an oversupply of 70,000 doctors by 1990 and 145,000 doctors by the year 2000.[3] The concept of oversupply is, of course, a fairly arbitrary one. In one sense, the number of

doctors one needs depends on the willingness to pay for services. Much evidence supports the belief that the nation is reaching a ceiling in its financial commitment to continuing growth in the medical care sector relative to other social priorities.

Though the total supply of physicians is estimated to be in excess, some specialties are expected to be in short supply, while others are seemingly in great abundance. Areas of anticipated undersupply include general and child psychiatry, preventive medicine and emergency medicine, and physical medicine and rehabilitation. Areas expected to have large oversupply include general surgery, obstetrics-gynecology, and many of the medical and surgical subspecialties such as nephrology, rheumatology, cardiology, endocrinology, pulmonary medicine, neurosurgery, and plastic surgery. Estimates of oversupply are uncertain to some degree because many subspecialists facing inadequate specialty work loads fill in their time doing general medicine,[4] because of unanticipated changes in science and technology, and because there are alternative ways of coping with excess supply, including cutbacks in medical school enrollment, retraining doctors for needed clinical areas, expanding the boundaries of medical work, and migration of physicians to underdoctored areas. Yet when all is said, it seems evident that physician supply will be very large as compared with prior decades.

Physicians are primarily organized in relation to three major dimensions: specialty, type of group organization, and form of remuneration. All of these are in a dynamic state, and it is difficult to clearly predict future trends. A major distinction is between doctors engaged in primary care as compared with those primarily practicing specialties and subspecialties. Most typically, the primary care disciplines are defined as family practice, general internal medicine, and general pediatrics. Despite many efforts on the part of government and private foundations to encourage primary care training and practice, the trend continues toward specialty training, with a very substantial growth of medical subspecialists. On average, generalists see many more patients than specialists, charge less for each encounter, and are less likely to order complex and expensive medical procedures and laboratory tests.

Physicians have traditionally worked in office-based solo practice, and rarely in large single-specialty or multispecialty groups or other organizational settings, but the trend is clearly toward larger practice groups. In 1983, excluding physicians employed by hospitals or government, approximately half of U.S. doctors practiced by themselves, but those practicing in groups of five or more increased from approximately 17 per cent in 1975 to 23 per cent in 1983. More than three-quarters of doctors in 1983 were self-employed, varying from 87 per cent in the surgical specialties and 83 per cent in general and family practice to 68 per cent in other specialties. Older doctors are more likely to be self-employed, varying from more than four-fifths among physicians older than 56 to 61 per cent among those younger than 36. While prepaid practice is growing at a rate of 18 to 21 per cent each year, it still only serves approximately 6 to 7 per cent of the population, and thus relatively few doctors work exclusively in such settings. A much larger proportion of doctors at least have some patients covered by prepayment plans, and such coverage is becoming increasingly common. Younger physicians and women are more receptive to practice in HMOs than their counterparts.

Most doctors receive their income through fees charged for visits and specific services and procedures performed. Third-party reimbursement for doctors' fees increased from 17 per cent in 1950 to 62 per cent in 1981. In 1983, three-quarters of all doctors' patients were covered by Medicare (21 per cent), Medicaid (9 per cent), Blue Shield (23 per cent), and other private insurers (23 per cent). In 1983, doctors reported that while Medicaid covered only slightly more than half their usual fee for a follow-up office visit, Medicare paid 68 per cent and Blue Shield 77 per cent.

Even doctors working in private settings have increasingly incorporated themselves for tax and other advantages, such as limiting their financial liability. Such incorporation increased from 31 per cent of physicians in 1975 to 54 per cent in 1983. More than half of physicians working with colleagues received their remuneration in the form of a salary, while approximately a third are paid on a fee-for-service basis. Approximately 10 per cent receive a proportion of either net or gross billings. These data reinforce an important but not widely appreciated point: how practices charge patients and insurers, and how physicians within these practices are paid, are two separable matters.

The Medicare program reimburses approximately 26 per cent of office visits and almost 31 per cent of all hospital visits. Thus, Medicare, and how it pays doctors, is of crucial importance to physicians and they feel very much threatened by impending changes. Medicare is particularly important for the medical specialties accounting for 44 per cent of all visits. Average net physician income before taxes in 1983 was $106,000. It varied a great deal by specialty from a low of $68,500 for family and general practitioners to $148,000 in radiology. Incomes were lower in nonmetropolitan areas and among those who were employees as compared with those self-employed. Both the youngest and more elderly doctors earned the lowest incomes, with income highest in the 46 to 55 age group.

In summary, doctors have done rather well in the context of growing government involvement in medical care, and particularly in the context of the Medicare program. Their current status, however, is unstable due to the vigorous efforts by the government to control expenditures for medical care, reduce the federal deficit, and contain increasing costs at the state level. There is little doubt that this is an area of impending tension and acrimony, and physicians' incomes are likely to erode to some degree.

In 1980, there were about 1.3 million active registered nurses (RNs) in the United States, one for about every 145 people. The availability of RNs more than tripled since 1950, reflecting not only population changes and the increased importance of hospital care, but also the growth of technology and intensity of treatment characterizing inpatient care. Approximately two-thirds work full time and one-third part-time. Nursing is primarily based in hospitals, where two-thirds of all nurses are employed. Although most do general nursing, in recent years there have been significant increases in more specialized roles—for example, clinical nurse specialists, nurse clinicians, nurse practitioners and midwives. While very important in leadership roles in clinical settings, their number remain relatively small. In 1980, there were about 8,000 nurse clinicians, 16,000 nurse practitioners and midwives, 18,000 clinical nursing specialists, and 14,000 nurse anesthetists. Other major settings for employment of registered nurses include nursing homes, public and community health agencies, physicians' and dentists' offices, and student health services.

Nursing has become increasingly professionalized, and while in earlier eras most nurses obtained three-year diploma degrees and two- and three-year associate degrees, most nurses are now educated in colleges and universities. While in 1980 only a third of all practicing nurses had baccalaureate degrees, a major goal of nursing is to eventually require the baccalaureate for entry into practice. Many nurses are also going on for graduate degrees as well.

Unlike physicians, nurses are primarily employees, paid through hospitals and other institutional or agency settings. Nursing salaries have been traditionally low, often on a par with secretaries and other female workers, but lower than teachers and social workers. While salaries vary to some extent depending on supply and demand for nurses and the ability of nurses to organize and conduct effective collective bargaining, nursing salaries are constrained both by the large potential supply and the cost pressures on hospital budgets. Nurses, despite their crucial importance to the sophisticated care of the critically ill, earn between one-fifth and one-sixth of physicians' incomes. Of even greater import is the absence of income-graded career structures in clinical nursing, allowing little income differentiation between the young starting nurse and the more experienced nurse. While various aspects of the economics of nursing are hotly debated, it seems clear that many nurses leave nursing or reduce their level of participation because of relatively low pay. This, in combination with responsibility for important on-the-spot clinical judgments but with little clinical autonomy, and gruelingly hard work, makes nursing less attractive to many talented and ambitious people who see better alternative career prospects, or to older nurses who may drop out as they find the physical and psychological demands too heavy for the rewards they receive.

While nursing care provided by RNs is the key to high-quality patient care in hospitals, their efforts are supported by large numbers of licensed practical nurses and nursing aides and orderlies. In 1978, half a million licensed practical nurses and 1.1 million aides and orderlies supplemented registered nursing. Hospitals in 1978 also employed 240,000 laboratory personnel, 104,000 workers in radiological services, 80,000 in medical records, 52,000 respiratory therapy workers, and innumerable others carrying out such varied functions as billing, speech therapy, physical therapy, dietary services, etc. Even a cursory examination of the range of hospital employees conveys the enormous complexity of hospitals, their technologies, and their managerial responsibilities and challenges. Dentistry constitutes a separate system to a considerable extent, but it is worth noting that by 1980 we had in excess of 144,000 dentists and 230,000 dental hygienists, assistants, and laboratory technicians.

THE HOSPITAL

With the emergence of intensive and sophisticated surgical and critical care technologies, the hospital has become the central focal point of the medical care system. Not only does the hospital provide the context, technology, and specialized personnel for a broad array of medical applications, it also often serves as the core element in a system that includes ordinary primary care services, specialized ambulatory clinics, home care programs, affiliated nursing homes, rehabilitation programs, and a wide array of other services. In 1983, there were 6,888 hospitals in the United States, accounting for 1,350,000 beds, almost 39 million hospital admissions, and more than 270 million outpatient visits. While the numbers of hospitals has not changed much in several decades, and the number of beds has been reduced by several hundred thousand in the past 20 years, the hospital's sophisticated capacities have accelerated rapidly, making the institutions of the 1950s and those of the present vastly different. As previously noted, two-fifths of all medical care expenditures—approximately $160 billion in 1984—are for hospital services.

The most typical component of the hospital system is the 5,789 community hospitals, acute short-stay institutions accounting for almost 900,000 beds in 1983, somewhat in excess of four beds per 1,000 persons in the population. Most of these hospitals have between 50 and 200 beds, although 613 hospitals have in excess of 400 beds. Because of both technology and the need for economies of scale, the average size of community hospitals has been growing, increasing from an average of 153 beds in 1972 to 176 beds in 1983. Other hospitals, in 1983, included

342 federal hospitals and 703 special hospitals, such as long-term care institutions, psychiatric hospitals, chronic disease hospitals, and hospitals for respiratory diseases, alcoholism, mental retardation, and so on.

In 1983, on any given day, there were 750,000 patients in community hospitals, an occupancy rate of 73.5 per cent, staying an average of 7.6 days. With aggressive cost-containment efforts, hospital admissions and length of stay have been falling, with occupancy rates dropping to 68 per cent by mid-1984. The average cost per day of providing inpatient care in 1982 was $369, of which more than half went for personnel other than interns, residents, and other trainees. Intensive and coronary care beds are about 6 per cent of all beds, but cost 2½ times the regular bed charge. In 1982, the average cost for an intensive care bed was $408 a day in contrast to $167 for a regular bed.[5] Averages, of course, hide extraordinary variations among institutions by geographic area, size, patient mix, type of sponsorship and control, as well as many other factors.

Although data beyond 1983 are limited, admissions to voluntary hospitals declined from 1983 to 1984 from more than 36 million to approximately 35 million, a drop of almost 4 per cent. Average length of stay also decreased from 7 to 6.7 days among the nonelderly population and from 9.6 days to 7.4 days among patients covered by Medicare. Despite a reduction in hospital beds, occupancy rates declined to about two-thirds of capacity, a rate sufficiently low to induce great alarm among hospital administrators. While it is too early to fully assess this trend, or to provide an adequate empirically substantiated explanation, one major change has been a shift in surgical procedures from the hospital to ambulatory surgi-centers. A major strategy of for-profit industries and major suppliers is to put emphasis on surgical procedures that can be used in ambulatory settings, thereby avoiding the necessity of hospitalization. American Hospital Supply, for example, has developed lasers and a special new eye lens that allows cataract removal on an outpatient basis. Such transfer of technologies from the hospital, involving several days of inpatient care, to outpatient settings has dramatic cost implications since cataract surgery is one of the most commonly used surgical procedures with the elderly population.

There is much speculation about the recent drop in hospital admissions and length of stay. While some attribute the effect to the initiation of a diagnostic-related group (DRG) methodology under the Medicare program, the drop preceded its implementation and is unlikely to explain the change. It is more likely that impending cost constraints in general, anticipation of DRGs, the tougher activities of peer review organizations that assess the necessity for hospital admission, and the overall influence of increased cost-consciousness have all contributed to a more thorough scrutiny of the necessity for inpatient care. Moreover, the profitability of ambulatory surgery and other technical procedures for health companies and physicians must be taken into account. Medicare data for the years 1977–1982 show astronomical increases in the numbers of services and procedures performed, ranging from routine urinalysis, blood sugar tests, and examination of the feces for occult blood to EKGs and their interpretation. Understanding changes in hospital patterns requires examining the changing mix between services provided in hospitals and in ambulatory settings.

Hospitals have traditionally been owned and operated by a variety of governmental, community non-profit, religious, and proprietary organizations. The dominant form has been the voluntary not-for-profit hospital, organized under the auspices of community groups, religious orders, and a variety of other groups—for example, unions and industrial organizations, cooperatives, and organizations such as the Shriners. A small segment of the industry has been owned by individuals, partnerships, and investors seeking profits and there has been a long and continuing debate about the contributions and costs of having a proprietary sector in health care. This debate has very much accelerated in recent years with the aggressive entry of large multihospital corporations and other large investor-owned facilities. Contentions vary greatly: some argue that these developments bring new services to populations presently lacking them and force greater efficiencies in hospitals specifically and the health industry more generally; others contend that these profit-oriented ventures "cream" the profitable illnesses and patients, leaving higher risk patients and those with nonprofitable conditions to the public sector. They also argue that the powerful profit motives of medical care corporations, and their potential influences over practitioners, will significantly alter the way medicine is practiced and decisions are made in the future.[6]

The debate will continue. One fact, however, is clear: profit corporations in health care operations are growing at a rapid rate. As of 1982, approximately 10 per cent of hospitals were owned and 4 per cent were managed by profit chains; another 5 per cent were independently owned proprietaries.[7] These numbers are less impressive than the fact that the number of hospitals owned or managed by for-profit chains doubled between 1976 and 1982 and such corporations are aggressively acquiring existing hospitals, constructing new ones, and taking over small proprietary enterprises. In 1985, Hospital Corporation of America (HCA), the largest such chain, owned or managed 431 hospitals accounting for in excess of 60,000 beds. In 1983, HCA had operating revenue of almost $4 billion and earnings per share that have increased for 15 straight years, yielding a compound annual earnings per share growth rate of 25 per cent.[8] In 1984, HCA had net income of almost $300 million on net revenue of $3.5 billion and was devoting considerable resources to acquire and build more hospitals. As of 1983, Humana Corporation averaged growth in earnings per share of 41 per cent, and American Medical International 26 per cent. In sum, as Richard Rosett has put it, whether or not these corporations "are doing good, they are certainly doing well."[9]

In addition to the growth of chains of institutions, known as horizontal integration, there are increasing efforts by the health industries to increase their span of involvement over the entire array of health services, facilitating greater control over their markets, sources of supply of patients and products, and interorganizational relationships. In April 1985, a merger was proposed between HCA and American Hospital Supply Corporation, the largest source of medical supplies, which makes and distributes 130,000 products. The combined revenues of these companies in 1984 totaled $7.6 billion.* HCA as of 1985 owned 17 per cent of shares in Beverly Enterprises, the largest nursing home chain, and it is

---

* The proposed merger between HCA and the American Hospital Supply Corporation failed when Baxter Travenol, a hospital supply company, offered a higher price for AHSC stock. Pressures from stockholders resulted in acceptance of the Baxter offer.

anticipated that the continuation of vertical integration will proceed by acquiring companies manufacturing drugs, medical technologies, and ambulatory services and products. Humana, the third largest hospital chain, is marketing health insurance—Humana Care Plus—which provides a patient population for the facilities they own. While mergers and integration of programs and facilities are a response to the changing and more constrained economic environment, and an aggressive effort to take advantage of new opportunities, it also characterizes the new and influential constellation of forces in the health care arena.

It is difficult to forecast future developments, but generally two rather different scenarios are predicted for the future. Some anticipate accelerated development of profit-oriented ventures with corporate chains taking over many more hospitals and other types of health care facilities, integrating them into systems, and setting the tone for the medical care marketplace overall. It is suggested that in a decade or two, six or seven large corporations will dominate hospitals and much of the industry, and physicians significantly will be proletariatized. Alternatively, others believe that such firms will control a stable segment of the market, but not dominate it, preferring to invest in selected areas where opportunities are more promising of profits in an environment increasingly characterized by cost-consciousness and cost-regulation.

AMBULATORY MEDICAL CARE

Ambulatory medical care is carried out in a variety of settings including doctors' offices, clinics, hospital outpatient departments, single-specialty and multispecialty group practices, prepaid group practices, independent practice organizations, health centers, and emergency rooms. A variety of factors affect where people come for care including the availability and accessibility of providers, ability to pay and insurance status, attitudes and knowledge, and personal taste. There is broad agreement that it is desirable that patients have a primary care service that monitors their continuing needs for care, provides basic services, and makes referrals when necessary. This service should provide most basic preventive and acute care, coordinate whatever specialty care is used, and serve as patients' ombudsmen, helping them negotiate the complexities of the system.

Only some ambulatory care settings provide primary care in the sense described. Many are simply points of first contact, making an initial assessment of the patient's complaint and referring the patient as needed. While the patient may or may not come back to this setting, the physicians involved do not necessarily view themselves as the patient's personal physician or has having responsibility for continuity of care. Other services of first contact, such as outpatient departments in hospitals or emergency rooms, typically provide episodic care with little continuity and with little assumption of the role of personal physician for coordinating the patients' medical needs. Patients using such sources of care may see different doctors each time or may be treated for a single condition with little attention to other problems and needs they may have. While such care may not be optimal, even patients having alternatives sometimes choose to seek care from these settings, suggesting the variability and complexity of patient preferences.

Some settings are organized to provide primary medical care services more consistent with the definition stated earlier. Among physicians, the specialties of family practice and general internal medicine espouse such philosophies, and for children and adolescents, many pediatricians typically take similar responsibilities. Among organized practices, those emphasizing a "gatekeeper" role for the physician of first contact, such as prepaid group practice and independent practice organizations, often have highly developed approaches to primary care, although much variation exists in how broadly the physician of first contact construes his or her responsibilities and the degree of continuity of care with a physician who knows the patient. In many large health maintenance organizations, for example, continuity of care may be more developed in theory than reality, and patients with a need for acute care may commonly see an "urgent care" physician other than their designated primary care doctor.

The National Ambulatory Medical Care Survey (NAMCS)[10] provides data on encounters with office-based physicians. Office-based general and family practitioners account for about one-third of all visits and internal medicine and pediatrics for approximately another 25 per cent. Specialists also provide much general care in addition to care in their special domains. Using estimates from NAMCS, the average patient made 2.6 office visits in 1981, varying from 2.1 visits among those under 15 years to 4.3 visits for those 65 and over. Women made more visits than men. Somewhat more than a third of the visits were for acute problems, 28 per cent for routine chronic problems, and about 18 per cent for nonillness care. Other major reasons were for flare-ups of chronic conditions (9 per cent) and postsurgical or postinjury care (9 per cent). The vast majority of patients seen were previous patients (86 per cent) with old problems (64 per cent). Twenty diagnoses accounted for two-fifths of all care. The five most common were: essential hypertension (4.9 per cent); normal pregnancy (4.3 per cent); health supervision of an infant or child (3.2 per cent); acute upper respiratory infection (2.5 per cent); and general medical exam (2.4 per cent). Other frequent diagnoses included ear infections and diabetes mellitus. The above data are based on diary studies completed by office-based doctors. An alternative approach is to survey the population to assess their access to and use of health services. Data collected in 1982 indicate that 90 per cent of those surveyed report a usual source of care, and 80 per cent saw a physician at least once in the previous 12 months.[11]

The data described earlier relate to visits in doctors' offices, but patients see doctors in other contexts as well. In 1981, 69 per cent of all visits with doctors were in their offices, 13 per cent were in hospital outpatient departments, and 12 per cent of consultations were over the phone. Using a broader definition of visits, including these three types, the average number for the population was 4.6, and was highest among children under six, the elderly, and women.[12] The most common complaints seen, of course, vary by specialty.[13] Among family practitioners, for example, the five most frequent reasons for a visit (examination, acute upper respiratory infection, hypertension, prenatal care, and diabetes mellitus) accounted for almost one-fifth of all visits. The five most common complaints seen by a gastroenterologist accounting for a comparable proportion of visits included chronic enteritis and ulcerative colitis, functional disorders of the intestines, diseases of the esophagus, cirrhosis of the liver, and ulcer of the duodenum.

HEALTH MAINTENANCE ORGANIZATIONS

Health maintenance organizations (HMOs) still serve only a small minority of the population, but they are growing rapidly and are commonly seen as a prevalent model for the future. A major advantage to consumers is its prepayment feature and the availability of comprehensive services with little or no out-of-pocket costs. Government advocates see the HMO as an attractive model because of its implicit incentives to maintain a low rate of hospital admissions. At last count there were almost 17 million enrollees in HMOs, and enrollments have been growing yearly at a hefty 18 to 21 per cent. Between June 1983 and June 1984, HMO membership increased by 21.2 per cent. In 1984, there were 28 plans with 100,000 or more subscribers, as compared with 19 plans in 1982.[14] As of June 1984, these plans accounted for 58 per cent of total HMO enrollment. Average (mean) plan size, in contrast, was just below 50,000 members as of 1985. The majority of plans are relatively small in membership but are expected to grow substantially in future years. HMOs develop more rapidly in large urban settings characterized by mobility of population, and have become particularly well established in California and the Northwest and in various Northcentral states, particularly Minnesota and Wisconsin.

HMOs come in a great variety of forms, making the term itself somewhat misleading. Though they all have prepayment in common, almost every other dimension varies from one to another. While traditional established plans, such as Kaiser-Permanente and the Health Insurance Plan (HIP) of New York, were organized around group practice—hence the rubric prepaid group practice—many independent practice associations have doctors providing services to enrollees in their private offices. Even among traditional prepaid practices, some, Kaiser-Permanente for example, build, own, and operate their own hospitals, while others, such as HIP, use community hospitals. Physicians in prepaid groups are organized as staff employees in some HMOs, while in others they constitute self-governing groups that contract with the health care plan. Some large prepaid groups almost exclusively serve enrollees, while others mix prepaid and fee-for-service patients. While many HMOs are nonprofit organizations, for-profit HMOs are now a growth industry. In short, knowing that an organization is an HMO conveys relatively little about its philosophy, structure, functioning, or quality.

HOSPITAL USE

Rates of admission to hospitals vary enormously from one area to another and cannot be explained by the populations served or patterns of need, illness, or disability. Criteria for hospital admission and length of stay are commonly ambiguous and depend as much on the experience and judgment of the individual physician and local practices as they do on established professional norms. Tougher criteria for hospital admission, earlier ambulation following surgery, reduced length of stay, and performance of many types of surgery on an outpatient basis, all attest to the ability to substantially change customary practice with few negative effects and often positive medical as well as economic benefits.

A major use of hospitals is for surgical procedures; in 1979, almost 30 million procedures were performed on almost 19 million patients in short-stay hospitals.[15] The most common surgical procedures, each performed at least half a million times were: episiotomy, diagnostic dilatation and curettage of the uterus, endoscopy of the urinary system, bilateral destruction or occlusion of the fallopian tubes, cesarean section, tonsillectomy, and repair of inguinal hernia. The average length of stay of patients receiving procedures was 7.2 days in 1979, with the hospital stay varying by type and number of procedures.

Surgical rates vary by age and sex, with the highest rates among the elderly and women. Young males under 15 have more surgery because of accidents and injuries, but in the age group 15 to 44, the rate among females is approximately four times that among men. Even if obstetrical procedures are excluded, the rate among women far exceeds that among men, largely due to procedures related to the female reproductive system. In the age group 45 to 64, the female rate is still higher but much closer to the male rate (1,746 as compared with 1,509 per 10,000 population). In the age group over 65, male rates are considerably higher (3,056 versus 2,256 per 10,000 population). These differences reflect the higher prevalence of procedures for men relating to the respiratory and cardiovascular systems. Older men also have more procedures than women affecting the urinary system. Procedures related to obstetrics or the reproductive system account for two-fifths of all female procedures, while male procedures predominate in the areas of the digestive system, the musculoskeletal system, and the urinary system.

Diagnostic procedures performed on inpatients are frequently performed on outpatients as well, and thus understate the total prevalence. In 1979, 2.4 million biopsies and endoscopies were performed on inpatients. Other common procedures were radioisotope scans, arteriography, myelograms, and intravenous pyelograms. In 1979, there were almost 200,000 CAT (computerized axial tomography) scans on inpatients; the frequency of such scans seem to be increasing rapidly as this type of radiography becomes a fairly conventional hospital technology. Such units are also increasingly available in offices of large medical practices.

Wennberg and Gittelsohn[16] have documented large variations in available resources and the amount of care given from one locality to another. In one analysis of variations among 13 hospital service areas in Vermont, for example, they documented extraordinary differences by area in hospital discharges (from 122 per 1,000 to 197), surgical procedures (from 36 to 69 per 1,000 population), available hospital beds per 10,000 persons (34 to 59), hospital personnel per 10,000 people (68 to 120), and so on. Their work suggests the importance of establishing clear norms within the medical profession describing reasonable ranges for resource need, hospital admission, and surgical intervention. Geographic, economic, and social differences would lead us to expect some variability, and uncertainty in medical practice is a reality we cannot wish away, but it is difficult to believe that with careful planning, education, and peer review we cannot more effectively limit the enormous range of these discrepancies. Some areas may have too few resources and fail to provide all the care needed, but most knowledgeable observers believe that these variations in large part reflect excess hospital beds, an overabundance of physicians and surgeons in particular areas, and incentives that encourage additional procedures and interventions at the margins.

LONG-TERM CARE

The long-term care industry and nursing homes as its dominant institution are not new, but they grew rapidly in response to the infusion of funds that followed the implementation of Medicaid in 1966. In 1960, only $500 million a year was expended in nursing home care, approximately 2 per cent of total personal expenditures for health care. In 1983, the comparable numbers were more than 9 per cent and approximately $29 billion. As of 1980, there were an estimated 23,000 facilities fitting the description of a nursing home, with approximately 1.5 million beds. As of the same year, the Government Accounting Office estimated the availability of 1,373,300 licensed nursing home beds.[17] Nursing homes are relatively small; the average in 1980 was 66 beds. Medicare only covers short-term skilled nursing and rehabilitative care and, in 1979, contributed only 3 per cent of nursing home expenditures. Medicaid, in contrast, has substantially become the nation's long-term care financing mechanism, contributing 45 per cent of all nursing home expenditures in 1979. In 1977, Medicaid supported to varying degrees between 48 and 75 per cent of all nursing home patients. Slightly less than half of all nursing home expenditures are privately financed.

The vast majority of nursing homes in the United States are proprietary institutions; of the 18,900 facilities included in the National Nursing Home Survey of 1977,[18] 14,500 were owned by private groups. These vary from the small "mom and pop" type operations, which are believed to constitute about 40 per cent of the total, to large corporate chains. For example, Beverly Enterprises as of 1985 owned 908 nursing homes. In 1984 Beverly earned almost $47 million on revenues of $1.4 billion.

The vast majority of patients in nursing homes are old and infirm and require assistance in many of the activities of daily living. In 1977, almost 600,000 patients had difficulties with incontinence, more than 400,000 required assistance in eating, and a majority required assistance in walking, in using the toilet, in dressing, and in bathing. Patients most commonly suffer from diseases of the circulatory system and mental disorders and senility. In 1977, only 4,200 facilities provided registered nurses on all shifts, and an additional 2,400 had registered nurses on duty for two shifts. Many institutions depend heavily or even exclusively on licensed practical nurses or even nurses' aides. While most institutions have an arrangement with a person who fills the title "medical director," most physicians spend little or no time in these institutions and the quality of care depends almost exclusively on the competence level and quality of the nurses who work there.

As they get older, the elderly are at much greater risk of institutionalization. The aging of the American population, and particularly the large increases in the population over age 85, suggests that we will need many more nursing home beds or must develop viable home care and other community alternatives if we are to escape significant expansions of the existing nursing home industry. Important alternatives are to convert unused or excess hospital bed capacity for long-term care; to develop grades of supervised housing in the community with adequate nursing, medical, and social service backup; and to develop and expand programs to enhance social functioning among the aged, to assist families who assume much of the ongoing care, and to remedy the social isolation of many frail elderly people. In coming years, long-term care considerations will increasingly dominate the nation's health and social services agenda.

SYSTEMS WITHIN SYSTEMS: FEDERAL HEALTH SERVICES

In addition to financing much of the public's health care, the federal government also owns, operates, or provides for relatively complete systems of services for veterans (Veteran's Administration), armed forces personnel and their dependents (Department of Defense), and American Indians (Bureau of Indian Affairs). This is not the context for any detailed discussion of these systems, but it is useful to provide some sense of their magnitude and scope.

The VA medical care system was originally developed to aid veterans with service-connected problems and disabilities, but over time, the system expanded to serve many others. In 1981, 84 per cent of VA patients were treated for health problems unrelated to military service. As of 1983, the VA operated 172 hospitals, 226 outpatient clinics, and 99 nursing home units.[19] Its department of medicine and surgery alone employed 194,000 persons. During 1981,

the VA served approximately 1.3 million inpatients, 42,000 nursing home patients, and provided almost 18 million outpatient visits. Its expenditures for 1983 were almost $8 billion, and large future increases are anticipated with the aging of our veteran population. The VA has developed a blueprint for meeting anticipated needs that would require increases of personnel by 70 to 150 per cent by the year 2000. With growing concern about government health budgets, various proposals have been made to integrate the VA system into our larger medical care system, to cut back on the scope of services offered to veterans with nonmilitary-related health problems, and to screen patients more carefully on the basis of their ability to pay their own medical care expenses. While some cutbacks and changes in service patterns are possible, veterans' groups constitute a powerful and effective lobby that have successfully thwarted such initiatives in the past.

The Department of Defense (DOD), in contrast, directly serves existing military personnel and provides for core dependents under the Civilian Health and Medical Program of the Uniformed Services (CHAMPUS), which authorizes care in non-DOD facilities when necessary services are not easily available in DOD installations. CHAMPUS operates like an insurance program with cost-sharing between the DOD and the recipient. It is estimated that the DOD provides service for 9 million persons, including both active and retired military personnel, their dependents, and survivors. In 1983, the DOD operated 161 hospitals and 310 clinics in the United States and abroad. Its medical care expenditures in 1982 were almost $7 billion, including the estimated provision of almost 900,000 hospital admissions and more than 51 million outpatient visits. The Indian Health Service, a considerably smaller program, operates 47 hospitals and 172 clinics for American Indians and Alaska natives.

THE HEALTH CARE RESEARCH ESTABLISHMENT, AMERICAN MEDICAL SCHOOLS, AND THE TEACHING HOSPITAL

The federal health research establishment, concentrated in the National Institutes of Health (NIH), and intimately linked with research efforts in medical schools, teaching hospitals, and universities is one of the most admired achievements of our national government. It has received sustained support from the public and the Congress, and the NIH alone has a budget in excess of $5 billion. In addition, extensive research and related efforts are supported by the Alcohol, Drug Abuse and Mental Health Administration (ADAMHA), consisting of three institutes relating to mental health, alcoholism, and drug abuse.

The NIH is organized around 12 bureaus and institutes that range widely over categorical disease areas and health concerns. The largest institutes include the National Cancer Institute, the National Heart, Lung and Blood Institute, and the National Institute of Arthritis, Diabetes and Digestive and Kidney Disease. The other institutes vary from broad general areas—such as aging, child health and development, the environmental health sciences, and general medical sciences—to more specific concerns—such as allergy, and infectious disease and dental research. Much of the basic and applied medical research in universities and medical schools is supported through the NIH extramural research program, involving a process where investigators submit requests for grants that are then evaluated by committees of peers rated on the basis of scientific merit. Proposals receiving the best priority scores are funded consistent with the availability of funds. In 1982, NIH contributed 20 per cent of all national basic research support, 37 per cent of all such federal support, and 48 per cent of all basic research support to universities and colleges.[20] The NIH also operates a vigorous intramural research program and supports research training and other research-related programs. More than half of all NIH funding goes to medical schools, and most of that goes to a relatively small group of elite institutions. In 1982, the top 20 medical schools accounted for half of all NIH support, and the top 10 for about one-third of all NIH support.

There are 127 medical schools in the United States. These schools have affiliation agreements with approximately 1,000 hospitals, but 100 of these hospitals account for about half of all residents trained. Thus, there are very major differences among institutions designated as teaching hospitals. Sixty-one hospitals share common ownership with medical schools, and for most purposes can be viewed as components of the same institution. Medical schools and major teaching hospitals also play an important part in the education of nurses, dentists, pharmacists, and other health professionals, and are important centers for research and training. The total effort is often given the title of Health Sciences Center.

Medical schools and teaching hospitals expanded rapidly in recent decades with the infusion of large sums of research support from the NIH. Seen as on the cutting edge of medical science, new technology, sophisticated patient care, and an investigatory mode, this perspective encouraged increasing specialization and subspecialization and a high dependence on the clinical laboratory and newly developed diagnostic procedures. Because of their sophistication, many teaching hospitals attracted a sicker and more complex mix of patients, and the process of training students and residents in these institutions contribute to a more expensive pattern of care than that found in the typical nonteaching community hospital.

As efforts are made to constrain expenditures for hospital care through rate regulation, diagnosis-related group methodologies, and other devices, there is growing concern among medical educators that new forms of reimbursement will not adequately pay teaching hospitals for their complex and sicker mix of cases, for their crucial role in training future generations of medical students, residents, and other health professionals, for the magnitude of uncompensated care they provide for the indigent without insurance, and for the intangible costs associated with maintaining sophisticated research operations. Our key teaching hospitals are a major national asset, and the way of reimbursing them fairly for their varied service, educational, and research functions are difficult issues. Balancing the preservation of their unique role in our health care system on the one hand, but also avoiding unnecessary costs on the other, will probably only evolve through a process of trial and error. We probably require a much more sophisticated classification of teaching hospitals, since many have only a modest teaching and research role.

There are those who believe that the technical orientation of our teaching hospitals, and their emphasis on the more rare and complex diseases, distort medical education and the health care system. They argue that the teaching hospital should play a larger and more central role in preventive medicine and primary medical care, assisting in better preparing young health professionals for the typical problems they are likely to confront in practice,[21] and teaching practice strategies that prevent illness and disability and promote functioning among the chronically ill. While these are all goals of much importance to our medical care system, it is unlikely that teaching hospitals will take a primary role in meeting these challenges; nor is it obvious that they should do so. Teaching hospitals serve a unique function in caring for the very sick, as well as expanding our knowledge of how to do so more effectively.

Medical care in America requires a better balance between prevention and treatment, promotion of function and cure, and educational as compared to technical approaches to care. We should not, however, confuse the need for a more sober balance with denigration of the search for more sophisticated treatments and better understanding of disease processes. It is the combined agenda of balance and scientific sophistication that offers us the greatest potential for a system of effective medical care for the future.

References

1. Aiken L, Bays K. The Medicare debate—round one. N. Engl. J. Med. 1984; 311:1196–1200.

2. Ginzberg E. Allied health resources. In: Mechanic D, ed. Handbook of health, health care, and the health professions. New York: Free Press, 1983:479–494.

3. U.S. Department of Health, Education and Welfare. GMENAC staff papers: supply and distribution of physicians and physician extenders. Washington, D.C.: Government Printing Office, 1978.

4. Aiken L, et al. The contribution of specialists to the delivery of primary care. N. Engl. J. Med. 1979; 300:1363–1370.

5. Congress of the United States, Office of Technology. News release, Nov. 29, 1984.

6. Starr P. The social transformation of American medicine. New York: Basic Books, 1982.

7. Gray B, ed. The new health care for profit: doctors and hospitals in a competitive environment. Washington, D.C.: National Academy Press, 1983:2.

8. Wohl S. The medical industrial complex. New York: Harmony Books, 1984.

9. Rosett R. Doing well by doing good: investor-owned hospitals. University of Chicago: Michael Davis Lecture, Center for Health Administration Studies, Graduate School of Business, 1984:3.

10. National Center for Health Statistics. Patients' reasons for visiting physicians: national ambulatory medical care survey, U.S. 1977–78. Hyattsville, Md.: National Center for Health Statistics, 1981. (DHHS publication no. 82–1717, Series 13, No. 56.)

11. Robert Wood Johnson Foundation. Special report, update on access to health care for the American people. Princeton, N.J.: Robert Wood Johnson Foundation, 1983, No. 1.

12. National Center for Health Statistics. Health—United States, 1983. Hyattsville, Md.: National Center for Health Statistics, 1983. (DHHS publication no. [PHS] 84–1232:137.)

13. Robert Wood Johnson Foundation. Special report, medical practice in the United States. Princeton, N.J.: Robert Wood Johnson Foundation, 1981.

14. National Industry Council for HMO Development. The health maintenance organization industry ten-year report, 1973–1983.

15. National Center for Health Statistics. Surgical and nonsurgical procedures in short-stay hospitals: United States, 1979. Hyattsville, Md.: National Center for Health Statistics, 1983. (DHHS publication no. [PHS] 83–1731, Series 13, No. 70:3.)

16. Wennberg J, Gittlesohn A. Small area variations in health care delivery. Science. 1973; 182:1102–1108.

17. U.S. General Accounting Office. Constraining national health care expenditures: achieving quality care at an affordable cost. Sept. 30, 1985.

18. National Center for Health Statistics. The national nursing home survey: 1977 summary for the United States. Hyattsville, Md.: National Center for Health Statistics, 1979. (DHEW publication no. [PHS] 79–1794, Series 13, No. 43.)

19. Veteran's Administration. Caring for the older veteran. Washington, D.C.: Government Printing Office, 1984.

20. National Institutes of Health. NIH data book. Bethesda, Md.: Office of Planning and Evaluation and the Division of Research Grants, June 1984.

21. Lewis I, Sheps C. The sick citadel: the American academic medical center and the public interest. Cambridge, Mass.: Oelgeschlager, Gunn and Hain, 1983.

Bibliographic Note

For the purposes of this introduction it is superfluous to document each of the figures or trends noted. Only occasional references are given. Much of the data in the chapter can be found in the following general data sources: National Center for Health Statistics, *Health—United States, 1983,* Washington, D.C.: U.S. Government Printing Office, DHHS Pub. No. (PHS) 84–1232, Dec. 1983; *Health—United States, 1984,* Washington, D.C.: U.S. Government Printing Office, DHHS Publ. No. (PHS) 85–1232, Dec. 1984; Center for Health Policy Research, *Socioeconomic Characteristics of Medical Practice 1984,* Chicago: American Medical Association, 1984; Daniel Waldo and Helen Lizenby, "Demographic characteristics and health care use and expenditures by the aged in the United States: 1977–1984," *Health Care Financing Review* 6:1–29, 1984; National Center for Health Statistics, *Patients' Reasons for Visiting Physicians: National Ambulatory Medical Care Survey, United States, 1977–78,* DHHS Pub. No. (PHS) 82–1717, 1981; National Center for Health Statistics, *Surgical and Nonsurgical Procedures in Short-Stay Hospitals: United States, 1979,*

DHHS Pub. No. (PHS) 83–1731, 1983; National Center for Health Statistics, *The National Nursing Home Survey: 1977 Summary for the United States,* DHHS Pub. No. (PHS) 79–1794, 1979; Eli Ginzberg, "Allied health resources," in David Mechanic (ed.) *Handbook of Health, Health Care, and the Health Professions,* New York: Free Press, 1983, pp. 479–494; Eugene Levine and Evelyn Moses, "Registered nurses today: a statistical profile," in Linda Aiken (ed.) *Nursing in the 1980's,* Philadelphia: Lippincott, 1982, pp. 475–494; National Center for Health Statistics, Annual Summary of Births, Deaths, Marriages and Divorces: United States, 1983, *Monthly Vital Statistics Report* 32, No. 13, Sept. 21, 1984; American Hospital Association, *Hospital Statistics,* Chicago, 1983; American Hospital Association, *Hospital Statistics,* Chicago, 1984; U.S. General Accounting Office, *Constraining National Health Care Expenditures: Achieving Quality Care at an Affordable Cost,* Sept. 30, 1985.

Irrationality as a Feature of Health Care in the United States

Howard D. Schwartz

To many observers of the American health care scene, the term "health care delivery system" is an inappropriate designation for the country's organization of health care services. Rather, they see a "nonsystem"—that is, an uncoordinated and often competing group of delivery mechanisms. In this view, the greatest failure is a lack of any overall health care planning. The lack of a comprehensive strategy directed toward defining the needs of the population and the best ways to meet them

has resulted in a massive lack of fit between the structure by which health care is provided and the health requirements of the nation. This "irrationality" in the provision of health care services is, to a large extent, the result of a social context of professional dominance in which the perogatives and vested interests of physicians and hospitals determine how and where health care is delivered. (The next chapter in *Dominant Issues* is devoted to the issue of professional dominance.)

Three manifestations of the irrationality embedded in the U.S. health care delivery system have been the focus of the most attention and will be

This is an original article written for this edition of *Dominant Issues in Medical Sociology.*

dealt with here. They are (1) the maldistribution of physicians, (2) the duplication of services, and (3) the incompatibility of the acute care capabilities of medicine with the increasingly chronic nature of illness.

Some Prefatory Remarks

In the last two to three decades, medicine has been undergoing an attack as to its usefulness. An example of this genre of argument is the McKinlay and McKinlay article that appears later in this book. Another is the work of Ivan Illich, which focuses on medicine as a "nemesis" and as frequently counterproductive to better health.[1] One writer has called this dismissal of medicine's contributions to health "therapeutic nihilism."[2] He argues that while it is true that modern medicine may have received too much credit for improved health status, it is overstating the case to dismiss it as having made virtually no contribution in this regard.

Since support of a policy of a better allocation of physician services assumes that this would bring health benefits to those currently deprived of those services, a look at some of the pertinent data would seem to be a prerequisite for the following discussion. A recent article by Crozier looks at several recent studies and concludes that medical care does have a beneficial effect on health.[3] The first, carried out by Hadley using 1970 data, included a large number of people who were older (the study was confined to those in the 45 to 65 age range) and found that medical care has a statistically significant effect on mortality rates. Overall, Hadley concluded that a 10 percent increase in per capita spending on medical care would decrease death rates by 1.57 percent. Another study cited was carried out by the Rand Corporation in 1984. It investigated the consequences of removing some 270,000 medically needy adults from MediCal (California's program for those receiving Medicaid). A comparison was made between 186 people who were removed from MediCal and a similar control group of people who were patients at an internal medicine practice at the University of California–Los Angeles. The researchers reported a "clinically meaningful deterioration" in the health status of the study group. In addition, although anecdotal in nature, three individuals died during the study period under circumstances that appeared to be related to the MediCal cut-off. In each case, the individual did not seek treatment for a treatable condition because of the belief that he or she was unable to afford it.

One of the most alarming statistics facing this nation is that the infant mortality rate (the number of babies dying within the first year of life for every 1000 live births) for black babies is twice as high as it is for white babies. One culprit in this case is the lack of quality medical care. As an illustration, we can look at the recent case of the Anacostia section within the District of Columbia. In 1980, this poorest area of the city had an infant mortality rate of 27.2 compared to a national average of 12.5. Within two years, the area had made a miraculous turnabout, cutting the rate in half to 13.7.

How can the dramatic drop in Anacostia's infant mortality rate be explained when the area itself changed so little? The answer lies in a multifaceted effort that was launched by the District. This all-out effort included better prenatal care for women as well as an upgrading of the quality of the care at the only local hospital that delivers babies. Prenatal care is critical because of the link between low birth weight and infant mortality. As far as the local hospital was concerned, it purchased more sophisticated equipment and intensified staff training to deal better with high-risk babies. Infant resuscitators were put into the delivery room for all high-risk pregnancies, and staff was added for resuscitation and neonatal monitoring (monitoring within the first month of life). Policies were also established for getting high-risk mothers and threatened newborns to higher intensity care available at other hospitals.

All of this is not meant to imply that criticisms of medicine's efficacy are totally unjustified, as will be made clear at various points in this paper. It is only to point out that there really are various sides to this issue, and more particularly as relates to the following discussion, that concerns over physician maldistribution have a substantial basis in fact.

THE MALDISTRIBUTION OF PHYSICIANS

One of the major problems of access to health care for the poor derives from a pattern of maldistributed health care resources. The extent of physician maldistribution has been well documented. It has been estimated that two-thirds of American physicians treat the one-third of the population that is most able to pay. Affluent towns and cities have an abundant supply, even an oversupply, whereas others—like those in rural areas—may not have even a single physician. The most wealthy states have over twice as many physicians as the least wealthy. In 1978, for example, Massachusetts and Connecticut were around the 250 physician per 100,000 residents mark, whereas Arkansas and Alabama each had about 120 doctors per 100,000. Differences among areas within states showed the same connection to socioeconomic class.

The geographical imbalance means that those Americans most in need of medical care are least likely to have it available to them. This is true because all measures of health status have shown that it is inversely related to social class. The poorer an individual, the more problematical that individual's good health. As can be seen from Table 1, black Americans have a higher risk of dying due to virtually all of the major factors related to mortality than do white Americans. (Here black–white is an imperfect but acceptable surrogate for social class.)

It can be seen from Table 1 that the relatively greater risk of mortality of blacks is highest for homicide-related deaths (black men are over six times more at risk than white men) and one and a half times greater for all of the conditions combined.

Something should also be said about the relationship between social class and hypertension. Blacks are more likely than whites to suffer from hypertension, but they are far less likely to get treated for it, despite the fact that the condition is controllable through proper treatment. Consequently, black males are about 10 times more at risk for death from hypertension than white males, and black females are about 13 times more at risk than their white counterparts. Hypertension itself accounts for more than 5 percent of the excess deaths in blacks as compared to whites.

There is no better illustration of the link between where a doctor locates and the financial pull of that area than the nation's capital. In 1981, Washington, D.C., had the nation's highest average household income, the nation's most educated population, and the nation's highest percentage of working women. As a result, Washington had a singular sufficiency of doctors. At that time, Washington's doctor to population ratio was 524 per 100,000 residents, a figure more than double that of the highest state. The obvious source of Washington's financial well being and consequent physician surplus is the presence of the nation's largest employer, the federal government, and the generous medical benefits it bestows on its workers. If Washington's general wealth of doctors is striking, its wealth of one particular type of specialist is astounding. In 1981, there were 1123 psychiatrists in Washington, more than any other kind of doctor. There were more psychiatrists than twice the combined number of all cardiovascular specialists, dermatologists, gynecologists, urologists, and proctologists. There were more psychiatrists than three times the number of all the psychiatrists in

TABLE 1 Age-adjusted death rates by selected cause, race, and sex in the United States in 1980 (rate per 100,000 population)

	BLACK MALE	WHITE MALE	RELATIVE RISK	BLACK FEMALE	WHITE FEMALE	RELATIVE RISK
Total deaths (all causes)	1112.8	745.3	1.5	631.1	411.1	1.5
Heart disease	327.3	277.5	1.2	201.1	134.6	1.5
Stroke	77.5	41.9	1.9	61.7	35.2	1.8
Cancer	229.9	160.5	1.4	129.7	107.7	1.2
Infant mortality	2586.7	1230.3	2.1	2123.7	962.5	2.2
Homicide	71.9	10.9	6.6	13.7	3.2	4.3
Accidents	82.0	62.3	1.3	25.1	21.4	1.2
Cirrhosis	30.6	15.7	2.0	14.4	7.0	2.1
Diabetes	17.7	9.5	1.9	22.1	8.7	2.5

Source: NCHS, Health: United States, 1983, Tables 9 and 15.

Nebraska, New Mexico, Idaho, Montana, South Dakota, and Alaska. There were even four times as many psychiatrists in one apartment building (known as the Freud Hilton) as in the entire state of Wyoming.[4] As already mentioned, the reason was insurance. In 1976, the federal government began providing generous outpatient mental health coverage under Blue Cross/Blue Shield. In the following four-year period, the number of psychiatrists mushroomed 50 percent, the sharpest such increase in the area's history.

One should not conclude from this brief profile, however, that all Washingtonians benefit equally from the physician oversupply. In fact, the distribution of doctors is very unbalanced over the eight political wards. In 1980, the ward with the highest ratio had 7.14 private physicians per 1000 ward residents, whereas the ward with the lowest ratio had 0.26 per 1000—meaning the former had 28 times the number of private doctors per capita as the latter.

In contrast to Washington, with its abundance of physician riches, some towns and cities in rural areas find it difficult to attract even a single physician. Their situation is made even more complicated by what several reports have labeled as an increasing recruitment problem for rural America. Physicians who have been found to be incompetent or impaired (e.g., those with personal problems stemming from such things as drug or alcohol abuse)—the estimate is that 10 percent of American physicians fall into the impaired category alone—find these rural areas handy havens for escaping their previous problems. At the present time, physicians who lose their licenses in one state are still able to practice in another. Newspaper stories have reported that Indian reservations and Veterans Administration hospitals have also become repositories for doctors with questionable backgrounds and competencies.

Geographical maldistribution is only one part of the physician maldistribution problem. The other is found in relation to specialty areas. In 1950, about one of every two physicians was a general practitioner; now about six out of seven are specialists (although some specialties, like internal medicine, are involved in the provision of general medical care). By the mid-1970s, it was clear that the balance had swung too far toward specialty medicine and more family practitioners—general practitioners in specialty robes—were needed. In 1981, the conclusions

of the Graduate Medical Education National Advisory Committee were published. The GMENAC report concluded, among other things, that there existed surpluses of surgeons in most surgical specialties and a shortage of family physicians.

The GMENAC report is most well known for its revelation concerning a doctor "glut" in the United States. The committee predicted that by 1990 there will be 70,000 excess physicians, and by the year 2000, an excess of 150,000. Given the existence of a doctor glut as well as the concentrations of physicians in certain geographical and specialty areas, one might ask, "How is it that the law of supply and demand does not seem to work in the case of physicians?" And that it does not work is abundantly clear. At least one major study has shown that where there are more doctors per capita, average physician fees are higher rather than lower. The study, a large national survey carried out by the Department of Health, Education and Welfare (now the Department of Health and Human Services) and published in 1977, confirmed earlier reports that had noted the same relationship. The HEW study found that in areas where there were fewer than 50 doctors per 100,000 patients, the average reported fee for an office follow-up visit was $9.20. The fee increased steadily to an average of $12.28 in areas where there were 150 to 200 doctors per 100,000.

One explanation for this contradiction of the law of supply and demand has been given by Uwe Reinhardt, who finds a partial answer in the phenomena that he calls "supply-induced demand."[5] He speculates that some doctors "target" their incomes by deciding how much they should make by using other doctors as benchmarks and then charge patients accordingly to meet their target goals. In order to raise income per patient, a physician may resort to inducing the patient to accept extra treatment.

It is not clear how prevalent supply-induced demand is since it is obviously very difficult to get the cooperation of physicians to gather information from them systematically. Nevertheless, the knowledge differential between physicians and their patients does leave the latter open to such exploitation. There is also substantial anecdotal evidence pointing to the existence of supply-induced demand. In the following excerpt from an interview with a *Washington Post* reporter, a young internist in Washington, D.C. discusses how physicians create a demand for their services among their clients.[6] The dialogue begins with the doctor responding to a question about how he keeps increasing competition and costs from cutting into his income:

Doctor: The way to overcome this was to increase the business some way, and the way to do that, I found, is to suggest to patients that they come in for an annual physical examination.

Reporter: How do you do that?

Doctor: I just told them that they either never had one, or that it had been at least a year since the last time they had one, and I think they ought to come in for one . . . in fact, there are a lot of patients that have never been in for a physical. This is very much like many other professions, even your own. I mean not every story you write gets published, but you get your salary. A doctor has to do this sort of thing in order to provide a base income so that he can continue to take care of his patients. Not every patient is going to be sick, not every patient is going to have a medical problem that warrants a complete physical but in a way that's sort of the dues of the population to their doctor.

Reporter: How do you go about determining what you charge?

Doctor: Well there is a certain amount of communication between doctors as to what our fees are . . . [I]n my case, I started working with another physician for a couple of years and I knew what he charged. . . . Then I moved on and set up my own practice. I knew that I needed a certain amount of income for the first year and figured out the number of patients I was intending to see a day and just multiplied and came up with a figure.

Reporter: This is the way the entire system operates?

Doctor: I talked to (another internist). . . . He was grossing $170,000 a year. He claims he was only seeing 12 patients a day. . . . His fees weren't that high; in fact, they were lower than mine. There was something going on, and I can't really tell you what it was.

Reporter: What do you think it was?

Doctor: I think it was X-rays. I think he was doing an enormous number of X-rays, absolutely outrageous and unnecessary X-rays.

Reporter: Just to make money?

Doctor: Yeah. . . . I know another guy who was charging far less than I charge, and he was grossing $190,000 a year . . . (because) he was seeing 50 patients a day.

Reporter: So he was busy.

Doctor: He was busy, but how do you see 40 or 50 patients in an eight-hour day or even longer? You can't see that many patients and really be taking care of a medical problem because it does take a little time and talking to. You can't zip in and out. . . . He created the need in his patients for weekly or biweekly vitamin shots.

Reporter: So in other words, he didn't have many patients, he was seeing them more frequently?

Doctor: For vitamin shots.

Reporter: And how much was he charging for vitamin shots?

Doctor: Just his office fee. A big bottle of vitamins only cost him a buck. I mean, they're cheap you know. . . . He was charging for a few minutes with his patient and the vitamin shot, $15.

Reporter: Was there any medical benefit from the vitamin shots?

Doctor: No.

Of all the possible consequences of supply-induced demand, none has received more attention than unnecessary surgery. An early and important study compared the United States with England and Wales in terms of the rate at which selected surgical procedures were performed.[7] It was found that twice as much surgery was performed for every 100,000 Americans as for every 100,000 residents of the United Kingdom countries. It was also found that there were twice as many surgeons per capita in the United States as in England and Wales. Although the existence of identically high relative rates of surgeons and surgery does not automatically lead to the conclusion of a cause and effect relationship between the two, these data are highly suggestive of one.

Since that early study, a number of published reports have linked the proliferation of surgeons in an area with high rates of surgery in that area. One such study, which is included in this volume, looked at surgery rates in 193 areas of New England.[8] In that study, which discovered that a physician's personal style in terms of a "surgical signature" can explain variations in the use of particular types of surgical procedures, it was also found that the total rate of surgery in a geographical area is correlated with the number of surgeons there. The more surgeons, the more surgery.

One group among whom "unnecessary surgery is widespread" is the elderly. This was the conclusion reached by a Senate special subcommittee in 1985. The unnecessary surgery included 23 to 36 percent of all cataract surgery, 17 to 43 percent of all hemorrhoid surgery, and 15 to 31 percent of all hernia repair surgery. The committee also reported that abuse of the Medicare system was partially responsible for the rate of surgery and that when second opinions are mandated, rates of unnecessary surgery are reduced by as much as 45 percent with no apparent threat to health. Reducing unnecessary cardiac pacemaker implants alone was seen as saving Medicare up to $358 million each year.

Rationality in the Distribution of Physicians

Given our definition of rationality in terms of fitting health policy to public need, other countries have, for a variety of reasons including political ideology, been far more rational in their approaches to the distribution of physicians. In the Soviet Union and its associated communist countries, most graduates of higher education—not only physicians—are assigned specific work locations after graduation. Some noncommunist countries, like Mexico, require physicians to do compulsory service for a limited time before going into normal practice. As far as specialty training is concerned, most physicians in Great Britain are confined to general as opposed to specialty practice, which is the reverse of what is found in the United States.

There are those who insist that it would be impossible to attack geographical and specialty maldistribution by means of a strongly interventionist governmental policy. For example, Blendon has discussed how difficult it would be to transplant the policies of Red China, where physicians have little independence compared to American physicians, to the United States without also transplanting China's economic policies.[9] It would be difficult to imagine American physicians submitting to the authority of the government as the Chinese physicians did when, in the late 1960s, two-thirds of the faculty of the Peking Medical College were assigned to the rural areas of Western China, where they were to serve in hospitals and clinics and on the faculties of local medical schools.

To be sure, the federal government has stopped far short of implementing policies mandating what kind of medicine American physicians should practice and where they should practice it. Instead, it has created a long line of programs employing various incentives to encourage physicians to voluntarily treat the underserved in physician-shortage areas and, most recently, to go into family practice. The Hill–Burton Act provided federal monies for the building of hospitals in areas where they were in short supply in the hope that physicians would follow the hospitals to these areas. Several programs were aimed at increasing the number of doctors so that competition would force some to go to underserved areas. For instance, medical schools were given grants for yearly increases in the number of students in the entering class. Loans were made available that would permit medical students to substitute working in specified high-need locations for repayment. (Many students "defaulted"—that is, they paid back the loans in full rather than fulfilling the service commitment.) Doctors were enlisted in a National Health Service Corps, which was entirely voluntary and met with only modest success. Fewer federal initiatives have been directed to creating a better distribution of doctors among specialties. Lately, however, medical schools have been strongly encouraged to produce fewer specialists and more primary care physicians such as family practitioners.

Not everyone believes that the voluntary approaches taken by the federal government are the only way to go. There are those who insist that, upon closer inspection, the situation demands that the government require physicians and other health workers to meet the distributional needs of the American public. A proponent of this view states:

> Medical training is even now to an increasing extent paid for by the public; it should be completely a public investment, at least up to a student population required to meet the anticipated public need for highly trained health workers. At the same time, it should be public policy to require of every graduated health worker that within the first ten years after graduation he or she spends as many years as required in servicing and teaching in disadvantaged communities, in remote areas, and in urban underpriviliged neighborhoods. "As required" here means whatever amounts of investments of service are needed to bring life and health expectancies, health standards, and medical knowledge in all communities up to national standards.[10]

A report in the *Journal of the American Medical Association* in late 1980 identified just how much of medical education is paid for by the public, concluding that, all in all, the public pays approximately 92 percent of the cost of educating its physicians.[11] Would not the possibility of the government's mandating a better geographical distribution of doctors warrant the public's also paying the small percentage of the cost of medical education left over? Some, such as the writers represented by the preceding quote, think so.

There is reason to believe that this policy might also impact on specialty maldistribution by eliminating medical student indebtedness. According to the Association of American Medical Colleges, medical students graduating in 1985 had incurred an average educational debt of $29,943. For some, of course, the debt can be astronomical—the tuition alone per year at the medical schools of George Washington and Georgetown Universities hovers around the $20,000 a year mark. As if payment of such accumulated debt were not difficult enough, medical students are prevented from seriously attacking their debt upon graduation from medical school since they are then obligated to multiyear residencies at modest pay. It should not be surprising, then, that there are many who feel medical student indebtedness may encourage students to choose high-paying specialties as opposed to lower-paying primary care ones. Elimination of debt might, the reasoning goes, result in

more physicians going into such fields as family practice.

Assuming that broad and direct governmental intervention to deal with the physician maldistribution crisis will not occur, the issue of affirmative action in recruiting members of minority groups to enter medical school takes on greater significance. The evidence strongly suggests that, on the whole, minority physicians are a better bet to fill the chronically unmet health care needs of less affluent Americans than are members of the majority. Two researchers who have studied the attitudes of black medical students assert that "it would be naive to think that health services in inner cities and rural areas (where most minorities reside) can be substantially increased without a significant increase of minority physicians."[12] Support for this position comes from a very recent study of the career patterns of a sample of several thousand graduates of the medical school class of 1975.[13] It was found that physicians from all racial and ethnic groups serve more people in their own groups. For example, black physicians had 57.4% black patients whereas white physicians had only 13.7% black patients. Black physicians were more likely to serve in areas officially designated as having a shortage of health professionals than were white physicians (12% to 6%), and black physicians served 31% Medicaid patients compared to the 14% served by white physicians. (Hispanic physicians served 24% Medicaid patients.) Additionally, 55% of minority physicians chose primary care fields (obstetrics, pediatrics, and family or general practice) compared to 41% of nonminority physicians.

Given these data, it should be of some concern that, due to federal cutbacks in support for medical education, there has been in recent years a steady decline in the percentage of blacks entering medical school. In late 1985, the figure was moving toward a low 5% of all entering freshmen.

DUPLICATION OF SERVICES

If one looks at the manner in which hospitals have been built and have gone about adding on specialized services and additional equipment and beds, an apparent lack of overall planning and coordination is very evident. A prime example of this is the enormous amount of unnecessary duplication of services that exists among hospitals. An oft-cited study showed that in 1972 one-third of the nearly 800 hospitals equipped to perform open-heart surgery had never performed such an operation; another third did less than twelve a year. Seven years later, a study was published concerning the approximately 15,000 open-heart operations performed yearly in California. Of the 91 hospitals performing open-heart surgery, 65% did less than 150 yearly whereas 48% did less than 100 each year. It was estimated that by confining the surgery to 30 major regional centers, the state could have saved $44 million or 24% of the total yearly cost of such surgery.

Money is not the only thing that would be saved through this kind of consolidation. A review of more than 800,000 operations in nearly 1500 hospitals published in *The New England Journal of Medicine* in 1979 confirmed that complicated surgery is far more risky when done at hospitals where doctors seldom perform it.[14] The researchers analyzed the death rates from 12 different kinds of procedures ranging from open-heart surgery to gall-bladder removals. They found that for operations on major blood vessels, such as open-heart surgery, and on surgery related to the prostate gland, the mortality rate was 25 to 41 percent lower in hospitals where 200 or more such procedures were done annually. The authors of the study estimate that if all such operations were done in these busy hospitals, the mortality rate would drop by 27 percent.

It has already been noted that, as a result of duplication of services, many hospitals face the potentiality of vastly underused specialized facilities. And used or not used, these facilities are costly to maintain because of such things as the long-term debt incurred in purchasing equipment and the need for the constant presence of a well-trained staff. In addition, hospitals depend on some specialized care units as moneymakers to offset losses in other areas. It is estimated, for example, that hospitals receive 20 percent of all their revenues from intensive care units alone. To ward off the disasterous consequences of underuse, hospitals may be subjecting many patients to a higher level of care than they need. A 1981 survey showed that the cost of care in intensive care wards rose 18 percent from the previous year and reached $356 a day. At about the same time, a *Journal of the American Medical Association* article

reported that a "substantial portion" of the patients in costly intensive care units need not be there.[15] An eight-month survey of 624 patients in the general-medical intensive care unit (ICU) in a major medical center, the study found that nearly half of those admitted were in stable condition and received only observation and minimal treatment. The researchers commented that this finding contrasts sharply with the traditional image of the ICU as a treatment location for critically ill patients who require a high level of specialized care and have a high probability of dying in the hospital. This study was considered the first of its kind involving general intensive care units. It did, however, support the conclusions of another study that found that more than 75 percent of patients in a coronary care unit were admitted for observation only and that only 10 percent required additional treatment.

Another major problem reflecting the lack of a coordinated hospital system is the problem of excess capacity. In short, there are too many hospital beds in the United States. It has been estimated that about one-quarter of the nation's nearly one million hospital beds are empty at any one time and 100,000 are completely unnecessary. As with specialized facilities, a hospital bed is costly whether it is used or unused. (The average cost of maintaining an unused hospital bed has been calculated to be between $10,000 to $20,000 a year.) One way hospitals have traditionally coped is through unnecessarily long stays. Although the patient pays the same basic rate per day, the costs to the hospital are greatest in the first few days, and less later on—the latter days of a stay are referred to in the trade as "gravy." Weekend admissions, where the patient often does not receive much medical attention until Monday, also fall into this category. (The federal government's recently implemented policy of paying hospitals set rates for each of about 450 disease categories should have an impact on reducing the length of stays of the hospitalized elderly.)

Overuse of a broad range of diagnostic tests is another way that hospitals, like physicians in private practice, increase revenues. In fact, there is a growing consensus that most of the technology-related costs for hospital care do not come from the use of very high-tech items such as CAT scanners and the like but from "low ticket" items like X-rays. In 1982, the council of the American College of Radiology estimated that one-third of the 45 million chest X-rays taken each year are a waste of time and money. They simply don't provide enough information to justify a patient's exposure to the radiation and the cost of the procedure. The council recommended ending routine X-rays for many groups admitted to hospitals with no symptoms.

Recent evidence suggests that for-profit hospitals that are part of large corporate chains are particularly adept at making profit from diagnostic tests. A review of 13 empirical studies found that for-profit hospitals do more tests and charge more for the tests they do than independent, nonprofit ones.[16]

Regionalization as a More Rational Form of Provision of Services

What can be done about the wasteful and sometimes dangerous duplication of services? What kind of system would provide better coordination among health care facilities? One answer, first seriously proposed by the Commission on the Cost of Medical Care in 1932, is a national system of regional medical care. A leading sociologist, Anselm Strauss, views regionalization as characteristic of the "ideal health care system."[17] A regionalized system would include a graded hierarchy of services within specified geographical areas as well as an overall integrated structure for decision making and fiscal management.

Sweden provides us with a good example of how such a system would look. (The regional system in Great Britain is discussed by Kaufmann in her article, which follows this one.) In the early 1960s, due to increasing health care costs, Sweden regionalized its medical services through the creation of seven health regions, each serving between 650,000 and 1.6 million people. Each region is further subdivided into counties with anywhere from 200,000 to 400,000 people. Finally, counties are broken up into health districts containing anywhere from 7,000 to 40,000 people. Within regions, health services are provided at each of the three levels—region, county, and district.

One description of the system of services provided within each region is as follows:

> The first level of care is provided in district health centers which have from one to fifteen doctors, as well as other medical personnel. It

has been estimated that district health centers could provide approximately 75 to 80 percent of all outpatient care—far more than they currently provide. Most of the physicians in district health centers are generalists, although the larger centers include specialists in, for example, pediatrics, obstetrics–gynecology, internal medicine and psychiatry.

> For the second level of care, most counties contain two or three district or "normal" hospitals which serve several health districts encompassing 75,000 to 100,000 people. These are general hospitals, with fewer than 600 beds, which provide care for emergencies, such as accidents, heart attacks and strokes, and also provide general hospital care, such as general surgery, internal medicine, anesthesiology and diagnostic X-rays. In addition, in each county there is one central county hospital with 500 to 1000 beds which provides both general hospital care for the immediately surrounding population and more specialized care for the county as a whole. For example, the county hospital not only provides care in internal medicine and surgery but also services in gynecology, ophthalmology and orthopedics, and sometimes in neurology, cardiology and urology.

> A third level of care is available at the regional level. Seven regional hospital centers have now been established, one in each of the seven health regions; six of these centers serve simultaneously as medical-college teaching hospitals. "Superspecialty" services such as neurosurgery, plastic surgery, thoracic surgery and radiation therapy are available at this level. There is, of course, no extra cost to patients who are referred from county hospitals to regional hospitals; the counties pay the cost of care to the region.

> A fourth, even more specialized level of care is available in a few regional hospitals where relatively rare special services—such as open-heart surgery, care of spinal injury patients, and transplantation work—are performed.[18]

In such a system, tertiary care—the most technologically sophisticated kind of care—is not done outside of major medical centers; at the same time, these centers do not provide basic primary care.

Thus, various facilities are confined to providing the care that they can best deliver. By comparison, in the United States, as we have already mentioned, smaller facilities often provide care with which they have little experience. On the other hand, major medical centers commonly provide primary care through the use of residents who are more interested in and primarily are trained in specialty medicine.

It is interesting to note that recent polls indicate that regionalization is supported by most Americans as a means of controlling health care costs. In a national poll in 1983, 74 percent said that they could support some kind of regionalization of high technology-related hospital care.

The reasonableness of regionalization has not been lost on health planners in the United States. In 1974, the federal government embarked on a program that emphasized regional planning within the existing system. Although little could be done about unnecessary duplication that already existed, legislation was passed by Congress in that year to prevent a continuation of this pattern of excess. Public Law 93–641, the National Health Planning and Resources Development Act, established regional agencies called health systems agencies (HSAs) to regulate the growth of health care services in specified regions. Each agency serves an area of from 500,000 to 3 million people. In order to have consumer input, the slightly over 200 HSAs must have between 50 and 60 percent of its board made up of consumer representatives. A major role of the HSAs is in granting or denying permission for hospitals to acquire new equipment or to increase the number of beds. Permission is granted by the issuance of a Certificate-of-Need (CON), a certification that the hospital growth is necessary to fulfill the needs of the population in that region.

HSAs face many barriers in carrying out their mandate. Most important, they are only advisory. Many decisions they have made have been overturned by other state agencies that had the final decision-making power. A Virginia hospital, for example, in applying for permission to buy a CAT scanner—a very expensive but very advanced piece of diagnostic equipment—claimed it would charge $220 per scan, or more than three times the anticipated per scan cost, to make up for the losses incurred in its obstetrical and emergency care services and for losses in revenue due to the opening of another hospi-

tal in the area. The local HSA disapproved the application but was overruled by the state health department.

It is also true that HSAs have jurisdiction over hospitals but not over office-based physicians. In New Haven, one of the two major hospitals applied for a CAT scanner. The situation was complicated by the fact that, besides the other hospital having two, a small, office-based physician group also had one. The HSA had had no control over this purchase.

Those HSAs that took tough stands against popular projects would frequently experience great pressure from local residents and politicians and could be tied up in law suits. A case in point is that of Oral Roberts and his City of Faith Medical Center. In a 22-page booklet mailed to all of his supporters, Roberts told how God commanded him to build a 60-story diagnostic clinic; a 30-story, 777-bed hospital; and a 20-story research center. Since research indicated that Tulsa already had a surplus of over 1000 beds, the HSA refused to grant a CON. In this case, the three-member Oklahoma Health Commission, which makes the final decision, upheld the HSA's decision. Roberts went to court and had his followers write thousands of letters. The City of Faith was built. Finally, hospital administrators and other representatives of medical care providers have frequently dominated board decisions on behalf of their own vested self-interests, as with the Los Angeles HSA.

Despite these obstacles, HSAs have made some notable contributions to the health care delivery system. Both opponents and proponents of regulation have agreed that they have had substantial impact. The American Enterprise Institute, an antiregulation, conservative think-tank, concluded that HSAs have had substantial success in blocking the construction of unnecessary beds. On the other side, proregulation Senator Edward Kennedy has estimated that, by 1980, every dollar spent on the planning process kept eight dollars from being spent on unneeded projects.

It is clear that the type of regulation of the growth of unnecessary duplication of services represented by the HSAs serves a critical function at this time of escalating health care costs. Nevertheless, health planning was not popular with the Reagan administration. The program was not reauthorized but Congress continued to appropriate money for the operation of HSAs on a year-to-year basis. In the Fall of 1986, however, Congress decided to end these appropriations. Without federal dollars HSAs must rely on state support so that their future is at present questionable.

An interesting system of coordinated hospital care, along the lines of regionalization, has developed in certain areas of the country. A good example of this can be found in Rochester, New York, where nine hospitals have joined together in a hospital cooperative. Each of the nine is given a fixed yearly budget within which it has to operate, and each receives a weekly check to cover its costs of operation. The cooperative also makes common decisions about such things as the need for new technologies and beds. The emphasis is on sharing. In New York City, a specialized hospital has decided to coordinate its activities with several area hospitals that it operates. The major effort will be to divert cases to the less specialized hospitals when specialized care is not called for.

ACUTE CARE VERSUS CHRONIC DISEASE: A "MISMATCH" OF SERVICES AND NEED

As David Mechanic points out in the lead article in this chapter, the mix of health care problems facing the nation has shifted dramatically during this century. Acute diseases have given way to chronic diseases, as illustrated in Table 2, which compares the leading causes of death at the turn of the century and at present.

TABLE 2   The ten leading causes of death in the United States, 1900 and 1985

1900	1985
Influenza and pneumonia	Heart disease
Tuberculosis	Cancer
Gastroenteritis	Cerebrovascular diseases
Heart disease	Accidents
Cerebral hemorrhage	Influenza and pneumonia
Chronic nephritis	Diabetes
Accidents	Cirrhosis of liver
Cancer	Arteriosclerosis
Diseases of early infancy	Suicide
Diphtheria	Diseases of early infancy

The change in the mix of diseases afflicting Americans stems from several factors. Public health initiatives in conjunction with medical discoveries have eliminated many of the major killer infectious diseases of yesteryear. The increasing age of the population has also played a major role. In 1900, 4% of the population was age 65 and over. By 1980, this had increased to 11.25%, and the projections for the years 2000 and 2050 are 12.2% and 21.7%, respectively. Moreover, the United States will see a dramatic increase in what is currently the fastest growing segment of the American population, the "oldest old"—those 85 and over. They now constitute about 1% of the population and are projected to increase to 1.9% by the year 2000 and to 5.2% by 2050. Chronic conditions are prevalent among the elderly: 44% have arthritis, 27% have heart conditions, 38% have hypertension, and 28% have a hearing impairment. Many have more than one condition. Some provocative articles have speculated that medical advances may result in an aging trajectory in which people may stay virtually disease free until they die, at which time the individual's biological system will simply cease functioning.[19] However, this is just speculation and it is likely that the inventory of degenerative conditions correlated with aging will continue to exist. In support of this point, it might well be wise to remind the reader of Lewis Thomas's characterization of much of current high technology as "half-way" technology.[20] Thus, coronary bypass surgery, a temporary panacea, is not the same as would be the discovery of a medicine to rid the occluded arteries, once and for all, of plaque. Lest we think of kidney dialysis as anything more than a "half-way" procedure, it should be noted that a recent study showed that 22 percent of the deaths of those receiving dialysis at a major dialysis center were of individuals who were withdrawn from the program by themselves or others when further treatment was deemed pointless.[21]

The increased incidence of chronic as opposed to acute disease has not been paralleled by a corresponding change in the health care delivery system. Attacks against illness are still being waged through the use of so-called clinical medicine, which centers around the curative services provided through the use of in-hospital, high-technology treatment. Many have noted the need for a new emphasis on post-clinical medicine relying on an expansion in services geared to supportive maintenance, patient management, and new kinds of preventive care. Before we elaborate on the meaning of post-clinical care, something must be said about the hold of clinical medicine on the reins of health care delivery and the difficulty of modifying its grasp. Several writers have noted that a predisposition to clinical medicine is embedded within the very fabric of American culture. Perhaps as good an indication as any that this is so is by reference to the language in which we couch our discussion of the problems and potential remedies related to health care delivery. The following excerpt from a paper by a leading medical ethicist looks at the implications of the "military metaphor" for our cultural perceptions of and prescriptions for health care and how it should be delivered.

Sociocultural Metaphors By James Childress[22]

Our health care policies are often shaped by our sociocultural images and metaphors. Metaphors involve "seeing as." In each use of metaphor, we see something as something else; we experience or understand one thing through another. For example, we see *X* as *Y,* human beings as wolves, love as a journey, and argument as warfare. In their exciting book, *Metaphors We Live By,* George Lakoff and Mark Johnson argue that our metaphors (often subconsciously) shape how we think, what we experience, and what we do.[23] Take their example: argument as warfare. We develop *strategies* of argument, *contend* with one another, *attack* positions as *indefensible,* and so on. Imagine how different our interactions would be if we viewed argument as a collaborative work of art through which people seek the truth. It is clear from this example that metaphors both highlight and hide, as Lakoff and Johnson note. For example, the metaphor of argument as warfare highlights the conflict involved in argument, but it hides the cooperation and collaboration that are also indispensable.

The metaphor of warfare is also prominent in health care, especially in medicine, where it largely (but not completely) shapes our conception of what we do. The language that follows is drawn from conversations and from the literature: The physician as the captain leads the battle against disease, orders a battery of tests, develops a plan of attack, calls on the armamentarium or arsenal of medicine, directs allied health personnel, treats aggressively, and expects compliance. Good patients are those who fight vigorously and refuse to give up. Victory is sought and defeat is feared. Sometimes there is even hope for a "magic bullet" or a "silver bullet." Only professionals who stand on the firing line or in the trenches can really appreciate the moral problems of medicine. As medicine wages war against germs that invade the body and threaten its defenses, so the society itself may also declare war on cancer under the leadership of its chief medical officer— the Surgeon General. Articles and books may even herald the "Medical–Industrial Complex: Our National Defense."[24]

The military metaphor clearly structures much, though by no means all, of our conception of health care, and it both illuminates and distorts health care. Because its positive implications are widely recognized, I only want to identify some of its negative implications, especially for the allocation of resources that affect the elderly in need of health care. It is no accident, for example, that two major terms for allocation and distribution of health care under conditions of scarcity emerged from, or have been decisively shaped by, military experiences: triage and rationing. As Richard Rettig and Kathleen Lohr note,

> *Earlier, policymakers spoke of the general problem of allocating scarce medical resources, a formulation that implied hard but generally manageable choices of a largely pragmatic nature. Now the discussion increasingly is of rationing scarce medical resources, a harsher term that connotes emergency—even war-time—circumstances requiring some societal triage mechanism.*[25]

The first negative implication of the military metaphor is that the society's health care budget tends to be converted into a *defense budget* to prepare for and to conduct warfare against disease, trauma, and death. As a consequence, the society may put more resources into health care than it could justify, especially under a different metaphor, in relation to other social goods.

Second, the military metaphor also implies patterns of allocation within health care by assigning priority to *critical care* over prevention and chronic care. It tends to view health in negative rather than positive terms, as the absence of disease rather than a positive state of affairs, and concentrates on critical interventions to cure disease. It tends to neglect care when cure is impossible. Recently Lawrence Pray noted that he originally tried to conquer his diabetes, but after futile and counterproductive struggles and battles, he came to see his diabetes not as an "enemy" to be "conquered," but as a "teacher."[26]

A third point is closely connected: the military metaphor may direct attention to certain diseases rather than others for research and treatment. In particular, it tends to assign priority to *killer diseases* rather than disabling diseases. As Franz Ingelfinger once noted, if we concentrated research and treatment more on disabling diseases, such as arthritis, than on killer diseases, then national health expenditures would reflect the same values that individuals affirm: "It is more important to live a certain way than to die a certain way."[27] Anne Somers has suggested that the stroke is "a metaphor for the most difficult problems and challenges of geriatric medicine."[28] Although strokes are not, of course, limited to the elderly, they are more common among the elderly. Each year in the United States there are between 500,000 and 600,000 victims of stroke, 80 to 90 percent of them surviving their initial catastrophe, often with paralysis and aphasia, which have a terrible impact on both the victim and the family. Approximately 2.5 million victims of stroke are alive today, 90 percent of them with varying degrees of incapacity and misery. Even though it has been called the single most costly disease in the United States, stroke received only $18 million in research expenditures in 1979 in contrast to cancer, which received $937 million, and heart disease, which received $340 million. A major reason for this pattern of allocation is that after the first acute phase, the stroke victim does not fit into the prevalent model of health care, which emphasizes the specialist who uses various technological weapons.

A fourth implication of the military metaphor—medicine as warfare—is its emphasis on *technological intervention* and on particular technologies, such as intensive care units, over other technologies such as prostheses. It downplays less technological modes of care.

A fifth implication is *overtreatment,* particularly of terminally ill patients, because death is the ultimate enemy even if disease is the immediate foe. It is difficult for physicians and families under the spell of this metaphor to let a patient die. "Heroic" actions befit the military effort that must be undertaken against the ultimate enemy. As Paul Ramsey notes, "A culture that defines death as always a disaster [I would add enemy] will be one that is tempted to resolve these (allocation) questions in terms of triage-disaster medicine [I would add military-triage medicine]."[29]

I do not propose that we abandon the military metaphor—it illuminates and directs much of health care in morally significant ways. But its negative implications can be avoided in part if we supplement it with other metaphors. The military metaphor tends to assign priority to health care (especially medical care) over other goods and, within health care, to critical interventions over prevention and chronic care, killer over disabling diseases, technological interventions over care, and heroic treatment of dying patients. One of the most promising supplementary metaphors is *nursing,* which some have even proposed as a paradigm of future health care. This metaphor is not adequate by itself just as the military metaphor (or any other metaphor, such as business) is not adequate by itself, but it could direct the society to alternative priorities in the allocation of resources for and within health care, particularly for the elderly.

Rationality in Matching Care to Chronic Illness

What the preceding excerpt suggests is the need for an overall shift from an emphasis on high-technology curing to one focusing on the maintenance of quality of life. Such a transition would bring us closer to a true "health care" provision of services from the presently existing "sickness care" provision of such services.

Health education initiatives concerning behaviors such as smoking, diet, and the like must receive ever-increasing priorities. The cost-effectiveness of lifestyle intervention has been brought out by a study that looked at the decline in mortality due to coronary disease from 1968 to 1976. Coronary-care units, drug therapy, treatment of high blood pressure, improved resuscitation, and coronary bypass surgery accounted for about 40 percent of the decline in mortality. But two simple lifestyle changes—reductions in fat consumption and cigarette smoking—had even more impact. Together, they accounted for over half the decline.

A prerequisite for health education is a priority on the continuation of epidemiological research identifying those factors that place people at risk, such as the link of increased smoking among women and the increase in lung cancer, the correlation between coronary disease and high-levels of cholesterol, the increased risk of mortality among black women due to hypertension, the increased risk of black Americans to hazards in the workplace (the average black worker is in an occupation 37 to 52 percent more likely to produce a serious accident or an illness than the white worker's),[30] and the large infant mortality differential between black and white infants.

Before leaving the issue of health education, mention should be made of those who fret about attempts to change lifestyle as "blaming the victim" and see them as diverting attention from the societal sources of diseases, such as those related to occupational and natural environments. A wide range of interventions, from anti-smoking campaigns in the workplace (see the article by Castillo-Salgado included in the last chapter of this book) to taking drugs for mild hypertension, have been looked at in this way. It should be obvious that what is needed is an eclectic approach to the problem. There is no reason that encouragement of individual responsibility for health must necessarily preclude societal responsibility to ameliorate disease-producing conditions under which people work and live.

A second major issue is one of allocating substantial resources to patient maintenance of the chronically ill. Since the elderly carry such a disproportionate share of disabling chronic illness, they will be the focus of the remaining remarks. A number of the points, of course, are relevant to the chronically ill regardless of age.

The development of services to allow those who wish to stay at home to do so should receive the highest priority. Community services must play an important supporting role here. Many states are, in fact, attempting to reduce the utilization of nursing home beds in favor of a variety of community-based alternatives. One illustration of this is South Carolina's effort to avoid using expensive nursing

home care for many of the poor disabled elderly. Nationally, nursing homes absorb 40 percent of Medicaid funds, and their cost is expected to rise further as the elderly increase their share of the population. In 1984, the elderly were paying for 49 percent of the cost of nursing home care out of their own pockets, an extraordinarily large financial burden. A year later, a Harvard study of a sample of single 75-year-olds found that 46 percent would be impoverished within three months of entering a nursing home and 72 percent would be bankrupt within a year. Under the South Carolina program, begun as an experiment in two counties and later made statewide, the state and families of the elderly share the responsibility, a solution particularly suitable for the South, where there are many large, close-knit families.

Most older people like to remain at home even when they are unable to care for themselves. But Medicaid has usually not provided home service on the grounds that it was too expensive. Under the South Carolina program, relatives take care of the elderly part of the time, and the state, through community-based health units, provides any medical care and other services when they are needed.

There are a whole range of community-based services that have sprung up throughout the country to serve the chronically ill, particularly the elderly. These include day care programs and sheltered work shops offering a vast array of services, such as nursing, occupational therapy, recreational services, and other rehabilitative services, in a community setting on less than a twenty-four hour basis. Also included are home health care, meals on wheels, and homemaker services as well as counseling and guidance services that can provide care and protection with respect to carrying out tasks of daily living.

As far as the elderly are concerned, there have been suggestions concerning the use of the "single agency" concept, in which one agency would coordinate the acute care needs (e.g., the need for hospitalization to deal with an infection) and chronic care needs (e.g., the need for maintenance support at home). The Canadian system employs case managers who perform just such a function for many elderly in that country. And case managers are not only important in their coordinating capacity. For various reasons, many elderly cannot be relied upon to initiate appropriate health care for themselves, particularly in the early stages of illness. Thus, the health system must act on their behalf by instituting periodic health checks and other types of active, casefinding initiatives, a role for which case managers are trained.

All of this is not to say that nursing home care will be rendered unnecessary. The Canadian experience indicates that available community services do not necessarily diminish the need for nursing home beds.[31] As regards future nursing home care need in the United States, a recent report of the General Accounting Office reviewed the characteristics leading to nursing home care and concluded that the need will grow. "Overall, unless major breakthroughs in the treatment of chronic disabling diseases occur, extended life expectancies with greater likelihood of chronic disabling diseases and a reduced number of family members able to provide informal care, will lead to a net increase in the population most likely to need intensive nursing home care." In 1980, there were 1.5 million nursing and related-care beds, or 60 beds per 1000 aged persons. If average lengths of stay do not change, 2.6 million nursing homes beds, or 74 beds per 1000 population 65 years and over, will be required in the United States in the year 2000.

Something must be done, then, to figure out a way to finance nursing home care so that the burden of payment will not fall so heavily on the shoulders of the elderly. It does not seem right that illness, after a life well spent, should leave a person destitute. One suggestion is that public funds, through Medicare, pay for some of the costs, just as it now pays for other services.

SUMMARY

A great deal of irrationality, defined as a lack of fit between the provision of services and public need, can be found in the U.S. health care delivery system. Much of the reason for this derives from the lack of a centralized system of health planning and services such as is found in most other nations of the world. Health care providers, like physicians and hospitals, have been able to mold many aspects of the system to their own vested interests and to their own perceptions of public need. As a result, health care providers and technical resources are often inappropriately and inefficiently allocated throughout

the society, and solutions tend to be piecemeal and short-term.

Although all three of the issues discussed in this paper are important, the last seems a bit more so. The fact of our society facing the inevitability of the rapid growth of a segment of the population whose needs are incompatible with the type of services being provided is a harsh reality and one that is begging for rational answers.

It may be, in the end, that because of the aging of our population, along with a greater public recognition of the uninsured and the underinsured, a greater public presence in the provision of health care will bring us closer to the rest of the world, and we will no longer be the odd person out in terms of the denial of necessary care for so many because they are unable to afford it. As this paper is being written, the administration in Washington is working on developing a plan to cover the costs of "catastrophic" illness for everyone. At the same time, a Harvard group has proposed and outlined such a plan for the elderly.

References

1. Illich, I., *Medical Nemesis: The Expropriation of Health,* New York: Pantheon, 1976.

2. Starr, P., *The Social Transformation of American Medicine,* New York: Basic Books, 1982.

3. Crozier, D. A., Health Status and Medical Care Utilization, *Health Affairs,* 1985, 4, pp. 114–127.

4. Harden, B., The City Shrinks Dream About, *Washington Post,* Nov. 22, 1981.

5. Reinhardt, U. E., *Physician Productivity and the Demand for Health Manpower,* Cambridge, Mass., Ballinger Publishing Company, 1975.

6. Meyer, L., My Share of the Pie, *Washington Post,* June 12, 1977.

7. Bunker, J. P., Surgical Manpower: A Comparison of Operations and Surgeons in the United States and in England and Wales, *New England Journal of Medicine,* 1970, 282, pp. 135–44.

8. Wennberg J., and Gittelsohn, A., Variations in Medical Care among Small Areas, *Scientific American,* 1982, 246, pp. 120–34.

9. Blendon, R. J., Can China's Health Care Be Transplanted without China's Economic Policies?, *New England Journal of Medicine,* 1979, 300, pp. 1453–1458.

10. Bay, J. E., and Bay, C., Professionalism and the Erosion of Rationality in the Health Care Field, *American Journal of Orthopsychiatry,* 1972, 43, pp. 55–64.

11. Staff, Annual Report on Medical Education: 1979–80, *Journal of the American Medical Association,* Dec. 26, 1980.

12. Bonnett, A., and Douglas, F. L., Black Medical Students in White Medical Schools, *Social Policy,* Summer, 1983, 14, pp. 23–26.

13. Keith, S. K., Bell, R. M., Swanson, A. G., and Williams, A. P., Effect of Affirmative Action in Medical School: A Study of the Class of 1975, *The New England Journal of Medicine,* 1985, 313, pp. 1520–1525.

14. Luft, H. S., Bunker, J. P., Enthoven, A. C., Should Operations Be Regionalized? The Empirical Relationship Between Surgical Volume and Mortality, *The New England Journal of Medicine,* 1979, 301, pp. 1364–1369.

15. Knaus, W. A., Wagner, D. P., Draper, E. A., Lawrence, D. E., and Zimmerman, J. E., The Range of Intensive Care Services Today, *Journal of the American Medical Association,* 1981, 246, pp. 2711–2718.

16. Light, D. W., Corporate Medicine for Profit, *Scientific American,* 1986, forthcoming.

17. Strauss, A., An Ideal Health Care System for America, in *Where Medicine Fails,* New Brunswick, N. J., Transaction Books, 1973.

18. Sidel, V. W., and Sidel, R., *A Healthy State: An International Perspective on the Crisis in United States Medical Care,* New York, Pantheon Books, 1977.

19. Fries, J. F., Aging, Natural Death, and the Compression of Morbidity, *The New England Journal of Medicine,* 1980, 303, pp. 130–135.

20. Thomas, L., The Future Impact of Science and Technology on Medicine, *Bulletin of the American College of Surgeons,* 1974, 59, pp. 25–35.

21. New, S., and Kjellstrand, C. M., Stopping Long-Term Dialysis: An Empirical Study of Withdrawal of Life-Supporting Treatment, *Milbank Memorial Fund Quarterly,* 1986, 314, 1, pp. 14–20.

22. Childress, J. F., Ensuring Care, Respect, and Fairness for the Elderly, 1984, *Hastings Center Report,* 14, pp. 27–31.

23. Lakoff, G., and Johnson, M., *Metaphors We Live By,* Chicago: University of Chicago Press, 1980.

24. For military metaphors in health care, see Warren, V., A Powerful Metaphor: Medicine as War (unpublished paper); Vaisrub, S., *Medicine's Metaphors: Messages and Menaces,* Oradell, N.J.: Medical Economics Company, 1977, chapt. 1; and Sontag, S., *Illness as Metaphor,* New York: Vintage Books, 1979.

25. Rettig, R., and Lohr K., Ethical Dimensions of Allocating Scarce Resources in Medicine: A Cross-National Case Study of End-Stage Renal Disease, unpublished manuscript, 1981.

26. Pray, L., *Journey of a Diabetic,* New York: Simon and Schuster, 1983; and How Diabetes Became My Teacher, *Washington Post,* July 31, 1983.

27. Ingelfinger, F., Editorial, *New England Journal of Medicine,* 1982, 287, pp. 198–199.

28. Somers, A., The "Geriatric Imperative" and Growing Economic Constraints, *Journal of Medical Education,* 1980, 55, pp. 89–98.

29. Ramsey, P., *The Patient as Person,* New Haven: Yale University Press, 1970.

30. Robinson, J. C., Racial Inequality and the Probability of Occupation-related Injury or Illness, *Milbank Memorial Fund Quarterly,* 1984, 62, pp. 567–590.

31. Kane, R. A., and Kane R. L., The Feasibility of Universal Long-Term-Care Benefits: Ideas from Canada, *The New England Journal of Medicine,* 1985, 312, pp. 1357–1363.

Rights and the Provision of Health Care: A Comparison of Canada, Great Britain, and the United States

Caroline Kaufmann

With the assistance of Howard D. Schwartz

Do human beings have a right to health care? The United States is currently debating this question and appears to be ambivalent about its answer. The problem lies partly in deciding what health care is and is not. Some see health care as a commodity to be sold to anyone who can pay the price. Others see health care as their livelihood—a way to make a living for themselves and their families. Many people see health care as a necessity arising from injury, disease, and human frailty.

In the United States, people who consider health care as a commodity tend to deny that people have a right to obtain it. If health care is distributed in a free market like other goods and services, they say, people have no more—and no less—right to health care than they do to food, clothing, housing, and other things they want or need. Those who see health care as a livelihood often regard it as personal property; they feel it is theirs to give or withhold as they see fit. Regulations or mandates requiring that it be provided to specified groups are seen as unjust intrusions on the right of health professionals to determine the conditions of their work. For most people, health care is seen as a necessity. People who are sick or injured demand treatment. Without it, they may recover, or languish, or die. For those in need, the right to health care is a matter of physical necessity.

This paper examines how the right to health care is defined in Canada, Great Britain, and the United States and how the health care delivery systems reflect those definitions. If a country states in written policy and through laws that people have a right to health care, then we expect to see a system that delivers health services to all citizens. Canada and Great Britain have rather clear-cut policies supporting the rights of Canadian and British citizens to health care. The United States does not. Canadian and British discussions concerning health care rights appear more coherent than those currently taking place in the United States. For Canadian and British scholars, the key questions concern how to provide health care for everyone who needs it, not whether the care should be provided at all. In the United States, statements about rights to health care are intermittent and conflicting. Although the United States is willing to acknowledge a need for health care, it appears confused about whether meeting that need is the responsibility of government or individuals.

Values are important when nations take action based on them. Canada and Great Britain established national systems of health care during a period of national consensus about rights to social services. Great Britain was the first to implement national health care in 1948. Canada began the process at about the same time but did not complete it until 1972. In the 1980s, the loudest and clearest public voices in both nations support universal rights to health care and the systems of delivery that translate those rights into reality. In Canada and Great Britain, consensus over the right to health care is re-

This is an original article written for this edition of *Dominant Issues in Medical Sociology*.

flected in unified, fairly coherent systems for health care delivery.

The United States lacks a national consensus about health care rights. In keeping with the disparities in public opinion, health care delivery is fragmented. There is no unified system of health care delivery in the United States. Programs are enacted in piecemeal fashion in efforts to "close the gaps" in a loosely connected set of health services.

Canada, Great Britain, and the United States are superficially similar in their political and economic systems. All are established democracies with well-developed systems of law. All have industrialized market economies. However, they differ radically in their approaches to health care. Canada and Great Britain have national systems for providing health care. Canadian National Health Insurance is an insurance program that provides a mechanism to pay for health services while preserving the independence of health professionals. The British National Health Service is a nationalized service industry. The British government employs physicians, nurses, and other professionals to provide health care to patients at public expense. In Canada, health care professionals are independent contractors, much like they are in the United States, though their fees are paid through a national insurance program. In Great Britain, health professionals are government employees. They work for a salary that they negotiate with the National Health Service. Both the Canadian and British systems are funded through general taxation. All citizens can use the system, and there are virtually no economic barriers in obtaining health care. In both systems, the government has a central role in planning and regulating health care.

In contrast, the United States has a mixed free market and social welfare system that uses private insurance, patient fees, public trust funds, and some general taxes to pay for health care. Health professionals have more independence than in Canada or Great Britain. There is relatively little centralized planning and regulation. The United States has experienced the most rapid growth in health care costs of all three countries.

There is growing concern in the United States over the cost and availability of health care. Canada and Great Britain face similar problems. Health care is expensive, and assuring access to needed services is not easy. Nevertheless, Canada and Great Britain may serve as examples for the United States in its attempts to improve health care delivery. Although it is unlikely that the United States will mimic either of these systems, Canada and Great Britain offer some valuable lessons in how to design and deliver comprehensive health care. As students of health services, we may look to Canadian National Health Insurance and the British National Health Service for ideas about how the current U.S. system may develop and improve.

NATIONAL HEALTH INSURANCE IN CANADA

Canada is an enigma to many citizens of the United States. It is our closest neighbor and political ally on the North American continent, yet its unique history and national character have distinguished it among the developed Western democracies. As a democratic society, Canada protects personal liberty. At the same time, Canadians are willing to accept limitations on their personal freedom in the interest of the common good.

Canada has always been a relatively weak confederation of provinces, each with unique ethnic and linguistic characteristics. The provinces are autonomous from the federal government to a degree far exceeding that of individual states in the U.S. Ethnic and language diversity is a source of tension between the provinces and the federal government of Canada. As late as 1983, the province of Quebec threatened to secede, not just from National Health Insurance, but from the country. National unity in Canada must be cultivated and is seldom taken for granted.

In health care, Canada is a "black swan"—contradicting the proposition that all swans are white (Evans, 1983). It has less wealth than the United States, but since 1972, it has eliminated virtually all economic barriers to health care. Unlike the United States, it has managed to control health care costs. In 1960, both the U.S. and Canada spent a little over 5% of their gross national product (GNP) on health care. This figure increased over the next twelve years. By 1972, both countries were spending about 7.5% of GNP on health care. Since 1972, Canada has stabilized health care expenditures at a little less than 8% of the Canadian GNP while expenditures in the U.S. continue to rise (Kane and Kane, 1986). In 1985, Canada spent 7.8% of its gross national product on health care, whereas the United States spent 10.8%. At the same time, Canada assures its citizens free comprehensive health care through National Health Insurance. The Canadians have established an efficient system. How did they accomplish this?

The Stormy History of National Health Insurance

National Health Insurance was constructed through a political process that began in earnest after World War II. In 1945, the Dominion-Provincial Conference drafted a set of proposals for social welfare in Canada. The proposals for health care outlined broad goals for health services in Canada. The proposals specified a uniform system of comprehensive care with cooperation between provincial and federal governments. The idea was to fund the system by small regular payments made by all taxpayers. Since all citizens were at risk for poor health at some time during their lives, and since the cost of health care could not always be met by the individual when he or she was sick, health care costs would be shared by everyone. The National Health Insurance system insured individuals against the universal risks of illness (Taylor, 1979).

Why was this system constructed? The need for publicly financed health care became obvious in the 1930s. During the Great Depression, many Canadians were "on relief" and many more narrowly escaped it. Traditional forms of charity placed primary responsibility for care of the indigent on local towns. With shrinking revenues and increasing joblessness, many cities and towns, especially those in rural areas of Canada, were nearly bankrupt. Medical care was not easily available to the growing number of poor and near poor. Most local municipalities were unable to pay for essential medical services. In 1933, The Canadian Medical Association reported that the majority of its physicians practicing in rural provinces were not paid adequately. They complained that physicians could not continue to provide free care for the growing population of poor people. It was impossible to maintain a fee-for-service system when so few patients could pay any fee at all (Taylor, 1979:4ff).

Innovations from Saskatchewan.   Public insurance for hospital care was the first form of national health insurance introduced in Canada. The province of Saskatchewan in western Canada set the trend for developing national health insurance for hospital care in 1914, as it did for comprehensive health insurance in 1948. This is not surprising in light of the political organization of this province (Taylor, 1979).

The political and economic life of Saskatchewan is one of rural socialism (Lipset, 1950). Saskatchewan is a large, agricultural province in western Canada. It was settled by pioneering farmers who established a one-crop economy based on the cultivation of wheat. The population is scattered over a large geographic area with an average density of three people per square mile. The social economy of the province is organized around a system of rural cooperatives that provide aid to farmers in purchasing seeds, equipment, and fertilizer and in marketing crops. The cooperatives also provide essential social and health care services.

In 1932, the province of Saskatchewan was the first to provide a cash subsidy to physicians who were unable to obtain payment for medical care from their patients. In response to the growing number of unemployed people who were unable to pay for health care and the growing number of physicians with unpaid bills, the Saskatchewan government approved a monthly stipend of $75 to be paid to each physician treating patients in the province. At the time, the cash payment for indigent care was viewed as a simple expedient to prevent physicians from leaving the province in search of more financially sound practices in the urban centers of eastern Canada.

The Saskatchewan hospital insurance system was a logical extension of the municipal doctor system that had been in operation since 1914. Under this plan, local towns contracted with physicians to provide basic medical services, including maternity care and minor surgery. Each physician was given a salary negotiated with the local government. By 1939, the system had evolved into a regional doctor system that allowed groups of smaller towns to contract for physician services. Physicians were paid through local property or personal taxes. Saskatchewan had a well-developed municipal hospital system and a hospital payment plan funded through general taxation. The extent of local government involvement in health care was unprecedented among the other Canadian provinces.

In 1946, while the Canadian national government debated the relative advantages of national health insurance, the Saskatchewan legislature enacted a hospital service plan that established universal, compulsory hospital care insurance paid for by individual taxation. The Saskatchewan plan succeeded even though plans for a national hospital insurance system failed. The 1945 Dominion-Provincial Conference proposed national health insurance but could not agree on how to pay for the system, especially with regard to the role of the federal government (Hatcher, 1981). Nevertheless, the idea of national health insurance had taken root in Canadian society. Hospital insurance schemes sprouted in the provinces and local municipalities. Saskatchewan's was the first to bear fruit.

From 1945 to 1961, the provinces of Alberta, British Columbia, Newfoundland, and Ontario each adopted some version of universal hospital insurance. The programs were not universally successful. An overriding tension developed concerning the role of the federal government in financing and administering the provincial systems. While a decentralized, province-by-province system was consistent with Canadian political experience, the expanding levels of service and growing costs encouraged local politicians to look to the federal government for relief. As one of the most densely populated and economically powerful provinces in Canada, Ontario pressured the federal government to take some financial responsibility for health care. The Ontario plan established a precedent for the federal government's financing medical care among all the provinces.

Universal Comprehensive Health Insurance in Canada. By 1961, Canada had a working system of public insurance for hospital care, and public support was growing for a comprehensive plan to cover all medical expenses—both hospital and office care. However, as comprehensive national health insurance became increasingly popular among citizens and political leaders, it became increasingly unpopular among physicians and insurance companies. By 1950, the Canadian Medical Association opposed further developments in national health care beyond the system of insured hospital care already in place. Physicians were wary of national health insurance

for outpatient services because it threatened their control over private practice. Although they were willing to accept reimbursements from national health insurance for hospital care, they feared that a comprehensive national program would give provincial and federal governments too much authority in controlling physician fees. Taking a negative lesson from their colleagues in Great Britain, they vehemently opposed a system that gave the appearance that Canadian physicians were employees of the federal government.

Insurance companies also opposed the plan because it superseded their administration. If the federal government became the ultimate insurer, it would drastically curtail the market for private health insurance in Canada. Their fears were well founded. Private insurance companies have no substantial role in administering National Health Insurance in Canada. The private companies now only provide insurance for added services, such as private hospital rooms and dental care, and health insurance for Canadians traveling abroad.

In 1968, Canada enacted the Medical Care Act, bringing all the provinces together under a comprehensive national insurance program. The plan covered all medically necessary health care, regardless of the setting in which services were provided. The benefits were paid from general revenues under a plan that shared costs between the provinces and the federal government. In the original design, the federal government paid for 50 percent of health care costs for each province, with the local provinces and municipalities paying the rest. Benefits were universal and transferable among the provinces. Participation in the plan was not mandatory. Some physicians chose to "opt out" of the system, though the proportion was small.

Organization and Finances in National Health Insurance

The Canadian National Health Insurance program is a confederation of provincial health insurance plans. The provincial plans are linked through a cost-sharing formula administered at the federal level. The plans differ slightly among the provinces, but the benefits are transferable among all the Canadian provinces.

National Health Insurance is a financial ar-

rangement to pay for health services. It is not a system for delivering those services. Unlike the British National Health Service, Canadian physicians are not employees of the government. They are private contractors. Some physicians are employed by the provinces or by municipalities to offer medical care in rural areas, although most physicians maintain their status as nonsalaried professionals. Although physicians are paid by National Health Insurance, they preserve their professional autonomy.

Canadian National Health Insurance pays for comprehensive health care from insurance premiums paid by all taxpaying citizens. Benefits include all medical expenses, both hospital and office visits, as well as other therapeutic services that are judged to be medically necessary. Hospital benefits include admission to a ward. Patients may purchase additional insurance through a private company if they want coverage for semiprivate or private hospital rooms. Dental services are not covered.

Most Canadian physicians accept payment from National Health Insurance as their entire fee, though they are not required to do so. Physicians who "opted out" of National Health Insurance bill patients directly for the entire fee. National Health Insurance then reimburses the patient for its percentage of the fee, and the patient pays the rest. Some physicians do bill patients for additional costs in excess of what they are paid through National Health Insurance. The practice of "extra billing" has been actively discouraged by the federal government (Minister of National Health and Welfare, 1983). Fewer than 10 percent of physicians "extra bill," and most of these are specialists practicing in urban centers. Under the Existing Program Financing arrangement (EPF), the federal government takes $1 from the federal allocation to the province for each dollar collected in extra billing in that province. This policy cost Ontario $52 million in federal money in 1985. At the time of this writing, physicians in Ontario have called a strike to improve their economic relationship with the federal and provincial governments. The majority of Canadian physicians are enrolled and almost all citizens of Canada rely on National Health Insurance to pay for most, if not all, of their medical care.

The Medical Care Act of 1968 paid little attention to controlling costs or monitoring efficiency. As in Great Britain and the United States, Canada un-derestimated the cost of the system and did not anticipate escalation in health care spending. The federal cost-sharing formula was popular with the provinces, particularly those in more rural areas, which saw it as a mechanism for redistributing wealth among the provinces (Veyda and Deber, 1984). However, the federal government had little control over health care costs incurred by the provinces and never received much political credit for funding the system. As a result, tensions mounted between the federal government and the provinces over the issues of cost control and political accountability for National Health Insurance.

In 1977, the federal and provincial governments agreed to a compromise. The federal government reduced its contribution to 25 percent across the board. In return, federal and corporate taxes were decreased so that the provinces could increase their taxes to make up for federal cuts. The revised formula provided incentives to the provinces to control costs. In Canada, the provinces are responsible for regulating and managing health care and also for financing the major portion of it (Veyda and Deber, 1984).

The provinces are largely self-regulating with regard to health care. Provincial governments negotiate contracts annually with physicians, and the levels of reimbursement are established for the period of that contract. The levels of care provided by each physician and health care facility are monitored. Physicians providing services in excess of an established level of care are subject to review. The monitoring system is designed to maintain quality and also to protect against fraud and abuse by health care professionals.

It appears that a combination of tighter regulation on service delivery and a centralized administrative structure have produced considerable savings in the cost of health care in Canada. With a lump-sum allocation for operating expenses and restrictions on capital investment, Canadian hospitals have relatively low administrative costs. Total overhead costs under National Health Insurance average about 2.5 percent of the cost of a program, compared to almost 16 percent overhead costs in the United States (Himmelstein and Woolhandler, 1986). Despite political and social pressures which escalate costs and increase demands for health care, Canada continually searches for ways to control the upward spiral of expenditures for health care (Evans, 1985).

National Health Insurance as Social Justice

The right to health care in Canada is a tangible benefit of Canadian citizenship, one that Canadians feel entitled to as a condition of life in a democratic society. The consensus that sustains National Health Insurance is grounded in the values of unity, equality, and prosperity, which are deeply rooted in the Canadian national character. Eliminating all economic barriers to health care assures that every citizen will be taken care of and that everyone has a stake in the well-being of all. The implications for Canadian society are significant. As the Canadian economist Robert Evans explains:

> The idea that one person's life and limb is more valuable than another's, more worth saving on the basis of his/her ability to pay, comes rather close to denying a fundamental "cherished illusion" of equality which underlies our [Canadian] political and judicial system. A society in which people come to see themselves as fundamentally different, as unequal, becomes if not ungovernable, at least very costly to uphold. People with no perceived stake in the social order do not strive to maintain it. . . .
>
> . . . Canadians (of both languages) see the country's health care system as a fundamental expression of social unity. This sense is not only political rhetoric; it is a genuine perception of equal status in confronting the common experience of illness and death. [Evans, 1983:30–31]

Canadians acknowledge national unity by recognizing a common need for health services and a mutual dependence among the provinces in meeting that need. The federal government links provincial health programs. Without federal support, the provincial plans would suffer. The federal government serves the provinces by making it easier for them to finance and administer health insurance, thereby providing an incentive that partly offsets the spirit of provincial independence.

Equality is a tangible by-product of national health in that all Canadians are given access to services that they feel are essential to physical well-being and are assured of care in times of illness or injury. The benefits of equality are more salient when

one is vulnerable. National Health Insurance assures that differences in income and social position need not translate into inequities in essential health services.

Prosperity is concrete for Canadians because National Health Insurance makes the best in Canadian health care available to all. Canada lies in the economic shadow of the United States, and may risk feelings of being a poor relative in view of the wealth of its prosperous neighbor to the south. However, Canada has surpassed the United States in the provision of comprehensive health care. While the United States argues about the relative costs of health care expenditures, Canada has decided it can "afford" comprehensive health care. It is a gift that a prosperous nation shares with all its citizens.

The need to provide citizens with concrete evidence of prosperity has also motivated Great Britain to provide comprehensive health care, as we will see in the next section.

HEALTH CARE IN GREAT BRITAIN: FROM ELITES TO EQUALITY

To the victor belong the spoils. At the end of World War II, Great Britain was victorious in name only. Major cities had been destroyed by the blitzkrieg, and the British economy was in shambles. There were shortages of housing, and the general health of the population was poor. As we have already seen in Canada, a national consensus in support of human services developed from the British experience during World War II. Health problems that had plagued the British population for centuries were brought to public attention (Armstrong, 1983). The forces of social cohesiveness and public awareness that seeded Canadian National Health Insurance burst into bloom in the British National Health Service.

British society has several distinct features that have worked to fashion its approach to health care. Social classes are defined more rigidly in Great Britain than in either the U.S. or Canada. Individuals are less likely to move up or down the social ladder through education or employment. As a result of this more rigid class structure, British people are more accepting of their position in society and are more tolerant of inequalities among social classes. The practice of waiting in line for one's turn—"queuing"—is characteristic of British willingness to cooperate in maintaining the social order. At the same time, the British expect that what they need will be provided when their turn comes. They accept adversity but insist on justice in its wake.

The British are more accepting of authority, particularly that of physicians, than are U.S. or Canadian citizens. They are more likely to accept unquestioningly a physician's judgement of their medical needs. The willingness to "queue up" for health care services and accept the authority of physicians in determining health needs are important factors in allocating health care resources in Great Britain. Compared to the United States, Britain is poor. It cannot afford to provide as much health care as the United States. Rationing is an essential feature of health care in Great Britain.

The National Health Service (NHS) was constructed during a period of political liberalism. The wartime experience had brought home the need for improved social and educational services. The push for improved health benefits was one element in the campaign to make Britain "a society fit for heroes to live in." The Beveridge report, published in 1942, outlined broad areas of reform in education, employment, and health benefits. The state government was to be used as a mechanism for planning and coordination. Universal free medical care was seen as an essential component in a complete system of public welfare (Gill, 1980).

Specific plans for a national health service developed over several decades. In 1911, Great Britain established a National Health Insurance system. Under this plan, general practice physicians were paid a salary to provide health care to the working poor and the indigent. This system was a carry-over from the seventeenth century. At that time, England enacted the Poor Laws to control vagrancy and force indigent families to work. The Poor Laws also established a rudimentary health care system under the assumption that improved health care would make the poor better workers. Poor Law health officers were salaried by local authorities to provide health care to indigent people in the community. The health officers were often less prosperous and had fewer professional credentials than physicians, and they did not have access to hospitals. Hospital care was controlled by elite members of the medical community (Hodgkinson, 1967).

National Health Insurance was administered through private insurance associations called "friendly societies." The societies offered insurance to individuals but reserved the right to refuse those who were poor health risks. This system functioned as partial assurance that British citizens would have access to the care they needed. By 1936, benefits under the National Health Insurance Act were extended to include dental care, skilled nursing, convalescent home treatment, and other services. However, coverage was spotty. Individuals who had greater medical needs were less attractive to the societies, and the cost of care was disproportionately born by those less able to pay (Lindsay, 1980).

The National Health Service has been described as Britain's reward to itself for having won World War II (Aaron and Schwartz, 1984). It was established in 1948 at the crest of a public consensus about the rights of human beings to basic services. While British society remains class conscious, with a clear division between elite and working class individuals, it maintains a system of universal free health care that assures that no financial barriers will prevent individuals from receiving the medical care they need. The National Health Service is a democratic counterbalance to the obvious elitism in British society. It is the "jewel in the crown" of the British welfare state.

In 1942, the Medical Planning Commission published a report outlining a plan for comprehensive health care in Britain. The organization of national health care preserved the essential features of British medicine from the nineteenth century. Medical doctors were divided into two general categories. The first, general practitioners, were community doctors who administered primary care, including obstetrics. General practitioners did not have direct access to hospitals, as they do in both Canada and the U.S. A second group of physician-consultants and surgeons provided hospital and specialty care. These individuals were the elite of the medical community. They controlled access to hospital care and enforced restrictions on the practice of surgery.

A Split-Level Health Care Delivery System

The National Health Service preserves the traditional distinction between general practice and specialization through a formal organization of primary and specialty care. The system is a "two-tiered" or split-level delivery system (Roemer, 1976). The general practitioner is the first level of contact for anyone seeking health care under the National Health Service. General practitioners practice exclusively in the communities. Each individual is assigned to a general practitioner who is responsible for meeting all the primary health care needs of that patient. The average general practitioner (GP) has approximately 2200 patients and is paid a fee based on the number of assigned patients. This eliminates any financial incentive to provide treatment in excess of medical need, since the GP receives the same amount of money regardless of the extent of treatment patients are given. The general practitioner is licensed to treat and prescribe medicines, although there are limitations imposed on the type of treatments he or she can prescribe. If the GP feels that more extensive care is needed, he or she refers the patient to a consultant.

Consultants are hospital-based physicians who are trained in a medical or surgical specialty. These physicians are paid a salary by the National Health Service. Their salary is negotiated as part of the annual budgetary process and is not dependent on the number of patients treated or the extent of care provided. They are the only physicians authorized to admit patients to hospitals. Consultants admit patients based on a priority system that divides patients into two classes—urgent and nonurgent. Urgent cases are supposed to be admitted to the hospital within one month. In fact, it takes up to three months in some cases. Nonurgent cases should be admitted within one year, but individuals have waited up to three years before being admitted. The private health care system siphons off some of the demand for hospital care from the National Health Service. Individuals who can pay for hospital care may bypass the waiting list and receive treatment for nonurgent conditions (Aaron and Schwartz, 1984).

The split-level delivery system has several advantages. First, it makes maximum use of the lower cost care provided by general practitioners. The GP channels the patient through the health care system so that the level of care is both appropriate and consistent. More expensive hospital and specialty care is reserved for more severe cases. The disadvantages of this system lie in restricted access to specialty care. Patients do not have direct access to specialist or inpatient hospital care. While they can and do make use of hospital emergency care, they must use general practitioners as the first point of contact in obtaining specialty treatment.

The existence of private practice medicine of any scope in Great Britain has been a source of contention within the National Health Service. While Canada has preserved the essential features of a private practice system, reimbursing physicians as private contractors, Britain has abandoned most private practice within the National Health Service. Some private practice medicine is preserved as a part of the original political compromise made between designers of the National Health Service and the medical profession. It is kept relatively small through tight regulations on the use of hospital facilities. Sophisticated medical and surgical treatments require laboratory facilities and skilled professional care that are only available through the National Health Service. Few if any privately-owned hospitals or clinics can maintain the minimal level of service required on their own. Because physicians in private practice are dependent upon the National Health Service for laboratory and other technical support, the NHS can effectively control the scope of private practice. Approximately 5 percent of hospital beds are set aside for private paying patients. This proportion is negotiated as part of the regular budgetary procedure.

As in Canada, hospital and nursing home care accounts for approximately two-thirds of national health care expenditures. Home care is provided by district nurses, home health visitors, and social workers. In addition, both general practitioners and consultants will make house calls for patients who are too sick to travel to a physician's office. Critics of the National Health Service have noted that a significant amount of the total expenditures for health care is spent on support services that are not directly related to medical services.

Bureaucracy and Health

The National Health Service is a bureaucracy. It has a defined set of departments organized into levels along a chain of command. However, it is also decentralized. This means that people working at a given level have the authority to make some decisions on their own without getting approval from higher levels. Authority is split between administrators and health care professionals, with physicians having the most authority among health care professionals. Physicians have a great deal of power to make decisions concerning medical services, but they have to take into account other professional groups. Nurses, physical therapists, dieticians, and health technicians all have some influence (Hunter, 1980).

The general organization of the NHS looks something like this. The Department of Health and Social Security is the highest level of organization in the NHS. The 14 Regional Health Authorities are next. Each region is responsible for planning, coordinating, and budgeting for the region. Within each region, there are Area Health Authorities. The Area Health Authorities are responsible for day-to-day operations. District Management Teams are organized within the Area Health Authorities and are responsible for planning, coordination, and management in the community (Owen, 1976).

A major issue in the NHS is resource allocation, deciding how money should be spent. Most of the money spent on health care in Britain comes from taxes. The British Treasury sets spending limits for the NHS based on how much was spent in the prior year with an adjustment for inflation. This budget is approved by the House of Commons. The Secretary of State for Health and Social Services distributes the money among the regions and districts. Regions and districts are at different levels of the bureaucracy and have different responsibilities, so how money is spent depends partly on who is authorized to spend it. Regions make decisions about the purchase of equipment or services that will cover more than one district. For example, CT scanners, blood banks, or changes in hospital services are all determined by the regions for the most part (Aaron and Schwartz, 1984). Districts are more concerned with direct delivery of care, so money allotted to the districts is more likely to be spent on primary health services.

Inequality, Scarcity, and Rationing

There are inequalities among regions in the National Health Service. Some regions have better equipped hospitals and more specialty services than others. In 1976, the Resource Allocation Working Party (RAWP) made recommendations on how to eliminate differences in the quantity and quality of health care

among the regions. However, critics of the RAWP plan felt that not all kinds of care can be offered in all regions and that some regional centers should be permitted to develop special centers for treatment of certain types of conditions—so-called "centers of excellence" (Aaron and Schwartz, 1984). Regional differences in the distribution of health services remain an issue.

Recently, the National Health Service has been concerned with inequities in health. A national survey—the "Black Report"—found that people who are in the lower social classes, that is, those whose jobs require low skills and little formal education, have a two-and-one-half greater chance of dying before the age of 65 than do people working in professional jobs. In addition, unskilled workers appear to use fewer health care services than might be expected. For example, although unskilled workers consult general practitioners more often, they have more health problems. Comparing their need for health care to their actual usage, lower skilled workers appear to be getting less health care than they need from the National Health Service. In addition, people from the lower classes do not tend to use as many family planning and preventive health services, such as birth control, annual check-ups, screening tests, and immunizations, as do people from middle and upper occupational groups (Townsend and Davidson, 1982).

Public concern over inequalities in health and health care has been a problem since the inception of the National Health Service. Health planners are sensitive to perceived inequities and work to assure that health services are distributed in a just and fair manner. However, in attempting to provide care for everyone, the NHS has encountered levels of need that exceed original expectations. The cost of meeting these needs may not be exorbitant, but it is higher than expected and is likely to be even more costly by the end of this century. The British spend approximately one third of the amount of money spent in the U.S. on health care. Yet, they aim to provide comprehensive care for all citizens. Can the British do more with less?

The British National Health Service is a classic example of explicit rationing of health care. Explicit rationing means the conscious allocation of limited resources so that some services are provided at the expense of others. The British ration some types of services and not others. Kidney dialysis is one example. In Britain, approximately 70 people per million receive dialysis. This compares to 230 per million in the United States, a three-fold difference. In contrast, rates of radiation therapy for cancer patients are equivalent to those in the United States. In Great Britain, kidney dialysis competes with other kinds of care for the scarce resources available (Aaron and Schwartz, 1984:34ff). However, the rate of kidney transplantation is about the same for both countries (Sells, Macpherson, and Salaman, 1985). The United States funds kidney dialysis under a special Medicare program. The National Health Service does not designate special funds for this procedure. It appears that when kidney dialysis must compete with other procedures, it is employed less often.

Ethics and Resource Allocation

Faced with the problem of a growing demand for health care and rising costs, British physicians learn first-hand about justice and the allocation of medical resources. They face crucial questions on a daily basis in deciding where scarce resources should be used. If five patients need kidney dialysis and only one machine is available, how should the physician decide whom to treat? In a system where all patients have a right to health care, the issue cannot be settled simply by appeal to rights. Some procedure for deciding who has the most "right" to treatment must be employed.

At least two ethical principles may be used in deciding whom to treat. The first is that the physician treats the patient who is in the greatest need. Following this rule, the patient who is most gravely ill will be treated. The second principle is to treat the patient who will benefit most from the procedure. On this basis, the physician will treat the patient who has the best chance of recovery or improvement in health—the best prognosis. British physicians regularly face clinical situations in which two equally ill patients with equally good prognoses need the same single piece of equipment. In such situations, all ethical principles become imperfect guides to action (Gillon, 1985).

The National Health Service was established to eliminate inequities in access to health care that arose from differences in the social and economic status of people within British society. The British hoped that eliminating differences in access to health care would eliminate differences in health among rich and poor people. After almost 30 years of nationalized health care, some differences remain.

The British National Health Service has confirmed the right to health care in principle and has designed a delivery system to realize that ideal. It now faces the problem of distributing those services. The principle of universal access to health care is tempered by the reality of short supplies. Health planners in Great Britain count on the willingness of British citizens to accept some degree of rationing in health care.

Public acquiescence to rationing is unlikely to occur in the United States, where people appear unwilling to accept scarcity as a justification for withholding health service. Allocating health care through explicit rules that selectively serve some groups over others is "politically explosive" in the United States (Aaron and Schwartz, 1984:126). The United States rations health care implicitly.

HEALTH CARE IN THE UNITED STATES: COMPREHENSIVE CARE IN PIECES

In the United States, the right to health care is played against the values of a free market. The U.S. has no system of national comprehensive health care, either in the form of national health insurance as in Canada or a national health service as in Great Britain. As Schwartz has already noted in this volume, there is no one system of health care delivery in the U.S. Instead, there are a variety of uncoordinated, often competing systems loosely connected through financial and regulatory mechanisms. In comparison to the British and Canadian systems, health care delivery in the U.S. is a complex and often bewildering process. However, with respect to national values toward health care, the U.S. differs from these nations in degree, but not in kind.

Most people in the U.S. feel that individuals have a right to some level of health care, though there is debate over how much. At the same time, significant segments of the health care industry feel that health care is a commodity to be allocated through a market system. Health care in the U.S. is provided through dual mechanisms, each consistent with one of these views. One mechanism relies on public subsidy; the other uses a regulated market. There is no centralized administrative or regulatory structure and no centralized system for allocating resources or controlling costs. The system mixes the best and worst in health care. It is flexible and innovative, but it is also expensive and piecemeal.

Health care delivery in the U.S. is guided by the values of personal liberty and free choice. However, there has always been a system of public welfare that has provided health care for the poor and other select groups of individuals. In the seventeenth century, Connecticut, Rhode Island, and Massachusetts enacted legislation to care for the indigent sick at public expense. These early plans were directed toward providing for the health needs of the very poor and may be considered transplants from the English Poor Law system we have already discussed. Individuals who worked paid for health care on a fee-for-service basis.

Providing health care for everyone regardless of their financial situation is not necessarily a new idea in the U.S. The U.S. Congress discussed this issue as early as 1914 and actively flirted with the notion of a national health care system during the Great Depression of the 1930s. However, unlike Great Britain and Canada, discussions of comprehensive national health care never resulted in an established system. With regard to health care, the U.S. is virtually alone among industrialized nations in its lack of a national system for financing and delivering health care services to its population.

There are several factors that explain this unique position. The United States is one of the most prosperous and politically stable nations on earth. It assumed this position with an almost absolute victory over the Axis nations in World War II. Unlike its European allies, the United States suffered no direct damage to its cities. With the exception of Pearl Harbor and the Pacific Islands, no battles were fought on U.S. soil. At the end of World War II, the U.S. emerged with an intact economy, abundant natural resources, and a young and healthy labor force. Poverty and poor health were not absent in the U.S., but they were less conspicuous in the context of national prosperity.

In Great Britain and Canada, the sense of national solidarity fostered through the war effort also nurtured public sentiment in favor of a comprehensive national health program. In the U.S., public opinion fixated more on prosperity than on poor health. The Veteran's Administration hospital system was enhanced through general revenues, and expanded services were provided for the victorious soldiers. The VA health care system remains a major provider of health care for individuals who have served in the U.S. armed services, but no successful effort has been made to extend these benefits to the entire civilian population.

The success of the U.S. economy bolstered American confidence in the virtues of free enterprise. The "free market" became an economic metaphor for the rights of individuals to liberty and opportunity. In the ethics of the marketplace, individuals purchased what they needed and laid claim to anything they could afford to buy that another offered for sale. Rights were defined by the ability to pay.

A casual observer of the United States might assume that the question of a right to health care plays almost no role in determining who receives health services. Such an assumption is simplistic. The right to health care has been a key element in the debate over the best way to allocate health services. However, in many ways, health care is viewed as a commodity bought and sold in a free market. The tension between these two views is reflected in a bifurcation in the delivery of health services— a two-tiered system of health care. One level provides health care to patients who are able to pay for it, and a second provides health care for indigent and elderly groups through public subsidy. As a result, health care is defined sometimes as a commodity and sometimes as a right, depending on which segment of the health care delivery system provides the care.

Health Care as a Right or a Commodity

Ethicists tend to support the notion of an absolute right to health care. The right is absolute because, it is argued, health care is essential to health, and health is necessary in all other aspects of human life. To deny anyone health care is to deny that person the conditions necessary to sustain him or her as a member of society. Treating health care in any other way places some individuals in the position of not having services that are essential to human well-being. Health care is different from other services because individuals risk death if they do not have it. A nation cannot deny its citizens the right to health care because it has a legally acknowledged responsibility to protect them from harm and preserve their lives.

In contrast, advocates of the market system define health care as a commodity. This view is supported by at least two lines of reasoning. The first challenges the equation of health and health care. In a major policy statement, Alain Enthoven suggests that health care may have little bearing on physical health, so providing health care may have very little to do with improving health. If the level of health care has a limited effect in improving health status, then there is no need for any society to guarantee health services to its citizens. Health care may be desirable, but it is not essential to human physical well-being. Therefore, there is no need to treat health care differently from any other commodity. In addition, Enthoven suggests that providing health care to everyone based on medically determined need may be detrimental to health. Citing cases of injury or disease that are directly caused by physicians—iatrogenic illnesses—he suggests that more health care is not necessarily better, but may be, at best, useless and, at worst, harmful (Entoven, 1980).

In the Enthoven view, the distinction between health and health care is one based on efficacy. The U.S. may want to guarantee each of its citizens the right to health, but if health services have little to do with actual health, then the expenses incurred in providing health care cannot be justified. People may want health care, but if health care is not tied directly to health, those desires are no more fundamental than the desire to have a new car.

The second argument is that health care is the property of health care providers, particularly physicians. In a pure market system, persons who provide goods and services have primary authority over their use. In the case of professional services, that authority is virtually absolute. Professional autonomy, supported by laws granting license to physicians and other health professionals, means that the professional person has almost exclusive rights to control health services. Health care professionals feel that their skills are their personal property, which they may sell, keep, or develop as they like.

One physician explained the situation in this way:

Medical care . . . is a service that is provided by doctors and others to people who wish to purchase it. It is the provision of this service that a doctor depends upon for his livelihood, and is his means of supporting his own life. If the right to health care belongs to the patient, he starts out owning the services of a doctor without the necessity of either earning them or receiving them as a gift from the only man who has the right to give them: the doctor himself [Sade, 1974].

There are several reasons why the U.S. does not regard health care as the exclusive property of physicians. First of all, the delivery of health care services depends upon the skill of a plethora of professional care givers. Physicians are outnumbered 12 to 1 by nonphysician professional staff, such as nurses, physical therapists, and other technical staff (Axelrod, Donabedian, and Gentry, 1976). The training required to become a physician is paid largely by public money. Medical schools and teaching hospitals are subsidized by state and federal taxes. The federal and state governments make funds available to finance tuition for medical school. In addition, physicians depend upon hospitals, laboratories, and clinics that are often built and operated with public money. As we have already seen in the British National Health Service, the private practice of medicine depends upon the investment of public money.

The ethical debate among those holding competing definitions of health care is important since it expresses the ambivalence underlying health care delivery in the U.S. Two alternative definitions are especially salient: one that defines health care as a right and a second that defines it as a commodity. If consensus develops around the notion of an absolute right to health care, the U.S. may move toward a comprehensive system of health care like those of Canada or Great Britain. If the definition of health care as a commodity is dominant, there is likely to be increased emphasis on markets with limited regulation and decreased services for the poor and the uninsured.

A pure market approach to the delivery of health services is unlikely to prevail in the U.S. Health care services have always been tightly regulated, both to protect patients against unscrupulous practices and to protect providers against encroachment into their professional domain. Health care is different from other commodities in that a patient is rarely free to make an informed choice over what operation, which set of pills, or what laboratory tests she or he should purchase. Patients seek medical services because they are sick and in need of help. Consumer choice is often limited to a simple veto of the doctor's decision—the patient either agrees to do what the doctor says or does not. Patients participate in the medical market out of necessity and ignorance. Competition among providers is minimal due to licensure and the social organization of professional associations.

A more pragmatic view of health care attempts to reconcile the difference between advocates of rights and advocates of the market by paying some attention to both. In the pragmatic approach, health care is neither a right nor a commodity, but an essential service. Some level of health care must be guaranteed to all people, but individuals cannot claim rights to any and all health services available. This perspective acknowledges a qualified right of all citizens to a minimally adequate level of care. The "decent minimum" level is provided to those who demonstrate clear need (Fried, 1976). Any services above the minimally acceptable level are allocated through the free market. The U.S. system does not guarantee a right to equality of care. That is, citizens who cannot pay for it may not be able to obtain all the health care they want or even all the health care a physician may feel is necessary. However, the U.S. does make a sincere effort to assure that no one will be left without some services in the face of illness or injury. Unfortunately, there is no consensus over what constitutes a "decent minimum" in health care. As we will see shortly, there are ongoing concerns over whether publicly subsidized care is of sufficient quality and quantity to meet minimum acceptable levels.

The compromise solution between competing definitions of health care is consistent with a two-tiered system of health care delivery. One level allocates health services based on the patient's ability to pay. A second level distributes care through public subsidy with little or no cost to the patient. These levels differ in terms of who is served and how services are provided.

Care at the First Level—Innovation in Health Care Delivery

The first tier of the two-tiered system in the U.S. operates as a regulated market, serving well-insured or affluent patients, including those using Medicare with supplemental insurance. Providers compete among one another for these consumers. Competition promotes innovation. This is apparent when we examine the variety of organizations offering health care services in the U.S. There are three broad types of health care organizations: ambulatory care facilities, hospitals, and long-term care facilities. Hospital care is by far the most expensive, accounting for 42 percent of all money spent on health care. Long-term care facilities, which include nursing homes and hospices, take up another 10 percent. The rest is spent on physician services, education, research, and other out-patient services provided in a variety of settings.

Ambulatory care is available to patients who do not need to be hospitalized. For the most part, health care in the United States is provided by physicians who work in some type of private practice (Roback, et al., 1984; Roemer, 1981). Over 90 percent of patients receive care in this setting (U.S. National Center for Health Statistics, 1978). Hospital outpatient departments also offer ambulatory care, and are frequently the primary source of routine outpatient treatment for people in lower income groups.

Prepaid group practice is a form of ambulatory care whereby the patient pays a set fee every month, regardless of his or her use of services. The earliest form of prepaid group practice is the health maintenance organization, or HMO, which began in the United States in the 1950s (Luft, 1981a). Currently, about 7 percent of the U.S. population is enrolled in an HMO (Interstudy, 1985). They are generally cheaper to operate than are fee-for-service practices (Newhouse et al., 1985). Families who enroll in HMOs are generally young, employed, and newly settled in the community (Buchanan and Cretin, 1986; Barr, 1983; Luft, 1981b). HMOs were first established to provide preventive health care, but recent studies show that patients enrolled in HMOs use them as sources of general ambulatory care (Maerki, Luft, and Hunt, 1986; Hibbard and Pope, 1986).

In the late 1970s, private, for-profit emergency

care centers began to compete with office practices and hospital emergency rooms for well-insured, paying patients. The majority of these centers are owned by physicians, and they have grown rapidly in the more affluent regions of the U.S. Walk-in clinics charge 30 to 50 percent less than hospital emergency rooms and have tended to drive down the cost of hospital emergency care in some cases. They tend to draw less ill, better insured patients away from the hospital emergency rooms. Ambulatory surgery centers are another recent innovation in outpatient treatment. Surgery at these centers is less expensive due to the lower costs of operations and no costs for an overnight stay in the hospital (Erman and Gabel, 1985).

U.S. Hospitals in a Competitive Market

Hospitals are the most expensive component of health care delivery in the United States. However, they have been the traditional source of care for the poor. The earliest form of charity care in the United States was provided at urban teaching hospitals, where the poor were treated at no cost so that medical students could obtain clinical experience. Hospital emergency rooms are still used as a source of primary care for the urban poor, and there is ongoing concern over the inappropriate use of hospital emergency rooms for nonemergency treatment (Schneider and Dove, 1983).

Although for-profit hospitals are relatively new to the U.S., they have had a dramatic effect on the health care industry. They provide high-quality, efficient care using the latest medical technology. They have generated innovations in hospital management and medical research. At the same time, they have had a devastating impact on public and charitable hospitals.

For-profit hospitals compete with other hospitals for well-insured, affluent patients. They are investor-owned and built and are accountable to their owners. In contrast, public hospitals are accountable to the taxpayers and the community. Many have been built with public money and are required as a condition of their charter to provide care to people who are indigent. Most public hospitals depend on the money they receive from paying patients, Medicare, Medicaid, and private insurance to cover the

operating expenses of treating nonpaying patients. They shift costs from the poor to the more affluent or well-insured patients. Survival for the public hospitals depends on generating sufficient income from paying patients so that they can absorb the cost of treating the poor. For-profit hospitals have been very successful in "skimming the cream" from the pool of patients who can pay for their care, leaving the public hospitals with primary responsibility for indigent care and no easy way to shift costs (Rogers, Rousseau and Nesbitt, 1984).

Public hospitals are mandated to provide free care to the poor, but how much free care and who will pay for it have not been decided. The public hospitals face severe financial difficulties, yet they continue to be the primary source of hospital care for poor people in many communities. The burden of free care is exacerbated through a common practice of selective transfer of patients to the public hospital. A recent study of patients transferred to a public hospital in Chicago found that the majority of patients transferred from other hospitals had either no insurance or received public assistance for medical care. Most of these patients were transferred to the public hospital because the transferring hospital did not want to assume the responsibility of providing free care for these patients (Schiff, et al., 1986). "Dumping" indigent patients onto the public hospitals has precipitated a financial crisis in hospital care for the poor. Recent legislation passed by the U.S. Congress would make transfer of patients, solely for economic reasons, illegal.

Publicly Subsidized Care— A Second Class System?

The second level of health care delivery is designed to provide services to individuals who are not able to pay for it. The two largest programs at this level are Medicare and Medicaid. These programs were designed to meet the health care needs of elderly and poor citizens. Medicare was enacted as an entitlement program, which means that all individuals are eligible regardless of their income. Medicaid is a "means tested" program in that individuals must demonstrate low income to qualify for benefits. Some observers in the U.S. see these programs as the beginnings of a national comprehensive health plan;

however, this has not developed in the 20 year history of these programs.

Medicare is a federally funded health insurance program for the elderly. It was enacted in 1965 as an amendment to the Social Security Act to provide health care for older citizens. As of 1972, Medicare also covers disabled people receiving Social Security and individuals with chronic kidney disease. Eligibility for Medicare does not depend on income. All individuals who reach the age of 65 are entitled to the benefits of the program. Medicare is paid for out of the Medicare Trust Fund and was intended to operate as a pay-as-you-go system. This is a significant factor, since most elderly in the U.S. do not see Medicare as a form of social welfare. Many people who receive Medicare benefits also purchase private insurance for services not covered under Medicare. Some elderly voluntarily deplete their financial resources so that they are eligible for Medicaid. The Medicare program overlaps both the market and welfare systems of health care.

The Medicare program has two parts. Part A is financed through a special tax levied on employers and employees. It pays for 90 days of hospital care with a deductible amount that the patient must pay himself. Part B is an optional coverage for 80 percent of doctors' fees and also has a deductible. Individuals pay a monthly premium to participate in this program.

Medicare was hailed as a major step in removing the fear of disease and destitution from older citizens in the U.S. However, there are specified limits on the amount and type of care for which Medicare will pay. It provides a broader range of benefits than most private insurance plans, yet an impressive list of services are not covered. Medicare does not pay for prescription drugs, routine eye and dental care, dentures, hearing aids, and routine physical examinations and immunizations. Deductibles, co-payments, and other expenses constitute substantial costs for the elderly. In 1977, Medicare covered 44 percent of the average $1745 per capita costs of health care. A significant portion of the cost of nursing home care is not covered by Medicare. In 1984, the elderly paid for 49.4 percent of the costs of nursing home care. It is not unusual for one year in nursing home care to cost $20,000. Such care poses an impossible financial drain on all but the most wealthy elderly citizens.

Medicaid is a public assistance program that uses state, local, and federal money to provide health care for the poor. Eligibility is tied to income. To qualify for Medicaid an individual must be eligible for public welfare under usually very restrictive state requirements. Both those who support and decry the right to health care point to Medicaid as proof that poor people have access to health care. Patients receiving Medicaid have approximately the same number of visits to physicians as do non-Medicaid patients, and slightly more in some cases. As we saw in the case of the Black Report in Great Britain, poor people may have more health care needs, so the number of their visits to physicians may be less than they require.

While Medicaid has been successful in improving access to care, there have been nagging questions over the quality of care Medicaid patients receive. A 1982 report by the National Academy of Sciences pointed to the lack of quality care afforded the poor. The report concluded that race and ethnic background influence both the nature and quality of health care. Specifically, black patients are concentrated in a limited number of inner-city hospitals. Blacks are less likely than whites to see a private physician and are more likely to see a general practitioner than a specialist. Blacks are more likely to use hospital emergency rooms and clinics. Differences in health status are cut along racial lines. For example, using infant mortality as an indication of health status, black infants are twice as likely as white babies to die within their first year of life (U.S. Department of Health and Human Services, 1985).

Physicians are not required to treat Medicaid patients, and only one-fourth of U.S. physicians do. This is analogous to "opting out," which we saw in the Canadian system, though it is much more common in the U.S. Some physicians refuse to accept Medicaid patients because of the lower levels of reimbursement. On the other hand, there are a number of clinics that try to attract Medicaid patients. These so-called "Medicaid mills" treat large numbers of poor patients in a very cursory fashion. The extent of this practice is unknown.

Uninsured workers are a significant group whose health care needs may be overlooked by the U.S. health care system. The paper by Davis and Rowland in this book deals extensively with the problem of uninsured workers in the U.S. In the present context, it is sufficient to point out that the number of uninsured people who are not covered under publicly subsidized health care plans appears to be growing. A recent survey of personal health care in the U.S. reported that 26.6 million citizens, or about 13 percent of the population, have no health insurance (Council on Medical Service, 1986). In periods of economic recession, many individuals lose their jobs, and with that, health insurance for themselves and their families. For example, during the recession of 1982, the Federal government reported that an additional 16 million people lost health insurance benefits due to unemployment. The American Medical Association has proposed that a system of state-subsidized insurance be established for unemployed workers and their dependents.

The existing two-tiered system of health care delivery operates on the assumption that the regulated market can provide adequately for the health care needs of the majority, supplemented by a publicly funded system for the minority who are poor, elderly, or disabled. As of 1982, Medicare has assumed some of the costs for hospice care. This alternative to hospital care for dying patients is one method for reducing health costs for individuals in their last months of life (Mor, Wachtel, and Kidder, 1985). While there is evidence that most individuals received health care through the market or by public subsidy, a sizable number of people are not adequately served by either system. The percentage of working people who lack adequate health insurance, either due to incomplete coverage or to no coverage, is estimated to be about 24 percent of the population (Council on Medical Services, 1986). The percentage of elderly people is increasing, and Medicare does not pay for all their health care needs. Although it is expected that the elderly will bear a significant part of the financial burden for nursing home and hospice care themselves, many are unable or unwilling to do so. In order to avoid a financial obligation that they feel is intolerable, many elderly individuals "spend down," that is, they make themselves destitute by transferring personal assets to family members or a nursing home so that they may qualify for medical and nursing home benefits under Medicaid. Many elderly citizens in the U.S. accept penury in order to assure that they will be provided with the health care they need.

Escalating Costs of Health Care

In 1950, health care costs accounted for about 5 percent of the U.S. gross national product (GNP). By 1984, this figure had risen to 10.6 percent. The prediction is that by 1990, health care costs will constitute over 11 percent of the U.S. GNP. The growth in health care expenditures is due largely to the growth in Medicare expenditures for the growing number of elderly citizens.

Burgeoning health care costs in the U.S. coincide with the enactment of the Medicare and Medicaid programs in 1965. The two programs are aimed at serving the health care needs of very different constituent groups. However, Congress has added disability, survivor benefits, and renal dialysis to the Medicare program. The inclusion of these groups has contributed to the mounting costs in the Medicare program.

The complexity in organizations providing health care is matched by the complexity of mechanisms that pay for it. Physicians are paid on a fee-for-service basis. This means that patients are charged individually for each treatment or procedure performed. An alternative type of payment is "capitation," in which the physician is paid a fee based on the number of patients seen, regardless of the level of care. This method of payment has been implemented in some health maintenance organizations in the U.S. Another method pays physicians based on the estimated cost of care, given the patient's diagnosis. This method, called diagnostic related groups or DRGs, is currently employed to determine reimbursements for hospital treatments under Medicare and Medicaid. Physicians have criticized the DRG systems because it is not sufficiently sensitive to differences in levels of care individuals may need. Several critics have indicated that patients with very different health problems are grouped in the same diagnostic category (Gonnella, 1986; Iezzoni and Moskowitz, 1986).

Both Medicare and Medicaid programs reimburse the patient for "reasonable fees" charged by the hospital and the physician. Fee-for-service is the primary method of billing. Government officials are concerned about abuse in the system, but there is no reliable information concerning the magnitude of abuse. Professional Service Review Organizations (PSROs) have been established to monitor the number of services provided under these programs and to report evidence of fraud by physicians. Few cases are reported. Whether this is due to the honesty of physicians or the weakness of the review system cannot be determined (Pontell et al., 1985).

Multiple payment methods and competing organizations appear to have added to the costs of administering health care in the U.S. For example, the DRG system used by Medicare requires a federal bureaucracy to administer the system. Approximately 6000 new fiscal personnel and millions of dollars in computer equipment are needed simply to run the DRG program.

In the absence of a centralized bureaucracy, each new program requires the creation of a new administrative structure, thereby increasing total administrative costs. It is estimated that in 1983, the U.S. spent 22 percent of its health care dollars, or almost $78 billion, in administrative costs for health care (including the 16 percent overhead mentioned on p. 495). This compares to estimates of 2.5 percent in Canada and 5.7 percent in Great Britain. The duplication of administrative costs is at least as noteworthy as the duplication of actual health services as a source of increased costs of health care in the U.S. (Himmelstein and Woolhandler, 1986).

A Future for Comprehensive Health Care?

The growing number of elderly, uninsured, and poor people who are unable to meet the cost of health care has refocused public attention on the issue of health care rights. Both the need for health care and the costs of providing it are increasing. In the absence of a universal public system of health care, the U.S. depends upon employers, patients, and public subsidy. None of these sources, alone or in combination, provide for comprehensive care.

All employers do not provide health insurance for their workers, and those that do are continually searching for ways to curtail the cost of health care benefits (Rublee, 1986). Two main strategies are available to employers in the private sector. They can either limit benefits, thus increasing the number of uninsured or underinsured workers, or they can limit reimbursement to providers. Both strategies limit the availability of health care for employed people and their dependents. In the late 1980s, the idea of reducing health care costs through prevention

of disease has attracted considerable attention. Employee Assistance Programs (EAPs) offer treatment for such problems as alcoholism, family distress, stress management, smoking, and weight control. These programs focus on changing the behavior of employees so that workers remain healthier. Professionals in the forefront of the "wellness" movement suggest that national health policy should be directed toward preventing health problems that are the result of environmental or behavioral factors (Foege, Amler, and White, 1985).

The public system of health care was designed to meet the needs of individuals not covered by either private insurance or personal wealth. However, there remain needs for which neither private nor public sector programs seem willing or able to provide. In the recent past, the U.S. has attempted to "fill the gaps" in health care delivery by developing programs targeted at specific areas of unmet needs.

For example, in 1983 an "orphan drug" bill was signed into law that provided $75 million in subsidies to commercial drug companies for the production of drugs to treat persons with rare diseases. Drugs effective in the treatment of such diseases as Touretts's syndrome, cystic fibrosis, and Huntington's chorea were not profitable for commercial manufacturers due to limited demand. The need for public subsidies to assure their supply is an excellent example of the failure of a market system alone to meet health care needs. More recently, there has been an effort to develop a public insurance program to cover "catastrophic illness" (Birenbaum, 1978). In mid-1986, the Reagan administration established a committee to develop a plan for catastrophic health insurance for all U.S. citizens. At about the same time, the Congress passed legislation requiring employers to continue health insurance for employees who are laid off.

States and municipalities are also taking a more active role in health care. South Carolina, a state not noted for its generosity in the provision of welfare services, has expanded its eligibility requirements for Medicaid and has established an assistance fund to reimburse hospitals who provide free care to the poor. Colorado has examined procedures for rationing health care services provided under the Medicaid program (Wright et al., 1985).

Many people in the United States assume that there are sufficient opportunities for people to provide for themselves, except for the very young, the old, and the disabled. In the land of plenty, there is enough for everyone. Yet, there is a growing recognition that all citizens will risk overwhelming costs in meeting the health care needs of themselves and their families at some time during their lives. The inevitability and universality of illness promotes public concern over the provision of care.

Through the 1970s, the U.S. Congress actively debated the question of national health insurance (U.S. Congress, 1978). By 1981, national health insurance of any kind had become unfeasible, given cutbacks in federal spending on domestic programs (Task Force on Academic Health Centers, 1985). Concern over access to health care, the right to treatment, and health care for the poor were replaced by debate about cost containment, competition, and the free market. The political rhetoric changed in the 1980s, but the underlying issues remain. How will the United States provide essential health care services for all its citizens?

CONCLUSION

This paper has sketched the systems of health care delivery in Canada, Great Britain, and the United States. It is a picture drawn with broad strokes in an attempt to portray the distinguishing features of each. Each nation has its own unique response to the issue of health care rights. Canada and Great Britain are similar in accepting the notion of health care as a right, but they are different in the mechanism they use to provide care. Canada has implemented a system of universal comprehensive health care that preserves some features of professional autonomy and patient choice. It has reorganized the method of paying for health services without drastic changes in the way health services are provided.

Great Britain has made the delivery of health services a function of government. The National Health Service is essentially a socialized industry for the provision of health care. This system may appear radical to a U.S. observer, but it is consistent with the British response to increasing demand and limited resources.

The Canadian and British systems demonstrate two different yet effective responses to the problem of comprehensive health care. If the U.S. is to take any lessons from these two nations, it is likely to be more comfortable with those offered by Canada in its establishment of National Health Insurance.

In 1977, it appeared that the United States was on the brink of establishing national health insurance. Public surveys show that the majority of the U.S. public favors some system of national insurance. Political opinion in the 1980s has discouraged the development of public services. However, opinions may change with changes in the composition of U.S. society. No one can predict the future, but an understanding of the past and present may make the future easier to apprehend.

References

AARON, HENRY J., and WILLIAM B. SCHWARTZ. 1984. *The Painful Prescription. Rationing Hospital Care.* Washington, DC: The Brookings Institution.

ARMSTRONG, DAVID. 1983. *Political Anatomy of the Body. Medical Knowledge in Britain in the Twentieth Century.* New York: Cambridge.

AXELROD, S. J., A. DONABEDIAN, and D. W. GENTRY. 1976. *Medical Care Chart Book.* Ann Arbor, Michigan.

BARR, JUDITH K. 1983. "Consumer Views of Prepaid Health Care: Perspectives on an Alternative System." Annual Meeting of the American Sociological Association, September, Detroit, MI.

BIRNBAUM, HOWARD. 1978. *The Cost of Catastrophic Illness.* Lexington, MA: Lexington Books.

BUCHANAN, JOAN L., and SHAN CRETIN. 1986. "Risk Selection in Families Electing HMO Membership." *Medical Care* 24(1):39–51.

COUNCIL ON MEDICAL SERVICE. 1986. "Closing the Gaps in Health Insurance Coverage." *JAMA* 255(6):790–793.

DOMINION-PROVINCIAL CONFERENCE. 1945. *Plenary Conference Discussions.*

ENTHOVEN, ALAIN. 1980. *Health Plan.* New York: Addison-Wesley.

ERMANN, DAN, and JON GABEL. 1985. "The Changing Face in American Health Care. Multi-hospital Systems, Emergency Centers, and Surgery Centers." *Medical Care* 23(5):401–420.

EVANS, ROBERT G. 1983. "Health Care in Canada: Patterns of Funding and Regulations." *Journal of Health Politics, Policy and Law* 8(1):1–43.

———. 1985. "Illusions of Necessity: Evading Responsibility for Choice in Health Care." *Journal of Health Politics, Policy and Law* 10(3):439–467.

FOEGE, WILLIAM H., ROBERT W. AMLER, and CRAIG C. WHITE. 1985. "Closing the Gap: Report of the Carter Center Health Policy Consultation." *JAMA* 254(10):1355–1358.

FRIED, CHARLES. 1976. "Equality and Rights in Medical Care." *Hastings Center Report* 6(1):30–32.

GILL, DEREK G. 1980. *The British National Health Service: A Sociologist's Perspective*. U.S. Department of Health and Human Services, National Institutes of Health.

GILLON, RAANAN. 1985. "Justice and Allocation of Medical Resources." *British Medical Journal* 291(6490):266–268.

GONNELLA, JOSEPH A. 1986. "Case Mix Classification: The Need to Reduce Inappropriate Homogeneity." *JAMA* 255(7):941–942.

HATCHER, GORDON H. 1981. *Universal Free Health Care in Canada, 1947–77*. Washington, D.C.: U.S. Department of Health and Human Services.

HIBBARD, JUDITH H., and CLYDE R. POPE. 1986. "Age Differences in the Use of Medical Care in an HMO: An Application of the Behavioral Model." *Medical Care* 24(1):52–66.

HIMMELSTEIN, DAVID U., and STEFFIE WOOLHANDLER. 1986. "Cost Without Benefit. Administrative Waste in U.S. Health Care." *New England Journal of Medicine* 314(7):441–445.

HODGKINSON, RUTH G. 1967. *The Origins of the National Health Services: The Medical Services of the Poor Law, 1834–1871*. London: Wellcome Historical Medical Library.

HUNTER, DAVID J. 1980. *Coping with Uncertainty. Policy and Politics in the National Health Service*. New York: John Wiley.

IEZZONI, LISA I., and MARK A. MOSKOWITZ. 1986. "Clinical Overlap Among Medical Diagnosis-Related Groups." *JAMA* 255(7):927–929.

INTERSTUDY. 1985. *National HMO Census: Annual Report on the Growth of HMOs in the U.S.* Excelsior, MN: Interstudy.

KANE, ROSALIE A., and ROBERT L. KANE. 1985. "The Feasibility of Universal Long-Term-Care Benefits. Ideas From Canada." *New England Journal of Medicine* 312(21):1357–1364.

LINDSAY, C. M. 1980. *National Health Issues. The British Experience*. Roche Laboratories.

LIPSET, SEYMOUR-MARTIN. 1950. *Agrarian Socialism*. Berkeley: University of California.

LUFT, HAROLD S. 1981a. *Health Maintenance Organizations, Dimensions of Performance*. New York: Wiley.

———. 1981b. *History of Health Maintenance Organizations*.

MAERKI, SUSAN C., HAROLD S. LUFT, and SANDRA HUNT. 1986. "Selecting Categories of Patients for Regionalization: Implications of the Relationship Between Volume and Outcome." *Medical Care* 24(2):148–158.

MINISTER OF NATIONAL HEALTH AND WELFARE. 1983. *Preserving Universal Medicare*. Canada: Minister of Supply and Services.

MOR, VINCENT, THOMAS J. WACHTEL, and DAVID KIDDER. 1985. "Patient Predictors of Hospice Choice." *Medical Care* 23(9):1115–1119.

NEWHOUSE, JOSEPH P., WILLIAM B. SCHWARTZ, ALBERT P. WILLIAMS, and CHRISTINA WITSBERGER. 1985. "Are Fee-For-Service Costs Increasing Faster than HMO Costs?" *Medical Care* 23(8):960–966.

OWEN, DAVID. 1976. *In Sickness and In Health*. London: Quartet Books.

PONTELL, HENRY N., PAUL JESILOW, GILBERT GEIS, and MARY JANE O'BRIEN. 1985. "A Demographic Portrait of Physicians Sanctioned by the Federal Government for Fraud and Abuse Against Medicare and Medicaid." *Medical Care* 25(8):1028–1031.

ROBACK, GENE, LILLIAN RANDOLPH, DIANE MEAD, and THOMAS PASKO. 1984. *Physician Characteristics and Distribution in the U.S.* Chicago: American Medical Association.

ROEMER, MILTON I. 1976. *Health Care Systems in World Perspective*. Ann Arbor: Health Administration Press.

———. 1981. *Ambulatory Health Services in America*. Rockville, MD: Aspen Systems Corporation.

ROGERS, SALLY J., ANN MARIE ROUSSEAU, and SUSAN M. NESBITT. 1984. *Hospitals and the Uninsured Poor: Measuring and Paying for Uncompensated Care*. New York: United Hospital Fund.

RUBLEE, DALE A. 1986. "Self-Funded Health Benefit Plans. Trends, Legal Environment, and Policy Issues." *JAMA* 255(6):787–789.

SADE, RICHARD M. 1974. "Medical Care as a Right: A Refutation." *New England Journal of Medicine* 285:1288–1289.

SCHIFF, ROBERT L., DAVID A. ANSELL, JAMES E. SCHLOSSER, AHAMED H. IDRIS, ANN MORRISON, and STEVEN WHITMAN. 1986. "Transfer to a Public Hospital. A Prospective Study of 467 Patients." *The New England Journal of Medicine* 314(9):552–557.

SCHNEIDER, KAREN. C., and HENRY G. DOVE. 1983. "High Users of VA Emergency Room Facilities: Are Outpatients Abusing the System or is the System Abusing Them?" *Inquiry* 20(1):57–64.

SELLS, R. A., S. MACPHERSON, and J. R. SALAMAN. 1985. "Assessment of Resources for Renal Transplantation in the United Kingdom. *Lancet* 8448:195–7.

TASK FORCE ON ACADEMIC HEALTH CENTERS. 1985. *Prescription for Change.* New York: The Commonwealth Fund.

TAYLOR, MALCOLM G. 1979. *Health Insurance and Canadian Public Policy. The Seven Decisions that Created the Canadian Health Insurance System.* Montreal: McGill-Queens.

TOWNSEND, PETER, and NICK DAVIDSON. 1982. *Inequalities in Health: The Black Report.* New York: Penguin.

U.S. CONGRESS, SENATE. 1978. *National Health Insurance Hearings Before the Subcommittee on Health and Scientific Research.* Washington, D.C.: Committee on Human Resources.

U.S. DEPARTMENT OF HEALTH AND HUMAN SERVICES, 1985. *Health United States 1984.* Hyattsville, MD: Public Health Service.

U.S. NATIONAL CENTER FOR HEALTH STATISTICS. 1978. "Access to Ambulatory Health Care: United States 1974." Advance Data No. 17.

VEYDA, EUGENE, and RAISA B. DEBER. 1984. "The Canadian Health System: An Overview." *Social Science and Medicine* 18(3):191–197.

WRIGHT, RICHARD A., DAVID GARR, FREDRICK ABRAMS, and STEFAN MOKROHISKY. 1985. "Conceptual Model for Allocation and Rationing Physical Health Services to Colorado's Medically Indigent. *Colorado Medicine* 82(10):169–172.

Uninsured and Underserved: Inequities in Health Care in the United States

Karen Davis
Diane Rowland

The United States has one of the highest quality and most sophisticated systems of medical care in the world. Most Americans take for granted their access to this system of care. In times of emergency or illness, they can call upon a vast array of health resources—from a family physician to a complex teaching hospital—assured that they will receive needed care and that their health insurance coverage will pick up the tab for the majority of bills incurred.

For a surprisingly large segment of the United States population, however, this ease of access to care does not exist. At any point in time, over 25 million Americans have no health insurance coverage from private health insurance plans or public programs (Kasper et al. 1978). Without health insurance coverage or ready cash, such individuals can be and are turned away from hospitals even in emergency situations (U.S. Congress, House Committee on Energy and Commerce 1981). Some neglect obtaining preventive or early care, often postponing care until conditions have become life-threatening. Others struggle with burdensome medical bills. Many come to rely upon crowded, understaffed public hospitals as the only source of reliable, available care.

The absence of universal health insurance coverage creates serious strains in our society. These strains are felt most acutely by the uninsured poor, who must worry about family members—a sick child, an adult afflicted with a deteriorating chronic health

condition, a pregnant mother—going without needed medical assistance. It strains our image as a just and humane society when significant portions of the population endure avoidable pain, suffering, and even death because of an inability to pay for health care. Those physicians, other health professionals, and institutions that try to assist this uninsured group also incur serious strain. Demands typically far outstrip available time and resources. Strain is also felt by local governments whose communities include many uninsured persons, because locally funded public hospitals and health centers inevitably incur major financial deficits. In recent years, many of the public facilities that have traditionally been the source of last-resort care have closed, thereby intensifying the stresses on other providers and the uninsured poor.

As serious as these strains have been in the last five years, the years ahead promise to strain the fabric of our social life even more seriously. Unemployment levels today are the highest since the Great Depression. With unemployment, the American worker loses not only a job but also health insurance protection. As unemployment rises and the numbers of the uninsured grow, fewer and fewer resources are available to fill the gaps in health care coverage. Major reductions in funding for health services for the poor and uninsured have been made in the last year; further reductions are likely. Deepening economic recession, high unemployment, and declining sales revenues are strapping the fiscal resources of state and local governments. Their ability to offset federal cutbacks seems limited. Nor can the private sector be expected to bridge this gap. The health industry is increasingly becoming an en-

Reprinted from the *Milbank Memorial Fund Quarterly/ Health and Society*, vol. 61, no. 2, 1983, pp. 149–176. Copyright © 1983 by the Milbank Memorial Fund Quarterly.

trepreneurial business endeavor—with little room for charitable actions.

It is especially timely, therefore, to review what we know about the consequences of inadequate health insurance coverage for certain segments of our population. The first section of this paper presents information on the number and characteristics of the uninsured, while the second section describes patterns of health care utilization by the uninsured. The third section assesses the policy implications of these facts and offers recommendations for future public policy to ensure access to health care for all.

WHO ARE THE UNINSURED?

The 1977 National Medical Care Expenditure Survey (NMCES) provides extensive information on the health insurance coverage of the U.S. population. Six household interviews of a nationwide sample of over 40,000 individuals were conducted over an 18-month period during 1977 and 1978. By following the interviewed population for an entire year, NMCES provided a comprehensive portrait of health insurance coverage, including changes in health insurance status during the course of that year.

Although the scope of the NMCES survey provides extensive information on the characteristics and utilization patterns of the uninsured, it should be noted that the profile of the uninsured presented here describes the portion of the population without insurance in 1977. Recent changes in health insurance coverage due to unemployment and cutbacks in eligibility for Medicaid have increased the size of the nation's uninsured population, but are not reflected in the statistics in this paper.

In the NMCES results, individuals classified as insured are those who were covered throughout the year by Medicaid, Medicare, the Civilian Health and Medical Program of the Uniformed Services (Champus), Blue Cross/Blue Shield or commercial health insurance, or who were enrolled in a health maintenance organization. Differences in scope of coverage among the insured were not available, although further analysis of the NMCES data will address this issue. Therefore, many individuals in the insured category may have actually had very limited health insurance coverage, leaving them basically uninsured for most services. For example, many individu-

als classified as insured have coverage for inpatient hospital care, but are not covered and are, therefore, essentially uninsured for primary care in a physician's office. In contrast, insured individuals also include those enrolled in a health maintenance organization offering comprehensive coverage for both inpatient and ambulatory care.

The uninsured fall into two groups: the always uninsured and the sometimes uninsured. The always uninsured are individuals without Medicare, Medicaid, or private insurance coverage for the entire year. Individuals using Veterans Administration hospitals and clinics or community health centers are classified as uninsured unless they have third-party coverage. The sometimes uninsured are those who were covered by public or private insurance part of the year but were uninsured the remainder of the year. The sometimes uninsured include the medically needy individuals who qualify for Medicaid coverage during periods of large medical expenses, but are otherwise uninsured. Changes in insurance status during the year are generally the result of loss of employment, change in employment, change in income or family situation that alters eligibility for Medicaid, or loss of private insurance when an older spouse retires and becomes eligible for Medicare.

A snapshot view of the uninsured at a given point in time understates the number of people who spend some portion of the year uninsured. At any one time, there are over 25 million uninsured Americans, but as many as 34 million may be uninsured for some period of time during the year. Approximately 18 million are without insurance for the entire year, and 16 million are uninsured for some portion of the year (Wilensky and Walden 1981; Wilensky and Berk 1982).

The 34 million uninsured are persons of all incomes, racial and ethnic backgrounds, occupations, and geographic locations. In some cases whole families are uninsured, while in others coverage is mixed depending on employment status and eligibility for public programs (Kasper et al. 1978). However, the poor, minorities, young adults, and rural residents are more likely than others to be uninsured. As noted in table 1, over one-quarter of all blacks and minorities are uninsured during the year—a rate 1 ½ times that of whites. This disparity holds across the demographic and social characteristics of the uninsured

(Wilensky and Walden 1981; Institute of Medicine 1981).

Age

The uninsured population, whether covered for all or part of a year, is almost entirely under age 65. Nearly one-fifth of the non-aged population is uninsured for some or all of the year. Less than 1 percent of the aged, barely 200,000 persons, are uninsured during the year (table 1). This is attributable primarily to Medicare which provides basic coverage for hospital and physician services to most older Americans. The success of Medicare in providing financial access to health care for the elderly is demonstrated by the extensive coverage of the elderly today in contrast to the dramatic lack of insurance prior to implementation of Medicare in 1966 (Davis 1982). Medicaid and private insurance help to fill the gap for those elderly persons ineligible for Medicare because they lack sufficient Social Security earnings contributions. The uninsured elderly are primarily individuals with incomes above the eligibility levels for welfare assistance and Medicaid.

Examination of the uninsured by age group reveals that young adults are the group most likely to be uninsured. As highlighted in table 2, almost one-third of all persons aged 19 to 24 are uninsured during the course of a year. Roughly 16 percent of this age group are without coverage all year, and an additional 14 percent lack coverage at least part of the year. This rate is nearly double that of other age groups. A variety of factors undoubtedly contribute to this situation. Young adults frequently lose coverage under their parents' policies at age 18. Many young adults may elect to forego coverage when it is available, since coverage is costly and they assume themselves to be relatively healthy. High youth unemployment, as well as employment in marginal jobs without health benefits, make insurance difficult to obtain or afford for this group.

Employment

Employment status and occupation are important factors in assessing the likelihood of being uninsured for all or part of a year. Most American workers receive their health care coverage through the workplace, but insurance coverage varies widely depending on the type of employer (Taylor and Lawson

TABLE 1   Insurance status during year by age and race, 1977

AGE AND RACE	TOTAL	ALWAYS UNINSURED	UNINSURED PART OF YEAR	ALWAYS INSURED
		NUMBER IN MILLIONS		
Total, all persons	212.1	18.1	15.9	178.1
Persons under age 65	189.8	18.0	15.8	156.0
White	163.7	14.5	12.5	136.7
Black and Other	26.1	3.5	3.3	19.3
Persons age 65 and over	22.3	0.1	0.1	22.1
White	20.2	0.07	0.09	20.0
Black and Other	2.1	0.03	0.01	2.1
		PERCENTAGE		
All persons	100%	8.6%	7.5%	83.9%
Persons under age 65	100	9.5	8.3	82.2
White	100	8.9	7.6	83.5
Black and Other	100	13.3	12.7	74.0
Persons age 65 and over	100	0.4	0.5	99.1
White	100	0.3	0.5	99.2
Black and Other	100	1.0	0.8	98.2

Source: Data from the U.S. Department of Health and Human Services, National Center for Health Services Research, National Medical Care Expenditure Survey.

TABLE 2   Percent uninsured during year by selected population
characteristics, 1977

POPULATION CHARACTERISTIC	PERCENT UNINSURED DURING YEAR	PERCENT ALWAYS UNINSURED	PERCENT UNINSURED PART OF YEAR
All persons	16.1%	8.6%	7.5%
Age			
Under age 65	17.8	9.5	8.3
less than 6 years	19.6	8.3	11.3
6 to 18 years	16.1	8.6	7.5
19 to 24 years	30.3	16.0	14.3
25 to 54 years	16.1	8.7	7.4
55 to 64 years	12.6	8.2	4.4
Age 65 and over	0.9	0.4	0.5
Occupation			
Farm	22.3	15.9	6.4
Blue collar	19.8	11.3	8.5
Services	20.8	11.9	8.9
White collar	12.6	5.6	7.0
Region			
Northeast	10.7	5.4	5.3
North Central	12.5	5.7	6.8
South	20.5	11.6	8.9
West	20.8	11.7	9.1

Source: Wilensky and Walden (1981), and data from the U.S. Department of Health and Human Services, National Center for Health Services Research, National Medical Care Expenditure Survey.

1981). Employees of small firms are less likely to be insured than employees of large firms. For example, 45 percent of employees in firms of 25 or fewer employees do not have employer-provided health insurance compared with only 1 percent in firms with more than 1,000 employees. Yet, small firms employ over 20 percent of all workers. Unionized firms are six times more likely to have employee health insurance than are nonunionized firms.

Insurance status varies by type of employment (table 2). Nearly one-quarter of all agricultural workers are uninsured during the year, with 16 percent uninsured for the entire year. As expected, white collar workers are the most likely to be insured, while blue collar and service workers fare only somewhat better than agricultural workers (Wilensky and Walden 1981). Among blue collar and service workers, insurance coverage is low in the construction industry, wholesale and retail trades, and service industries, and high in manufacturing. Of manufacturing employees, 96 percent have health insurance through their place of employment (Davis 1975).

Residence

These trends in coverage by employment are reflected in the regional picture of insurance status. In the heavily industrial and unionized Northeast and north central regions of the country, the percentage of uninsured during the year is half that of the South and the West. In these areas where agricultural interests are strong and unionization less extensive, over 20 percent of the population is uninsured during the course of a year. Of those living in the South and West, 11 percent are uninsured throughout the year compared with 5 percent in the Northeast and north central regions. Similarly, people in metropolitan areas are more likely to be insured than people living outside metropolitan areas (Wilensky and Walden 1981).

Income and Race

However, while nature of employment and unionization may explain some of the regional variations, a critical underlying factor in the analysis is the distribution in the population of poverty and minorities. Residents of the South comprise 32 percent of the total population under age 65. Yet 48 percent of the nation's minorities live in the South (Department of Health and Human Services 1982a). The higher concentration of poor and minority persons in the South in comparison with other parts of the country helps explain the high level of uninsured individuals.

Poverty and lack of insurance are strongly correlated. Of poor families with incomes below 125 percent of the poverty line, 27 percent are uninsured. The near-poor, with incomes between 125 and 200 percent of poverty, fare only slightly better, with 21 percent uninsured during the year. The poor are always more likely to be uninsured than the middle and upper income groups (table 3) (Wilensky and Walden 1981).

The limited health insurance coverage for the poor and near-poor demonstrates the limits of coverage of the poor under Medicaid (Wilensky and Berk 1982). Many assume that Medicaid finances health care services for all of the poor. However, many poor persons are ineligible for Medicaid due to categorical

requirements for program eligibility and variations in state eligibility policies. Two-parent families are generally ineligible for Medicaid and single adults are covered only if they are aged or disabled (Davis and Schoen 1978). Moreover, many states have established income eligibility cutoffs well below the poverty level. Many states have not adjusted income levels to account for inflation, resulting in a reduction in the number of individuals covered over the last few years (Rowland and Gaus 1983). As a result of the restrictions on Medicaid coverage, about 60 percent of the poor are not covered by Medicaid. Of the 35 million poor and near-poor in 1977, almost 5 million or about 15 percent had no insurance throughout 1977. Approximately 35 percent were on Medicaid for at least part of the year (Wilensky and Berk 1982). This situation can only be expected to worsen as the recession swells the numbers of poor and near-poor while cutbacks in social programs and Medicaid further erode the health coverage available to some of the poor.

Thus, while the poor are obviously the least able to pay for care directly, they are the most likely to be without either Medicaid or private insurance. The

TABLE 3 Percent uninsured during year by ethnic/racial background and income, 1977*

ETHNIC/RACIAL BACKGROUND	PERCENT UNINSURED DURING YEAR	PERCENT ALWAYS UNINSURED	PERCENT UNINSURED PART OF YEAR
White, all incomes	14.0	7.0	7.0
Poor	27.1	13.5	13.6
Other low income	21.0	10.9	10.1
Middle income	12.6	6.3	6.3
High income	8.8	4.2	4.6
Black, all incomes	23.2	9.7	13.5
Poor	32.2	10.6	21.6
Other low income	26.6	11.9	14.7
Middle income	17.4	8.6	8.8
High income	12.4	7.1	5.3
Hispanic, all incomes	24.3	12.8	11.5
Poor	29.6	9.5	20.1
Other low income	32.0	18.2	13.8
Middle income	17.7	12.4	5.3
High income	20.0	12.3	8.0

Source: Wilensky and Walden (1981).

* In 1977, the poverty level for a family of 4 was $8,000. Poor are defined as those whose family income was less than or equal to 125 percent of the 1977 poverty level. Other low income includes those whose income is 1.26 to 2 times the poverty level; middle income is 2.01 to 4 times the poverty level; and high income is 4.01 times the poverty level or more.

poor are twice as likely to be uninsured as the middle class and three times as likely as those in upper income groups. Lack of insurance is inversely related to ability to bear the economic consequences of ill health.

Blacks, Hispanics, and other minorities are also more likely to be uninsured than whites regardless of their income; poor blacks are the most likely to be uninsured. As noted in table 3, nearly one-third of poor blacks are uninsured during a year. If you are poor and a member of a minority group, your chances of being uninsured are four times as great as for a high income white.

Yet this relationship between race and income (table 3) actually understates the situation because the aged are included in the population analyzed. The aged are overrepresented in the lower income groups, but, as noted in table 1, almost all of the aged are insured. Thus, inclusion of the aged in table 3 tends to overstate the insured status of the nonelderly poor.

Regional and racial differences in insurance coverage for the population under age 65 are enumerated in table 4. When the aged are excluded from the analysis, the differentials become even more striking. Southerners are nearly 1½ times as likely

to be uninsured as those from other parts of the country. But blacks in the South are 1½ times more likely to be uninsured as are whites from the South or nonsouthern blacks. Southern blacks are twice as likely to be uninsured as nonsouthern whites.

Similarly, when differences in insurance status are assessed from the perspective of metropolitan versus nonmetropolitan areas, blacks fare much worse than whites. Over 16 percent of nonelderly residents of Standard Metropolitan Statistical Areas (SMSAs) are uninsured compared with over 21 percent of those residing in non-SMSA areas. But, for minorities living outside SMSAs, almost 40 percent are uninsured—a rate twice that of whites residing in non-SMSA areas and 2½ times that of whites in SMSAs.

Thus, health insurance coverage in the U.S. is to some extent a matter of luck. Those fortunate enough to be employed by large, unionized, manufacturing firms are also likely to be fortunate enough to have good health insurance coverage. Those who are poor, those who live in the South or in rural areas, and those who are black or minority group members are more likely to bear the personal and economic effects of lack of insurance and the consequent financial barriers to health care.

TABLE 4   Percent of persons under age 65 uninsured during year by race and residence, 1977

RACE AND RESIDENCE	POPULATION (IN MILLIONS)	PERCENT UNINSURED DURING YEAR	PERCENT ALWAYS UNINSURED	PERCENT UNINSURED PART OF YEAR
Total, all persons under 65	189.8	17.8%	9.5%	8.3%
South	60.5	24.4	12.7	9.7
White	47.9	20.4	11.8	8.6
Black and Other	12.6	30.0	16.2	13.8
Non-South	129.3	15.7	8.0	7.7
White	115.8	14.9	7.7	7.2
Black and Other	13.5	22.2	10.7	11.5
SMSA	132.6	16.3	8.2	8.1
White	111.3	14.9	7.6	7.3
Black and Other	21.3	23.2	11.1	12.1
Non-SMSA	57.2	21.4	12.5	8.9
White	52.5	19.9	11.6	8.3
Black and Other	4.7	38.2	23.3	14.9

Source: Data from the U.S. Department of Health and Human Services, National Center for Health Services Research, National Medical Care Expenditure Survey.

UTILIZATION OF HEALTH SERVICES BY THE UNINSURED

With the investment in primary care made by federal programs in the late 1960s and 1970s, significant progress in improving access to primary care for the poor and other disadvantaged groups was achieved. Virtually all of the numerous studies examining trends in access to health care conclude that differentials in utilization of physician services and preventive service by income have narrowed (Davis et al. 1981).

In the early 1960s the nonpoor visited physicians 23 percent more frequently than the poor even though the poor, then as now, were considerably sicker than the nonpoor. By the 1970s the poor visited physicians more frequently than the nonpoor, and more in accordance with their greater need for health care services. Blacks and other minorities also made substantial gains over this period. Utilization of services by rural residents also increased relative to urban residents (Davis and Schoen 1978).

However, use of preventive services by the poor, minorities, and rural residents continues to lag well behind use by those not facing similar barriers to health care. Some studies have also found that these differentials continue to exist for all disadvantaged groups even when adjusted for the greater health needs of the disadvantaged (Davis et al. 1981).

The major difficulty with past studies, however, is that they have not examined insurance coverage of subgroups of the poor to detect the cumulative impact of lack of financial and physical access to care. How do uninsured blacks in rural areas fare in obtaining ambulatory care services? Can nearly all disadvantaged persons get care from public hospitals or clinics, or do those facing multiple barriers to care simply do without?

Data and Methodology

New data from the 1977 National Medical Care Expenditure Survey (NMCES) shed some light on the cumulative effect of multiple barriers to care. Insured persons are those covered during the entire year; the uninsured are those uninsured for the entire year. Those insured for part of the year are excluded; presumably their utilization resembles that of the insured for the portion of the year in which they are insured and that of the uninsured for the portion of the year in which they are uninsured.

The NMCES sample was designed to produce statistically unbiased national estimates that are representative of the civilian noninstitutionalized population of the United States. Since the statistics presented here are based on a sample, they may differ somewhat from the figures that would have been obtained if a complete census had been taken. Tests of statistical significance are indicated in the tables included below (see Department of Health and Human Services 1982d, Technical Notes, for further detail on methodology). Particular caution should be taken in interpreting those data items for which the noted relative standard error is equal to or greater than 30 percent.

The statistics presented here show utilization differentials between insured and uninsured individuals under age 65. Analysis of age-specific differentials between the insured and uninsured showed patterns similar to the general pattern of the nonelderly population. The elderly were excluded from the analysis since the majority of the elderly population is insured.

Ambulatory Care

Most striking is the extent to which insurance coverage affects use of ambulatory care. Table 5 presents data on use of physicians' services from NMCES for the population under age 65; the insured average 3.7 visits to physicians during the year compared with 2.4 visits for the uninsured. That is, the insured receive 54 percent more ambulatory care from physicians than do the uninsured. However, the differential between the insured and uninsured for physician visits may understate the actual differential because variations in scope of coverage among the insured population are not accounted for. Some of the insured may only have insurance coverage for inpatient hospital care, not ambulatory care. Thus, although their utilization pattern is considered in the insured category, such individuals are actually uninsured for physician visits. Better data on ambulatory-care insurance coverage of the insured population therefore might indicate even greater differentials in use of ambulatory care.

Residence and race also affect utilization of am-

TABLE 5 Physician visits per person under age 65 per year, by insurance status, residence, and race, 1977

INSURANCE STATUS, RESIDENCE, AND RACE	UNINSURED	INSURED	RATIO
Total	2.4	3.7	1.54*
South	2.1	3.5	1.67*
White	2.3	3.7	1.61*
Black and Other	1.5	2.8	1.87*
Non-South	2.6	3.8	1.46*
White	2.7	3.8	1.41*
Black and Other	1.9	3.5	1.84*
SMSA	2.4	3.8	1.58*
White	2.6	3.9	1.50*
Black and Other	1.7	3.2	1.88*
Non-SMSA	2.3	3.3	1.43*
White	2.4	3.4	1.42*
Black and Other	1.6	2.9	1.81

* Indicates values for insured and uninsured are significantly different at the .05 level.

Source: Data from the U.S. Department of Health and Human Services, National Center for Health Services Research, National Medical Care Expenditure Survey.

bulatory services. The lowest utilization of ambulatory care occurs for uninsured blacks and other minorities, including Hispanics. These persons use far less than more advantaged groups. For example, uninsured blacks and other minorities in the South make 1.5 physician visits per person annually, compared with 3.7 physician visits for insured whites in the South. That is, to be advantaged multiply leads to a utilization rate almost 2.5 times that of individuals who are disadvantaged multiply.

These data point to the importance of financial and physical barriers to access. It is not the case that the uninsured manage to obtain ambulatory care comparable in amount to that obtained by the insured by relying on public clinics, teaching hospital outpatient clinics, nonprofit health centers, or the charity of private physicians. Without insurance, many simply do without care.

The patterns of utilization for different groups provide some insight into the relative importance of financial, physical, and racial barriers to care. Financial access to care is clearly the most important factor affecting use. Insurance coverage reduces much but not all of the differential in use of ambulatory services. Insured blacks in the South, for example, average 2.8 physician visits annually, compared

with 3.7 for insured whites in the South. That is, whites average about 30 percent more ambulatory care than blacks and other minorities even if both are insured. But this differential is substantially smaller than the 2½ times greater use of physicians between insured southern whites and uninsured southern blacks.

Location remains an important determinant of use of physician services. Lack of insurance coverage is more predominant in rural areas; however, even among the insured, urban residents are more likely to receive ambulatory care than are rural residents, whether white or black (see table 5). Among insured groups, rural whites receive 3.4 physician visits annually compared with 3.9 visits for urban whites. Rural blacks and other minorities with insurance make 2.9 physician visits compared with 3.2 visits for their insured counterparts in urban areas. That is, a 10 to 15 percent differential in use between urban and rural areas occurs even when financial access to care is not a problem. It should be noted, however, that the quality of insurance for ambulatory care may not be as good in rural areas as in urban areas.

Racial differentials in utilization of ambulatory care are also ameliorated with insurance coverage.

Insurance is particularly helpful in improving access to care for minorities. Insured minorities receive 80 to 90 percent more ambulatory care than do uninsured minorities, in both rural and urban areas. But even with insurance, strong racial differences persist.

Hospital Care

Despite the common perception that all disadvantaged persons can obtain hospital care from some charity facility, tremendous differentials in use of hospital care also exist by insurance status, residence, and race. The insured receive 90 percent more hospital care than do the uninsured (see table 6). Differentials by insurance status are particularly marked in the South and in rural areas. In the South, insured persons receive three times as many days of hospital care annually as uninsured persons, regardless of race or ethnic background.

These hospital utilization differentials clearly demonstrate that the insured fare much better than the uninsured in obtaining health care services. Since those with insurance are likely to have basic coverage for hospitalization, the hospital utilization

data provide a more accurate assessment of the role of insurance coverage in the use of health care services than do the ambulatory care differentials in the previous section.

These differentials remove any complacency about the accessibility of inpatient care. They reinforce similar findings by Wilensky and Berk (1982) who find that the insured poor use more hospital care than the uninsured poor. They find the biggest differences between those always uninsured and those on Medicaid all year. Those on Medicaid part of the year used fewer hospital services than those on Medicaid all year. The uninsured also used less hospital care than those privately insured. The analysis here extends these results to examine racial and regional differentials.

More disaggregated information is essential on the types of conditions for which the insured receive inpatient care and the uninsured do not. Standards for appropriate utilization of hospital services are still the subject of wide debate. Some of the differential between the insured and uninsured seen here may be the result of overutilization of hospital services by the insured. However, this is unlikely to explain the entire differential.

TABLE 6 Hospital patient days per 100 persons under age 65, by insurance status, residence, and race, 1977

INSURANCE STATUS, RESIDENCE, AND RACE	UNINSURED	INSURED	RATIO
Total	47	90	1.91*
South	35	104	2.97*
White	33	100	3.03*
Black and Other	40†	119	2.98*
Non-South	56	84	1.50
White	51	81	1.59*
Black and Other	89†	114	1.28
SMSA	50	86	1.72*
White	44	83	1.89*
Black and Other	70†	106	1.51
Non-SMSA	42	99	2.36*
White	43	94	2.19*
Black and Other	39†	175	4.49*

* Indicates values for insured and uninsured are significantly different at the .05 level.

† Indicates relative standard error in equal to or greater than 30 percent.

Source: Data from the U.S. Department of Health and Human Services, National Center for Health Services Research, National Medical Care Expenditure Survey.

Some of the greater utilization of hospital care by the insured may represent self-selection. Those who expect to be hospitalized may obtain such coverage. Hospitalization may itself result in Medicaid coverage of some of the poor and near-poor. However, this should affect primarily those who are insured part of the year and uninsured the remainder of the year. Such partially insured persons are excluded from this analysis. These explanations are unlikely to account for a three-fold differential in use.

Some of the results by region and race are surprising. It is interesting to note that outside the South uninsured blacks receive more hospital days per 100 persons than insured whites. Insured blacks have the highest use. This may reflect greater health problems among blacks, or the tendency of blacks to receive care in public hospitals which have longer stays. Another unexpected result is high hospitalization among insured blacks in nonmetropolitan areas. This is one of the smallest population groups in the study and results, in this case, may simply be statistically unreliable.

Barriers to access to hospital services for the uninsured need to be explored. To what extent do hospitals require preadmission deposits for the uninsured? What are the consequences of such policies on access to care? Which hospitals serve the uninsured and the insured? Do the differences between metropolitan and nonmetropolitan areas reflect the role of teaching hospitals and public hospitals in caring for the uninsured in the inner city? Do the uninsured have to travel sizeable distances to obtain services? What are the health problems of the insured and uninsured, for what conditions are the insured hospitalized but not the uninsured, and what are the health consequences of lack of hospital care for the uninsured? To what extent do any or all of these factors influence the use of hospital care by the uninsured? Further exploration is certainly warranted.

Health Status and Use of Services

Lower utilization of ambulatory and inpatient care by the uninsured is not a reflection of lower need for health care services. Instead, as measured by self-assessment of health status, the uninsured tend to be somewhat sicker than the insured. Fifteen percent of the uninsured under age 65 rate their health as fair or poor, compared with 11 percent of the insured. Blacks and other minorities in the South systematically rate their health the worst. Of insured blacks and other minorities in the South, 19 percent assess their health as fair or poor, compared with 9 percent of insured whites outside the South.

One possible explanation of the higher rate of poor or fair health among the uninsured is that the lack of insurance is itself related to health status. Those who rate their health as poor or fair are more likely to be unable to work because of illness than those who rate their health good or excellent. Since insurance coverage in the United States is related to employment, those who are unemployed due to poor health are also likely to be without insurance. Under an employment-based insurance system, the working population enjoys both good health and insurance coverage, while those too ill to work suffer both lack of employment and lack of insurance.

The sick who are uninsured use medical care services less than their insured counterparts. Utilization of ambulatory services, adjusted for health status, shows that the insured in poor health see a physician 70 percent more often than the uninsured in poor health. Physician visits per person under age 65 in fair or poor health average 6.9 among the insured, compared with 4.1 visits for the uninsured with similar health problems (table 7). Blacks and other minorities with fair or poor health who are insured receive twice as much care as their uninsured counterparts.

Among the uninsured in poor or fair health, the differentials in physician visits by race and residence are especially noteworthy. Uninsured whites have greater access to physician services than do uninsured minorities. A southern white in fair or poor health sees a physician twice as often as a southern minority person in fair or poor health. The same relationship exists for utilization of physician services in metropolitan areas. However, the utilization differential between whites and minorities narrows in areas outside the South and in nonmetropolitan areas.

The number of physician visits by the uninsured versus the insured in fair or poor health warrants further examination. It is expected that the individual in fair or poor health would require frequent physician visits for diagnosis and treatment of the

TABLE 7 Physician visits per person under age 65 in fair or poor health per year, by insurance status, residence, and race, 1977

INSURANCE STATUS, RESIDENCE, AND RACE	UNINSURED	INSURED	RATIO
Total	4.1	6.9	1.68*
South	3.8	6.1	1.61*
White	4.4	6.4	1.45*
Black and Other	2.2†	5.0	2.27
Non-South	4.5	7.4	1.64*
White	4.6	7.6	1.65*
Black and Other	3.5†	6.5	1.86
SMSA	4.1	7.2	1.76*
White	4.7	7.6	1.62*
Black and Other	2.3†	5.9	2.57
Non-SMSA	4.2	6.3	1.50
White	4.3	6.4	1.49
Black and Other	3.2†	5.4	1.69

* Indicates values for insured and uninsured are significantly different at the .05 level.

† Indicates relative standard error is equal to or greater than 30 percent.

Source: Data from the U.S. Department of Health and Human Services, National Center for Health Services Research, National Medical Care Expenditure Survey.

condition. The average of five to seven visits annually by the insured would appear to provide a reasonable level of physician contact. But for uninsured minorities in the South in fair or poor health, the average number of visits is two per year. This rate would provide no more than an initial visit and one follow-up visit, which might be insufficient to treat serious or complex illnesses. Thus, lower rates of physician visits could impair adequate treatment and follow-up to promote a rapid recovery.

Dental Care

Dental care, unlike hospital care and most physician services, is not covered under most insurance plans. Therefore, differentials in dental visits between the insured and uninsured are not meaningful. However, the NMCES data do show a striking contrast between dental visits by whites and minorities.

Whites obtain dental care twice as often as minorities, averaging 1.5 visits per year compared to 0.7 visits for minorities. Nonsouthern whites had two times the number of visits as nonsouthern minorities and over three times the number of visits as

southern minorities. Rural minorities appear to have the least access to dental services.

The significant differential between access to dental services for minorities and whites warrants further examination. The extent to which this differential reflects differences in health practices and attitudes toward dental care or differences in availability and accessibility to dental care should be explored.

Usual Source of Care

The NMCES data confirm other studies that have found that disadvantaged groups are less likely to have a usual source of ambulatory care and more likely to receive their care from a hospital outpatient department or a clinic than from a physician's office. Table 8, for example, enumerates that 84 percent of the insured have a physician's office as their usual source of care compared with 67 percent of the uninsured. About 50 percent of uninsured blacks and other minorities have a physician's office as their usual source of care. While this percentage is quite low in comparison with other groups, it does not fit the stereotype that all minorities in urban areas

TABLE 8   Percent of persons under age 65 whose usual source of care is a physician's office, by insurance status, residence, and race, 1977

INSURANCE STATUS, RESIDENCE, AND RACE	UNINSURED	INSURED	RATIO
Total	67	84	1.25*
South	66	81	1.22*
White	70	82	1.16*
Black and Other	53	76	1.41*
Non-South	68	85	1.25*
White	70	86	1.22*
Black and Other	45	69	1.53*
SMSA	63	82	1.31*
White	66	84	1.27*
Black and Other	49	71	1.43*
Non-SMSA	73	86	1.19*
White	76	87	1.15*
Black and Other	52	79	1.53*

* Indicates values for insured and uninsured are significantly different at the .05 level.

Source: Data from the U.S. Department of Health and Human Services, National Center for Health Services Research, National Medical Care Expenditure Survey.

receive the bulk of their care from public facilities or hospital outpatient departments.

Uninsured residents of nonmetropolitan areas are more likely to have a physician as a usual source of care than are residents of a metropolitan area. In nonmetropolitan areas, 73 percent of the uninsured have a physician as a usual source of care in contrast to only 63 percent of the uninsured in metropolitan areas. However, nonmetropolitan residents are still likely to have fewer physician visits than their metropolitan counterparts (see table 5). The nonmetropolitan uninsured get more of their care from physicians but receive less total care. These differences in utilization among the uninsured undoubtedly reflect differences between metropolitan and nonmetropolitan areas in the availability of alternatives to physician care. Residents of metropolitan areas are more likely to have access to clinic and outpatient hospital services that can substitute for care in physicians' offices.

The metropolitan and nonmetropolitan differential for physicians as a usual source of care is markedly reduced among the insured. As seen in table 8, 86 percent of insured nonmetropolitan residents and 82 percent of insured metropolitan residents have a physician as a usual source of care. Insurance coverage significantly increases the proportion of minorities who have a physician's office as their usual source of care. Among the minority uninsured 49 percent of those living in metropolitan areas and 52 percent of those in nonmetropolitan areas have a physician as a usual source of care. In contrast, for insured minorities, 71 percent in metropolitan areas and 79 percent outside of metropolitan areas have physicians as a usual source of care. This would suggest that Medicaid and private health insurance coverage enable a substantial number of minorities to obtain care in a physician's office.

Convenience of Care

When they are able to obtain care, the uninsured must travel longer distances than the insured to obtain it. As enumerated in table 9, 25 percent of the uninsured travel 30 minutes or more to obtain care compared with 18 percent of the insured. Differentials in travel time between the insured and uninsured are somewhat more marked in rural areas than in urban areas, but travel time is a problem for uninsured persons everywhere. These data sug-

TABLE 9   Percent of persons under age 65 traveling more than 29 minutes to receive medical care, by insurance status, residence, and race, 1977

INSURANCE STATUS, RESIDENCE, AND RACE	UNINSURED	INSURED	RATIO
Total	25	19	1.39*
South	29	21	1.39*
White	30	20	1.48*
Black and Other	28	26	1.09
Non-South	21	16	1.29*
White	22	16	1.35*
Black and Other	17	21	.81
SMSA	22	17	1.27*
White	21	16	1.32*
Black and Other	24	24	1.00
Non-SMSA	29	20	1.46*
White	30	20	1.50*
Black and Other	23	19	1.24

* Indicates values for insured and uninsured are significantly different at the .05 level.

Source: Data from the U.S. Department of Health and Human Services, National Center for Health Services Research, National Medical Care Expenditure Survey.

gest not only that the uninsured receive less care, but also that when they do obtain care they do so by searching over a longer distance for providers willing to see them. The effort involved in such a search for care may discourage the use of preventive services, resulting in the uninsured only seeking care for serious illness or in crises. This would help explain the lower utilization levels of the uninsured.

When the uninsured arrive at a care provider, they generally have to wait longer for care to be delivered. Regardless of residence, the waiting time for insured blacks and other minorities is longer than the waiting time experienced by uninsured whites. Waiting times are longer in the South. Uninsured southern minority persons experience the longest waiting times. The NMCES data show that they wait one-third longer than do insured southern whites (Department of Health and Human Services 1982a).

POLICY IMPLICATIONS

The utilization differentials between the insured and uninsured underscore the importance of financial barriers to health care. Lack of insurance coverage is the major barrier. It markedly affects the amount of both ambulatory and inpatient care received. Without insurance coverage, many individuals obviously do without care. Those able to obtain care incur substantial travel and waiting times.

Lack of insurance coverage has three major consequences: it contributes to unnecessary pain, suffering, disability, and even death among the uninsured; it places a financial burden on those uninsured who struggle to pay burdensome medical bills; and it places a financial strain on hospitals, physicians, and other health care providers who attempt to provide care to the uninsured.

Research is limited on both the health of the uninsured and the health consequences of having no insurance. Extensive data on utilization patterns by the uninsured disaggregated by residence and race are presented for virtually the first time in this report. But a number of recent studies have shown that medical care utilization has a dramatic impact on health. A recent Urban Institute report by Hadley (1982) explores the relation between medical care utilization and mortality rates. It contains persuasive evidence that utilization of medical care services leads to a marked reduction in mortality rates. A recent study by Grossman and Goldman (1981) at the National Bureau of Economic Research has found that infant mortality rates have dropped significantly in communities served by federally funded community health centers. This growing body of evidence does provide considerable support to the importance of medical care utilization in assuring a healthy population—and at least indirectly provides a basis for concern that the lower medical care utilization of the uninsured contributes to unnecessary deaths and lowered health status.

Lack of insurance coverage also imposes serious financial burdens on those who try to make regular payments to retire enormous debts incurred in obtaining medical care. With the average cost of a hospital stay in the United States now in excess of $2,000, few individuals can afford to build payments for hospital care into their monthly living allowance (Department of Health and Human Services 1982b). Yet, since the uninsured are more likely to be poor, the economic consequences of lack of insurance fall heaviest on those least able to bear the burden.

In addition to its consequences for the uninsured, lack of insurance also takes its toll on the health care system. One result is that the financial stability of hospitals and ambulatory care providers willing to provide charity care for those unable to pay is jeopardized. Health care providers serving the uninsured—particularly inner city community and teaching hospitals, county and municipal clinics, and community health centers—absorb much of the cost of this as charity care or a bad debt. Yet this burden is not evenly distributed among hospitals and other providers. A recent study by the Urban Institute found that one-seventh of a national sample of hospitals studied provided over 40 percent of the free care (Brazda 1982).

Recent policy measures are likely to exacerbate this situation. The Omnibus Budget Reconciliation Act of 1981 reduced federal financial participation in Medicaid and curtailed eligibility under the Aid to Families with Dependent Children (AFDC) program. Actions by state governments in response to this legislation could swell the ranks of the uninsured poor by over 1 million people. Coupled with the highest rate of unemployment since the Great Depression and the loss of health insurance coverage frequently occurring with unemployment, the number of unin-

sured continues to rise. Undoubtedly the situation has worsened rather than improved since the NMCES study in 1977. Today, the access problems of the uninsured should be a pressing concern on the nation's health agenda.

For many of the uninsured, community health centers and migrant health centers have helped to fill the gap in access created by the lack of insurance. This was especially important for those ineligible for Medicaid. However, simultaneously with the cutbacks in Medicaid, major reductions were made in these service delivery programs. Overall funding was reduced by 25 percent in absolute dollars, which may lead to 1.1 million fewer people being served than the 6 million served in 1980. The National Health Service Corps, while not as seriously affected now, will be substantially reduced in future years since no new scholarships are being awarded with commitments for service in underserved areas (Davis 1981).

Financial strains on public hospitals and clinics supported by state and local governments are leading to further curtailment of services. Preadmission deposits, often sizeable in amount, impose serious barriers for many of the uninsured seeking hospital care. Teaching hospitals that have for years maintained an open-door policy are reevaluating the fiscal viability of continuing such a policy. In many areas, hospitals are beginning to transfer nonpaying patients to public facilities, further expanding the charity load of those facilities and reducing their ability to remain solvent (Brazda 1982).

Public hospitals, traditionally the care provider of last resort, are under new pressures to close or reduce services as local governments respond to shrinking revenues. Yet, shifting the responsibility of public hospitals to community hospitals will not solve the problem of caring for the uninsured. Recent hearings have documented the refusal of community hospitals to take uninsured patients, even in emergency situations. This has led to documented cases of deaths that could have been avoided with prompt medical attention (U.S. Congress, House Committee on Energy and Commerce 1981).

Such disparities in access to care are unacceptable in a decent and humane society. Several actions are required to assure progress toward adequate access for all. Medicaid coverage should be expanded to provide basic insurance coverage for all low-income individuals. The Medicaid programs in southern states have tended to have very restrictive eligibility policies leaving many of the poor uncovered (Department of Health and Human Services 1982c). Expanded coverage of the poor through Medicaid would improve the scope of coverage in the South and could help to alleviate some of the extreme utilization differentials between the South and non-South. A minimum income standard set at some percentage of the poverty level would be an important first step. In 1979, 23 states, including most of the southern states, had income eligibility levels for Medicaid below 55 percent of the poverty level. Texas, Alabama, and Tennessee had the lowest standards in the nation—less than $2,000 for a family of four. Coupled with implementation of a minimum income standard, Medicaid coverage should be broadened to include children and ultimately adults in two-parent families. Such steps would help assure access to care for the nation's poorest families.

Yet, the near-poor and working poor without insurance cannot be forgotten. Today, under Medicaid, only 29 states cover the medically needy to provide health coverage for those with large medical expenses. In effect, this catastrophy coverage provides some measure of protection to working families and is undoubtedly the source of care for many of the "sometimes insured." Coverage for the medically needy is currently very limited in the South; implementation of coverage for the medically needy would be another step toward reducing the disparities between the South and the rest of the country. Expansion of this coverage option is an important component of a positive health care agenda.

Finally, the extensiveness of unemployment in today's economy underscores the need to refine the link between employment and health insurance coverage. "Out of work" ought not to translate to "without health care services." Often, health needs are greatest during periods of stress related to unemployment (Brenner 1973; Lee 1979). Health insurance coverage should be extended through employer plans for a period following unemployment, and guaranteed through public coverage until reemployment. Employers should also be encouraged to provide comprehensive coverage, including prevention and primary care services, to all workers and their families.

These measures would help to provide protection and improved access to care for the 34 million or more Americans now without health care insurance. However, as the metropolitan and nonmetropolitan differentials among the insured demonstrate, financing alone is not enough to correct access differentials. Resources development must be coupled with improved financing in underserved areas to assure that needed providers are available. Continued funding and expansion of the community and migrant health center programs to assure physical access to services for residents of high poverty, medically underserved communities is an essential adjunct to broadened financing for low-income populations. Other important ways to provide expanded insurance coverage without perpetuating the cost inefficiencies of the existing system include: reform of Medicaid, Medicare, and private health insurance plans to encourage ambulatory care in cost-effective primary care programs; and experimentation with capitation payments to individual primary care centers, networks of centers, hospitals, or other major primary care providers for providing ambulatory and inpatient services to Medicaid beneficiaries.

This agenda of improved financing and resource development represents a positive strategy that can be employed to reduce major inequities in American health care. Today, some will argue that this agenda is too ambitious and costly and would instead opt for a more targeted and incremental approach. For example, instead of expanding Medicaid coverage, advocates of the incremental approach would favor renewed support to public hospitals and financial aid to hospitals serving large numbers of uninsured to mitigate the worst problems. These approaches are piecemeal, however, and do not address the fundamental problems identified in this paper. Such targeted approaches focus on protecting institutions serving the uninsured rather than protecting the uninsured themselves. Thus, they provide for the continued existence of a source of care for the uninsured seeking care, but do not provide comprehensive coverage to the uninsured to encourage early and preventive services. The poor and uninsured who do without care either because they do not live near an "aided facility" or do not know they could obtain free care from a hospital with a financial distress loan would still suffer inequitable health care differentials.

This paper demonstrates that lack of insurance

makes a difference in health care utilization. Studies such as the recent work by Hadley (1982) point out the positive impact of medical care on mortality. Society ultimately bears the burden for care of the uninsured. The choice is between paying up front and directly covering the uninsured or indirectly paying for their care through subsidies to fiscally troubled health facilities, higher insurance premiums, and increased hospital costs to cover the cost of charity care and pay for the ill health caused by neglect and inadequate preventive and primary care. Thus, the best and most pragmatic approach is to provide health insurance coverage to the uninsured and to use targeted approaches to improve resource distribution and to remove remaining differentials. The inequities in health care in the United States described here will deepen unless a positive agenda is pursued.

References

BRAZDA, J., ed. 1982. Perspectives: Who Will Care for the Uninsured? (September 27) *Washington Report on Medicine and Health* 36 (38, Sept. 27): unpaged insert.

BRENNER, H. 1973. *Mental Illness and the Economy*. Cambridge: Harvard University Press.

DAVIS, K. 1975. *National Health Insurance: Benefits, Costs, and Consequences*. Washington: Brookings Institution.

———. 1981. Reagan Administration Health Policy. (December). *Journal of Public Health Policy* 2(4):312–32.

———. 1982. Medicare Reconsidered. Paper presented at Duke University Medical Center Private Sector Conference on the Financial Support of Health Care of the Elderly and the Indigent, March 14–16.

DAVIS, K., and C. SCHOEN. 1978. *Health and the War on Poverty: A Ten Year Appraisal*. Washington: Brookings Institution.

DAVIS, K., M. GOLD, and D. MAKUC. 1981. Access to Health Care for the Poor: Does the Gap Remain? *Annual Review of Public Health* 2:159–82.

DEPARTMENT OF HEALTH AND HUMAN SERVICES. 1982a. National Medical Care Expenditure Survey, 1977. Unpublished Statistics. Hyattsville, Md.: National Center for Health Services Research.

———. 1982b. *Health Care Financing Trends*, June. Baltimore: Health Care Financing Administration.

———. 1982c. *Medicare and Medicaid Data Book 1981*. Baltimore: Health Care Financing Administration.

———. 1982d. Usual Sources of Medical Care and Their Characteristics, Data Preview 12. Hyattsville, Md.: National Center for Health Services Research.

GROSSMAN, M., and F. GOLDMAN. 1981. The Responsiveness and Impacts of Public Health Policy: The Case of Community Health Centers. Paper presented at the 109th Annual Meeting of the American Public Health Association, Los Angeles, November.

HEALTH CENTERS. Paper presented at the 109th Annual Meeting of the American Public Health Association, Los Angeles, November.

HADLEY, J. 1982. *More Medical Care, Better Health?* Washington: Urban Institute.

INSTITUTE OF MEDICINE. 1981. *Health Care in a Context of Civil Rights*. Washington: National Academy Press.

KASPER, J. A., D. C. WALDEN, and G. R. WILENSKY. 1978. *Who Are the Uninsured?* National Medical Care Expenditures Survey Data Preview no. 1. Hyattsville, Md.: National Center for Health Services Research.

LEE, A. J. 1979. *Employment, Unemployment, and Health Insurance*. Cambridge, Mass.: Abt Books.

ROWLAND, D., and C. GAUS. 1983. Medicaid Eligibility and Benefits: Current Policies and Alternatives. In *New Approaches to the Medicaid Crisis*, ed. R. Blendon and T. W. Moloney. New York: Frost and Sullivan.

TAYLOR, A. K., and W. R. LAWSON. 1981. Employer and Employee Expenditures for Private Health Insurance. National Medical Care Expenditures Survey Data Preview 7. Hyattsville, Md.: National Center for Health Services Research, June.

U.S. CONGRESS. House. Committee on Energy and Commerce, U.S. House of Representatives. 1981. *Hearings on Medicaid Cutbacks on Infant Care*. Washington, 27 July.

WILENSKY, G. R., and M. L. BERK. 1982. The Health Care of the Poor and the Role of Medicaid. *Health Affairs* 1(4):93–100.

WILENSKY, G. R., and D. C. WALDEN. 1981. Minorities, Poverty, and the Uninsured. Paper presented at the 109th Meeting of the American Public Health Association, Los Angeles, November. Hyattsville Md.: National Center for Health Services Research.

Life and Death in a Welfare State: End-stage Renal Disease in the United Kingdom

Thomas Halper

We die with the dying:
See, they depart, and we go with them.

(T. S. Eliot, "Little Gidding")

This is a case study of how a national health system in an advanced Western democracy confronts an affliction which poses a life or death issue for thousands of its citizens every year. The health system is the National Health Service, the democracy is the United Kingdom, and the affliction is end-stage renal disease. This case is not unique; if it were, it could hardly serve as an illustration. Nor is it without the ambiguities that real life attaches to phenomena, like bits of fried fish sticking to a pan. But at its center is a rather unusual starkness, for the life or death question is less often whether the medically indicated therapies will succeed than whether they will even be tried.

END-STAGE RENAL DISEASE

The kidneys are the body's main organs of excretion. They are, however, subject to serious, progressive, and irreversible deterioration, usually as a result of glomerulonephritis (Bright's disease), pyelonephritis (scarring from reflux and infections), polycys-

tic kidney disease, and vascular disease (chiefly, hypertension). This condition is called chronic renal failure, and is marked, among other consequences, by the kidneys' decreased ability to extract excess fluids and poisonous wastes from the blood. Anemia, edema, and infection frequently accompany the condition, and the functioning of the brain, intestine, heart, skin, and other organs is impaired. Eventually, chronic renal failure nearly always reaches the point where it is termed end-stage renal disease (ESRD), which, as the name suggests, is invariably fatal.

By the 1960s, two principal treatments for ESRD had been developed. One utilizes a dialysis machine, at first called an artificial kidney. A continuous flow of the patient's blood is diverted to a semipermeable membrane, which permits excess fluids and wastes to pass through its tiny holes like water through a sieve. The blood, now with tolerable fluid and waste levels, is then returned to the patient.

For patients using the kidney machine, dialysis is typically necessary three times a week for approximately three to six hours per session. Enervating side effects, in addition to profound emotional and interpersonal strain and debilitating physiological disorders, are common (Czaczkes and Kaplan De-Nour 1978, chaps. 5–6; Rosa, Fryd, and Kjellstrand 1980; Levy 1979; Farmer, Snowden, and Parsons 1979).

At first, it was believed that dialysis was so complicated and dangerous that it required a hospital setting (de Wardener 1966, 115–17), but after the feasibility of dialysis at home was demonstrated (Merrill et al. 1964; Baillod et al. 1965), many physi-

Reprinted from the *Milbank Memorial Fund Quarterly/ Health and Society*, vol. 63, no. 1, 1985, pp. 52–93. Copyright © 1985 by the Milbank Memorial Fund Quarterly.

527

cians and patients began to conclude that where appropriate, it was preferable. Though preparation, operation, and clean-up are time consuming and sometimes stressful, the risk of infection is less and the patient's convenience, comfort, and sense of control over his own life are greater. Home dialysis patients tend to have superior survival and rehabilitation rates.

From the outset, machine dialysis, whether performed in the patient's home or in a hospital or dialysis center, has remained by a large margin the most widely utilized therapy for ESRD in the world.

In the late 1970s, a variant, the less grueling continuous ambulatory peritoneal dialysis (CAPD), began to appear as an alternative treatment in certain cases. Here, a catheter is inserted into the patient's abdominal cavity, and wastes and excess fluid pass through the cavity's natural lining, the peritoneum, into a bag, which, when full, is simply discarded and replaced. This procedure is repeated four times a day and, in all, consumes about two and a half hours.

The second major treatment is kidney transplantation. It began with identical twin donors (Merrill et al. 1956), and became feasible for genetically different donors with the development of drugs that successfully suppressed the body's normal rejection of foreign tissue. Even today, however, 25 per cent of United Kingdom first cadaveric kidney transplants fail during the first three months, and 40 per cent do not survive two years (Broyer et al. 1982, 16a), a success rate about half that of the United States (Krakauer et al. 1983). Despite this, its promise of far greater physical and mental vigor (Kaplan De-Nour and Shanan 1980)—as well as its freedom from the oppressive dialysis routine—has meant that from the earliest days, patient demand for transplantation has vastly exceeded the supply of available kidneys.

There is some dispute as to the incidence of treatable ESRD. In the United Kingdom, the "often quoted" rule of thumb (Laing 1978, 16) is that forty new patients per million population (PMP) are suitable for treatment (Branch et al. 1971; Pendreigh et al. 1972; McGeown 1972). Many contend that in excluding those under age 5, over age 60, or with complicating diseases, this figure is much too low, and even a former chief medical officer of the Department of Health and Social Security (DHSS) conceded

that it is "now regarded as an underestimate" (Yellowlees 1982, 116). American nephrologists generally give 100 PMP as their estimate (Luke 1983, 1593), and if age and the presence of complicating disease were ignored completely, the number might soar to 150 (Laing 1978, 18; Berlyne 1982, 189). ESRD must be termed an uncommon, if not precisely a rare condition.

THE UNITED KINGDOM RESPONSE

Of those ESRD patients undergoing treatment in the U.K. in 1982, 24.8 percent were on home dialysis, 16.7 percent on hospital dialysis, and 12.7 percent on CAPD; 44.7 percent had had successful transplants. Compared to other nations, the U.K. is unique in its stress upon transplantation and home dialysis, and relies upon nonhospital-based therapies over hospital-based therapies by a ratio of nearly 5:1 (Broyer et al. 1982, 7). In contrast, in France hospital-based therapies are preferred by 2:1, in West Germany by 3:1, and in Italy by almost 4:1. While it is widely acknowledged that nonhospital-based therapies are medically preferable in many instances, it is also generally conceded that their dominance in the U.K. is due more to the extreme pressures of ESRD cost-control imposed by years of chronic underfunding. In this context, the stress on nonhospital-based therapies, as one American analyst put it, "is simultaneously an escape from the small number of dialysis centers and also a rationing mechanism, since only the 'best' of the terminally ill ESRD patients do well at home."

It is hardly surprising, then, that this emphasis upon less expensive nonhospital-based treatments is accompanied by a more generally selective approach toward treatment in general. Thus, in contrast to France, West Germany, and Italy, where in 1982 from 250 to 234.5 ESRD patients PMP were treated, in the U.K. only 159.8 were treated. And while those countries admitted from 47.3 to 37.9 new patients PMP to treatment in 1982, the U.K. added only 29.5, a rate exceeded by the poorer Spain and virtually equalled by the far poorer Portugal and Greece (Broyer et al. 1984, 8).

The burden of the U.K.'s low treatment rates falls almost entirely upon those over age 45 or suffering from complicating diseases (like diabetes), for these kinds of patients are ordinarily considered less suitable for transplantation and home dialysis. There are also marked discrepancies among the regions—North West Thames, for example, treats patients at almost three times the rate of Wessex—and a common if unsubstantiated belief that the lower classes are disadvantaged, in that home dialysis places a premium upon certain middle-class attributes, like education and self-discipline (Fox 1975, 710; Simmons 1979, 202; Bryan 1981, 412).

The Office of Population Censuses and Surveys (1983, 38) reports that well over 3,000 persons die from ESRD in England and Wales each year and that another 2,000 die from unspecified renal failure, which is almost certainly very largely ESRD. It is generally conceded, however, that death from ESRD is frequently—perhaps, usually—ascribed to some more proximate cause, like ischemic heart disease, cerebral hemorrhage, or pulmonary infection. "Death certification," as one nephrologist put it, "is notoriously unreliable as a source of . . . data." True ESRD mortality rates are unknown, then, though they clearly far exceed official figures.

MACROALLOCATION: HOW SOCIETY ASSIGNS RESOURCES

Virtually all patients in the U.K. suffering from ESRD are wholly dependent upon the National Health Service (NHS), a comprehensive, centrally financed health care system that provides for the entire population with little or no charge at the point of service. It is the NHS that, at least ostensibly, is in command of the macroallocation of health resources.

Despite the apparent primacy of the NHS and its parent organization, the DHSS, the ESRD treatment pattern in the U.K. does not derive from a formal national policy, which in an explicit sense simply does not exist. This is not, however, to deny the central office a major policy role, particularly in the early 1960s when the new ESRD technologies were developing and gaining acceptance.

Most important was the spectacular development of dialysis, which created, as one official of the Ministry of Health (the DHSS's predecessor), who observed matters at first hand, put it, "intense pressure to provide this life-saving measure" (Dennis

1971, 144). At the same time, however, the Ministry saw that if not carefully controlled, dialysis (and transplantation) could become a bureaucrat's nightmare. For it was immediately apparent to the Ministry's sophisticated civil servants that the new technologies combined three incendiary ingredients: they were fairly reliable, they were lifesaving, and they were expensive. If they had incorporated only two of these characteristics, no great problem would have been posed. If, for example, they had been reliable and lifesaving but not expensive (like, say, the Heimlich maneuver), they might have been adopted without frightening allocative consequences. Or if they had been lifesaving and expensive but not reliable (like heart transplants), they might have been assigned a low priority. Or if they had been reliable and expensive but not lifesaving (like cosmetic facelifts), they might simply have been put aside as a luxury. But dialysis and transplantation each had all three qualities.

It was probably equally obvious to the Ministry that in an era of rapid advances in medical technology that tend to generate a "technological imperative" to use them (Mechanic 1979), dialysis and transplantation would before long be joined by other therapies that would also be reliable, lifesaving, and expensive, and have their own articulate advocates (see, e.g., Sherlock 1983; Timmins 1983). The new renal technologies, therefore, could not be viewed in isolation, but rather had to be seen as prototypes of a new kind of treatment that would threaten existing financial patterns, even as it provided hope to patients and their families.

How was the Ministry of Health to respond? The new technologies seemed both too valuable to ignore and too costly to embrace. The answer plainly was a policy lying somewhere between these two poles. Since the Ministry was perennially short of funds, was at this time dominated by "an ideology of efficiency" (Klein 1983, 64), and could hardly have welcomed the prospect of reallocation that a major ESRD effort would have involved, the policy it chose did not lie exactly halfway between the two extremes. Instead, the decision was for an understandably rather cautious beginning, coupled with no firm commitments about the future. . . .

. . . the expensiveness of ESRD treatment raises questions about the individual's right to health care that do not emerge with comparable impact in most other conditions. This is not the place to rehearse the familiar ethical arguments, pro and con. They have been addressed at great length in appropriate forums (e.g., Rescher 1969; Katz and Capron 1975; Almeder 1979; Winslow 1982), and doubtless will be discussed at even greater length in the future. It is enough to say here that in the U.K. it has traditionally been accepted that, in the words of Guido Pincherle, a DHSS senior medical advisor, "there is no right to treatment" (Parsons and Ogg 1983a, 113).

In West Germany, France, Italy, and Spain, on the other hand, ESRD treatment is funded through insurance schemes, and so the ruling assumption is that the patient is entitled to whatever treatment is medically indicated. The United States, which funds ESRD treatment under Medicare, has taken essentially the same view, though a number of significant costs are not covered (Campbell and Campbell 1978; Greenberg 1978).

The notion that ESRD patients ought legally to be entitled to treatment, however, is regarded by U.K. policy makers with a mixture of contempt and horror. Indeed, it is the American experience that is looked to as the chief cautionary example. In interview after interview, both administrators and physicians decried it as medically absurd—with tales of senile patients with metastatic cancer being dialyzed—and financially "out of control," attributing it to naively idealistic Congressmen and greedy proprietary dialysis center owners. America, it was always pointed out, was wealthy enough to afford such foolish extravagance; the U.K. was not. The fear of treating too many, in short, inspired much more passion than the fear of treating too few.

It would be too facile, however, to attribute this attitude simply to America's greater wealth, for what is involved are also certain highly pertinent choices. If the British have been rather parsimonious with the NHS, in other words, this partially reflects decisions taken after the war to allocate large sums on schools, housing, and social services; even as Tocqueville noted ([1840] 1961, 153–55), Americans put unusual value on health. Equally, perhaps, the U.K. practice may stem from an almost reflexive horror of welfare state extravagance. "Value for money" is a phrase a visitor soon learns, and "value" here implies a reasonable return not only to the patient but also to the public. This attitude, embedded long ago in the notorious Elizabethan Poor Laws, lies near the core of the benevolent NHS, too. The present reluctance to dialyze older ESRD patients, for example, finds a clear parallel in the late 1950s, when full rehabilitation services were offered pretty much only to those under age 65 (with first priority to those under age 50 or 55), to those with a prior history of gainful employment, and to those for whom reemployment was certain. Similarly, cataract surgery for a while was also restricted to patients under age 65. Given this tradition and what has become an almost universal pessimism regarding a near-term end to significant scarcity in Britain, the ESRD budgetary restraints must have seemed not only sensible but necessary—and in a patently obvious way. . . .

MICROALLOCATION: HOW PATIENTS ARE SELECTED FOR TREATMENT

The importance of the microallocative level is directly attributable to the macroallocative patterns that have emerged. If sufficient resources had been provided to treat virtually all ESRD patients, as in the United States, the microallocative decision as to whether to treat would have long since faded away, like the background in an old snapshot. Because such resources have not been made available—because, indeed, a condition of hyperscarcity has prevailed from the outset—the microallocative decision has retained immense significance and continues to raise a number of rather disturbing issues.

In the microallocative decision as to which ESRD patients are to receive treatment, the key actors are the patient, his general practitioner and general medicine hospital consultant, and his nephrologist.

The Patient

The patient's importance, it must be said at the outset, lies almost entirely in his condition and rarely is a function of effective efforts on his part to influence outcomes. Partly, this may simply be a function of the nature of most health care in advanced societies. Health care, of course, is unusual in that after the initial patient decision to see a physician, it is producers who determine demand far more than consumers. In the first place, that is, it is normally the physician who determines whether and what tests, drugs, surgery, and so forth are required by the patient, not the patient himself.

More than that, it is a producers' elite that helps to shape the working physicians' demands. These are the individuals who are invariably given credit: Scribner and his associates (Quinton, Dillard, and Scribner 1960), who made dialysis a viable treatment for ESRD; Cimino and Brescia (1966), whose forearm fistula made the procedure capable of many more repetitions; Tenckhoff and Schechter (1968), whose improved catheter made CAPD feasible; and so on. The patient's inarticulate plea to "help me," in other words, would remain a mere pitiful noise without innovators to create the technological possibility to help and without physicians to utilize that technology actually to help. The innovators saw a need and responded to it, and so did the physicians; the patients benefit from the technology but do not bring it into being or apply it to individuals, though their compliance with physicians' instructions (particularly, if they dialyze at home) does make them, in a sense, junior partners in the implementation of treatment.

Partly, also, the patient's relative unimportance may reflect the physician's natural dominance, commonly attributed to his vast advantages in knowledge, skills, and experience and to the potent scientific life-or-death mystique surrounding his role. There is some evidence that the traditionally passive British patients are more assertive and knowledgeable today than in the past, but the differences are small, and since the hospital specialist may be the most prestigious of professions, patient deference to him is likely to be very great indeed (Cartwright and Anderson 1981, 115, 186; Schwartz and Aaron 1984, 56). ESRD patients, often fatigued, confused, and vulnerable, may seem particularly helpless and aware of their own dependency and limitations.

Partly, too, as several physicians who were interviewed suggested, the passivity of the patient may be a function of the more general British deference to official authority. "The English tend to be rather docile," as one consultant phrased it. Another spoke of the "British quality of 'up-puttingness'" (i.e., the predilection for putting up with adversity and viewing complaining as bad form). This, he felt, was reinforced by a "rather stratified class structure" that in the medical context encourages the belief that

the "doctor knows best." Similarly, other doctors interviewed observed that though when patients complained about the decision not to treat, the decision was sometimes reversed, the overwhelming proportion of patients denied treatment simply acquiesced without protest (cf., Schwartz and Aaron 1984, 56).

Clearly, however, it would be a mistake to exaggerate the extent of this docility; the U.K. is a nation not only of considerable class deference but also of class conflict, and the modern history of the society could not be told without reference to the rise of the Labour Party, the actions of militant trades unions, the intellectual generation of *Look Back in Anger,* the persistent disaffection of significant strata of the youth, and so on (Hart 1978, 193–202; Kavanaugh 1980, 156–58; Beer 1982, chap. 4). Yet the sheer, almost overwhelming stability of the U.K. certainly suggests that respect for authority has long been a potent factor.

The relative passivity of U.K. patients may also be traced to a greater capacity to cope with pain and discomfort. Less likely to complain, they may be more likely to accept both their illness and their physician's decision as to what ought to be done about it (though not focusing upon ESRD, see Zborowski 1952; Sternbach and Tursky 1965; Zola 1966; but cf., Koopman, Eisenthal, and Stoeckle 1984).

Additionally, the patients' passivity appears to be accentuated by certain structural constraints built into the National Health Service; for they cannot consult a specialist on their own but only upon a specific referral from their general practitioner. And if the general practitioner concludes that a specialist is required, he selects the specialist. In such a context, the patients' passivity can be said to be one of the system's ruling assumptions, for if dissatisfied, they may perceive their options as exceedingly limited. They can accept their lot, perhaps grumbling to themselves about their bad luck. Or they can complain to their general practitioner, risking alienating him during this time of crisis. Or they can try to replace their general practitioner, a task entailing obtaining permission from their local Family Practitioner Committee and then finding a new general practitioner who will accept them. But though Family Practitioner Committees usually grant permission, their involvement ordinarily is so intimidating and time consuming that most patients are deterred from this option—and for those patients not so deterred, the difficult job of securing another, more compliant general practitioner is a prospect sufficient to scare most of them. Patient "shopping around" for physicians that is so widespread in the United States is far less common in the U.K., where convenience and tradition rather than medical evaluation tend to determine the patient's choice of a general practitioner. Usually, in fact, the British patient does not even perceive a choice to be made; either he knows no other doctor or has no reason to believe that a change would bring an improvement. It is hardly surprising, then, that only 4 percent of patients surveyed in 1977 had changed general practitioners as a result of dissatisfaction (Cartwright and Anderson 1981, 8).

The General Practitioner

Far more important than the patient as a microallocative actor is his general practitioner. It is his responsibility to reach a preliminary diagnosis and to decide whether the patient should be sent on either to a nephrologist or, as is more often the case, to a general medicine department at a local hospital, which may then refer the patient to a renal unit.

The general practitioner's significance, therefore, is more commonly negative than positive; by misdiagnosing or deciding against referral, he effectively closes the door to treatment, while by sending the patient to a nephrologist or a general medicine department, he merely passes the decision onto a higher level. His relative inexperience with ESRD, however, may hamper his efforts, for many general practitioners identify only a single case every ten years (Parsons, in Parsons and Ogg 1983b, 245), and most lack all ties with nephrologists and are without personal access to the biochemical facilities that ESRD diagnosis requires. General practitioners may also be quite unacquainted with prevailing treatment patterns, and fail to refer patients for reasons that have long since become procedurally obsolete. Thus, one general practitioner, when presented with sixteen hypothetical cases, observed ruefully that "under present circumstances probably none would be accepted" for treatment (Challah et al. 1984, 1122), though such extreme resource scarcity had not existed for many years. No wonder that among nephrologists, general practitioner apathy and ignorance concerning ESRD is proverbial (e.g.,

Little, Cattell, and Dowie, in Parsons and Ogg 1983b, 242–43).

Although the general practitioner may reject referral for treatment of some ESRD patients, this negative decision is more likely to be made by a general medicine consultant from a nearby hospital (Challah et al. 1984, 1120). The consultant, however, typically has "limited experience in renal medicine" (Gabriel 1983, 36), and may be prone to make referral decisions on moral or other nonmedical grounds. "I have always referred on merit," one consultant reported, "but I have made the value judgment as to who is meritorious myself" (Challah et al. 1984, 1122). There is also reason to believe that out-of-date clinical selection criteria may sometimes be used. As one nephrologist put it, "New developments have not really percolated to the consultant level," and so their practice tends to reflect what they learned a decade or more earlier. But since the patient cannot ordinarily see the nephrologist on his own, it is frequently the view of the general medicine consultant that prevails (cf., Chantler, paraphrased by Lupton 1979, 3–4).

Both the general practitioner and the general medicine consultant, then, illustrate some of the strengths and weaknesses of the so-called "gatekeeper" approach to medical cost-containment. On the one hand, by minimizing the role of the specialist, the more expensive styles of practicing medicine are restrained. Costs, as a result, certainly are kept down. On the other hand, however, some medical decisions that might better be made by specialists are left to physicians with less relevant expertise and experience. The problem, of course, is exacerbated if the physician is overloaded with patients or is the kind of doctor who requires external stimulation (competition, colleague pressure, etc.) to keep current and provide personalized service. For a comprehensive, taxpayer-supported system like the NHS, the cost-containment imperative probably will always dominate. Nonetheless, as the case of ESRD demonstrates, there are medical costs in ascribing the gatekeeper role to nonspecialists, and these costs are borne primarily by the patient.

The Nephrologist

It is with the third actor, the nephrologist, that the most carefully considered microallocative decision ordinarily rests. His decision context, to be sure, may be far from ideal. The nature of renal failure is such that symptoms are not usually reported until the disease has progressed quite far, and referral procedures may sometimes add to the delay. As a consequence, by the time the nephrologist sees the patient, it may be "too late for there to be time for a carefully considered plan of investigation leading to a carefully constructed strategy for treatment" (Knapp 1982, 484). It may even in some rare cases be "too late to treat the patient at all" (*British Medical Journal* 1978, 1449).

Whether confronted in an optimal context or not, the decision as to treatment must be made. How is it reached? The usual answer given by physicians—general practitioners, general medicine consultants, or nephrologists—is that it is a clinical judgment found by applying sound medical criteria to the individual patient's case. These criteria are not always clearly spelled out, but generally seem to entail at least an implicit calculation of the probability that the treatment will succeed and, if successful, that the patient could then expect a satisfactory quality of life. Thus, the physician asks, for example, whether the patient is otherwise healthy or suffers from a complicating illness; or whether he is psychologically able to cope with the stress the treatment will impose or is likely to fail to comply adequately with the prescribed regimen or even to drop out of the treatment program entirely.

Despite the apparent straightforward reasonableness of such questions, however, the exclusive emphasis upon the medical character of patient selection appears undermined by several major problems. The first is that physicians' clinical judgments need not agree with one another. Error and disagreements regarding observations and evaluations are hardly unique to ESRD (see, e.g., Graham, de Dombal, and Goligher 1971; Bennett 1979, 165–75). In ESRD cases, though, there is evidence that the extent of the disagreement may be quite astonishing. In one study, for example, 25 British nephrologists were asked to reject 10 out of 40 hypothetical ESRD "patients." Only 13 "patients" received unanimous judgments—all acceptances—and 6 of the "patients" most frequently rejected were actually modeled after real patients who had been successfully treated (Parsons and Lock 1980). Similarly, in another study, 8 Glasgow clinicians in a renal unit were asked to classify

the suitability of 100 hypothetical ESRD "patients" for treatment; in only 32 cases did the physicians all agree either to treat or not to treat the patients (Taylor et al. 1975).

Moreover, different physicians apparently rely upon different key indicators to aid their judgments. Some physicians, for instance, may predict medical outcomes on the basis of early patient reactions to dietary restrictions (Czaczkes and Kaplan De-Nour 1978, 154–56); others report this to be of little help (Robinson 1978, 16). Some may tend to turn away diabetics (Medical Services Study Group of the Royal College of Physicians 1981, 285); others may accept them (Berger, Alpert, and Longnecker 1983; Legrain 1983). Some may be doubtful about treating children under age 5; others may treat infants (Trompeter et al. 1983; Hodson et al. 1978). Some may automatically reject patients over age 65; others may treat those in their 80s (Chester et al. 1979) or even a senile patient of 90 (H. Gurland in *Controversies in Nephrology* 1979, 133). For certainty of death in the absence of treatment is countered by the uncertainty of the efficacy of treatment in specific cases. As one prominent nephrologist concluded, "When treatment is provided for patients with an apparently poor prognosis, surprisingly often those expected to fare badly may do well. There are, in fact, few objective measurements to predict the response to treatment" (Knapp 1982, 848).

To some extent, these differences among physicians may reflect differences in levels of ability and conscientiousness. And as one analyst argued, "Although U.K. consultants have more freedom than most [specialists in other countries], they also are more isolated and have fewer means of knowing how their performance compares with others. . . . Consultants," he adds, "may be appointed at thirty-five and for the next thirty years have no real scrutiny of their work" (Dick 1983, 899).

More than this, however, differing medical judgments also flow from what one physician who was interviewed called the "inherent subjectivity" of the process. Though some patients clearly have excellent prognoses and others poor ones, a number of patients fall in the gray area in between. Whether they will be assigned to the "accept" or "reject" tracks are difficult, complex, problematical questions. In answering them, physicians naturally proceed analogically. That is, they compare the patient before them with similar patients they have treated, observed, or otherwise learned about through the literature or from colleagues. The physician assumes that identical patients with identical diseases will respond identically to identical therapies. But he knows, too, that in the real world "identical" is merely an analytical construct and that in the real world he must content himself with "similar." This realization, however, necessarily generates uncertainty: Is the patient before me, he must ask, so like another patient I am familiar with that I should treat him in the same way or so different that I should treat him in a different way—and if he is different, how different is he? To such questions, there may be several answers, for a single response is compelled neither by science nor by logic. Instead, reasonable, thoroughly competent physicians will differ, some stressing the similarities, others the differences. No ambiguous, objective methodology can be relied on to yield infallible answers.

Lacking such a methodology, physicians must be presumed to be influenced by their knowledge, experience, and training, and probably also by the prevailing practices at their hospitals, their own personalities, pressures from the patient's family, and any number of other factors which will be unique to each individual physician. Whatever the explanation, though, the data on physician disagreements on ESRD patients would seem to leave in tatters any pretense that the uttering of "clinical judgment" can banish doubts behind a curtain of consensus.

The Limitations of Clinical Judgment

Is "clinical judgment," then, uniquely subjective in cases of ESRD? Clearly not. All clinical judgments are, after all, *judgments,* a word that implies a recourse to a subjective best estimate. Moreover, since untreated chronic renal failure almost uniformly results in death, the consequences of a decision not to treat are quite predictable. This element of virtual certainty, however distressing, is lacking in the vast majority of other diseases. Furthermore, inasmuch as the U.K. nephrologist is not employed on a fee-for-service basis, he lacks the "personal financial incentive to treat more patients" (*British Medical Journal* 1978, 1449; Schwartz and Aaron 1984, 54), and thus may work with greater detachment than his colleagues in other countries. (It is easy to exaggerate

the significance of this point; the financial is only one of a vast tangle of incentives and disincentives [see, e.g., Grist 1981]).

By the same token, however, it may be more difficult to forecast patient response to ESRD treatment than is true in many other diseases. For, to an uncommon degree, success depends not only upon physiological factors, but also upon psychological and even domestic factors. The physician's ability to predict the effects of these variables, let alone to influence them, may be much less than he would desire.

A second problem with an exclusive reliance upon clinical judgment is that many pertinent medical criteria that underlie it have not been systematically tested empirically. One pioneering figure in the development of home dialysis, for example, stressed the importance of the patient's being of average intelligence (Shaldon 1968a, 522). If he were below average, it was argued, he might be unable to learn and perform all his tasks; and if he were above average, he might have difficulty accepting his role and become extremely anxious. Presumably, some patients considered to be outside the intelligence limits were denied treatment on that account and consequently died. But was the hypothesis on intelligence ever tested? Was the intelligence of the patients precisely determined? Was intelligence itself, notoriously an ambiguous and vague concept, satisfactorily defined? The record is barren of answers.

Of course, the intelligence hypothesis appears plausible, but plausibility cannot be confused with confirmation, particularly when life or death decisions are being taken. Psychological denial, for example, may not at first glance seem a good predictor of successful patient adjustment to home dialysis, but, by inducing patients to see themselves as only marginally ill and thus quite able to resume their normal roles, it is (Glassman and Siegel 1970; Short and Wilson 1969; Richmond et al. 1982).

Some hypotheses, though, lack even surface plausibility. In the early years of dialysis, for example, one of the most widely respected of U.K. nephrologists assured his colleagues that "gainful employment in a well-chosen occupation is necessary to achieve the best results" in hemodialysis, since "only the minority wish to live on charity" (Parsons 1967, 623). This extraordinary proposition—that the unemployed make poor patients because most would literally rather die than become public charges—was simply announced, despite the fact that large numbers of dialysis patients have always found the treatment too debilitating or time consuming to permit them to work.

A third problem is that medical criteria incorporated into the judgment process often become entangled with clearly nonmedical considerations. Another major pioneering nephrologist, for instance, declared that in selecting patients for dialysis, preference would be given not only to those with "the qualities of reliability, common sense, and stoicism"—all of which arguably would increase the likelihood of successful treatment—but also to patients with young children (Ogg 1970, 412). This consideration bears on the worthiness of the patient to receive treatment, and is really not medical in character at all. While physicians may for good and obvious reasons claim authority to devise and apply medical criteria, however, their nonmedical judgments would not appear to deserve special weight. Indeed, given what one philosopher of medicine who was interviewed characterized as the average physician's rather shallow acquaintance with systematic work in medical ethics, his implicit assumption of competence in this area must strike some observers as deeply disturbing.

A fourth problem with an exclusive reliance upon clinical judgment is that even if the first three problems were to vanish, the number of patients deemed medically suitable for treatment would substantially exceed the number whom the system could accommodate (but cf., Medical Services Study Group of the Royal College of Physicians 1981; Abram and Wadlington 1968). In such a situation, what should the physician do? The platitudinous reply (drawn here from a non-ESRD context) is that the "individual physician in his effort to save the individual patient, cannot, and cannot be expected to, consider the allocation of resources" (Bendixen 1977, 383; Beauchamp and Childress 1979, 195; Hiatt 1975, 235–41).

But if this represents the ideal, the real world extorts the precise opposite answer: "What constitutes 'good' medical practice and 'right' clinical decision will be determined by cost-effective analysis as well as by scientific correctness and by humanitarian content" (Wing 1979, 152). With this in mind, two doctors deplored "the extent to which physicians'

professional expertise and position of trust is being used to translate economic and political decisions into the selection of patients, without those presenting with renal disease, their relatives or the public necessarily being aware of the process" (Parsons and Lock 1980, 175). The *Lancet* (1981, 595) echoed this conclusion, editorializing, "Economic necessity dictates clinical decisions but is not always seen to do so."

Even if, for the sake of argument, we assume that wholly objective medical criteria simply await the physician's automatic application, a larger question persists: Ought medical criteria to be the only legitimate criteria utilized in patient selection? In the U.K., the prevailing answer is clearly "yes." As one distinguished nephrologist put it, "If we cannot treat all, then those left to die will be chosen because, in the opinion of doctors, they are likely to do less well on treatment than others" (Wing 1979, 163). Though some dispute may attach to the nature and application of these medical criteria, almost no one dissents from the proposition that medical criteria are the best (if not the only) guide to patient selection. The sole criticism emanating from the medical community would seem to be that implementation of the ideal has been, like all human endeavors, imperfect.

It is not difficult to speculate as to why such a view should have become so universal. After all, physicians make the actual choices, and their authority and expertise extend only to medical matters. Moreover, to speak exclusively of medical criteria is to suggest to the lay public an objective, rather mechanical reasoning procedure, whose very impersonality may seem a reassuring protection against favoritism and abuse. Of course, this view may be quite naive and misleading, but it is no less widespread for that.

Yet, the judgment that only medical criteria should be applied is also a normative judgment. It is true, of course, that treating only patients with the best prognoses is the most efficient use of scarce resources; more patients per unit of resources can be treated in this way than in any alternative approach. Some observers might retort, however, that efficiency is not the highest value. Ought dialyzing ten Antonio Salieris be preferred to five Amadeus Mozarts merely because the Salieris have better prognoses? Upon such questions, the consensus supporting exclusive reliance upon medical criteria must founder. Even physicians appear on occasion to share this kind of reservation. When one consultant wrote that "one would have to rank on the positive side—ability to help the community by working" (Challah et al. 1984, 1122), he was clearly uttering an ethical, not a clinical judgment.

The problem is that, to the extent that microallocative decisions reflect macroallocations, they are true tragic choices (Calabresi and Bobbitt 1978). Society spares only some ESRD patients from suffering and death, finds it awkward to face the fact of its abandoning many helpless and blameless citizens, and prefers that physicians make the selections according to their own divinations—and do so privately. Medical criteria, if they were widely discussed, doubtlessly could be revealed as inadequate, but it is the nature of tragic choices that no criteria can receive near universal acceptance. However much a detached analyst may deplore it, therefore, there may be an irresistible tendency to transmute certain kinds of normative decisions about resources into technical decisions about treatment. "Human kind cannot bear very much reality" (Eliot 1958, 118).

If the prime victims of these microallocative pressures are the ESRD patients, hyperscarcity takes a heavy toll from nephrologists and other medical personnel, as well. For the process of selection, according to some observers, forces physicians to act as judges, sometimes in the face of fears about their own imperfect knowledge and objectivity. Rejecting patients desiring treatment may be particularly difficult, as it may seem contrary to the physicians' medical training and to the ethic of the welfare state into which they have been socialized. That the nephrologist ordinarily makes the decision alone (though typically after consultation with other members of his renal unit) also makes for a certain stressful ambivalence; an unconscious wish for omnipotence may produce some enjoyment from the exercise of power, while the decision to say no may generate feelings of guilt often accompanied by an emotional withdrawal from the patients under care (Kaplan De-Nour and Czaczkes 1968; Shaldon 1968b). Such feelings are probably not uncommon among all kinds of physicians responsible for the longterm care of patients with potentially fatal diseases.

On the other hand, another observer, who for many years has been committed to viewing patient selection from the patient's viewpoint, claimed that a more ominous development was more typical. At the beginning, she said, young physicians were "appalled" at letting treatable patients die; after a while, "they learn to stomach it"; within a couple of years, it had "become part of their lives," an accepted element in the routine. In this sense, she argued, most participating physicians may be compared to the "good Germans," who gradually accommodated themselves to the "final solution" and whose active cooperation in the annihilation of much of European Jewry was essential to the success of the enterprise. Far from being burdened with guilt, the physician, in order to cope with the perceived necessity of rejecting treatable patients, instead hardens his heart, she maintains. Meanwhile, easing the doctor's rejection decision somewhat is the "clinical myth" that renal failure "is a pleasant way to die" (Knapp 1982, 847; Challah et al. 1984, 1122; but cf. Roher 1959).

Yet even this view must find a place for the terrible anguish repeatedly and publicly expressed by many of the U.K.'s leading nephrologists. Unwilling simply to exit and make a bad situation worse, a number have given voice to their frustration over macroallocation in an effort that outsiders can only find moving and heroic (cf. Hirschmann 1970).

For others, however, the prospect of becoming or remaining a nephrologist in the U.K. evidently seems simply too daunting. Thus, while in Italy there are 2,500 accredited nephrologists, in the U.K. there are only 117 senior and 207 junior staff (Royal College of Physicians, College Committee on Renal Disease, Executive Committee of the Renal Association 1983, tables 1–2). Constricted opportunities arising from budgetary restraints, furthermore, may also be contributing to the fact that, among new physicians, only 0.1 percent list nephrology as their first choice and only 0.2 percent as their second or third choice (Parkhouse et al. 1983). Nor is the impact confined only to physicians. For the paucity of dialysis centers has sometimes led to very tightly packed dialysis schedules and very heavy workloads for the support staff; this, in turn, has resulted in difficulty in obtaining and keeping staff (McGeown 1978, 418; more generally, Kaplan De-Nour 1984).

The picture that emerges is of a physician whose theoretical autonomy—constrained only by sound medical considerations and legal and contractual obligations—is seriously limited by practical considerations. He routinely prefers nonhospital-based therapies not because they are necessarily superior, but because their lower cost renders them the only ones available. As a consequence, some patients will receive optimal treatment, some suboptimal, and some none at all.

In this, the physician is not submitting to cynicism. On the contrary, he is likely to be acting in what he himself perceives as a highly ethical manner. But it is a hard-headed utilitarian ethic of choosing to treat many low-cost patients, rather than fewer high-cost ones.

Medical and Political Roles in Conflict

The physician, however, is not merely a philosopher, declaring and defending certain ethical preferences. He is also an actor with dual roles: medical and political. He must not only make "clinical judgments" and practice "good medicine," but must also authoritatively allocate resources (Easton 1953, 130). Faced with a situation of rather oppressive scarcity, he must decide who gets what, when, and how—classic political questions (Lasswell 1936). And if relatively few persons will be affected by his decisions, the impact for these few will be difficult to exaggerate, for nothing less than life or death is involved. What makes a physician "political," then, is not merely partisan or pressure-group activity; his role as a clinician, in which he must grant and withhold resources with considerable discretion, is profoundly political, even if not ordinarily recognized as such.

Of course, this political role is nowhere explicitly acknowledged. This is not a trivial answer, for it helps to ensure that the vast majority of patients and their families—and even a few physicians themselves—will be blind to the true nature of the situation. Thus blind, they will mistake political judgments for medical ones and be far more likely to acquiesce in the decisions. The fiction that the selection process is purely medical, in other words, is clearly functional as a powerful legitimator of rejection. It is important for its acceptance by patients and their families, that is, that the selection process not only be just but appear to be just, and this requires that it appear intelligible and patently reasonable to ordinary people (Rescher 1969, 176–86; cf. Powell 1976, 38). The ritualistic pronouncement of "clinical judgment" evidently fulfills that need,

though sometimes at the cost of honesty and candor.

The unacknowledged political character of the physician's role also forces upon him an agonizing conflict of interest. His manifest function as healer entails his primary obligation as being to his patient's welfare; his latent function as resource allocator entails his primary obligation as being to the DHSS (cf. Merton 1949, 21–81). Though it implicitly recognizes the problem, DHSS policy is more platitude than solution:

> Hospital consultants have clinical autonomy and are fully responsible for the treatment they prescribe for their patients. They are required to act within the broad limits of acceptable medical practice and within policy for the use of resources, but they are not held accountable to NHS Authorities for their clinical judgments (Committee of Inquiry into Normansfield Hospital 1978, 424–25).

But what if the physician's clinical judgment, for which he cannot be "held accountable," conflicts with "policy for the use of resources," within which he is "required to act"? What, in other words, if his manifest and latent functions are incompatible? In cases of severe scarcity (as in ESRD), both functions can be made to appear to be honored only through serious misrepresentation. Of course, it is much easier to deceive patients than bureaucrats. As one nephrologist, A. J. Wing, told the *Times*:

> Some of us have to tell lies to older patients, partly to make the patients more comfortable and partly to make ourselves more comfortable. We have to say to them that their hearts are too dodgy to stand the strain of dialysis (Ferrimann 1980).

To the other burdens of the physician, then, must sometimes be added the demeaning necessity of lying (cf. Calabresi and Bobbitt 1978, 24–26).

Not only the *individual* patient and his *particular* physician suffer from this conflict of interest. There is a larger *societal* interest in protecting the integrity of the doctor-patient relationship, an interest enshrined in such devices as the physician's freedom from coercion to testify about his patient's medical affairs in a court of law. That relationship depends upon trust, and trust, in turn, depends upon the physician's not being seen as serving any master before the patient, an appearance evidently maintained only through occasional resort to subterfuge and manipulation.

The refusal openly to acknowledge the physician's political role has also meant that the decision-making process has escaped serious outside scrutiny, for allocative decisions have been treated as if they were conventional medical decisions. Thus, the kinds of questions regarding dialysis and transplantation that were raised in the United States in the 1960s have never been explicitly and publicly addressed by U.K. political or bureaucratic leaders; instead they have been left implicitly to the private decisions of physicians.

Consider some of the questions that have been ignored. Who selects the selectors? Shall they operate singly, in ad hoc groups, or in a more institutionalized structure? What are their qualifications to be (medical competence, of course, but what of societal representativeness or philosophical expertise)? Should the social worth of competing patients be weighed and, if so, how (past performance? future potential? personal decency? responsibility for dependents?)? Is the selection process so strewn with imponderables that the only sensible course is to throw up one's hands and call for a lottery, which at least would respect the value of equality (Gorovitz 1966, 7; Childress 1979, 138; Siemsen 1978, 88)? So completely have U.K. physicians monopolized the microallocative decision-making process that virtually everyone concerned has taken the monopoly for granted, accepted it as a "given," and never seriously considered the merits of different systems.

This is not to argue that the U.K. adopt an earlier American practice, in which hospitals often relied upon selection committees composed of laymen and physicians, who were given no guidelines and developed no fixed criteria themselves (Murray et al. 1962, 315; Fox and Swazey 1974). The result, it is generally conceded, was not really satisfactory (see, e.g., Sanders and Dukeminier 1968, 377–78), despite the unquestionably earnest, good intentions of those who took part.

Nor is it to argue for the institutionalized presence of other interests. Their representatives, lacking the authority bases of physicians, would likely be dominated by them and rendered ineffective. And if not ineffective, they might be naive or wrong-headed and greatly complicate an already nearly impossibly complex situation. Almost certainly, in any case, these interests would tend to press for treatment, for who else but representatives of patient, nurse, social worker, or other caring groups would feel intensely enough about the matter to get involved and seek a position of influence?

But it is to argue that the decision-making process often seems to exhibit a formless, almost casual character that hardly appears in keeping with its life or death significance. Greater structure, it is true, might prove a little less convenient and a little more costly than current practices. Yet it is hard to see why a refusal to treat should not require at least one nephrologist's opinion. In the United States, it is generally accepted (and for some purposes required) that a patient obtain a second medical opinion before undergoing some surgical procedures; it may not be presumptuous to suggest the need of a second opinion in the U.K. before an ESRD patient is denied treatment.

Should the patient himself participate in the discussion? Certainly, it is difficult to imagine any discussion a patient would find more stressful. Desperate, arguing for his life, not knowing exactly what information may be of help and, therefore, feeling compelled to bare his soul and plead for pity, the patient may find himself denuded of privacy and self-respect. Even if his efforts succeed, he may retain scars from the confrontation; if he fails, his bitterness may well blight much of his remaining time.

Nor is it even clear that the decision itself would necessarily be improved by his presence, for in place of medical expertise his main contribution might well be an issue-clouding emotionalism. The discomfort all this might generate for physicians, moreover, might be hard to exaggerate. Indeed, in order to avoid such agonizing confrontations, some physicians might even decide to treat patients where medical indications would seem to suggest the reverse (cf. Schwartz and Aaron 1984, 56).

At the same time, however, it *is* the patient's life that is on the line, and though many patients may prefer passively to distance themselves from the decision making, others might desire an opportunity actively to defend their own interests. Accused criminals have such a right, of course, and while it may be objected that the doctor-patient relationship ought not to be made into an adversarial proceeding, the fact remains that a physician's decision may so profoundly conflict with a patient's wishes that it is disingenuous to speak as if doctor and patient must perforce be on the same side. There is a place for paternalism in medicine, of course, but in a democracy premised upon the individual's pursuit of his own interests, a heavy burden must fall to those claiming to represent another's interests so fully that he himself can be banished from the proceedings that may determine his life or death.

And it is to argue, too, that there is a fundamental lack of congruence between the physician's medical role, which is built on clinical autonomy, and his political role as an allocator, which implies effective accountability. As a medical actor, in the words of a former DHSS chief medical officer, "each consultant is the monitor of his own work and that of his junior" and, indeed, need not even "submit it to collective review, which is therefore poorly developed" (Godber 1982, 371). As a result, the "final arbiter of a doctor's conduct is his conscience, influenced in turn by his personal ethical code" (Warren 1979, 25).

Such heavy reliance upon internal restraints may suffice for medical actors. Indeed, all the physicians interviewed stressed that individual variations among patients made individual clinical judgment by the doctor in charge indispensable. The alternative, as they all pointed out, was clinical judgment by some physician-bureaucrat, who never examined the patient and whose rules would inescapably be so rigid as to be unworkable.

Yet physicians are political actors, too, and in democracies we normally expect the added presence of institutionalized external restraints when political actors are involved. No mechanisms—no formal statements on treating young children, persons over age 45, diabetics, those unable to speak English or of low intelligence, or other controversial patient populations—in fact, virtually no explicit policy statements whatever have been forthcoming either from the DHSS or from the Regional Health Authorities. But as these difficult, often personally wrenching decisions are remanded to the physicians on the line, effective accountability is sacrificed.

Of course, resolving such problems through criteria that determine which ESRD patients shall be treated, and procedures that govern how this determination shall be reached, would involve trade-offs. The doctor-patient relationship would become more formal and legalistic; physician morale and perhaps patient confidence would suffer; the responsiveness of regions and districts to local interests would be compromised; most obviously, the criteria and procedures devised (particularly, at first) would not fit all circumstances satisfactorily. Nor would the implementation of criteria and procedures cause the awkward and painful necessity of saying "no" to some patients to disappear. Indeed, rejecting patients would only become more difficult for all concerned.

And yet the current system—or nonsystem—has costs, too, though they are not always noted. The lack of accountability. The conflicts of interest. The white and not so white lies. The pretense that ethical issues can be ignored, as if the exclusive rhetorical reliance upon medical criteria were not itself an unexamined ethical judgment. The unrestrained power over life and death, especially in the hands of general practitioners and internists with only modest ESRD expertise and experience. The inequity of similar patients granted treatment here but denied there. To all this, it hardly seems sufficient for bureaucrats to observe that patient selection is left to the physicians and for physicians to reply that resource allocation is left to the bureaucrats.

Obviously, this is not the place to prescribe microallocative criteria and procedures. The issues, of course, are complex, and both the incrementalists and the expansionists can point to major strengths of their own and major weaknesses in the opposition. Moreover, however the issues are resolved, they will be resolved in the unique British context and thus cannot depart too sharply from the congeries of values, tradition, and practices that characterize that context. It may, therefore, be reckless to predict precisely what such criteria and procedures might emerge. But given the widespread dissatisfaction with microallocation among those with the greatest expertise and experience, it would be more reckless still to pretend that no such examination is necessary.

CONCLUSIONS

It is possible to view the ESRD microallocative process as a natural consequence of the tradition of clinical autonomy interacting with the multitudinous variations among physicians. That is, physicians are granted vast discretionary authority to determine which patients to treat, and different physicians produce different treatment patterns, depending upon training, biases, interests, and a number of other medical and nonmedical factors (cf. Wennberg, Barnes, and Zubkoff 1982). Underlying this is the recognition that many key physician decisions are not compelled by an indisputable logic, but instead are choices presented by analogical reasoning on which experts may differ. Viewed from this perspective, disparities in treatment patterns are likely to persist so long as physicians retain their autonomy and distinctive individuality—in short, certainly for the foreseeable future.

In another sense, though, the ESRD microallocative process reflects larger macroallocative pressures. For the scarcity of resources allocated to ESRD patients is not irremediable (like, say, the scarcity of Rembrandt portraits), but rather is a function of an implicit policy decision against reallocating resources in sufficient quantities to relieve it. Put differently, the scarcity is not so much imposed on society as imposed by society, or at least by its agents. Clearly, if enough resources were made available (perhaps, less than £10 per taxpayer per year) virtually all patients would be treated. With the necessity of denying treatment effectively eliminated, the significance of clinical autonomy and physician variation as determinators of patient selection would effectively be eliminated, too.

Seen from this vantage, the U.K. experience with ESRD is simply that of a welfare state endeavoring to live within its means. In the larger view and measured in terms of direct costs, the U.K. has been remarkably successful; it devotes a smaller percentage of its gross national product to health care, and operates under a lower rate of health care cost inflation, than does almost any other industrialized nation. At the same time, though, its ESRD treatment patterns remind all other Western democracies caught up in the quest for cost-containment and cutbacks in entitlements that this involves sacrifices not only from prosperous physicians and inefficient hospitals, but also from vulnerable patients.

Yet, to acknowledge that the U.K. must live within its means is not to concede the justice of every decision made in this name, even the most carefully considered and well-intentioned of decisions. For like a sore that will not heal, the question just will not go away: in order for the U.K. to live within its means, must so many ESRD patients be abandoned to die? The obvious answer is no; so trifling a burden could hardly be thought to exceed the U.K.'s capacity nor to be excessive, given the vastly incommensurate benefit of prolonging useful life for thousands of persons.

A less obvious answer, however, must also intrude. For if ESRD is seen as an exemplar of a larger problem—must living within its means compel a society to consign some treatable patients to death?—the response is not quite so plain. There are never enough resources to treat or aggressively to seek the cure for every malady; there are always more potentially beneficial claims (and claimants) than can be met at any level of health care funding. Moreover, individuals and governments will always conclude that as important as health is, there are other goals (sometimes, unhealthy goals) on which they also desire to expend resources. Health care, as a consequence, is not invariably the first claimant on resources, but must compete with thousands of other mundane, heroic, dangerous, or trivial goods and services in the public and private sectors. For good health may be perceived as necessary, but it is certainly not perceived as sufficient. There are many other things we also demand, and so good health is seen not as an end, but rather as a means, or a precondition, to their enjoyment. Barring the imposition of a rigid ranking placing health care first, therefore, the answer would seem to be: Perhaps ESRD patients need not be left to perish, but some sizable number of treatable patients afflicted with other diseases probably will be ignored. It is easy to deplore this conclusion and to argue for a health-dominated priority system, of course, but a free people, mostly healthy and given to focusing upon the near term, has never supported such a system. Nor does it seem likely to change its mind.

That many treatable patients will continue to perish is a very sobering conclusion. For some observers, however, a pair of other considerations may somewhat mitigate its impact. First, the problem of scarcity appears inherent in the human condition. There have never been enough resources to go around, and even as resources increase, so, too, do demands. The founders of the NHS may have believed that once the pent-up demand for health care had been met public demand would recede, but with hindsight their naiveté is exposed. From this perspective, what is noteworthy is not how many treatable ESRD patients perish but how many are saved —more today than ever before and doubtlessly even more tomorrow than today. Scarcity remains, to be sure, but major progress has been made.

Second, health care is not the only (or even the chief) determinant of health. Public funds spent on sanitation, pollution control, and police and fire protection, and private funds spent on food, clothing, exercise, and auto repair may all compete with health care for their share of the resource pie. Yet since each of these other claimants may promote good health, though they may divert resources from health care, this diversion need not lower actual levels of health. Indeed, as one analyst sarcastically phrased it, "If health status is primarily determined by socioeconomic conditions, why bother to spend money on health care in the first place instead of devoting it to improved housing, nutrition, and so on?" (Klein 1984, 90).

In the last analysis, though, such reassurances may seem to some observers too facile to persuade. For they cannot erase the image of a treatable ESRD patient drifting inexorably toward death or cancel the indelible realization that there, but for the grace of God, go us all.

References

ABRAM, H. S., and W. WADLINGTON. 1968. Selection of Patients for Artificial and Transplanted Organs. *Annals of Internal Medicine* 69:615–20.

ALMEDER, R. F. 1979. The Role of Moral Considerations in Reallocation of Exotic Medical Life Saving Therapy. In *Biomedical Ethics and the Law,* ed. J. M. Humber and R. F. Almeder, 543–55. New York: Plenum Press.

BAILLOD, R. A., C. COMTY, M. ILAHI, F. I. D. KONOTEY-AHOLU, L. SEVITT, and S. SHALDON. 1965. Overnight Haemodialysis in the Home. In *Proceedings of the European Dialysis and Transplant Association,* ed. D.N.S. Kerr, 99–103. Amsterdam: Excerpta Medica Foundation.

BEAUCHAMP, T. L. and J. F. CHILDRESS. 1979. *Principles of Biomedical Ethics.* New York: Oxford University Press.

BEER, S. H. 1982. *Britain against Itself: The Political Contradictions of Collectivism.* London: Faber and Faber.

BENDIXEN, H. H. 1977. The Cost of Intensive Care. In *Costs, Risks and Benefits of Surgery,* ed. J. P. Bunker, B. A. Barnes, and F. Mosteller, 372–84. New York: Oxford University Press.

BENNETT, G. 1979. *Patients and Their Doctors.* London: Ballière Tindall.

BERGER, P. S., B. E. ALPERT, and R. E. LONGNECKER. 1983. Dialysis Therapy for Diabetics. *Diabetics Nephropathy* 2:22–25.

BERLYNE, G. M. 1982. Over 50 and Uremic Equals Death. *Nephron* 31:189–90.

BRANCH, R. A., G. W. CLARK, A. L. COCHRANE, J. H. JONES, and H. SCARBOROUGH. 1971. Incidence of Uraemia and Requirements for Maintenance Dialysis. *British Medical Journal* 1:249–54.

BRESCIA, M. J., J. E. CIMINO, K. APPEL, and B. J. HORWICH. 1966. Chronic Hemodialysis Using Venopuncture and a Surgically Created Arteriovenous Fistula. *New England Journal of Medicine* 275:1089–92.

BRITISH MEDICAL JOURNAL. 1978. Editorial. 2:1449–59.

BROYER, M., F. P. BRUNNER, H. BRYNGER, R. A. DONCKERWOLCKE, C. JACOBS, P. KRAMER, N. H. SELWOOD, and A. J. WING. 1982. Combined Report on Regular Dialysis and Transplantation in Europe, 1981. In *Proceedings of the European Dialysis and Transplant Association,* ed. A. M. Davison, 2–59. London: Pitman Books.

———. 1984. Combined Report on Regular Dialysis and Transplantation in Europe, 1982. In *Proceedings of the European Dialysis and Transplant Association,* ed. A. M. Davison, 2–108. London: Pitman Books.

BRYAN, F. A., JR. 1981. The Patient and Family in Home Dialysis. *Controversies in Nephrology* 3:406–25.

CALABRESI, G., and P. BOBBITT. 1978. *Tragic Choices.* New York: Norton.

CAMPBELL, J. D., and A. R. CAMPBELL. 1978. The Social and Economic Costs of End-Stage Renal Disease. *New England Journal of Medicine* 289:386–92.

CARTWRIGHT, A., and R. ANDERSON. 1981. *General Practice Revisited: A Second Study of Patients and Their Doctors.* London: Tavistock Publications.

CHALLAH, S., A. J. WING, R. BAUER, R. W. MORRIS, and S. A. SCHROEDER. 1984. Negative Selection of Patients for Dialysis and Transplantation in the United Kingdom. *British Medical Journal* (288): 1119–22.

CHESTER, A. C., T. A. RAKOWSKI, W. P. ARGY, A. GIACALONE, and G. E. SCHREINER. 1979. Hemodialysis in the Eighth and Ninth Decades of Life. *Archives of Internal Medicine* 139:1001–5.

CHILDRESS, J. F. 1979. A Right to Health Care? *Journal of Medicine and Philosophy* 4:132–47.

COMMITTEE OF INQUIRY INTO NORMANSFIELD HOSPITAL. 1978. *Report.* Cmnd. 7537. London: Her Majesty's Stationery Office.

CONTROVERSIES IN NEPHROLOGY. 1979. 1:123–35.

CZACZKES, J. W., and A. KAPLAN DE-NOUR. 1978. *Chronic Hemodialysis as a Way of Life.* New York: Brunner/Mazel.

DENNIS, C. N. 1971. Regular Haemodialysis and Renal Transplantation. In *Portfolio for Health: The Role and Program of the DHSS in Health Services Research,* ed. G. McLachlan, 143–47. London: Oxford University Press for the Nuffield Provincial Hospitals Trust.

DE WARDENER, H. E. 1966. Some Ethical and Economic Problems Associated with Intermittent Haemodialysis. In *Ethics and Medical Progress: With Special Reference to Transplantation,* ed. G. E. W. Wolstenholme and M. O'Connor, 104–18. London: J. & A. Churchill.

DICK, D. 1983. How Long Can NHS Ignore Quality Control? *Health and Social Services* 93 (July 28):898–99.

EASTON, D. 1953. *The Political System: An Inquiry into the State of Political Science.* New York: Knopf.

ELIOT, T. S. 1958. Burnt Norton. In *The Complete Poems and Plays, 1901–1950.* New York: Harcourt, Brace.

FARMER, C. V., S. A. SNOWDEN, and V. PARSONS. 1979. The Prevalence of Psychiatric Illness among Patients on Home Dialysis. *Psychological Medicine* 9:509–14.

FERRIMAN, A. 1980. 1000 Kidney Patients Die "Because Treatment Unavailable." *The Times* (London), March 20, p. 4, col. 1.

FOX, R. C. 1975. Long-Term Dialysis. *American Journal of Medicine* 59:702–12.

FOX, R. C., and J. P. SWAZEY. 1974. *The Courage to Fail.* Chicago: University of Chicago Press.

GABRIEL, R. 1983. Chronic Renal Failure in the UK: Referral, Funding and Staffing. In *Renal Failure—Who Cares?,* ed. F. M. Parsons and C. S. Ogg, 35–40. Lancaster: MTP Press.

GLASSMAN, B. M., and A. SIEGEL. 1970. Personality Correlates of Survival in a Long Term Hemodialysis Program. *Archives of General Psychiatry* 22:566–74.

GODBER, G. 1982. The British Health System: Achievements and Limitations. *Israeli Journal of Medical Sciences* 18:365–73.

GOROVITZ, S. 1966. Ethics and the Allocation of Medical Resources. *Medical Research Engineering* 5:5–7.

GRAHAM, N. G., F. T. DE DOMBAL, and J. C. GOLIGHER. 1971. Reliability of Physical Signs in Patients with Severe Attacks of Ulcerative Colitis. *British Medical Journal* 2:746–48.

GREENBERG, D. S. 1978. Washington Report: Renal Politics. *New England Journal of Medicine* 298:1427–28.

GRIST, L. 1981. Are Some Doctors Pulling the Plug? *General Practitioner* 11 (October 16):73.

HART, V. 1978. *Distrust and Democracy: Political Distrust in Britain and America.* Cambridge: Cambridge University Press.

HIATT, H. 1975. Protecting the Medical Commons: Who Is Responsible? *New England Journal of Medicine* 293:235–41.

HIRSCHMANN, A. O. 1970. *Exit, Voice, and Loyalty: Responses to Decline in Firms, Organizations, and States.* Cambridge: Harvard University Press.

HODSON, G. M., J. S. NAJARIAN, C. M. KJELLSTRAND, R. L. SIMMONS, and S. M. MAURER. 1978. Renal Transplantation in Children Aged 1–5 Years. *Pediatrics* 66:454–64.

KAPLAN DE-NOUR, A. 1984. Stresses and Reactions of Professional Hemodialysis Staff. *Dialysis and Transplantation* 13:137–49.

KAPLAN DE-NOUR, A., and J. W. CZAZCKES. 1968. Emotional Problems and Reactions of the Medical Team in a Chronic Haemodialysis Unit. *Lancet* 2:987–91.

KAPLAN DE-NOUR, A., and J. SHANAN. 1980. Quality of Life of Dialysis and Transplanted Patients. *Nephron* 25:117–20.

KATZ, J., and A. M. CAPRON. 1975. *Catastrophic Diseases: Who Decides What?* New York: Russell Sage Foundation.

KAVANAUGH, D. 1980. Political Culture in Great Britain: The Decline of the Civic Culture. In *The Civic Culture Revisited,* ed. G. Almond and S. Verba, 124–76. Boston: Little, Brown.

KLEIN, R. 1983. *The Politics of the National Health Service.* London: Longmans.

———. 1984. The Politics of Ideology vs. the Reality of Politics: The Case of Britain's National Health Service in the 1980s. *Milbank Memorial Fund Quarterly/ Health and Society* 62:82–109.

KNAPP, M. S. 1982. Renal Failure—Dilemmas and Developments. *British Medical Journal* (284):847–50.

KOOPMAN, C., S. EISENTHAL, and J. D. STOECKLE. 1984. Ethnicity in Reporting Pain, Emotional Distress and Requests of Medical Outpatients. *Social Science and Medicine* 18:487–90.

KRAKAUER, H., J. S. GRAUMAN, M. R. MCMULLAN, and C. C. CREEDE. 1983. The Recent U.S. Experience in the Treatment of End-Stage Renal Disease by Dialysis and Transplantation. *New England Journal of Medicine* 308:1558–63.

LAING, W. 1978. *Renal Failure: A Priority in Health?* London: Office of Health Economics.

———. 1979. Cost Effectiveness. *Journal of Medical Engineering and Technology* 3:113.

LANCET. 1981. 1:594–96.

LASSWELL, H. D. 1936. *Politics: Who Gets What, When, How.* New York: McGraw-Hill.

LEGRAIN, M. C. 1983. Diabetics with End-Stage Renal Disease: "The Best Buy." *Diabetic Nephropathy* (August). 2:1–3.

LEVY, N. B. 1979. Psychological Problems of the Patient on Hemodialysis and Their Treatment. *Psychotherapy and Psychosomatics* 31:260–66.

THE TIMES (London). 1981. February 9. p. 3, col. 5.

LUKE, R. C. 1983. Renal Replacement Therapy. *New England Journal of Medicine* 308:1593–95.

LUPTON, R. 1979. *Caring for Children in Renal Failure: Report of the Conference Held at the King's Fund Center,* London, October 9.

McGEOWN, M. G. 1972. Chronic Renal Failure in Northern Ireland. *Lancet* 1:307–10.

———. 1978. Selection of Patients: Integration between Dialysis and Transplantation. In *Replacement of Renal Function by Dialysis,* ed. W. Drukker, F. M. Parsons, and J. F. Maher, 418–25. The Hague: Martinus Nijhoff Medical Division.

MECHANIC, D. 1979. *Future Issues in Health Care.* New York: Free Press.

MEDICAL SERVICES STUDY GROUP OF THE ROYAL COLLEGE OF PHYSICIANS. 1981. Deaths from Chronic Renal Failure under the Age of 50. *British Medical Journal* (283):283–86.

MERRILL, J. P., J. E. MURRAY, J. W. HARRISON, and W. R. GUILD. 1956. Successful Homotransplantation of the Human Kidney between Identical Twins. *Journal of the American Medical Association* 160:277–82.

MERRILL, J. P., E. SCHUPAK, E. CAMERON, and C. L. HAMPER. 1964. Hemodialysis in the Home. *Journal of the American Medical Association* 190:468–70.

MERTON, R. K. 1949. *Social Theory and Social Structures: Toward the Codification of Theory and Research.* Glencoe: Free Press.

MORRIS, G. P. 1983. Enforcing a Duty to Care: The Kidney Patient and the NHS. *Law Society's Gazette* 80(December 7):3156, 3164–65.

MURRAY, J. S., W. H. TU, J. B. ALBERS, J. M. BURNELL, and B. H. SCRIBNER. 1962. A Community Hemodialysis Center for the Treatment of Chronic Uremia.

Transactions of the American Society for Artificial Internal Organs 8:315–20.

OFFICE OF POPULATION CENSUSES AND SURVEYS. 1983. *Mortality Statistics, Cause.* London: Her Majesty's Stationery Office.

OGG, C. 1970. Maintenance Haemodialysis and Renal Transplantation. *British Medical Journal* 4:412–15.

PARKHOUSE, J., M. G. CAMPBELL, B. A. HAMBLETON, and P. R. PHILIPS. 1983. Career Preferences of Doctors Qualifying in the UK in 1980. *Health Trends* 20:12–14.

PARSONS, F. M. 1967. A True "Doctor's Dilemma." *British Medical Journal* 1:623.

PARSONS, F. M., and C. S. OGG. 1983a. Discussion. In *Renal Failure—Who Cares?,* ed. F. M. Parsons and C. S. Ogg, 110–18. Lancaster: MTP Press.

———. 1983b. Discussion. In *Renal Failure—Who Cares?,* ed. F. M. Parsons and C. S. Ogg, 239–46. Lancaster: MTP Press.

PARSONS, V. and P. M. LOCK. 1980. Triage and the Patient with Renal Failure. *Journal of Medical Ethics* 6:173–76.

PENDREIGH, D. M., M. A. HEASMAN, L. F. HOWITT, A. C. KENNEDY, A. I. MACDOUGALL, M. MACLEOD, J. S. ROBSON, and W. K. STEWART. 1972. Survey of Chronic Renal Failure in Scotland. *Lancet* 1:304–7.

POWELL, J. E. 1976. *Medicine and Politics: 1975 and After.* Tunbridge Wells: Pitman Medical.

QUINTON, W. E., D. H. DILLARD, and B. H. SCRIBNER. 1960. Cannulation of Blood Vessels for Prolonged Hemodialysis. *Transactions of the American Society for Artificial Internal Organs* 6:104–9.

RESCHER, N. 1969. The Allocation of Exotic Lifesaving Therapy. *Ethics* 79:173–86.

RICHMOND, J. M., R. M. LINDSAY, H. J. BURTON, J. CONLEY, and L. WAI. 1982. Psychological and Physiological Factors Predicting the Outcome of Home Dialysis. *Clinical Nephrology* 17:109–13.

ROBINSON, H. B. 1978. Selection of Patients for Dialysis and Transplantation. In *Living with Renal Failure,* ed. J. L. Anderson, F. M. Parsons, and D. E. Jones, 9–18. Lancaster: MTP Press.

ROHER, M. 1959. *Days of Living.* Toronto: Ryerson Press.

ROSA, A. A., D. S. FRYD, and C. M. KJELLSTRAND. 1980. Dialysis Symptoms and Stabilization in Long Term Disease. *Archives of Internal Medicine* 140:804–7.

ROYAL COLLEGE OF PHYSICIANS OF LONDON, COLLEGE COMMITTEE ON RENAL DISEASE, EXECU-

TIVE COMMITTEE OF THE RENAL ASSOCIA-
TION. 1983. Manpower and Workload in Renal
Medicine in the United Kingdom, 1975–1983. July.
(Unpublished.)

SANDERS, D., and H. DUKEMINIER. 1968. Medical Advances and Legal Lag: Hemodialysis and Kidney
Transplantation. *U.C. L. A. Law Review* 15:357–413.

SCHWARTZ, W. B., and H. J. AARON. 1984. Rationing
Hospital Care. *New England Journal of Medicine*
310:52–56.

SHALDON, S. 1968a. Independence in Maintenance Haemodialysis. *Lancet* 1:520–23.

———. 1968b. Emotional Problems in a Chronic Haemodialysis Unit. *Lancet* 2:1347.

SHERLOCK, S. 1983. Hepatic Transplantation. *Lancet*
2:778–79.

SHORT, M., and W. P. WILSON. 1969. Roles of Denial
in Chronic Hemodialysis. *Archives of General Psychiatry* 20:433–37.

SIEMSEN, A. W. 1978. Experience in Self-Care and Limited Care Haemodialysis. In *Living with Renal Failure,* ed. J. L. Anderson, F. M. Parsons, and D. E. Jones,
87–97. Lancaster: MTP Press.

SIMMONS, R. G. 1979. Discussion. *Controversies in Nephrology* 1:202–3.

STERNBACH, R. A., and TURSKY, B. Ethnic Differences
among Housewives in Psychophysical and Skin Potential Responses to Electric Shock. *Psychophysiology*
1:241–46.

TAYLOR, T. R., J. AITCHESON, L. S. PARKER, and
M. F. MOORE. 1975. Individual Differences in Se-
lecting Patients for Regular Haemodialysis. *British
Medical Journal* 2:380–81.

TENCKHOFF, H., and H. SCHECHTER. 1968. A Bacterio-
logically Safe Peritoneal Access Device. *Transactions
of the American Society for Artificial Internal Organs*
14:181–86.

TIMMINS, N. 1983. Transplant Cash "a Sop" Specialist
Says. *The Times* (London), November 3, p. 2, col. 6.

TOCQUEVILLE, A. DE [1840] 1961. *Democracy in America,* 2 vols., H. Reeve, trans. New York: Schocken
Books.

TROMPETER, P. S., M. BEWICK, G. B. HAYCOCK, and
C. CHANTLER. 1983. Renal Transplantation in Very
Young Children. *Lancet* 1:373–75.

WALTERS, V. 1980. *Class Inequality and Health Care:
The Origins and Impact of the National Health Service.*
London: Croom Helm.

WARREN, D. 1979. The Doctor's Freedom under Authority.
In *Decision Making in Medicine: The Practice of Its
Ethics,* ed. G. Scorer and A. J. Wing, 25–37. London:
Edward Arnold.

WENNBERG, J. E., B. A. BARNES, and M. ZUBKOFF.
1982. Professional Uncertainty and the Problem of
Supplier Induced Demand. *Social Science and Medicine* 16:811–24.

WING, A. J. 1979. The Impact of Financial Constraint.
In *Decision Making in Medicine: The Practice of Its
Ethics,* ed. G. Scorer and A. J. Wing, 151–64. London:
Edward Arnold.

WINSLOW, G. R. 1982. *Triage and Justice.* Berkeley: University of California Press.

YELLOWLEES, H. 1982. *On the State of the Public Health.*
London: Her Majesty's Stationery Office.

ZBOROWSKI, N. 1952. Cultural Components in Response
to Pain. *Journal of Social Issues* 8:16–30.

ZOLA, I. K. 1966. Culture and Symptoms: An Analysis of
Patients Presenting Complaints. *American Sociological Review* 31:615–30.

The Consequences of Professional Dominance

In the context of American health care, professional dominance refers to the control that physicians have traditionally had over the provision of health care. The term was coined by Eliot Freidson and discussed in *Professional Dominance: The Social Structure of Medical Care,* which was published in 1970. According to Freidson, a most important condition resulting in professional dominance has been the unprecedented degree of autonomy that American society has bestowed upon the medical profession. More recently, the importance of professional dominance to an understanding of the American system of health care has been articulated by Paul Starr in his Pulitzer-prize winning book *The Social Transformation of American Medicine.*

Caroline Kaufmann has shown in her comparative article in the previous chapter that U.S. physicians have a far greater degree of control over health care services than physicians in most other nations. Through the use of the following tables, Donald Light, in a clear and concise fashion, contrasts the physician-controlled "professional" (i.e., professional dominance) model and government-controlled "state" model of a health care system.

In the professional model the core value, according to Light, is to "enhance the power and effectiveness of the medical profession." While health care is a professional responsibility, the individual has the responsibility for maintaining his or her own health. In the state model, physicians are state employees. Also, the state does involve itself in maintaining individual health through programs of prevention and health promotion

TABLE 1   The professional model of a health care system*

Inherent Values and Goals	*To provide the best possible clinical care to every sick patient.*
	To develop scientific medicine to its highest level.
	To protect the autonomy of physicians and keep the state or others from controlling the health care system.
	To increase the power and wealth of the profession.
	To generate enthusiasm and admiration for the medical profession.
Organization	A loose federation.
	Administratively collegial and decentralized.
	Services and recruitment follow the stratification of the society.
	Emphasis on acute, hi-tech intervention and specialty care.
	Organized around hospitals and private offices.
	Weak ties with other social institutions.
	Organized around clinical cases and doctors' preferences.
Key Institutions	Physicians' associations.
	Autonomous physicians and hospitals.
Power	Profession the sole power.
	Uses state powers to enhance its own.
	Protests state interferences.
	Protests, boycotts all competing models of care.
Finance and Cost	Private payments, by individual or through private insurance plans.
	Doctors' share of costs more.
Image of the Individual	A private individual. Chooses how to live and when to use the medical system.
Division of Labor	Proportionately more physicians.
	More specialists.
	More individual clinical work by the physician; less delegation.
Medical Education	A private and/or autonomous system of schools with tuition.
	Disparate, loosely coupled continuing education.

* From D. Light, 1986.

to a much greater extent than does the professional model system. A further difference between the two models lies in the degree of control physicians have over such decisions as the nature of professional education, the proportion of specialists and their distribution, and the proportion of non-physicians and how they are employed. Physician control over these kinds of decisions are much greater in the health care system characterized by the professional model.

This chapter consists of four articles that, taken together, look at the nature and consequences of professional dominance in the United States. In the first article, Paul J. Feldstein debates the question of whether the American Medical Association has used its virtual freedom from outside regulation for self-interest or with the interest of the public

TABLE 2   The state model of a health care system**

Inherent Values and Goals	*To strengthen the state via a healthy, vigorous population.* To minimize illness via preventive medicine, public health, and patient education. To control the health care system. To minimize the cost of health care to the state. To provide good, accessible care to all sectors of the population. * To indoctrinate, through health care; and enhance loyalty to the state. * To increase the power of the state.
Organization	A national, integrated system. Administratively decentralized * (or hierarchical). Egalitarian services and recruitment patterns. Organized around primary care units. Strong ties with health programs in other social institutions. Organized around epidemiological patterns of illness.
Key Institutions	The Ministry of Health. Regional/district councils (or regional/district health officers).
Power	* State the sole power. * Professor associations prohibited. OR Tiers of representative councils. Active partnership with medical associations.
Finance and Cost	All care free, from taxes. Doctors' share of costs less.
Image of the Individual	A member of society. Thus the responsibility of the state, but also responsible to stay healthy.
Division of Labor	Proportionately fewer physicians and more nurses, etc. Fewer specialists. More middle-level providers (nurse-clinicians); more delegation; more teamwork.
Medical Education	A state system for all providers and extensive continuing education.

* Features of the autocratic state model.

** From D. Light, 1986.

in mind. His examination of a good number of AMA policies leads him to the conclusion that self-interest is a distinct priority.

The remaining three articles deal with the ramifications of organized medicine's control of the health care system for other groups of health professionals. Howard D. Schwartz, Peggy L. deWolf, and James K. Skipper, Jr. look at the professionalization of nursing. They first provide the historical background that led to the subordination of nursing to medicine and discuss the importance, in this regard, of the fact that nursing is predominantly female. They then analyze the impact of the growing assertiveness of American women on nursing's push for fuller professional status and show how this process of professionalization has resulted in a profession with two distinguishable views of itself.

Although not female dominated, pharmacy has often been used as an example of a "semi-profession" because of its lack of ultimate control over the key element defining its place in the provision of services. It is physicians who prescribe drugs and pharmacists who function in the much more routinized role of filling the prescriptions. In the third article in this chapter, Arnold Birenbaum describes how, due to a number of factors outside of its control, pharmacy is facing a real loss of its traditional role. In response, the profession is trying to take over a new role. However, opposition mainly from the medical profession, but other groups as well, will make this a difficult task. One path being taken to gain increased recognition is the same one doctors have taken and nurses are taking— increased education. In the last paper, Paul Root Wolpe describes how physicians have wrested control of acupuncture from practitioners who frequently have far more experience and expertise than they have. His description of the medical profession's rejection of acupuncture reminds one of the profession's past rejection of chiropractic. For a variety of reasons, chiropractors were successful in becoming duly recognized by the AMA in 1980. Wolpe also shows how, over time, the medical profession brought acupuncture in line with its biomedical model of health and disease (that model discussed in Chapter 8) in the process of laying claim to the use of the technique.

References

FREIDSON, E. 1970. *Professional Dominance: The Social Structure of Medical Care*. New York: Aldine Publishing Company.

LIGHT, D. 1986. Comparing health care systems: Lessons from East and West Germany in *The Sociology of Health and Illness* (edited by P. Conrad and R. Kern). New York: St. Martin's Press.

STARR, P. 1982. *The Social Transformation of American Medicine*. New York: Basic Books.

Policies of the American Medical Association: Self-Interest or Public-Interest?

Paul J. Feldstein

. . . Three entry barriers to the physician's market have been suggested: licensure, graduation from an approved medical school, and continual increases in training, such as the movement to a three-year residency program. There is, however, an alternative hypothesis to explain why barriers in medicine exist: rather than serving to increase the economic returns to physicians, the barriers increase the quality and competence of practicing physicians. It is rationalized that these entry barriers enhance the public interest in a variety of ways. Consumers have very little information on the quality and competence of physicians. Because gathering this information is costly and the consumer may be irreparably injured if the physician is incompetent, licensure provides consumer protection by reducing the uncertainty as to the provider's training. Occupational licensure has also been rationalized on grounds of "neighborhood effects"; preventing an incompetent physician from practicing because he or she may cause an epidemic is an example, because an incompetent physician may harm persons other than the patient being treated. Licensure is thus a means of protecting others from bearing the costs of incompetent practitioners; that is, the social costs exceed the private costs (1).

Given these alternative hypotheses to explain the reasons for entry barriers to becoming a physician—namely, to increase physician incomes or to provide consumer protection from incompetent practitioners—which is the more accurate justification? If the barriers are reduced because they are believed

This article originally appeared as Chapter 14, "The Market for Physician Manpower," in *Health Care Economics*, second edition, by Paul Feldstein, pp. 380–395. Copyright © 1983 by John Wiley and Sons, Inc.

to provide physicians with monopoly incomes, then will the public lose its protection from incompetent providers? Similarly, if it is public policy to maintain such entry restrictions in the belief that they reduce consumer uncertainty and protect society from incompetent providers, but in truth such barriers are meant to provide physicians with monopoly incomes, then is the public really protected from incompetent practitioners? Could the public be better protected using other approaches and at a lower cost?

To determine which hypothesis best describes the reasons for entry restrictions in medicine one must determine how consistent each of these hypotheses is with regard to the assurance of quality or the achievement of monopoly power. If the restrictions that have been developed in medicine are for consumer protection, then the medical profession should also favor other measures that have the effect of improving quality and/or offering consumers protection from incompetent practitioners. If, on the other hand, the entry restrictions are meant to provide a monopoly to physicians and to increase their incomes, then the profession would only favor those quality measures that are in the economic interests of physicians and would oppose quality measures that would adversely affect physicians' incomes.

BARRIERS TO ENTRY IN MEDICINE

The first step in controlling entry into a profession is to establish a licensure requirement. Each state has the authority to license occupations under the power granted to it to protect the public's health. A license to practice medicine, therefore, can be granted only by a state. Beginning in the mid-1800s, when the American Medical Association (AMA) was formed, and extending until 1900, the medical profession sought and received licensure in each state (2). The states, in turn, delegated this licensure authority to medical licensing boards, which have the authority to determine the requirements for licensure. These state licensing boards also have the authority to set the conditions for suspending or revoking a license once it has been granted. The conditions for licensure and for maintaining a license can be set to place the emphasis on the quality of care that the physician provides, or they can be used to impose restrictions on who can practice so as to limit the number of persons entering the profession. The membership of the medical licensing boards in each state is composed of physicians who are either nominated by or representatives of the state and county medical associations. It is in this manner that the county and state medical associations have influenced the conditions for licensure in each state.

The earliest requirement for licensure was an examination. Examination by itself, however, is a weak barrier to entry if a person may try to pass the examination many times and if the number of people who may take the examination is not limited (3). A more effective barrier is one which raises the cost to those wishing to take the examination. Not everyone would be willing to bear this cost, particularly if there was uncertainty as to whether they would pass the licensure exam. The second barrier to entry into the medical profession, therefore, became the imposition of an educational requirement and a limit on the number of institutions that could provide such an education.

This second stage began in 1904 with the AMA's founding of its Council on Medical Education. This group had the task of upgrading the quality of medical education offered by existing medical schools. Of the 160 medical schools in 1906, the Council on Medical Education found only 82 offering a fully acceptable medical education (4). To achieve greater recognition of its findings, the Council on Medical Education induced the Carnegie Commission to survey the existing medical schools and publish a report. The resulting report, popularly known as the Flexner report, recommended the closing of many medical schools and an upgrading of the educational standards in the other schools. "Flexner forcefully argued that the country was suffering from an overproduction of doctors and that it was in the public interest to have fewer doctors who were better trained" (5).

The result of the Flexner report was that state medical licensing boards instituted an additional requirement for state licensure: before taking an examination for licensure, an applicant had to be a graduate of an approved medical school. The approval of medical schools was conducted by the AMA's own Council on Medical Education. In the years that followed, as expected, the number of medical schools decreased, from 162 in 1906, to 85 in 1920, to 76 in 1930, to 69 in 1944. The graduates of those medical schools that were closed continued to practice. No attempts were made to rectify any supposed inadequacies in their educational backgrounds. Whenever standards are raised, grandfather clauses protect the rights of existing practitioners, regardless of their abilities. The AMA now had control over entry into the profession in two ways: first, through its Council on Medical Education, the AMA was able to limit the number of approved medical schools and, hence, the number of applicants for licensure exams; second, entrants into the profession then had to pass state licensure exams and any other prerequisites promulgated by the individual state medical licensing boards. Thus the AMA, through its Council on Medical Education, was able to determine the "appropriate" number of physicians in the United States.

The third method used by the medical profession to restrict entry, which is also meant to increase the competence of the new physician, is to lengthen the training time required for the student to become a practicing physician. Before entering medical school, a student has to have four years of undergraduate education. The time spent in internship and residency programs after graduation from medical school continually increases; medical school graduates usually take a three-year residency program. For students desiring to enter certain specialties, more than three years is required. The effect of continually increasing the training required before entering a profession is to raise the costs to the entering student. Not only are tuition costs higher the longer are the requirements for undergraduate and medical school education, but more importantly, the income foregone because of the additional years of training is very large. These increased costs reduce the rate of return to someone entering the medical profession. The emphasis in terms of quality is always on the *entering* physician and not on those currently in the profession. It is in the economic interests of current practitioners that the costs of entering the profession continually increase; since their training occurred in the past at a lower cost, they will receive higher prices and higher incomes in the form of economic rent (6).

If the market for physician services were a competitive one, then the more highly trained physicians could advertise their increased training and more recent knowledge and receive a higher price for their services than physicians without this additional training. In such a competitive situation there would be little economic incentive for current physicians to promote higher training requirements for new physicians; therefore, to prevent new physicians from receiving higher returns than current physicians with less training do, it is necessary for the medical profession to maintain the fiction that *all* physicians are of uniform quality. To enforce this impression among patients, the medical profession discourages any intraprofessional criticism and, until recently, prohibits the advertisement of differences in training or any other quality differentials among physicians. Whether or not persons can perform certain medical tasks depends upon whether they are licensed as physicians, thereby being provided with an unlimited scope of practice, rather than whether they have had certain specialized training. Anesthesiologists, for example, can be physicians who are board certified in anesthesiology, or they can be physicians with additional training but who are not board certified, or they can be physicians without any additional training in anesthesia. It appears that merely being licensed is sufficient to allow physicians to undertake most tasks performed by other physicians who may have additional training.

This third barrier to entry, which takes the form of continual increases in the training costs for entering physicians, suggests that measures to increase the quality of physician services are independent of demands by consumers for increased quality and instead are related to the income considerations of the medical profession.

In addition to barriers to entry, another condition is necessary if physicians are to be able to secure monopoly profits. Unless productivity increases among physicians can be controlled, it would be pos-

sible for some physicians to greatly increase their output and thereby decrease the price and output and, consequently, the rate of return to competing physicians. Productivity increases are limited in two ways. First, only licensed physicians are allowed to perform certain tasks, thereby severely limiting the ability of physicians to greatly increase their output by delegating tasks to other personnel. Second, when new types of health personnel, such as physician's assistants, are permitted to undertake certain tasks which were formerly the sole prerogative of the physician, the state boards of medical examiners retain the authority to certify their use on an individual physician-by-physician basis. In this manner, a particular physician would not be able to hire a large number of such personnel and greatly increase his or her output. The medical licensing boards' control over physician's assistants can be used to approve their use in situations where demand for physician services has increased, or where no physicians are available, such as in rural areas; their employment can be limited in cases where physician's practices, from the standpoint of the physicians, are underutilized.

The foregoing methods, which have been used successfully by the medical profession to restrict entry into the profession, have been adapted by other health professions as well. The American Dental Association (ADA), after successfully achieving state licensure of dentists, had a study conducted on dental education, which resulted in the Gies report in the early 1920s. As a result of this report, applicants for state dental examinations had to be graduated from approved dental schools, with the accreditation being conducted by the ADA's own Council on Dental Education. The number of dental schools declined as standards, mandated by the ADA and carried out by its Council, were increased. The length of the training time to become a dentist has also increased; however, the dental profession has not yet instituted any residency requirements such as exist in medicine.

Increased educational requirements increase the investment cost of becoming a physician, thereby decreasing the rate of return to entering physicians. The extent to which the price of physician services and physicians' incomes will rise in response to higher entry costs and fewer physicians will depend upon the elasticities of the demand and supply of physician services. Barriers to entry in the physician market are consistent with a monopoly model which would confer higher incomes on physicians.

We now turn to an examination of these barriers as a means of protecting the consumer from incompetent providers. For this hypothesis to be an accurate description of the justification for such restrictions, the medical profession, through its representatives in county, state, and national organizations, should favor *all* policies, not just entry barriers, to protect the consumer from incompetent practitioners. If the AMA is not consistent in its support of quality measures and only favors those that favorably affect its members' incomes, while opposing those that adversely affect its members' incomes, then we must conclude that the real motivation for such measures is to enhance the monopoly power of its members.

If the AMA were in favor of protecting consumers from incompetent physicians, then one measure the AMA would be expected to favor would be reexamination and relicensure of physicians. One justification given for increased training requirements for new physicians is that there has been an explosion of medical knowledge. Some physicians received their medical education 30–40 years ago; reexamination and relicensure would insure that existing physicians have kept up with this increase in knowledge. Reexamination for relicensure is required in other areas, such as for renewal of driver licenses, or for commercial airline pilot licenses. There can be little justification for favoring increased training for new physicians but not for existing physicians if improving quality is at issue. Yet the AMA is opposed to reexamination and/or relicensure. If reexamination and relicensure were required, then unless the passing level were set so low that everyone always passed, either large numbers of physicians would fail the reexamination and be unable to practice, or different levels of licensure would be established to recognize what exists in practice.

Not all physicians should be permitted to undertake all tasks even though they are licensed. With the realization that licensure should exist by tasks or levels would come the recognition that it is possible to prepare for different levels by using different educational requirements. It should be possible to have lower training requirements for some tasks; as the complexity of the task to be performed increased, so would the training requirements. One would expect, therefore, that the number of entrants would

be greater, the lower the training requirements. If different levels of licensure were to exist, barriers to entry would be lowered and the incomes of practicing physicians would be decreased. Since such an approach to increasing quality among physicians would decrease the monopoly power of physicians, we would therefore expect the AMA to oppose reexamination and licensure by task.

The emphasis on quality control in medicine is on the "process" of becoming a physician and not on the care that is provided ("outcome") once a person has become a physician. Controlling quality and competency of physicians through process measures which require an undergraduate education, four years of education in an approved medical school, a minimum of three years in residency, and, throughout this period, a series of examinations, is consistent with constructing barriers to entry and raising training costs, which thereby lower the entering physician's rate of return. Once the physician has met all of these requirements, then there is no monitoring of the care he or she provides. Physicians may be well trained at at least one point in time, but this does not mean that they will be ethical. A number of studies document the amount of "unnecessary" surgery; other studies show that more than one-half of all surgery is undertaken by unethical or unqualified practitioners. Virtually no quality control programs have been instituted by the medical profession that are directed toward practicing physicians. It was for precisely this reason that Congress passed the Professional Standards Review Organizations (PSROs) legislation in an attempt to develop peer review mechanisms to monitor the quality of care provided by physicians. The AMA opposed this legislation. If the medical profession were concerned primarily with quality rather than with monopoly power, then one would expect that there would be at least some emphasis on the quality of care provided by practicing physicians.

Requiring citizenship for licensure, as a number of states did (it is now unconstitutional), is another example of the use of entry barriers to becoming a physician to achieve monopoly power instead of promoting quality. If a prospective physician has met all the educational and licensure requirements, then a citizenship requirement can *only* be viewed as a means of preventing entry into the profession by foreign-trained physicians. Although the quality of foreign-trained physicians varies greatly, examinations and other procedures, such as monitoring of care, would be more direct and accurate measures of quality than whether or not the individual is a U.S. citizen.

Similar to the citizenship requirement is the requirement by some professional associations (e.g., state dental associations) of residency in a state before the individual is permitted to practice. A year's residency is imposed on dentists who wish to locate in Hawaii. Such a requirement, in forcing the practitioner to be without income for a year, decreases the attractiveness of locating in that particular location. Such a barrier to entry is unrelated to quality, since it does not differentiate among the educational or performance backgrounds of the individuals wishing to locate there. It is solely a device to enhance the monopoly power of the practicing professionals in that location.

It would appear, therefore, that the concern of the medical profession (as well as of other health professions) with quality is selective. Quality measures that might adversely affect the incomes of their members are opposed, such as reexamination, relicensing, continuing education, and any measures that attempt to monitor the quality of care delivered. The hypothesis that quality measures are instituted to raise the rate of return of practicing physicians appears to be consistent with the positions on quality taken by the medical profession.

It has been claimed that the selective approach to quality favored by the medical profession may have served to actually *lower* the quality of care available to the U.S. population (7). Once entry into a profession is restricted, there is an increase in the growth and use of substitutes for that profession. As entry into medicine is restricted, substitutes for medicine such as chiropractic and faith healers are used.

With higher prices for physician services, people also substitute self-diagnosis and treatment for the physician's services. Some of these alternatives may be of lower quality than if the restrictions on medicine were lower. Fewer, more highly trained physicians means that a smaller percentage of the population will have access to medical care. If only physicians are permitted to perform a number of tasks, even though other trained personnel might be equally capable of performing them, this will again mean that a smaller percentage of the population will have access to such services. A relevant measure

of the quality of care in society should not be confined to the care received by only those persons receiving physician services; it should also incorporate the size of the population that does not receive any (or much fewer) physician services or use poorer substitutes.*

The current system of medical licensure, with its attendant requirements and emphasis on entry into the profession, imposes certain "costs" on society. The presumed successes of such a system of licensure in protecting consumers against unethical and incompetent practitioners are uncertain. What is desirable is the least costly system for alleviating consumer uncertainty and for meeting society's demand for protection. Several proposals in this regard will be discussed at the conclusion of this article.

THE PHYSICIAN AS A PRICE-DISCRIMINATING MONOPOLIST

(Editor's Note: Here Feldstein focuses on the motives of physicians as relates to the cost to the public of their services. First, he looks at the fact that physicians price discriminate—that is, charge different prices to persons of varying abilities to pay—and weighs two alternatives hypotheses as to why price discrimination exists. Hypothesis one is that physicians are price-discriminating monopolists who wish to exact as much profit as possible from those most able to pay. A second hypothesis is that in price discrimination physicians are acting charitably by charging the affluent more in order to be able to provide care for those with less ability to pay. Feldstein provides evidence which results in his rejecting the notion that the pricing of services by physicians is done for charitable reasons.)

---

* Milton Friedman also states that quality has been adversely affected because there is less experimentation in treatment, which tends to reduce the rate of growth in medical knowledge, since a person desiring to experiment in treatment must be a member of the medical profession. The profession also encourages conformity in medical practice. The medical profession has also discouraged malpractice suits against physicians by discouraging physicians from testifying against one another. This action has also limited the consumer's protection against unethical and incompetent practitioners. The possibility of high malpractice awards against them would discourage incompetent practitioners from practicing, thereby providing protection to future patients.

In his classic article entitled "Price Discrimination in Medicine," Reuben Kessel claimed that control over physician pricing behavior was related to the AMA's control over medical education (8). The AMA's control over postgraduate medical training and control over which physicians may take specialty board exams was the source of its control over physicians.

Internship and residency programs are offered only in hospitals approved by the AMA. Physicians want the hospitals they are associated with to be approved for such programs, since interns and residents increase the physician's productivity and income; the availability of interns and residents in a hospital frees up a physician's time both to see more patients and to have more leisure time. Interns and residents are thus demanded by physicians. The hospital pays the salaries of interns and residents, and the physicians receive the benefits of their services as they care for the physicians' patients in the hospital. The Mundt resolution, which was declared unconstitutional in the mid-1960s, required that the entire attending medical staff in the hospital be members in the county medical society if the hospital were to be approved for intern and residency training. Membership in the county medical society thus became important to physicians if they wished to have the hospital privileges which are a necessity for almost all specialties of medicine. Similarly, membership in the county society was a prerequisite for a physician to take examinations for various specialty boards. If a physician engaged in any form of competitive behavior which was branded "unethical," the county medical society, which determines its own rules for membership, could deny such a physician membership in the society and thereby deny hospital privileges.

Those physicians who potentially offer the greatest threat to the existence of price discrimination are new physicians in the community. To establish a market, new firms must advertise their availability, competence, and specialty, and they also must offer lower prices to attract consumers away from established firms. To prevent such competitive behavior from occurring, county medical societies gave new physicians probationary membership. If the new physician engaged in any of the above "unethical" activities to become established in the community, the county medical society would revoke membership and thereby deny hospital privileges to that physician. Probationary status was granted, not just to recent graduates, but also to physicians who had been in practice for a long time in another area (and were members of another county medical society) and had recently moved into the community.

More recently, the sanctions available to the medical societies for use against physicians who wish to compete on price have been state laws which delegate authority to medical licensing boards to determine the conditions for medical licensure. Included in such state laws were severe penalties for advertising and fee splitting. Although the mechanism for inhibiting price competition among physicians has shifted from control over hospital privileges by county medical societies to state laws which prohibit such behavior, the effect has been the same. Strong sanctions and penalties were available to organized medicine (which may be viewed in this instance as a cartel) to inhibit price competition, which would have eroded the physician's ability to price-discriminate.

What is the evidence to support the price-discrimination hypothesis of physician pricing? Does the evidence indicate that the foregoing sanctions were consistently imposed on physicians who attempted to engage in price competition rather than imposed for "quality" reasons? The AMA's position with regard to health insurance is the first evidence Kessel examines in his test of the price-discrimination hypothesis. Insurance coverage to pay for physician services would generally be favored by physicians, since it increased both the demand for physician services and the patient's ability to pay for those services. Health insurance varies with regard to the manner in which the physician is reimbursed. Indemnity plans reimburse the patient a certain dollar amount and allow the physician to charge the patient whatever he or she believes the patient can pay. Such plans are the most conducive to price discrimination by physicians. Health insurance plans that guarantee medical services rather than dollars if the consumer becomes ill would be opposed by the medical profession because they are sold at the same price to consumers regardless of their incomes. Such plans are a form of price competition, since a person with a high income can purchase the same medical services at the same price as could a person with a low income. If the charity hypothesis were the more accurate explanation of physician pricing behavior, then medical societies would not be expected to oppose such plans. The only conceivable reason for the medical profession's opposition to such medical service plans is that they undercut the ability of physicians to price-discriminate in the communities where such plans exist. Examples of such medical service plans are prepaid group practices (PPGPs) where the consumer pays a yearly capitation fee, regardless of family income, and is then entitled both to hospital and medical services when ill. It is interesting, therefore, to examine the sanctions that local medical societies have applied to prevent the development of PPGPs.

The opposition mounted by organized medicine against PPGPs was unaffected by the location of these plans or their sponsorship. The first type of sanction aimed at putting such plans out of business was to deny the physicians associated with them hospital privileges. If the physician was already a member of the county medical society, the medical society would disband and reestablish itself without including the particular physician. New physicians entering the area with the intention of joining a PPGP in the community would not be permitted to join the county medical society. Whether or not a PPGP had its own hospital determined whether it was able to survive. It is for this reason that Kaiser Foundation, a well-known PPGP on the West Coast, operated its own hospitals; otherwise, it could not have offered hospital care to its subscribers and would not have been able to compete. The county medical societies tried other tactics against the Kaiser Foundation. The State Board of Medical Examiners in California tried Dr. Garfield, the medical director of Kaiser, for unprofessional conduct and suspended his license to practice. In subsequent legal rulings the suspension was overruled; the board's action was considered arbitrary in that Dr. Garfield did not have a fair trial.

Another approach used by the medical societies to inhibit the development of PPGPs was to have a higher proportion of physicians who belonged to PPGPs drafted during World War II. (The medical society played a strong role with regard to the drafting of physicians at that time.) A number of physicians serving during World War II were unable to qualify as officers in the Navy and had to serve as enlisted men because they could not obtain a let-

ter from their county medical society stating that they were members in good standing. These physicians believed they were discriminated against because they were associated with PPGPs. In other instances where the local medical societies ousted physicians belonging to PPGPs, successful lawsuits were brought against the medical societies under the Sherman Anti-Trust Act (9).

In addition to attempting to terminate PPGPs through the use of sanctions against physicians associated with them, medical societies attempted to legislate them out of business. State medical societies sponsored legislation in many states, and were successful in more than 20 of them, which placed restrictions on PPGPs, thereby inhibiting their growth. Such restrictive statutes permitted only the medical profession to operate or to control prepaid medical plans. (Federal legislation on health maintenance organizations specifically preempted such restrictive statutes if the HMO qualified under the federal HMO law.)

Another example of the medical profession's interest in maintaining the physician's ability to price-discriminate among patients is the type of medical insurance plan favored by organized medicine. Blue Shield plans, which were developed and controlled by state medical societies, offered physician coverage to consumers under the following terms: if a subscriber's income was less than a certain amount, generally $7,500 a year, then the participating physician would accept the Blue Shield fee as full payment for services provided to the patient; however, if the patient's income was in excess of the stated amount, then the physician could bill the patient an amount in excess of the Blue Shield fee for that service. The medical profession favored Blue Shield because physicians would be assured of payment from low-income subscribers and would still be able to price-discriminate among higher-income subscribers. If the physicians were charitable agencies, then they would not need to charge higher-income patients an additional amount once the lower-income patient was able to pay the full fee for their services. Some medical societies have recently dropped their sponsorship of Blue Shield plans because the plans wished to raise the income limits below which the Blue Shield fee would represent full payment for the patient's use of physician services.

Additional evidence that the charity hypothesis

is inapplicable to explain physician pricing behavior is provided in the following statement by Kessel:

> Most of the "free" care that was traditionally provided by the medical profession fell into three categories: (1) work done by neophytes, particularly in the surgical specialties, who wanted to develop their skills and therefore require practice; (2) services of experienced physicians in free clinics who wish to develop new skills or maintain existing skills so they can better serve their private, paying patients; and (3) services to maintain staff and medical appointments which are of great value financially. The advent of Medicare has reduced the availability of "charity" patients used as teaching material, and has led to readjustments in training procedures, particularly for residents. (10)

The sanctions available to the medical profession to prevent price competition have changed over time. Advertising can no longer be prohibited by state practice acts. That the medical profession had been successful in inhibiting price competition is evidenced by the recently successful suit brought by the Federal Trade Commission (FTC) against the AMA and several medical specialty societies. The FTC claimed that the AMA's "Principles of Medical Ethics," which banned advertising, price competition, and other forms of competitive practices, resulted in a situation in which "prices of physician services have been stabilized, fixed, or otherwise interfered with; competition between medical doctors in the provision of such services has been hindered, restrained, foreclosed and frustrated; and consumers have been deprived of information pertinent to the selection of a physician and of the benefits of competition" (11).

The medical profession, then, has been successful in acting in the economic interest of its members. The continually high rates of return to an investment in a medical education and the excess of applicants to acceptances in medical schools are evidence that there has been a static shortage of physicians. To ensure monopoly profits over time, the medical profession has constructed barriers to entry into the profession. Under the guise of controlling quality of care and eliminating unqualified professionals the medical profession emphasized "process" measures of quality control. Quality assurance was present only at the point of entry into the profession by means of requiring attendance at an approved medical school, licensure examinations, and longer minimum times spent in postgraduate training programs; virtually no quality control measures were directed at practicing physicians.

With the authority delegated to it by the state, the medical profession was then able to go beyond establishing a simple monopoly. The medical profession, acting as a cartel to protect the economic interests of its members, was able to establish and enforce the necessary conditions to enable physicians to price-discriminate among their patients. The sanctions used by the medical profession against members who participated in prepaid medical plans were severe enough to retard the development of such organizations for many years. The consequences to society of these actions by organized medicine are that prices of medical services are higher than they would otherwise be, the availability of such services is lower, and, importantly, consumers are not as well protected from unqualified and unethical practitioners as they have been led to believe.

PROPOSED CHANGES IN THE PHYSICIAN MANPOWER MARKET

The objective of proposing changes in the market for physicians is twofold: first, the demand for consumer protection should be achieved in the least costly manner possible, and second, the market for physicians should perform efficiently. The key to improving market performance is to deal first with the concern for consumer protection.

Entry into the Medical Profession

If a prospective physician can pass the licensing examination, it is not clear why he or she also has to have attended an approved medical school to be licensed. The only logical reason for also requiring attendance at an approved medical school is that the licensing examination is not a sufficient assurance of the physician's knowledge. If this is the case, then the examination process should be improved and less emphasis placed on the number of years of education required and on attendance at approved schools.

A second approach to lowering the cost of licensure, while also achieving a certain performance level of entering physicians, is to have "task" licensure. Currently physicians are either licensed or they are not, and, once licensed, they are permitted to undertake many tasks, the full scope of medical practice, a number of which they might not be well trained for, such as in the case of the family practitioner who performs general surgery. Instead of such a "zero–one" level of licensure, physicians should be licensed to perform specific tasks. Such task or specific-purpose licenses would recognize what exists in the real world; namely, even though physicians are licensed, the public would be better protected if they performed only those tasks which they are qualified to perform. Task licensure would mean that all physicians would not need to take the same educational training; it might be possible to provide alternative levels of training (or train certain types of physicians) in a much shorter period, which would lower the costs of producing them, since both their educational and opportunity costs would be reduced. If physicians wanted to receive additional specific-purpose licenses, they could return to school to receive additional training before taking the licensure examination for that license. (In this way a career ladder could be developed for medicine.) Under such a proposal, the training requirements to enter the medical profession would not be determined by the medical profession itself but would be related to the *demand* for different types of physicians and the least costly manner of producing them.

Continuing Assurance of the Quality of Physician Services

As discussed earlier, beyond the licensing of a physician the medical profession undertakes virtually no quality assurance mechanisms. Several proposals to deal with the issue of unethical and unqualified physicians should be considered. First, periodic reexamination and relicensure would require physicians to keep up with their field of practice. Rather than mandating a certain number of hours of continuing education, reexamination would determine the appropriate amount of continuing education on an individual basis. It would also be a more direct measure of whether or not the physician has achieved the objectives of continuing education. Periodic reexami-

nation and relicensure would be consistent with the earlier proposal of task or "specific-purpose" licensure.

If physicians were reexamined and relicensed every few years for specific-purpose licenses, we would have greater assurance that physicians were practicing in the fields of medicine for which they were qualified. There would still be a concern, however, regarding the physician who may be qualified but is unethical in performing services that are not needed and in charging for services not performed. Continual monitoring of the care provided by physicians, with a state agency taking responsibility (with the cooperation of the medical profession), would help to ensure that a minimum of unethical and unqualified actions were undertaken. Penalties assessed by state quality review agencies should be financial and should vary according to the severity of the misbehavior. Penalties that remove or suspend the physician's license are usually considered to be so severe that they are rarely undertaken. Financial penalties would be more likely to be imposed for actions that are not sufficiently flagrant to call for removal of the physician's license but are in need of redress.

Another approach that was developed to safeguard consumers is recourse to the courts, but because malpractice premiums have risen so rapidly recently, proposals have been made to remove the threat of malpractice. Suggestions have been made that the government should pay malpractice premiums for those physicians participating in government programs such as Medicare and Medicaid. The desired effect of such a proposal is to increase physician participation in government medical programs; however, it would negate the relationship between physicians' performance and their malpractice premiums. There are problems associated with the current system of malpractice, such as the uncertainty of future awards, but it would be preferable to improve the current malpractice system rather than do away with it. A well-functioning malpractice system would serve as an incentive to physicians to confine themselves to tasks they are qualified to perform (12).

Now that advertising among physicians and other health professions has been made possible as a result of the FTC action, consumers should begin to have access to greater information on physician qualifications, fees, and availability. One other reform that would improve the performance of the medical profession is to allow productivity increases to occur independent of the permission of the medical profession. Productivity increases through the use of physician's assistants and other paraprofessionals would increase the supply of physician services at a lower cost and in a shorter period than if all tasks had to be performed by highly trained physicians with training requirements in excess of those required for competency. Such productivity increases, occurring at a time of increased supply of physicians, would be strongly resisted by organized medicine. Some physicians will have excess capacity while other physicians will seek to expand their services by employing nonphysician personnel.

Advertising and unlimited productivity increases should create a competitive atmosphere among physicians that should improve the level of consumer protection while increasing the availability of physician services and lowering prices. In conjunction with these proposals, permitting the corporate practice of medicine through HMOs and PPGPs and experimenting with the concept of institutional responsibility for quality of care should result in far-reaching changes leading to improvement in the organization and delivery of medical care.

References

1. Thomas G. Moore, "The Purpose of Licensing," *Journal of Law and Economics,* October 1961.

2. Reuben Kessel, "Price Discrimination in Medicine," *Journal of Law and Economics,* October 1958, pp. 25–26.

3. Milton Friedman, *Capitalism and Freedom* (Chicago: The University of Chicago Press, 1962), p. 151.

4. Kessel, "Price Discrimination," p. 27.

5. *Ibid.*

6. This aspect of licensing board behavior is discussed in Simon Rottenberg, "Economics of Occupational Licensing," in *Aspects of Labor Economics,* National Bureau of Economic Research (Princeton, N.J.: Princeton University Press, 1962).

7. Friedman, *Capitalism and Freedom,* pp. 155–158.

8. Kessel, "Price Discrimination," p. 29.

9. This example of Group Health Association in Washington, D.C., and the other examples cited are from Kessel, "Price Discrimination," pp. 30–41.

10. Reuben Kessel, "The AMA and the Supply of Physicians," *Law and Contemporary Problems* (Chapel Hill, N.C.: Duke University Press, 1970), p. 273.

11. United States of America Before Federal Trade Commission in the Matter of the American Medical Association, a corporation, The Connecticut State Medical Society, a corporation, The New Haven County Medical Association, Inc., Docket No. 9064, p. 3, December 1975.

12. For some readings on malpractice, see: Simon Rottenberg, ed., *The Economics of Medical Malpractice* (Washington, D.C.: American Enterprise Institute for Public Policy Research, 1978). Also see: William B. Schwartz and Neil K. Komesar, *Doctors, Damages and Deterrence: An Economic View of Medical Malpractice,* Rand Corporation Publication, R-2340-NIH/RC, June 1978; and Clark C. Havighurst, "Medical Adversity Insurance—Has Its Time Come?," *Duke Law Journal* 6 (1975).

Gender, Professionalization, and Occupational Anomie: The Case of Nursing

Howard D. Schwartz
Peggy L. deWolf
James K. Skipper, Jr.

A common observation in the literature on occupational stratification concerns the prestige of Soviet physicians. Members of that profession in the Soviet Union—75 percent of whom are female—are accorded a rank similar to that of school teachers and social workers in the United States. What this tells us, in a comparative perspective, is that gender has great impact on the prestige of an occupation and, consequently, on the relative rewards received by its members.

In the United States, one of the occupational categories most affected by gender has been that of the "female semiprofessions," a designation that refers to the four occupations of school teacher, social worker, librarian, and nurse. Table 1, which presents the percentages of women in each of the four female semiprofessions, shows that they have been, and still are, dominated by women.

The link between the "professional marginality" of the semiprofessions and gender is summarized by Ritzer and Walczak (1986) as follows:

> Put in simplest terms, males have won the most prestigious, powerful, and highest paying established professions for themselves and have relegated females with professional aspirations to the less prestigious, less powerful, and less paying semiprofessions. In other words, the existence of male-dominated professions and female-dominated semiprofessions is illustrative of a patriarchal society. [p. 238]

This is an original article written for this edition of *Dominant Issues in Medical Sociology*.

The final sentence represents a recognition that "male and female professions are stratified on the occupational continuum according to how the sexes are ranked in the society" (Ritzer and Walczak, 1986, p. 239). Given this fact, questions arise as to if and how the current women's movement in America is influencing the status of the female semiprofessions.

The focus in this paper is on only one of the female semiprofessions—the one that has, perhaps, been the most prominent in attempting to recast its self-image. Nursing was once anathema to the feminist movement. According to four nurses, all prominent observers of the nursing scene, "nursing has been seen as one of the ultimate ghettos from which women should be encouraged to escape" (Vance et al., 1985, p. 282). The same authors go on to say that although

> nursing has not always embraced feminist ideology [feminist is used here to refer to advocating the same rights for women accorded men, particularly in the areas of economics and politics] . . . more and more nurses are identifying with feminist goals. They are beginning to view their profession as an important career, rather than seeing it as simply preparation for marriage and motherhood. [p. 282]

Nursing schools are teaching not only about nursing but also about its relationship with "womanpower." For example, many baccalaureate nursing programs assign the highest priority to courses in nursing leadership. Students learn that they are no longer to acquiesce to the "handmaiden" image that has defined physicians' reactions to them in the past.

TABLE 1   Female semiprofessions: 1972 and 1982 (% female)

YEAR	LIBRARIANS*	NURSES (REGISTERED)	SOCIAL WORKERS**	ELEMENTARY SCHOOL TEACHERS
1972	82%***	98%	55%	85%
1982	81	96	66	82

* Also includes archivists and curators.

** Also includes recreation workers.

*** Percentages are rounded.

Source: U.S. Bureau of the Census, *Statistical Abstract of the United States,* 104th ed. (Washington, D.C., 1983), p. 419.

They are exposed to the details of their relative deprivation, such as the fact that whereas nurses have one-half the education of physicians they get about one-fifth the pay, and are urged to be more demanding in the marketplace.

Just as the feminist movement in America has accelerated dramatically in the last two decades, so has nursing been undergoing a pronounced period of professionalization within the same short period. The rapidity of this change—and the eminent sociologist Emile Durkheim (1951) might well have predicted this—has resulted in a condition of "occupation anomie" in which the contemporary nurse is being exposed to differing, if not competing, definitions of what a nurse should be and what the appropriate domain of her or his activity should encompass.

NURSING PAST AND PRESENT: THE FLIGHT FROM PROFESSIONAL BONDAGE

The role of nurse as "handmaiden," or at best "technical assistant," to the physician parallels the traditional role of the wife as "handmaiden" to her husband. It goes back to the very beginning of nursing when it was created by Florence Nightingale in the mid-nineteenth century during the Crimean War. The development of nursing was vigorously opposed by the all-male medical corps, who considered the idea of female health care providers of this kind a violation of social norms regarding appropriate behavior for women.

In the face of this adversity, Nightingale achieved her mission by allowing nursing to be subordinated to the authority and direction of the medical profession. Ironically, while this tactic was successful in circumventing established medicine's resistance to a professional female nursing corps, it left a legacy of dependency on medicine that continues to plague nursing to this day.

Well past the turn of the century, graduates of nursing schools were primarily employed outside the hospital as private duty nurses. Some have viewed private duty nursing as an indicator of professional autonomy and have seen in the decline of the private duty nurse a "proletarianization" of nursing, resulting in a weakening of its claim to professional status (Wagner, 1980). Yet, as Reverby (1986) notes, private duty nurses "were still expected to kowtow and cover for the physicians and their mistakes" (p. 189). Elaborating on the nurse's subordinate position, she states:

> Dr. William L. Richardson, for example, told the graduating class at the Boston Training School for Nurses on June 18, 1886, to "always be loyal to the physician." He warned them not to be "tempted" to impress the doctor with their knowledge because "what error can be more stupid?" Although the private duty nurse was technically working "independently," she was in fact dependent on the physicians for her reputation and often for her actual case loads. The difference in the situation for nurses and physicians was clearly reflected in the language used to describe their respective positions: a doctor out on his own was in private practice, the nurse was working on private duty. [p. 189]

Historically, the use of nurses in hospitals also reveals a process through which the nursing role was subordinated to the roles of the physician and administrator. At first, student nurses provided most of the nursing care in American hospitals. For a variety of reasons, nursing students were easier to dominate than nursing graduates. During the depression, when most individuals had little money to employ private duty nurses, that type of nursing went into a permanent decline. In addition to the economic misfortunes of the country, an oversupply of nurses resulted in a high proportion of private duty nurses desiring hospital work. Hospitals were at first reluctant to employ a substantial number of graduate nurses (as opposed to nursing students). In 1927, a questionnaire was sent to 500 supervisors asking about which type of worker they preferred: 76 percent wanted students whereas only 24 percent wanted graduate nurses. The fear of employing nurses who were accustomed to their independence in their work was explicit in the statement of one nursing supervisor who rejected the use of graduate nurses on the grounds that ". . . they find even kindly direction irksome" (Reverby, 1986, p. 192).

In the end, graduate nurses were employed in the hospital, but the nursing role was subordinated within the hospital hierarchy. A major strategy for doing this was to separate the nurse from her potential source of power—the paying patient. The nurse's relationship with the patient became more and more dictated by and limited by hospital rules and regulations. As late as the 1950s, deference to physicians was still a major dictum of the socialization process undergone by student nurses. Wessen, in a study of a large New England hospital, noted that nursing instructors in a course entitled "Professional Adjustment" would teach deference to physicians because they are older than the nursing students and "contribute more to the community than [they] will" (Wessen, 1972, p. 321).

Initiatives to develop teamwork and a more collegial relationship between physicians and nurses have been generally unsuccessful due in large part to the lack of commitment of physicians. A recent report concerning interdisciplinary teamwork at a large medical center and teaching hospital, considered to be highly supportive of the concept, found that the physician on the team continues to view himself as the "Lone Ranger" as far as diagnosis and treatment is concerned. In addition, physicians view teamwork as a nursing concept being used to "usurp" the traditional authority of medicine in health care provision (Temkin-Greener, 1983).

Obviously, as others point out, many physicians continue to see nurses as their inferiors and subordinates. However, this is not true of all physicians. There are indications that younger physicians are more adaptable to a colleague-oriented view of nurses than are older ones. Some prominent medical journals, such as the *Journal of the American Medical Association,* have included articles by physicians exhorting the medical profession to reconsider its traditional stance toward the nurse as "handmaiden" (e.g., Berman, 1981).

For its part, the nursing profession has been subsumed, along with many other women's groups, within the women's movement. A comparison of contemporary courses on nursing leadership with those of the past dealing with the proper decorum for women certainly bears this out. In fact, politicized nursing graduates of today face a reality shock when they find a gap between the view of the highly professional, independent nurse promoted in nursing school and the realities of hospital life that they face on their first encounter with the real world. As evidenced in the turmoil surrounding the "nursing shortage" days of 1981, nurses are no longer willing to accept limitations on what they perceive as an extended role for nursing.

Several current studies suggest a considerable change in the perception that nurses have of themselves. Among the most interesting is one carried out by Rank and Jacobsen, the results of which were reported in 1977. The study involved an experiment in which an assistant, using the name of a little known staff surgeon at the hospital with his permission, telephoned 18 nurses who were on duty and ordered them to administer a nonlethal overdose of Valium to appropriate patients. (Safeguards were taken to insure that no dosage was actually administered to a patient.) Of the 18 subject-nurses, 16 refused to administer the Valium. One nurse said, "Whew! 30 mg.—he (the doctor) doesn't want to sedate her (the patient)—he wants to knock her out" (Rank and Jacobsen, 1977, p. 191). The authors suggest that the high rate of noncompliance was due principally to an increased willingness among hospital personnel to challenge a doctor's orders within the contemporary medical system and to the rising self-esteem of nurses. What is particularly significant to the present argument is that an earlier study, published a little over a decade before, found that 21 out of 22 nurses were willing to give such an overdose (Hofing, 1966).

Perhaps the strongest evidence of a significant effort on the part of nursing to raise its occupational status is the existence of a clearly defined process of professionalization. It is to a discussion of this process that the remainder of this paper will be devoted.

THE PROFESSIONALIZATION OF NURSING

Several attributes have been identified with an occupation's gaining professional status. They are (1) a service orientation, (2) control over the determination of standards and training, (3) a practice regulated by licensure, (4) a code of ethics, (5) a professional organization, (6) a prolonged period of specialized training, and (7) a distinct body of knowledge (Goode, 1960; Greenwood, 1966).[1] It is in regard to the latter two characteristics that nursing, in aspiring to full professional status, has been most lacking. Not suprisingly, then, a key strategy in the professionalization process relates to eliminating these deficits. In addition, still another initiative relates to extending nursing's boundaries into the domain of medicine.

Raising the Minimum Level of Education for the Registered Nurse: The Baccalaureate Degree Requirement

The educational degree proposal concerning the requirement of a baccalaureate degree (graduation from a four-year college with a Bachelor of Science in Nursing degree) evolved from the American Nurses' Association's (ANA) own 1965 resolution that the BSN be the minimal requirement for registered nurses by 1985. It is important to note that the push for this came from the leadership of the profession and not from the membership, the majority of whom had less than bachelor's degrees. In 1986, the first two states to do so, Maine and North Dakota, adopted the BSN requirement. And throughout the country, many nurses, anticipating that the BSN will become the minimal "union card" for a

job, are returning to school to get it. At the same time, the number of three-year hospital-related diploma schools is declining rapidly.

Traditionally, American nursing has had three avenues of access: the two-year associate degree from community colleges, the three-year hospital diploma program, and the four-year baccalaureate degree. Each avenue has had different time investments as well as different levels of orientation to clinical practice, yet each has served as a legitimate route to the status of registered nurse. It is this diversity—some may say confusion—of pathways to nursing practice that has contributed to the failure of nursing to achieve full professional status. In the words of Stevens (1985), "No field in the history of this country has achieved professional status outside of traditional academic structures" (p. 124); that is, without limiting all training to the confines of traditional four-year colleges and universities.

The "1985" push for raising the minimal educational standard for RNs reflects a naturally occurring trend in the direction of more formal education among nursing graduates over the past 20 years. In 1961, 83.6 percent of those entering the field did so via the hospital diploma route. By 1981–82, their proportion had diminished to a scant 15.8 percent. In contrast, there has been a surge in the number of students entering nursing from associate and baccalaureate degree programs. In 1961, these programs together accounted for only 16.4 percent of nurses entering the field. In 1981–82, 84.2 percent were coming from these programs (Cockerham, 1986). In sum, whereas hospital diploma nurses prevailed as entrants to nursing in 1961, holders of associate and bachelors degrees prevail in the 1980s.

The implications of raising the minimal educational level of nursing to that of the BSN degree are far reaching. It represents an effort to buoy nursing's professional status through a newly-defined hierarchy based on education. In the future, it is likely that professional nurse status will be accorded only those with a BSN degree. The practical or technical nurse with an associate or hospital degree will probably be accorded the lower status of associate nurse. Eventually, the three-year hospital programs will probably be phased out entirely.

In the preceding article in this chapter of *Dominant Issues*, Feldstein argues that increased barriers into medicine, including an extended period of training, derive more from professional self-interest than from concern with public-interest (see also Freidson, 1970). The same is true of nursing's drive to institute a baccalaureate degree requirement. Dolan (1978) makes it clear that the elevated educational requirements did not evolve from any recognized problem in the quality of care provided by those with less than a BSN degree. In fact, he notes that in one poll, hospital heads of nursing were of the opinion that it is the more academically trained baccalaureate nurses who are emerging from training deficient in some aspects of primary patient care.

That the aim of educational reform is, first and foremost, a mechanism for status enhancement is brought out further by a strikingly revealing article that appeared in *Nursing Outlook* (cited from previously) that was written by a leading figure in the movement to professionalize nursing. Noting that the increased education of nurses may not be cost effective for consumers of health care, the author writes, "[F]irst, what is best for nursing may or may not coincide with what is best for society at large" (Stevens, 1985). She then goes on to the main thrust of her argument concerning the advantages of the BSN minimal requirement with reference to the New York State debate over the issue, known in brief as "1985":

> The debate on "1985" has tended to focus on the BSN as a professional degree which represents a general upgrading of the nursing discipline. Nursing can be compared with other fields for an historical perspective. A master's degree is required for social work or speech pathology. A bachelor's degree is required for physical therapists, pharmacists, and occupational therapists. However, a non-academic program of studies will suffice for a position as dental hygienist or masseuse.
>
> No field in the history of this country has achieved full professional status outside of traditional academic structures and there is no reason to assume that nursing is so powerful or so profound as to achieve this status outside the system. In that sense, "1985" is essential if nursing is to be recognized as a profession by society at large. If nurses want their discipline—or some portion of it—to be accorded professional status

> by society, nursing must pay its academic dues. [*Stevens, 1985, p. 124*]

Should the BSN actually become the legally legislated minimal requirement throughout the country, several questions would need to be addressed. First of all, to what extent do these proposed educational reforms meet the prevailing market conditions for nurses? Are there established employment niches for both professional and technical nurses; that is, will they be in competition for the same jobs, or will one or the other be forced to create a new niche for itself? A related question pertains to the reward system that may or may not be built into the job market. Will there be sufficiently enhanced autonomy, prestige, and salary to pull students to the more rigorous, time-consuming, and costly professional nurse route? Finally, and perhaps most importantly, have curricula been devised so as to justify this bifurcation of the profession? Will professional nurses in fact function at a discernibly different level than so-called technical nurses?

The Development of a Distinct Body of Knowledge

Another key element of a profession that does not yet characterize nursing is its own body of research and theory. In the case of nursing, this refers to research and theory that is distinct from that of medicine. Once again, a key ingredient in the motivation to correct this deficiency is the desire for professional status. In an article appearing in *Nursing Research*, entitled "Development of Theory: A Requisite for Nursing as a Primary Health Profession," a leading nurse–researcher writes, "If nursing is indeed an emerging profession, nurses must be able to identify clearly and develop continually the theoretical body of knowledge upon which practice must rest" (Johnson, 1974, p. 372). Even more strident is the following statement, which places the issue in a feminist context:

> Nursing can no longer exist in the shadows of medicine but must become an entity in its own right. It is time that nursing move away from its sexist self-identity problem and begin to assume full responsibility and authority as an equal participant in the health care arena. This can only be achieved through the authority of

knowledge and through scholarly discipline, coupled with a clear sense of history and purpose. [*Grace, 1978, p. 122*]

A content analysis of articles in nursing journals over the last 25 years would no doubt show a great increase in those dealing with the lowly but improving state of the present knowledge base and the pressing need for the development of sophisticated and rigorously scientific research and theory. Perhaps, the greatest indication of the fact that the development of a knowledge base in nursing is now only in its infancy is the fact that so many articles deal with the process of research and theory development per se. How to do research or what theory should be are as much a focus of the literature as are specific studies. Issues dealt with range from the more general ones to the more pedestrian, such as how to assign credits for collaborative research.

To some extent, as already indicated, research and theory building are viewed, in and of themselves, as important since they are preconditions for professional status. But there is also recognition that knowledge so developed must be seen by outsiders as having some practical application at the level of the practicing nurse.[2] Evidence of this can be found in the creation of nursing diagnosis, a combination of nomenclature and definitions of appropriate nursing actions, the teaching of which is now found in many BSN programs.

Nursing diagnosis is an attempt to bring nursing knowledge to bear on defining what it is that separates nursing and medical care of patients. It is thereby also an attempt to separate nursing from the past, when both nurses and doctors employed the diagnostic language and models of the latter.

Given its very short history, the definition of nursing diagnosis is still unclear. As one writer puts it, "Nurses vary in their opinions as to what constitutes the essential feature of nursing diagnosis. Their definitions of a diagnosis vary from stating it is a symptom, or a need, or a problem, to a concern and/or a prescription. In addition, other nurses interchange the terms *needs, problems,* and *concerns*" (Soares, 1978, p. 270). Notwithstanding this ambiguity, nursing seems to have arrived at some relative degree of consensus about the difference between nursing and medical diagnosis. Medical diagnosis can be considered as "comprising a statement about the pathological state of a person's anatomical structure and/or pathological organ functioning that can be alleviated or corrected by surgery or pharmacodynamics" (Soares, 1978, p. 270). In short, it looks at the underlying, medically-defined nature of the problem. Nursing diagnosis, on the other hand, looks at the symptoms of an illness and how these might be managed on a moment-to-moment, day-to-day basis. Table 2 distinguishes between the medical and nursing diagnosis in relation to a patient in a diabetic coma.

TABLE 2 Medical and nursing diagnoses

	NORMAL CRITERIA	ABNORMAL FINDINGS	MEDICAL DIAGNOSIS	APPROPRIATE ACTION
Medicine	Pancreatic structure and physiological function	Deterioration of beta cells of Langferhan and inability to produce insulin and metabolize carbohydrates with resulting acidosis	Diabetic coma	Administration of insulin
Nursing	Balanced circadian rhythm in rest/ wake patterns	Disruption in rest/ wake pattern; inability to sleep	Altered state of consciousness	Helping patient to breathe, eat, etc.

Source: Adapted from Soares, 1978, p. 271.

Of all the nursing functions, diagnosis may rely most greatly on clinical specialists; that is, those specializing in an area of nursing frequently associated with the use of high technology. (The articles in Part III of *Dominant Issues* concerning high technology in the hospital setting deal with the clinical specialist nurse.) The technology provides them with a distinguishable identity within the context of the team concept that is so central to high-technology medicine as found in, for example, the neonatal intensive care unit.

The growth of theory and research in nursing is tied to the increased number of nurses getting advanced degrees, particularly doctorates. In 1959, there were less than 150 practicing nurses who had earned doctoral degrees. Under the sponsorship of various governmental programs and incentives in the 1960s and 1970s, the number increased to approximately 1000 by 1973 (Pitel and Vian, 1975). By 1977, there were over 2000 practicing nurses with doctoral degrees, of which a little over 1000 were Ph.D.s in nursing (Roth et al., 1977). The number of doctoral degrees continued to increase to over 4000 by 1980 (U.S. Department of Health and Human Services, 1982).

These nurses with advanced credentials now comprise the emergent leadership within nursing. The profession's recognition of this new leadership is illustrated by the name change that occurred in the prominent nursing journal *Nursing Outlook* in late 1985. In the last issue of that year, the magazine introduced the subtitle *The Journal for and by Nursing Influentials*. An editorial explained the title change in terms of nursing's emergent quest for influence on health care policy. Equally important, the editorial referenced a study of the profiles of identified leaders within the profession: 95 percent were authors of articles, 75 percent were authors of books, and 65 percent were members of editorial boards. What is most significant here is that the criteria used to define leadership is so closely linked to those generating the current knowledge base within nursing.

Congruent with Stevens' observation that professional status cannot be achieved outside of traditional academic settings, a disproportionate amount of research in nursing is being done by academic nurses. Although only about 40 percent of the faculty of schools of nursing with graduate programs engage in research, this relatively small group of individuals has been responsible for an ever increasing body of published reports (Craig, 1985). Perhaps this increase in published reports can best be understood in terms of the rapid growth of nursing journals. Of 44 journals available in 1982 (McCloskey and Swansen, 1982), whose date of origin we were able to determine, 4 predated 1950, 6 were founded during the 1950s, 10 during the 1960s, 22 during the 1970s, and 4 more during the first two years of the 1980s.

Before proceeding to a discussion of the nurse practitioner, a point mentioned earlier must be reaffirmed. The emerging leadership in nursing about whom we have been talking—those with advanced academic degrees, who are often members of college and university faculties—desire that nursing achieve professional status by upgrading within the traditional boundaries of nursing. As discussed in reference to nursing diagnosis, the nursing role in patient care is seen as patient maintenance and concern with the psychosocial needs of the patients, not diagnosis and treatment of the underlying medical problem. Other roles identified as important in nursing's future include home care, public health, and patient advocacy.

The Nurse Practitioner—Enlarging the Boundaries of Nursing

One of the newest roles in nursing is that of the nurse practitioner (NP), commonly referred to in the literature as a "bridge occupation," denoting its perceived intermediate position between medicine and nursing. This occupation developed in the 1960s, with the first NPs being graduated around 1970.

Two important factors during this period were catalysts to the creation of the NP role: the development of physician assistants (PA) programs, beginning with Duke University in 1965, tailored specifically to retrain some of the 30,000 men who had served in the military as medical corpsmen; and a labor force of nurses who had had a hand in running federally subsidized health clinics during the days of the antipoverty programs but were facing unemployment due to federal cutbacks in the late 1960s. The PA role provided a viable model for those nurses who, in the spirit of feminism, sought a new niche in the health care system, and the NP program allowed them to compete for this. It has also been observed that nurses perceived the physician's assistant as encroaching on their territory and that the NP role was developed, in part, as a buffer against this encroachment.

Additionally, the nurse practitioner concept emerged at a time when consumerism in American health care took a more assertive turn. To some, the nurse practitioner has been the answer to the public's demand for a less elitist system of health care that might also help to correct imbalances in health care delivery across communities.

The success of the NP movement is illustrated by the rapid growth in its numbers during the past 10 years. In 1977, there were approximately 8000 trained NPs (Mumford, 1983). In 1984, that number had increased to 15,000 (Backup and Molinaro, 1984). The Congressional Budget Office projects the number to increase to 30,000 by 1990 (Mumford, 1983). In addition, there have been no documented cases of litigation against NPs by clients, and reports of client satisfaction have been uniformly positive. Several studies have suggested that NPs are perceived by the public to be just as able to execute a variety of medical functions as physicians and at considerably less cost. A national poll taken in late 1985, the first large-scale study of Americans' views of the nursing profession, found that the majority of Americans felt that nurses were being underemployed (*USA Today,* July 22, 1985). In the area of services, 68 percent said that nurses are actually trained to play a larger role than they are presently allowed to play. A very high percentage, between 85 and 96 percent, believed that, with specialized training, nurses would be qualified to do such things as prescribe routine prescription drugs, give general physical exams, deliver babies, and administer psychotherapy to individuals and families.

On the one hand, there appears to be wide agreement that the nurse practitioner constitutes an expanded role for nurses and that this role should move in the direction of responsibilities traditionally assumed by physicians. On the other hand, the scope of practice of the NP is limited by the various states on a state-by-state basis. Currently, NPs are lobbying state legislatures for the passage of legislation supportive of their entrepreneurial ambitions.

To a number of legal experts, the Missouri case of *Sermchief* v. *Gonzales* represents a judicial landmark in supporting the expanded role of the NP (Wolff, 1984; Greenlaw, 1984). The case involved a suit brought by the medical establishment against two nurses in a federally funded program serving rural areas in southeastern Missouri. The nurses performed a variety of medical diagnostic and treatment functions, including performing breast and pelvic examinations, pregnancy testing, Pap smears, gonorrhea cultures, and blood serology; the administration of all kinds of contraceptive methods, including intrauterine devices and oral contraceptives; and the counseling and education of clients. The suit complained that the nurses were practicing medicine without a license to do so. At issue was how broad the statutory definition of nursing should be. An earlier decision (1980) by the Missouri Attorney General's Office had ruled that nurses could not engage in the delivery of primary care that included diagnosis and treatment. In *Sermchief* v. *Gonzales,* the court ruled that what the nurses were doing did fall within a broad definition of nursing and that an expanded description of nursing can legally include two important rights—the right to diagnose and the right to administer medications as prescribed by a licensed person.

Diagnosing and prescribing are at the core of the expanded role of the nurse as embodied in the NP. One commentator observes that the Missouri decision gives recognition to the fact that "the act of diagnosis is not the exclusive domain of the medical or osteopathic professions" (Wolff, 1984, p. 27). NPs have now expanded their practices to health maintenance organizations (HMOs) and private practice (sometimes solo, sometimes in partnership with each other or with physicians).

Equally important, authority for nurses to prescribe drugs has been broadened in several states. In Tennessee, for example, the State Board of Nursing originally required that an NP who wants to prescribe medications complete an educational program with specified curriculum hours devoted to pharmacology. This requirement was changed to graduation from a master's degree program in a nursing clinical specialty area that includes three quarter hours of pharmacology instruction.

Nursing has also fought to gain access to direct insurance reimbursement, which would allow such agencies as Blue Cross to pay nurses directly for services rendered to clients. In the state of Washington, for example, free-choice legislation adopted in

1981 requires that health insurers pay benefits for health care services when performed by professional nurses if such services are within the lawful scope of the professional nurse.

The Link Between Gender and Occupational Anomie Within Nursing

As described in the foregoing pages, the profession of nursing can be characterized in terms of a bifurcation of pathways to fuller professional status. The two routes being taken lead in two somewhat different directions. The first route moves the profession to a higher level within the traditional boundaries of nursing. Here, clinical nursing specialists with MA degrees, for example, work to become more respected members of the health care team while academic nurses with advanced degrees generate theory and research to provide a basis for the claims of the clinical specialists to a fuller professional status. The second route, taken by nurse practitioners, moves in the direction of medicine by assuming some of the physician's routine duties.

What we have, then, is what every student who has had at least an introductory course in sociology will recognize as a condition of anomie—in this case, occupational anomie. In Durkheim's classic analysis, which was alluded to at the very beginning of the paper, anomie represents a condition where a multiplicity of norms creates a social situation of ambiguity. In the case of nursing, there are now two significantly varying but equally legitimate views of what nurses can do and what they should strive to be. This is not to say, however, that there is not considerable overlap between the two views.

As was also stated at the outset, it is impossible to understand what has happened within nursing since the 1960s without understanding what has happened to women in American society during that same period. Nursing, as well as other occupations and professions, have felt the impact of a broadening reassessment of what it is to be female. Thus, the changes within nursing must be looked at in concert with changes taking place, for example, in medicine, where more and more women—about 35 percent of medical students are now women—are opting to become physicians.

What is striking about these changes in the occupational world is how the pace of change has quick-ened in the last two decades. While much is still to be accomplished, it is precisely the rapidity of this change that Durkheim identified 80 years ago as a condition leading to the development of a collective anomie.

FINAL COMMENT

The final outcome of nursing's initiatives toward fuller professional status is still anyone's guess. There are those like Oakley (1984) who question any movement toward medicine and see in it a loss of identity of what nursing is. There are just as many, in and outside of the profession, who extol the virtue of what it is doing and expect it to persist. In a larger sense, it may be that occupations and professions are always in a process of becoming as they respond to contingencies from within and without. We have described in this paper where nursing stands today in its quest to achieve professionalization. Other efforts are likely to arise in the future. While the continuation of the quest is predictable, the directions yet to be taken are not. And these directions will undoubtedly be influenced by what occurs in the future regarding the status of American women.

Notes

1. It is our contention that these attributes will not lead automatically to professional status, although they may be used to convince others that self-regulative autonomy ought to be granted. In a sense, they may be considered steps toward that goal. They are ammunition, so to speak, to be used in the process of negotiation and persuasion in gaining autonomy over a professed area of expertise. Yet, it is the right to control its own work that best distinguishes a profession from an occupation. Autonomy is the *sine qua non* (Skipper and Hughes, 1983).

2. For extended discussion and examples of the relationships among nursing theory, nursing research and methodology, and nursing practice, see the following: Skipper and Leonard, 1968; Wooldridge, et al., 1968; Wooldridge et al., 1978; Wooldridge and Schmitt, 1983; Wooldridge et al., 1983.

References

BACKUP, MOLLY, and JOHN MOLINARO
1984 "New health professionals: Changing the hierarchy." In Victor Sidel and Ruth Sidel (eds.), *Reforming Medicine: Lessons of the Last Quarter Century.* New York: Pantheon Books, pp. 201–219.

BERMAN, LEONARD
1981 "The generation gap." *Journal of the American Medical Association.* 246:872.

COCKERHAM, WILLIAM C.
1986 *Medical Sociology,* 3rd ed. Englewood Cliffs, N.J.: Prentice-Hall.

CRAIG, BEVERLY
1985 *"Climate and research productivity of collegiate and nursing faculty: Implications for educational and administrative interventions.* Unpublished Ph.D. dissertation. Blacksburg: Virginia Polytechnic Institute and State University.

DOLAN, ANDREW K.
1978 "The New York State Nurses Association 1985 proposal: Who needs it?" *Journal of Health, Politics, Policy and Law,* pp. 508–527.

DURKHEIM, EMILE
1951 *Suicide.* New York: The Free Press.

FREIDSON, ELIOT
1970 *Professional Dominance:* The Social Structure of Medical Care. New York: Atherton Press.

GOODE, WILLIAM J.
1960 "Encroachment, charlatanism, and the emerging profession: psychology, sociology, and medicine." *American Sociological Review* 25:902–914.

GRACE, HELEN
1978 "The development of doctoral education in nursing: A historical perspective." In Norma L. Chaska (ed.), *The Nursing Profession: Views Through the Midst,* New York: McGraw-Hill, pp. 112–123.

GREENLAW, JANE
1984 *"Sermchief* v. *Gonzales* and the debate over advanced nursing practice legislation." *Law Medicine and Health Care,* February, pp. 30–31.

GREENWOOD, ERNEST
1966 "The elements of professionalization." In Howard Vollmer and Donald Mills (eds.), *Professionalization.* Englewood Cliffs, N.J.: Prentice-Hall, pp. 9–18.

HOFING, C. K., E. BROTZMAN, S. DALRYMPLE, et al.
1966 "An experimental study in nurse–physician relationships." *Journal of Nervous and Mental Disease,* 143:177–180.

JOHNSON, DOROTHY
1974 "Development of theory: A requisite for nursing as a primary health profession." *Nursing Research* 23(5):372–377.

McCLOSKEY, JOANNE, and ELIZABETH SWANSEN
1982 "Publishing opportunities for nurses: A comparison of 100 journals." *Image XIV* 2:50–56.

MUMFORD, EMILY
1983 *Medical Sociology.* New York: Random House.

OAKLEY, ANN
1984 "The importance of being a nurse." *Nursing Times,* December 12, pp. 24–27.

PITEL, MARTHA, and JOHN VIAN
1975 "Analysis of nursing doctorates: Data collected for the International Directory of Nurses with Doctoral Degrees." *Nursing Research* 24:340–351.

RANK, STEVEN G., and CARDELL K. JACOBSEN
1977 "Compliance with medication overdose orders: A failure to replicate." *Journal of Health and Social Behavior* 18:188–193.

REVERBY, SUSAN
1986 "Re-forming the hospital nurse: The management of American nursing." In Peter Conrad and Rochelle Kern (eds.), *The Sociology of Health and Illness,* 2nd ed. New York: St. Martin's Press, pp. 187–195.

RITZER, GEORGE, and DAVID WALCZAK
1986 *Working: Conflict and Change,* 3rd ed. Englewood Cliffs, N.J.: Prentice-Hall.

ROTH, ALEDA, et al.
1979 1977 National Sample Survey of Registered Nurses. Washington, DC. NT1S Publication #HRP-0900630.

SKIPPER, JAMES K., JR., and JAMES HUGHES
1983 "Podiatry: A medical care specialty in quest of full professional status and recognition." *Social Science and Medicine* 17(20):1541–1548.

SKIPPER, JAMES K., JR., and ROBERT C. LEONARD
1968 "Children stress and hospitalization: A field experiment," *Journal of Health and Social Behavior* 9:275–287.

SOARES, CAROL A.
1978 "Nursing and medical diagnosis: A comparison of variant and essential features." In Norma L. Chaska (ed.), *The Nursing Profession: Views Through the Midst.* New York: McGraw-Hill, pp. 269–286.

STEVENS, BARBARA J.
1985 "Does the 1985 nursing education proposal make any sense?" *Nursing Outlook* 33:124–127.

TEMKIN-GREENER, HELENA
  1983 "Interprofessional perspectives on teamwork in health care: A case study." *Milbank Memorial Fund Quarterly/Health and Society* 61:641–657.

U.S. DEPARTMENT OF HEALTH AND HUMAN SERVICES
  1982 *Third Report to the President and Congress on the Status of Health Professions Personnel in the United States.* Washington, DC: DHHS Publication #(HRA) 82–2.

VANCE, CONNIE, SUSAN TALBOTT, ANGELA McBRIDE, and DIANA MASON
  1985 "An uneasy alliance: Nursing and the women's movement." *Nursing Outlook* 33:281–285.

WAGNER, DAVID
  1980 "The proletarianization of nurses in the United States: 1932–1946." *International Journal of Health Services* 10:271–290.

WESSEN, ALBERT F.
  1972 "Hospital ideology and communication between ward personnel." In E. Gartley Jaco (ed.), *Patients, Physicians and Illness,* 2nd ed. New York: The Free Press, pp. 315–332.

WOLFF, MICHAEL A.
  1984 "Court upholds expanded practice roles for nurses." *Law, Medicine and Health Care,* February, pp. 26–29.

WOOLDRIDGE, POWHATAN, JAMES K. SKIPPER, JR., and ROBERT C. LEONARD
  1968 *Behavioral Science, Social Practice, and the Nursing Profession.* Cleveland: Press of Case Western Reserve University.

WOOLDRIDGE, POWHATAN, ROBERT C. LEONARD, and JAMES K. SKIPPER, JR.
  1978 *Methods of Clinical Experimentation Improve Patient Care.* St. Louis: Mosby.

WOOLDRIDGE, POWHATAN, and MADELINE SCHMITT
  1983 "Examining research for its contributions to nursing practice." In Powhatan Wooldridge, Madeline Schmitt, James K. Skipper, Jr., and Robert C. Leonard, *Behavioral Science and Nursing Theory.* St. Louis: Mosby, pp. 265–300.

WOOLDRIDGE, POWHATAN, MADELINE SCHMITT, JAMES K. SKIPPER, JR. and ROBERT C. LEONARD
  1983 *Behavioral Science and Nursing Theory.* St. Louis: Mosby.

Reprofessionalization in Pharmacy

Arnold Birenbaum

Traditional sociological analyses of the professions rarely have considered how, and under what conditions, an established profession seeks to change its position within a single industry. In the *structural-functional* perspective [1–3] an occupation becomes a profession when granted autonomy and receives recognition from society for possessing a technical knowledge-base, demonstrating effective performance, developing a lengthy and superior education, and espousing ethical commitments to the common good. This list of attributes does not take into account that new technology can take functions away from established professional practitioners, new market and organizational structures may delegate tasks to lesser trained occupations, and other occupations may try to encroach on a profession by increasing educational requirements and adopting a code of ethics.

An alternative approach (but within the same tradition) is suggested by Wilensky [4], in which professionalization is designated a *social and political* process. Herein some occupations (with particular attributes) actively take on the task of getting societal recognition, usually through creating full-time educational programs which are connected with universities, national organizations to represent the interests of the occupation, and codes of ethics. Professionalization movements within an occupation are usually led by elites capable of taking risks to bring about the future desired legal support and social recognition. But how does it come to be that these groups emerge within a profession? And what kinds of responses do they receive internal to the profession and from other professions with which a division of labor is shared?

Reprinted from *Social Science and Medicine,* vol. 16 (1982), pp. 871–878.

Whether structural-functional or processual, the available theoretical frameworks fail to recognize the interactive and contextual nature of the development of the professions. In both views there is a tacit recognition of societal design, with each depicting licensure by government as the culmination of professionalization. Autonomy and recognition by society are not guaranteed, and under certain conditions, a profession can *lose* autonomy and recognition while still being licensed. A more dynamic orientation is suggested by the often cited observation of Marx [5] that "Men make their own history, but they do not make it just as they please; they do not make it under circumstances chosen by themselves, but under circumstances directly found, given and transmitted from the past." Consistent with this dictum is Klegon's [6] focus on both "concrete occupational strategies as well as wider social forces and arrangements of power." It is the interplay, then, between these two sets of factors which influence the capacity of a profession to maintain or expand its status in an industry.

There have been a few empirical studies of professions of the kind suggested by Klegon. The changing division of labor, technology, social organization, and economic support of the health professions have received little investigation. Kronus [7] has examined the historical evolution of pharmacy and medicine in the differing social contexts of nineteenth century England and the United States. Informal efforts by apothecaries in England to take care of the health care needs of the middle-class client population were rewarded by social support, eventually culminating in the evolution of this role into the medical general practitioner. In contrast, pharmacists in the United States were relegated to technical support roles to medicine because the profession of medicine was successful in controlling health care delivery. Using a more quantitative approach, Begun and Feldman [8] examined the actual political activities of optometrists in four states with widely different economic, political and social characteristics, in their study of how this profession was and was not successful in limiting competition.

When an occupation seeks to change its position in society it may be an unsettling experience, challenging traditional beliefs held by those inside the vocation and outsiders as well. It may come as no surprise that support for acquiring more education and new responsibilities may vary within the occupational community. Not all practitioners of the vocation seek change, and elite groups or segments within the occupation may be identified as the 'carriers' of the seeds of new roles [9]. Professionalization, even where peer control over licensing exists, may be conceived of as a militant process, a drive for higher standards of performance, and greater recognition by the public of services performed [10].

Professionalization drives are further complicated by the existence of other professions which control the delivery of related services. The elites of American medicine, for example, did not have to contend with already established and licensed professions, only reluctant members of their own professional community. The early elite-sponsored drive for professionalization among physicians, and engineers as well, focused on the acquisition of peer regulation in order to improve overall standards of training and performance, creating uniformity where none existed [11]. Upgrading was performed to secure state licensing under the control of the professional associations.

Reprofessionalization must be considered as a possibility for a licensed profession as well as the initial drive for licensure. Given the existence of the established profession of medicine, the contemporary drive among pharmacists to upgrade their educational standards and also acquire new clinical responsibilities, often manifests a strong consciousness of mission. Alternatively, many pharmacists in practice express dissatisfaction with current work situations [12–14].

Some segments of pharmacist are better educated today than in the past and capable of assuming new responsibilities. Therefore, this effort to upgrade the status of pharmacy in the health care delivery system can be characterized as reprofessionalization. Yet those who seek upgrading must convince the medical profession, reluctant members of their own profession, health planners, and the public of the need for these services. Why are these efforts being made now? What are the possible outcomes?

This paper is a case study of efforts to reprofessionalize in the profession of pharmacy. It is a thesis of this paper that the contemporary movement in pharmacy is a reaction to developments in technology, social organization, the division of labor and financing of health care services and pharmaceuticals. These developments have imposed greater uniformity and predictability in the work situation of the pharmacist, mainly through increased bureaucratic organization and specialization.

There is a spectre haunting the profession of pharmacy, manifest in the fear of displacement and downgrading of the craft. This concern is strikingly similar to the fears expressed by English artisans in the late eighteenth century when faced with the rise of the factory system of production [15]. The honorable craft of pharmacy is facing a loss of power or control over scarce resources, including the utilization of learned skills, and the loss of status or the social approval accorded by others.

This paper examines (1) the origins of this crisis in pharmacy, (2) the new beliefs about the field which were generated in response to the crisis and (3) the possible consequences of the new beliefs. The purpose of this analysis is to see what happens when a field is subject to stress and to make predictions about the tendencies of particular beliefs or solutions to the general problem of the field to produce stability of roles.

Reprofessionalization is advocated by elites in pharmacy but it is met with resistance inside and outside the field. The goal of upgrading pharmacy into a clinical profession involves the acquisition of qualitatively different roles from those performed by members of the profession in the past. Simply to view pharmacy as smoothly changing from craft to profession ignores the new consciousness of those members of the profession who see themselves as clinicians–possessing knowledge which directly benefits patients, and services which deserve respect from both patients and physicians. A need for intervention for patients is brought about by universal recognition that adverse drug interactions can lead to death and is one of the ten leading causes of hospitalization. The pharmacist, by virtue of careful record keeping and knowledge of drug interactions, is able to warn patients and physicians when a drug therapy is prescribed which can adversely interact with a drug now being taken by a patient. A new practice has been created which goes far beyond filling a prescription; it is called clinical pharmacy.

The justification for this new practice is expressed in the priorities of Jere E. Goyan, both former head of the Food and Drug Administration and the dean of a college of pharmacy.

> . . . we need to devote more time to . . . the effect that as many as eight different drugs taken concurrently might have on those persons who might be taking them all [16].

However, the recognition of the need and the opportunity to keep drug profiles on patients does not automatically produce the appropriate clinical behavior by pharmacists. Dr. Goyan conceded that clinical pharmacy is far from a standard practice in every community or hospital pharmacy. His admission that there is still a "long way to go" before all pharmacists were clinicians reveals some of the built-in tensions in the profession [17]. The clinical pharmacy segment is seeking to change the knowledge, ability and motivation of pharmacists, and convince outsiders, e.g. physicians and hospital administrators, that pharmacists should be allowed to consult with patients and physicians. Having complete control over entry into the profession—physicians do not sit on the state pharmacy licensing boards—has been an insufficient basis for acquiring new responsibilities.

Medicine is not the only source of resistance. The clinically oriented members of the profession are also critical of the lack of unity in pharmacy. They note that community and hospital pharmacists have few common professional interests; that many older pharmacists have shown no interest in acquiring new knowledge and responsibilities; that there is a great deal of direct competition between community pharmacies. Further, the clinically oriented also find that physicians and patients do not give them enough respect, claiming that the entire profession is judged by the worst aspects of pharmacy, i.e. high prices, steering patients to over-the-counter drugs,

lavish gifts to physicians and the filling of illegal prescriptions.

THE ORIGINS OF THE CRISIS

The traditional organization of the field permitted pharmacists to combine professional and business orientations [18–20]. The community locations of retail pharmacies allowed the sale of patent medicines and sundries as well as filling prescriptions. Unlike physicians who were constrained by the ongoing character of relationships with patients, pharmacists could devote considerable time, both publicly and privately, to building up the business part of their practice. This mixed image of the pharmacist and the community pharmacy ('the drug store') as half profession, half business is rejected by the faculties of colleges of pharmacy, who view themselves and the recent graduates as militant upholders of complete professionalization, mixing enthusiasm for change with challenges to existing social arrangements in community and hospital pharmacy.

This tentative characterization of the field of pharmacy is supported by editorials and articles in pharmacy journals and interviews with practicing pharmacists. Hospital pharmacists are perceived as well suited to the role of change agent [21]. Pharmacists are running special clinics in hospitals to increase the rates of patient compliance with physicians' medication regimens [22]. Pharmacy is perceived by authors as "changing from a response oriented . . . to an active, participatory system . . ."[23].

The reaction of physicians to the changing role of the pharmacist is of equal concern to those who advocate change. An assessment of physicians' attitudes toward pharmacists as drug information consultants is also reported [24]. Finally new skills needed for pharmacists to play clinical roles, such as interviewing techniques, are demonstrated to be important in establishing the right to play these roles [25].

There are five structural changes in the organization and delivery of pharmaceutical services which have encouraged reprofessionalization. These factors are threats to the power and status of pharmacists, and reprofessionalization is a collective response to occupational displacement.

The Decline of Community Pharmacy

There has been a reduction in the number of small retail pharmacies in the United States, with many larger discount drug stores replacing several pharmacist-owned stores in any given area. Observers of the field note that

> Aggressive chain operators are dispensing prescriptions at lower cost to the patient. They are charging roughly $3 to $3.25 a prescription, whereas a typical independent pharmacy averaged $3.60 per prescription in 1966. These lower charges are possible due to purchase economies and increased promotion of the prescription department [26].

Independent owners who operated pharmacies found this arrangement a satisfactory way of earning a livelihood and even provided opportunities for employing other pharmacists. As of 1972, slightly over 50% of all 103,340 pharmacists in the United States were working in or were owner/operators of independent community pharmacies [27]. Like many other small businesses, independent community pharmacies depended on fair trade legislation which allows manufacturers to set minimum retail prices for which their products will be sold. Organized in 1898, the National Association of Retail Druggists led this struggle and encouraged protective state legislation on pricing. Consequently the proliferation of chain stores which could afford to give discounts on prescriptions and sundries was limited [28]. State courts, however, have declared some fair trade agreements as illegal and large discount drug outlets have grown over the past 15 years.

The strong roots of pharmacy in entrepreneurial activities is also reflected in the lack of appeal that purely professional associations have had for pharmacists, as compared to physicians and dentists. Relatively few pharmacists belong to professional associations such as the American Pharmaceutical Association and the American Society of Hospital Pharmacists, or even the National Association of Retail Druggists [29]. Membership in the APhA totaled 34,692 in 1974 or about one third of all practicing pharmacists [30]. The more purely professional atmosphere of hospital pharmacy is reflected in the high proportion of pharmacists working in those organizations who belong to ASHP. While hospital pharmacy employment constituted 14,425 members of the profession in 1972, or roughly 14% 1975 membership figures for the ASHP were over 12,500 [31]. While it is not possible to determine whether every member of the ASHP was employed in a hospital, it seems unlikely that community based pharmacists would join an organization designed to further the development of that speciality and protect the interests of the membership. Merton [32] has hypothesized that one function of a professional association is to reduce power and status differences which occur in the workplace and make communication among various professional associations possible, perhaps even convincing other professions that high standards of training and performance are insured.

The decline of opportunities for ownership has also produced concern about developing organizations which can protect pharmacists working for others both in hospital and community pharmacy. In 1970 there were 19,820 'small independent' retail pharmacies in the United States and estimates in the field predict that there will be far fewer such businesses in the future [33]. Regardless of whether such a diminution of opportunities for ownership actually occurs, a projection of this kind provides little comfort for those who wish to 'be my own boss.'

Automation

Pharmacy is a field that is threatened by automation, both in manufacture of drugs and in dispensing in hospitals and nursing homes. Mechanic [34] noted that pharmacy was facing a crisis of purpose brought about when manufactured drug combinations made compounding unnecessary. Today some state licensing examinations for pharmacists have eliminated questions on compounding techniques. As a result of this development in technology, the pharmacist provides consumers with a service in which craftsmanship related to product formulation does not take place.

The enormous expansion of hospitals and nursing homes has created many employment opportunities in the pharmacy but hardly requires the performance of traditional crafts. In the future even the traditional role of dispensing medication may be limited since automated dispensing and packaging equipment is already being used to fill individualized prescriptions for hospitalized patients where large demand takes place. The equipment combines computerized prescriptions with vending machine-like equipment that can be programmed and licensed pharmacists do not need to perform these tasks. Pharmacy technicians and assistants can perform these machine tending functions under the supervision of a single licensed pharmacist. This separation of decision making from the performance of routine tasks takes place in the design of work and work settings, a process that is often noted in American industry [35].

Physician Extenders

The development of middle level health care provider roles, namely physician assistants and nurse practitioners, has created a great deal of interest on the part of pharmacists to upgrade their responsibility and authority in hospitals, both in relation to other health care providers and patients. Pharmacists would like to receive greater honor and recognition for the work that they do as medication control agents, educators of other health care providers and monitors of patient compliance with physician's prescriptions. While demanding clear delegation of these responsibilities, hospital pharmacists are also experiencing a loss of status brought about by technological displacement and exacerbated by new practices and regulations which permit nurse practitioners and physician assistants to prescribe for minor illnesses, under the standing orders written by a physician. Consequently, pharmacists must now take orders from providers who they may regard as not well trained. Furthermore, this close clinical contact between nurse practitioners or physician assistants and both patients and physicians, is a source of envy for the pharmacist. The new literature in pharmacy speaks of the clinical role of the pharmacist and the right to charge a fee for the service, both in hospital and community practices [36, 37]. In one experiment at the University of Southern California's School of Pharmacy, clinical pharmacists are permitted to prescribe under standing orders.

New Patterns of Recruitment

Recent attrition of vocational opportunity in the natural sciences, particularly in university and college research and teaching positions, may have attracted more academically minded students to the profession of pharmacy. Since pharmacy training in the United States is now part of 5 and sometimes 6 year baccalaureate degree programs, the field is more interesting to students who wish a scientific education with some potential for following a research career. While in the past pharmacists interested in academic careers or opportunities to do research in commercial laboratories acquired Ph.D. degrees, the newly created Pharm. D. degree reflects efforts to upgrade the field both educationally and clinically. The new degree makes pharmacy a field with people who have received advanced training *as* pharmacists, combining scholarly potential with immediate economic opportunity. Compared to vocational opportunities for biologists and chemists, recent graduates who acquire state licences have found a great deal of employment. A survey of 5000 graduates of colleges of pharmacy conducted in 1974 found only 10 failing to find employment [38].

Communication among Pharmacists

The generalized fear of being dispossessed and displaced would not have been possible if the disgruntled could not find out that their dissatisfaction was shared with others. The numerical expansion of the field of pharmacy is dependent on the continued use of drugs in treatment, making for growth in the area of hospital and nursing home pharmacy; the number of hospital pharmacists doubled in the 1970s [39]. There is far more interaction among pharmacists in larger departments and they are less isolated than in the past. Pharmacy colleges attempt to maintain tight control over preceptor programs to maintain the students clinical interests. Recent graduates of first pharmacy degree programs are encouraged to maintain contact with schools of pharmacy, even when employed, through the use of preceptorship programs where the newly licensed give on-the-job training to future pharmacists. As a result, linkages are maintained with the more idealistic and elite representatives of the field who advocate increased professionalization of the field through performance of clinical roles in health care. Opportunity for interaction around these goals and others helps to create an atmosphere of a commitment to a cause, a strong sense of shared fate, and personal obligation to others who are similarly situated. These socially structured conditions promote the development of ideas that pharmacy can and should undergo reprofessionalization.

NEW BELIEFS AND REPROFESSIONALIZATION

Reprofessionalization represents both a problem (status and power loss) and an opportunity (new roles and recognition). Larson [40] considers professionalization a form of social mobility. The success of a profession's organizational efforts determines whether mobility is going to occur, and such an effort must be cooperative among those similarly situated.

> . . . the professional project of social mobility is considered as a collective project, because only through a joint organizational effort could roles be created—or redefined—that would bring the desired social position to their occupants [41].

Unlike medicine or engineering, pharmacy is not seeking to enhance its status as much as it seeks to avoid being dispossessed. Moreover, reprofessionalization must be accomplished within a highly complex health care system. Given the structural changes discussed above, and the idiom by which status is expressed in the medically dominated health care field in the United States, the direction pharmacy is compelled to take is away from the technical and business components and toward the clinical service ideal. Redefinition of technical functions as clinical services has occurred in the health care field in the past. The specialities of anesthesiology, radiology and pathology which were once outside of medicine, became defined as clinical services and increased their prestige by joining it. Pharmacy has no such goals at this time but does demand more responsibility.

The goals of the advocates of clinical pharmacy reflect confidence in pharmacists as professionals who can work directly with patients; they also are viewed as information specialists. The increased education of pharmacists has made them more knowledgeable about drugs and adverse drug interactions. They can now not only observe other health care

practitioners make mistakes in prescribing or administering medications but also explain to them *why* these procedures are in error. Such encounters confirm beliefs among pharmacists that they are rightfully drug experts.

Pharmacists are aware of their contribution to health care but are also dismayed at the lack of recognition for what they do. An independently derived report urges reforms in education and practice of pharmacy to make pharmacists better able to communicate their skills as clinicians and providers of information. The American Association of Colleges of Pharmacy commissioned a study directed by a noted scholar, John Millis, to evaluate the state of practice and education in pharmacy. The American Foundation for Pharmaceutical Education, an offshoot of the APhA, helped to fund the commission [42]. The director of the commission had performed a similar study on graduate education in medicine a few years earlier.

The Mills report, like the Flexner report on medicine 60 years ago, focuses on the need to remove the noted entrepreneurial character to the field. Moreover, the end of compounding is not considered as the removal of the technical basis of the craft but rather as a way of freeing the pharmacist to do more professional tasks. This theme has been echoed in various professional publications, pointing to the ". . . widespread and serious problems related to the use of therapeutic drugs . . ." [43]. The advocates of reform argue that the pharmacist does not simply sell a product but provides an essential service, using the knowledge and training acquired to help the patient.

The tasks of removing drugs from a larger to smaller container and the typing of a label may be all there is to filling a prescription, as seen from the perspective of the ordinary citizen. For the professionally committed, there is no such thing as a simple prescription and the routine is symbolically transformed into a sacred trust.

> The trouble is that every prescription, every situation, every question from a physician, nurse or patient, is potentially crucial. The pharmacist's response, his action, his answer can do the utmost good or cause the utmost harm or even death as a result. A major question for pharmacy and for pharmaceutical educators is how to ori-

*ent the individual practitioner to view his prac-
tice in such a light [44].*

Clearly, this statement reflects a strong sense of responsibility. There are two dimensions to responsibility. First, there is the idea of careful work based on conscientiousness and avoiding unethical conduct, such as fee splitting with physicians who steer patients and illegal dispensing of desired medications. Second, there is the idea of sharing meaningful authority in providing health care, an authority now monopolized by the dominant profession of medicine. Some pharmacists seek increased responsibilities commensurate with their training, arguing that they be permitted to make generic drug substitutions for name brands, unless otherwise specified by the prescribing physician, to countersign the prescription after making sure that no medication error has been made, to advise all health care providers, including physicians, on the merits of new drugs, and to instruct and followup patients to insure medication compliance.

NEW DIRECTIONS

The two meanings of responsibility discussed above direct the field of pharmacy to enhancing the status of the field through self-improvement based on ethical behavior or to gaining power by being delegated meaningful responsibility. These two dimensions also represent two structural problems of all professionalization and reprofessionalization drives, namely, (1) how to gain recognition and approval for upgrading by demonstrating professional self-improvement (i.e. increased education and ethical conduct) and (2) how to gain control over resources so that members or adherents to the movement are sufficiently rewarded by participation to remain loyal (i.e. increased opportunity to receive higher pay and promotions for performing clinical roles). All modifications of pharmacy as a profession, it is hypothesized, will result from efforts to make the extraordinary behavior of pacemakers in pharmacy a part of the work of garden variety pharmacists and health care organizations.

The following predictions are made, based on the assumption that reprofessionalization in pharmacy will be in the direction of institutionalization,

a social process which creates stabilized roles for the various leadership groups in efforts of professionals to gain power and status [45]. It is not assumed that institutionalization through solving one problem (recognition or approval vs a stable reward system) will end all competition and conflict within the profession.

I. A strong emphasis on inculcating professional values and techniques without acquiring opportunities to reward members through clinical practice will result in an inward looking effort to construct a more meaningful culture, similar to revitalization movements identified [46].

Wallace claims that these types of responses occur among dispossessed peoples and

. . . always originate in situations of social and cultural stress and are in fact, an effort on the part of the stress-laden to construct systems of dogma, myth, and ritual which are internally coherent as well as true descriptions of a world system and which thus will serve as guides to efficient action [47].

The specific form this direction will take in the field of pharmacy will be a strong emphasis on receiving deference and respect from patients, doctors and other significant role partners. Pharmacies both in the community and in hospitals will be so constructed to display the clinical concerns of practitioners, with consulting rooms and reference texts available. Public debate will focus on the ethical purity of the profession, manifested in discussions in professional journals and other forums of what is professional and unprofessional conduct.

II. Alternatively, strong emphasis on sharing authority with physicians in health care organizations such as hospitals is likely to result in a process of segmentation within the field between the clinical pharmacists holding the rare Pharm. D. degree and the many licensed pharmacists with the bachelor's degree. Therefore, clinical pharmacy will be a special practice within the field, limited to clearly clinical settings.

To reach this outcome, there would have to be an opportunity for educated and trained clinical pharmacists to perform an expanded role in health care delivery, demonstrating effectiveness in terms of higher quality care than before and being able to save money in some other area of service.

Leadership from hospital pharmacy will focus on the organizational contribution that clinical pharmacy can make, particularly in the area of reducing the costs of care. Clinical pharmacists who improve patient compliance will reduce the likelihood of rehospitalization. Further, clinical competency will be based on holding the doctoral degree, a way of convincing the medical profession that pharmacy has a right to shared authority. Consequently, the Master's degree in clinical pharmacy, currently a popular advanced degree, will not be considered sufficient training for clinical responsibilities. Furthermore, the hospital-based leadership will seek to make their branch of pharmacy a doctoral-led profession, aided by pharmacy technicians and assistants. These efforts will further the process of segmentation in pharmacy.

It is also possible that the hospital-based segment will actively work within professional associations to upgrade the entire profession, creating in-service training programs for baccalaureate pharmacists, with the legal right to practice as a clinician dependent on the doctoral degree and internship: in addition, the current conventional role of the community pharmacist would produce great strain among those practitioners because they would be subject to some downgrading by the rise of the more credentialed (Pharm. D.) clinical pharmacist.

Clinical pharmacy cannot demonstrate this effectiveness in helping patients unless resources are allocated to support this practice. A number of studies which have appeared over the past 10 years justify the expanded role of pharmacists in increasing patient compliance, but there is little evidence suggesting that hospitals save money as a result of these activities. For example, a controlled study of compliance among hypertensive patients showed a significant improvement in the number of patients who complied with prescribed therapy and a significant increase in the number of study patients whose blood pressures were kept within normal range during the study period, when clinical services were provided by a pharmacist [48]. Deviation from prescribed drug regimens among discharged hospital patients were found among a control group receiving no consultation prior to going home while two study groups showed 90% compliance [49]. However, one study

of efforts to teach a study group of patients about their medications and labeling their drug containers with the contents did not significantly decrease the number of medication errors made at home [50].

There is a great deal of evidence that medications are not always administered correctly, particularly by elderly people with chronic illnesses:

> *Two studies of elderly patients receiving care in clinical settings revealed that 59 per cent of the patients had made one or more errors in taking medications and roughly one quarter had made errors that could be classified as potentially serious [51].*

Currently, other clinical health care providers do not see the pharmacist's major role as involvement with patients on a direct or regular basis. The pharmacist was perceived in one survey as having very little patient involvement and was encouraged to become more involved. Reviewing drug utilization was considered by clinical providers as the major clinical activity for pharmacists and should remain as such [52]. Despite this limited acceptance by other health care providers, as of 1978, at least one clinical service was offered by pharmacists in 23% of the nationally surveyed acute care hospitals [53].

Evaluations of new modes of clinical participation continue to be performed and reported by pharmacists; these efforts serve to document their capacity to perform useful clinical services. Specific studies have compared the readability of patient information materials in order to learn how to more effectively reduce patient medication errors [54–56]. Direct clinical interventions were compared in a project which used patient counseling and special medication containers to see whether compliance among 100 hypertensive patients could be improved. Each intervention was measured in combination and separately in this controlled study. Rehder *et al*. [52] reported that combined interventions had an additive effect in increasing compliance.

Therapeutic pharmacy consultations with patients were also evaluated. Clinical pharmacists in a family practice office worked with physicians in providing information about a patient's drug therapy, and in some instances, making specific recommendations for immediate implementation. Sixteen physicians independently evaluated these consultations, concluding that the pharmacist's recommendations were appropriate and had favorable effects on patient care [58]. In an unrelated study, patients in a family care practice were asked to evaluate the quality of health care received both with and without pharmacy consultations [59]. Those patients who had encounters with pharmacists were significantly more satisfied with their health care than the control groups. Finally, McKenney, *et al.* [60] compared drug therapy assessments for ambulatory patients made by pharmacists and primary physicians. Pharmacists were able to detect drug therapy problems and recommend appropriate actions for resolving them. The differences between the pharmacist's assessment and physician agreement were not significant.

Reprofessionalization in pharmacy faces considerable resistance because of three structural features of the carriers of this drive. First, the strongest advocates of the clinical role are among pharmacists who are most vulnerable to retaliation because they are young, are not well known to other health care providers at the workplace, and not protected by bureaucratic rules or seniority. Secondly, the strongest concentration of advocates for clinical roles are in academic posts and are not in direct practice. The Pharm. D. who educates does not face the day-to-day resistances found in hospitals. Finally, pharmacy students, by virtue of the location of their colleges on campus which often do not have medical colleges, have little opportunity to interact with physicians in training. Therefore, they only come into contact with physicians in superior-subordinate relationships, making it difficult for them to convince doctors that they can make a clinical contribution. Moreover, they cannot influence new generations of physicians when they are easily influenced and before they professionally close ranks as practicing physicians.

That the carriers of the ideas of clinical pharmacy may influence a new generation of graduates of colleges of pharmacies, there can be no doubt. Whether they will produce the results they intend may have more to do with their way of solving problems of adaptation in a stressful environment.

EDITOR'S NOTE

In recent years, some states have passed laws allowing pharmacists to prescribe certain drugs directly to patients. As of May 1986, druggists in Florida are allowed to prescribe more than 30 medicines in 14 categories for treatment of minor illnesses, and they are permitted to charge for writing these prescriptions. At the time the Florida law went into effect, California and Washington state already allowed hospital pharmacists to prescribe some medicines.

References

1. Goode W. J. Encroachment, charlatanism and the emerging profession: Psychology, sociology, and medicine. *Am. Soc. Rev.* **25,** 902–914, 1960.
2. Greenwood E. The elements of professionalization. In *Professionalization* (Edited by Volmer H. M. and Mills D. L.), pp. 10–19. Prentice-Hall, Englewood Cliffs, NJ, 1966.
3. Parsons T. Professions. *Int. Encycl. Soc. Sci.* **12,** 536–547, 1968.
4. Wilensky H. L. The professionalization of everyone? *Am. J. Sociol.* **70,** 137–158, 1964.
5. Marx K. *The Marx-Engels Reader* (Edited by Tucker R. C.), 2nd Edition, 595 pp. Norton, New York, 1978.
6. Klegon D. The sociology of professions: An emerging perspective. *Sociol. Work Occup.* **5,** 259–283, 1978.
7. Kronus C. The evolution of occupational power: An historical study of task boundaries between physicians and pharmacists. *Sociol. Work Occup.* **3,** 3–37, 1976.
8. Begun J. W. and Feldman R. D. *A Social and Economic Analysis of Professional Regulation in Optometry*. National Center for Health Services Research. Washington, DC, 1981.
9. Bucher R. and Strauss A. Professions in process. *Am. J. Sociol.* **66,** 324–334, 1961.
10. Corwin R. G. *Militant Professionalism: A Study of Organizational Conflict in High Schools*. Appleton-Century-Crofts, New York, 1970.
11. Larson M. S. *The Rise of Professionalism: A Sociological Analysis*. University of California, Berkeley, 1977.
12. Robbins J. Pharmacy's unfulfilled status as a profession. *Am. Drug.* **176,** 34–37, 1977.
13. Curtiss F. R., Hammel R. J. and Johnson C. A. Psychological strain and job satisfaction in pharmacy practice: Institutional vs community practitioners. *Am. J. Hosp. Pharm.* **35,** 1516–1520, 1978.
14. Donehew G. R. and Hammerness F. C. Pharmacists' job feelings. *Contemp. Pharm. Pract.* **1,** 22–24, 1978.

15. Thompson E. P. *The Making of the English Working Class.* Vintage, New York, 1963.

16. Lyons R. C. Incoming chief of drug agency. *New York Times* September 12, 1979.

17. Lyons R. C. *ibid.*

18. Denzin N. Incomplete professionalization: The case of pharmacy. *Sociol. Forces* **16,** 375–381, 1968.

19. Mechanic D. Social issues in the study of the pharmaceutical field. *Am. J. Pharm. Educ.* **34,** 536–543, 1970.

20. Kronus C. Occupational values, role orientations and work settings: The case of pharmacy. *Sociol. Q.* **16,** 171–183, 1975.

21. Kormel B. Hospital pharmacist: master of victim of the environment. *Am. J. Hosp. Pharm.* **35,** 151–154, 1978.

22. Schneider P. and Cable G. Compliance and clinical opportunity for an expanded practice role for pharmacists. *Am. J. Hosp. Pharm.* **35,** 288–295, 1978.

23. Lamy P. O. Pharmacy—Today and tomorrow. *Contemp. Pharm. Pract.* **1,** 1, 1978.

24. Nelson A. A., Meinhold J. M. and Hutchinson R. A. Changes in physicians' attitudes toward pharmacists as drug information consultants following implementation of clinical pharmacy services. *Am. J. Hosp. Pharm.* **35,** 1201–1206.

25. Love D. W. *et al.* Teaching interviewing skills to pharmacy residents. *Am. J. Hosp. Pharm.* **35,** 1073–1074, 1978.

26. Knapp D. A. and Knapp D. E. An appraisal of the contemporary practice of pharmacy. *Am. J. Hosp. Pharm.* **32,** 749, 1968.

27. Smith M. and Knapp D. A. *Pharmacy, Drugs and Medical Care,* 2nd edition, 122 pp. Williams & Wilkins, Baltimore, 1976.

28. Smith M. and Knapp D. A. *ibid.*

29. Akers R. L. and Qinney R. Differential organization of health professions: A comparative analysis. *Am. soc. Rev.* **33,** 104–121, 1968.

30. Smith M. and Knapp D. A. *Pharm. Drugs Med. Care* **114,** *op. cit.*

31. Smith M. and Knapp D. A. *ibid.* 120.

32. Merton R. K. The functions of the professional association. *Am. J. Nurs.* **58,** 50–54, 1958.

33. Anderson J. *et al. Remington's Pharmaceutical Sciences* p. 36. Mack Publishing Co., Easton, PA, 1975.

34. Mechanic D., *op. cit.* 536.

35. Braverman H. *Monopoly Capital and Labor.* Monthly Review Press, New York, 1972.

36. Provost C. P. Clinical pharmacy—speciality or general direction? *Drug Intelligence and Clinical Pharmacy* **6,** 235, 1972.

37. Anonymous Communicating the value of comprehensive pharmaceutical services to the consumer. *J. Am. Pharm. Ass.* **NS13,** 23, 1973.

38. Smith M. and Knapp D. A. *op. cit.* 33.

39. Zellmer W. A. Reviewing the 1970s: Hospital pharmacy practice. *Am. J. Hosp. Pharm.* **36,** 1490, 1979.

40. Larson M. S. *The Rise of Professionalism. op. cit.*

41. Larson M. S. *ibid.* 67.

42. Millis J. *Pharmacists for the Future: The Report of the Study Commission on Pharmacy.* Health Administration Press, Ann Arbor, MI, 1975.

43. Editorial. Effect of upgraded pharmacy education on pharmacy practice. *Am. J. Hosp. Pharm.* **34,** 929, 1977.

44. Knapp D. A. and Knapp D. E. *op. cit.* 755.

45. Parsons T. *op. cit.* 545.

46. Wallace A. F. C. *Religion: An Anthropologic View,* p. 30. Random House, New York, 1966.

47. Wallace A. F. C. *ibid.*

48. McKenney J. M. *et al.* The effect of clinical pharmacy services on patients with essential hypertension. *Circulation* **48,** 1104, 1973.

49. Cole D. and Emmanuel S. Drug consultation: Its significance to the discharged hospital patient and its relevance as a role for the pharmacist. *Am. J. Hosp. Pharm.* **23,** 960, 1971.

50. Malahy B. The effect of instruction and labeling on the number of medication errors made by patients at home. *Am. J. Hosp. Pharm.* **23,** 292, 1966.

51. Smith D. B. A cooperative pharmacy project: An autopsy on a community health intervention. *J. Comm. Hlth* **2,** 223, 1977.

52. Lambert E. L. *et al.* The pharmacist's clinical role as seen by other health workers. *Am. J. Publ. Hlth* **67,** 253, 1977.

53. Stolar M. M. National survey of hospital pharmaceutical services—1978. *Am. J. Hosp. Pharm.* **36,** 316–325, 1979.

54. Spadaro D. C., Robinson L. A. and Smith L. T. Assessing readability of patient information materials. *Am. J. Hosp. Pharm.* **37,** 215–221, 1980.

55. Eaton M. L. and Holloway R. L. Patient comprehension of written drug information. *Am. J. Hosp. Pharm.* **37,** 240–243, 1980.1

56. Morris L. A., Myers A. and Thilmen D. G. Application of the readability concept to patient-oriented drug information. *Am. J. Hosp. Pharm.* **37,** 504–508, 1980.

57. Rehder T. *et al.*, Improving medication compliance by counseling and special prescription container. *Am. J. Hosp. Pharm.* **37,** 379–385, 1980.

58. Brown D. J., Helling D. K. and Jones M. E. Evaluation of clinical pharmacist consultation in a family practice office. *Am. J. Hosp. Pharm.* **36,** 912–915, 1974.

59. Helling D. K., Hepler C. D. and Jones, M. E. Effect of direct clinical pharmaceutical services on patients' perceptions of health care quality. *Am. J. Hosp. Pharm.* **36,** 325–329, 1979.

60. McKenney J. M. *et al.*, Drug therapy assessments by pharmacists. *Am. J. Hosp. Pharm.* **37,** 824–828, 1980.

The Maintenance of Professional Authority: Acupuncture and the American Physician

Paul Root Wolpe

A profession's power rests on its consensually granted authority over a specific cultural tradition. Knowledge and maintenance of that tradition is the profession's social capital, and it must guard that capital from challenges while projecting an aura of confidence, competence, trust, and self-criticism. Professions institutionalize control over social capital by establishing licensing procedures, internally-run educational institutions, and self-regulation. But institutional legitimacy, while somewhat self-sustaining, also depends on ongoing public acceptance of a profession's claim of exclusive expertise over a realm of specialized knowledge. Lacking broad coercive powers, professions have developed strategies to protect their socially granted right to interpret their particular cultural tradition.

Paul Starr recently suggested the term "cultural authority" to describe a profession's ability to construct "particular definitions of reality and judgments of meaning and value [that] will prevail as true" (1982:13). Cultural authority complements Weber's social authority, which Starr describes as control of action through commands. The distinction is important, as a profession uses different strategies to maintain each type of authority. *Social* authority can be legislated and built into the formal structure of institutions; *cultural* authority cannot be as effectively decreed, for, as history has shown, it is extremely difficult to coerce belief. A profession must use more subtle means to insure that its definitions of reality and judgments of value will continue to prevail in the social realm.[1]

[1] As Starr (1982) points out, the physician's cultural authority is legally binding in some cases, as when a physician assesses fitness for an employer, pronounces death, or adduces insanity. However, these cases are predicated on the acceptance of the profession's broader cultural authority to define illness, which is the concern of this discussion.

Reprinted from *Social Problems*, vol. 32 (June, 1985), pp. 409–424. Copyright © by The Society for the Study of Social Problems.

Since professionals usually control or have close ties with agencies that produce knowledge, their institutionalized cultural authority is protected. For example, medical researchers, if not physicians themselves, typically have been indoctrinated into the biomedical model that lies at the heart of the medical profession's cultural authority in Western society. Researchers define their role, at least partially, as providing the data and methods necessary for the physician to improve biomedical practice. Research findings that seem to refute basic tenets of the biomedical "disciplinary matrix," to use a Kuhnian phrase, generate unease and great efforts to bring the aberrant data back under a biomedical rubric.

Part of the success of the biomedical model has been due to its resilience in the face of anomalous data. Michael Polanyi (1964) has suggested that belief systems are tenacious and virtually invulnerable to external criticism. Marxism, psychoanalysis, theosophy, and other totalistic models provide elaborate systems of theories, comprehensive interpretive frameworks that absorb seemingly contrary data and defuse their threat to the belief system. Both science and its offspring, biomedicine, fit Polanyi's description of tenacious belief systems. Each normally exists in a state that Kuhn calls "normal science," where a prevailing ideology is ingrained through a reiterated and reinforced methodology (Kuhn, 1962). Revolutions in science occur when the theoretical framework cannot cope with internally generated anomalies. Kuhn implies that these anomalies seem to hover ominously while scientists struggle to cope with them by creating ad hoc theories and articulations that avoid disruption of the prevailing "paradigm." However, anomalies may evoke crises not only by calling into question fundamentals of a paradigm, but simply by "the mere length of time" that an anomaly persists (Kuhn, 1962:82). Therefore, it becomes important to minimize the time that such threats are allowed to remain unincorporated into the theoretical structure of the belief system.

Science, as a sprawling, multifaceted, and somewhat insulated and hidden institution, can afford to allow anomalies a long lag time before coping with them. A profession does not have that luxury; being always in the public eye and responsible for application of a cultural model on a large scale, a profession cannot appear self-contradictory or baffled as it strives to interpret and define facts and values within its cultural jurisdiction.

On occasion, a profession confronts a sudden, unexpected challenge to its cultural (and, potentially, its social) authority. When the situation develops slowly, the profession can plan responses and strategies to protect itself. When unanticipated contingencies arise, the dynamics of its response process are often revealed as the profession scrambles to assess the challenge and protect its interests.

Such a situation occurred in 1972 with the rediscovery of acupuncture in the United States,[2] a therapeutic modality that seemed to defy anatomical, neurophysiological, and philosophical principles of Western biomedicine. The appearance of acupuncture was so sudden, and media attention so overwhelming, that the medical profession was caught off guard by an onslaught of questions and eyewitness accounts for which it had no available response. Yet it *was* to the medical profession that the public turned for interpretation of a technique that seemed to fall under the physician's cultural jurisdiction. How did the medical profession—initially unable to assess acupuncture—assert, maintain, and interpret professional ownership of this emergent phenomenon? How did physicians protect the biomedical model against a modality that did not seem to conform to that model? Before addressing these questions, I must review the history of the arrival of acupuncture in the United States that set the stage for professional and lay reactions to an alien medical philosophy.[3]

[2] I use the term "rediscovery" because acupuncture had been periodically introduced to American medicine by physicians training in France, where the practice has been used since the eighteenth century (see Quen, 1975; Wolpe, 1982).

[3] This paper is based on a search of all articles published in U.S. and Canadian journals on acupuncture in both the professional medical literature and the popular media from 1970 to the present. The search was conducted by consulting the medical, social science, and lay media indices, and then using a snowball technique from the references found. Over 250 relevant articles on acupuncture were found, mostly published between 1971 and 1975. I attempt to present quotes that are representative of opinions expressed in the literature.

ACUPUNCTURE ARRIVES IN TWENTIETH CENTURY AMERICA

In the history of medicine, at least in our lifetimes, no other development, including the antibiotic era, has so captured the interest of the public, and so confounded and confused the health professionals, as has the introduction into Western medicine of the ancient Oriental practice of acupuncture. When confronted on one hand with the philosophy, art, and indeed, science thousands of years old, and on the other hand with modern scientific theory and medical knowledge, and to find, initially and superficially, the two in diametric conflict, it is easy to understand why acupuncture is being considered with mixed emotions (Riddle, 1974:289).

This observation by Jackson W. Riddle, Chairman of The New York State Acupuncture Commission, reflects the state of opinion almost three years after the initial reports of acupuncture emerged from China when Nixon began lifting the bamboo curtain in 1971. The acupuncture explosion began in earnest in July 1971 when James Reston of the *New York Times* was rushed to the "Anti-Imperialist Hospital" in Peking. His appendix was removed by a surgical team using conventional anesthesia (Xylocain and Benzocane). The next night, however, he experienced considerable abdominal discomfort, and Li Changyuan, the hospital acupuncturist, relieved his distress by inserting three needles into Reston's right elbow and below his knees. Relief was immediate and lasting.

Reston told his story on the front page of the *New York Times* a few days later (Reston, 1971). From that moment on, every visitor to China seemed to return with tales of acupuncture wonders. In September 1971, four distinguished physicians were month-long guests of the Chinese Medical Association; a few months later, President Nixon visited China and brought his personal medical and osteopathic physicians. These physicians all filed astonished reports of witnessing acupuncture anesthesia, a procedure that seemed to allow major operations to be performed with nothing more than thin needles in earlobes and distant limbs. Patients were fully awake, talking, and even sipping liquids during major surgery! For the first time in modern American history, acupuncture was taken seriously. The American Medical Association (AMA) delegation to China reported: "Although authenticating statistical information is not readily available, [acupuncture] invites serious attention and further investigation" (quoted in Davis, 1975:18).[4] American physicians concentrated their glowing reports on acupuncture anesthesia and usually ignored therapeutic or "traditional" acupuncture, which had been developed over 5,000 years based on traditional Chinese theories of etiology, diagnosis, and treatment.[5]

The impact of acupuncture on the United States in 1972 would be difficult to exaggerate. This miracle cure for everything from baldness to frigidity was reported in all the popular media, from *Life* (Saar, 1971) to *Vogue* (Topping, 1972) to the *National Review* (Hazelton, 1972). *Newsweek* (1972) ran a lead story with a cover picture of a woman whose smiling face was studded with acupuncture needles. One reporter called acupuncture "a darling of the American media" due to its potential for dramatic photography, tales of miracle cures, and accusations of quackery (Africano, 1975:657).

Meanwhile, Chinese newspapers hailed Reston's cure and the U.S. reception as "a great victory for the proletarian medical line of Chairman Mao and the great Cultural Revolution" (*New York Times*, 1971). The New York State Board of Medicine encouraged serious investigation. The federal govern-

---

[4] The resurgence of acupuncture in the 1970s is an interesting example of the politics of medicine—the new fraternity between East and West demanded a delicate treatment of issues that each considered culturally sensitive. Acupuncture, seen as an ancient and "venerable" medical modality restored to prominence by Mao's revolution, was therefore accorded respect by Western politicians, journalists—and physicians.

[5] E. Grey Dimond, one of the four physicians to visit China in 1971, noted explicitly that he had no method of evaluating the claims of traditional acupuncture, and wrote primarily of acupuncture anesthesia. This is interesting, as James Reston's operation was performed under conventional anesthesia, and what he reported in the *New York Times* was his experience with traditional acupuncture. I discuss in more detail below the tendency of physicians to slight traditional acupuncture.

ment recommended the establishment of research projects through grants from the National Institute of General Medical Sciences (NIGMS), and the National Institutes of Health (NIH) announced it would conduct a major study of acupuncture (*New York Times,* 1972a). The Internal Revenue Service (1972) ruled that fees for acupuncture services qualified as medical expenses, and the Food and Drug Administration exerted quality control regulations over acupuncture needles (Riddle, 1974). The American Society of Chinese Medicine was formed, and the *American Journal of Chinese Medicine* was begun. In 1974 Hahnemann Medical School graduated the first American resident in acupuncture anesthesia (Davis, 1975). There was also an exponential increase in the American scientific and medical journal articles on acupuncture: the United States, which had almost no published articles on acupuncture in 1970, accounted for about one-fifth of all printed scientific research on the subject by 1974 (Davis, 1975). NIGMS sponsored a two-day national conference on acupuncture, bringing together approximately 100 scientists and physicians to discuss potential research directions. Research centers were established, conferences were organized, and articles gushed forth.

On May 26, 1972, a patient at the Albert Einstein College of Medicine in New York underwent a skin graft operation with acupuncture as the sole anesthesia, offering the press the first reported use of acupuncture anesthesia in the United States (*Medical World News,* 1972). At a hastily called press conference the next day, a group from Downstate Medical Center in Brooklyn announced that they had removed a papilloma from a medical student's tonsil using acupuncture anesthesia ten days before the Einstein group. The race to claim the first successful use of acupuncture anesthesia in the United States was finally put to rest when a letter appeared in the *Journal of the American Medical Association* (*JAMA*) from a physician at Weiss Memorial Hospital in Chicago, announcing that a tonsillectomy had been performed there on a 31-year-old male nurse anesthetist on April 21, 1972 (Liu, 1972). A report in the *Medical World News* (1972) on the rush to perform acupuncture anesthesia in the United States began: "Acupuncture anesthesia has made a highly theatrical debut in America. Without an Actors

Equity card, a number of doctors turned thespian, starting last month. They did the procedure on each other . . . and they did it presurgically on patients. They even did it on reporters." The article ended by noting the American Society of Anesthesiologists' "grave concern" over acupuncture anesthesia's "hasty application with little thought of safeguards or hazards."

The lay public was equally mobilized as the fascination with this exotic new therapy spread. In September 1972, Roman Gabriel, the popular quarterback for the Los Angeles Rams, underwent acupuncture treatment for his injured elbow. He reported a 60 to 70 percent improvement of motion and relief from pain (*New York Times,* 1972b). Organized sports perked its collective ear as professional athletes began to hire acupuncturists (Blount, 1972), and acupuncture was soon a household word. The American Society of Chinese Medicine had to hold a secret conference in New Haven because curiosity seekers had disrupted a similar conference in New York City (*New Haven Register,* 1972). American acupuncturists, most of whom were Oriental lay practitioners trained in the Far East, were swamped with patients. The first acupuncture clinic in New York City opened in July of 1972; one week later, when it was shut down by the State Health Department for practicing medicine without a license, 500 patients had been served and the clinic was booked solid for months in advance (*New York Post,* 1972a, 1972b; *Time,* 1972).[6]

By 1974 all the conditions seemed to exist for acupuncture's development as part of organized medicine in the United States: it had attained basic medical legitimacy, had developed a large, enthusiastic patient pool, and had begun licensure, a professional literature, and research programs. Davis (1975), in an analysis of the exponential growth of acupuncture publications in the United States from 1970 to 1974, speculated that scientific research on the technique would probably cease maintaining its growth curve

---

[6] In the *Time* magazine report (1972) about the closing of the clinic, the growing conflict between lay practitioners and organized medicine is pointed out. One patient is quoted as saying that no acupuncture clinics had been closed "until people started leaving their regular doctors and seeking out acupuncturists."

within "one human generation."[7] The only question appeared to be whether acupuncture would become a subdiscipline of physician practice or an allied medical profession with its own practitioners, as in nursing or physical therapy. Yet, within five years of its introduction, acupuncture research reached the end of its growth curve in the United States, almost no physicians included acupuncture in their treatment regimen, and practically no medical schools had instituted acupuncture as a normal part of their curriculum. Why did acupuncture fail to become firmly established in American medicine?

THE PHYSICIANS REACT

The overwhelming media and lay interest in acupuncture quickly became anathema to most of organized medicine. Physicians had no expertise in acupuncture and no knowledge of physiological mechanisms that could account for it. Indeed, it seemed to violate laws of anatomy and neurophysiology. Acupuncture was an alien treatment with an alien philosophical basis imported as a package from the East; it was not an indigenous alternative modality that reacted to (and thus was informed by) the biomedical model. Yet, it became apparent to medical professionals that the maintenance of their cultural authority over definitions of health and illness demanded that they provide the laity with a reasonable explanation of acupuncture's effects, and that the explanation fit the biomedical tradition that supported that authority. Eyewitness accounts from reputable physicians (e.g., Dimond, 1971b) and movies of Chinese operations using acupuncture anesthesia precluded dismissing acupuncture as fakery; but biomedicine had no ready explanation for the analgesic effects of needling distant loci. An explanation was needed that would account for acupuncture but conform to the theoretical basis of biomedicine.

Biomedicine, like most resilient belief systems, contains mechanisms that absorb anomalies and in-

corporates them into existing theoretical structures. However, the process of reinterpreting and redefining data takes time, and professions cannot allow aberrant data to remain unexplained for extended periods. To mitigate the threat posed to its cultural authority by lingering anomalous data, biomedicine has created residual categories that can temporarily absorb such aberrations.

These biomedical "holding cells" are used as tentative explanations for anomalous data while researchers work to create new areas of orthodox theory to account for enigmatic findings. The most commonly used surrogate theories are the "placebo" or "psychosomatic" explanations of phenomena, and the related categories of "hypnosis" and "suggestability." Any nonconventional treatment that is shown to be effective—and for which biomedicine has no existing categorization or relevant theory—is almost always initially credited to one of these categories.

Therefore, it is not surprising that these explanations were immediately called upon to explain acupuncture. The mechanistic theories of biomedicine are weakest in their attempts to connect the categorizations of "mind" or "psyche" and physiology; any phenomenon that can be banished to the former realm cannot threaten the latter, upon which the bulk of biomedical theory rests. Thus E. Grey Dimond, one of the original members of the medical delegation to China, wrote in the *Saturday Review* that the majority of claims for traditional acupuncture (not, as we shall see, acupuncture anesthesia) were "based on the simple fact that most patients have complaints that will get well with time or else need the solace of a 'doctor's' attention. Placing a sharp needle in the skin for a few minutes could well be impressive psychosomatic therapy" (Dimond, 1971a:19). However, in his report to *JAMA* (Dimond, 1971b), he was more circumspect; there was less need to protect cultural authority among colleagues.

Other physicians were less prudent in assessing the new therapy. Robert J. White, professor of neurosurgery at Case Western Reserve University, commented that acupuncture anesthesia was "basement neurophysiology . . . basically to distract the patient" and "overload the circuits." The operations must include "a very high element of hypnotic suggestion." He concluded that acupuncture anesthesia would never replace, or even "take its place alongside of," classical anesthesia (*Medical World News,*

---

[7] Davis cites 21 acupuncture citations in 1970, 43 in 1971, 29 in 1972, 202 in 1973, and about 250 in 1974, more than a four-fold increase in five years. By 1974, one-third of all research was published in English, and one-fifth of all research came from the United States, almost all of it from within the previous two years.

1972:13). The seriousness of much of the medical profession's concern over acupuncture can be gauged by the vehemence of some physicians' denunciations of the practice in the popular media and professional journals. One physician castigated his colleagues who took acupuncture seriously as bowing to the pressures of "non-scientific weirdos and the high priests of folk medicine," and advocated the hypnosis theory to account for reports of its efficacy (Goldstein, 1972:15). Arthur Taub (1972), a Yale University neurosurgeon, responded to the announcement that the National Institutes of Health was committed to funding acupuncture research with a letter to *Science* stating "neither the diagnostic nor the therapeutic technique has any basis." He continued:

> It would be tragic if the announcement of such a premature "commitment" to the funding of research in acupuncture were to be interpreted by the public as an endorsement of the technique. While placebo effects have their place in therapy, the absence of adequate diagnosis before treatment may lead to needless suffering and, in some cases to avoidable death (Taub, 1972).

Dr. Taub was not alone. Physician reaction to acupuncture was so strong that a September 1972 poll revealed that 41 percent of physicians polled were opposed to any further clinical research into acupuncture at all (*Modern Medicine,* 1972).

Another explanation cited for the efficacy of acupuncture in China was "Chinese stoicism" and the patriotic zeal of the Cultural Revolution (see, for example, *JAMA,* 1973a). This placebo explanation was enhanced by the image of Chinese patients who "seemed to derive courage for their operations and emotional sustenance from having the famous 'Red Book' next to their heads on the operating table," as one physician described it (Veith, 1972:109; see also Dimond, 1971b; Goldstein, 1972; *Newsweek,* 1971). An editorial in the *Canadian Medical Association Journal* (1974) concurred; after stating that "however satisfactory this type of anesthesia may be in the Orient it just does not work on most Occidentals," the article concluded with its explanation of the phenomenon: "If Mao's teaching and the rest of the preoperative ritual is not operant conditioning, what is it?" Yet, the prestige of medical eyewitnesses, the few hurried operations using acupuncture anesthesia in the United States, and reports of vet-

erinary acupuncture (see Riddle, 1974:295; Wei, 1979:54–55) challenged the permanent dismissal of acupuncture to the residual categories of placebo and hypnosis.[8]

Medical organizations were perplexed about what stand to take on acupuncture. The Secretary General of the Canadian Medical Association, in an article entitled "The Acupuncture Mess" (Wallace, 1975), complained that acupuncture remained unregulated in Canada partially because the medical licensing authorities who viewed it as a legitimate medical therapy were in conflict with spokesmen for the voluntary medical association, who referred to acupuncture as "hocuspocus with knitting needles."

Physicians were also concerned about distancing themselves from the untrained "quackupuncturists" who were rushing to provide acupuncture services.[9] *JAMA* (1973b) warned against the "quick quacks" who were practicing acupuncture and offering physician training programs lasting three days for large enrollment fees. The *Journal of the American Osteopathic Association* (*JAOA,* 1974:69) also decried the fact that "acupuncture has become a medical fad and the money changers of the medical market place are trying to capitalize on it while 'it still works.'" However, biomedical research needed the skills of trained acupuncturists, and the only practitioners in the United States were the lay practitioners, mostly Oriental, who had been practicing illegally for years in the Chinatowns of major cities. Physicians had to draw on their expertise without seeming to associate themselves with such marginal groups.

Strong physician reaction to acupuncture was partly due to the changing nature of public opinion about organized medicine in general. The early 1970s marked the beginning of what Paul Starr (1982) calls the "decline of professional sovereignty." Confidence in professionals of all types was eroding. "Establish-

---

[8] Despite conclusive evidence that acupuncture has physiological effects, placebo and hypnosis advocates have maintained their position (see Finzi, 1974; Kroger, 1973; Mendelson, 1981; Sweet, 1981).

[9] Using placebo and hypnosis effects as explanations to account for the efficacy of alternative therapies also may serve to delegitimize the lay practitioner, opening the way for later takeover of the technique by physicians once research has demonstrated its effectiveness.

ment" medicine was a primary target of the women's movement, special interest groups for the handicapped and the mentally ill, and a spate of lawsuits by patients demanding rights over their health care. Such assaults were a blow to a profession that prided itself on being the patient's advocate. The reaction to institutional medicine took the form of a revival of self-help groups and the expansion of a therapeutic counterculture including lay midwives, "holistic" practitioners of every ilk, chiropractic, homeopathic, etc. It was in that milieu that acupuncture had arrived and became a visible symbol of the battle being fought along many fronts by organized medicine.

ACUPUNCTURE MEDICALIZED

Acupuncture had become problematic to the American physician. The medical establishment had to protect its cultural authority against its admitted inability to explain acupuncture and respond to the growing number of patients attracted to lay acupuncture practitioners. A twofold strategy was initiated: (1) *research* was needed to incorporate acupuncture into the biomedical belief system, and large-scale medical research projects—many federally funded— were begun; and (2) acupuncture *practice* had to be wrested from lay practitioners, and so legislative and propagandist strategies began to appear.

Acupuncture Research

Acupuncture's potential impact on biomedical beliefs was expressed by Dr. Gerald Looney of the UCLA medical school in 1973:

> If these reports can be confirmed and the autonomic theory of acupuncture validated, then the astounding implications of acupuncture from the patient's point of view may well be surpassed by the physician's point of view: an entirely new look will have to be taken at human physiology in general and the nervous system in particular. The simple and comfortable concepts from the past may have to be re-defined as we find the central nervous system/autonomic nervous system axis actually seems more comprehensible when viewed as a highly integrated and unified system, and that this unitary nervous system,

in turn, is involved intimately in the dysfunction and pathology of all other body systems (quoted in Riddle, 1974:296).

The biomedical cultural model was not to crumble so easily, however, as medical research had begun a concentrated campaign to force acupuncture into a Western mold. To do so, the entire theoretical framework of *traditional* Chinese acupuncture had to be replaced. To support the integrity of ancient yin-yang polarity theory, "five element" or phase theory, and the existence of the meridians,[10] medical researchers would have to relinquish any claim that acupuncture was part of biomedicine and thus was under their exclusive control. Biomedicine had no means of assessing the validity of these cultural models.[11] Traditional acupuncture theory and treatment philosophy was therefore all but discarded, and acupuncture analgesia/anesthesia—a very small part of traditional acupuncture's therapeutic claims (acupuncture anesthesia was not used in China until the 1960s)—was presented as acupuncture's only true potential contribution to Western medicine.[12] NIH's "commitment" to fund research into acupuncture's effects was expressly limited to surgical anesthesia and the treatment of pain in chronic syn-

[10] Traditional acupuncture is based on a belief in the balancing of life energy, called "ch'i," which flows mainly through fourteen parasagittal lines or meridians. The quality of the flow of this energy was determined by reference to yin-yang and the five "elements" or phases (or, alternatively, the "eight principles") which provide a blueprint for assessing types of energy blockages, flows, and quality. The interested reader is referred to Porkert (1974) for the definitive scientific analysis of this medical philosophy in English.

[11] Manfred Porkert's (1974) book on the philosophical and theoretical foundations of traditional Chinese medicine stresses the rational, empirical, and scientifically derived basis of these concepts. However, traditional Eastern science has certain premises that are not shared by Western science, which make cross-cultural testing extremely difficult.

[12] This is not to say that research was not carried out on other aspects of acupuncture. Steiner's (1983) article, for example, cites many studies by American researchers. However, few of the experimenters tried to incorporate traditional acupuncture's claims into their research, their reports were published in minor journals, and positive findings have been largely ignored by organized medicine.

dromes (*Science*, 1972). *Pain* was a phenomenon familiar to biomedical research.

Traditional acupuncture does not lend itself to Western scientific study, for the biomedical research model assumes that people react similarly to similar stimuli and that statistical generalizations can be based on their reactions. This mechanistic assumption is antithetical to traditional acupuncture and its philosophy of etiology, diagnosis, and treatment—all of which are extremely individualistic. Traditional diagnosis is a complex procedure, involving sphygmology (pulse diagnosis), patient history, the patient's circadian and seasonal rhythms, color, odor, energy balance, diet, emotional framework, and so on. Acupuncture is foremost a philosophy of preventive medicine, of intervention to correct the body's energy balance before pathology becomes manifest. To restore correct energy flow, the Chinese employ a variety of needles of varying widths, lengths, and metals, and base the correct depth, rotation, and duration of needle use on the diagnosis. Traditional diagnosis and treatment differ profoundly for two patients with a common Western diagnosis. Traditional acupuncturists also assert that needles placed in the same locus in two people will have different effects depending on the particular configuration of energy balance in each individual, which would negate much of the scientific research performed in the United States. Reducing the complex diagnostic procedure developed over thousands of years to static point-equals-effect needling would remove acupuncture technique from its traditional rationale.

Most researchers quickly discarded traditional acupuncture without any serious attempts to evaluate its merits clinically. The New York Commission on Acupuncture, on the whole unabashedly enthusiastic about the unlimited possibilities of acupuncture, wrote:

> There has been general concurrence that if the subject of pulse diagnosis is not considered, and modern Western medical diagnosis procedures used, and if the other ancient philosophical explanations are not studied, the simple techniques of needle insertion and stimulation can be readily learned and incorporated into the body of Western medicine. . . . If one does not have to learn all of the archaic Oriental theory and philosophy, and simply concentrates on the appropriate loci

> and technique . . . acupuncture can be practiced very successfully for relief of pain and the treatment of certain diseases. . . . In our own civilization, that which has outlived its usefulness is rapidly discarded and replaced by new material, or new theories, or new practices (*Riddle, 1974:303*).

Teruo Matsumoto, a surgeon at Hahnemann Hospital in Philadelphia who was trained in acupuncture in Japan, also suggested abandoning the five element theory for "electrophysiologic concepts, Reverse Head-Mackenzie Theory, and the gate control system theory proposed by Melzack and Wall" (Matsumoto, 1972).[13] In an issue of the *Bulletin of the New York Academy of Medicine* devoted entirely to acupuncture in September 1975, William Dornette, an anesthesiologist, wrote that "one of the great disadvantages of acupuncture—an impediment to its acceptance among scientists in the United States—is that it is often associated with the philosophy, mysticism, and magic of the East. Clearly, too, the study of anatomy as applied to acupuncture will reveal that neural and vascular structures are truly involved" (Dornette, 1975:895). And, as recently as 1981, a physician wrote in *JAMA:* "It now becomes no [more] necessary to learn ancient rituals and practice complicated by Oriental hocus-pocus to locate and stimulate motor points on appropriate dermatome levels than it is to burn down a Chinese farmhouse to prepare roast pork" (Ulett, 1981:769). Almost all Western researchers agreed on these points, independent of their belief in acupuncture's efficacy, which led the American Osteopathic Association to note: "It is curious that there seems to be a great rush to separate acupuncture from its philosophy. And somehow an uneasy feeling grows that in throwing away some of the myths and philosophy, an inte-

---

[13] Reverse Head-Mackenzie Theory refers to a "sensory zone" in the skin which radiates visceral pain to certain parts of the skin and shows some relationship to acupuncture points. Melzack and Wall's "Pain gate" theory was frequently called upon to explain acupuncture analgesia. It postulates that there are "gates" (originally one was proposed, then two) through which impulses flow to the brain. When stimulated by minor impulses (such as the acupuncture needle) major pain impulses cannot get through. (This purportedly explains why we put pressure on a sore spot, as in clutching our toe when we stub it.)

gral part of the understanding of the therapy may be lost" (*JAOA,* 1974:69). Of course, in order for physicians to accomplish their goal of subjugating acupuncture to an alien Western medical model, it was necessary and desirable that the tenets of traditional acupuncture be excluded.

Before physicians could translate acupuncture into conventional medical terms, they had to simplify the technique and minimize its claims. By downgrading acupuncture to analgesic needling, physicians could claim to show that: (a) acupuncture was not as effective as had originally been claimed; (b) acupuncture was not a threat to biomedical models, because it is based on stimulus-response reactions of a neurophysiological type; (c) the physician was best suited to evaluate, explain, and ultimately, practice acupuncture; and (d) since there were physiological, experimentally demonstrated analgesic reactions to loci needling, all claims of acupuncture were reducible to this analegsic effect. Thus the physician could credit the Chinese with using a real modality, while maintaining that the original explanatory system and its claims could be dismissed.

Acupuncture Practice

As the medical profession fought to assert *cultural* authority over acupuncture by subjugating it under a biomedical interpretive framework, it also sought to assert *social* authority by pressing for restriction of acupuncture practice to physicians or, alternatively, to strict medical supervision. Since Western research decreed that acupuncture was for symptom relief only and that its rationale conformed to the biomedical model, the years of training and study of the Oriental acupuncturists could be discounted as "an example of big investment for little intellectual return" (Feibel, 1974:525).

In 1974 the House of Delegates of the AMA resolved:

> *that it is the current judgment of the American Medical Association that since the practice of acupuncture in the United States is an experimental medical procedure, it should be performed in a research setting by a licensed physician or under his direct supervision and responsibility, and therefore the A.M.A. urges its constituent state and territorial associations*

> *to seek appropriate legislation and rules and regulations to confine the performance of acupuncture to such research settings (quoted in Schwartz, 1981:5).*

The New York State Commission on Acupuncture's final report, which recommended research into acupuncture's use for a variety of disorders, also proposed that acupuncture practice be regulated by the state board of medicine or dentistry and rendered only under strict medical supervision (Riddle, 1974). The American Osteopathic Association, after lamenting the quickness with which acupuncture was separated from its traditional philosophy, adopted a resolution that read, in part:

> *RESOLVED that the AOA go on record as favoring the acceptance of acupuncture as part of the armamentarium of its qualified and licensed physicians and so recognizes acupuncture as an adjunctive and beneficial modality and be it further*

> *RESOLVED that the AOA go on record as favoring the practice of acupuncture only by qualified physicians* (JAOA, *1974:70*).

It must be remembered that in the early 1970s there were practically no American-trained physicians practicing acupuncture in the United States, though there were a number of often highly trained Oriental practitioners, many of whom were licensed physicians in their native countries. McRae (1982) has suggested that ethnic prejudice was not an insignificant part of the medical establishment's opposition to these practitioners. In order to legitimize their claim that acupuncture should and could be practiced competently only by physicians, the technique had to be simplified to a degree that the average physician could learn it without an excessive investment of time and energy. A. J. Webster (1979) describes how the medical profession carefully parceled acupuncture out among its subspecialties so that each had its share without unduly intruding on specialty boundaries. For example, dentists only did research on the technical efficiency of acupuncture for pain relief and avoided neurophysiology's domain of *how* acupuncture worked. Webster suggests that dentists minimized the challenge of acupuncture by insisting that it required little time to master while they rushed to gain proficiency and to be recognized as "experts" in this new field. In order to protect their monopoly on medical practice, the profession not only instituted efforts to control acupuncture research, but was careful to regulate its internal dissemination to the appropriate specialties to allow a new array of experts the financial and prestige benefits of medical expertise.

Those medical spokesmen who recognized the need, at least initially, to employ non-physician acupuncturists in practice, invariably assumed medical supervision was a necessity. Ginger McRae (1982:167) argues that:

> State regulation limiting the practice of acupuncture to physicians exhibits excessive deference to orthodox medicine. . . . There is no evidence that such regulation has ever been necessary to protect the public health, and in view of its deleterious effects on acupuncture's growth and availability, it should be overturned.

She continues:

> Supervised-practice regulation entails the same monopolistic and anti-competitive effects as regulation limiting acupuncture practice to physicians. . . . [I]t, too, views acupuncturists in a Western medical context, mistrusts the safety and effectiveness of acupuncture, greatly restricts its availability, may fail to insist that practitioners have adequate training and experience, and frequently discourages highly qualified persons—especially Orientals—from practicing (1982:172).

In addition, since acupuncture was (and is) viewed with suspicion by many physicians, and since physicians assume primary liability for allied health professionals under their supervision, it is difficult to find physicians willing to sponsor acupuncture practitioners. One Oriental practitioner remarked: "I practiced long before there was a law. Now they say I can only practice under medical supervision in medical schools. So I work with doctors at the University. It's unfair, but what can I do? The thing I don't understand, though, is how can American doctors supervise acupuncture if they don't know anything about it?" (quoted in Koenig, 1973:37–8).

A number of court cases have challenged physicians' effective monopoly of acupuncture. The most controversial is undoubtedly *Andrews v. Ballard* (1980). In this celebrated Texas case, a group of people filed suit against an edict restricting acupuncture practice to licensed physicians, claiming that the lack of qualified physician acupuncturists effectively denied them access to their choice of treatment and thus denied their constitutional right to privacy. The court ruled: (1) "Whatever the best explanation is for how acupuncture works, one thing is clear: it does work." (2) "Moreover, acupuncture has been practiced for 2,000 to 5,000 years. It is no more experimental as a mode of medical treatment than is the Chinese language as a mode of communication. What is experimental is not acupuncture, but Westerners' understanding of it and their ability to utilize it properly." (3) Denial of acupuncture may force the patient to resort to much riskier Western techniques. (4) Qualified lay practitioners pose no threat to the health of the community. (5) Therefore, the rule limiting acupuncture to licensed physicians makes it effectively unavailable in Texas and is therefore unconstitutional (*Andrews v. Ballard,* 1980). The court also agreed with the plaintiffs that there was a paradox in the existing legislation: "[The state] has prohibited the formally trained from practicing, but has allowed the formally untrained, who it admits [in its brief] 'are not schooled enough in acupuncture to effectively supervise acupuncturists,' . . . to proceed without any showing of skill or knowledge" (quoted in Schwartz, 1981:7). The suit was filed against the Texas State Board of Medical Examiners and the Attorney General of the State of Texas. The verdict, not surprisingly, was opposed by organized medicine (e.g., Curran, 1981).

As of 1982, three states limited acupuncture practice to physicians by statute, while 30 limited it based on medical board rule, regulation, or policy. Most others allow non-physician acupuncturists to practice only under direct supervision of a physician, usually as a type of physician's assistant, though seven states do allow independent practice by non-physician acupuncturists (see McRae, 1982). In California, 500 people, mostly trained lay practitioners, had been certified as acupuncturists by 1978, and were declared primary health care practitioners by 1979; acupuncture is also covered by California's Medicaid program, Medi-Cal. So physicians have been successful in severely restricting acupuncture practice in all but a handful of states.[14]

DISCUSSION

The tactics pursued by the medical profession in the United States to monopolize acupuncture have effectively restricted its large-scale use as a therapeutic tool by physicians in the United States. After the initial confusion,. acupuncture was brought firmly under control by the medical profession, and public (and professional) interest declined. One indication of the waning interest in acupuncture is noted by McRae (1982), who reports that, after the flurry of legislative activity from 1972 to 1975, acupuncture's legal status has stagnated in most states. There are also indications that acupuncture research still maintains an ambiguous status in the medical community. The editors of a journal containing a recent favorable review of acupuncture research in the United States (Steiner, 1983) felt the need to preface the piece with a paragraph justifying the decision to print it. Despite articles such as Steiner's exhaustive review, and despite international conferences in other countries dealing exclusively with acupuncture research (Ulett, 1985), only one article at all favorable to acupuncture (Ulett, 1981) has appeared in *JAMA* since 1974, and acupuncture research and practice has been ignored altogether by the *New England Journal of Medicine*. In Britain, the President of the British Acupuncture Association claims that the *British Medical Journal* will not publish research reports submitted by traditional acupuncturists (Webster, 1979:137).

One reason for the medical profession's unease with acupuncture may be that, despite ongoing attempts to emerge with a mechanistic, predictable, Western acupuncture, the traditional framework has not been easily discarded. The acupuncture points are arranged in an ancient pattern, and the sophisti-

cated system of loci and their specific effects is intimately tied to the very background that the profession has dismissed as superstition. Acupuncture is not an herb or root from which the effective chemical can be extracted and synthesized.

Research does continue in the United States, primarily being reported in specialty journals like the *American Journal of Chinese Medicine* (*AJCM*). However, in the 1975 volume of *AJCM*, 71 percent of the articles had a U.S. or Canadian contributor; by 1980, that had dropped to 27 percent; and by the 1984 and 1985 volumes, only 8 percent of the articles had North American contributors.[15] Recent advances in pain management have lessened the attraction of acupuncture analgesia to American researchers (Bonica, 1979) and confusion and stigma are attached to its practice. Articles expressing opposite opinions about acupuncture's use and effectiveness can still be found in the American medical literature (see, for example, Sweet, 1981 and Ulett, 1981).[16]

Since acupuncture is too complex a modality to master quickly and efficiently, or to subjugate easily to biomedical explanations, it has been more expedient to discredit it. Rather than repudiate acupuncture and thus relinquish control over the modality, organized medicine claimed jurisdiction over the therapy and then severely circumscribed its claims. For example, in 1977 *JAMA* reported the failure of acupuncture anesthesia as a reliable modality (de Jong, 1977). Despite the fact that the article itself included reports of five thyroidectomies, five of six intrathoracic operations, and eight of nine dental extractions successfully performed with acupuncture

---

[14] It is interesting that much of the lay acupuncture that is attracting clients today is not the Western analgesic type, but an adapted traditional acupuncture which uses Oriental diagnosis and treatment. Schools of traditional acupuncture across the U.S. are graduating students and acupuncture survives as an alternative modality. Many of these practitioners still practice illegally.

[15] In 1975 (volume 3) 22 of 31 articles had American contributors; in 1980 (volume 8), it was 9 of 33; and by 1984 and 1985 (volumes 12 and 13, combined) it had fallen to 2 of 24. Authors who appeared more than once in a single volume were counted as a single contributor.

[16] It is ironic that the article by Sweet, which is a polemic against acupuncture, was first given as the second annual John J. Bonica lecture. Bonica, the President of the International Association for the Study of Pain, and chairman of the NIH Ad Hoc Committee on Acupuncture, was a strong supporter of acupuncture research. In an article included in a White House Report on pain therapies, he encouraged further research into acupuncture which "produces short term relief of chronic pain in about 40 to 60% of patients" (Bonica, 1979; see also Bonica, 1974).

anesthesia,[17] the author concluded that its use "loses much of its immediate appeal." Similarly, an anesthesiologist concluded in 1981 that "for Western anesthesiologists, acupuncture is useless. It is too difficult and too chancy" (Hassett, 1981:89). Yet the World Health Organization reported in 1980 that, even though Chinese anesthesiologists usually use Western-style anesthesia, 15 to 20 percent of all surgical procedures in China are done with acupuncture anesthesia (*WHO Chronicle,* 1980). Acupuncture anesthesia would seem to be indicated for patients who are at risk under conventional anesthesia; with acupuncture the patient remains conscious, has no post-operative nausea, no systemic depression, and recovery time is greatly shortened. Nonetheless, acupuncture anesthesia is not practiced regularly in any major American hospital.

The World Health Organization recommends acupuncture highly for at least 47 disorders, including the common cold, bronchial asthma, childhood myopia, and dysentery (*WHO Chronicle,* 1980). Acupuncture is a fully accepted and practiced therapy in Argentina, Austria, Belgium, Brazil, England, Finland, Germany, Italy, Switzerland, and other Western countries; acupuncture research has also progressed rapidly in the Soviet Union (Riddle, 1974; *WHO Chronicle,* 1980). In France, a significant number of physicians practice acupuncture, which is officially recognized by L'Academie de Medicine and is covered by the French National Health Insurance as a form of minor surgery (Bowers, 1978).[18] In contrast, as late as 1981, the AMA still labeled acupuncture an "unproved modality of therapy" (Ulett, 1983).

In one sense, acupuncture has been less of a threat to the cultural authority of physicians than chiropractic or osteopathy. Since acupuncture was "foreign" and had almost no non-Oriental practitioners, its takeover by physicians was unopposed by any powerful special interest groups, and even pro-vided physicians with the opportunity to portray their openness to "folk" medicines. Indigenous modalities like chiropractic, on the other hand, involve a greater power struggle of both social and cultural authority (see Firman and Goldstein, 1972). In the case of osteopathy, the House of Delegates of the AMA recommended in 1953 that "so little of the original concept of osteopathy remains that it does not classify . . . as the teaching of 'cultist' healing" (*JAMA,* 1953:739). Osteopathy was only accepted as a reasonable healing modality after its cultural model conformed sufficiently to that of orthodox medicine.[19]

Nurses have been more accepting of traditional acupuncture than physicians. Lacking the cultural authority of physicians and thus the need to protect their cultural model as vigorously, nurses generally are more receptive to unconventional modalities. An article in the *American Journal of Nursing* described traditional acupuncture and its philosophical and theoretical perspectives in great detail and concluded:

> *Several principles of traditional acupuncture are akin to ideas nursing has been advocating for many years; the importance of preventive health measures, active involvement of the individual patient, detailed observations, patient teaching . . . the importance of the whole man, in whom nothing happens in isolation but in relationship to other events occurring in his internal or external environment (Armstrong, 1972:1588).*

CONCLUSION

In describing the overwhelming opposition by the medical elite to Mesmerism in mid-nineteenth century England, Parssinen (1979:107–8) argues that

---

[17] It should be noted that all of these operations were performed in the neck or above, which are the areas most conducive to acupuncture anesthesia.

[18] French physicians have been more successful in monopolizing acupuncture without unduly restricting its availability; this may be due to the fact that acupuncture has been practiced there since the eighteenth century, and was established before biomedicine became the prevailing French medical belief system.

[19] Due partially to the pressure of constant antitrust lawsuits by chiropractors, the AMA changed its code of ethics in 1981, which now states that physicians are "free to choose whom to serve, with whom to associate, and the environment in which to provide medical services" (*Medical World News,* 1980). No longer can they be censured by the AMA for associating with those who do not practice a "method of healing founded on a scientific basis." Thus the formal barriers to association with nonconventional practitioners have been removed, but informal pressures and stigma still exist.

there were two main reasons that the response was more intense than in previous importations of alien therapies into Britain: first, "[Mesmerism] contradicted so completely the contemporary theory and practice of medicine";[20] and second, "It threatened the social and professional aspirations of medical men during a critical period of their history."[21] Much the same could be claimed for acupuncture in the 1970s. The theoretical basis of the modality was antithetical to biomedicine, and the physician confronted acupuncture at a time of waning prestige and increasing challenge to the professional sovereignty that had been built up since the early part of the century.

The medical profession has been singularly successful in asserting social authority in the United States (Starr, 1982). In order to protect that stature, the explicit basis upon which physician practice is founded—biomedical science—must be protected as the sole legitimizing cultural model of American medical practice. (No authors in the medical literature suggested that there might not *be* a Western scientific explanation for acupuncture.) To subjugate acupuncture under the cultural authority of medicine, acupuncture was stripped of its theoretical framework and most of its technique, and declared part of biomedicine. Thus training in medicine was deemed sufficient background to prepare a physician for practice with only minimal additional training—and most states do not require *any* special training in acupuncture for physicians to be allowed to prac-

[20] Most techniques in the nineteenth century which were outside scientific medicine as it then existed were performed by "empirics," who claimed that a specific remedy worked without understanding why. Mesmerists, on the other hand, advocated a "fluidist" interpretation of illness, and thus presented a theoretical basis for its effects that contradicted the current theories of scientific medicine (Parssinen, 1979).

[21] In the 1840s, the British medical community was trying to reform the profession by petitioning Parliament to create a central medical organization which would register all practitioners and administer a qualifying examination. The petition also advocated standardizing medical education and instituting criminal sanctions against unlicensed practitioners (Parssinen, 1979). In other words, physicians were trying to professionalize medicine, and Mesmerism was a popular, lay practice that resembled the medico-magical techniques that the medical community was trying to eliminate.

tice it. As McRae (1982:167) comments, "The refusal of state medical boards to protect the public from licensees [physicians] untrained in acupuncture may rest less on negligence than on an illogical, unproved, and even arrogant assumption that Western medical training is adequate preparation for acupuncture practice."

Since acupuncture could not easily be subjugated to biomedicine, it has been relegated to minor, auxiliary status. Since there was too much evidence that acupuncture does work, it has been restricted on the basis that Western research has not been able to make it work on its own terms. Physicians have successfully coped with a threat to their cultural authority while retaining the appearance of a willingness to explore and evaluate new therapies.

References

AFRICANO, LILLIAN
  1972 "Acupuncture, child of the media." The Nation (May):657–60.

ARMSTRONG, MARGARET E.
  1972 "Acupuncture." American Journal of Nursing 72: 1582–88.

BONICA, JOHN J.
  1974 "Therapeutic acupuncture in the People's Republic of China: implications for American medicine." Journal of the American Medical Association 228:1544–54.
  1979 "Current status of pain theory." In The Interagency Committee on New Therapies for Pain and Discomfort: Report to the White House. U.S. Department of Health, Education, and Welfare.

BOWERS, JOHN Z.
  1978 "Reception of acupuncture by the scientific community: from scorn to a degree of interest." Comparative Medicine East and West 6:89–96.

BLOUNT, ROY
  1972 "Quick Nagayana, the needle." Sports Illustrated 36:36–40.

Canadian Medical Association Journal
  1974 "Does acupuncture work?" 110:257.

CURRAN, WILLIAM J.
  1981 "Acupuncture, the practice of medicine, and the right to demand medical service." New England Journal of Medicine 305:439–40.

DAVIS, DEVRA LEE
1975 "The history and sociology of the scientific study of acupuncture." American Journal of Chinese Medicine 3:5–26.

DE JONG, RUDOLPH H.
1977 "Acupuncture anesthesia: pricking the balloon." Journal of the American Medical Association 237:2530.

DIMOND, E. GREY
1971a "More than herbs and acupuncture." Saturday Review (December):17–19, 71.

1971b "Acupuncture anesthesia: Western medicine and Chinese traditional medicine." Journal of the American Medical Association 218:1558–63.

DORNETTE, WILLIAM H. L.
1975 "The anatomy of acupuncture." Bulletin of the New York Academy of Medicine 51:893–4.

FEIBEL, ARIE
1974 "Acupuncture: dilemmas, problems, perspectives." Archives of Physical Medicine and Rehabilitation 55:524–5.

FINZI, DAVID B.
1974 "A mini-symposium on acupuncture." Journal of the American Medical Association 227:1122.

FIRMAN, G. J. and MICHAEL GOLDSTEIN
1975 "The future of chiropractic: a psychosocial view." New England Journal of Medicine 293:639–42.

GOLDSTEIN, DAVID N.
1972 "The cult of acupuncture." Wisconsin Medical Journal 71:14–6.

HASSETT, JAMES
1981 "Acupuncture is proving its points." Psychology Today 14:81–9.

HAZELTON, NIKA
1972 "Acupuncture, anyone?" National Review (July): 808–9.

Internal Revenue Service
1972 Rev. Rul. 72–593, IRB 1972 -51,7.

Journal of the American Medical Association
1953 "Report of the committee for the study of the relations between osteopathy and medicine." 152:734–9.

1973a "Acupuncture." 223:77–8.

1973b "Acupuncture and the acuchiropractors." 223: 682–3.

Journal of the American Osteopathic Association
1974 "American acupuncture." 74:68–70.

KOENIG, PETER
1973 "The Americanization of acupuncture." Psychology Today 7:37–8.

KROGER, WILLIAM S.
1973 "Hypnosis and acupuncture." Medical World News 14:a.

KUHN, THOMAS
1962 The Structure of Scientific Revolutions. Chicago: University of Chicago Press.

LIU, WEI-CHI
1972 "Acupuncture anesthesia: a case report." Journal of the American Medical Association 221:87–8.

MATSUMOTO, TERUO
1972 "Acupuncture and U.S. medicine." Journal of the American Medical Association 220:1010.

McRAE, GINGER
1982 "A critical overview of U.S. acupuncture regulation." Journal of Health Politics, Policy and Law 7:163–96.

Medical World News
1972 "Acupuncture explained: or is it?" (June):11–13.

1980 "Ethics: an opening to chiropractic?" (August):10.

MENDELSON, GEORGE
1981 "Effectiveness of acupuncture." Journal of the American Medical Association 246:1900.

Modern Medicine
1972 "A message from the editorial director." (September 18):6.

New Haven Register
1972 "Conference could speed use of acupuncture." (August 6):1.

New York Post
1972a "Acupuncture center opens here." (July 13).

1972b "State shuts acupuncture center here." (July 19).

New York Times
1971 "When in Peking . . ." (July 20):38.

1972a "U.S. to evaluate acupuncture for safety and effectiveness." (July 28):1.

1972b "Personalities." (September 30):23.

Newsweek
1971 "The Chinese surgeons." (June 7):78.

1972 "All about acupuncture." (August 14):48–52.

PARSSINEN, TERRY M.
1979 "Professional deviants and the history of medicine: medical mesmerists in Victorian Britain." In Roy Wallis (ed.), On the Margins of Science: The Social Construction of Rejected Knowledge. Sociological Review Monograph 27:103–20.

POLANYI, MICHAEL
1964 Personal Knowledge: Towards a Post Critical Philosophy. New York: Harper and Row.

PORKERT, MANFRED
  1974 The Theoretical Foundations of Chinese Medicine. Cambridge, MA: MIT Press.

QUEN, JACQUES
  1975 "Acupuncture and Western medicine." Bulletin of the History of Medicine 49:196–205.

RESTON, JAMES
  1971 "Now, about my operation in Peking." New York Times (July 26):1,6.

RIDDLE, JACKSON W.
  1974 "Report of the New York State commission on acupuncture." American Journal of Chinese Medicine 2:289–318.

SAAR, JOHN
  1971 "A visit to a friendly neighborhood sorcerer." Life (August 13):34.

SCHWARTZ, ROBERT
  1981 "Acupuncture and expertise: a challenge to physician control." Hastings Center Reports 11:5–7.

Science
  1972 "Acupuncture: fertile ground for faddists and serious NIH research." 177:592–93.

STARR, PAUL
  1982 The Social Transformation of American Medicine. New York: Basic Books.

STEINER, R. PRASAAD
  1983 "Acupuncture: cultural perspectives." Postgraduate Medicine 74:60–7.

SWEET, WILLIAM H.
  1981 "Some current problems in pain research and therapy (including needle puncture, 'acupuncture')." Pain 10:297–309.

TAUB, ARTHUR
  1972 "Acupuncture." Science 178:9.

Time Magazine
  1972 "Acupuncture crackdown." (September 18):55.

TOPPING, AUDREY
  1972 "Acupuncture." Vogue (January):94–5, 115–6.

ULETT, GEORGE A.
  1981 "Acupuncture treatments for pain relief." Journal of the American Medical Association 245:768–9.
  1983 "Acupuncture—time for a second look." Southern Medical Journal 76:421–3.
  1985 "Acupuncture update." Southern Medical Journal 78:237–8.

VEITH, ILZA
  1972 "Acupuncture: ancient enigma to East and West." American Journal of Psychiatry 129:333–6.

WALLACE, J. D.
  1975 "The acupuncture mess." Canadian Medical Association Journal 112:203.

WEBSTER, A. J.
  1979 "Scientific controversy and socio-cognitive metonymy: the case of acupuncture." In Roy Wallace (ed.) On the Margins of Science: The Social Construction of Rejected Knowledge. Sociological Review Monograph 27:121–37.

WEI, LING Y.
  1979 "Scientific advance in acupuncture." American Journal of Chinese Medicine 7:53–75.

WHO Chronicle
  1980 "Use of acupuncture in modern health care." 34:294–301.

WOLPE, PAUL ROOT
  1982 "Acupuncture and the American medical profession: a historical review." Unpublished paper.

Case Cited
Andrews v. Ballard, 498 F. Supp. 1038 (S.D. Texas, Houston Div.), 1980.

The Medical–Industrial Complex

This chapter deals with an issue to which the reader has already been exposed in bits and pieces. It is the problem arising from physicians having financial interests in the tests and remedies they provide for patients and in the facilities where these tests and remedies are provided.

As this introduction was being written, a physician in a highly publicized case was sentenced to 10 years in jail and fined heavily for implanting pacemakers unnecessarily in patients in order to receive income from the companies manufacturing the devices. And this is not the only individual engaged in this activity. A few years ago, it was estimated that almost $400 million a year could be saved by eliminating the unwarranted implanting of pacemakers.

The lead article is, most appropriately, the seminal article by Arnold S. Relman, the editor of *The New England Journal of Medicine,* written in 1980. Relman describes the medical–industrial (MI) complex, discusses the problems associated with it, and makes recommendations about what he feels must be done to protect the public. In a postscript written in 1986 for this book, Relman looks at what has happened to the MI complex in the almost six years since the publication of the original article. Gwen Kinkaid then describes how the Humana Corporation runs its chains of for-profit hospitals. She notes, among other things, that doctors have financial arrangements with these hospitals that place pressure on them to provide the hospitals with patients.

In the third article, Howard Waitzkin, a very prominent Marxist-sociologist, applies the Marxist approach to the development of coronary care units. According to Waitzkin, much of what he sees as the unnecessary development of these units can be traced to the fact that this development has served the financial interests of several important groups, including corporations and medical centers. In an addendum to Waitzkin's article, Bernard S. Bloom argues that Waitzkin is far too cynical in imputing only financial motives to the medical profession. He also argues that public demand for new technologies is a variable that Waitzkin has failed to recognize in his equation. And there would seem to be, at the very least, a kernel of truth to this contention. The mass media consistently reports of instances when a "promising" but untested drug or procedure is made public and doctors are inundated with requests to try it. Most recently, this happened with the publicity surrounding a new drug related to AIDS. Although only a few hundred could be accepted for a clinical test of the drug's effectiveness, thousands called, wanting to be included.

Mark Dowie and Tracy Johnston end this chapter with a rendering of the history of the Dalkon Shield, a history implicating a physician in a series of events that, in the end, led to tragic medical consequences for tens of thousands of women who used the device.

The New Medical–Industrial Complex

Arnold S. Relman

In his farewell address as President on January 17, 1961, Eisenhower warned his countrymen of what he called "the military-industrial complex," a huge and permanent armaments industry that, together with an immense military establishment, had acquired great political and economic power. He was concerned about the possible conflict between public and private interests in the crucial area of national defense.

The past decade has seen the rise of another kind of private "industrial complex" with an equally great potential for influence on public policy—this time in health care. What I will call the "new medical-industrial complex" is a large and growing network of private corporations engaged in the business of supplying health-care services to patients for a profit—services heretofore provided by nonprofit institutions or individual practitioners.

I am not referring to the companies that manufacture pharmaceuticals or medical equipment and supplies. Such businesses have sometimes been described as part of a "medical-industrial complex," but I see nothing particularly worrisome about them. They have been around for a long time, and no one has seriously challenged their social usefulness. Furthermore, in a capitalistic society there are no practical alternatives to the private manufacture of drugs and medical equipment.

The new medical-industrial complex, on the other hand, is an unprecedented phenomenon with broad and potentially troubling implications for the future of our medical-care system. It has attracted remarkably little attention so far (except on Wall Street), but in my opinion it is the most important

recent development in American health care and it is in urgent need of study.

In the discussion that follows I intend to describe this phenomenon briefly and give an idea of its size, scope, and growth. I will then examine some of the problems that it raises and attempt to show how the new medical-industrial complex may be affecting our health-care system. A final section will suggest some policies for dealing with this situation.

In searching for information on this subject, I have found no standard literature and have had to draw on a variety of unconventional sources: corporation reports; bulletins and newsletters; advertisements and newspaper articles; and conversations with government officials, corporation executives, trade-association officers, investment counselors, and physicians knowledgeable in this area. I take full responsibility for any errors in this description and would be grateful for whatever corrections readers might supply.

THE NEW MEDICAL–INDUSTRIAL COMPLEX

Proprietary Hospitals

Of course proprietary hospitals are not new in this country. Since the past century, many small hospitals and clinics have been owned by physicians, primarily for the purpose of providing a workshop for their practices. In fact, the majority of hospitals in the United States were proprietary until shortly after the turn of the century, when the small doctor-owned hospitals began to be replaced by larger and more sophisticated community or church-owned nonprofit institutions. The total number of proprietary hospitals in the country decreased steadily during the first half of this century. In 1928 there were

Reprinted from *The New England Journal of Medicine*, vol. 303 (1980), pp. 963–970. Copyright © 1980, Massachusetts Medical Society.

2435 proprietary hospitals, constituting about 36 per cent of hospitals of all types; by 1968 there were only 769 proprietary hospitals, 11 per cent of the total.[1] However, there has been a steady trend away from individual ownership and toward corporate control. During the past decade the total number of proprietary hospitals has been increasing again, mainly because of the rapid growth of the corporate-owned multi-institutional hospital chains.

There are now about 1000 proprietary hospitals in this country; most of them provide short-term general care, but some are psychiatric institutions. These hospitals constitute more than 15 per cent of nongovernmental acute general-care hospitals in the country and more than half the nongovernmental psychiatric hospitals. About half the proprietary hospitals are owned by large corporations that specialize in hospital ownership or management; the others are owned by groups of private investors or small companies. In addition to the 1000 proprietary hospitals, about 300 voluntary nonprofit hospitals are managed on a contractual basis by one or another of these profit-making hospital corporations.

The proprietary hospitals are mostly medium-sized (100 to 250 beds) institutions offering a broad range of general inpatient services but few outpatient facilities other than an emergency room. Some are smaller than 100 beds and a few are larger than 250 beds, but none would qualify as major medical centers, none have residency programs, and few do any postgraduate teaching. Most are located in the Sunbelt states in the South, in the Southwest, and along the Pacific Coast, in relatively prosperous and growing small and medium-sized cities and in the suburbs of the booming big cities of those areas. Virtually none are to be found in the big old cities of the North or in the states with strong rate-setting commissions or effective certificate-of-need policies.

Although there are no good, detailed studies comparing the characteristics and performance of proprietary and voluntary hospitals, there is a generally held view that proprietary hospitals have more efficient management and use fewer employees per bed. It is also said that fewer of the patients in proprietary hospitals are in the lower income brackets and that fewer are funded through Medicaid. One prominent hospital official told me that proprietary hospitals generally have per diem rates that are comparable to those in the voluntary hospitals, but that

their ancillary charges are usually higher. However, this official stressed the lack of good data on these questions.

Last year the proprietary-hospital business generated between $12 billion and $13 billion of gross income—an amount that is estimated to be growing about 15 to 20 per cent per year (corrected for inflation). A major area of growth is overseas—in industrialized Western countries as well as underdeveloped countries—where much of the new proprietary-hospital development is now taking place. Of the two or three dozen sizable United States corporations now in the hospital business the largest are Humana and Hospital Corporation of America, each of which had a gross revenue of over $1 billion last year. Others are American Medical International (AMI) and Hospital Affiliates International (a unit of the huge INA Corporation), with gross revenues last year of approximately $0.5 billion each.

Proprietary Nursing Homes

Proprietary nursing homes are even bigger business. In 1977 there were nearly 19,000 nursing-home facilities of all types, and about 77 per cent were proprietary. Some, like the proprietary hospitals, are owned by big corporations, but most (I could not find out exactly how many) are owned by small investors, many of them physicians. The Health Care Financing Administration estimates that about $19 billion was expended last year for nursing-home care in the United States. Assuming that average revenues of proprietary and nonprofit facilities are about equal, this means that about $15 billion was paid to proprietary institutions. This huge sum is growing rapidly, as private and public third-party coverage is progressively extended to pay for this kind of care.

Home Care

Another large and rapidly expanding sector of the health-care industry, but one that is even less well defined than the nursing-home business, is home care. A wide variety of home services are now being provided by profit-making health-care businesses. These services include care by trained nurses and nurses' aides, homemaking assistance, occupational and physiotherapy, respiratory therapy, pacemaker monitoring, and other types of care required by chronically ill house-bound patients. The total expenditures for these services are unknown, but I have been told that the market last year was at least $3 billion. Most of these services are provided by a large array of small private businesses, but there are about 10 fairly large companies in this field at present, and their combined sales are probably in excess of $0.5 billion. The largest corporate provider of home care is said to be the Upjohn Company. About half the total cost of home health care in this country is currently paid by Medicare. As Medicare and private third-party coverage broadens, this health-care business can be expected to grow apace.

Laboratory and Other Services

Last year, about $15 billion was spent on diagnostic laboratory services of all kinds. The number of laboratory tests performed each year in this country is huge and growing at a compound rate of about 15 per cent per year.[2] About a third of the diagnostic laboratories are owned by profit-making companies. Most of these are relatively small local firms, but there are a dozen or more large corporations currently in the laboratory business, some with over $100 million in sales per year. Some of these corporations operate laboratories in the voluntary nonprofit hospitals, but most of the proprietary laboratories are outside hospitals and use an efficient mail or messenger service. Including all proprietary laboratories, large and small, in and out of hospitals, probably some $5 billion or $6 billion worth of services were sold last year.

A large variety of services are being sold by newly established companies in the medical-industrial complex. Included are mobile CAT scanning, cardiopulmonary testing, industrial health screening, rehabilitation counseling, dental care, weight-control clinics, alcohol and drug-abuse programs, comprehensive prepaid HMO programs, and physicians' house calls. Two markets that deserve special mention are hospital emergency-room services and long-term hemodialysis programs for end-stage renal disease.

With the decline in general practice and the virtual disappearance of physicians able and willing to make house calls, the local hospital emergency room has become an increasingly important source of walk-in medical and psychiatric services in urban and suburban areas. The use of emergency rooms has increased rapidly in the past two decades and has stimulated the development of emergency medicine as a specialty. Most third-party payers reimburse for services rendered in hospital emergency rooms at a higher rate than for the same services provided by physicians in their private offices. The result has been a vigorous new industry specializing in emergency services. Many large businesses have been established by entrepreneurial physicians to supply the necessary professional staffing for emergency rooms all over the country, and this has proved to be a highly profitable venture. In some cases, large corporations have taken over this function and now provide hospitals with a total emergency-care package. Once an appropriate financial arrangement is made, they will organize and administer the emergency room, see to its accreditation, recruit and remunerate the necessary medical and paramedical personnel, and even arrange for their continuing education. At least one large corporation that I learned about has such arrangements with scores of hospitals all over the country and employs hundreds of emergency physicians. I do not know exactly how much money is involved or how many physicians and hospitals participate in such schemes around the country, but I am under the impression that this is a very large business.

Hemodialysis

Long-term hemodialysis is a particularly interesting example of stimulation of private enterprise by public financing of health care. In 1972 the Social Security Act was amended to bring the treatment of end-stage renal disease under Medicare funding. When the new law was enacted, only about 40 patients per million population were receiving long-term hemodialysis treatment in this country, almost entirely under the auspices of nonprofit organizations. Forty per cent of these dialyses were home based, and renal transplantation was rapidly becoming an alternative form of treatment. The legislation provided for reimbursement for center-based or hospital-based dialysis without limit in numbers. The result was an immediate, rapid increase in the total number of patients on long-term dialysis treatment and a relative decline in home dialysis and transplantations. The number of patients on dialysis treatment in the United States is now over 200 per million population (the highest in the world), and only about 13 per cent are being dialyzed at home.

Proprietary dialysis facilities began to appear even before public funding of end-stage renal disease but the number increased rapidly thereafter. These facilities were usually located outside hospitals and had lower expenses than the hospital units. Many were purely local units, owned by nephrologists practicing in the area, but one corporation, National Medical Care, soon became preeminent in the field.[3] This company was founded by nephrologists and employs many local nephrologists as physicians and medical directors in its numerous centers around the country. It currently has sales of over $200 million annually and performs about 17 per cent of the long-term dialysis treatments in the country. It has recently expanded into the sale of dialysis equipment and supplies and the provision of psychiatric hospital care, respiratory care, and centers for obesity treatment, but its main business is still to provide dialysis for patients with end-stage renal disease in out-of-hospital facilities that it builds and operates. According to data obtained from the Health Care Financing Administration, nearly 40 per cent of the hemodialysis in this country is now provided by profit-making units. This figure suggests that total sales are nearly $0.5 billion a year for this sector of the health-care industry.

INCOME AND PROFITABILITY

This, in barest outline, is the present shape and scope of the "new medical-industrial complex," a vast array of investor-owned businesses supplying health services for profit. No one knows precisely the full extent of its operations or its gross income, but I estimate that the latter was approximately $35 billion to $40 billion last year—about a quarter of the total amount expended on personal health care in 1979. Remember that this estimate does not include the "old" medical-industrial complex, i.e., the businesses concerned with the manufacture and sale of drugs, medical supplies, and equipment.

The new health-care industry is not only very large, but it is also expanding rapidly and is highly profitable. New businesses seem to be springing up all the time, and those already in the field are diversifying as quickly as new opportunities for profit can be identified. Given the expansive nature of the health-care market and the increasing role of new technology, such opportunities are not hard to find.

The shares of corporations in the health-care business have done exceedingly well in the stock market, and many Wall Street analysts and brokers now enthusiastically recommend such investments to their clients. According to an article in the *Wall Street Journal* of December 27, 1979, the net earnings of health-care corporations with public stock shares rose by 30 to 35 per cent in 1979 and are expected to increase another 20 to 25 per cent in 1980. A vice-president of Merrill Lynch appeared a few months ago on "Wall Street Week," the public television program, to describe the attractions of health-care stocks. According to this authority, health care is now the basis of a huge private industry, which is growing rapidly, has a bright future, and is relatively invulnerable to recession. He predicted that the health business would soon capture a large share of the health-care market and said that the only major risk to investors was the threat of greater government control through the enactment of comprehensive national health insurance or through other forms of federal regulation.

WHY HAVE PRIVATE BUSINESSES IN HEALTH CARE?

Let us grant that we have a vast, new, rapidly growing and profitable industry engaged in the direct provision of health care. What's wrong with that? In our country we are used to the notion that private enterprise should supply most of the goods and services that our society requires. With the growing demand for all kinds of health care over the past two decades and the increasing complexity and cost of the services and facilities required, wasn't it inevitable that businesses were attracted to this new market? Modern health-care technology needs massive investment of capital—a problem that has become more and more difficult for the voluntary nonprofit institutions. How appropriate, then, for private entrepreneurs to come forward with the capital needed to build and equip new hospitals, nursing homes, and laboratories, and to start new health-care businesses. The market was there and a good profit ensured; the challenge was simply to provide the necessary services efficiently and at an acceptable level of quality.

In theory, the free market should operate to improve the efficiency and quality of health care. Given the spur of competition and the discipline exerted by consumer choice, private enterprise should be expected to respond to demand by offering better and more varied services and products, at lower unit costs, than could be provided by nonprofit voluntary or governmental institutions. Large corporations ought to be better managed than public or voluntary institutions; they have a greater incentive to control costs, and they are in a better position to benefit from economies of scale. We Americans believe in private enterprise and the profit motive. How logical, then, to extend these concepts to the health-care sector at a time when costs seem to be getting out of control, voluntary institutions are faltering, and the only other alternative appears to be more government regulation.

That, at least, is the theory. Whether the new medical-industrial complex is in fact improving quality and lowering unit cost in comparison with the public or private voluntary sectors remains to be determined. There are no adequate studies of this important question, and we will have to suspend judgment until there are some good data. But even without such information, I think that there are reasons to be concerned about this new direction in health care.

SOME ISSUES

Can we really leave health care to the marketplace? Even if we believe in the free market as an efficient and equitable mechanism for the distribution of most goods and services, there are many reasons to be worried about the industrialization of health care. In the first place, health care is different from most of the commodities bought and sold in the marketplace. Most people consider it, to some degree at least, a basic right of all citizens. It is a public rather than a private good, and in recognition of this fact,

a large fraction of the cost of medical research and medical care in this country is being subsidized by public funds. Public funds pay for most of the research needed to develop new treatments and new medical-care technology. They also reimburse the charges for health-care services. Through Medicare and Medicaid and other types of public programs, more and more of our citizens are receiving tax-supported medical care.

The great majority of people not covered by public medical-care programs have third-party coverage through private insurance plans, most of which is provided as a fringe benefit by their employers. At present almost 90 per cent of Americans have some kind of health insurance, which ensures that a third party will pay at least part of their medical expenses. Federal programs now fund about 40 per cent of the direct costs of personal health care, and a large additional government subsidy is provided in the form of tax exemptions for employee health benefits. Thus, a second unique feature of the medical-care market is that most consumers (i.e., patients) are not "consumers" in the Adam Smith sense at all. As Kingman Brewster recently observed,[4] health insurance converts patients from consumers to claimants, who want medical care virtually without concern for price. Even when they have to pay out of their own pockets, patients who are sick or worried that they may be sick are not inclined to shop around for bargains. They want the best care they can get, and price is secondary. Hence, the classic laws of supply and demand do not operate because health-care consumers do not have the usual incentives to be prudent, discriminating purchasers.

There are other unique features of the medical marketplace, not the least of which is the heavy, often total, dependence of the consumer (patient) on the advice and judgment of the physician. Kenneth Arrow, in explaining why some of the economist's usual assumptions about the competitive free market do not apply to medical care, referred to this phenomenon as the "informational inequality" between patient and physician.[5] Unlike consumers shopping for most ordinary commodities, patients do not often decide what medical services they need— doctors usually do that for them. Probably more than 70 per cent of all expenditures for personal health care are the result of decisions of doctors.[6]

All these special characteristics of the medical market conspire to produce an anomalous situation when private business enters the scene. A private corporation in the health-care business uses technology often developed at public expense, and it sells services that most Americans regard as their basic right—services that are heavily subsidized by public funds, largely allocated through the decisions of physicians rather than consumers, and almost entirely paid for through third-party insurance. The possibilities for abuse and for distortion of social purposes in such a market are obvious.

Health care has experienced an extraordinary inflation during the past few decades, not just in prices but in the use of services. A major challenge—in fact, *the* major challenge—facing the health-care establishment today is to moderate use of our medical resources and yet protect equity, access, and quality. The resources that can be allocated to medical care are limited. With health-care expenditures now approaching 10 per cent of the gross national product, it is clear that costs cannot continue to rise at anything near their present rate unless other important social goals are sacrificed. We need to use our health-care dollars more effectively, by curbing procedures that are unnecessary or inefficient and developing and identifying those that are the best. Overuse, where it exists, can be eliminated only by taking a more critical view of what we do and of how we use our health-care resources.

How will the private health-care industry affect our ability to achieve these objectives? In an ideal free competitive market, private enterprise may be good at controlling unit costs, and even at improving the quality of its products, but private businesses certainly do not allocate their own services or restrict the use of them. On the contrary, they "market" their services; they sell as many units as the market will bear. They may have to trim their prices to sell more, but the fact remains that they are in business to increase their total sales.

If private enterprise is going to take an increasing share of the health-care market, it will therefore have to be appropriately regulated. We will have to find some way of preserving the advantages of a private health-care industry without giving it free rein and inviting gross commercial exploitation. Otherwise, we can expect the use of health services to continue to increase until government is forced to intervene.

THE ROLE OF THE MEDICAL PROFESSION

It seems to me that the key to the problem of overuse is in the hands of the medical profession. With the consent of their patients, physicians act in their behalf, deciding which services are needed and which are not, in effect serving as trustees. The best kind of regulation of the health-care marketplace should therefore come from the informed judgments of physicians working in the interests of their patients. In other words, physicians should supply the discipline that is provided in commercial markets by the informed choices of prudent consumers, who shop for the goods and services that they want, at the prices that they are willing to pay.

But if physicians are to represent their patients' interests in the new medical marketplace, they should have no economic conflict of interest and therefore no pecuniary association with the medical-industrial complex. I do not know the extent to which practicing physicians have invested in health-care businesses, but I suspect that it is substantial. Physicians have direct financial interests in proprietary hospitals and nursing homes, diagnostic laboratories, dialysis units, and many small companies that provide health-care services of various kinds. Physicians are on the boards of many major health-care corporations, and I think it is safe to assume that they are also well represented among the stockholders of these corporations. However, the actual degree of physician involvement is less important than the fact that it exists at all. As the visibility and importance of the private health-care industry grow, public confidence in the medical profession will depend on the public's perception of the doctor as an honest, disinterested trustee. That confidence is bound to be shaken by any financial association between practicing physicians and the new medical-industrial complex. Pecuniary associations with pharmaceutical and medical supply and equipment firms will also be suspect and should therefore be curtailed.

What I am suggesting is that the medical profession would be in a stronger position, and its voice would carry more moral authority with the public and the government, if it adopted the principle that practicing physicians should derive no financial benefit from the health-care market except from their own professional services. I believe that some statement to this effect should become part of the ethical code of the AMA. As such, it would have no legal force but would be accepted as a standard for the behavior of practicing physicians all over the country.

The AMA's former Principles of Ethics, which has just been superseded by the new set of principles adopted by the House of Delegates at its last meeting,[7] did include a declaration on physicians' financial interests, but it was directed primarily at fee-splitting and rebates. The old Section 7 of the Principles said: "*In the practice of medicine* a physician should limit the source of his *professional* income to medical services actually rendered by him, or under his supervision, to his patients [italics mine]." Although at first glance this statement might appear to have proscribed any involvement of physicians in health-care businesses, it actually did not. The italicized words in effect restricted the application of Section 7 to income derived directly from the care of a physician's own patients. In the Opinions and Reports of the Judicial Council, a more detailed commentary that supplements and interprets the Principles of Ethics, this restriction is made quite clear. The council says that "It is not in itself unethical for a physician to own a for-profit hospital or interest therein," provided that the physician does not make unethical use of that ownership. With respect to ownership of nursing homes and laboratories or interest in them, the council's position is much the same. Similarly, there is no proscription of ownership of a pharmacy or of financial interest in pharmaceutical corporations—only of improper professional behavior on behalf of such economic interests. In the revised new Principles of Medical Ethics just adopted, there is no statement about economic conflicts of interest, but the council's previous Opinions and Reports on this matter will presumably stand.

The position of the Judicial Council seems to be that although physicians must always place the welfare of their patients above their own financial interests, there is nothing inherently improper in physicians' owning or investing in health-care businesses. If they act on their financial interests by overusing services or through kickbacks and rebates, that would be considered improper; but only actual abuses are of concern, not hypothetical or potential conflicts of interest.

The trouble with that policy is that it ignores the public responsibilities of the medical profession. Physicians evaluate drugs, devices, diagnostic tests, and therapeutic procedures in the public interest. Their opinions—expressed publicly in articles, speeches, and committee reports—not only influence the practices of their colleagues but carry weight in the councils of government and directly affect the fortunes of health-care businesses. That is why the *Wall Street Journal* and the financial sections of the major newspapers carry so many news items about medical developments. The medical-industrial complex depends heavily on the favorable public judgments of physicians, individually and collectively. Doctors may not be able to affect the profits of large companies by what they do in their own practices, but they can easily do so through published articles, public statements, or committee reports. The Judicial Council, in commenting on the potential abuse of laboratory services, rightly declared that a physician "is not engaged in a commercial enterprise . . ." (Opinions and Reports, Section 4.40(2)). That statement should apply to all of a physician's professional activities in the health-care field, not just to personal practice.

If the AMA took a strong stand against any financial interest of physicians in health-care businesses, it might risk an antitrust suit. Its action might also be misconstrued as hostile to free enterprise. Yet, I believe that the risk to the reputation and self-esteem of the profession will be much greater if organized medicine fails to act decisively in separating physicians from the commercial exploitation of health care. The professional standing of the physician rests no less on ethical commitment than on technical competence. A refusal to confront this issue undermines the moral position of the profession and weakens the authority with which it can claim to speak for the public interest.

A brochure published by Brookwood Health Services, Inc., one of the many new corporations that owns and operates a chain of proprietary hospitals, says that it "views each physician as a business partner." (In evidence of this commercial partnership, the company recruits young physicians and subsidizes their start in private practice.) That sentiment may make for good working relations between hospital administration and medical staff, but it sounds precisely the wrong note for a private market in which the hospital is the seller, the physician is the purchasing agent for the patient, and the public pays the major share of the bill.

Critics of the position argued here will probably point out that even without any investment in health-care businesses, physicians in private fee-for-service practice already have a conflict of interest in the sense that they benefit from providing services that they themselves prescribe. That may be true, but the conflict is visible to all and therefore open to control. Patients understand fee-for-service and most are willing to assume that their doctor's professional training protects them from exploitation. Furthermore, those who distrust their physicians or dislike the fee-for-service system have other alternatives: another physician, a prepayment plan, or a salaried group. What distinguishes the conflict of interest that I have been discussing are its invisibility and a far greater potential for mischief.

OTHER PROBLEMS

The increasing commercialization of health care generates still other serious problems that need to be mentioned. One is the so-called "cream-skimming" phenomenon. Steinwald and Neuhauser discussed this problem with reference to proprietary hospitals 10 years ago, when the new health-care industry was just appearing on the scene. "The essence of the cream-skimming argument," they said, "is that proprietary hospitals can and do profit by concentrating on providing the most profitable services to the best-paying patients, thereby skimming the cream off the market for acute hospital care and leaving the remainder to nonprofit hospitals."[1] According to these authors, there are two types of "cream-skimming": elimination of low-frequency and unprofitable (though necessary) services, and exclusion of unprofitable patients (e.g., uninsured patients, welfare patients, and those with complex and chronic illnesses). The nonprofit hospitals could not employ such practices, even if they wished to do so, because they have community obligations and are often located in areas where there are many welfare patients. Another form of "skimming" by proprietary hospitals, whether intentional or not, is their virtual lack of residency and other educational programs. Teaching programs are expensive and often oblige hospitals to maintain services that are not economically viable, simply to provide an adequate range of training experience.

Although these arguments seem reasonable, there are no critical studies on which to base firm conclusions about the extent and implications of the skimming phenomenon in the proprietary sector. One has the sense that the larger teaching institutions, particularly those that serve the urban poor, will be feeling increasing competitive economic pressure not only from the proprietary hospitals but also from the medium-sized community hospitals in relatively well-to-do demographic areas. Their charges are generally lower than those of the teaching centers, they take patients away from the centers, and they put the centers in a difficult position in negotiating with rate-setting agencies.

Another danger arises from the tendency of the profit-making sector to emphasize procedures and technology to the exclusion of personal care. Personal care, whether provided by physicians, nurses, or other health-care practitioners, is expensive and less likely to produce large profits than the item-by-item application of technology. Reimbursement schedules are, of course, a prime consideration in determining what services will be emphasized by the health-care industry, but in general the heavily automated, highly technical procedures will be favored, particularly when they can be applied on a mass scale. Just as pharmaceutical firms have tended to ignore "orphan" drugs, i.e., drugs that are difficult or expensive to produce and have no prospect of a mass market,[8] the private health-care industry can be expected to ignore relatively inefficient and unprofitable services, regardless of medical or social need. The result is likely to exacerbate present problems with excessive fragmentation of care, overspecialism, and overemphasis on expensive technology.

A final concern is the one first emphasized by President Eisenhower in his warning about the "military-industrial complex": "We must guard against the acquisition of unwarranted influence." A private health-care industry of huge proportions could be a powerful political force in the country and could exert considerable influence on national health policy. A broad national health-insurance program, with the inevitable federal regulation of costs, would be anathema to the medical-industrial complex, just as a national disarmament policy is to the military-industrial complex. I do not wish to imply that only vested interests oppose the expansion of federal health-insurance programs (or treaties to limit armaments), but I do suggest that the political involvement of the medical-industrial complex will probably hinder rather than facilitate rational debate on national health-care policy. Special-interest lobbies of all kinds are of course a familiar part of the American health-care scene. The appearance of still one more vested interest would not be a cause for concern if the newcomer were not potentially the largest, richest, and most influential of them all. One health-care company, National Medical Care, has already made its political influence felt, when Congress was considering a revision of the legislation supporting the end-stage renal disease program in 1978.[3,9]

SOME PROPOSALS

The new medical-industrial complex is now a fact of American life. It is still growing and is likely to be with us for a long time. Any conclusions about its ultimate impact on our health-care system would be premature, but it is safe to say that the effect will be profound. Clearly, we need more information.

My initial recommendation, therefore, is that we should pay more attention to the new health-care industry. It needs to be studied carefully, and its performance should be measured and compared with that of the nonprofit sector. We need to know much more about the quality and cost of the services provided by the profit-making companies and especially the effects of these companies on use, distribution, and access. We also must find out the extent to which "cream-skimming" is occurring and whether competition from profit-making providers is really threatening the survival of our teaching centers and major urban hospitals.

I suspect that greater public accountability and increased regulation of the private health-care industry will ultimately be required to protect the public interest. However, before any rational and constructive public policies can be developed, we will need a much greater understanding of what is happening. A vast amount of study is still to be done.

The private health-care industry is primarily interested in selling services that are profitable, but patients are interested only in services that they need, i.e., services that are likely to be helpful and are relatively safe. Furthermore, everything else being equal, society is interested in controlling total expenditures for health care, whereas the private health-care industry is interested in increasing its total sales. In the health-care marketplace the interests of patients and of society must be represented by the physician, who alone has the expertise and the authority to decide which services and procedures should be used in any given circumstance. That is why I have urged that physicians should totally separate themselves from any financial involvement in the medical-industrial complex. Beyond that, however, physicians must take a more active interest in assessing medical procedures. Elsewhere I have argued for a greatly expanded national program of evaluation of clinical tests and procedures.[10] Such a program would provide an excellent means by which to judge the social usefulness of the private health-care industry, which depends heavily on new technology and special tests and procedures.

If we are to live comfortably with the new medical-industrial complex we must put our priorities in order: the needs of patients and of society come first. If necessary services of acceptable quality can be provided at lower cost through the profit-making sector, then there may be reason to encourage that sector. But we should not allow the medical-industrial complex to distort our health-care system to its own entrepreneurial ends. It should not market useless, marginal, or unduly expensive services, nor should it encourage unnecessary use of services. How best to ensure that the medical-industrial complex serves the interests of patients first and of its stockholders second will have to be the responsibility of the medical profession and an informed public.

POSTSCRIPT, APRIL 1986

In the more than five years since my article on "The New Medical–Industrial Complex" was published, much has happened in this field.

Investor-ownership has continued to expand rapidly, but the direction of this expansion has taken some new and unexpected directions. The total number of proprietary hospitals in the United States has increased by about 25 percent in the past five years and now is approximately 1300, or nearly a quarter of all the nonpublic hospitals in the country. The fraction owned or leased by large chains has increased to about two-thirds. The large hospital chains have not only acquired many small community hospitals, but in recent years, they have become interested in larger teaching hospitals. At the moment, only a few such hospitals have been taken over, but negotiations for the transfer of several others are currently in progress.

In general, however, the rapid expansion of investor-owned hospital facilities seems to have slowed down, and the large companies are now seeking to extend and diversify their activities in other sectors of the health-care system. This undoubtedly reflects the recent decline in the demand for hospital beds and the new restrictions on the payments for hospital services. Utilization of inpatient services has fallen off dramatically with the past few years as a result of the expansion of HMOs, the pressure from third-party payers to reduce unnecessary hospitalization, and the rapid shift of services to outpatient facilities.

The large investor-owned companies have increasingly been seeking new opportunities outside of traditional hospital care. They are now investing more of their resources in nursing homes, home health-care services, freestanding ambulatory facilities (such as ambulatory surgery centers, imaging centers, and walk-in clinics), special treatment programs (in mental health, alcoholism, etc.), and HMOs. Most recently, there has been considerable interest in establishing health insurance programs tied in to existing investor-owned facilities. Thus, the trend is toward vertical integration, i.e., the development of integrated and diversified corporate health systems that are capable of selling insurance and then providing all the health services covered by that insurance.

The trend toward physician investment in health-care businesses noted in the 1980 article has also continued. There are still no hard data, but there is a generally held opinion that increasing numbers of physicians have equity or other kinds of economic interests in various types of facilities and services, including facilities to which the investing physicians refer their own patients. Physicians are also participating in joint ventures with hospitals or other business entities. To date, few physicians have become full-time employees of the investor-owned corporations, but that development seems inevitable. As HMOs come increasingly under for-profit ownership, physician groups will contract with corporations even if they do not become employees.

In my original article, I estimated that in 1979 the combined revenues of the proprietary health-care businesses, large and small, amounted to about a quarter of all the money spent on personal health-care services. Today, that fraction must be larger, perhaps approaching a third. Total annual revenues of this now vast and highly diversified industry are probably at least 80 or 90 billion dollars.

What have we learned about the performance of investor-owned hospitals? Since 1980 several comparative studies of the economic operations of for-profit and nonprofit hospitals have been published that have dissolved the previously prevailing opinion that investor-owned hospitals were more efficient—and therefore probably less expensive—than nonprofit hospitals. These studies have shown that operating costs have been a few percent higher in the investor-owned hospitals, whereas patient charges have been 10 to 15 percent higher. After-tax, net operating income (called "profit" in the for-profit hospitals and "operating surplus" in the nonprofit institutions) has been about the same: approximately five percent of revenues. However, since the for-profit sector generally operates with much higher debt-to-equity ratios, its profit expressed as a percent of equity is also much higher. In short, these studies have shown that for-profit hospitals have been, if anything, slightly less efficient than their nonprofit competitors, and they have charged the users of their services considerably more. As money-making enterprises, they have been highly effective, thus accounting for their remarkable past performance in the stock market. Very recently, the value of hospital company stocks has declined, a reaction to the slackening of demand for hospital beds nationwide.

Investor-owned hospitals have, in general, provided proportionately less uncompensated care than the nonprofit, nonpublic hospitals. This is not surprising, since they have generally taken the position that their tax liability exempts them from any social responsibility to provide free care. It should be understood, however, that "uncompensated" care includes uncollected debts as well as free care. Differences in "uncompensated" care between the for-profit and nonprofit sectors are therefore blurred by the frequent inability of hospital accounting methods to make the distinction between true charity and bad debts. Although these differences are relatively modest when averaged over the entire country, they are more striking in those states (such as Florida, Texas, Tennessee, and Kentucky) where for-profit hospitals have a large market share. In Florida, for example, uncompensated care in the voluntary sector, expressed as a percentage of total revenues, is approximately twice as large as in the for-profit sector (eight percent versus four percent). Furthermore, most of the uncompensated care in the investor-owned hospitals represents bad debts rather than charity, whereas charity generally represents nearly half of the uncompensated care provided by the voluntary hospitals.

All of these data were obtained before the recent dramatic change in hospital payment from a cost- or charge-reimbursement system to a competitive prospective-payment system. Under the old system, investor-owned hospitals had no economic incentives to be efficient and reduce operating costs. Now that a substantial fraction of patients are paid for under the DRG system, and now that hospitals are competing on the basis of price, profits will accrue to those institutions that can deliver acceptable services at the lowest cost. Advocates of the for-profit sector are therefore predicting that investor-owned hospitals will soon demonstrate their greater efficiency by providing satisfactory services at lower costs than their nonprofit competitors. For-profit partisans can also point out, with some justification, that in the new economic climate the nonprofit hospitals will be—and in fact, are being—forced to act just like their for-profit competitors or else face economic disaster.

To date, however, I believe it is fair to say that the only advantages for-profit hospitals seem to have demonstrated is their greater ability to finance new services and facilities and their greater responsiveness to economic incentives. Viewed strictly as businesses, i.e., as institutions designed to generate profits and increase capital, they have been successful. The big investor-owned chains have had the resources to maintain or expand services when public and private nonprofit institutions have been faltering. They have not, on the other hand, discernibly improved the quality or efficiency of hospital services, nor have they contributed to a solution of the indigent care problem. Quite the contrary, their record so far seems to suggest that they have been financially successful simply because they have been able to exploit an open-ended reimbursement system and have used their resulting financial power to acquire an ever-increasing market share.

With the recent change in the economic climate of health-care institutions, it remains to be seen how successful the for-profit sector will be in delivering good quality care at competitively low prices. What will also need to be watched closely is the changing impact of an increasingly commercialized market on the access of the poor and the uninsured to the health services they need. Another area of concern will be the effects of the increasing vertical integration of the health-care system in the hands of the giant hospital chain companies. When a single investor-owned corporation sells the insurance, owns all the facilities and services covered by the insurance, and employs or contracts with the physicians who deliver the services, what will happen to the quality, accessibility, and cost of health care? Who will protect the interests of patients enrolled in these closed, proprietary systems, and how will those who cannot afford to buy the insurance be cared for?

These questions and many other issues related to the development of "the new medical-industrial complex" are attracting increasing attention from government, the media, the public, and professional students of the health-care system. They will ultimately be resolved in the political arena, for they basically involve social policy decisions.

The medical profession is becoming concerned about the increasing power of the health-care corporations, which threatens the autonomy of physicians and their economic freedom to practice in the traditional fee-for-service mode. There is also growing concern about the ethical and legal issues raised by the burgeoning entrepreneurialism of practicing physicians and by the increasing tendency for hospitals and other health-care institutions to involve physicians in joint business ventures. Professional societies are beginning to warn physicians about the risks of commercial involvement, but none has yet flatly declared such involvement unethical. However, two states have already passed laws preventing physicians from holding financial interests in facilities to which they refer their patients, and this issue is being more widely debated.

The Institute of Medicine of the National Academy of Sciences has been studying the general problem of for-profit health care, with a particular focus on the hospital sector. Its final report is due to be published in May, 1986.

References

1. Steinwald B, Neuhauser D. The role of the proprietary hospital. Law Contemp. Prob. 1970; 35:817–38.

2. Bailey RM. Clinical laboratories and the practice of medicine: an economic perspective. Berkeley, Calif.: McCutchan, 1979.

3. Kolata GB. NMC thrives selling dialysis. Science. 1980; 208:379–82.

4. Brewster K. Health at any price? Proc. R. Soc. Med. 1979; 72:719–23.

5. Arrow KJ. Uncertainty and the welfare economics of medical care. Am. Econ. Rev. 1963; 53:941–73.

6. Relman AS. The allocation of medical resources by physicians. J. Med. Educ. 1980; 55:99–104.

7. Alsofrom J. New ethical principles for nation's physicians voted by AMA house. Am. Med. News. August 1/8, 1980; 23(30):1,9.

8. Finkel MJ. Drugs of limited commercial value. N. Engl. J. Med. 1980; 302:643–4.

9. Greenberg DS. Renal politics. N. Engl. J. Med. 1978; 298:1427–8.

10. Relman AS. Assessment of medical practices: a simple proposal. N. Engl. J. Med. 1980; 303:153–4.

Humana's Hard-Sell Hospitals

Gwen Kinkaid

Since their emergence in 1968, for-profit hospital chains have grown even faster than the computer and drug industries. By buying up doctor-owned hospitals and building scores of new ones, the industry now boasts revenues of $12.4 billion a year and owns 11% of America's hospital beds. It has also stirred up a bitter name-calling controversy about whether it is luring away the most lucrative patients, leaving institutions that are supported by taxpayers and charities with the losers.

Among the top six companies, which control a third of the business, the one whose meteoric rise and pugnacious management most inspire fear and envy among rivals is strapping Humana Inc. of Louisville, Kentucky. Its 90 hospitals, tied together by cost and quality controls, have a mission: in the words of the co-founder and chairman, David Jones, it is "to be the hospitals of choice in their communities and to provide unexcelled, measurable care at the lowest possible cost." Toward this end, Humana thinks of itself as serving not patients but "customers," and it woos them aggressively with newspaper ads, elaborate food, fast service, and Holiday Inn-like private rooms with bath and color TV. Jones has given up tactlessly comparing his hospitals to McDonald's hamburger franchises, but he still aims to offer a product standardized from California to Florida. . . .

A LESSON FROM THE FLU

Most managers would view Humana's leverage as tantamount to walking the gangplank. But going for broke suits the combative, quick-witted, self-assured "Gold Dust Twins," as business associates sometimes call Jones and Cherry. In 1961, the pair, then Louisville law associates, took their first gamble and borrowed to build a nursing home. Seven years later, after they'd expanded to ten, a flu epidemic struck New Haven, Connecticut. When an overburdened hospital placed flu sufferers in their local nursing home, Jones and Cherry discovered that hospitals earned six times as much per patient from Medicare and Medicaid as nursing homes. After that eye-opener, the convalescent-care field began to look a little congested.

So Jones and Cherry gambled again. In 1968, a boom year for nursing-home stocks, they took their company public. For the following three years, they bought a hospital a month, all moneymakers, by swapping stock with the doctors who owned them. Then they went on a construction binge. Between 1972 and 1975, they built 27 hospitals in rapidly growing southern and southwestern towns. Some of these were limited partnerships set up with doctors who owned the real estate. The doctors provided a stream of patients, some shared in the profits, and all got tax shelters. Voluntary hospitals and the press roundly attacked arrangements, common in the early Seventies, that gave doctors a financial interest in steering patients to particular institutions. But Humana was in a hurry.

The National Health Planning and Resources Development Act, passed in 1974, threatened to slow the company down. The law virtually prohibited renovation, construction, or purchase of equipment costing more than $100,000 unless state and local health-planning agencies approved it as necessary. But it

took a couple of years for the agencies to get set up, and Humana overbuilt many hospitals before then to escape review. In most locations, that made sense. The federal law would keep new competitors out, and Humana's extra beds could be put to use as the patient roster grew.

But the tactic backfired in some towns where Humana should have known it would face tough competition. In Springfield, Illinois, for instance, Humana built a 200-bed facility in the middle of a cornfield that turned out to be on the wrong side of a highway interchange. Patients trying to find the hospital often drove right past it. An anticipated population surge fizzled, and local doctors effectively boycotted the place, resenting it as unneeded and profit-mongering. "Our feasibility study didn't show the medical community's conspiracy against us," says Cherry. To this, a leading Springfield doctor retorts, "You bet we don't support their hospital. We never wanted it here. It's draining the lifeblood off our local facilities." Five years after opening, the hospital has just 27% of its beds filled.

BEDS AT HALF PRICE

The likelihood that federal planning laws would practically halt new construction convinced Jones and Cherry that the only way to grow was to acquire competitors. In 1978, when the company ranked third among the major chains, it took over No. 2, American Medicorp, which owned 40 hospitals. It was a masterful coup. The $304-million deal averaged out to $57,000 a bed, half what it costs to build from scratch today. Says one chief executive, fearful that his company might be next, "Humana borrowed itself up to the hilt and then hit so fast and with such animosity that Medicorp couldn't defend itself. That move scared the liver out of the industry."

All Medicorp's hospitals have received Humana's cost-cutting treatment. Changes at Medicorp's Clinch Valley, Virginia, hospital illustrate the process. Since labor costs represent 50% to 60% of a hospital's budget, industrial engineers used computers to compare each department with those in Humana hospitals. The study found 53 employees, mostly nurses' aides and cleaning staff, who could be dismissed, saving $225,000 a year. Since Humana's purchases of supplies are larger than Medicorp's were, the company got higher volume discounts under nationwide contracts, saving $171,500. Tough billing and collection procedures, including a requirement that patients put down deposits if their insurance won't cover their bills, help hold down bad debts. All in all, Humana has raised Clinch Valley's profits by $1.5 million since 1978.

What makes or breaks a for-profit hospital is the kinds of patients it attracts. Medicare and Medicaid reimburse only a hospital's costs, as opposed to its normal prices; private insurance and most Blue Cross plans in the Sunbelt, where 70% of Humana's hospitals are situated, pay full rates. Privately insured patients can be charged whatever the market will bear. When a hospital has empty beds, Medicare and Medicaid patients are better than cold sheets, and Humana charges off every penny of overhead on them that the government will allow. But if it isn't trying to fill a lot of empty beds, Humana treats as few of those patients as possible. As Wendell Cherry allows, "We can't turn them away, but if we don't have the beds . . ."

Humana prefers to own facilities in suburbs where young working families are having lots of babies. Though young people use hospitals less than the elderly, they are more likely to be privately insured and in need of surgery, which makes the most money. The babies provide a second generation of customers.

This strategy outrages the directors of nonprofit hospitals, who charge that investor-owned chains skim off the moneymakers, leaving them with poor people and the costliest ailments. Routine operations—appendectomies, hysterectomies, and gallbladder operations—make money by efficiently using the facilities. The patients are otherwise healthy people who can be quickly treated and released.

M.D.s SUPPLY THE FEED

In general, the shorter the stay, the more profitable the case. Diagnostic tests, operating-room services, and intensive-care facilities are used during the first few days of hospitalization and produce the highest revenues. After that, a hospital charges patients mainly for room and board. By attracting young, privately insured customers, Humana lowers the chance of having to deal with multisystemic or chronic diseases like leukemia or cancer that are

four and five times more expensive to treat than a hernia.

To attract the "right" patients, Humana tries to sell the "right" doctors on its services. Doctors usually decide where patients are to be hospitalized. Family doctors are the first feeders: they see the most potential patients. Specialists are the second source, and Humana tries to influence the decisions of specialists with the greatest number of young, privately insured patients—gynecologists, neurologists, general surgeons, and so on. But choosing which specialists to attract can be tricky. By nosing around town, Humana discovers which orthopedists work with sports injuries (young patients apt to be privately insured) and which replace hips (older Medicare patients).

Humana often puts up office buildings next to its hospitals and offers doctors space at a discount— as much as a year's free rent. It readily approves doctors' requests for the latest diagnostic and therapeutic gadgetry and urges administrators to help physicians find office staff, furnishings, and even partners. Humana recruits doctors from Canada and all over the U.S., encouraging them to settle down near its hospitals and use the facilities. . . .

"THE PRESSURE'S A PROBLEM"

Doctors subsidized by Humana are free to send their business wherever they like, but the company counts on their feeling beholden and acting accordingly. "If the patient has no preference," a doctor from Rochester, Illinois, says, "I refer him to Humana's hospital because Humana helped me get started." The company keeps records on every doctor's monthly admissions and the revenues these produce. "They let you know if you're not keeping up to expectations," says Dr. John Kreml, who has privileges at Springfield. "The pressure's a problem, but I've no contractual obligation to send them patients." Still, if the doctors don't produce for Humana, Cherry says, "I'm damn sure I'm not going to renegotiate their office leases. They can practice elsewhere."

As owner of the newest hospitals in many towns, Humana frequently faces strenuous competition. Only 16 of the company's 90 hospitals monopolize their markets, and just two others rank No. 1 in competitive situations. The rest try to establish themselves by supplying services that capitalize on the oversights of rival hospitals and the frustrations of the doctors who use them. . . .

Consider Humana's Lucerne General Hospital in Orlando, Florida. Located to grow along with nearby Walt Disney World and opened in 1974, it quickly went nowhere in an overbedded city crowded with five established competitors. So Lucerne's administrators left obstetrics, ophthalmology, pediatrics, neurosurgery, and otolaryngology to the others, and dedicated an entire floor to serving the needs of family doctors. G.P.'s, who had complained of getting low priority at other hospitals, stampeded to Lucerne.

Then Humana urged a local orthopedist, eager to head his own spinal-injury clinic, to set one up at Lucerne. Its reputation soon attracted complicated cases from all over Florida. Spinal injuries affect mostly young people, who are apt to be privately insured. The hospital set up an open-heart-surgery unit to draw business from doctors dissatisfied with another facility. Coronary-bypass operations, the kind that are usually performed at the unit, rarely involve Medicare or Medicaid patients. Exults Paul Gross, Humana's regional administrator for Florida: "That spinal-injury unit is not something every hospital can create, and it sets ours apart. Now the open-heart—that really legitimizes you as a real acute-care hospital. You can't get any closer to acuteness than the heart!" Today, Lucerne is Orlando's third-largest hospital and Humana's eighth most profitable.

Besides selling the doctors on its services, Humana descends aggressively on the public. Virtually all the hospitals have expensive, labor-intensive emergency rooms, which provide the only avenue a customer can take into a facility without a doctor's referral. At Sunrise Memorial in Las Vegas, the nation's largest for-profit and Humana's most lucrative outpost (it earned $10 million last fiscal year—8% of corporate pretax profits), more than one out of four emergency-room visitors wound up as inpatients.

CARDS THAT MAKE YOU FEEL GOOD

Humana advertises one-minute emergency care and sends out Insta-Care cards that play on people's fears of helplessness in a crisis: the promotion stresses that since card-carriers are considered financially

sound, they receive faster treatment without the delay of filling out forms. Jones thought up the program after market research showed that people judge a hospital largely by its emergency care. But he concedes that the cards are a selling tool that entitle patients to next to nothing. "Hopefully you get 60-second treatment whether or not you have them," he says. "But people don't know that and the cards make them feel good."

Humana will treat all genuine emergencies. But if an uninsured person can be stabilized and safely moved, it will transfer him to a municipal hospital to be treated at public expense. Company executives bristle at suggestions that this amounts to turning away the poor, but it's hard to see the practice any other way. This year, Humana's charity and bad-debt bill amounted to $33.6 million, or 2.5% of revenues. The typical community hospital's losses are closer to 4.5%.

In Las Vegas . . . , John Grego, a 56-year-old former parking-lot attendant, was internally hemorrhaging when he arrived at the emergency room of Humana's Sunrise Hospital. Dr. Karl Fazekas, an internist with privileges at Sunrise, worked on Grego for three hours until he believed the man was stabilized. Told that Grego lacked insurance, Dr. Fazekas ordered an ambulance to transfer him to the county-owned Southern Nevada Memorial Hospital four miles away.

Grego died the following day. Says Dr. Charles Zumpft, co-chief of Memorial's emergency room, "Grego shouldn't have been sent." Dr. Fazekas says: "My conscience is 100% clear. If he had been in such bad shape he wouldn't have arrived alive. These freebies cost $2,000 or $3,000 a day. Who's going to pay for them?" The hospital has the case under investigation. Though such extreme incidents are rare, voluntary hospitals argue that by transferring indigents the for-profits save money by shirking their ethical duty.

ARE THEY MORE EFFICIENT?

Does Humana measure up to its goal of providing unexcelled care at the lowest possible cost? Interviews with doctors in several communities where Humana operates indicate that the quality of care equals or exceeds that of other area hospitals. But by several standard industry measures, Humana's hospitals do not stand out as the most efficient providers of that care.

In fiscal 1979, . . . Humana's operating costs per inpatient day averaged $234. For the same 12 months, all hospitals averaged $218—and that figure drops to $190 when the 800-odd hospitals affiliated with medical schools are subtracted. Humana acknowledges that its expenses are higher but says this is because it pays taxes. However, income taxes added only $10 to the operating costs, not enough to make up the difference. The hospitals' heavy debt and below-average occupancy, concomitants of being relatively new, provide a more logical explanation. . . .

Humana prefers to talk about expenses *per case* as proof of efficiency. In fiscal 1979, its average cost per inpatient case came to $1,453 vs. the community hospitals' average of $1,564. Humana's patients are released one day earlier than the national average, and the shorter stays yield lower costs per case. There's no way of telling whether Humana does a better job of getting patients on their feet fast or whether it treats illnesses that require shorter stays. Given the company's marketing strategy, the latter would seem likely. But neither Humana nor the nation's hospitals as a whole have statistics on the mix of ailments in their wards.

How do the patients make out financially? Again, the answer varies. On average, Humana's customers paid $241 per day vs. $217 in all community facilities. When the length of stay is factored in, Humana's customers forked over $1,487 per case, against $1,554 in the community hospitals. The inconclusiveness of the numbers allows both sides of the debate about hospital care to conclude what they will. "The chains claim they're more efficient," notes Donald Giffen, head of Blue Cross in Humana's home state of Kentucky. "But I don't see it in their daily costs and I don't see it in their patient bills." Another expert counters: "Again and again I hear that for-profits should be chastened for making unwarranted claims. Unwarranted? They can't prove them and no one else can disprove them. Nothing in America has ever prevented anyone from tooting his own horn."

A HARD CASE TO ARGUE

The ultimate question about the for-profits has to do with their effect on hospital care. Assuming that Humana skims off the most profitable patients, is that sufficient reason to indict? Voluntary hospitals partially subsidize charity cases from what they make on profitable business. It is hard to argue that supporting indigents with the profits earned on insured patients is morally superior to supporting them on taxpayer dollars.

Humana's chairman views the charges of cream skimming as nothing more than competitors' protectionism. "If we accomplish our mission," he says, "the record will stand on its own." If all those newly built hospitals fill up with patients, Jones may one day be able to demonstrate that he is providing "unexcelled, measurable care at the lowest possible cost." In the meantime, he'll have to settle for the kind of achievement most businessmen would be more than satisfied with—unexcelled measurable profits in the shortest possible time.

A Marxian Interpretation of the Growth and Development of Coronary Care Technology

Howard Waitzkin

The financial burden of health care has emerged as an issue of national policy. Legislative and administrative maneuvers purportedly aim toward the goal of cost containment. New investigative techniques in health services research, based largely on the cost-effectiveness model, are entering into the evaluation of technology and clinical practices. My purposes in this paper are to document the analytic poverty of these approaches to health policy and to offer an alternative interpretation that derives from Marxian analysis.

In the Marxian framework, the problem of costs never can be divorced from the structure of private profit in capitalist society. Most non-Marxian analyses of costs either ignore the profit structure of capitalism or accept it as given. But the crisis of health costs intimately reflects the more general fiscal crisis, including such incessant problems as inflation and stagnation, that advanced capitalism is facing worldwide. Wearing blinders that limit the level of analysis to a specific innovation or practice, while not perceiving the broader political-economic context in which costly and ineffective procedures are introduced and promulgated, will only obscure potential solutions to the enormous difficulties that confront us.

In this paper I focus on coronary care, having selected this topic merely as one example of apparent irrationalities of health policy that make sense when seen from the standpoint of the capitalist profit structure. The overselling of many other technologic advances such as computerized axial tomography and fetal monitoring (which have undeniable usefulness for a limited number of patients) reflects very similar structural problems.

Reprinted from the *American Journal of Public Health*, vol. 69, no. 12 (December, 1979), pp. 1260–1268.

One cautionary remark is worthwhile. The Marxian framework is not a conspiratorial model. The very nature of capitalist production necessitates the continuing development of new products and sales in new markets. From the standpoint of potential profit, there is no reason that corporations should view medical products differently from other products. The commodification of health care and its associated technology is a necessary feature of the capitalist political-economic system.[1-3] Without fundamental changes in the organization of private capital, costly innovations of dubious effectiveness will continue to plague the health sector. It is the structure of the system, rather than decision-making by individual entrepreneurs and clinicians, that is the appropriate level of analysis.

HISTORICAL DEVELOPMENT OF INTENSIVE CORONARY CARE

Early Claims

Intensive care emerged rapidly during the 1960s. The first major reports of coronary care units (CCUs) were written by Day, who developed a so-called "coronary care area" at the Bethany Hospital in Kansas City, with financial help from the John A. Hartford Foundation.[4] From these early articles until the mid-1970s, claims like Day's were very common in the literature. Descriptions of improved mortality and morbidity appeared, based totally on uncontrolled data from patients with myocardial infarction (MI) admitted before and after the introduction of a CCU. Until the 1970s, no major study of CCUs included a randomized control group.

However, Day's enthusiasm spread. In 1967, the classic descriptive study by Lown's group at the Peter Bent Brigham Hospital in Boston appeared.[5] This study was supported by the U.S. Public Health Service, the Hartford Foundation, and the American Optical Company, which manufactured the tape-loop recall memory system that was being used in the CCU. The CCU's major objective, as the article pointed out, was to anticipate and to reduce early heart rhythm disturbances, thereby avoiding the need for resuscitation. The paper cited several other articles showing before-after decreases in mortality with a CCU, but never with randomization or other forms of statistical control introduced, and certainly never with a random controlled trial.

This publication led to a conference in 1968, sponsored by the Department of Health, Education, and Welfare (HEW), in which greater development and support of CCUs were advocated, despite clear-cut statements within the conference that the effectiveness of CCUs had not been demonstrated. For example, at the conference the Chief of the Heart Disease Control Program of the Public Health Service claimed: "An attempt was made a few years ago to make some controlled studies of the benefits of CCU efforts, but it was not possible to carry out those investigations for many reasons, some of them fiscal. Therefore, we do not have proper studies for demonstrating the advantages of CCUs. But now that these opportunities and occasions to prevent heart rhythm disturbances have become a great deal more common, we can be assured that our efforts are worthwhile. . . . Upon advice of our colleagues in the profession, we have not considered it ethically acceptable, at this time, to make a controlled study which would necessitate shunting of patients from a facility without a CCU (but with the support that CCUs provide) to one with a CCU."[6]

So, despite the lack of controlled studies showing effectiveness, there were many calls for the expansion of CCUs to other hospitals and increased support from the federal government and private foundations. In 1968 HEW also issued a set of Guidelines for CCUs.[7] Largely because of these recommendations, CCUs grew rapidly in the following years. Table 1 shows the expansion of CCUs in the United States between 1967 and 1974.[8]

TABLE 1   Growth of coronary care units in the United States, by region, 1967–1974

REGIONS	CORONARY CARE UNITS (% OF HOSPITALS)	
	1967	1974
United States	24.3	33.8
New England	29.0	36.8
Mid-Atlantic	33.8	44.2
East North Central	31.0	38.2
West North Central	17.0	25.3
South Atlantic	23.3	38.2
East South Central	13.4	30.1
West South Central	15.3	24.3
Mountain	21.4	29.3
Pacific	32.7	37.8

Source: Reference 8

Later Studies of Effectiveness

Serious research on the effectiveness of CCUs did not begin until the 1970s. As several critics have pointed out, the "before-after" studies during the 1960s could not lead to valid conclusions about effectiveness, since none of these studies had adequate control groups or randomization.[9–13]

Several later studies compared treatment of MI patients in hospital wards vs. CCU settings.[14–17] Patients were "randomly" admitted to the CCU or the regular ward, simply based on the availability of CCU beds. Ward patients were the "control" group; CCU patients were the "experimental" group. Table 2 reviews the findings of these studies, which are

TABLE 2   Recent studies comparing coronary care unit and ward treatment for myocardial infarction

STUDIES	NO CCU		CCU	
	N	% MORTALITY	N	% MORTALITY
Prospective				
Hofvendahl[14]	139	35	132	17
Christiansen[15]	244	41	171	18
Hill[16]				
<65 yrs	186	18	797	15
≥65 yrs	297	32	200	31
Retrospective				
Astvad[17]	603	39	1108	41

TABLE 3 Recent studies comparing hospital and home care for myocardial infarction

STUDIES	HOSPITAL		HOME	
	N	% MORTALITY	N	% MORTALITY
Prospective Randomized				
Mather[18,19]				
<60 yrs	106	18	117	17
≥60 yrs	112	35	103	23
TOTAL	218	27	220	20
Hill[20]	132	11	132	13

	HOSPITAL CCU		HOSPITAL WARD		HOME	
	N	% MORTALITY	N	% MORTALITY	N	% MORTALITY
Epidemiologic						
Dellipiani[22]	248	13	296	21	193	9

very contradictory. From this research it is unclear, at this late date, that CCUs improve in-hospital mortality.

More recent research contrasted home vs. hospital care (Table 3). One major study was the prospective, random controlled trial by Mather and his colleagues in Great Britain.[18,19] This was an ambitious and courageous study, of the type that was not considered possible by HEW in the 1960s.[6] Although some methodologic problems arose concerning the randomization of patients to home vs. hospital care, the cumulative 1-year mortality was not different in the home and hospital groups, and there was no evidence that MI patients did better in the hospital. A second random controlled trial of home vs. hospital treatment tried to correct the methodologic difficulties of the Mather study by achieving a higher rate of randomization and strict criteria for the entry and exclusion of patients from the trial. The preliminary findings of this later study, conducted by Hill's group in Great Britain, confirmed the earlier results; the researchers concluded that for the majority of patients with suspected MI, admission to a hospital "confers no clear advantage."[20] A third study of the same problem used an epidemiologic approach in the Teesside area of Great Britain. This investigation was not a random controlled trial but simply a 12-month descriptive epidemiologic study of the incidence of MIs, how they were treated in practice, and the outcomes in terms of mortality. Both the crude and age-standardized mortality rates were better for patients treated at home.[21, 22]

In summary, these issues are far from settled even now. The thrust of recent research indicates that home care is a viable treatment alternative to hospital or CCU care for many patients with MI. Early CCU promotion used unsound clinical research. More adequate research has not confirmed CCU effectiveness. One other question is clear—if intensive care is not demonstrably more effective than simple rest at home, how can we explain the tremendous proliferation during the past two decades of this very expensive form of treatment?

From a Marxian perspective, these events cannot be chance phenomena. Nor are they simply another expression of the Pollyanna-like acceptance of high technology in industrial society. People are not stupid, even though the enormously costly development of CCUs occurred without any proof of their effectiveness. Therefore, we must search for the social, economic, and political structures that fostered their growth.

THE POLITICAL ECONOMY OF CORONARY CARE

The Corporate Connection

To survive, capitalist industries must produce and sell new products. Expansion is an absolute necessity for capitalist enterprises. The economic surplus (defined as the excess of total production over "socially essential production") must grow continually larger. Medical production also falls in this category, although it is seldom viewed in this way. The economist Mandel emphasizes the contradictions of the economic surplus: "For capitalist crises are incredible phenomena like nothing ever seen before. They are not crises of scarcity, like all pre-capitalist crises; they are crises of over-production."[23] This scenario also includes the health-care system, where an overproduction of intensive care technology contrasts with the fact that many people have little access to the most simple and rudimentary medical services.

Large profit-making corporations in the United States participated in essentially every phase of CCU research, development, promotion, and proliferation. Many companies involved themselves in the intensive care market. Here I consider the activities of two such firms: Warner-Lambert Pharmaceutical Company and the Hewlett-Packard Company. I selected these corporations because information about their participation in coronary care was relatively accessible and because they have occupied prominent market positions in this clinical area. However, I should emphasize that many other firms, including at least 85 major companies, also have been involved in coronary care.[24]

Warner-Lambert Pharmaceutical Company (W-L) is a large multinational corporation, with $2.1 billion in assets and over $2.5 billion in annual sales during recent years.[25] The corporation comprises a number of interrelated subsidiary companies: Warner-Chilcott Laboratories, the Parke-Davis Company, and Warner-Lambert Consumer Products (Listerine, Smith Brothers [cough drops], Bromo-Seltzer, Chiclets, DuBarry, Richard Hudnut, Rolaids, Dentyne, Certs, Cool-ray Polaroid [sunglasses], and Oh Henry! [candy]).[26] Warner-Lambert International operates in more than 40 countries. Although several divisions of the W-L conglomerate participated actively in the development and promotion of coronary care, the most prominent division has been the American Optical Company (AO), which W-L acquired during 1967.

By the early 1960s, AO already had a long history of successful sales in such fields as optometry, ophthalmology, and microscopes. The instrumentation required for intensive coronary care led to AO's diversification into this new and growing area. The profitable outcomes of AO's research, development, and promotion of coronary care technology are clear from AO's 1966 annual report: "In 1966, the number of American Optical Coronary Care Systems installed in hospitals throughout the United States more than tripled. Competition for this market also continued to increase as new companies, both large and small, entered the field. However, we believe that American Optical Company . . . will continue a leader in this evolving field."[27]

After purchasing AO in 1967, W-L maintained AO's emphasis on CCU technology and sought wider acceptance by health professionals and medical centers. Promotional materials contained the assumption, never proven, that the new technology was effective in reducing morbidity and mortality from heart disease. Early products and systems included the AO Cardiometer, a heart monitoring and resuscitation device; the first direct current defibrillator; the Lown Cardioverter; and an Intensive Cardiac Care System that permitted the simultaneous monitoring of 16 patients by oscilloscopes, recording instruments, heart rate meters, and alarm systems.[28] In 1968, after introducing a new line of monitoring instrumentation and implantable demand pacemakers, the company reported that "acceptance has far exceeded initial estimates" and that the Medical Division was doubling the size of its plant in Bedford, Massachusetts.[29] By 1969, the company introduced another completely new line of Lown Cardioverters and Defibrillators.[30] The company continued to register expanding sales throughout the early 1970s.

Despite this growth, W-L began to face a typical corporate problem: the potential saturation of markets in the United States. Coronary care technology was capital-intensive. The number of hospitals in the United States that could buy coronary care systems, although large, was finite. For this reason, W-L began to make new and predictable initiatives to assure future growth. First, the company expanded coronary care sales into foreign markets, especially the Third World. Subsequently, W-L reported notable gains in sales in such countries as Argentina, Canada, Colombia, France, Germany, Japan, and Mexico, despite the fact that during the early 1970s "political difficulties in southern Latin America slowed progress somewhat, particularly in Chile and Peru."[31]

A second method to deal with market saturation was further diversification within the coronary care field with products whose intent was to open new markets or to create obsolescence in existing systems. For example, in 1975 the AO subsidiary introduced two new instruments. The "Pulsar 4," a lightweight portable defibrillator designed for local paramedic and emergency squads, created "an exceptionally strong sales demand." The Computer Assisted Monitoring System used a computer to anticipate and control changes in cardiac patients' conditions and replaced many hospitals' CCU systems that AO had installed but that lacked computer capabilities. According to the company's 1975 annual report, these two instruments "helped contribute to record sales growth in 1975, following an equally successful performance in the previous year."[32]

A third technique to assure growth involved the modification of coronary care technology for new areas gaining public and professional attention. With an emphasis on preventive medicine, AO introduced a new line of electrocardiogram telemetry instruments, designed to provide early warning of MI or rhythm disturbance in ambulatory patients. In addition, AO began to apply similar monitoring technology to the field of occupational health and safety, after the passage of federal OSHA legislation in 1970.[33]

W-L is only one of many companies cultivating the coronary care market. Another giant is the Hewlett-Packard Company (H-P), a firm that in 1977 held more than $1.1 billion in assets and reported over $1.3 billion in sales. Since its founding in 1939 II-P has grown from a small firm, manufacturing analytical and measuring instruments mainly for industry, to a leader in electronics. Until the early 1960s, H-P's only major product designated for medical markets was a simple electrocardiogram machine. Along with pocket computers, medical electronic equipment has since become the most successful of H-P's product groups. During the 1960s, H-P introduced a series of innovations in coronary care (as well as perinatal monitoring and instrumentation for respiratory disease) that soon reached markets throughout the world.

Initially the company focused on the development of CCU technology. H-P aggressively promoted CCU equipment to hospitals with the consistent claim that cardiac monitors and related products were definitely effective in reducing mortality from MI and rhythm disturbances. Such claims as the following were unambiguous: "In the cardiac care unit pictured here at a Nevada hospital, for example, the system has alerted the staff to several emergencies that might otherwise have proved fatal, and the cardiac mortality rate has been cut in half."[34] Alternatively, "hundreds of lives are saved each year with the help of Hewlett-Packard patient monitoring systems installed in more than 1,000 hospitals throughout the world. . . . Pictured here is an HP system in the intensive care ward of a hospital in Montevideo, Uruguay."[35]

Very early, H-P emphasized the export of CCU technology to hospitals and practitioners abroad, anticipating the foreign sales that other companies like W-L also later enjoyed. In 1966, the H-P annual report predicted that the effects of a slumping economy would be offset by "the great sales potential for our products, particularly medical instruments, in South American, Canadian and Asian markets. These areas should support substantial gains in sales for a number of years."[36] In materials prepared for potential investors, H-P made explicit statements about the advantages of foreign operations. For example, because H-P subsidiaries received "pioneer status" in Malaysia and Singapore, income generated in these countries remained essentially tax-free during the early 1970s: "Had their income been taxed at the U.S. statutory rate of 48 per cent in 1974, our net earnings would have been reduced by 37 cents a share."[37] By the mid-1970s, H-P's international medical equipment business, as measured by total orders, surpassed its domestic business. More than 100 sales and service offices were operating in 64 countries.

Like W-L, H-P also diversified its products to deal with the potential saturation of the coronary care market. During the late 1960s, the company introduced a series of complex computerized systems that were designed as an interface with electrocardiogram machines, monitoring devices, and other CCU products. For example, a computerized system to analyze and interpret electrocardiograms led to the capability of processing up to 500 electrocardiograms per 8-hour day: "This and other innovative systems recently introduced to the medical profession contributed to the substantial growth of our medical electronics business during the past year. With this growth has come increasing profitability as well."[38] Similar considerations of profitability motivated the development of telemetry systems for ambulatory patients with heart disease and battery-powered electrocardiogram machines designated for regions of foreign countries where electricity was not yet available for traditional machines. In 1973, H-P provided a forthright statement of its philosophy: "Health care expenditures, worldwide, will continue to increase significantly in the years ahead, and a growing portion of these funds will be allocated for medical electronic equipment. Interestingly, this growth trend offers the company . . . the unique opportunity to help shape the future of health care delivery."[39] From the corporate perspective, spiraling health-care expenditures, far from a problem to be solved, are the necessary fuel for desired profit.

The Academic Medical Center Connection

Academic medical centers have played a key role in the development and promotion of costly innovations like those in coronary care. This role has seldom attracted attention in critiques of technology, yet both corporations considered here obtained important bases at medical centers located in geographic proximity to corporate headquarters.

Before its purchase by W-L, American Optical—with headquarters in Southbridge, Massachusetts—had established ties with the Peter Bent Brigham Hospital in Boston. Specifically, the company worked with Bernard Lown, an eminent cardiologist who served as an AO consultant, on the development of defibrillators and cardioverters. Lown pioneered the theoretical basis and clinical application of these techniques; AO engineers collaborated with Lown in the construction of working models. As previously discussed, AO marketed and promoted several lines of defibrillators and cardioverters that bore Lown's name.

AO's support of technologic innovation at the Peter Bent Brigham Hospital is clear. The CCU developed in the mid-1960s received major grants from AO that Lown and his group acknowledged.[5] AO also used data and pictures from the Brigham CCU in promotional literature distributed to the medical profession and potential investors.[40] Lown and his group continued to influence the medical profession through a large number of publications, appearing in both the general medical and cardiologic literature, that discussed CCU-linked diagnostic and ther-

TABLE 4 Publications concerning coronary care from Peter Bent Brigham Hospital and Stanford University Medical Center Groups, 1965–1975

YEAR	PETER BENT BRIGHAM HOSPITAL	STANFORD UNIVERSITY MEDICAL CENTER
1965	1	1
1966	3	1
1967	3	4
1968	7	4
1969	11	3
1970	6	1
1971	7	2
1972	3	4
1973	4	5
1974	3	5
1975	2	4

Source: Index Medicus, citations listing B Lown or DC Harrison as author or co-author and dealing specifically with diagnostic or therapeutic techniques in coronary care units.

apeutic techniques (Table 4). In these papers, Lown emphasized the importance of automatic monitoring. He also advocated the widespread use of telemetry for ambulatory patients and computerized data-analysis systems, both areas into which AO diversified during the late 1960s and early 1970s. AO's relationships with Lown and his colleagues apparently proved beneficial for everybody concerned. The dynamics of heightened profits for AO and prestige for Lown were not optimal conditions for a detached, systematic appraisal of CCU effectiveness.

H-P's academic base has been the Stanford University Medical Center, located about one-half mile from corporate headquarters in Palo Alto, California. For many years William Hewlett, H-P's chief executive officer, served as a trustee of Stanford University. In addition, as I will discuss later, a private philanthropy established by Hewlett was prominent among the University's financial benefactors.

Since the late 1960s, Donald Harrison, professor of medicine and chief of the Division of Cardiology, has acted as H-P's primary consultant in the development of coronary care technology. Harrison and his colleagues at Stanford collaborated with H-P engineers in the design of CCU systems intended for marketing to both academic medical centers and community hospitals. H-P helped construct working models of CCU components at Stanford University Hospital, under the direction of Harrison and other faculty members. Stanford physicians introduced these H-P systems into clinical use.

Innovations in the treatment of patients with heart disease had a profound impact on the costs of care at Stanford. As documented in a general study of the costs of treatment for several illnesses at Stanford, Scitovsky and McCall stated: "Of the conditions covered by the 1964–1971 study, the changes in treatment in myocardial infarction had their most drastic effect on costs. This was due principally to the increased costs of intensive care units. In 1964, the Stanford Hospital had a relatively small Intensive Care Unit (ICU). It was used by only three of the 1964 coronary cases. . . . By 1971, the hospital had not only an ICU but also a Coronary Care Unit (CCU) and an intermediate CCU. Of the 1971 cases, only one did not receive at least some care in either the CCU or the intermediate CCU."[41]

During the late 1960s and early 1970s, many articles from the Harrison group described new technical developments or discussed clinical issues tied to intensive care techniques (Table 4). Several articles directly acknowledged the use of H-P equipment and assistance. These academic clinicians also participated in continuing medical education programs on coronary care, both in the United States and abroad. The Stanford specialists thus played an important role in promoting technology in general and H-P products in particular.

Private Philanthropies

Philanthropic support figured prominently in the growth of CCUs. Humanitarian goals were doubtless present, but profit considerations were not lacking, since philanthropic initiatives often emerged from the actions of corporate executives whose companies produced medical equipment or pharmaceuticals.

Primary among the philanthropic proponents of CCUs was the American Heart Association (AHA). The AHA sponsored research that led to the development of CCU products, especially monitoring systems. In addition, the AHA gave financial support directly to local hospitals establishing CCUs. "The underlying purpose" of these activities, according to the AHA's 1967 annual report, was "to encourage and guide the formation of new [CCU] units in both large and small hospitals."[42] Justifying these expenditures, the AHA cited some familiar "data": "Experi-

ence with the approximately 300 such specialized units already established, mostly in large hospitals, indicated that a national network of CCUs might save the lives of more than 45,000 individuals each year."[42] The source for this projected number of rescued people, though uncited, presumably was a "personal communication" from an HEW official to which Day referred in his 1963 article.[4] Later in the 1960s, the AHA's annual number of estimated beneficiaries rose still higher, again with undocumented claims of effectiveness. According to the 1968 annual report, "only about one-third of hospitalized heart attack patients are fortunate enough to be placed in coronary care units. If all of them had the benefits of these monitoring and emergency service facilities, it is estimated that 50,000 more heart patients could be saved yearly."[43] This unsubstantiated estimate, raised from the earlier unsubstantiated figure of 45,000, persisted in AHA literature into the early 1970s. During this same period the AHA cosponsored, with the U.S. Public Health Service and the American College of Cardiology, a series of national conferences on coronary care whose purpose was "the successful development of the CCU program" in all regions of the United States.[42]

Other smaller foundations also supported CCU proliferation. For example, the John A. Hartford Foundation gave generous support to several hospitals and medical centers during the early 1960s to develop monitoring capabilities. The Hartford Foundation's public view of CCU effectiveness was unequivocal; the Kansas City coronary care program "has demonstrated that a properly equipped and designed physical setting staffed with personnel trained to meet cardiac emergencies will provide prophylactic therapy which will materially enhance the survival of these patients and substantially reduce the mortality rates."[44] Another foundation that supported CCU growth, although somewhat less directly, was the W. R. Hewlett Foundation, founded by H-P's chief executive officer. The Hewlett Foundation earmarked large annual grants to Stanford University which chose H-P equipment for its CCU and other intensive-care facilities.[45]

The commitment of private philanthropy to technologic innovations is a structural problem that transcends the personalities that control philanthropy at any specific time. The bequests that create philanthropies historically come largely from funds generated by North American industrial corporations, that are highly oriented to technologic advances. Moreover, the investment portfolios of philanthropic organizations usually include stocks in a sizable number of industrial companies. These structural conditions encourage financial support for technological advances, like those in coronary care.

In addition, it is useful to ask which people made philanthropic decisions to fund CCU development. During the mid-1960s, the AHA's officers included eight physicians who had primary commitments in cardiology, executives of two pharmaceutical companies (L. F. Johnson of American Home Products Corporation's drug subsidiaries and Ross Reid of Squibb Corporation), a metals company executive (A. M. Baer of Imperial Knife Associated Companies), a prominent banker (W. C. Butcher, president of Chase Manhattan Bank), and several public officials (including Dwight Eisenhower). At the height of CCU promotion in 1968, the chairman of the AHA's annual Heart Fund was a drug company executive (W. F. Laporte, president of American Home Products Corporation, former chief of its pharmaceutical subsidiaries, and director of several banks).[43] During the 1960s and early 1970s, bankers and corporate executives also dominated the board at the Hartford Foundation. The Hewlett Foundation remained a family affair until the early 1970s, when R. W. Heyns— former chancellor of the University of California, Berkeley, and also a director of Norton Simon, Inc., Kaiser Industries, and Levi-Strauss—assumed the Foundation's presidency. It is not surprising that philanthropic policies supporting CCU proliferation showed a strong orientation toward corporate industrialism.

The Role of the State

Agencies of government played a key role in CCU growth. Earlier I discussed the financial support that the U.S. Public Health Service provided to clinicians in the early 1960s for CCU development. An official of HEW provided an "estimate" of potential lives saved by future CCUs[4]; without apparent basis in data, this figure became a slogan for CCU promotion. Conferences and publications by HEW during the late 1960s specified guidelines for adequate CCU equipment, even though the effectiveness of this approach admittedly remained unproven by random controlled trial.

In these activities, three common functions of the state in capitalist societies were evident.[2] First, in health policy the state generally supports private enterprise by encouraging innovations that enhance profits to major industrial corporations. The state does not enact policies that limit private profit in any serious way. Recognizing the high costs of CCU implementation, state agencies could have placed strict limitations on their number and distribution. For example, HEW could have called for the regionalization of CCU facilities and restrictions on their wider proliferation. Subsequently, studies of CCU mortality rates generally have shown better outcomes in larger, busier centers and have suggested the rationality of regionalized policies.[46] HEW's policies supported just the opposite development. By publishing guidelines that called for advanced CCU technology and by encouraging CCU proliferation to most community hospitals, HEW assured the profitability of corporate ventures in the coronary-care field.

A second major function of the state is its legitimation of the capitalist political-economic system.[2, 3] The history of public health and welfare programs shows that state expenditures usually increase during periods of social unrest and decrease as unrest becomes less widespread. The decade of the 1960s was a time of upheaval in the United States. The civil rights movement called into question basic patterns of injustice. Opposition to the war in Indochina mobilized a large part of the population against government and corporate policies. Labor disputes arose frequently. Under such circumstances, when government and corporations face large-scale crises of legitimacy, the state tends to intervene with health and welfare projects. Medical technology is a "social capital expenditure" by which the state tries to counteract the recurrent legitimacy crises of advanced capitalism.[47] Technologic innovations like CCUs are convenient legitimating expenditures, since they convey a message of deep concern for the public health, while they also support new sources of profit for large industrial firms.

Thirdly, government agencies provide market research that guides domestic and foreign sales efforts. The Global Market Survey, published by the

U.S. Department of Commerce, gives a detailed analysis of changes in medical facilities, hospital beds, and physicians throughout the world. The Survey specifies those countries that are prime targets for sales of biomedical equipment. For example, the 1973 Survey pointed out that "major foreign markets for biomedical equipment are expected to grow at an average annual rate of 15 per cent in the 1970s, nearly double the growth rate predicted for the U.S. domestic market."[48] The same report predicted that West Germany (which would emphasize CCU construction), Japan, Brazil, Italy, and Israel would be the largest short-term markets for products manufactured in the United States. According to the report "market research studies identified specific equipment that present [sic] good to excellent U.S. sale opportunities in the 20 [foreign] markets"; "cardiological-thoracic equipment" headed the list of products with high sales potential.[48] Market research performed by state agencies has encouraged the proliferation of CCUs and related innovations, whose capacity to generate profits has overshadowed the issue of effectiveness in government planning.

Changes in the Health Care Labor Force

Intensive care involves workers as well as equipment. Throughout the twentieth century, a process of "deskilling" has occurred, by which the skilled trades and professions have become rationalized into simpler tasks that can be handled by less skilled and lower paid workers.[49] In medicine, paraprofessionals take on rationalized tasks that can be specified by algorithms covering nearly all contingencies. This deskilling process applies equally to CCUs and other intensive care facilities, where standard orders—often printed in advance—can deal with almost all situations that might arise.

The deskilling of the intensive care labor force has received support from professional, governmental, and corporate planners. During the late 1960s and early 1970s, the training of allied health personnel to deal with intensive care technology became a priority of educators and administrators. According to this view, it was important to train a "cadre of health workers capable of handling routine and purely functional duties."[50] The linkage between allied health workers and new technology was a clear

assumption in this approach. There were limits on "the extent to which a markedly greater delegation of tasks can be achieved without the introduction of new technology" that compensates for aides' lack of "decisional training."[51] The availability of monitoring equipment in CCUs made this setting adaptable to staffing partly by technicians who could receive lower wages than doctors or nurses.[52] Paramedical training programs, focusing on intensive care, became a goal of national policy makers, even though they recognized the "built in obsolescence of monitoring equipment" and the tendency of industrial corporations to "capitalize" in this field.[53, 54]

CONCLUSIONS

Although not exhaustive, an overview helps clarify the history of CCUs and other technologic "advances" (Figure 1). Corporate research and development lead to the production of new technology, pharmaceuticals, and related innovations. The guiding motivation for corporations is profit; in this sense the commodification of health care resembles non-medical goods and services. Closely linked to corporations, philanthropies support research and clinical practices that enhance profits. Agencies of the state encourage innovations by grants for investigation, financial assistance to medical centers adopting new technology, and advocacy of new practices. While state intervention benefits private enterprise, it also enhances the faltering legitimacy of the capitalist political-economic system. Academic clinicians and investigators, based in teaching hospitals, help develop technology and foster its diffusion through professional publications and pronouncements in the public media. Corporate sales efforts cultivate markets in health institutions, both domestic and foreign. Technologic change generates the need for allied health workers who are less skilled than professionals. The cyclical acceptance of technologic innovations by medical institutions involves capital expenditures that drive up the overall costs of health care.

Cost containment activities that do not recognize these dynamics of the capitalist system will remain a farce. During the last decade, sophisticated methodologies to analyze costs and effectiveness have emerged in medical care research. These techniques

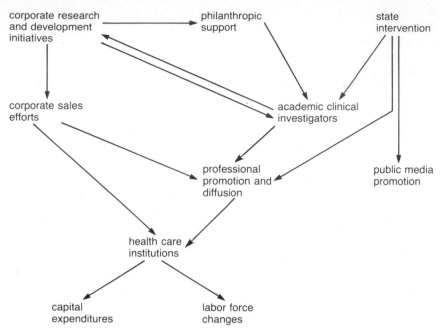

Figure 1 Overview of the Development, Promotion, and Proliferation of CCUs and Similar Medical Advances

include clinical decision analysis and a variety of related methods.[55-58] Ironically, economists first developed this type of analysis at the Pentagon, to evaluate technologic innovations like new missiles.[59] This methodology led to disastrous policy decisions in Indochina, largely because the cost-effectiveness approach did not take into account the broader, so-called "imponderable" context. This analysis did not predict accurately the political response of the Indochinese people to such technologies as napalm and mechanized warfare. Ironically, many of the same people who developed cost-effectiveness research at the Department of Defense now are moving into the health field, where this approach has become quite fashionable.[60]

In health care as in other areas, cost-effectiveness methodology restricts the level of analysis to the evaluation of specific innovations.[61-65] Studies using this framework generally ignore, or make only passing reference to, the broader structures of capitalism.[66] As a result, this approach obscures one fundamental source of high costs and ineffective practices: the profit motive. Because of this deficiency, cost-effectiveness analysis mystifies the roots

of costly, ineffective practices in the very nature of our political-economic system.

Defects of research, however, are less dangerous than defects of policy. Cost containment has become a highly touted national priority. In a climate of fiscal crisis, an ideology of austerity is justifying cutbacks in health and welfare programs. Services whose effectiveness is difficult to demonstrate by the new methodologies are prime candidates for cutbacks and therefore face a bleak future. Poor people and minority groups, historically victimized by the free enterprise system, will be the first to suffer from this purported rationalization of policy. Meanwhile, private profit in health care, a major fuel for high costs, continues unabated. Just as it eludes serious attention in research, the structure of profit evades new initiatives in health policy.

Cost containment will remain little more than rhetoric in the United States unless we begin to address the linkages between cost and profit. It is foolish to presume that major restrictions on profit in the health system can succeed without other basic changes in the political-economic system. On the other hand, working toward progressive alternatives in health care is part of longer-term efforts aimed at social reconstruction.

An initial step involves support for policies that curtail private profit. Unlimited corporate involvement in medicine must end. The corporations that develop and successfully promote ineffective innovations like those in coronary care must cease these activities. Because this will not happen voluntarily, we need compulsory restriction of profit in health care and eventual public ownership of medical industries, especially pharmaceutical and medical equipment manufacturing.[67] A national formulary of permitted drugs and equipment, like that established in several socialist countries, would reduce costs by eliminating the proliferation of unneeded products. Socialization of medical production is no more fanciful than public ownership of utilities, transportation facilities, or schools.

In summary, CCU development and promotion may seem irrational when analyzed in terms of proven medical effectiveness. These trends appear considerably more rational when viewed from the needs of a capitalist system in crisis. By questioning what capitalism does with our hearts, we get closer to the heart of many of our other problems.

References

1. Waitzkin H, Waterman B: The Exploitation of Illness in Capitalist Society. Indianapolis, Bobbs-Merrill, 1974.
2. Waitzkin H: A Marxist view of medical care. Ann. Intern. Med. 89:264–278, 1978.
3. Navarro V: Medicine Under Capitalism. New York, Prodist, 1976.
4. Day HW: An intensive coronary care area. Dis Chest 44:423–427, 1963.
5. Lown B, Fakhro AM, Hood WB, et al: The coronary care unit: new perspectives and directions. JAMA 199:188–198, 1967.
6. United States Department of Health, Education, and Welfare: Heart Disease Control Program: Proceedings of the National Conference on Coronary Care Units. DHEW Pub. No. 1764. Washington, DC, Govt Printing Office, 1968.
7. United States Department of Health, Education, and Welfare: Heart Disease and Stroke Control Program: Guidelines for Coronary Care Units. DHEW Pub. No. 1824. Washington, DC, Govt Printing Office, 1968.
8. Geographical distribution of coronary care units in the United States. Metropolitan Life Insurance Company Statistical Bulletin 58:7–9, July-August 1977.
9. Peterson OL: Myocardial infarction: unit care or home care? Ann. Intern. Med. 88:259–261, 1978.
10. Martin SP, Donaldson MC, London CD, et al: Inputs into coronary care during 30 years: a cost effectiveness study. Ann. Intern. Med. 81:289–293, 1974.
11. Anti-dysrhythmic treatment in acute myocardial infarction (editorial). Lancet 1:193–194, 1979.
12. Coronary-care units—where now? (editorial). Lancet 1:649–650, 1979.
13. Waitzkin H: How capitalism cares for our coronaries: a preliminary exercise in political economy. In The Doctor-Patient Relationship in the Changing Health Scene, Gallagher EB (ed.) DHEW Pub. No. (NIH) 78–183. Washington, DC, Govt Printing Office, 1978.
14. Hofvendahl S: Influence of treatment in a CCU on prognosis in acute myocardial infarction. Acta. Med. Scand. (Suppl) 519:1–78, 1971.
15. Christiansen I, Iversen K, Skouby AP: Benefits obtained by the introduction of a coronary care unit: a comparative study. Acta. Med. Scand. 189:285–291, 1971.
16. Hill JC, Holdstock G, Hampton JR: Comparison of mortality of patients with heart attacks admitted to a coronary care unit and an ordinary medical ward. Br. Med. J. 2:81–83, 1977.
17. Astvad K, Fabricius-Bjerre N, Kjaerulff J, et al: Mortality from acute myocardial infarction before and after establishment of a coronary care unit. Br. Med. J. 1:567–569, 1974.
18. Mather HG, Morgan DC, Pearson NG, et al: Myocardial infarction: a comparison between home and hospital care for patients. Br. Med. J. 1:925–929, 1976.
19. Mather HG, Pearson NG, Read KLQ, et al: Acute myocardial infarction: home and hospital treatment. Br. Med. J. 3:334–338, 1971.
20. Hill JC, Hampton JR, Mitchell JRA: A randomized trial of home-versus-hospital management for patients with suspected myocardial infarction. Lancet 1:837–841, 1978.
21. Colling A, Dellipiani AW, Donaldson RJ: Teesside coronary survey: an epidemiological study of acute attacks of myocardial infarction. Br. Med. J. 2:1169–1172, 1976.
22. Dellipiani AW, Colling WA, Donaldson RJ, et al: Teesside coronary survey—fatality and comparative severity of patients treated at home, in the hospital ward, and in the coronary care unit after myocardial infarction. Br. Heart J. 39:1172–1178, 1977.
23. Mandel E: An Introduction to Marxist Economic Thought. New York, Pathfinder, 1970.

24. DeSalvo RJ: Medical marketing mixture—update. Med Marketing & Media 13:21–35, September 1978.

25. Warner-Lambert Pharmaceutical Company: Annual Report. Morris Plains, NJ, 1977.

26. Idem: Annual Report. Morris Plains, NJ, 1969, p 8.

27. American Optical Company: Annual Report. Southbridge, MA, 1966, p 9.

28. Warner-Lambert Pharmaceutical Company: Annual Report. Morris Plains, NJ, 1967, p 7.

29. Idem: Annual Report. Morris Plains, NJ, 1968, p 25.

30. Idem: Annual Report. Morris Plains, NJ, 1969, pp 18–19.

31. Idem: Annual Report. Morris Plains, NJ, 1970, p 19.

32. Idem: Annual Report. Morris Plains, NJ, 1975, p 5.

33. Idem: Annual Report. Morris Plains, NJ, 1970, p 16.

34. Hewlett-Packard Company: Annual Report. Palo Alto, CA, 1966, p 11.

35. Idem: Annual Report. Palo Alto, CA, 1969, p 11.

36. Idem: Annual Report. Palo Alto, CA, 1966, p 4.

37. Idem: Annual Report. Palo Alto, CA, 1974, p 2.

38. Idem: Annual Report. Palo Alto, CA, 1971, p 5.

39. Idem: Annual Report. Palo Alto, CA, 1973, pp 18–19.

40. Warner-Lambert Pharmaceutical Company: Annual Report. Morris Plains, NJ, 1967, p 7.

41. Scitovsky AA, McCall N: Changes in the Costs of Treatment of Selected Illnesses, 1951–1964–1971. DHEW Pub. No. (HRA) 77–3161. Washington, DC, Govt Printing Office, 1977.

42. American Heart Association: Annual Report. New York, 1967, p 11.

43. Idem: Annual Report. New York, 1968, pp 2, 13–14.

44. John A. Hartford Foundation: Annual Report. New York, 1963, p 58.

45. W. R. Hewlett Foundation: Annual Report to the Internal Revenue Service. Palo Alto, CA, 1967, 1971.

46. Bloom BS, Peterson OL: End results, cost and productivity of coronary-care units. N Engl J Med 288:72–78, 1974.

47. O'Connor J: The Fiscal Crisis of the State. New York, St. Martin's Press, 1973.

48. United States Department of Commerce, Domestic and International Business Administration: Global Market Survey: Biomedical Equipment. USDC Pub., unnumbered. Washington, DC, Govt Printing Office, 1973.

49. Braverman H: Labor and Monopoly Capital. New York. Monthly Review Press, 1974.

50. Rosinski EF: Impact of technology and evolving health care systems on the training of allied health personnel. Milit. Med. 134:390–393, 1969.

51. Moore FJ: Information technologies and health care: the need for new technologies to offset the shortage of physicians. Arch. Intern. Med. 125:351–355, 1970.

52. Foster FL, Casten GG, Reeves TJ: Nonmedical personnel and continuous ECG monitoring. Arch. Intern. Med. 124:110–112, 1969.

53. Sanazaro PJ: Physician support personnel in the 1970s. JAMA 214:98–100, 1970.

54. Barnett GO, Robbins A: Information technology and manpower productivity. JAMA 209:546–548, 1969.

55. McNeil BJ, Keeler E, Adelstein SJ: Primer on certain elements of medical decision making. N. Engl. J. Med. 293:211–215, 1975.

56. Schoenbaum SC, McNeil BJ, Kavet J: The swine-influenza decision. N. Engl. J. Med. 295:759–765, 1976.

57. Costs, Risks, and Benefits of Surgery. JP Bunker, BA Barnes, F Mosteller (eds.) New York, Oxford University Press, 1977.

58. Abrams HL, McNeil BJ: Medical implications of computed tomography ("CAT scanning"). N. Engl. J. Med. 298:255–261, 310–318, 1978.

59. Hitch CJ, McKean RN: The Economics of Defense in the Nuclear Age. New York, Atheneum, 1967.

60. Enthoven AC: Consumer-choice health plan. N. Engl. J. Med. 298:650–658, 709–720, 1978.

61. Cochrane AL: Efficiency and Effectiveness: Random Reflections on Health Services. London, Nuffield Hospitals Trust, 1972.

62. Illich I: Medical Nemesis. New York, Pantheon, 1976.

63. Rose G: The contribution of intensive coronary care. Br. J. Prev. Soc. Med. 29:147–150, 1975.

64. Mechanic D: Approaches to controlling the costs of medical care: short-range and long-range alternatives. N. Engl. J. Med. 298: 249–254, 1978.

65. United States Congress, Office of Technology Assessment: Development of Medical Technology: Opportunities for Assessment (OTA Pub. unnumbered). Washington, DC, Govt Printing Office, 1976.

66. Stevenson G: Laws of motion in the for-profit health industry: a theory and three examples. Internat. J. Health Serv. 8:235–256, 1978.

67. Dellums RV, et al: Health Service Act (H.R. 11879). Washington, DC, Govt Printing Office, 1978.

Addendum: Stretching Ideology to the Utmost: Marxism and Medical Technology

Bernard S. Bloom

There is a great temptation to analyze critically the article by Dr. Howard Waitzkin[1] . . . by weighing all the relative merits and demerits of the democratic, capitalist, free enterprise political and economic system against that of state capitalism practiced in Eastern Europe and the Soviet Union. It is particularly tempting because Dr. Waitzkin has interpreted the development and growth of coronary care units (CCUs) in the United States in terms of a wider political and economic structure, rather than as an unusually good example of technological development with rapid, uncritical dispersion, a phenomenon common to medical care systems under any political and economic system.

Dr. Waitzkin has wisely chosen coronary care units as a dramatic example of our inability to contain costs. He ascribes this failure to the relationship between health care costs and private profit in the general U.S. economic system. In addition, he tries to show that CCU proliferation was part of a complex process initiated by private industrial organizations with the full and knowing cooperation of clinicians and research workers, primarily at academic medical centers, and with the support of private philanthropic foundations and government agencies, mainly federal.

It is important to have published Dr. Waitzkin's analysis even though his framework of analysis appears to me to be inappropriate. Irrespective of framework, it is useful to present multiple analyses of problems so that we may learn from events by studying them from as many points of view as possible. Hopefully, this will help us not to repeat too many of our past mistakes. We may also learn from the uncomfortable stimulus he applies to the half-formed economic theories most of us hold.

Where I think Dr. Waitzkin is directly on target is in his analysis of CCU development. He shows, in detail, that there was rapid growth in the United States without benefit of controlled investigations that could have determined efficacy, effectiveness and cost. CCUs were accepted unquestioningly for the treatment of acute heart disease. They have now increased to a level where approximately one-half of U.S. acute care hospitals have such units.[2] At the present time in the U.S. there is no possibility of being able to perform a well-controlled trial of CCU efficacy and cost-effectiveness. The randomized clinical trials done in Great Britain have had little effect here.[3–5] Perhaps skepticism of CCU effectiveness has increased, but CCU use has also increased since the first random clinical trial by Mather, et al., was published in 1971.[3] Other studies of output and cost,[6] cost-effectiveness,[7] and oversupply, rational planning and regionalization[8] have also had little impact.

This is an unfortunate, but all too common occurrence in our health and medical care system. Therapies are often devised, accepted and proliferate rapidly on the weakest of evidence. When a well-controlled investigation finally is conducted, some therapies are found to be less effective or entirely without merit. Some, fortunately, have been rapidly abandoned, as shown by the recent dramatic examples of gastric freezing for peptic ulcer[9] and internal

Reprinted from the *American Journal of Public Health,* vol. 69, no. 12 (December, 1979), pp. 1269–1271.

625

mammary artery ligation for angina pectoris.[10] In other cases, when a technology may be of benefit to only a minority of patients with specific characteristics (as with CCUs), it has proved difficult to prevent its indiscriminate (hence costly and ineffective) application. Fetal monitoring seems to be another example.[11]

In a field with scientific pretensions, it is a curious phenomenon that so much medical care is prescribed, based upon a belief in its efficacy and effectiveness, without having subjected the belief to controlled clinical trial. Not uncommonly, when someone suggests a randomized clinical trial to determine efficacy, the ground shifts and the trial becomes unethical because physicians believe the therapy to be effective, use it widely, and claim that it is immoral to withhold it from their patients. Thus, belief becomes equivalent to efficacy. In this Alice in Wonderland situation, Dr. Waitzkin has unwittingly fallen into the trap of allowing an ideology to shape an explanation for a curious phenomenon which he has correctly observed.

Dr. Waitzkin presents an informative review of how the American Optical Division of Warner-Lambert Pharmaceutical Company, and Hewlett-Packard Company early became involved in the development and sales of this new technology. Among questions that immediately arise are:

- Did these corporations (as Waitzkin intimates) "foist off" equipment on gullible physicians or did they merely meet demand for this equipment generated by physicians themselves? The latter seems more likely.
- Are physicians so easily duped into purchasing expensive technology (as Waitzkin implies) or did they only purchase what they thought they needed for good patient care? Again, the latter appears to be closer to the truth.
- Are similar techniques for implementing medical technology used in Marxist countries where CCUs are also popular although less widespread? This, too, seems probable. I suspect that physicians in those countries firmly believe in the efficacy of CCUs and, being the prime clinical decisionmakers just as they are in capitalist countries, seek to acquire the technology that they believe useful in diagnosis

and efficacious in therapy. Budgetary rather than clinical judgmental factors prevent their acquiring them.

Dr. Waitzkin has also presented an interesting thesis regarding the relationship between American Optical, Hewlett-Packard, academic medical centers, private foundations, and government agencies. Although this relationship may be open to charges of conflict of interest when it comes to an objective evaluation of the technology, it seems hard to believe that a conspiracy existed. It is more likely that a desire to tackle a grave problem rather than cupidity led to the ready acceptance of CCUs. We must not forget that in 1960 when the first CCU was opened, heart disease was (as it is today), *the* major cause of death and that it was logical as an hypothesis lending itself to a technological approach. American Optical and Hewlett-Packard were only among the first to discover the connection and exploit its marketing potential. Other corporations in the U.S., soon followed by those of Europe, began to sell CCU monitoring equipment. Today, the German Democratic Republic, Czechoslovakia, and the Soviet Union are all busily marketing their own CCU equipment. The fault lies not with the hypothesis but with the failure to subject its ramification to scientific study.

The fact, often overlooked, is that Communist countries also need new products and markets to keep their economies expanding so that ever-increasing fruits of labor can accrue to the proletariat, as well as to earn the necessary foreign exchange to buy capitalist technologies, blue jeans and Elton John records. Marxist countries are also open to the vagaries of economic cycles as witnessed by the current inflation and economic stagnation in many Eastern European countries including the Soviet Union. Some Marxist countries are again using monetary and other incentives to raise worker productivity, and profit incentives to managers and supervisors for more efficient resource allocation and to meet consumer demand; on the surface this is anathema to Marxist doctrine. The individual's desire for more—irrespective of the economic or political system—is a powerful motivating force, as Marxist economists and planners are rediscovering.

In short, one need not resort to Marxian ideology to explain the development of CCUs and the medical profession's uncritical and enthusiastic acceptance of a technology that was not adequately evaluated. The profit motive may have helped accelerate the speed of the technology's dispersion but is not the villain pulling the strings behind the scene.

An alternative analysis of this development and growth could be based on a theory of foolishness— that cardiologists, third-party payors and policy makers accepted weak evidence for CCU effectiveness and incorporated it as one of their fundamental beliefs. An analysis postulating a capitalist, profit-oriented basis for CCU implementation and growth has little to do with making sense of therapeutic or medical policy nonsense.

How then can the uncritical dispersion and widespread use of diagnostic and therapeutic interventions be controlled? Cochran has suggested that no medical intervention should be paid for unless subjected to rigorous clinical investigation by the most appropriate statistical technique, preferably by double-blind, random-controlled trial, or, if this is not possible, then the next best statistical study design.[12] The suggestion could become the focus of a serious public policy debate. In essence, this policy now holds for drugs. No drug is allowed for general use unless the Food and Drug Administration is convinced of its efficacy and safety. Some may feel that the FDA is not a very good model in that many useful drugs are kept out of use or that it takes too long for a drug to wind its way through the bureaucracy for approval. However, the original idea is still a good one despite faulty execution.

For all the ills of a capitalist society, the profit system still is the most efficient, i.e., lowest unit cost, allocator of scarce resources; and, as is being brought dramatically to our attention every day, all resources are ultimately scarce. One strength of the free enterprise system lies in the fact that there is an impersonal market which allocates these scarce resources. Conversely, a weakness of Marxist economics is that resource allocation decisions are more likely to be inefficient because they are made by individuals whose judgments may be fallible. Even the high income Western European countries that are termed "socialist" (Great Britain and the Nordic countries) are, in fact, not very socialist. Only a minor part of economic activity, the production and distribution of goods and services, are owned by the government. In Sweden only about 30 per cent of the economic output is owned by the government.[13] These socialist countries, too, recognize many of the strengths of the free and open market. Gunnar Adler-Karlson has noted that:

> It is my conviction that much of the present ideological debate in terms of socialism versus capitalism is not only outdated but even outright dangerous as it blurs our deeper understanding of the ideological problems of our societies, and as it makes us less efficient in our fight for the socialist ideals. The debate is still largely centering around the formal ownership, private or by the state, of the means of production. Actually, the formal ownership of the means of production is a secondary issue, as has been amply proved by Swedish socialist experience. What is of prime importance is the distribution in society of the economic and political functions which are hidden beneath formal ownership.[14]

Thus, if we accept Adler-Karlson's argument, ownership of the means of production and distribution are not necessary in order to control the economy. And, by inference, it is fair to assume that the strengths of the capitalist system, including the profit motive, can even be used to achieve a more equitable distribution of income. It is also fair to assume that political power, which is often closely related to money, can theoretically also be more equitably distributed. There is nothing inherent in the capitalist, free enterprise economic system that precludes this. It is still the democratic political system that has ultimate control and can change or modify the economic system, as it has done continuously throughout our history. Whether economic system changes wrought by the political system have been too few or too many is not an argument that will be explored here.

Dr. Waitzkin certainly has a point in his thesis that medical technology is oversold to both physicians and the public. The benefits of this untested technology are lauded, which give rise to unrealizable expectations by the public. As a physician, Dr. Waitzkin no doubt is aware of the overselling of much of medical care and also of the indiscriminate consumption of over-the-counter drugs, nostrums, and aids that hold promise of longer life, greater desirability by the opposite sex, and relief from the vagaries and minor irritations of daily living. Should government, as society's voice, forbid the manufacture, advertising, sale, and purchase of these preparations if they really are relatively harmless, even though their efficacy is unproven? I think not, for the rights of individuals to be fools is no doubt just as important, and human, as are their Constitutional rights. It is primarily when great harm is possible, when the market fails, as in medical care, or when public monies are spent, that government can and should effectively intervene to control, modify, own, or regulate. In medical care all these criteria are met.

In medical care, the market system does not work like that of other industries. In fact, it works perversely at times. However, there are aspects of the free market that might be utilized to bring about desired changes. Market characteristics, such as monetary and other incentives, could be used to reward greater efficiency (without loss of efficacy) in those areas of the health industry that are clearly amenable to these incentives. Such incentives might cause inefficiently used resources (such as CCU resources) to be employed for more worthwhile purposes: providing services of known and proven value in health care or other social arenas, or accruing directly to consumers as tax reductions which will allow them greater disposable income to use as they desire.

According to Waitzkin, "Cost containment will remain little more than rhetoric in the United States, unless we begin to address the linkages between cost and profit."[1] I agree with this statement but not with Waitzkin's interpretation. I believe that in order to achieve cost containment we must change the structure of the industry, restructure control of the industry, of provider payments and incentives, and introduce a healthy dose of competition including the profit motive. It seems to me that it is not a desire for profit that is linked to rising costs, but the lack of competition among providers, and the absence of a link between profits and the efficient (lowest unit cost) use of resources and technologies whose effectiveness has been proven. These links, together with the impact on the system of an enhanced consumer voice and choice, may be our most effective tools in the struggle to contain costs. Minor tinkering will produce few results; although unpopu-

lar with providers, major restructuring is required to bring order out of the present chaos.

For the first time the United States is feeling the pinch of constrained resources. Other high income countries have long realized that resources are finite. In many cases other countries have been more effective than the US in distributing scare resources and national income. Perhaps the growing realization of the finiteness of resources will serve as a catalyst for a more equitable distribution of health resources, making best use of free enterprise capitalism as well as public control and accountability.

References

1. Waitzkin H: A Marxian interpretation of the growth and development of coronary care technology. Am. J. Public Health, 69:1260–1268, 1979.

2. Guide to the Health Care Field. 1978 Edition. Chicago: American Hospital Association, 1978.

3. Mather HG, Pearson NG, Read KLQ, et al: Acute myocardial infarction: home and hospital treatment. Brit. Med. J. 3:334–338, 1971.

4. Mather HG, Morgan DC, Pearson NG, et al: Myocardial infarction: a comparison between home and hospital care for patients. Brit. Med. J. 1:925–929, 1976.

5. Hill JD, Hampton JR, Mitchell JRA: A randomized trial of home versus hospital management for patients with suspected myocardial infarction. The Lancet. 2:837–841, 1978.

6. Bloom BS, Peterson OL: End results, cost and productivity of coronary care units. N. Engl. J. Med. 286:189–194, 1972.

7. Martin SP, Donaldson MC, London CD, et al: Inputs into coronary care during 30 years: a cost effectiveness study. Ann. Intern. Med. 81:289–293, 1974.

8. Bloom BS, Peterson OL: Patient needs and medical care planning: the coronary care unit as a model. N. Engl. J. Med. 290:1171–1177, 1974.

9. Miao LL: Gastric freezing: an example of the evaluation of medical therapy by randomized clinical trials, in Costs, Risks and Benefits of Surgery. Bunker JP, Barnes BA, Mosteller F (eds.). New York: Oxford University Press, 1977.

10. Barsamian EM: The rise and fall of internal mammary artery ligation in the treatment of angina pectoris and the lessons learned, in Costs, Risks and Benefits of

Surgery. Bunker JP, Barnes BA, Mosteller F (eds.). New York: Oxford University Press, 1977.

11. Banta HD, Thacker SB: Policies toward medical technology: the case of electronic fetal monitoring. (commentary). Am J. Public Health 69:931–935, 1979

12. Cochrane AL: Effectiveness and Efficiency: Random

Reflections on Health Services. London: Nuffield Provincial Hospitals Trust, 1972.

13. Statistical Abstract of Sweden 1974. Stockholm: National Central Bureau of Statistics, 1974.

14. Adler-Karlson GL: Functional Socialism. Stockholm: Prism, 1969.

A Case of Corporate Malpractice and the Dalkon Shield

Mark Dowie
Tracy Johnston

In 1971, Dr. Hugh J. Davis, associate professor of gynecology at Johns Hopkins, decided to write up his experiments with a new intrauterine device he had been using at the university's family planning clinic. He heads the clinic, which is part of one of the country's most prestigious medical schools. The clinic, like the Johns Hopkins Medical School, is in the middle of one of the worst ghettos in Baltimore, and Davis spends a lot of his time prescribing pills, inserting IUDs and advising poor black and Latin American women how to prevent unwanted children. One of the many lawyers who do the talking for him now says Davis thinks of pregnancy as "a social evil—contributing to poverty, unhappiness and unrest."

Although Davis's book, a slim volume sprinkled with charts and graphs and called *The Intrauterine Device for Contraception,* was not stacked up alongside the cash registers of bookstores across the country, many doctors read it eagerly. The results of research performed under the auspices of Johns Hopkins could certainly be trusted, and doctors everywhere were anxious for information about the various plastic loops and squiggles and paper-clip-like things they had inserted in over three million women in America. They still know almost nothing about intrauterine devices, except that somehow a foreign object in the uterus usually prevents pregnancy.

At that time, the entire subject of contraception was especially controversial. Pill men and IUD men were known to exchange bitter comments at conventions and engage in primitive avoidance rituals if they discovered each other at the same party. The Davis book, since it came from Hopkins, was discussed by most everyone in the field and widely reported on in women's magazines.

In his book, Davis gives evidence that the IUD is a better birth-control device than the Pill—almost as efficient and much safer. More important, he indicates that a certain new IUD recently put on the market works better than any of the old ones.

To be sure, Davis doesn't directly recommend the Dalkon Shield over the Lippes Loop, the Saf-T-Coil, the Copper-7 or its other competitors; such recommendations in medical texts are considered highly unprofessional. The Shield's experimental results just look a lot better. The comparisons appear to be thorough, scientific and convincing. On every graph, on every chart and in every analysis, the Dalkon Shield is first.

The only thing the book does not say about the Dalkon Shield—and the full story has not been told before—is that Davis had not only tested it, he had invented it, along with his good friend Irwin Lerner, and he was making money on every new Shield sold. At the time the book was published, Davis had already made $250,000 on the sale of the Shield to the A. H. Robins Company, one of the largest pharmaceutical houses in the United States. In five years' time, before the Shield would be removed from the market amid increasing publicity about deaths and injuries to women who used it, Davis would earn well over $300,000 more in royalties and consultants' fees.

No one knows exactly how many women have been killed by the Dalkon Shield. As of last January, seventeen American women had died. There have been a number of deaths since, but the government totals and releases such figures only once a year. Statistics from the dozens of other countries where the Shield has been in use—mostly in the Third World—are fragmentary or nonexistent. In other ways, too, the full story of the device that has left untold hundreds of women sterile, and that is still in use by more than a million women around the world, has been hard to get. Doctors do not easily reveal secrets about each other. Also, all the principal characters in this story are under orders from their lawyers not to speak, for the Dalkon Shield has become one of the most litigated products in pharmaceutical history.

Since Davis would not talk to us, it was difficult to get a full picture of this paradoxical man, who teaches at a leading university and runs a clinic for the poor, yet who succumbed to the temptation of making big money by the most unethical means. We could assemble only a fragmentary picture of him from others' reports. Thomas Kemp, a lawyer handling many of the cases for Robins, describes Davis as "tall," "neat" and a man of "overwhelming heart." Davis's wife says she hopes the true story about her husband will get out, but she doesn't know what it is. "Work is work and home is home," she says on the phone over the sounds of children giggling, and Davis doesn't mix the two. Still another picture of him comes from a woman who once worked in his clinic, who described him as "the most efficient man I ever met." She said he once used a vacation to have his appendix taken out, just so that he would lose no work time if he ever got appendicitis.

Luckily for our story, though, there are sworn depositions in the Dalkon case, and although Davis is cagey and doesn't reveal a thing when he talks to lawyers, Irwin Lerner is a garrulous guy and tells the story of the Dalkon Shield with relish.

"Win" Lerner is an inventor, really. He started off in 1948 as an electrical engineer in oil development. He went on to computers and then typewriters, where, he claims, he developed the Selectric. In 1960 he got interested in the medical supplies field and started working for a company making polyethylene tubing, bloodtest equipment, automatic pipettes and all sorts of things a burgeoning medical market could use. He met Hugh Davis in 1964, while trying to push one of his inventions, and the two men liked each other right away. Also, they realized, according to Lerner, how they "could use each other's expertise."

The Davis-Lerner association started out as business (they worked on several products together from 1964 to 1967) but it soon turned into friendship. In fact, it was on Christmas Day 1967, while the two families were opening presents and sitting around Davis's home in Baltimore, that the idea for inventing a new IUD came to them.

Each man claims it was the other who first came up with the idea, but whatever the case, both were very excited about it. The two men would call each other up at midnight and three o'clock in the morning to discuss the project. Davis would tell Lerner the little that was known about IUDs and the failures of the ones already on the market: they caused pain, cramps and bleeding; they didn't work; they came out. And Lerner would discuss ways of solving each problem. For the expulsion problem, they had a unique solution: a disk-like IUD with stubby tentacles whose barb effect would hold the device in the uterus. Within a few months Lerner had his first model of the Dalkon Shield, and in August, Davis took a few of them fresh from the Pee Wee Plastic Company, where they had been manufactured, and inserted them into some patients at his clinic. Patients had heard about dangers from the Pill and were quite willing to try a different contraceptive. Initial results looked good, and one month later Lerner applied for a patent.

Instead of donating the device to a medical institution for study, Lerner and Davis decided to market it themselves and to get private physicians across the country to test it for them. Lerner says Davis had some money from Hopkins, which he used to buy Dalkon Shields, and over a one-year period, Davis inserted 640 of them into women (558 clinic patients, 82 private patients) and carefully noted down the "results." He wrote them up and published them in February 1970 in the *American Journal of Obstetrics and Gynecology,* the leading journal in the field. They were remarkable to say the least, especially the pregnancy rate—the lowest among all IUDs (1.1 per cent). The article concluded, "Taken all together, the superior performance of the Shield intrauterine device makes the technique a first choice method of contraception control."

Meanwhile, other doctors across the nation were beginning to hear about the device that had impressive Johns Hopkins statistics behind it, and many were sending for it to try out on their own patients.

One of the people who read of Dr. Davis's exciting discovery was Mary Bolint. She was a junior at the University of Arizona in Tucson at the time and was engaged to Ned Ripple. She planned to go to law school after college, so she wanted to wait to have children until after she finished four more years of school. Contraception was an important factor in her life, and so she informed herself about such things. "What makes me angriest now," she says today, "is that I didn't just go to my doctor and let him put whatever he wanted in my body, I studied all the statistics carefully." She read glowing reports of the Dalkon Shield in a feminist health book and asked her doctor if she should have one. Since he too had heard favorable reports, and since a model had been specially designed for women who had never had children, he inserted a Dalkon Shield into Mary's uterus. Carefully following the instructions that accompanied the product, he warned her that she might experience some minor discomfort and slightly heavier bleeding with her period. The pain, however, was immediate and acute. Mary returned to her doctor, who told her it would subside. It did, but her first period was profuse and painful. Again, her doctor promised that once her system grew used to the device all would be well.

After a few months the pain during her period became tolerable. Mary and Ned were married, and she was accepted into law school during her senior year. She continued to study hard and became an avid modern dancer.

The rise of the Dalkon Shield really began with Davis's research at Hopkins, and the more closely you look back on it, the less scientific it appears. For one thing, the women tested didn't sign any consent forms, so no one knows what Davis told them about the fresh-off-the-drawing-board gadgets he was putting into their uteri. Also, many people claim that Davis regularly told his IUD patients to use spermicidal foam during the tenth to seventeenth days of their cycle, which would leave it unclear whether his study reported the contraceptive effects of the Dalkon Shield or of the foam. Davis said the people who came to his clinic wouldn't use foam even if they were told to, but that is questionable. In any case, Davis admits that at least some of the 82 private patients in his study might have taken his suggestion to use foam, and that makes his research findings dubious. It is as if, in studying a new headache remedy, he had told patients to take aspirin as well. Also, the study sounds less impressive when you realize there was an average of only 5.5 months testing per woman—not much time to get a reliable pregnancy figure.

Hindsight aside, however, after the *Journal of Obstetrics and Gynecology* article was published, the Dalkon Shield began to take off. Additional help had come to Lerner and Davis on New Year's Eve 1969, in the form of Dr. Thad Earl. He was a small-town practitioner from Defiance, Ohio, and had inserted the Shield into some of his own patients and thought it was a great idea. He offered Lerner, Davis and their lawyer, Robert Cohn, $50,000, and got a 7.5 per cent interest in what became "The Dalkon Corporation." (The name was probably an amalgam of Davis, Lerner, and Cohn.)

Lerner had been the inventor, Davis the scientist whose research at a famous institution had validated the invention, Cohn the lawyer who had put together a corporate framework that would allow everyone to get rich, and now, finally The Dalkon Corporation had what it needed to get off the ground: Thad Earl, the enthusiastic salesman willing to go on the road drumming up publicity. If you don't have a large marketing organization or the capital to advertise, about the only effective way to sell a new medical product is to set up demonstration booths at medical conventions. Earl proved to be an energetic salesman. IUDs were not, at the time, classified as drugs, so Dalkon Shields could be hawked just like new office furniture to doctors browsing in convention hallways. Earl passed out the Shields from his booth and showed everyone the impressive testing results of Dr. Hugh Davis of Johns Hopkins.

One warm spring day toward the end of her senior year in college, while Mary Bolint was shopping for dinner, she began to feel uneasy. Suddenly an enormous wave of nausea swept over her. She left her groceries and walked as fast as she could to her car, where she lay down in the back seat. She had been dancing all afternoon, preparing for a summer arts festival, and hoped that she was simply overtired. She remained dizzy and confused, however, and had to ask a friend to drive her home. Her main worry was appendicitis. That would have spoiled her summer of dancing and working. She worked as a nurses' aide in the local hospital and was saving her money for law school.

She made it home, cooked a small dinner and went to bed early—tired and sore. The pain grew worse through the night and at six A.M. she woke her husband Ned. She barely had enough strength left to ask him to take her to the hospital, and he rushed her to the emergency ward, where her condition was quickly diagnosed as appendicitis. When the doctors opened her up, however, they found a healthy appendix, but large abscesses on her ovaries. They drained the abscesses, took out her appendix and sewed her up. When she awoke she told her doctor she was using a Dalkon Shield and asked him if he thought it should be taken out. He said he didn't think it was necessary since he had never heard of IUDs causing infection, but that he would remove

it if she wanted. She decided to leave it in and was released from the hospital in a few days. She returned home satisfied that she had made the right decision. The infection was gone and, even if the Dalkon Shield was uncomfortable, it couldn't be as dangerous as the Pill.

It was 1970, and the scene was a medical convention in Ohio. Thad Earl was there selling Dalkon Shields and found himself set up in a booth next to one run by John McClure, a salesman for A. H. Robins Company. The two men began talking; their chitchat quickly turned to business talk, and suddenly the promoters of the Dalkon Shield had a big break beyond their greatest dreams.

Robins is headquartered in Richmond, Virginia, and has assets of $186 million and subsidiaries in more than a dozen foreign countries. Tranquilizers and appetite suppressants are among the best-selling products of its large line of drugs; it also makes cosmetics, Robitussin cough syrup, Chapstick and Sergeant's Flea Collar, which *Forbes* business magazine accused of killing pets.

At the time Thad Earl and John McClure got to talking outside their convention booths, Robins was looking for an entry into the growing contraceptive market. Its rivals Schmidt and Ortho had captured the Pill business and were beginning to reap enormous profits from their own IUDs. When McClure started chatting with Earl, he didn't waste time. Within a few days after their meeting, Robins acquisition manager flew to Defiance, Ohio, to watch Earl make a few insertions of the Dalkon Shield and to talk medicine and markets. A week later the company's medical director, Dr. Fred Clark, flew to Baltimore to meet Hugh Davis.

Davis told him, by Clark's account, "that the company that takes the Dalkon Shield must move fast and distribute much merchandise and really make an inroad 'in the next eight months.'" Several other people Davis knew were working on similar devices. The courtship quickly intensified; both sides were eager to consummate.

Within a few days Lerner and Cohn, Dalkon's lawyer, flew to Richmond to work out a deal. After three days of negotiating, everyone returned home richer. Robins paid The Dalkon Corporation $750,000 for the patent, which was split among Lerner, Davis, Earl and Cohn according to their interests in the Corporation. Also, an agreement was made (and this is where the big money comes in) that the four men would split ten per cent royalties on all gross sales of the Shield by Robins in the U.S. and Canada. Finally, Earl was retained by Robins as a $30,000-a-year consultant for three years; Davis consulted at $20,000 a year for five years; and Lerner consulted for one year at $12,500 and two more at $2,500.

As the deal was being made, however, something was discovered that proved to be a portent of troubles ahead. Dr. Fred Clark, the Robins official who had flown up to Baltimore to meet Hugh Davis, dictated a three-page memorandum to the files on his return to Richmond. In it he said that of the 832 patients Davis had tested so far, 26 had become pregnant. This would raise the pregnancy rate from the previously published 1.1 per cent to close to three per cent. The dates on the Clark memo show that Hugh Davis was aware of this new, less impressive result back in February when his *Journal* article was published.

(Robins' lawyers claim that Fred Clark's memo about a higher pregnancy rate is merely a typo. They say Clark never read the typed version of the notes he dictated and that he meant to say "an additional six" rather than "26." But their claim sounds weak, for there is other material in the subpoenaed files that indicates Clark did not believe Davis's figures were as impressive as he had first heard.)

Although not quite the corporate equivalent of a smoking gun, the memo has become an important document in the Dalkon affair. It indicates that both Davis and Robins are guilty of promoting the Dalkon Shield with false statistics. The crucial importance of the pregnancy rate becomes clear when you imagine a fetus having to share a uterus with a small crab-shaped piece of plastic. Most of those 17 deaths were due to blood poisoning caused by infection and spontaneous abortion among women who got pregnant while wearing the Dalkon Shield.

Readers of five national medical journals in December 1970 found themselves looking at a remarkable two-page advertisement. It became known in Robins' ad department as the "flying uterus" ad, and it was Robins' way of beginning the vigorous promotion of the Dalkon Shield it had bought only six months earlier. The ad's art page is a painting by a prominent medical artist, Arthur Lidov. It shows a cross-sectioned uterus floating through the sky toward the reader with a Dalkon Shield nestled in it. The Shield looks like some sort of space bug out of the pages of Ray Bradbury—it's about the size of a small fingernail, is made of white plastic and its most notable feature is the little spines or legs surrounding it to keep it from slipping out of the womb. It also has a "tail" or piece of string attached to facilitate medical removal.

It turns out that the string is more important than it would seem. In fact, technically speaking, it is the culprit of the Dalkon affair. According to most researchers (although not Robins) who have since studied it, its construction (which is multifilament, meaning several threads wound together) acts like the wick of a kerosene lamp and allows bacteria from the vagina to creep up and enter the uterus, where massive infections leading to blood poisoning, and eventually death, can result.

The copy on the companion page of the advertisement, with the "scientific" findings from Dr. Hugh Davis's earliest research, boasts of the 1.1 per cent pregnancy rate, and says nothing about the women in the study also using foam or being tested for an average of less than six months. Davis is impressively footnoted as a research physician with citations from the articles he published. He is not cited as a businessman who had just collected $250,000 from his share of the sale of the Shield to Robins.

For the next few years, everything went wonderfully for Robins. The Dalkon Shield was inserted into 3.3 million women in the U.S. and overseas. Robins reaped huge profits from it (each device had only a few cents' worth of plastic in it, but sold for $4.35 retail). The Shield was hailed as the latest thing in IUDs, particularly good for women who had not yet had children. E. Claiborne Robins, Sr., chief executive officer of the company started by his grandfather in 1878, was proud of his officers and was looking forward to the day when the Dalkon Shield would be as familiar a product as Chapstick.

Not long after her "appendectomy," when the abscesses on her ovaries had been discovered and drained, Mary Bolint again began feeling pain and nausea. She went directly to the gynecologist in the hospital where she was working for the summer. He tried in his office to remove her Dalkon Shield but was unable to do it, and so she was put in an operating room where it was removed surgically. For two days after the operation Mary remained in the hospital, running a temperature of 104 degrees and experiencing almost constant dreamlike hallucinations. When her temperature returned to normal several days later, she was sent home with antibiotics. She was still too weak to work or dance, so she stayed home to cook for Ned, who was working. She grew weaker day by day, and finally her parents convinced her to come home to Louisiana, where they could take care of her. Her mother flew to meet her and took Mary to the plane. When they arrived in New Orleans, a flight attendant had to carry Mary off. After she had been home for a few days the fever returned and again she was rushed to the hospital, where she was found to have septicemia, or blood poisoning. For ten days she was kept in intensive care, receiving intravenous antibiotics. During that time, her appendectomy scar burst open from new abscesses on her ovaries, which were again drained. When she finally regained her strength after a month, she flew to San Francisco to join Ned and begin law school. She hoped at last that she could put the painful memories behind her and look ahead to law school, a career, a good marriage, and someday, children.

Up to this time all the characters on the corporate side of the Dalkon history have been men. (One wonders how different this story might be had the subjects of their experiments and sales been men also: would it have taken 17 deaths and hundreds of painful operations on male genitalia before a new variety of condom, say, was taken off the market?) But one woman played a role in the discovery of the Dalkon Shield's dangers, although, unfortunately, her warnings were ignored by higher-ups.

She is Dr. Ellen (Kitty) Preston, a Southern woman who got her M.D. in 1950. She had worked as a physician in private practice and for the State of Virginia Health Department before coming to Robins to be chief of the Antibacterial and Miscellaneous Division (the Shield came under Miscellaneous). In 1971, Preston wrote a memo to medical director Fred Clark (the same Robins official who had flown to Baltimore to meet Hugh Davis and had discovered Davis had been using inflated statistics). In her memo, Preston said that she and Daniel French, president of Robins' Chapstick Division, were concerned that the Dalkon's multifilament tail might display "wicking qualities." She was predicting the source of the very problem that was to lead to so many injuries and deaths among women who used

the Shield. On August 20, 1971, Clark replied with a curt letter saying that it was not up to Drs. Preston and French to test the Shield. He indicated in the letter that he was passing the problem to Dr. Oscar Klioze, the company microbiologist. But did he ever do so? In a sworn deposition four years later, Dr. Klioze said he had never heard of the Preston and French memos, and when he was shown them he swore he had never seen them.

It was one of Dr. Ellen Preston's duties to answer medical inquiries from doctors regarding the Shield. After her rebuff by Clark, she responded to at least one doctor who wrote asking about the possibility of "wicking," saying that as far as Robins knew, such a problem did not exist.

Robins must have been having some second thoughts about the Shield's safety, for around this time it did its own testing, came up with a pregnancy rate of 2 per cent, somewhat higher than Davis's, and cited the new figure as well in its ads. However, some other studies done at the same time that showed vastly greater pregnancy rates—one by Dr. Johanna Perlmutter at Beth Israel Hospital in Boston (10.1 per cent) and one by the Kaiser Medical Center in Sacramento (5.6 per cent)—Robins simply chose to ignore.

Two weeks after she had arrived in California to enter law school, Mary Bolint again began experiencing fever and nausea. She went to a doctor and told him her history. He examined her and said she had a new large abscess on her left ovary and that if it burst she might die. Very scared and sick, Mary decided to fly back to Lancaster, Pennsylvania, where her father-in-law, a doctor, could supervise her medical care. On the plane east she began to wonder if it would ever end. She was going in for her fourth operation in four months.

While she was under anesthesia, the surgeon made a six-inch incision from her navel down to the top of her pubic bone and two 1½-inch incisions on either side of her abdomen to drain the infection. The doctors were working to save her reproductive organs, but cautious not to give her too many pain-killing drugs because her nervous system was by now so weak. Mary lay in bed for two weeks with tubes and needles running in and out of her body and was in constant excruciating pain.

When she recovered and again flew home to Louisiana to recuperate, she was badly scarred all over her abdomen, emotionally drained but dimly grateful that she would still be able to have children.

Let us backtrack in time a little to take up another strand of the Dalkon story. It is an important one, for it involves a slip for which—in the unlikely event that the law is enforced justly—one of the principals could go to jail.

In January 1970 the controversy over the damaging side effects of oral contraceptives was at its height, and a Senate Subcommittee headed by Senator Gaylord Nelson was holding hearings on the subject. One of the experts on contraception they called in to testify was Dr. Hugh Davis. Davis took a stand against birth-control pills with high estrogen content and for IUDs, especially "the new ones" that have been developed. He disapproved of the collection of information regarding the side effects of the Pill, saying that they were vastly "underreported." He said information regarding contraception supplied to women is not adequate, and that gynecologists aren't all that informed about it either. "They are busy," he said. "They read the brochures and information that the drug houses tend to pump into them, I am sorry to say."

It is true that IUDs are generally safer than the Pill, but, sensing that Davis might have some special stake in his strong case for the IUDs, one of the committee members asked if he had a patent on any intrauterine device. Davis mentioned an IUD (not the Dalkon Shield) he had co-invented ten years earlier that was never marketed. The time to tell it straight came, however, when the question was put more bluntly.

"Then you have no particular commercial interest in any of the intrauterine devices?"

"That is correct," replied Dr. Davis.

For the first time in the whole murky history of the Dalkon Shield, someone had clearly and indisputably broken the law: Davis had committed perjury. In flatly lying under oath to the Senate Subcommittee, Davis had committed a felony—one that carries a prison sentence of up to five years and one for which a whole host of people, from Alger Hiss to one or two of the lesser Watergate defendants, have done time in prison. To date, Davis has not been indicted or charged.

The first hint of trouble for Robins in the Dalkon matter came in 1973, and it came, surprisingly, from a man in an Army uniform. He was a witness at a federal hearing called to discuss whether or not medical devices should be subject to the same kind of controls as regular drugs. The hearings dealt with every device imaginable, from pacemakers to artificial kidneys, but on May 30 Army Major Russel Thomsen stole the show by recounting his experiences with the Dalkon Shield. Like so many doctors, he said, he had trusted his medical journals and assumed their editors made sure their authors and advertisers were responsible. On the strength of Robins' advertisements and Davis's article, he had convinced his patients to switch to the Dalkon Shield, only to see them go through a great deal of suffering because of it. Thomsen described cases of septic abortion, pelvic inflammatory disease, massive bleeding, incessant cramps. Some of his patients had almost died. He said he was "revolted" by the gap between the glossy advertising claims and the occurrence of serious and even fatal complications. His testimony about the gruesome effects of the Dalkon Shield was in most major American newspapers the following morning.

After the Dalkon Shield became a public issue, a flood of reports like Thomsen's began coming in from throughout the country. After a year of such information-gathering, Robins got word, finally, of a death in Arizona due to the Shield. From this point on, Robins at last began to act responsibly. The company went to the Food and Drug Administration with the information, and when four more deaths were reported soon after, Robins decided to send out a strongly worded "Dear Doctor" letter to every physician in the country. The letter warned doctors about possible septic abortion and death from the Dalkon Shield and recommended that women who got pregnant with the Shield be given therapeutic abortions. Similar warnings were printed on the packages of new Shields being manufactured. All this seems reminiscent of the Surgeon General's warning on cigarette packs, with one difference: as with prescription drugs, the ultimate recipient never gets to see the label.

Things began looking bad for Dalkon sales. Within weeks of the Dear Doctor letter, the Planned Parenthood Federation sent a memorandum to its 700 membership clinics. It suggested that they immediately cease prescribing the Shield and recommended that they call in all patients then wearing it, advise them of the dangers and offer a substitute contraceptive. They also said the 26.4 per cent of the women in their clinics fitted with the Dalkon Shield experienced severe cramps and bleeding.

Davis was interviewed by the press around this time. He was known as the Shield's co-inventor, but not as someone who still owned a piece of the action. "The whole thing has been blown out of proportion by a certain amount of deliberate design," he reportedly said. "There are large commercial forces that are quite interested in selling new IUDs."

While all the fuss was going on, the Food and Drug Administration began hearings on the Dalkon Shield. Robins executives were frightened, and the highway from its headquarters near Richmond to Washington was soon filled with scouts and lobbyists it was sending to the hearing. According to Dr. Richard Dickey, a member of the FDA's Ob/Gyn Committee, which conducted the hearing, "throughout the entire proceedings the halls and offices of the FDA were crawling with the Robins men. It was disgusting."

Finally, though, before the FDA committee made its recommendations, Robins itself suspended sale of the Shield. It was a difficult decision for the company, as Dalkon had recently moved into the lead in national IUD sales. But in 30 short days, the deaths reported to the FDA had risen from four to seven and the septic abortions from 36 to 110. By this time, also, many people were pointing to the possibility of "wicking," which was the subject of the Preston/Clark memos written back in 1971. Now, in 1975, Robins knew its product was commercially dead, and wanted to forget it. Only, as things turned out, it couldn't.

The day Mary Bolint was scheduled to leave Louisiana to fly back to California for another try at law school and a normal life with her husband, she came down with a high fever. Despairingly, she checked into the hospital again. When doctors opened up her abdomen this time, they found that the infection was everywhere. To save her life they performed a complete hysterectomy and rinsed her peritoneal cavity with antibiotic fluid. During recovery, the intern told Mary that for a while he couldn't get a blood pressure on her and her pulse measured 150.

"I knew from working as a nurses' aide," she says, "that it meant death, but you know, I didn't care. In fact I was relieved. My skin was gray, my

hair was falling out and I weighed about 100 pounds."

Throughout the rise and fall of the Dalkon Shield, one irony is how seldom anyone actually broke the law. Hugh Davis did, when he perjured himself by telling senators he had no commercial interest in any IUD. But his having that interest in the first place in a harmful device he and the Robins Company were vigorously promoting by questionable means was not really illegal.

Most doctors we talked to either avoided comment on the Dalkon controversy or seemed to genuinely consider it business as usual. Even Dr. John Brewer, editor of the *American Journal of Obstetrics and Gynecology,* sidestepped the issue. We asked him if he considered it unethical for Davis to have published an article in his journal praising the IUD Davis co-owned, without revealing his financial stake.

"I don't know what you're talking about and I consider it no business of mine."

"But we know lawyers have been taking depositions from you," we persisted.

"I just answer their questions," Brewer replied. "Until you told me this minute, I had no idea of what it was all about, and I don't want to know."

Others in the medical profession say this kind of conflict of interest is fairly common. Many medical researchers are paid by drug companies to test new products and don't mention that fact in their statistical write-ups. Aside from his distortion of statistics, the main thing medical people consider unusual about what Davis did is that he developed the Dalkon Shield while using the clinic and the prestige of Johns Hopkins. Doctors who are out to make big money in the medical market are usually not at medical schools.

A 1976 law (passed largely because of the Dalkon controversy) will make it somewhat harder for anyone to profiteer from a new medical device in precisely the same manner Davis and the Robins Company did. Medical devices are now subject to many of the same kinds of government monitoring and approval as drugs have been.

Nonetheless, we can still expect drug companies to rush new drugs and devices onto the market as fast as whatever the current law allows. Not because the companies mean harm, but because they have no choice. If a drug or device is tested more cautiously or for a longer time than the law requires, or advertised with less distortion or oversell than the law permits, someone else will corner the market with a competing product. That's why Hugh Davis warned Robins the company had to "move fast and distribute much merchandise."

As long as there is a free market for medical products, that's the way business will be done. Indeed, though there have been civil lawsuits aplenty as a result of the Dalkon Shield, the whole affair has been considered so normal a way of conducting free-enterprise medicine that Johns Hopkins took no action against Davis, state medical authorities censured neither Davis nor Earl and the government left the A. H. Robins Company and The Dalkon Corporation alone.

A product that has been heavily promoted and advertised gathers a certain kind of momentum, a momentum that can carry it right over obstacles like bad publicity, studies of its dangers and the like. In the case of the Dalkon Shield, this momentum brought a curious coda to its story: throughout the entire controversy over the Shield, long past the time Major Thomsen had testified before the Senate committee, past the time Robins sent out its "Dear Doctor" letter, past the time Planned Parenthood and HEW clinics stopped using them and right up to the moment Robins took the Shield off the market, the U.S. foreign aid program was busily sending huge quantities of the device to more than 40 countries throughout the world.

The Agency for International Development's population control program is in the hands of Dr. R. D. Ravenholt, a man whose enthusiasm for birth control as a solution to the world's problems borders on the fanatical. When one of us visited his office several years ago she found it filled with charts of female reproductive organs, packages of condoms, and models of a small vacuum cleaner-like device Ravenholt was promoting at the time as the latest in birth-control techniques. When she got up to leave, he said "Here, take these," reaching into a small box overflowing with little packets of Pills.

"But I don't use Pills," she replied.

"That's all right," he said. "Give them to your friends."

Only when the FDA ruled the Shield unsafe (which was some time *after* Robins had stopped selling it) did Ravenholt and AID try to recall any Shields. They managed to get back fewer than half of the 769,000 Shields they had given away.

Today Mary Bolint has regained her health, but her entire abdomen is a mass of scar tissue. She can never have children. For a long time, she says, she could not think about the Dalkon Shield. Now she is one of many women engaged in lawsuits against the A. H. Robins Company and Hugh Davis, Irwin Lerner, Thad Earl and Robert Cohn.

Robins spent $5 million in litigation costs over the Shield last year, and more suits are yet to come. The company is setting aside a reserve from its profits to cover future lawsuits, and its stock value has dropped sharply. All told, though, Robins' corporate health is not bad: profits were up 26 percent in the first half of 1976.

Hugh Davis still teaches at Johns Hopkins and still heads the university's Family Planning Clinic. He does not return phone calls from the press. Thad Earl is still in private practice, although he has moved to Arizona. "Win" Lerner is still an engineer, working for himself at "Lerner Labs." Like the others, he had been told by his lawyers to say nothing, but he is the only one who sounds frustrated with this prohibition. Lerner would like to tell the whole story, he says, but he can't. The Dalkon Corporation still exists, he adds, and maybe someday it will come up with a new product.

Dr. Ellen Preston, the woman whose memo about "wicking" first pinpointed the danger of the Dalkon Shield, still works for A. H. Robins in Virginia. She has been forbidden by company lawyers to talk about the case with anyone.

Some 800,000 women in the United States and an estimated 500,000 in other countries are still wearing the Dalkon Shield as a birth-control device. Planned Parenthood and several similar groups have considered recommending that all women wearing Shields have them removed immediately. But these organizations have decided not to do so, for recently it has been discovered that removal of the Shield frequently causes lesions of the cervix, followed by serious infection.

CHAPTER 15 _____

Social Epidemiology

Social epidemiology attempts to determine who in a particular population develops a disease, when it is developed, and under what influences. The study of the circumstances relating to illness in a single person may contribute very little to the understanding of the cause of disease. Social epidemiology, however, assumes that each illness follows a fairly characteristic pattern that is in some part determined by social influences. Thus, the social epidemiologist examines cases of an illness as they occur throughout a population in the attempt to determine (1) which social groups have high susceptibility to the illness and which do not, and (2) the circumstances or influences that distinguish the sick from the well. Ultimately, the social epidemiologist hopes that the increased understanding of the environment within which the disease occurs will be followed by an understanding of the causes and the development of effective methods of disease prevention. In the meantime, social epidemiological research may be particularly useful in suggesting to physicians in their diagnoses the likelihood of members of a particular group having a particular illness.

The relationship between race and blood pressure is a good case in point. A large number of studies have shown that blacks in the United States have higher blood pressures in all age–sex groups than do whites (Boyle 1970; Comstock 1957; McDonough et al. 1964; U.S. Department of Health and Human Services 1985). Generally speaking, the causes of these racial differences are unknown. There is some speculation in the literature that unfavorable factors, such as the conflict between people's aspirations and their opportunities and experiences, may be responsible (Henry and Cassel 1969; Kagan and Levi 1974).

In a previous article by Howard D. Schwartz concerning irrationality in the American health-care system, the link between health and the factors of social class, race, age, and occupation were touched upon. In this chapter the relationships between health and both occupation and social class are discussed in more depth. In addition, the influences of gender and general life stresses upon health status are explored.

Moving away from the most commonly studied variables that impact upon health status, social epidemiologists have carried out some of the most interesting and provocative research in social science.

One factor that is receiving increasing attention is the effect of social support and social networks. One of the first studies of the health effects of different support systems looked at army wives who delivered children (Nuckolls, Cassel, and Kaplan 1972). It was found that among those wives who had undergone many changes in their lives, those with a great deal of social support had one-third the pregnancy complication rate of those who were low on social support. In their study of residents of Alameda County, California, Berkman and Syme (1979) found that an individual's social and community ties were related to risk of dying. One of the social ties considered by Berkman and Syme was marriage. Other studies support their finding that those who are married have lower mortality rates than those who are single, widowed, or divorced (Ortmeyer 1974; Pelletier 1981). This mortality risk seems to be greater for men than women and seems to decrease with age.

The relationship between death of a spouse and both morbidity (sickness) and mortality (death) is particularly dramatic. Taylor (1981) has found, for example, that widows, especially in the first year following bereavement, report an increased number of psychological and physical symptoms and have a higher risk of dying themselves. Parkes, Benjamin, and Fitzgerald (1969) studied almost 4500 widowers 55 years of age and older and found that 213 had died during the first six months following bereavement. This is 40 percent above the expected rate for married men of the same age. After six months, the rates gradually returned to the level of married men and stayed at that level.

Social and cultural change is also associated with many disease consequences. Industrialization, urbanization, migration, and occupational and geographical mobility have all been shown to increase the risk of coronary heart disease. A number of studies have shown, for example, how "modernization" and "westernization" can adversely affect health. Zulus in South Africa (Scotch 1963) and Polynesians in the Cook Islands (Prior 1974) have been observed as having increased blood pressure levels as they live in more "modern" social settings. Marmot and Syme (1976) found that among Japanese-American men in California, those who were most acculturated (i.e., westernized) were three to five times more likely to have coronary heart disease than were those who had retained traditional Japanese ways.

Something should also be said about the social epidemiological research directly bearing on mental health. Perhaps the most well known studies are those that were carried out by Leo Srole, and his colleagues. In the original study carried out in the 1950s (Srole et al. 1962), 1160 people living in the midtown Manhattan area of New York City were interviewed. Most of these people had never been in a mental hospital and were not considered to be mentally ill. Yet the researchers found that 80 percent of the sample had at least one psychiatric symptom and that 75 percent of the entire community showed "significant" pathological anxiety. In the second study some twenty years later, Srole, Fisher, and colleagues (1978) restudied residents of midtown Manhattan. Looking at those from the original sample again (they were able to contact about one-half of the original sample), the researchers found that 40.9 percent were rated the same, 32.5 percent were rated better, and only 26.6 percent showed lower mental health scores. Thus, contrary to what one might expect, overall mental health seemed to have improved with age among those who were restudied. In addition, it was found that individuals in the 1970s seemed to feel better than those who were of the same age in the 1950s. Moreover, while women were more severely mentally impaired in the 1950s study, the 1970s follow-up showed that the mental health gap between men and women was narrowing.

Finally, the existence of two very important, on-going epidemiological studies should be noted. The first is the Framingham Heart Study, which has been going on now for more than three decades and is the first study in which the science of epidemiology, traditionally used to investigate epidemics of infectious disease, has been applied to a chronic illness. It is a longitudinal study, so it is following the same people through their whole lives. This approach has enormous advantages over studies where people are asked to recollect previous health-related experiences. Perhaps Framingham's most important contribution has been the discovery of the link between the risk of cardiovascular disease and the level and kind of cholesterol in a person's blood. One of the more surprising findings of the study was that women in clerical occupations have a much higher rate of heart disease than women in other kinds of occupations.

A second study of note is more short-term. Beginning in 1982, partly because of criticism that not enough research was being done in terms of lifestyle and environmental (both social and physical) correlates of cancer, the American Cancer Society has been studying the effects of these factors. Over a six-year period, the lives of over one million people will be scrutinized in order to determine the extent to which cancer is associated with air and water pollution, long-term exposure to radiation, diet, drugs, jobs, and other factors. Some of the findings that have already been reported show that obese men have increased risks of colon-rectum and prostate cancer whereas obese women have a five-fold increase in the risk of dying of uterine cancer.

The selections in this chapter review some important social epidemiological research. The first article, by S. Leonard Syme and Lisa F. Berkman, summarizes a large number of studies of the relationship between social class and sickness. Generally, the lower class is found to have consistently higher death, illness, and disability rates than the middle and upper classes. Syme and Berkman discuss the various explanations of these findings and generate questions concerning further research in the area. The next article, by Theodore J. Jacobs and Edward Charles, presents the conclusions of their study that explores the effects of disruptive life events on the onset of cancer in children. The chapter closes with Lois M. Verbrugge's compilation of data and hypotheses that have been gathered in an attempt to explain differences in health status, therapeutic health behaviors, and longevity between men and women.

References

BERKMAN, L. F., and S. L. SYME   1979. Social Networks, Host Resistance, and Mortality: A Nine-Year Follow-Up Study of Alameda County Residents. *American Journal of Epidemiology* 109:186–204.

BOYLE, E.   1970. Biological Patterns in Hypertension by Sex, Body Weight and Skin Color. *Journal of the American Medical Association* 213:1637–1643.

COMSTOCK, G. W.   1957. An Epidemiologic Study of Blood Pressure Levels in a Biracial Community in the Southern United States. *American Journal of Hygiene* 65: 271–315.

HENRY, J., and J. CASSEL   1969. Psychosocial Factors in Essential Hypertension. *American Journal of Epidemiology* 90:171–200.

KAGAN, A., and L. LEVI   1974. Health and Environment—Psychosocial Stimuli: A Review. *Social Science and Medicine* 8:225–241.

MARMOT, M., and S. L. SYME   1976. Acculturation and Coronary Heart Disease in Japanese-Americans. *American Journal of Epidemiology* 104:225–247.

McDONOUGH, J., G. GARRISON, and C. HAMES   1964. Blood Pressure and Hypertensive Disease Among Negroes and Whites: A Study in Evans County, Georgia. *Annals of Internal Medicine* 61:208–228.

NUCKOLLS, K. B., J. C. CASSEL, and B. B. KAPLAN   1972. Psychosocial Assets, Life Crisis, and Prognosis of Pregnancy. *American Journal of Epidemiology* 95:431–441.

ORTMEYER, C. F.   1974. Variations in Mortality, Morbidity, and Health Care by Marital Status. In C. F. Erhardt and J. E. Berlin (eds.), *Mortality and Morbidity in the United States*. Cambridge, Mass.: Harvard University Press, pp. 159–188.

PARKES, C. M., B. BENJAMIN, and R. G. FITZGERALD   1969. Broken Heart: A Statistical Study of Increased Mortality Among Widowers. *British Medical Journal* 2:274–279.

PELLETIER, K. R.   1981. *Longevity: Fulfilling Our Biological Potential*. New York: Delacorte and Elta.

PRIOR, I. A.   1974. Cardiovascular Epidemiology in New Zealand and the Pacific. *New England Medical Journal* 80:245–252.

SCOTCH, N. A.   1963. Sociocultural Factors in the Epidemiology of Zulu Hypertension. *American Journal of Public Health* 53:1205–1213.

SROLE, L., T. S. LANGNER, S. T. MICHAEL, M. K. OPLER, and T. A. C. RENNIE   1962. *Mental Health in the Metropolis: The Midtown Manhattan Study*. New York: McGraw-Hill.

SROLE, L., and A. FISCHER   1978 (April 11). Generations, Aging, Gender and Well-Being: The Midtown Manhattan Follow-Up Study. Presented to the Eastern Sociological Society Annual Meeting—Philadelphia.

TAYLOR, R. L.   1981. The Widowed: Risks and Interventions. *Wellness Resource Bulletin*. California Department of Mental Health, Mental Health Promotion Branch 2:1.

UNITED STATES DEPARTMENT OF HEALTH AND HUMAN SERVICES 1985. *Report of the Secretary's Task Force on Black and Minority Health*. Volume I.

Social Class, Susceptibility, and Sickness

S. Leonard Syme
Lisa F. Berkman

ocial class gradients of mortality and life expectancy have been observed for centuries, and a vast body of evidence has shown consistently that those in the lower classes have higher mortality, morbidity, and disability rates. While these patterns have been observed repeatedly, the explanations offered to account for them show no such consistency. The most frequent explanations have included poor housing, crowding, racial factors, low income, poor education and unemployment, all of which have been said to result in such outcomes as poor nutrition, poor medical care (either through nonavailability or nonutilization of resources), strenuous conditions of employment in nonhygienic settings, and increased exposure to noxious agents. While these explanations account for some of the observed relationships, we have found them inadequate to explain the very large number of diseases associated with socioeconomic status. It seemed useful, therefore, to reexamine these associations in search of a more satisfactory hypothesis.

Obviously, this is an important issue. It is clear that new approaches must be explored emphasizing the primary prevention of disease in addition to those approaches that merely focus on treatment of the sick.[1] It is clear also that such preventive approaches must involve community and environmental interventions rather than one-to-one preventive encounters.[2] Therefore, we must understand more precisely those features of the environment that are etiologically related to disease so that interventions at this level can be more intelligently planned.

Of all the disease outcomes considered, it is evident that low socioeconomic status is most strikingly associated with high rates of infectious and parasitic diseases[3-7] as well as with higher infant mortality rates.[8,9] However, in our review we found higher rates among lower-class groups of a very much wider range of diseases and conditions for which obvious explanations were not as easily forthcoming. In a comprehensive review of over 30 studies, Antonovsky[10] concluded that those in the lower classes invariably have lower life expectancy and higher death rates from all causes of death, and that this higher rate has been observed since the 12th century when data on this question were first organized. While differences in infectious disease and infant mortality rates probably accounted for much of this difference between the classes in earlier years, current differences must primarily be attributable to mortality from noninfectious disease.

Kitagawa and Hauser[11] recently completed a massive nationwide study of mortality in the United States. Among men and women in the 25–64-year age group, mortality rates varied dramatically by level of education, income, and occupation, considered together or separately. For example, as shown in Table 1, white males at low education levels had age-adjusted mortality rates 64 percent higher than men in higher education categories. For white women, those in lower education groups had an age-adjusted mortality rate 105 percent higher. For nonwhite males, the differential was 31 percent and, for nonwhite females, it was 70 percent. These mortality differentials also were reflected in substantial differences in life expectancy, and, as shown in Table 2, for most specific causes of death. In Table 2, it can be seen that white males in the lowest education groups have higher age-adjusted mortality rates for every cause of death for which data are available. For white females, those in the lowest education group have an excess mortality rate for all causes

Reprinted from the *American Journal of Epidemiology*, vol. 104, no. 7 (July, 1976), pp. 1–8.

TABLE 1 Mortality ratios by education level for whites and nonwhites, 25–64 years of age, United States, 1960*

EDUCATION LEVEL	MALES		FEMALES	
	WHITE	NON-WHITE	WHITE	NON-WHITE
Lowest	1.15	1.14	1.60	1.26
Highest†	.70	.87	.78	.74
Differential	64%	31%	105%	70%

* Adapted from Kitagawa and Hauser,[11] pp. 12–14. The mortality ratios in this table measure the range of education differentials in mortality within each age-color-sex subgroup of the population. They were derived from the ratios of actual to expected deaths by setting the ratio for each subgroup total equal to 1.00.

† For whites, highest education level was defined as "four or more years of college"; for nonwhites, it was defined as "high school or college."

except cancer of the breast and motor vehicle accidents.

These gradients of mortality among the social classes have been observed over the world by many investigators[12–18] and have not changed materially since 1900 (except that nonwhites, especially higher status nonwhites, have experienced a relatively more favorable improvement). This consistent finding in time and space is all the more remarkable since the concept of "social class" has been defined and measured in so many different ways by these investigators. That the same findings have been obtained in spite of such methodological differences lends strength to the validity of the observations: it suggests also that the concept is an imprecise term encompassing diverse elements of varying etiologic significance.

In addition to data on mortality, higher rates of morbidity also have been observed for a vast array of conditions among those in lower-class groups.[19–28] This is an important observation since it indicates that excess mortality rates among lower status groups are not merely attributable to a higher case fatality death rate in those groups but are accompanied also by a higher prevalence of morbidity. Of special interest in this regard are data on the various mental illnesses, a major cause of morbidity. As shown by many investigators,[29–35] those in lower as compared to higher socioeconomic groups have higher rates of schizophrenia, are more depressed,

TABLE 2 Percentage difference in mortality ratio between highest and lowest education level, by cause of death, for whites, 25–63 years, United States, 1960*

CAUSE OF DEATH	PERCENTAGE DIFFERENCE IN MORTALITY RATIO	
	WHITE MALES	WHITE FEMALES
Tuberculosis	776	†
Malignant neoplasms	31	23
Stomach	123	†
Intestine, rectum	21	66
Lung, bronchus, trachea	93	37
Breast	†	22
Uterus	†	109
Other neoplasms	5	12
Diabetes	45	332
Cardiovascular-renal diseases	33	109
Vascular lesions of the CNS	27	103
Rheumatic fever	24	26
Arteriosclerotic	25	139
Hypertensive	79	158
Other cardiovascular	71	72
Influenza pneumonia	159	†
Cirrhosis of the liver	2	16
All accidents	127	24
Motor vehicle accidents	84	4
Other accidents	163	
Suicide	74	
Other causes of death	100	48

* Adapted from Kitagawa and Hauser,[11] pp. 76–77. See note in Table 1 for definition of ratios. Mortality ratios for nonwhites are not shown due to insufficient data. In this table, the percentage differential in mortality ratio is computed by dividing the *difference* in ratios by the ratio at the lowest education level. Any given percentage figure in the table may be read as the percentage by which the ratio at the lowest education level is *higher* than the ratio at the highest education level.

† Insufficient data to calculate ratios.

more unhappy, more worried, more anxious, and are less hopeful about the future.

In summary, persons in lower-class groups have higher morbidity and mortality rates of almost every disease or illness, and these differentials have not diminished over time. While particular hypotheses may be offered to explain the gradient for one or another of these specific diseases, the fact that so many diseases exhibit the same gradient leads to speculation that a more general explanation may be more appropriate than a series of disease-specific explanations.

In a study reported elsewhere,[36] it was noted that although blacks had higher rates of hypertension than whites, blacks in the lower classes had higher rates of hypertension than blacks in the upper classes. An identical social class gradient for hypertension was noted among whites in the sample. In that report, it was concluded that hypertension was associated more with social class than with racial factors, and it was suggested that the greater prevalence of obesity in the lower class might be a possible explanation. The present review makes that earlier suggestion far less attractive since so many diseases and conditions appear to be of higher prevalence in the lower-class groups. It seems clear that we must frame hypotheses of sufficient generality to account for this phenomenon.

One hypothesis that has been suggested is that persons in the lower classes either have less access to medical care resources or, if care is available, that they do not benefit from that availability. This possibility should be explored in more detail, but current evidence available does not suggest that differences in medical care resources will entirely explain social class gradients in disease. The hypertension project summarized above was conducted at the Kaiser Permanente facility in Oakland, California which is a prepaid health plan with medical facilities freely available to all study subjects. The data in this study showed that persons in lower-status groups had utilized medical resources more frequently than those in higher-status categories.[37] To study the influence of medical care in explaining these differences in blood pressure levels, all persons in the Kaiser study who had ever been clinically diagnosed as hypertensive, or who had ever taken medicine for high blood pressure, were removed from consideration. Differences in blood pressure level between those in the highest and lowest social classes were diminished when hypertensives were removed from analysis, but those in the lowest class still had higher (normal) pressures. Thus, while differences in medical care may have accounted for some of the variation observed among the social class groups, substantial differences in blood pressures among these groups nevertheless remained. Similar findings have been reported from studies at the Health Insurance Plan of New York.[38]

Lipworth and colleagues[39] also examined this issue in a study of cancer survival rates among various income groups in Boston. In that study, low-income persons had substantially less favorable one- and three-year survival rates following treatment at identical tumor clinics and hospitals: these differences were not accounted for by differences in stage of cancer at diagnosis, by the age of patients, or by the specific kind of treatment patients received. It was concluded that patients from lower-income areas simply did not fare as well following treatment for cancer. While it is still possible that lower-class patients received less adequate medical care, the differences observed in survival rates did not seem attributable to the more obvious variations in quality of treatment. Other studies support this general conclusion but not enough data are available to assess clearly the role of medical care in explaining social class gradients in morbidity and mortality: it would seem, however, that the medical care hypothesis does not account for a major portion of these gradients.

Another possible explanation offered to explain these consistent differences is that persons in lower socioeconomic groups live in a more toxic, hazardous, and nonhygenic environment resulting in a broad array of disease consequences. That these environments exert an influence on disease outcome is supported by research on crowding and rheumatic fever,[5] poverty areas and health,[40] and on air pollution and respiratory illnesses.[41] While lower-class groups certainly are exposed to a more physically noxious environment, physical factors alone are frequently unable to explain observed relationships between socioeconomic status and disease outcome. One example of this is provided by the report of Guerrin and Borgatta[16] showing that the proportion of people who are illiterate in a census tract is a more important indicator of tuberculosis occurrence than are either economic or racial variables. Similarly, the work of Booth[42] suggests that perceived crowding which is not highly correlated with objective measures of crowding may have adverse effects on individuals.

There can be little doubt that the highest morbidity and mortality rates observed in the lower social classes are in part due to inadequate medical care services as well as to the impact of a toxic and hazardous physical environment. There can be little doubt, also, that these factors do not entirely explain the discrepancy in rates between the classes. Thus, while enormous improvements have been made in environmental quality and in medical care, the mortality rate gap between the classes has not diminished. It is true that mortality rates have been declining over the years, and it is probably true also that this benefit is attributable in large part to the enormous improvements that have been made in food and water purity, in sanitary engineering, in literacy and health education, and in medical and surgical knowledge. It is important to recognize, however, that these reductions in mortality rates have not eliminated the gap between the highest and the lowest social class groups: this gap remains very substantial and has apparently stabilized during the last 40 years. Thus, while improvements in the environment and in medical care clearly have been of value, other factors must be identified to account for this continuing differential in mortality rate and life expectancy.

The identification of these new factors might profitably be guided by the repeated observation of social class gradients in a wide range of disease distributions. That so many different kinds of diseases are more frequent in lower class groupings directs attention to generalized susceptibility to disease and to generalized compromises of disease defense systems. Thus, if something about life in the lower social classes increases vulnerability to illness in general, it would not be surprising to observe an increased prevalence of many different types of diseases and conditions among people in the lower classes.

While laboratory experiments on both humans and animals have established that certain "stressful events" have physiologic consequences, very little is known about the nature of these "stressful events" in nonlaboratory settings. Thus, while we may conclude that "something" about the lower class environment is stressful, we know much less about what specifically constitutes that stress. Rather than attempting to identify *specific* risk factors for *specific* diseases in investigating this question, it may be more meaningful to identify those factors that affect *general* susceptibility to disease. The specification of such factors should rest on the identification of variables having a wide range of disease outcomes. One such risk factor may be life change associated with social and cultural mobility. Those experiencing this type of mobility have been observed to have

higher rates of diseases and conditions such as coronary heart disease,[43–46] lung cancer,[47] difficulties of pregnancy,[48,49] sarcoidosis,[50] and depression.[30] Another risk factor may be certain life events; those experiencing what are commonly called stressful life events have been shown to have higher rates of a wide variety of diseases and conditions.[51–57]

Generalized susceptibility to disease may be influenced not only by the impact of various forms of life change and life stress, but also by differences in the way people cope with such stress. Coping, in this sense, refers not to specific types of psychological responses but to the more generalized ways in which people deal with problems in their everyday life. It is evident that such coping styles are likely to be products of environmental situations and not independent of such factors. Several coping responses that have a wide range of disease outcomes have been described. Cigarette smoking is one such coping response that has been associated with virtually all causes of morbidity and mortality;[58] obesity may be another coping style associated with a higher rate of many diseases and conditions;[59,60] pattern A behavior is an example of a third coping response that has been shown to have relatively broad disease consequences.[61] There is some evidence that persons in the lower classes experience more life changes[62] and that they tend to be more obese and to smoke more cigarettes.[63,64]

To explain the differential in morbidity and mortality rates among the social classes, it is important to identify additional factors that affect susceptibility and have diverse disease consequences; it is also important to determine which of these factors are more prevalent in the lower classes. Thus, our understanding would be enhanced if it could be shown not only that those in the lower classes live in a more toxic physical environment with inadequate medical care, but also that they live in a social and psychological environment that increases their vulnerability to a whole series of diseases and conditions.

In this paper, we have emphasized the variegated disease consequences of low socioeconomic status. Any proposed explanations of this phenomenon should be capable of accounting for this general outcome. The proposal offered here is that those in the lower classes consistently have higher rates of disease in part due to compromised disease defenses and increased general susceptibility. To explore this proposal further, systematic research is needed on four major problems:

1. The more precise identification and description of subgroups within the lower socioeconomic classes that have either markedly higher or lower rates of disease: Included in what is commonly called the "lower class" are semiskilled working men with stable work and family situations, unemployed men with and without families, the rural and urban poor, hard core unemployed persons, and so on. The different disease experiences of these heterogeneous subgroups would permit a more precise understanding of the processes involved in disease etiology and would permit a more precise definition of social class groupings.

2. The disentanglement of socio-environmental from physical-environmental variables: It is important to know whether high rates of illness and discontent in a poverty area, for example, are due to the poor physical circumstances of life in such an area, to the social consequences of life in such an area, or to the personal characteristics of individuals who come to live in the area.

3. The clarification of "causes" and "effects": The implication in this paper has been that the lower-class environment "leads to" poor health. Certainly, the reverse situation is equally likely. Many measures of social class position may be influenced by the experience of ill health itself. Further research is needed to clarify the relative importance of the "downward drift" hypothesis. One way of approaching such study is to use measures of class position that are relatively unaffected by illness experience. An example of one such measure is "educational achievement" as used by Kitagawa and Hauser.[11] In this study, educational level was assumed to be relatively stable after age 20 and was felt to be a measure relatively unaffected by subsequent illness experience.

4. The more comprehensive description of those psycho-social variables that may compromise bodily defense to disease and increase suscep-

tibility to illness: The possible importance of life events, life changes, and various coping behavior has been suggested but systematic research needs to be done to provide a more complete view of the factors involved in this process. Of particular interest would be research on the ways in which social and familial support networks[48,55] mediate between the impact of life events and stresses and disease outcomes.

The research that is needed should not be limited to the study of the specific risk factors as these affect specific diseases. Instead, the major focus of this research should be on those general features of lower class living environments that compromise bodily defense and thereby affect health and well-being in general. This research should go beyond the superficial description of demographic variables associated with illness and should attempt the identification of specific etiologic factors capable of accounting for the observed morbidity and mortality differences between the social classes.

The gap in mortality and life expectancy between the social classes has stabilized and may be increasing; the identification of those factors that render people vulnerable to disease will hopefully provide a basis for developing more meaningful prevention programs aimed toward narrowing the gap.

References

1. Winkelstein W Jr, French FE: The role of ecology in the design of a health care system. Calif. Med. 113:7–12, 1970

2. Marmot M, Winkelstein W Jr: Epidemiologic observations on intervention trials for prevention of coronary heart disease. Am. J. Epidemiol. 101:177–181, 1975

3. Tuberculosis and Socioeconomic Status. Stat. Bull., January 1970

4. Terris M: Relation of economic status to tuberculosis mortality by age and sex. Am. J. Public Health 38:1061–1071, 1948

5. Gordis L, Lilienfeld A, Rodriguez R: Studies in the epidemiology and preventability of rheumatic fever. II. Socioeconomic factors and the incidence of acute attacks. J. Chronic Dis. 21:655–666, 1969

6. Influenza and Pneumonia Mortality in the U.S., Canada and Western Europe. Stat. Bull., April 1972

7. Court SDM: Epidemiology and natural history of respiratory infections in children. J. Clin. Pathol. 21:31, 1968

8. Chase HC (ed): A study of risks, medical care and infant mortality. Am. J. Public Health 63: supplement, 1973

9. Lerner, M: Social differences in physical health. *In:* Poverty and Health. Edited by J Koza, A Antonovsky, IK Zola. Cambridge, Harvard University Press, 1969, 69–112

10. Antonovsky A: Social class, life expectancy and overall mortality. Milbank Mem. Fund Q. 45:31–73, 1967

11. Kitagawa EM, Hauser PM: Differential Mortality in the United States. Cambridge, Harvard University Press, 1973

12. Nagi MH, Stockwell EG: Socioeconomic differentials in mortality by cause of death. Health Serv. Rep. 88:449–465, 1973

13. Ellis JM: Socio-economic differentials in mortality from chronic disease. *In:* Patients, Physicians and Illness. Edited by EG Jaco. Glencoe, Il, The Free Press, 1958, pp. 30–37

14. Yeracaris J: Differential mortality, general and cause-specific in Buffalo, 1939–1941. J. Am. Stat. Assoc. 50:1235–1247, 1955

15. Brown SM, Selvin S, Winkelstein W Jr: The association of economic status with the occurrence of lung cancer. Cancer 36:1903–1911, 1975

16. Guerrin RF, Borgatta EF: Socio-economic and demographic correlates of tuberculosis incidence. Milbank Mem. Fund Q. 43:269–290, 1965

17. Graham S: Socio-economic status, illness, and the use of medical services. Milbank Mem Fund Q 35:58–66, 1957

18. Cohart EM: Socioeconomic distribution of stomach cancer in New Haven. Cancer 7:455–461, 1954

19. Socioeconomic Differentials in Mortality. Stat. Bull., June 1972

20. Hart JT: Too little and too late. Data on occupational mortality, 1959–1963. Lancet 1:192–193, 1972

21. Wan T: Social differentials in selected work-limiting chronic conditions. J. Chronic Dis. 25:365–374, 1972

22. Hochstim JR, Athanasopoulos DA, Larkins JH: Poverty area under the microscope. Am. J. Public Health 58:1815–1827, 1968

23. Burnight RG: Chronic morbidity and socio-economic characteristics of older urban males. Milbank Mem. Fund Q. 43:311–322, 1965

24. Elder R, Acheson RM: New Haven survey on joint diseases. XIV. Social class and behavior in response to symptoms of osteoarthritis. Milbank Mem. Fund Q. 48:499–502, 1970

25. Cobb S: The epidemiology of rheumatoid disease. *In:* The Frequency of Rheumatoid Disease. Edited by S Cobb. Cambridge, Harvard University Free Press, 1971, pp. 42–62

26. Graham S: Social factors in the relation to chronic illness. *In:* Handbook of Medical Sociology. Edited by HE Freeman, S Levine, LG Reeder. Englewood Cliffs, NJ, Prentice-Hall Inc, 1963, pp. 65–98

27. Wan T: Status stress and morbidity: A sociological investigation of selected categories of working-limit conditions. J. Chronic Dis. 24:453–468, 1971

28. Selected Health Characteristics by Occupation, U.S. July 1961–June 1963. National Health Center for Health Statistics, Series 10 21:1–16, 1965

29. Abramson JH: Emotional disorder, status inconsistency and migration. Milbank Mem. Fund Q. 44:23–48, 1966

30. Schwab JJ, Holzer CE III, Warheit GJ: Depression scores by race, sex, age, family income, education and socioeconomic status. (Personal communication, 1974)

31. Srole L, Langner T, Michael S, et al: Mental Health in the Metropolis: the Midtown Study. New York, McGraw-Hill, 1962

32. Jackson EF: Status consistency and symptoms of stress. Am. Sociol. Rev. 27:469–480, 1962

33. Hollingshead AB, Redlich FC: Social Class and Mental Illness. New York, John Wiley and Sons Inc, 1958

34. Gurin G, Veroff J, Feld S: Americans View their Mental Health. New York, Basic Books Inc, 1960

35. Langner TS: Psychophysiological symptoms and the status of women in two Mexican communities. *In:* Approaches to Cross-cultural Psychiatry. Edited by AH Leighton, JM Murphy. Ithaca, Cornell University Press, 1965, pp. 360–392

36. Syme SL, Oakes, T, Friedman G, et al: Social class and racial differences in blood pressure. Am. J. Public Health 64:619–620, 1974

37. Oakes TW, Syme SL: Social factors in newly discovered elevated blood pressure. J Health Soc Behav 14:198–204, 1973

38. Fink R, Shapiro S, Hyman MD, et al: Health status of poverty and non-poverty groups in multiphasic health testing. Presented at the Annual Meeting of the American Public Health Association, November 1972

39. Lipworth L, Abelin T, Connelly RR: Socioeconomic factors in the prognosis of cancer patients. J. Chronic Dis. 23:105–116, 1970

40. Hochstim JR: Health and ways of living. *In:* Social Surveys, The community as an Epidemiological

Laboratory. Edited by I Kessler, M Levine. Baltimore, Johns Hopkins Press, 1970, pp. 149–176

41. Winkelstein W Jr, Kantor S, Davis EW, et al: The relationship of air pollution and economic status to total mortality and selected respiratory system mortality in men. I. Suspended particulates. Arch Environ Health 14:162–171, 1967

42. Booth A: Preliminary Report: Urban Crowding Project. Canada, Ministry of State for Urban Affairs, August 1974 (mimeographed)

43. Syme SL, Hyman MM, Enterline PE: Some social and cultural factors associated with the occurrence of coronary heart disease. J. Chronic Dis. 17:277–289, 1964

44. Tyroler HA, Cassel J: Health consequences of cultural change. II. The effect of urbanization on coronary heart mortality in rural residents. J. Chronic Dis. 17:167–177, 1964

45. Nesser WB, Tyroler HA, Cassel JC: Social disorganization and stroke mortality in the black populations of North Carolina. Am. J. Epidemiol 93:166–175, 1971

46. Shekelle RB, Osterfeld AM, Paul O: Social status and incidence of coronary heart disease. J. Chronic Dis. 22:381–394, 1969

47. Haenszel W, Loveland DB, Sirken N: Lung-cancer mortality as related to residence and smoking histories. I. White males. J. Natl. Cancer Inst. 28:947–1001, 1962

48. Nuckolls KB, Cassel J, Kaplan BH: Psychosocial assets, life crisis, and the prognosis of pregnancy. Am. J. Epidemiol. 95:431–441, 1972

49. Gorusch RL, Key MK: Abnormalities of pregnancy as a function of anxiety and life stress. Psychosom. Med. 36:352–362, 1974

50. Terris M, Chaves AD: An epidemiologic study of sarcoidosis. Am. Rev. Respir. Dis. 94:50–55, 1966

51. Rahe RH, Gunderson EKE, Arthur RJ: Demographic and psychosocial factors in acute illness reporting. J. Chronic Dis. 23:245–255, 1970

52. Wyler AR, Masuda M, Holmes TH: Magnitude of life events and seriousness of illness. Psychosom. Med. 33:115–122, 1971

53. Rahe RH, Rubin RT, Gunderson EKE, et al: Psychological correlates of serum cholesterol in man: A longitudinal study. Psychosom. Med. 33:399–410, 1971

54. Spilken AZ, Jacobs MA: Prediction of illness behavior from measures of life crisis, manifest distress and maladaptive coping. Psychosom. Med. 33:251–264, 1971

55. Jacobs MA, Spilken AZ, Martin MA, et al: Life stress and respiratory illness. Psychosom. Med. 32:233–242, 1970

56. Kasl SV, Cobb S: Blood pressure changes in men undergoing job loss; A preliminary report. Psychosom. Med. 32:19–38, 1970

57. Hinkle LE, Wolff HG: Ecological investigations of the relationship between illness, life experiences, and the social environment. Ann. Intern. Med. 49:1373–1388, 1958

58. US Dept. of Health, Education, and Welfare: The Health Consequences of Smoking. National Communicable Disease Center. Publication No 74–8704, 1974

59. US Public Health Service, Division of Chronic Diseases: Obesity and Health. A Source Book of Current Information for Professional Health Personnel. Publication No 1485. Washington DC, US GPO, 1966

60. Build and Blood Pressure Study. Chicago, Society of Actuaries, Vol I and II, 1959

61. Rosenman RH, Brand RJ, Jenkins CD, et al: Coronary heart disease in the Western collaborative group study: Final follow-up experience of 8½ years. (Manuscript)

62. Dohrenwend BS (ed): Stressful Life Events: Their Nature and Effects. New York, Wiley-Interscience, 1974

63. US Dept of Health, Education, and Welfare: Adult Use of Tobacco 1970. Publication No HSM-73–8727, 1973

64. Khosla T, Lowe CR: Obesity and smoking habits by social class. J. Prev. Soc. Med. 26:249–256, 1972

Life Events and the Occurrence of Cancer in Children

Theodore J. Jacobs
Edward Charles

It is over twenty years ago that Greene and Miller (1), in a pioneering study, investigated the role of emotional and psychological factors in the development of leukemia in children and adolescents. This study extended and expanded prior work done by Greene and his associates on the relationship of such factors to the onset of leukemia and lymphoma in adults (2–4).

The study of the pediatric age group, consistent with the earlier findings, suggested that experiences of separation and loss played a role as one of the multiple conditions determining the development of leukemia in children. Of the thirty-three patients with lymphocytic and myelogenous leukemia investigated, thirty-one were said to have experienced one or more losses or separations in the two-year period prior to the onset of their illness, with half of these experiences occurring in the six months prior to that time. These events, which included such experiences as a change of residence or school, the death of a parent and separation or threat of separation from grandparents, often involved as well "a separation, loss, or change for the mother, father or other members of the family." A subsequent investigation by Greene and Swisher (5) of monozygotic twins discordant for leukemia lent weight to the idea that major psychological stress may constitute one of the precipitating factors in the onset of the manifest symptoms of leukemia.

Since that time a number of studies (6–10) have investigated the relationship of life change experiences, including real or threatened loss, to the onset of a variety of disease states. Despite the potential significance of Greene's work to the field of pediatric cancer, however, there has been no systematic study that has attempted to carry forward the investigation of the relationship of psychological factors to the occurrence of cancer in children. Nonetheless, a considerable amount of anecdotal material, based primarily on individual case records, has suggested that the kind of life experiences reported by Greene in his group of patients are not infrequently met with in the recent history of children and adolescents with cancer. It was because the senior author, quite by chance, came across such instances in the course of obtaining the social and family histories of pediatric cancer patients, that we decided to undertake this study.

METHOD

Utilizing a questionnaire (The Holmes and Rahe Schedule of Recent Events), a semistructured interview schedule, and an open-ended format, one or both parents of twenty-five children and adolescents with cancer were interviewed over a two-year period. An equal number of youngsters who were brought to a medical facility for a variety of physical complaints served as a comparison group. The children with malignancies were diagnosed as having either leukemia, a lymphoma, or other form of cancer, and were being treated on one of the two pediatric services associated with the Albert Einstein College of Medicine.

Neoplastic diseases of several kinds were included for two reasons. The first was a practical one. The number of cancer patients seen on the pediatric services in any one year is not large and it would have required several more years of study to accumulate a sufficient number of cases of any one kind. The authors also felt that the inclusion of neoplasms of several kinds would be of interest from the point of view of the setting in which they arose. As it turned out, the majority of cases were diagnosed as having leukemia, with lymphomas being the next most frequently encountered group.

The comparison group, which was matched for sex, age, and socioeconomic background, was drawn from children who were brought to the general pediatric clinic. The great majority of these children suffered from minor ailments such as sore throats or upper respiratory infections, although some more serious conditions, e.g., asthma, were also diagnosed. There was no effort on the part of the researchers to select the children on the basis of their diagnoses or the seriousness of their complaints. The only criteria used were that the comparison group be matched in the parameters mentioned and that they be brought by their families to see a physician. A group of children who were considered to be physically ill were chosen for comparison rather than normal, healthy children because research in recent years has shown that life changes such as those cited by Greene in relation to leukemia are likely to precede the onset of a variety of illnesses in children (11–13).

The semistructured interview schedule included a detailed medical history of the patient and his family; a history of the mother's pregnancy and delivery; a developmental history of the child, including personality characteristics and psychological symptoms; a history of exposure to known carcinogens; information on the quality of the child's relationship to family and friends prior to the onset of the illness; a history of psychological symptoms in other members of the family; questions pertaining to assessment of the marriage and the parents' relations to each other, their own parents, and children; a history of the illness, including its onset, course, and treatment; and, finally an exploration of life changes within the family one year prior to the apparent onset of the disease.

For the last purpose, the Holmes and Rahe Life Schedule of Recent Events was included (14, 15).

The use, in this way, of a standardized instrument, whose forty-three items have been assigned a weighted value, measured in life change units, allowed for some quantification of the data obtained and for a more meaningful comparison between the two groups. The fact that the Holmes and Rahe Scale includes a broad spectrum of questions pertaining to events that have involved the entire family, as well as the child, made it suitable for our purposes.

To obtain a more thorough picture of the family's experience in the two years prior to the onset of the disease, more extensive, open-ended interviewing was also undertaken. The material thus obtained provided some insight into the quality of life and coping styles of the child and his family as well as providing information on experiences and social supports not touched on in the Life Events Scale. Although not all of this material could be quantified, as in the Holmes and Rahe weighted scoring system, the clinical data thus obtained supplemented and enriched our understanding of the recent experiences of the families that we studied.

RESULTS

Patient and Comparison Group Characteristics

The patient group ranged in age from three to seventeen years with a Mean age of 9.5 years (see Table 1). There were fifteen cases of leukemia, four of non-Hodgkin's lymphoma, and three of Hodgkin's disease. Other types of cancer diagnosed and represented by one case each were: Ewing's sarcoma, Wilm's tumor, and a sarcoma of the brain. The diagnoses and demographic characteristics of both the patient and the comparison group are shown in Table 1.

Information pertaining to several factors of importance in the study of pediatric cancer was obtained from the semistructured interview schedule and compared for the two groups (see Table 2). There were five first born children in the patient group (20%) compared with 9 (36%) in the comparison group. Thus the high percentage of first born children reported by Greene (55%) was not confirmed in the present study. Eighty percent of the children in the patient group and 84% in the comparison had

TABLE 1 Characteristics of the child and adolescent sample (*N* = 50)

	PATIENT GROUP (*N* = 25) (%)	COMPARISON GROUP (*N* = 25) (%)
Sex		
Female	56	56
Male	44	44
Age		
1–5 years	20	24
6–10 years	44	40
11–17 years	36	36
Religion		
Catholic	68	56
Protestant	20	28
Jewish	12	16
Education		
Preschool	16	20
<8th grade	60	60
High School	24	20
Socioeconomic Class (Hollingshead Scale)		
Class I	4	4
II	12	8
III	56	60
IV	20	20
V	8	8
Symptoms and/or Diagnosis		
Leukemia	60	
Lymphoma	16	
Other cancer	12	
Upper respiratory/sore throat and fever		56
Stomach virus		16
Asthma		12
Eczema		8
Kidney disease		4
Deafness		4

TABLE 2 Characteristics of the patient and comparison groups on the semistructured interview schedule (*N* = 50)

	PATIENT GROUP (*N* = 25) (%)	COMPARISON GROUP (*N* = 25) (%)
Birth order		
Only child	20	16
1st born	20	36
Later born	60	48
History of cancer in the family[a]	60	32
Planned pregnancy[a]	32	90
Somatic and/or emotional problems reported during pregnancy[a]	56	28
Difficult birth[a] (cesarean, forceps, etc.)	20	4
Frequency of illness during childhood		
Common infectious diseases	44	36
Upper respiratory and colds	60	44
Ear, eye, urinary infections[a]	24	8

[a] Statistical significance between patient and control groups with Yates correction for discontinuity, χ^2 tests, $p < 0.01$.

siblings. Some pediatric oncologists, noting the occurrence of cancer in certain later born children with older parents, have speculated about the possible significance, from a genetic point of view, of maternal age. In our study, only 8 mothers in the patient group and 6 of the comparison group mothers were over the age of thirty at the time of the birth of their children.

The incidence of known cancer in the families of the patient group was 60% as compared with 32%

in the comparison group families. This included both the immediate and the more extended families. In one case, the older sibling of a five-year-old boy had died of Hodgkin's disease several years before the boy developed a Wilm's tumor. In two cases of children with acute lymphocytic leukemia (ALL), siblings of their fathers had died in early adolescence of leukemia. In the cases of two other children, one with Hodgkin's disease and one with ALL, the patients' own fathers had developed thyroid and lung cancer as young adults. This high incidence of cancer, both in the immediate family and in close relatives, while not unexpected, is nevertheless noteworthy.

The incidence of other known illnesses in the families of both groups were similar with the exception of heart disease, which occurred more frequently in the comparison group families. There was no difference in the reported incidence of diabetes, hypertension, asthma, or blood disorders.

Data on the pregnancies of mothers of both

groups of children were obtained. In the patient group, 56% of the mothers reported either somatic or emotional problems during their pregnancies. Sixty-eight percent of the pregnancies in this group were unplanned. In the comparison group, 28% of the mothers reported similar problems, and 10% of these pregnancies were unplanned. Seventy-two percent of the mothers in the comparison group gave a history of nonproblematic pregnancies. The kinds of difficulties reported were as follows: acute viral illnesses, vaginal and kidney infections, intermittent bleeding, drug allergies, and severe depression and anxiety in some women as a consequence of family and marital problems and unplanned pregnancies.

It was not possible to pinpoint with sufficient accuracy the time during the pregnancies that these events occurred for us to comment on the temporal relationship between them and phases in the prenatal development of the hematopoietic system. Greene's interesting idea that physical or emotional stress occurring at a specific time in that development could affect the blood forming elements in such a manner as to pave the way for the later development of malignant changes could not, in this study, be investigated.

No difference was found between the patient and comparison groups with regard to the common infectious diseases of childhood, nor was there any difference in the amount of immunization received or in the reaction of the children to these procedures. There were, however, six children (24%) who had a history of having had rather severe ear, eye, or urinary infections in the patient group as compared with two (8%) in the comparison group. In several instances, the mothers of children with leukemia reported that their youngsters were diagnosed as anemic by physicians several years before the apparent onset of the disease. In addition, parents of the patient group reported a higher number of colds, sore throats, and upper respiratory infections in their children than did the parents of the comparison group children.

There was a small number of children in the patient group who were said to be unusually healthy prior to their developing cancer. This was also true, however, of a number of children in the comparison group. As there was no way of documenting the minor illnesses reported in the patient group neither their nature nor severity could be ascertained.

Life Events

Results obtained by use of the Holmes and Rahe Schedule of Recent Events revealed significant differences between the patient and the comparison groups. Each item on this scale has been assigned a weighted value that is based on extensive testing carried out in the general population. For example, "death of a spouse" is assigned a value of 100, "marital separation" a value of 65, and "son or daughter leaving home" a value of 29. In our interviews of the families of both groups of children, information was obtained about life events occurring in the one year prior to the apparent onset of illness in the child. On many items it was also of interest to use a two-year period prior to onset as the basis for comparison.

Mean "Life Change Units" (LCU), i.e., total weighted scores, and the mean number of life events were contrasted in the two groups. In addition, the individual life events were compared. Use of the first method resulted in a LCU score of 197.0 for the patient group as compared with a mean of 91.8 for the comparison population. This is a highly significant difference at the $p < 0.001$ level of confidence and suggests that the patient group experienced both a greater number of the designated life change events and, by the standards of this instrument, events of greater emotional significance than did the comparison group.

Figure 1 graphically compares the matched patient and comparison groups for each of the 25 cases. The difference in the groups are clearly seen. The actual emotional impact on the children of the events may, however, vary quite widely from child to child and is very much an individual matter. Experiences that have been assigned a low value on the scale may, for a given youngster, be of great emotional significance and vice versa. Only a study of the individual cases provides insight into such situations.

Calculation of the mean number of life events included in the scale that had actually occurred in each group showed an average of 5.7 for the patients and 2.8 for the comparison population. This indicates that the number of designated events which took place in the lives of the children with cancer in the one year prior to their becoming ill was approximately twice that of the comparison group. The number of such events experienced by individuals is

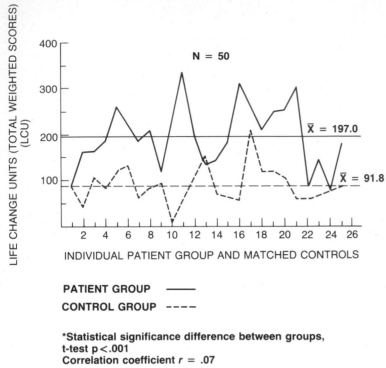

*Statistical significance difference between groups,
t-test p < .001
Correlation coefficient r = .07

Fig 1 Comparison Life Change Units of the Individual Patients and the Matched Controls (Comparison Group).

considered by Holmes and Rahe to be the single most important measure by which meaningful comparisons can be made between such groups. This might suggest, then, that the emotional setting in which illness may develop is characterized not so much by the single stressful experience, as by the accumulative effect of a number of such experiences.

Of particular interest are some of the individual items (see Table 3). A marital separation occurred in 32% of the patients' families and, in an additional 20% there was a loss by death of a family member (other than a parent). The average parent age in both groups was approximately 33 years, and in no case was there a report of a parent's death. In the comparison group, 12% experienced a marital separation, and 4% reported the death of a close family member.

With regard to a change of school, 56% of the youngsters in the patient group had that experience as compared to 32% in the comparison group. Other findings of interest were as follows: 60% of the patient group reported a major change in the health or behavior of a family member (not including the patient) as opposed to 24% in the comparison group. Examples of such changes were: serious illness of a parent, sibling, or grandparent; alcoholism in one of the parents or grandparents; hostility and alienation between parents and grandparents; and marital discord between parents.

Forty-eight percent of the patients' families reported a major change in their financial state (in all it was worse) as compared to 22% in the comparison families. In 32% of the patients and 12% of the comparison group a major personal injury or illness was experienced by a member of the family other than the patient. Twenty percent of the patient group also reported "a major change in the number of arguments with spouse," compared to 4% in the

TABLE 3 Frequency of occurrence of individual life events[a] ($N = 50$)

LIFE EVENT	PATIENT GROUP ($N = 25$) (%)	COMPARISON GROUP ($N = 25$) (%)
Marital separation	32	12
Death of close family member	20	4
Change in residence	72	24
Change in schools	56	32
Change in health or behavior of a family member (other than patient or control)	60	24
Change in financial state	24	22
Personal injury or illness (other than patient or control)	32	12
Change in the number of arguments with spouse	20	4
Major change in social activities	16	8
Wife beginning or stopping work	20	44
Son or daughter leaving home	12	20
Gain of new family member	4	12

[a] Statistical significance between groups over all items, χ^2 test, $p < 0.001$.

comparison group. In all instances there was an increase in such arguments. In addition, 16% of the patients' families reported a major change in social activities as compared to half that percentage in the comparison population.

There were some differences, too, on the other side of the ledger. In 44% of the comparison group there was a change in the mother's work status (most often with her beginning to work) as compared to 20% in the families of patients. Also, 20% of the comparison families reported a son or daughter leaving home and 12% reported the birth of a new child, in contrast to the patient group (12% and 4%, respectively).

A surprising 72% of the families in the patient group had moved within two years of the onset of the illness. This compared with 24% of the families in the comparison group. The figures for the one-year period prior to the apparent onset of the disease were 60 and 12%, respectively. In many instances, it is quite clear that moving was associated in a youngster with strong feelings of anxiety or depression. In others, however, there was no clear evidence that such reactions played a significant role in the child's life.

These differing reactions are illustrated by the following two children both of whose families moved in the year prior to the apparent onset of leukemia.

Case 1. The first patient was four and a half years old at the time that his disease was diagnosed. When he was two, his father left the family and he was taken care of by his mother and maternal grandparents who lived in the same two-family house. In the year before he became ill, his mother ended her relationship with a boyfriend and felt very depressed. Then, rather suddenly, she developed the idea of moving to Las Vegas. This she did abruptly, taking the boy away from his grandparents and the familiar home environment. In Nevada the child seemed sad and unhappy. He whined and cried a great deal and was interested in nothing. The mother, too, was unhappy with her decision, felt even more depressed than before, and after approximately five months in the new environment, decided to return home. Just before she could make final arrangements to do so, the boy developed numerous bruises and the diagnosis of ALL was made.

Case 2. The second case concerns a three-year-old girl with leukemia. In the year prior to her becoming ill, her father was obliged, for business reasons, to be away from home for several weeks at a time. He was quite unhappy about this, as was his wife. The youngster became sad and agitated every time her father left on a business trip. She also became, in that year, a poor and finicky eater. A few months before the diagnosis was made, the father was transferred by his firm and, on short notice, the family was obliged to move to a small Southern city. The mother was distressed by the change, but tried to take it philosophically and to see something positive in the move. The father was also quite unhappy about this change of residence but accepted it as a necessity for his career. Following the move, the youngster reacted with some regressive behavior, acted like a baby, and seemed depressed. Her reaction, though, was not sustained and after a week or two she seemed her old self. A few months later, however, during a period in which the father was away from home a good deal, the child developed fever and recurrent abdominal pain and the diagnosis was made.

Further clinical material from the open-ended interview illustrates some of the conflicts, as well as the feelings of anxiety and depression, experienced by two children in the months prior to the appearance of cancer.

Case 3. M. was 10 when her family moved from the city to the suburbs. For some months prior to the decision being made, she protested the idea vigorously and showed considerable apprehension about the change. After it had taken place she was, for two or three months, visibly anxious and depressed. Gradually these symptoms dissipated, and the child showed signs of making a reasonable adjustment both socially and in school. While this adaptation was taking place, her class went on a five-day outing to a nature camp. The child was fearful about sleeping away from home and the prospect of going on such a trip with new and untried classmates produced in her the greatest conflict. On the one hand, she felt she should go. On the other hand, she was terrified to do so. For several weeks while this conflict raged she lived in a state of torment. And finally, when the situation was resolved by her not going with the class, her feeling of being an outsider was increased and her depression returned. Approximately a month later, the patient developed a low grade fever and malaise. Some weeks after that, cervical adenopathy appeared and the diagnosis of malignant lymphoma was ultimately made.

Case 4. The parents of R, a twelve-year-old boy, had been having marital difficulty for some years. About a year before he became ill, however, the mother insisted on a separation. The father resisted this, but, finally, was forced to agree. The boy was extremely unhappy about this situation, became visibly depressed, and felt torn between his parents and their conflicting wishes. Shortly before his father actually moved out of the home, he developed fever and lympho-

denopathy and was diagnosed as having Hodgkin's disease.

Another vignette concerns a youngster in the control group, and, in light of the above examples, is a case of particular interest.

Case 5. The parents of a fourteen-year-old girl were involved in an acrimonious divorce. In the course of this turmoil, the mother, with whom the girl lived, was forced to sell her suburban home and to move into an apartment near the city. Initially, the youngster protested this change and was extremely unhappy about it. Once the move was accomplished, however, the girl showed signs of adjusting to the new situation, but was very much troubled by the divorce and began to act out her conflicts by becoming hostile and rebellious towards both parents. In this setting she developed a persistent sore throat, was taken to see a local physician, and was found to have developed a premalignant lesion in the tonsillar area. For some time thereafter, the girl's emotional turmoil continued unabated and, six months later, she came down with a severe case of mononucleosis.

DISCUSSION

In a study such as this, certain methodologic and interpretive problems inevitably arise and require comment. Not the least of these is presented by the nature of cancer itself. It is impossible, for example, to determine with certainty either just when in a given individual the cancerous process has been initiated or the length of time between the occurrence of such an event and the clinical manifestations of disease. Much depends on the nature of the cancer and its rate of growth, as well as on resistance factors in the host.

In an attempt to cope with these difficulties we have followed Greene and Miller in utilizing the concept "apparent onset" to designate the time at which either a clear-cut manifestation of the disease was observed by a parent or the diagnosis was actually established. In Greene's study, as in ours, these two events usually occurred within a week or two of one another and the time of their occurrence could be distinguished from the time at which the vaguer and more diffuse signs of illness were first noticed by the parents. In Greene's study the median time for the onset of such general complaints was four months prior to the apparent onset of disease, while in our own study it was two months, with the longest interval between these two events being four months and the shortest two weeks.

The implications of such inevitable uncertainties concerning the time of origin of the cancerous change and even, in certain instances, the time of its clinical appearance for a study which purports to investigate the relationship of life events to the onset of cancer is obvious. It is conceivable that a given life event taking place even as long as two years prior to the apparent onset of cancer may have occurred within the context of already existing disease. For that reason no attempt has been made, in this report, to associate the life events experienced by patients with the later development of cancer. We have noted only that cancer arose in a context in which certain life events took place and, where known, we have described the emotional response of the child to these events. Whether such life circumstances played any role in the initiation of the neoplastic transformation, enhanced or retarded the growth of malignant cells, or had no effect on this process, remains a matter of conjecture.

Another problem of importance concerns the meaning to the individual child of the life changes that he has experienced. While emphasizing, in a number of studies, the importance of the affects of helplessness and hopelessness in providing the emotional context in which illnesses of various kinds may arise, Engel (16) has, however, made clear that one cannot, with accuracy, judge whether a given event has been experienced as one of loss from the nature of the external event itself. Much depends on the meaning of the event to the individual, both in reality and in fantasy, and on the particular manner in which he copes with it. Rabkin and Streuning (17) point out the importance of available social supports in addition to the individual's ability to cope with stress. Theorell et al. (18) have shown that life changes and social supports are reciprocally related, and that even when significant life changes have occurred, the existence of supports and surrogates within a family may help protect an individual against the subsequent development of illness. To

make, therefore, an accurate assessment of the impact of any event on a given child requires access to information about all of these matters.

In many instances in the present study it was not possible to gain as comprehensive a view as we would have liked of the patient's emotional reactions, the meaning to them of the events experienced, and the supports available. For one thing, we were relying primarily on the memory of parents at a time, for them, of extreme stress. Moreover, the parents' view, even if accurate, could not provide an adequate view of the youngster's inner, private experiences and reactions. To obtain such information, one would have to observe a child both at the time of, and subsequent to, the occurrence of the event in question. When it was possible to interview the child as well as the parents, a more complete picture of his life experiences and reactions to events in his world was obtained, but this was not feasible in every case.

We did not feel, then, that it was possible to designate any of the life changes experienced by the children as losses in the psychological sense without access to this observational data. Where a clear-cut separation existed, one could, perhaps, speak of a presumed loss, but in only relatively few cases was the evidence obtained from parents and children sufficient to warrant such an outright designation.

In light of these considerations, interpretation of the data we obtained is not without difficulty. What, for instance, is one to make of the rather startling findings that 72% of the children who developed cancer experienced a change of residence within the two years prior to its onset? This was three times the rate in the comparison group and far higher than one would ordinarily expect. It also supports an earlier finding, of the Greene study, in which 57% of the leukemic children were found to have moved within a two-year period.

It might be assumed that moving is an emotionally disruptive experience for a child and that whatever link there could conceivably be between such an event and the later onset of cancer would occur as a consequence of the impact that the negative affects aroused by it have on the immunological, endocrine, or other biological systems.

In the first case example cited, it seemed clear that the child had a strong reaction to the move and to being separated from his grandparents. The mother was able to give a good description of the boy's behavior which was, unquestionably, that of a depressed child. It might be pointed out that the boy may already have had leukemia at the time of the move, and that the disease contributed to his emotional state. This of course, is a possibility, but evidence obtained both from the mother and from the child himself, through play therapy and story telling techniques, left no doubt that the experience of moving and the separation it entailed had a profound effect on him.

In the second situation, case 2, the evidence was less clear. Both parents were clearly disturbed by the move, but their adaptation was relatively rapid and there was no sign of severe or prolonged depression or anxiety in either. The same seemed to be true of the child despite the evidence of emotional upset which surrounded the father's leaving and the family's move. Such reactions are difficult to evaluate, particularly in retrospect, but, from the mother's description, the child did not seem to experience severe distress. One fact of note in this case, however, is that the separations from her father were, for the child, repeated events rather than a single experience. Data from the Holmes and Rahe questionnaire indicates that repeated stressful experiences were far more commonly found in the children who later developed cancer.

Thus, in these two cases, although moves preceded by some months the apparent onset of cancer in both children, the reaction of each child to the change was quite different. Nothing meaningful about such reactions could be inferred from the fact of the move alone. The same could be said about the finding that in 60% of the patient group there occurred a major change in the health or behavior of a family member, whereas such changes occurred in less than half that number of children in the comparison group. While such experiences may have had a strong emotional impact on the children involved, understanding the nature of that impact and how it interdigitated with other life experiences would have required a study of each individual child. While it was possible to acquire quite specific information on several children, in the case of others only a general description of their reactions could be obtained.

In certain cases, however, not only had separations taken place and clear-cut anxiety developed in the children, but it was evident that intense feelings of conflict were present as well. This seems noteworthy because previous reports on psychological factors associated with cancer have stressed such reactions as feelings of depression and loss, as well as a tendency to suppress and internalize emotions. There has been relatively little emphasis on the role that intense emotional conflict may play, through its impact on the immunologic and endocrine system, as an antecedent stress.

In cases #3 and #4, there was no doubt that both the children experienced intense feelings of conflict and anxiety. It is also true that, in each instance, separations played a significant role, and feelings of loss and depression were also important. It would seem, then, that the role of conflict as well as of certain negative affects, in creating a setting in which malignant change may occur, especially in certain biologically predisposed children whose defenses against painful emotions may be ineffective, is worthy of further investigation.

Although, since the time of Galen, physicians have speculated about a possible link between man's emotional life and cancer, it is only within the past few years that research has focused on the mechanisms by which such an influence might be mediated and has pointed out promising areas for investigation. It has been known for some time that bereaved widows and widowers have a higher incidence of illness and of mortality than do their contemporaries who have not experienced the loss of a spouse. Studies carried out in Australia (19), have shed new light on this problem by showing that impairment of cell-mediated immunity could be demonstrated in a group of such bereaved individuals. This was one of the first studies in humans to show that an experience of loss could be associated with a defect in the functioning of the immune system.

In another study, Locke (20), in Boston, has shown that the efficacy of an individual's psychological defenses may be related to certain capacities of the immune system. Working with a group of college-age students, he has demonstrated greater antileukemic activity in the lymphocytes of individuals who were able to cope with stress without becoming symptomatic as compared to those who, under such circumstances, developed psychological symptoms.

Studies such as these and others cited by Rogers in his excellent review article on the influence of the brain and psyche on immunity (21) are pointing the way to greater understanding of the impact of emotions on the functioning of the immune system. They suggest the possibility that in children, too, psychological and emotional factors may have a significant effect on this system. Such alterations in immune status could, theoretically, prepare the way either for the initiation of, or tolerance to, neoplastic change. It seems likely that certain children, genetically, are more predisposed to the development of malignancies than others. In our study, the number of close family members who had a history of cancer was striking. In addition, a history of cancer in somewhat more distant relatives was not uncommon. Whether certain children who are predisposed to cancer may be so by virtue of defects or variations of their immune system which, in turn, make the system more vulnerable to stresses of various kinds, including emotional stress, is a possibility that requires further investigation.

It is well-known, too, that experiences of severe anxiety as well as those leading to feelings of loss and depression may be associated with a significant increase, in certain individuals, in specific hormonal levels, particularly those of the corticosteroids. The impact of such shifts in hormonal levels on the immune system is a matter of current investigation and might provide a link to understanding the way in which emotions can affect that system.

Open to investigation, too, is the way in which hormonal levels in children and adolescents are affected, both by normal psycho-physiologic processes of growth and maturation, and by experiences of anxiety, stress, or depression. Particularly interesting would be the study, from a hormonal and immunologic point of view, of children who have a strong family history of cancer, both under conditions of ordinary living and at times when significant changes have occurred.

The relationship of viruses and viral illnesses to the process of neoplasia is currently one of great interest as well as controversy in the field of cancer research. Recent statistical evidence pointing to the existence of contact, possibly through an asymptomatic carrier, among cases of Hodgkin's disease and the occasional outcropping of clusters of such cases, as well as of ALL, has given fresh impetus to the theory that an infectious component may play a role in these illnesses. Some years ago Gross (22) suggested the idea of the vertical transmission of a virus, and, in more recent years, the Epstein-Barr virus has been thought to be associated with pharyngeal cancer and Burkitt's lymphoma in certain predisposed African children as well as with mononucleosis in this and other countries (23).

Although still controversial, some virologists (24) have postulated mechanisms by which infection with this virus could lead, on the one hand, to the benign proliferation of lymphocytes and, on the other, to the malignant transformation of affected cells. Epidemiologists have suggested that the Epstein-Barr virus, or one like it, could be implicated in Hodgkin's disease. Such a virus, they hypothesize, could be harbored by asymptomatic carriers and affect only those individuals who, for immunologic or genetic reasons, have a high degree of susceptibility.

The role that psychological and emotional factors play in increasing the susceptibility of youngsters to this and other forms of cancer is not known. The impact that such factors can have on rendering children susceptible to a variety of diseases, including viral illnesses, has been appreciated since the work of Spitz and others showed the vulnerability of emotionally deprived children to serious, and often fatal, infections. The possibility that life events such as those reported here can stimulate, in certain children, emotional reactions which make them more vulnerable to the activity either of latent or exogenous viruses that may, on rare occasions, have an oncogenic effect, can not be dismissed.

Many of the ideas that we have touched upon in this article await clarification by further research. They were stimulated by the new and intriguing vistas being opened in cancer research by the growing recognition of the impact that emotions can have on various bodily systems, including immunologic processes at the cellular level. In a recent interview concerning the role of viruses in cancer, Dr. Fred Rapp (25), of Pennsylvania State University of Medicine, expressed the widely held view that cancer occurs as a result of a number of factors acting in concert. When the conditions are right and these several factors come together, a malignant transformation may ensure. Whether one of these factors, or, alternatively, one of the underlying conditions that fosters the operation of these factors, relates to an individual's emotional state is not known with certainty, but seems, on the basis of recent studies, to be a strong possibility. The idea that cancer, like many other illnesses, may, in fact, be a psychobiological phenomenon in the broadest sense; a disease process whose complexity may require for its ultimate comprehension contributions from fields as divergent as molecular biology and depth psychology, is not a new one. It is, however, an idea whose potential is just beginning to be explored.

References

1. Greene WA Jr, Miller G: Psychological factors and reticuloendothelial disease. IV. Observations on a group of children and adolescents with leukemias: an interpretation of disease development in terms of mother-child unit. Psychosom. Med. 10:124–144, 1958

2. Greene WA Jr: Psychological factors and reticuloendothelial disease. III. Further observations on psychological and somatic manifestations in patients with lymphomas and leukemias. Presented at the Annual Meeting, American Psychosomatic Society, Chicago, 1952

3. Greene WA Jr: Psychological factors and reticuloendothelial disease. I. Preliminary observations on a group of males with lymphomas and leukemia. Psychosom. Med. 16:220–230, 1954

4. Greene WA Jr, Young LE, Swisher SN, Miller G: Psychological factors and reticuloendothelial disease. II. Observations on a group of females with lymphomas and leukemias. Psychosom. Med. 18:284–303, 1955

5. Greene WA Jr, Swisher SN: Psychological and somatic variables associated with the development and course of monozygotic twins discordant for leukemia. Ann. NY Acad. Sci. 164:394–408, 1969

6. Adler R, MacRitchie K, Engel GL: Psychologic processes and ischaemic stroke (occlusive cerebrovascular disease). I. Observations on 32 men and 35 strokes. Psychosom. Med. 31:1–29, 1971

7. Brown GW, Birley JLT: Crises and life changes and the onset of schizophrenia. J. Health Soc. Behav. 9:203–214, 1968

8. DeFaire U: Life change patterns prior to death in ischaemic heart disease: a study on death-discordant twins. J. Psychosom. Res. 19:273–278, 1975

9. Rahe RH, Bennett L, Romo M: Subjects' recent life changes and coronary heart disease in Finland. Am. J. Psychiatry 130:1222–1226, 1973

10. Theorell T, Rahe RH: Psychosocial factors and myocardial infarction. I. An inpatient study in Sweden. J. Psychosom. Res. 15:25–31, 1971

11. Heisel JS: Life changes as etiologic factors in juvenile rheumatoid arthritis. J. Psychosom. Res. 16:411–420, 1972

12. Marx MB, Garrity TF, Bowers FR: The influence of recent life experiences. J. Psychosom. Res. 19:87–98, 1975

13. Stein SP, Charles E: Emotional factors in juvenile diabetes mellitus: A study of early life experiences of adolescent diabetics. Am. J. Psychiatry 128:56–60, 1971

14. Holmes TH, Meyer M, Smith M et al: Social stress and illness onset. J. Psychosom. Res. 8:35–44, 1964

15. Rahe RH, Arthur RJ: Life change and illness studies: past history and future directions. J. Human Stress March 3–15, 1978

16. Engel GL: Studies of ulcerative colitis: the nature of the psychologic processes. Am. J. Med. 19:231–255, 1955

17. Rabkin JG, Streuning EL: Life events, stress and illness. Science 194:1013–1020, 1976

18. Theorell T, Lind E, Floderus B: The relationship of disturbing life changes and emotions to the early development of myocardial infarctions and other serious illnesses. Int. J. Epidemiol. 4:281–292, 1975

19. Bartrop RW, et al: Depressed lymphocyte function after bereavement. The Lancet 1:834–836, 1977

20. Locke SE: The influence of stress and emotions on immune response. Biofeedback Self-Regulation, 2, 1977

21. Rogers MP, Dubey D, Reich P: The influence of the psyche and the brain on immunity. Psychosom. Med. 41:147–164, 1979

22. Gross SJ: Human blood groups. A substance in human endometrium and trophoblast. Am. J. Obstet. Gynecol. 1149–1159, 1966

23. Holden G: Cancer and the mind—How they are connected. Sci. News 20, June 3, 1978

24. Klein G: The Epstein-Barr virus. The Herpes Viruses. Edited by AS Kaplan, New York, Academic Press, pp. 521–555

25. Rapp F: Ca—A Cancer Journal for Clinicians Vol 28, No. 6, 1978

Gender and Health: An Update on Hypotheses and Evidence

Lois M. Verbrugge

INTRODUCTION

The far-reaching differences between men and women have inspired curiosity, poetry, romance, and polemics for centuries, but they have only recently prompted scrutiny by social scientists. A key reason is that the social lives of men and women used to be more predictable; men typically behaved in certain ways and women in others. Gender differences in activities, goals, and longevity were taken for granted, being the persistent outcomes of quite predictable lives. At best, social statistics in this century reported data separately for men and women, but the fundamental scientific question "Why are there differences?" was not voiced.

This situation has changed markedly in the past few decades. As options expand for both sexes, men and women are varying more in their roles, attitudes, and behaviors than before, and gender differences are open to more change. In tandem with this, scientists have become more interested in those differences and they are now asking: "What makes males and females choose different social paths, and what are the consequences for their physical, mental, and material-well being?" "Do contemporary changes result in more similar life styles, health risks, and social resources for women and men than before?"[1]

Some of the most striking and persistently documented differences concern men's and women's health and mortality. As long as vital statistics, health surveys, and medical/hospital records have been available for the United States population, they have shown higher mortality rates for men but higher rates of morbidity and health services use for women. Why is the pace of death quicker for men? Why are illnesses more frequent for women? Is higher morbidity the sole reason for women's higher restricted activity, greater use of medical drugs, and more frequent medical care? Do reproduction events and problems account for most of the difference? Are sex differences in morbidity and mortality narrowing in recent decades?

This article aims to consolidate social scientists' thinking and research on gender and health in the past 10–15 years. It presents the key hypotheses about sex differences that have been proposed and condenses the findings of research, especially sociological research, to date. Some excellent and detailed reviews of sex differences in health indicators and risk factors already exist, and we shall point to them rather than repeat them. Instead, our aim is to discuss the "state of the issue" and offer a context for research in the next decade or two. References will typically be listed at the end of each section rather than throughout it.

The discussion focuses on health and mortality of contemporary American (U.S.) adults. The rationale is: First, adults' rates of chronic disease, disability, and mortality are much higher than children's, and their inputs into health are more personal and cumulative. Both aspects increase the potential for sex differences in health outcomes. The chance that such differences are due to social and psychological factors also rises. Second, research on gender differences is most prolific for the United States. Findings for European and other developed countries are generally parallel. By contrast, data for developing countries are sparse, and because acute conditions and pregnancy constitute a larger share of serious morbidity and mortality, the factors that propel sex

Reprinted from the *Journal of Health and Social Behavior*, vol. 26 (1985), pp. 157–177.

differences in health are probably quite different. The basic theoretical design of this article can be adapted to developing countries, but we leave that to researchers with pertinent expertise.

We consider three facets of health: (1) morbidity, (2) health actions taken to treat or prevent morbidity, and (3) mortality. Morbidity is the presence of illness or injury, measured by incidence and prevalence rates. Health actions include short-term disability such as staying in bed during illness, long-term disability due to chronic conditions, health services use, medical drug use, and other self-care actions.

Sociologists and psychologists use the terms sex and gender to denote causes of behavior. While sex indicates that solely biological factors are responsible, gender indicates the presence of social, psychological, and cultural ones as well as biological. We will use the term gender in that manner. Sex will be used in the demographic sense to denote the population groups of interest, with no presumption about causes of any observed differences. The words male(s) and female(s) refer to people of any age, while the words men and women indicate adults. Thus, where the text says sex, males and females, or men and women, it is simply designating population groups for comparison.

SEX DIFFERENCES IN HEALTH OF AMERICAN MEN AND WOMEN

We begin with a capsule summary of sex differences in health, relying on national statistics except where noted.

Sex differences in mortality are well known and can be summarized simply. Based on current death rates, females have a life expectancy seven years longer than males. Risks of death are higher for males than females at all ages and for all leading causes of death (Table 1).[2]

Health statistics look quite different. They routinely show higher morbidity from acute conditions and nonfatal chronic diseases for women and also more short-term disability, medical services use, and medical drug use by women (Table 2). We review the myriad indicators of worse health for women first, then the few that show worse health for men.

The sex difference in incidence of acute conditions is on the order of 20–30% overall. Women are

in excess for all key groups: infective/parasitic diseases, respiratory conditions, digestive system conditions, injuries (at ages 45+ but not younger), and all other acute conditions. The last group encompasses reproductive conditions (deliveries and disorders of pregnancy and the puerperium), ear diseases, headaches, genitourinary disorders, and skin and musculoskeletal diseases. Even when the reproductive conditions are excluded, a sizable sex difference still persists in all other acute conditions.

Most nonfatal chronic diseases are also more prevalent among women. The excess is especially large, by twofold or more, for: varicose veins, frequent constipation, gallbladder conditions, chronic enteritis and colitis, corns and callosities, bunion, thyroid conditions, anemias, migraine, and chronic urinary diseases. Also more common for women are: hypertensive disease, hemorrhoids, chronic bronchitis, chronic sinusitis, diverticula of intestine, arthritis, and synovitis/bursitis/tenosynovitis.

Women restrict their activities for health problems (acute and chronic combined) about 25% more days each year than men do, and they spend about 40% more days in bed per year on the average. The differences are largest (30–50% for restricted activity, 70–85% for bed disability) at ages 17–44, the reproductive years for women. Problems of pregnancy and the puerperium are counted as acute conditions. They constitute only about 10% of the short-term disability women 17–44 take for all their acute conditions; so even when reproductive conditions are excluded, a sizable sex difference still remains in short-term disability.

Some long-term disabilities are also more prevalent among women. More women in middle and older ages report trouble doing their secondary activities (such as shopping, going to church, recreation) due to chronic health problems, than same-age men.

Sex differences in health services use are largest for young adults and narrow as age advances. In the age range 17–44 women have twice as many physician visits and hospital stays as men do. When reproductive and other sex-specific conditions are excluded, there is still a gap of about 30% for ambulatory care, but the gap for hospitalization virtually disappears. After age 45, again excluding all sex-specific conditions, women continue to have more physician visits by about 10–20%, but men exceed them in frequency of hospital stays.

TABLE 1 Death rates for males and females, by age and by cause of death, United States, 1980

AGE-SPECIFIC DEATH RATES	(RATES PER 100,000 POPULATION)		SEX DIFFERENCE	SEX RATIO
	MALE	FEMALE	(M-F)	(M/F)
All Ages	977	785	192	1.24
Under 1	1428	1142	286	1.25
1–4	73	55	18	1.33
5–14	37	24	13	1.54
15–24	172	58	114	2.97
25–34	196	76	120	2.58
35–44	299	159	140	1.88
45–54	767	413	354	1.86
55–64	1815	934	881	1.94
65–74	4105	2145	1960	1.91
75–84	8817	5440	3377	1.62
85+	18801	14747	4054	1.27

CAUSE-SPECIFIC DEATH RATES FOR LEADING CAUSES[a]	(AGE-ADJUSTED RATES PER 100,000 POP.)[b]		SEX DIFFERENCE	SEX RATIO	RANKS[c]			
	MALE	FEMALE	(M-F)	(M/F)	M		F	
All causes	777.2	432.6	344.6	1.80				
Diseases of heart	280.4	140.3	140.1	2.00	1	(1)	1	(1)
Malignant neoplasms	165.5	109.2	56.3	1.52	2	(2)	2	(2)
Cerebrovascular diseases	44.9	37.6	7.3	1.19	4	(4)	3	(3)
Accidents	64.0	21.8	42.2	2.94	3	(3)	4	(4)
Motor vehicle	34.3	11.8	22.5	2.91				
Other	29.6	10.0	19.6	2.96				
Chronic obstructive pulmonary diseases	26.1	8.9	17.2	2.93	5	(5)	7	(8)
Pneumonia and influenza	17.4	9.8	7.6	1.78	7	(6)	6	(5)
Diabetes mellitus	10.2	10.0	0.2	1.02	10	(10)	5	(6)
Chronic liver disease and cirrhosis	17.1	7.9	9.2	2.16	8	(8)	9	(9)
Atherosclerosis	6.6	5.0	1.6	1.32	11	(12)	12	(7)
Suicide	18.0	5.4	12.6	3.33	6	(7)	11	(12)
Homicide	17.4	4.5	12.9	3.87	7	(9)	13	(13)
Conditions originating in perinatal period	11.1	8.7	2.4	1.28	9	(11)	8	(11)
Nephritis and nephrosis	5.7	3.6	2.1	1.50	13	(13)	14	(10)
Congenital anomalies	6.5	5.6	0.9	1.16	12	(14)	10	(12)
Septicemia	3.2	2.2	1.0	1.45	14	(15)	15	(14)
All other causes	83.1	52.1	31.0	1.60				

Sources: For age-specific rates, Monthly Vital Statistics Report, Vol. 31, No. 13: Table 6. 5 October 1983. For cause-specific rates, Monthly Vital Statistics Report, Vol. 32, No. 4, Supplement: Table 9. 11 August 1983. Published by National Center for Health Statistics. Hyattsville, MD.

[a] Causes are listed on left in rank order of 1980 crude rates for the total population.

[b] Computed by the direct method, using as the standard population the age distribution of the 1940 total U.S. population.

[c] Ranks outside parentheses are based on the age-adjusted rates; those inside are based on crude rates (Table 8 of source). The 15th rank age-adjusted cause for males is: Hypertension with or without renal disease (2.4) and ulcer of stomach and duodenum (2.4).

TABLE 2 Health statistics for American men and women. (Rates and sex ratios (F/M) based on national health surveys)

INCIDENCE OF ACUTE CONDITIONS (1981 AND 1977–78)	NO. OF CONDITIONS PER 100 PERSONS PER YEAR					
	MEN 17–44	WOMEN 17–44	F/M	MEN +45	WOMEN +45	F/M
All acute conditions (1981)	190.8	243.1	1.27	107.6	131.3	1.22
Infective and parasitic diseases	17.5	25.5	1.46	5.8	9.7	1.67
Respiratory conditions	98.2	123.6	1.26	61.0	70.9	1.16
Upper resp. cond.	46.1	56.7	1.23	24.3	30.1	1.24
Influenza	48.0	59.9	1.25	32.6	34.8	1.07
Other resp. cond.	4.1	7.0	1.71	4.1	5.9	1.44
Digestive system conditions	9.7	11.4	1.18	4.5	5.6	1.24
Injuries	47.1	29.3	0.62	20.4	22.2	1.09
All other acute conditions	18.3	53.3	2.91	15.9	23.0	1.45
All other acute conditions (1977–78)[a]	21.8	50.3	2.31	15.7	26.0	1.66
—Excluding reproductive conditions	21.8	40.4	1.85	15.7	26.0	1.66

PREVALENCE OF CHRONIC CONDITIONS (1979) (SELECTED TITLES)[b]	NO. OF CONDITIONS PER 1,000 POPULATION								
	AGES 17–44			45–64			65+		
	M	F	F/M	M	F	F/M	M	F	F/M
Heart conditions#	33	41	1.24	132	126	0.95	266	281	1.06
Coronary heart disease#	4*	1*	0.25	76	34	0.45	145	96	0.66
Hypertensive disease[c]	60	57	0.95	203	225	1.11	315	434	1.38
Cerebrovascular disease#	1*	2*	2.00	14	17	1.21	40	40	1.00
Atherosclerosis#	1*	1*	1.00	28	15	0.54	122	125	1.02
Varicose veins	5*	32	6.40	23	77	3.35	37	126	3.41
Hemorrhoids	45	52	1.16	60	69	1.15	52	76	1.46
Chronic bronchitis	18	35	1.94	34	37	1.09	36	52	1.44
Emphysema	2*	.5*	0.25	29	18	0.62	68	24	0.35
Asthma, with or without hay fever	22	26	1.18	28	40	1.43	22*	20	0.91
Chronic sinusitis	120	176	1.47	164	212	1.29	135	171	1.27
Ulcer of stomach and duodenum	19	18	0.95	34	26	0.76	21*	39	1.86
Frequent constipation	2*	19	9.50	13	40	3.08	42	80	1.90
Gallbladder conditions	1*	12	12.00	9*	17	1.89	13*	22	1.69
Diverticula of intestine	.2*	1*	5.00	14	16	1.14	16*	37	2.31
Chronic enteritis and colitis	4*	13	3.25	8*	20	2.50	10*	23	2.30
Eczema, dermatitis, and urticaria	26	48	1.85	32	44	1.38	30	24	0.80
Corns and callosities	14	21	1.50	23	57	2.48	30	74	2.47
Arthritis	37	58	1.57	188	312	1.66	355	504	1.42
Bunion	2*	8	4.00	8*	23	2.88	5*	42	8.40
Synovitis, bursitis, and tenosynovitis	14	20	1.43	46	56	1.22	19*	43	2.26
Gout	4*	1*	0.25	28	11	0.39	34	22	0.65
Thyroid conditions	3*	21	7.00	8*	43	5.38	12*	37	3.08
Diabetes#	8	9	1.13	56	60	1.07	74	84	1.14
Anemias	2*	27	13.50	3*	17	5.67	10*	36	3.60
Migraine	16	48	3.00	17	63	3.71	8*	20	2.50
Diseases of urinary system[d]	10	42	4.20	17	45	2.65	36	71	1.97
Visual impairments	42	18	0.43	74	43	0.58	120	118	0.98
Hearing impairments	56	34	0.61	148	93	0.63	327	250	0.76
Absence of extremities or parts of extremities	7	1*	0.14	34	7*	0.21	42	12*	0.29

(Chronic bronchitis, Emphysema, and Asthma, with or without hay fever are bracketed together with the symbol #)

(continued)

TABLE 2 (*Continued*)

PREVALENCE OF CHRONIC CONDITIONS (1979) (SELECTED TITLES)[b]	NO. OF CONDITIONS PER 1,000 POPULATION								
	AGES 17–44			45–64			65+		
	M	F	F/M	M	F	F/M	M	F	F/M
Paralysis, complete or partial, of extremities or parts of extremities	4*	1*	0.25	8*	5*	0.63	20*	18	0.90
Deformities or orthopedic impairments	103	88	0.85	122	114	0.93	145	174	1.20

TOTAL SHORT-TERM DISABILITY (FOR ACUTE AND CHRONIC CONDITIONS COMBINED) (1981)	DAYS OF DISABILITY PER PERSON PER YEAR											
	AGES 17–24			25–44			45–64			65+		
	M	F	F/M	M	F	F/M	M	F	F/M	M	F	F/M
Restricted activity days[e]	9.6	14.2	1.48	14.7	18.7	1.27	26.5	28.4	1.07	37.6	41.5	1.10
Bed disability days	3.4	6.3	1.85	4.2	7.0	1.67	7.8	10.1	1.29	13.9	14.0	1.01

SHORT-TERM DISABILITY FOR ACUTE CONDITIONS (1977–78)	DAYS OF DISABILITY PER 100 PERSONS PER YEAR					
	MEN 17–44	WOMEN 17–44	F/M	MEN +45	WOMEN +45	F/M
Restricted activity days[a]						
For all acute conditions (total)	800	1083	1.35	798	1150	1.44
For all other acute conditions (subcategory)	78	288	3.69	160	244	1.53
—Excluding reproductive conditions from restricted activity						
For all acute conditions	800	978	1.22			
For all other acute conditions	78	183	2.35			
Bed disability days[a]						
For all acute conditions (total)	318	536	1.69	331	476	1.44
For all other acute conditions (subcategory)	25	141	5.64	61	107	1.75
—Excluding reproductive conditions from bed disability						
For all acute conditions	318	478	1.50			
For all other acute conditions	25	83	3.32			

LIMITATION OF ACTIVITY DUE TO CHRONIC CONDITIONS (1981)	PERCENTS								
	AGES 17–44			45–64			65+		
	M	F	F/M	M	F	F/M	M	F	F/M
With any activity limitation	8.9	7.9	0.89	24.9	23.1	0.93	49.6	43.1	0.87
Limitation in major activity[f]	5.7	5.1	0.89	20.5	17.9	0.87	44.7	35.3	0.79
Limitation in secondary activities only	3.2	2.8	0.88	4.4	5.2	1.18	4.9	7.8	1.59

HEALTH SERVICES USE (1979)	VISITS OR DISCHARGES PER 1,000 POPULATION								
	AGES 15–44			45–64			65+		
	M	F	F/M	M	F	F/M	M	F	F/M
Visits to office-based physicians	1667	3068	1.84	2544	3367	1.32	3583	4239	1.18
—Excluding reproduction diagnoses[g]	1659	2505	1.51	2543	3364	1.32	3583	4239	1.18

(*continued*)

TABLE 2 (Continued)

	VISITS OR DISCHARGES PER 1,000 POPULATION								
	AGES 15–44			45–64			65+		
HEALTH SERVICES USE (1979)	M	F	F/M	M	F	F/M	M	F	F/M
—Excluding all sex-specific diagnoses	1631	2209	1.35	2461	3053	1.24	3438	4107	1.19
Discharges from short-stay hospitals	97	213	2.20	193	199	1.03	410	374	0.91
—Excluding reproduction diagnoses[g]	97	118	1.22	193	197	1.02	410	374	0.91
—Excluding all sex-specific diagnoses	95	88	0.93	186	167	0.90	381	355	0.93

	AGES 19–34			35–49			50–64			65+		
DRUG PRESCRIPTIONS (1977)	M	F	F/M	M	F	F/M	M	F	F/M	M	F	F/M
Persons receiving at least one medical drug prescription during the year[h] (percent)	42.2	70.4	1.67	50.2	65.8	1.31	59.0	74.0	1.25	70.9	78.3	1.10
No. of prescriptions per person												
For all people	1.6	4.1	2.56	3.3	5.6	1.70	5.7	9.0	1.58	8.8	12.0	1.36
For people with at least one prescription	3.7	5.9	1.59	6.6	8.4	1.27	9.7	12.2	1.26	12.4	15.3	1.23
Persons receiving at least one psychotropic drug prescription during the year[h,l] (percent)	3.6	8.2	2.28	8.0	17.5	2.19	12.9	23.0	1.78	14.3	23.3	1.63
No. of psychotropic prescriptions												
For all people (per 1,000 pop.)	122	263	2.16	374	739	1.98	613	1220	1.99	692	1132	1.64
For people with at least one psychotropic prescription (per person)	3.3	3.2	0.97	4.7	4.2	0.89	4.8	5.3	1.10	4.8	4.8	1.00

	AGES 18–34			35–49			50–64			65–79		
DRUG USE (1979)	M	F	F/M	M	F	F/M	M	F	F/M	M	F	F/M
Persons who used any psychotherapeutic drug in past year[j] (percent)	6.1	13.3	2.18	9.7	21.4	2.21	18.3	26.5	1.45	16.2	27.5	1.70

	PERCENTS								
	AGES 17–44			45–64			65+		
SELF-RATED HEALTH STATUS (1978)	M	F	F/M	M	F	F/M	M	F	F/M
Excellent[k]	56.8	48.3	0.85	39.4	33.3	0.85	29.1	27.3	0.94
Good	35.9	41.5		39.3	43.9		39.7	42.1	

(continued)

TABLE 2 (Continued)

SELF-RATED HEALTH STATUS (1978)	PERCENTS								
	AGES 17–44			45–64			65+		
	M	F	F/M	M	F	F/M	M	F	F/M
Fair	5.8	8.4		14.4	16.6		21.0	21.9	
Poor	1.3	1.5		6.4	5.6		9.6	7.8	

Sources: For acute condition incidence, Vital and Health Statistics, Series 10, Nos. 132, 141. National Center for Health Statistics, Hyattsville, MD. For chronic condition prevalence, Vital and Health Statistics, Series 3, No. 24 (Hing et al., 1983). For short-term disability, Vital and Health Statistics, Series 10, Nos. 132, 141. For limitation of activity, Vital and Health Statistics, Series 10, No. 141. For health service use, Vital and Health Statistics, Series 3, No. 24 (Hing et al., 1983). For drug prescriptions, unpublished data from the National Medical Care Expenditures Survey. (See also Kasper, 1982.) For psychotropic drug prescriptions, National Medical Care Expenditures Survey, Data Preview No. 14 (Cafferata and Kasper, 1983). National Center for Health Services Research, Rockville, MD. For psychotropic drug use, (Mellinger and Balter, 1981). For self-rated health status, Vital and Health Statistics, Series 10, No. 142.

A leading cause of death.

* Figure has relative high sampling error.

ᵃ All other acute conditions include diseases of the ear, headaches, genitourinary disorders, deliveries and disorders of pregnancy and the puerperium (ICDA-8 630–678), diseases of the skin, diseases of the musculoskeletal system, and a residual group. Published estimates for the fourth group are not age-specific; they were attributed to age group 17–44 and rates for "Excluding reproductive conditions" were then calculated by the author.

ᵇ Ratios based on * rates should be viewed with caution. Source presents additional decimal place for all rates.

ᶜ Hypertension without heart involvement. Commonly called high blood pressure.

ᵈ Includes nephritis/nephrosis (a leading cause of death) but many other nonfatal conditions as well.

ᵉ The first item is: days a person cuts down his/her typical activities for the whole day due to illness or injury. The second item is a subset, namely, days a person spends in bed all or most of the day due to illness or injury.

ᶠ The first item is: unable to have a job/keep house or limited in amount or kind of job/housework. Men are asked about job, and women about job or housework depending on their usual activity in the past year. The second item is: problems in going to church, clubs, shopping, etc.

ᵍ Complications of pregnancy/childbirth/puerperium, normal pregnancy, postpartum care and exam, and contraceptive and procreative management (including sterilization procedures and deliveries in the hospital discharge rates). The reproductive diagnoses for men 15–44 and 45–64 are mostly for contraceptive/procreative counseling and male sterilization.

ʰ The medicines could be obtained directly from physicians or purchased by prescription.

ⁱ Includes antianxiety agents, sedatives and hypnotics, antidepressants, and antipsychotics.

ʲ Includes antianxiety agents, hypnotics, daytime sedatives, antidepressants, and antipsychotics. Data shown refer to use of drugs prescribed by physicians to respondents. Excluded are over-the-counter sleeping pills/tranquilizers and prescription-type drugs obtained from friends and relatives. The exclusions are a small fraction of total use (see data in Source).

ᵏ "Compared to other persons [NAME]'s age, would you say his health is excellent, good, fair, or poor?" The categories add to slightly less than 100.0 because of N.A. (health status not ascertained) cases. Sex ratio is shown for "excellent" category only.

Women obtain substantially more prescription medicines per year than men at all ages, but especially in young reproductive ages (19–34). The overall difference is based on two factors: First, a larger percent of women get a prescription for any type of drug in a year's time and, second, more drugs are prescribed to women recipients on the average than to men recipients. Differences are especially large for psychotropic drugs, with women twice as likely to receive a prescription for such drugs in a year. But among recipients, men and women get similar numbers of psychotropics prescribed.

Sex differences in actual use of drugs are of similar magnitude. Women's use of prescription and over-the-counter drugs is about 50% higher than men's. The sex difference and psychotropic drug use is especially high, on the order of twofold higher for women than men.[3]

Men show health disadvantages in fewer but more serious respects. They suffer 50–60% more injuries at ages 17–44. Most types of impairment are also more common among men: Their rates of visual and hearing problems, absence of extremities, and paralysis typically exceed women's at all ages, but especially for young and middle age groups. More importantly, men have higher prevalence rates for key life-threatening chronic diseases: coronary heart disease, atherosclerosis, and emphysema. (Reported experiences of cerebrovascular events and diabetes are similar for men and women; data on malignant neoplasm experience are difficult to obtain in population health surveys.) Long-term disability in one's major activity (job or housework) due to chronic health problems is more common among men. The difference increases from about 10% at young ages to about 25% at older ones.

Summary

In sum, women have more frequent illness and disability, but the problems are typically not serious (life threatening) ones. In contrast, men suffer more from life threatening diseases, and these cause more permanent disability and earlier death for them. One sex is "sicker" in the short run, and the other in the long run. There is no contradiction between the health and mortality statistics since both point to more serious health problems for men.

Over the adult life course, the size and components of sex differentials change. Gaps tend to be largest in young adulthood and smallest for elderly people. For adults 17–44, reproduction events are a prominent (but *not* sole) factor in women's excess morbidity and health care. At older ages, women's excess in such conditions persists, and women have more short-term disability and minor limitations. But older men catch up to them in health services use because their problems are more severe and pose immediate threats to life.

It is important not to stereotype these sex differences. Obviously, men as well as women suffer from headaches and arthritis; women as well as men experience emphysema and die from it. In fact, when the leading problems (acute conditions, chronic conditions, or causes of death) are ranked for men and women, their lists are very similar. This means that men and women essentially suffer the same *types* of problems; what distinguishes the sexes is the *frequency* of those problems and the *pace* of death. The same conclusion emerges from measures of impact for illness and injury. That is, the leading problems that spur limitation, ambulatory care, and hospital episodes for men and women are very similar. What differs most are the rates, not the ranks.[4]

References. For discussions and data on sex differentials in morbidity and mortality, see Hing et al. (1983), Nathanson (1977a, 1984), Nathanson and Lorenz (1982), Verbrugge (1976a, 1976b, 1982a, 1983a, 1984a, 1985), Verbrugge and Wingard (1986), Waldron (1982, 1983a), and Wingard (1984). For data on drug obtaining and use, see Cafferata and Kasper (1983), Kasper (1982), Mellinger and Balter (1981), and Rossiter (1983).

THE ICEBERG OF MORBIDITY

Health statistics emphasize severe health problems and publicly visible health actions. Acute condition rates for the U.S. population, which come from the National Health Interview Survey, are based on only those problems which cause people to cut back their regular activities for whole days or which result in medical care. Until recently, chronic condition rates were based on problems which inhibit performance of a person's major (job/housework) or secondary activities; now rates are based on simply presence of conditions. The health actions most commonly measured are contacts with medical services. Drug data typically deal with how often people obtain medications and expenditures for them, not about actual use. Largely ignored are help from nonmedical health professionals, and the great variety of self-care actions possible besides restricted activity. In sum, the aches and discomforts that people endure without taking any action, or with entirely personal action, are missed in health statistics. This is the majority of ill health experience, not the minority.

This has a fascinating implication for sex differences: Problems which women experience more than men—the bothersome symptoms of nonfatal chronic conditions and acute conditions—are not captured well by national health statistics. These may be minor from a medical viewpoint, but they are not so in women's daily lives. Furthermore, because of more frequent minor symptoms, women probably take even more therapeutic actions than national statistics measure, especially self-care actions.

A visual metaphor may help: Only a small part of the "iceberg of morbidity" is visible in health statistics or in clinical practice (White et al., 1961). Its gender hue varies, most likely being deeply feminine at the bottom and gradually fading until it is intensely masculine at the very top. The bulk of the iceberg is a feminine shade.

These are speculations, but they are scientific rather than whimsical ones. Existing health statistics offer direct evidence that health experiences differ substantially for men and women, and they give clues about facets of health which are not measured. The full picture of lifetime health is not known, especially about symptoms of daily life and self-care actions for illness.

WHY ARE THERE SEX DIFFERENCES IN HEALTH?—HYPOTHESES

This question is the crux of social scientists' work on gender and health. Social science starts with an important question, proceeds with a fair-minded overview of possible answers, chooses some for empirical testing, and secures the best possible data to do so. In the past decade, sociologists and psychologists have suggested many hypotheses to explain why women are more troubled by acute and nonfatal chronic problems; why men have fewer but more serious conditions; and why women are more active in virtually all aspects of therapeutic care. Their hypotheses emphasize risks from roles and stresses, and also attitudes underlying symptom perception, health actions, and the reporting of health problems. Those hypotheses are organized and presented here, together with hypotheses derived from biology and epidemiology. After that, evidence on the hypotheses is considered.

There are five categories of explanation for sex differences in health: (1) biological risks of disease, (2) acquired risks of illness and injury, (3) psychosocial aspects of symptoms and care, (4) health reporting behavior, and (5) prior health care. Biological and acquired risks determine the occurrence of illness and injury. Psychosocial factors are involved in the social experience of illness that ensues; namely, the perception of symptoms, evaluation of their cause and severity, choice of therapeutic actions, continuation of treatment regimens, and role accommodations made for long-term problems. Further, when people report their health to others, there are added psychosocial inhibitors and inducers to discuss fully their discomforts. Lastly, health care for a current problem can influence one's future health experiences and health attitudes.

These differences between men and women in health risks, attitudes, reporting, and prior care have been proposed.

Biological Risks

These are intrinsic differences between males and females based on their genes or reproductive physiology which confer differential risks of morbidity. It is generally thought that males are less durable biologically than females, offset only during females' reproductive years by pregnancy-related and breast / genital-tract morbidity. Specific hypotheses are:

1. Women have greater genetic resistance to infectious diseases and also to some rare X-chromosome linked diseases.

2. Women are protected from cardiovascular morbidity by sex hormones up to the time of menopause.

3. The reproductive events of pregnancy, childbirth, and the puerperium give women unique morbidity risks not experienced by men. In addition, women's more complex reproductive system increases their risks of other female-specific disorders (these are neoplasms of breast /genital and genitourinary disorders such as cervicitis, menstrual and menopausal symptoms).

4. The pathology of some diseases—their symptoms and developmental course—may differ for men and women.

Acquired Risks

These are risks of illness and injury encountered in a person's work and leisure activities, from one's life style and health habits, psychological stress, and social milieu. It is generally thought that men have more risks from their jobs and household tasks, recreation pursuits, life style behaviors, health habits, self-imposed stress, reactions to stress, and social ties over a lifetime. Women have more risks in two respects, from more contact with young children and from more emotional distress. Specific hypotheses are:

1. Women have lower morbidity risks from their work tasks (job and housecare activities) because of (a) less employment, (b) safer jobs, and (3) safer housecare activities. First, homemaking poses relatively few risks of serious illness and injury compared to jobs. Second, employed women tend to have less

exposure to physical hazards (chemicals, noise, lifting and carrying, vibration, etc.) than employed men. Hypotheses vary about which sex finds more psychological hazards in their job tasks (due to repetitive actions, nonstop workload, little discretion in time allocation or decision making, etc.). Third, considering the types of household tasks men and women generally perform (whether homecare is their principal activity or not), men usually encounter more risks of serious injury than women do.

2. Men's choices of hobbies and sports boost their risks of injury, compared to risks women encounter in comparable activities.

3. Mothers generally have more contact with their children than fathers do, and this heightens women's risks of developing infectious diseases transmitted by children.

4. Men tend to smoke, drink, and drive more than women, and these behaviors markedly elevate their risks of some chronic diseases and injuries.

5. Women adopt more preventive health practices such as vitamin supplements, seat belt use, moderate alcohol consumption, and routine screening exams than men do.

6. Women feel more psychological distress (anxiety, depression, guilt, conflicting demands) on a day-to-day basis and over their lifetimes than men do, and this may decrease their physiological resistance to acute and chronic conditions. Women tend to be less delighted about life than men, and this may make them more vulnerable to stress-related illnesses. But women also buffer the route from stress to disease by reacting in more benign ways to disrupting life events and upsets. They turn to other people and to medical drugs for relief, whereas men opt more often for quiet brooding or overt behaviors like alcohol, smoking, and illicit drugs.

The most popular reasons offered for greater female distress concern women's social roles. Homemakers of this era are thought to feel unchallenged, bored, and undervalued. Employed women are believed to have excessive demands on their time and attention, since they relinquish few responsibilities for childcare or home management when they work.[5] Thus, because of too little social involvement or too much, contemporary women are presumed to feel frequently upset. In addition, some scientists posit that women's nurturant orientation—their attentiveness to others' problems and efforts to help—

places continual emotional burdens on their lives. All in all, it is argued that contemporary women have more stressed lives than men, no matter what they do.

7. Men may stress their bodies more by time pressures, drive to achieve, impatience, and other tensions. This array of self-imposed stresses is called the Type A behavior pattern.

8. Over their lifetimes, women maintain stronger emotional ties with more people. This hypothesis is about quality of informal ties, not about simple quantity. Intimate ties with friends, colleagues, and neighbors offer social support and deter loneliness. They may act as a buffer for disease—reducing its occurrence, severity, and especially its duration.

Psychosocial Aspects of Symptoms and Care

People vary in their perception of symptoms, assessment of symptom severity, readiness to take curative actions, and ability to do so. This collection of predispositions is often subsumed in the concept "illness behavior" in medical sociology. It is believed that psychosocial factors encourage greater awareness of physical symptoms among women, and also earlier and more persistent care by women for their symptoms.

The following hypotheses about psychosocial differences have been proposed:

1. *Perception:* Women are more sensitive to body discomforts than men are. This may come about because of childhood socialization (e.g., discouragement for boys to complain about bumps and bruises), more attention given to menarche and girls' puberty, and the body awareness that menstruation and reproduction provoke.

2. *Evaluation:* Women are more apt to label their symptoms as physical illness, and, after so labeling, assess their illnesses and injuries as more severe and serious than men do. Lower estimation of illness by men could come about because men tolerate physical discomfort better, are less interested in or concerned about their personal health, have less knowledge about signs of serious illness, feel it is not "masculine" to be ill, or wish to ignore the implications of symptoms for their usual activities.

3. *Action:* Given similar evaluations of illness

and injury, women more readily decide their symptoms warrant care. Once they decide action is needed, women are more likely to take it at all, and to take it sooner (with less delay). Women are more likely than men to favor professional help in their initial care for a problem.

Women's propensity to take actions for symptoms—to adopt the sick role—is based on greater willingness and ability to do so. Willingness hinges on numerous specific factors, such as (1) beliefs about the cause of a health problem, (2) beliefs about efficacy of different actions, (3) social pressures and dispensations for the sick role, and (4) psychological needs. Ability depends on (1) how readily people can take the time for care, (2) if they can incur financial costs of care, and (3) how accessible professional help is to them.

Taking each "willingness" factor one-by-one, we note:

First, there are no prominent hypotheses about how men and women differ in causation beliefs—whether health problems are due to one's own behavior, chance, God, family history, etc. One might hazard the hypothesis that women consider themselves responsible for health problems more readily than men do.

Second, women, more than men, may believe that bed rest, other activity restrictions, and medical care help a person become well.

Third, being sick and taking care of one's illnesses and injuries is more socially acceptable for women. This is a subtle aspect of gender roles stemming from long-term socialization into womanhood and manhood. Men may sometimes feel reluctant to care for their physical symptoms without knowing precisely why they feel that way.

Fourth, basic psychological traits may urge women toward medical care. They may be more dependent and help-seeking for any kind of personal problem than men, have less tendency to deny life troubles, and have more trust in authority. The notion of "learned helplessness" as more typical of women than of men fits here.

Looking at each "ability" factor separately, we note:

First, women may typically have more discretion in their time schedules and incur fewer costs for taking time off for curative actions. The argument about time is not that women have fewer objective time constraints, but that their schedules are more flexible and can be changed to accommodate health problems. (Time discretion may vary sharply among groups of women, so that homemakers have more than men, but women with job plus family roles have less.) Sociologists who note how the sick role is "compatible" with women's other roles are essentially pointing to time flexibility. A further note: Gender differences in objective time flexibility should be mirrored in men's and women's subjective views of time and time pressures.

Second, although married women and men have similar financial access to care, nonmarried women have less than male peers due to less adequate health insurance and lower incomes to purchase services.

Third, women have easier access to medical services because they have a regular physician more often than men do.

4. *Continued Care:* Women show more persistence in caring for their health problems—by purchasing drugs prescribed to them, complying with medical regimens, making followup visits or recommended referral visits, and even changing their roles permanently to accommodate health problems. Sex differentials for continued care have two facets: Not only do women take followup actions sooner than men, but they are more likely to take them at all.

Propensity to take protracted care depends, once again, on willingness and ability. Willingness stems from attitudes about prognosis and the recuperative effect of therapies, legitimacy of the sick role, and compliant personality traits. Ability stems from time flexibility, financial supports to purchase services and to permit job reduction, and familiarity with medical services. Some of these were previously discussed; they uniformly point toward greater motivation for continued care by women.

An especially important aspect of continued care is how employed people change their labor force activity in the face of chronic health problems. Married women with serious problems may drop out of the labor force more easily than married men do, because it is more likely that their spouse works and is the principal contributor to family income. For nonmarried people, the reverse may be true: Nonmarried women who have children at home to support and less adequate pensions and disability payments than their male peers may feel greater pressure to continue working when ill.

Summary of Psychosocial Aspects. In informal terms, the stages of illness behavior are: "I do not feel good," "I am ill/injured and it is very uncomfortable," "I am going to do something about this problem," and "I will continue to care for this problem until it disappears or abates." This is a typical sequence of stages, reflecting the discretionary aspect of illness behavior. Individuals can stop at any point; for example, deciding that a symptom is not worth mental attention or scrutiny, or going on a business trip despite the flu. Stages may be skipped when nondiscretionary factors intrude, that is, when someone else makes the decision about the ailment and care. For example, people may have an asymptomatic disease diagnosed during a general physical examination or they may find themselves admitted to a hospital after a heart attack.

The psychosocial hypotheses stated above are quite simple. In real life, assessing and caring for health problems are more complex. For example, the distinction between physical and mental distress that scientists make is probably not one that people make so clearly in their daily lives. Men and women may differ in how they ascribe symptoms to physical or emotional problems (and also in the actual interpenetration of the two). Further, people differ in the whole course of care and the continuity of care for a problem. Men and women may differ substantially in the sequencing of care for illness episodes and lifelong chronic ailments.

The many psychosocial differences between men and women do not "just happen"; rather, they have two key sources. First, childhood socialization about health differs for boys and girls, and it later underlies their adult health perceptions and attitudes. Second, adult role commitments are important factors in how readily men and women decide they have a serious health problem and in how they choose therapeutic care. In sum, broad cultural and social forces act to separate the sexes in their personal health ethos and their sick role propensity.

Health Reporting Behavior

When people talk about their symptoms and diseases, they do not always tell the full story: They commonly forget some actions taken in the past for their problems, and the words they choose to describe a discomfort may vary. Moreover, when people dis-

cuss the health of another household member, they may have limited information about that person's problems and health actions. It is generally thought that women are more complete and detailed reporters in interview settings, and also in clinical ones, than men. Specific hypotheses for sex differentials in health reporting behavior are the following:

1. Women are more willing to tell their symptoms to others—whether the "others" are interviewers, physicians, friends, or employers. This may be especially true for conditions considered embarrassing or fearsome; for example, genitourinary problems, hemorrhoids, cancer. The willingness may be due to greater social acceptance of sickness among women, and also to greater compliance in the interview task.

2. Women recall minor health problems and minor health actions better than men do. The presumed reason is that women are more interested in health matters and also more often involved in them as a health helper for children and kin, and this greater salience enhances their memory. It is less likely that women and men differ in recall of major health problems such as life-threatening chronic diseases or major health care such as hospital episodes.

3. The "vocabulary of illness" differs for women and men. Women may use different words than men do for the same physical symptom. They may elaborate more, giving more details about how a symptom feels. Women may discuss more often the psychological effects of their physical symptoms; thus their presentation includes both somatic and psychological content more often.

4. Women are more commonly proxy respondents for household members than men are, and this might affect health statistics by reducing some rates for men. Proxy respondents for absent adults can be unaware of asymptomatic chronic conditions or some acute conditions those individuals had, and of their drug-taking or activity restrictions. Proxies may also forget what they do know about the other adults more easily than their own health experiences.

Prior Health Care and Caretakers as Causes

So far, we have discussed health care as the outcome of symptoms and motivations, but health care can also act as their cause.

Health actions (restricted activity, drug use, etc.) are done with the intention of influencing the course of current disease. How well they succeed for a given person affects his/her likelihood of trying them again for flareups or new problems. When medical care is sought, physicians become important factors in determining the actions for current symptoms, long-term programs of treatment, and future attitudes about medical care. In sum, health care can influence the course of current illness, future risks of illness and injury, and even future illness perceptions and attitudes. As a result of their lifetime experiences of self-care and medical care, women may derive more benefits than men for long-term health risks and also get more reinforcement to be attentive to symptoms and take remedies for them. Specific hypotheses are:

1. Women's more active care for symptoms speeds their recovery from current problems, slows the progress of chronic problems, and enhances their resistance to new diseases.

2. Women's more frequent medical care boosts their chances of early diagnosis of asymptomatic problems and of effective treatment for them.

3. Experience with the sick role can change health perceptions, knowledge, and attitudes. Women develop keener recognition of important signs of diseases, more familiarity with medical services available, more trust (or distrust) of medical therapy, better understanding of what relieves symptoms, and more (or less) willingness to use medical drugs. In turn, these changes affect their future health care experiences and prognoses. Psychosocial aspects of health may be more dynamic over women's lifetimes than men's.

4. Physicians sometimes respond differently to men and women patients who present the same complaint, offering different diagnoses and treatments. Differential care can reflect sound medical practice since a given symptom often signals a variety of diseases, which can vary in frequency for the two sexes. Further, personal consideration of patients' social and psychological circumstances can also lead to some systematic differences in care for men and women; this too can be sound medical practice. But differential care based on inflexible attitudes about men and women (their ailments, time constraints, treatment preferences, psyches, etc.) is not legitimate; this is called physician sex bias. Some scientists and writers argue that sex bias is a common feature of medical care, leading to more psychologically toned diagnoses, unnecessary diagnostic services, and excess drug prescribing for women patients.

Summary of Hypotheses

The purpose of this section has been to present a comprehensive list of hypotheses advanced by social scientists, and to arrange them in a simple and coherent fashion. Readers will find some very familiar hypotheses here, while others are new or are now integrated into a larger scheme. The framework readily allows additional hypotheses to be added in the future.

References. Some of the hypotheses above have been elaborated at length in prior theoretical papers. Readers are referred especially to Mechanic (1976), Nathanson (1975, 1977a), and Verbrugge (1976a, 1979), which have a broad scope of hypotheses.

WHY ARE THERE SEX DIFFERENCES IN HEALTH?—THE EVIDENCE

What do we now know about the hypotheses on gender and health? In the past decade, social researchers have scrutinized available biological, epidemiological, and social evidence and they have designed analyses to test specific hypotheses. This section aims to distill research findings and then to compare the weight of the five key factors for gender differences (namely, inherited risk, acquired risk, psychosocial, health reporting, and prior care). After discussion of each factor, we will cite references that offer the most extensive reviews and most pertinent tests. (Numbers used below refer to our prior Hypotheses section.)

Inherited Risks

1 & 2. Women's intrinsic protection through genes and hormones is well documented. But the mechanisms by which sex hormones buffer cardiovascular disease are not fully known.

3. Reproductive conditions (pregnancy, childbirth, disorders of puerperium) account for a substantial amount, but not all, of women's excess morbidity and health care at ages 17–44. When re-

productive conditions are removed from the data, large sex differences persist in acute condition incidence and in discretionary (nonhospital) health care. Sex-specific problems cause more short-term morbidity for women than men until elderly ages, when men's prostate troubles ascend sharply in prevalence.

4. There is as yet no evidence to suggest that men and women differ in the pathology of particular diseases.

References.   Biological factors are discussed extensively in Nathanson and Lorenz (1982) and Waldron (1938b).

Acquired Risks

1 & 2. That men's jobs, household work, and leisure activities generally pose greater risks of illness and injury than women's is usually taken for granted rather than demonstrated. For example, to the author's knowledge, there has been no comparative analysis of the male and female work forces to measure the extent of hazards each sex confronts and the length of lifetime exposure to those hazards. Current interest in occupational hazards for women, especially in jobs where they are the majority work force, offsets the historical focus on men and gives better overall balance to our knowledge about job hazards. But overt comparative research on risks in men's and women's activities is still needed.

3. Risks of common respiratory infections have been shown to be higher among women in several longitudinal studies of family illness. This is, however, a small facet of the total health picture for men and women.

4. Men are more likely to engage in certain behaviors antithetical to health. Men's higher lifetime intake of tobacco products is now considered the foremost reason for their higher cancer morbidity and mortality, and a principal reason for their higher cardiovascular disease rates. Men's greater alcohol intake also contributes to excess morbidity and mortality from cardiovascular diseases and cirrhosis of liver; and their driving frequency and style, to injury and deaths from motor vehicle accidents.

5. There is no consistent gender difference in preventive health behaviors. Women excel in many respects, such as vitamin use, frequency of brushing teeth, and physical checkups when not sick. Men

excel in a few, such as strenuous exercise and chest X-rays. Sleep, eating routine, fluid intake, regular exercise habits, seat belt use, and eye exams are quite similar. Because preventive health practices are highly changeable in society and within an individual's lifetime, these gender differences may not endure. The central research issue now is whether preventive practices confer a health benefit to individuals; longitudinal surveys indicate the answer is yes. This may not go far in explaining sex differentials in morbidity and mortality, however, since women do not consistently engage in more healthful habits.

6 & 7. Research is very active on men's and women's levels of stress and their reactions to it. Findings indicate that contemporary women feel more daily and long-term emotional distress, and they are less happy about life and less satisfied with their roles. By contrast, men have more intense self-drive. How adults cope with stress and low morale, and if women cope in less health damaging ways, is still uncertain. Also, how stress is physiologically transformed into acute and chronic disease is not fully known, but evidence of causal links is accumulating.

In the past decade, there has been active research on how social roles (job, marriage, parenthood) are linked to health status of men and women. It offers some indirect clues about stress. Employment and marriage are consistently associated with good health for both sexes, and people with both roles are healthiest. Nonmarried women who work and also have children have poorer health than their peers without children; but children make no health difference for employed married women. Such findings inspire the following questions: Is marriage an important protector for women, offering a context in which they can safely manage both a job and children? Do active social roles and multiple roles offer enough satisfactions and rewards to offset stresses, for both sexes, so that they help maintain or even enhance health? By contrast, does inactivity pose great stresses (financial, social, emotional) for contemporary adults and ultimately harm their health? The fact that contemporary women are less often employed or married than men may be key explanatory factors for women's higher morbidity and health care.

8. Women's informal social networks tend to be

larger than men's, and their ties are also more intimate and active. Evidence is growing that social ties favor health and longevity, possibly by buffering the impact of social stress on health. If further research sustains this relationship, then it would seem that contemporary women gain more health benefits from their social supports and ties than men do.

References.   There are many review articles on sex differences in acquired risks. Readers are especially referred to Nathanson (1977a, 1977b), Ortmeyer (1979), Verbrugge (1976a, 1982a), Waldron (1976, 1982, 1983a), and Wingard (1984). These offer ample reference lists.

We shall point out some key references for specific risks here: For occupational hazards encountered by women, see Stellman (1977, 1978). For research on family health, see Dingle et al. (1964). For the importance of men's smoking, see Waldron (1985). For data on health habits of men and women, see Danchik et al. (1981), Mechanic and Cleary (1980), National Analysts Inc. (1972), and Schoenborn et al. (1981); and for links between preventive health habits and subsequent health or mortality, Belloc (1973), Branch and Jette (1984), and Wiley and Camacho (1980). For sex differences in distress and role stress, see Al-Issa (1982); Aneshensel et al. (1981), Gove (1985, but see critique by Marcus et al., 1985), Guttentag et al. (1980), and Veroff et al. (1981); for links between stress and health, Cohen (1979), Cooper (1983), Elliott and Eisdorfer (1982), House (1981), Rabkin and Struening (1976), and Stroebe and Strocbc (1983); and for links between happiness/satisfaction and health, Maddox and Douglass (1974), Palmore (1969a, 1969b), and Verbrugge (1982b). For research and reviews on roles and health, see Haw (1982), Haynes and Feinleib (1980), Nathanson (1980), Sorensen and Mortimer (1985), Verbrugge (1983b, 1983c), Verbrugge and Madans (1985), and Waldron (1980). For research and reviews on gender differences in social ties, and the links between social ties and health, see Berkman (1984), Berkman and Syme (1979), Broadhead et al. (1983), Fischer and Oliker (1983), and Kaplan et al. (1977). For overview of risk factors for diseases which women often experience, see Gold (1984).

Empirical research papers on how acquired risks help explain sex differentials in morbidity and mortality are Gove and Hughes (1979, but see critiques by Marcus and Seeman, 1981a; Mechanic, 1980; and Verbrugge, 1980a), Marcus and Seeman (1981b), Marcus et al. (1983), Retherford (1972), Verbrugge and Depner (1980), Waldron (1985), Wingard (1982), and Wingard et al. (1983).

Psychosocial Aspects of Symptoms and Care

Despite the plethora of hypotheses, there are few answers. Our review will accordingly indicate absence as well as presence of evidence.

1. Whether women are more body sensitive and symptom sensitive than men is unknown. Symptom perception may be an important cause of gender differences in day-to-day health experiences. But it is resistant to study, being almost intractable in respondent reports and heavily veiled in projective data.

2, 3 & 4. Reactions to perceived symptoms, especially behavioral ones, are much easier to study. In line with this, almost no evidence exists about how men and women label feet symptoms and assess their severity. Instead, research has focused on whether symptomatic men and women restrict their activities, how long they do so, if they seek medical care for the problem, how much they use drugs, and if they change their roles for serious chronic illness. The evidence suggests that women and men with comparable health problems and work roles seek out medical care and restrict their activities at the same pace. Thus, men are not delayers compared to women. But women take more time off for the problem, and they are more likely to abandon employment in response to a serious health problem. Drug use by women remains higher even when morbidity is controlled; this is partly explained by their greater access to care, attitudes about symptom care, and psychological traits. In sum, the clues are that the sexes do not differ in tendency to take some care of their health problems or even in the timing of care, but that women take more extensive and prolonged care of them.

Studies of reactions to perceived symptoms have two basic designs—either choosing a single health problem and comparing men's and women's reactions to it, or choosing a health behavior (done for all kinds of health problems in a period of time) and finding predictors that explain sex differences. Both approaches lead to the same general conclusion.

To date, studies of the first kind have considered actions for life threatening chronic conditions such as cancer and heart disease. The timing of medical care and job continuation may not be very discretionary for these, especially if the problem develops rapidly. The same is true for severe infections or trauma. In such cases, gender differences in actions are likely to be quite small, and psychosocial factors not very important. By contrast, it is nonfatal chronic diseases with bothersome symptoms and milder acute problems that are most likely to reveal gender differences, due to psychosocial factors, in the timing and extent of health actions. Gender differences for these have not been studied yet. We shall come back to this point later.

Looking at the central precursors of health actions, we note: First, willingness to care for health problems has had surprisingly little empirical attention. Although community surveys often query adults' health attitudes and sick role propensity, gender differences have not been pooled and reviewed.[6] Several studies of children indicate that attitudes begin to differ very early in life. Boys and girls differ in their responses to pain, willingness to talk about symptoms, rejection of the sick role, and use of school health services. With respect to adult personality, "learned helplessness" is more typical for women, but how that specifically affects health behavior is not known. Second, ability to get care has been studied more than willingness to take care. Women have an advantage over men by having a regular physician more often. However, women also have the obstacle of fewer financial resources to cover medical expenses. Whether women have more time flexibility to take care of symptoms is not known now.

References. A fine, and isolated, sociological analysis of symptom perception and evaluation is in Davis (1981). Psychological research on health perceptions is reviewed in Pennebaker (1982). Analyses of how men and women differ in their behavioral responses to health problems are in Brown and Rawlinson (1977), Chirikos and Nestel (1982, 1984, 1985), Chirikos and Nickel (1984), Cleary et al. (1982), Hibbard and Pope (1983), Marcus and Seeman (1981b), Marcus and Siegel (1982), Marcus et al. (1983), Marshall et al. (1982), and Verbrugge and Depner (1980). Psychosocial reasons for gender differences in drug use are studied in Bush and Osterweis (1978), Cafferata

et al. (1983), Svarstad (1983), Svarstad et al. (1985), and Verbrugge (1982c).[7] Research on boys' and girls' health dispositions is reported in Campbell (1978), Gochman (1970), Lewis et al. (1977), Mechanic (1964), and Nader and Brink (1981). "Learned helplessness" is discussed in Garber and Seligman (1980).

Health Reporting Behavior

Hypotheses on this topic are common, but research is not. There is no convincing evidence yet that health reporting contributes to measured sex morbidity differences.

1 & 2. Willingness to report health problems, and memory about them, are difficult to study in a direct fashion. An indirect approach, comparing medical records with interview reports, shows no difference in how often women and men report their diagnosed chronic conditions, medical visits, and hospitalizations. (Any differences in the first item are presumed to reflect willingness; for the other two, memory.) Such research excludes the many acute and chronic symptoms people have which are not medically diagnosed and also the many minor health actions people take. We have no idea if men and women differ in their readiness to discuss these or in their keenness of memory about them.

3. "Vocabulary of illness" is an unstudied area with rich potential. Gender differences may not influence health interview data and statistics much. Their importance lies in clinical practice. Do men's and women's vocabularies influence the diagnoses and medical care they receive? It is especially important to learn if women's reports to physicians have more emotional content than men's, and if so, whether this leads to different care.

4. Evidence is still out about whether, and how much, proxy reporting depresses health statistics for men. In any case, it is an undesirable artifact of data collection procedures, and social scientists try to eliminate it whenever possible by securing self-reports.

References. For a review of research comparing medical records and interviews, see Waldron (1983a). Clues about vocabulary differences are in Verbrugge (1980b). Current issues about proxy reporting are in Mathiowetz and Groves (1985); additional discussion and references are in Nathanson (1978) and Verbrugge (1982a).

Prior Health Care and Caretakers as Causes

Speculation far exceeds evidence for these hypotheses, and they will be very difficult to test scientifically.

1 & 2. Statements that women benefit more from medical care than men do are buttressed more by presumption than by empirical proof.

3. To learn how health care influences future health and health attitudes requires prospective panel data for many years, and even with the best data it would be difficult to extricate the answer. We simply do not know if women's active responses to illness in the short-run help them in the long-run, though the hypothesis is frequently advanced.

4. There is limited evidence that physicians' images of men and women patients do differ, but no compelling evidence so far that different diagnoses and treatments ensue from such images. The findings about sex bias to date are based on small projective studies and on reviews of ambulatory care records. The data of choice are tape/video-recorded encounters of physicians and patients, but such data are difficult to gather in abundance and laborious to code. Furthermore, with even the finest observation data, separating the components of differential care given to men and women into legitimate medical factors and less desirable nonmedical ones is difficult.

References. Clues about how earlier health actions influence mortality risks can be found in Berkman (1975). Empirical research pertinent to physician sex bias is in Bernstein and Kane (1981), McCranie et al. (1978), Verbrugge and Steiner (1981, 1985), and Wallen et al. (1979).

A VIEWPOINT: WHY THERE ARE GENDER DIFFERENCES IN HEALTH

Based on the accumulating evidence and social science theorizing reviewed to this point, the author offers a summary view of gender differences in health. The first section takes sides on the hypotheses, and the second reflects on the relative importance of causal factors. These are personal summations with which readers may agree or not. The new hypotheses offered in the last section are especially important for future studies.

A View on the Hypotheses

The author subscribes to the following hypotheses:

First, due to both biological and acquired risks, men have higher incidence and prevalence of serious morbidity than women. Women have higher rates for most nonfatal chronic conditions, but the specific risks that cause this excess are unknown, largely because scientific attention has been aimed at life-threatening diseases. Nonfatal conditions accumulate over time and women end up with more chronic conditions on the average than same age men. Women also experience higher rates of most acute diseases and disorders. Apart from the obvious (that is, reproductive conditions), the biological or acquired risks that underly this excess of acute problems have not been systematically examined. Altogether, women have more real health problems in any time frame—daily, annual, lifetime—than men do.

Second, women's attentiveness to body discomforts increases their felt symptom experience and their evaluation of symptoms as illness. For *major* problems such as life threatening chronic diseases and severe acute conditions, women and men are similar in willingness and ability to take initial health actions. But women do take more extensive care for episodes (for example, more drugs or more kinds of actions) and more protracted care (such as more bed days per episode or earlier job retirement) for such problems. For *minor* health problems such as nonfatal chronic conditions and mild acute ones, women have stronger predispositions to take both initial and continued care.

Third, the sexes have similar recall ability and motivation to report major health problems and care. But women are better reporters of minor problems, because of both memory and willingness. Health reporting by men and women often differs in vocabulary and style, and women do include emotional content more often. Proxy reporting causes undercounting of minor health problems and actions, but it is a small factor in current health surveys (which focus on major events, not minor ones) and sex differences derived from them.

Lastly, women's greater health care in early years diminishes the severity of their problems compared to same age men, and it ultimately helps extend their lives.

The Relative Weight of Causes

What is the relative importance of biological risk, acquired risk, psychosocial, reporting, and prior care factors for the sex differences? The author offers this view:

The foremost reasons for sex differences in health are epidemiological—the outcome of *risks acquired* from roles, stress, life styles, and long-term preventive health practices. Differences measured in health surveys mainly reflect physiological, or medical, reality.

Psychosocial factors rank next. They are pervasive aspects of illness experience and behavior, and they operate to boost women's perception of symptoms and their health care for symptoms. Women's more active health care of all kinds is due primarily to more experienced and perceived symptoms, and secondarily to the psychosocial factors that encourage care. For recent research evidence on this point, see Cleary et al. (1982), Hibbard and Pope (1983), and Verbrugge (1982c).

For long-term health, *prior health care* ranks in the middle as a cause. It acts to change acquired risks and psychosocial factors over a lifetime. The more efficacious medical and personal therapies are, the more women's long-term risks are reduced and their motivation to care for new problems is reinforced.

Biological factors rank next as an overall cause of sex differences in morbidity and mortality. They have obvious importance in reproductive ages for women, and for sex-specific conditions at all ages for both sexes. Apart from that, their impact on sex differences is quite small over the life course. Overall they act to give an advantage to women.

Reporting factors nudge morbidity statistics in small ways. Their principal effect is to color interviews and medical histories.

Caretaker factors such as physician sex bias are of little importance in differential diagnosis and treatment. Though it occurs in some individual cases, its aggregate importance for sex differentials is small.

New Hypotheses

Even if the condensed summary above is sound, the specific risks that propel people toward specific dis-

eases and injuries vary. So do the attitudes and opportunities that determine how specific symptoms are experienced and treated. This implies that for illness behavior, (1) the relative importance of psychosocial factors versus risks will vary for different conditions, and (2) the relative importance of psychosocial factors as causes of gender differences will also vary.

Both of the foregoing depend on three key characteristics of the health problem: its temporal nature (acute vs. chronic), its ultimate threat to life (fatal vs. nonfatal), and its severity (stage of disease or degree of bother).[8] We hypothesize that:

1. Psychosocial factors are more important in responses to chronic, nonfatal, and low severity conditions than they are for acute, life threatening, and high severity ones. Taking each factor one-by-one: Chronic conditions give people repeated opportunities to try different therapies; the timing, types and duration of care will differ widely among people with a given problem. For nonfatal conditions like headcolds and osteoarthritis, individuals' discretion about care is great; it is much less for heart attacks and skull fractures. Similarly, occasional mild headaches and static moles permit plenty of discretion in response (doing nothing, personal care, medical care), but anemia and deep cuts propel most people toward medical care.

2. Diseases and injuries which allow psychosocial factors to operate strongly will also show greater differences in men's and women's illness behavior. Thus, the sexes will react *less* similarly to chronic, nonfatal, and low severity conditions than they do to acute, life threatening, and high severity ones. Conditions with all of the first-named characteristics inspire the greatest differences; those with none prompt the least. Thus, men and women will differ notably in their reactions to mild arthritis; less so for bruised elbows or persistent hemorrhoids, and they will react very similarly to advanced colon cancer and spine fractures.

These hypotheses center on the characteristics of *conditions* and urge research that controls for them. But social scientists often want to study particular *actions* instead, such as physician visits or drug use in a time period, hoping to locate reasons for sex differences in these general behaviors. Every type of action has a filtrate of conditions; that is, it tends to have limits in the nature/life threat/severity dimensions. The most discretionary actions have the broadest compass (for example, nonprescription drugs can be used for any kind of problem); the least discretionary ones have the narrowest (for example, hospitalization generally occurs for life threatening and high severity problems). We offer a third hypothesis:

3. The more discretionary a health action is, the more it allows psychosocial factors to operate (as determinants of its occurrence, timing, duration, frequency, etc.), and the larger sex differences will be.

A SOCIAL SCIENCE AGENDA

Social scientists' particular contributions to research on gender and health are to identify some of the acquired risks for specific diseases and overall health status, to study especially the psychosocial aspects of illness—how people perceive, evaluate, and care for symptoms, and to search for reporting effects in health surveys and medical offices. I offer here several general thoughts and strategies:

First, the essence of explaining gender differences is to find factors which (1) differ between men and women and (2) are important causes of illness, injury, or health actions. The two criteria must be kept in mind in the design of a study. Ignoring them at the outset inevitably clutters data and results.

Second, the simplest reasons for a phenomenon (which usually come first to mind) are often the most important ones in real life. Social science curiosity about psychosocial facets of gender differences in health must not lead to forgetting the more basic ones, namely the environmental and role exposures that lead to disease occurrence and subsequent care. Tests of psychosocial factors should control for acquired risk factors identified in epidemiological and social research, whenever possible.

Third, although the hypotheses about gender differences can be usefully tested for general measures of health (such as number of acute conditions or of prescription drugs in the past month), the best tests will come through study of specific symptoms and diseases. Such evidence will admittedly be more difficult to collate into generalizations, but that may be an acceptable price for the clarity of explanation gained.

Fourth, comparative analysis of conditions cho-sen on the basis of their nature/life threat/severity is needed to determine whether men and women differ in their reactions to "minor" and "major" health problems. *Single* studies which apply one theoretical design to *several* diseases will be more informative than trying to pool results from diverse studies of single diseases.

Fifth, reproduction events should be removed when analyzing general measures of health. Removing all sex-specific conditions (reproduction, prostate cancer, disorders of menstruation, etc.) should also be considered. What remains in that case are health problems for which both sexes are biologically eligible, and comparing risks and reactions for them is more illuminating as to psychosocial and other non-biological factors.

Sixth, unveiling the reasons for the strong links between role occupancy and health will go a long way to revealing the reasons for sex differences in health. The link between employment and health is very strong for both sexes; to a lesser extent, marriage is also related to good health. These are cardinal results for sex morbidity differentials because women have less lifetime employment experience and a larger percent of them are nonmarried. But precisely what risks and psychosocial factors are contained in "employment" and "marriage" are not known. Both quantity and quality aspects may be important in how adult roles influence disease vulnerability and people's attitudes about health actions. Social selection—how health influences roles—must also be addressed empirically, using long-term prospective data. For some evidence on selection, see Chirikos and Nestel (1985) and Waldron et al. (1982).

Seventh, a wide variety of data can be used; the important features are the quality of a data set and the good fit of hypotheses being tested. Prospective data that trace stages of illness behavior from symptom perception through the entire course of care are needed to see how men and women differ in all the psychosocial processes. Prospective data are also important for testing the causal efficacy of risk factors. Cross-section data are appropriate for many hypotheses about health attitudes and predispositions of men and women. They can also shed light on causal hypotheses about risks but not prove them. Combining self-reports and medical records offers especially good opportunity to study men and women with comparable clinical stages of a disease—their symptoms, evaluation, self-care, and medical treatments.

Lastly, many "women's health issues" can be addressed in the context of gender differences. More can be learned about women by comparing their illness experience and responses to men's than by studying them alone. To be sure, there are important research questions about sex-specific problems that do not permit comparative analysis. But for studies of other problems and of global health, men should ideally be included.

THE LONG PERSPECTIVE—TIME TRENDS AND THE FUTURE

We have focused on contemporary sex differences in health. Now we put them into a time perspective. What has happened to sex differentials in health and mortality in this century, especially the past few decades? What can be said about the future?

Time Trends

Throughout this century, American females have had a sizable longevity advantage over males. Around 1920 that advantage began to increase sharply, and each decade thereafter showed a widening gender gap. Over the same period, mortality rates dropped for both sexes—rapidly from the 1920s to the early 1950s, then more slowly for women and not for men until the late 1960s, when they began to drop rapidly again. In sum, risks of death have declined for both sexes but faster for females than for males.

There are new signs of change. The gender gap in mortality has stabilized in the past decade. Since 1975, the Male/Female ratio for age-adjusted rates is positioned at 1.79–1.80. In contrast to prior decades of increase, sex differentials for some leading causes of death have become stable; others have started to decrease; and some continue to widen but more slowly than before. These are important clues that the American population may be shifting toward greater equality in mortality for the sexes.

Because death generally occurs at older ages in the United States, the timing and cause of death reflect risks that individuals experienced over many years. Changes in risk factors for the population or a sex group do not show up immediately in mortality rates or sex mortality differentials. There has been energetic discussion about how women's increasing labor force participation will affect their longevity. Whether that effect is propitious or detrimental will not be known soon. To find the answer requires statistical patience until the cohorts of women who have been making these changes die, and also better knowledge of how role commitments influence health.

In the meantime, health statistics can offer information about changes in population health closer to the time that population habits and exposures change. Statistics from the National Health Interview Survey show signs that American men's and women's health has worsened since the late 1950s, especially since about 1970. The indicators of this are increased short-term disability rates, longer-lasting restrictions per acute condition, rising rates of chronic activity limitation, and higher prevalence rates for most fatal and nonfatal chronic conditions. The most likely reasons for the trends are *not* increased disease risks over the period, but instead: (1) falling mortality rates since the late 1960s, so that ill people are staying alive longer, (2) earlier medical diagnosis of chronic diseases, so that people are more likely to know about their problems, make accommodations to them, and report them, and (3) greater willingness and ability to suspend normal activities (especially job) for illness or injury. More people are wending their way through life with chronic health problems that are managed but never cured. In brief, the key factors for the trends are (we believe) psychosocial and prior care, not acquired risks.

For American women, the worsening health profile is concentrated among those with few roles (nonemployed nonmarried), whereas employed married women have had stable or improving health in the past two decades. (Trends for role groups of men are similar.) There is no indication, therefore, that multiple roles are impairing American women's health.

What has happened to sex differences in health in recent decades? From the late 1950s through the 1960s, there were signs of greater worsening for men than women, especially in chronic conditions and limitations. But in the 1970s, some new dynamics appeared. There are indications that health is worsening faster for women than men.[9] Again, this probably does *not* mean that acute and chronic disease risks have increased more for women. Instead, we wonder if the changes in diagnosis timing and sick role propensity noted above are truer (faster) for women? We can only speculate now and watch the health statistics as the time series lengthens to see if the new dynamics continue.

It is important to document recent trends in sex morbidity and mortality differentials, acknowledging that their stability and interpretation are uncertain. We cannot expect large changes in these differentials in short time frames (a decade is "short"). Observed changes may evanesce when more decades of data are available. The reasons for observed changes are uncertain and undoubtedly complex, and they may never be known.

A critical caution must be added: There is no simple equation between mortality and morbidity changes. For example, precisely how recent mortality declines have affected the health profile of Americans is not known. As a second example, the recent stasis of the sex mortality differential on the one hand, and worsening of women's health relative to men

on the other, might seem compatible trends. But their co-occurrence is not logically necessary. Manton (1982) proposes a "dynamic equilibrium" between population mortality and morbidity—a basic assertion that they causally influence each other. A formal theory for these interrelationships is needed but very difficult to develop; see Manton and Stallard (1982) for one approach. Such a theory would help us interpret trends better and also make better forecasts.

References.   For trends in U.S. mortality and in sex mortality differentials, see Crimmins (1981), McMillen (1984), McMillen and Rosenberg (1983), and Verbrugge (1980c, 1984b). For trends in health of the U.S. population, and trends in sex morbidity differentials, see Colvez and Blanchet (1981), Verbrugge (1976a, 1984b, Footnote 9 of this article), and Verbrugge and Madans (1985).

The Future

To think about the future health of American women and men, we need some theoretical banisters. Consider the rudimentary model in Figure 1. It states

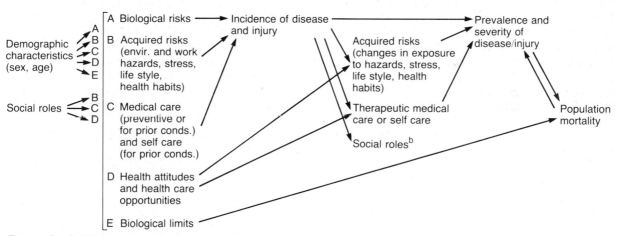

Figure 1 A Model of the Precursors of Population Morbidity and Mortality.[a]

[a] The model adapts readily to individual-level analysis by removing the arrow from Population mortality to Prevalence, and by eliminating Biological limits (E). It can then be expanded to include other psychosocial factors (perception, evaluation, reporting behavior): Incidence and prevalence are replaced by Reported incidence and Reported

prevalence; two new arrows come directly to them from Health attitudes; and Reporting behavior is added as a predictor (F) with arrows to them as well.

[b] Social selection effects are shown by the arrow from Incidence to Social roles. The ensuing possible reciprocal effects from changed roles to changed risks and therapeutic care are not shown.

that population mortality depends on the incidence, prevalence, and severity of diseases and injuries. Levels of morbidity, in turn, are influenced by biological risks, acquired risks, prior health care, health attitudes, and access to care. We are familiar with all of these from earlier sections of this article. One additional factor affecting mortality is proposed, called biological limits. These are intrinsic aging processes of humans which influence the timing and cause of death in the absence of disease.

This model is relevant for understanding population morbidity and mortality in the past, present, or future. The diagram is heuristic; it simply names the key variables we must consider and shows their temporal order of impact. It urges us to make overt statements about those factors, based on empirical knowledge or reasoned hypotheses, when we try to explain past trends, or understand current differentials, or foresee future changes.

We do not know enough about this model to make confident forecasts about future levels of mortality or sex differentials. (We must nevertheless respect the amount we do know already, especially about acquired risks for specific diseases.) So let us use it as a guide for thinking about an ideal scenario:

The most desirable future course is one with declining morbidity and mortality rates for both sexes and a narrowing of sex differences. This situation is feasible (1) if fatal and nonfatal chronic diseases can be prevented more effectively than now, and (2) if males and females have more similar lifetime risks and attitudes. On the first point, recent decades show great strides in disease treatment for people who already have a disease; the result is lower mortality but *higher* morbidity rates. To lower both rates requires disease prevention. This in turn will depend on major individual and societal changes and on further knowledge about risks so we know what changes to make. On the second point, men and women now have more options for their roles, leisure pursuits, and attitudes than 30 years ago. This is creating more variety within each sex group and, most likely, more similarity overall between them in health risks and attitudes. Over the long run, this should narrow sex differentials in morbidity and mortality.

References. For thoughts about future health of Americans, see Fries (1983), Ibrahim (1980), Lewis and Lewis (1977), Manton (1982), and Verbrugge (1984b).

We have used the model to discuss population rates of morbidity and mortality. It can be easily adapted to studies of individual-level health events (see Figure notes). It serves as a pictorial scheme for the hypotheses and thinking in this article.

Filling in the pieces of the model is the endeavor of many scientists in many disciplines. Answers will come by blending skill, imagination, and common sense in individual research efforts and also by vigorous communication and collaboration among biologists, epidemiologists, and social scientists. Only through such cooperation will we learn the full story about why men and women differ in their physical wellbeing and longevity.

Notes

1. This same history occurred for age differences. Once seen as fixed and therefore unremarkable by scientists, age differences are now thought to be more changeable across time as birth cohorts vary more in their attitudes and life experiences. Reflecting this dynamism, social scientists are devoting energetic attention to age differences and psychosocial reasons for them.

2. Table 1 uses 1980 data because that year is close to the years of health indicators shown in Table 2. Sex mortality differentials for years after 1980 are very similar (see recent Annual Summary issues and Advance Report of Final Mortality Statistics issues and Advance Report of Final Mortality Statistics issues of Monthly Vital Statistics Report, National Center for Health Statistics).

3. To the author's knowledge, national data on prescription (all types) and nonprescription drug use are not available. There have been several national studies of psychotropic drug use, and data from the most recent one are in Table 2. The 50% differences reported here are culled from several community studies (Baltimore, Detroit, and Marshfield, WI). Age-sex rates and ratios for these sites are available from the author.

4. Support for these conclusions is in another article (Verbrugge, 1985). Leading causes of acute illness, chronic illness and impairment, limitation due to chronic conditions, ambulatory care, hospitalization, and death are presented for American men and women in three age groups. Table 1 here has a small piece of the evidence,

showing how similar men's and women's ranks are for causes of death.

5. Pessimistic views about employed women have been countered by sociologists who point to the positive aspects of jobs for people. They suggest that the satisfactions and resources derived from paid work offset the stresses of multiple roles, so on balance employed women are less distressed and less vulnerable to illness than nonemployed women. Empirical data confirm greater happiness and role satisfaction among employed women.

6. The author's Health In Detroit survey shows surprisingly small gender differences in health attitudes. They are in hypothesized directions; for example, women feel more vulnerable to illness and believe more in the efficacy of self-care and medical care (Depner, 1981). Some gender differences are also reported in Cleary et al. (1982) and Hibbard and Pope (1983).

7. For several of these studies, gender differences in drug use were not the principal focus, but reasons behind the reported differences can be determined from the data.

8. Marshall et al. (1982) have suggested another characteristic, the specificity/identifiability of symptoms. This means whether symptoms can be readily diagnosed or not. We concur with their suggestion but believe this facet is less important than the three discussed. Hypotheses 1 and 2 can be augmented: 1. Psychosocial factors are more important in responses to ambiguous (low specificity) symptoms than nonambiguous (high specificity) ones. Individuals and physicians experiment more when they are not sure what the problem is. 2. Sex differences will be larger in responses to ambiguous symptoms than nonambiguous ones.

9. The author has reviewed annual data for 1957–81 from the National Health Interview Survey. These indications of faster health decrements for women during the 1970s appear: (1) Injury rates have risen slightly faster for women than for men, and women 45+ now show higher rates of injury than men 45+. (2) The impact of acute conditions increased for women in several ways. The average number of bed days per injury used to be smaller for women than men, but this has reversed so the number is now larger among them. The same reversal occurred for respiratory conditions at ages 45+; at younger ages, women have had more bed days per condition for the whole period but this disadvantage has increased recently. (3) Chronic limitations for major and secondary activities possibly increased faster for women ages 45–64 than for men these ages. (4) At ages 45–64, total disability days rose slightly faster for women than men. Further comments on recent trends in sex morbidity differentials are in Verbrugge (1983c).

References

AL-ISSA, IHSAN
1982 "Gender and adult psychopathology." Pp. 84–103 in Ihsan Al-Issa (ed.), Gender and Psychopathology. New York: Academic Press.

ANESHENSEL, CAROL S., RALPH R. FRERICHS, and VIRGINIA A. CLARK
1981 "Family roles and sex differences in depression." Journal of Health and Social Behavior 22:379–393.

BELLOC, NEDRA B.
1973 "Relationship of health practices and mortality." Preventive Medicine 2:67–81.

BERKMAN, LISA F.
1984 "Assessing the physical health effects of social networks and social support." Pp. 413–432 in Lester Breslow, Jonathan E. Fielding, and Lester B. Lave (eds.), Annual Review of Public Health. Volume 5. Palo Alto, CA: Annual Reviews Inc.

BERKMAN, LISA F., and S. LEONARD SYME
1979 "Social networks, host resistance, and mortality: A nine-year follow-up of Alameda County residents." American Journal of Epidemiology 109:186–204.

BERKMAN, PAUL L.
1975 "Survival, and a modicum of indulgence in the sick role." Medical Care 13:85–94.

BERNSTEIN, BARBARA, and ROBERT KANE
1981 "Physicians' attitudes toward female patients." Medical Care 19:600–608.

BRANCH, LAURENCE G., and ALAN M. JETTE
1984 "Personal health practices and mortality among the elderly." American Journal of Public Health 74:1126–1129.

BROADHEAD, W. EUGENE, BERTON H. KAPLAN, SHERMAN A. JAMES, EDWARD H. WAGNER, VICTOR J. SCHOENBACH, ROGER GRIMSON, SIEGFRIED HEYDEN, GOSTA TIBBLIN, and STEPHEN H. GEHLBACH
1983 "The epidemiologic evidence for a relationship between social support and health." American Journal of Epidemiology 117:521–537.

BROWN, JULIA S., and MAY E. RAWLINSON
1977 "Sex differences in sick role rejection and in work performance following cardiac surgery." Journal of Health and Social Behavior 18:276–292.

BUSH, PATRICIA J., and MARIAN OSTERWEIS
1978 "Pathways to medicine use." Journal of Health and Social Behavior 19:179–189.

CAFFERATA, GAIL LEE, and JUDITH A. KASPER
  1983 Psychotropic Drugs: Use, Expenditures, and Sources of Payment. Data Preview 14. National Medical Care Expenditures Survey. DHHS Pub. No. PHS 38–3335. Rockville, MD: National Center for Health Services Research.

CAFFERATA, GAIL LEE, JUDITH A. KASPER, and AMY BERNSTEIN
  1983 "Family roles, structure, and stressors in relation to sex differences in obtaining psychotropic drugs." Journal of Health and Social Behavior 24:132–143.

CAMPBELL, JOHN D.
  1978 "The child in the sick role: Contributions of age, sex, parental status, and parental values." Journal of Health and Social Behavior 19:35–51.

CHIRIKOS, THOMAS N., and GILBERT NESTEL
  1982 "The economic consequences of poor health, by race and sex." Proceedings of the American Statistical Association (Social Statistics Section) 473–477.
  1984 "Economic determinants and consequences of self-reported work disability." Journal of Health Economics 3:117–136.
  1985 "Further evidence on the economic effects of poor health." Review of Economics and Statistics 67: 61–69.

CHIRIKOS, THOMAS N., and JENNIE L. NICKEL
  1984 "Work disability from coronary heart disease in women." Women and Health 9:55–74.

CLEARY, PAUL D., DAVID MECHANIC, and JAMES R. GREENLEY
  1982 "Sex differences in medical care utilization: An empirical investigation." Journal of Health and Social Behavior 23:106–119.

COHEN, FRANCES
  1979 "Personality, stress, and the development of physical illness." Pp. 77–111 in George C. Stone, Frances Cohen, and Nancy Adler (eds.), Health Psychology—A Handbook. San Francisco: Jossey Bass.

COLVEZ, ALAIN, and MADELEINE BLANCHET
  1981 "Disability trends in the United States population 1966–76: Analysis of reported causes." American Journal of Public Health 71:464–471.

COOPER, CARY L. (ed.)
  1983 Stress Research. New York: Wiley.

CRIMMINS, EILEEN M.
  1981 "The changing pattern of American mortality decline, 1940–77, and its implications for the future." Population and Development Review 7:229–254.

DANCHIK, KATHLEEN M., CHARLOTTE A. SCHOENBORN, and JACK ELINSON
  1981 Highlights from Wave I of the National Survey of Personal Health Practices and Consequences: United States, 1979. Vital and Health Statistics. Series 15, No. 1. DHHS Pub. No. PHS 81–1162. Hyattsville, MD: National Center for Health Statistics.

DAVIS, MARADEE A.
  1981 "Sex differences in reporting osteoarthritic symptoms: A sociomedical approach." Journal of Health and Social Behavior 22:298–310.

DEPNER, CHARLENE E.
  1981 Predictor Variables. Technical Report No. 2. Health in Detroit Study. Ann Arbor, MI: Survey Research Center, Institute for Social Research, The University of Michigan. (Available from author of this article.)

DINGLE, JOHN H., GEORGE F. BADGER, and WILLIAM S. JORDAN
  1964 Illness in the Home. Cleveland: The Press of Case Western Reserve University.

ELLIOTT, GLEN R., and CARL EISDORFER (eds.)
  1982 Stress and Human Health. New York: Springer-Verlag.

FISCHER, CLAUDE S., and STACEY J. OLIKER
  1983 "A research note on friendship, gender, and the lifecycle." Social Forces 62:124–133.

FRIES, JAMES F.
  1983 "The compression of morbidity." Milbank Memorial Fund Quarterly/Health and Society 61: 397–419.

GARBER, JUDY, and MARTIN E. P. SELIGMAN (eds.)
  1980 Human Helplessness: Theory and Applications. New York: Academic Press.

GOCHMAN, DAVID S.
  1970 "Children's perceptions of vulnerability to illness and accidents." Public Health Reports 85:69–73.

GOLD, ELLEN B. (ed.)
  1984 The Changing Risk of Disease in Women: An Epidemiologic Approach. Lexington, MA: D.C. Health and Co.

GOVE, WALTER R.
  1985 "Gender differences in mental and physical illness: The effects of fixed roles and nurturant roles." Social Science and Medicine 19:77–84. (See critique by Marcus et al., 1985.)

GOVE, WALTER R., and MICHAEL HUGHES
  1979 "Possible causes of the apparent sex differences in physical health: An empirical investigation." American Sociological Review 44:126–146. (See cri-

tiques by Marcus et al., 1981a; Mechanic, 1980; Verbrugge, 1980a.)

GUTTENTAG, MARCIA, SUSAN SALASIN, and DEBORAH BELLE (eds.)
1980 The Mental Health of Women. New York: Academic Press.

HAW, MARY ANN
1982 "Women, work and stress: A review and agenda for the future." Journal of Health and Social Behavior 23:132–144.

HAYNES, SUZANNE G., and MANNING FEINLEIB
1980 "Women, work and coronary heart disease: Prospective findings from the Framingham Heart Study." American Journal of Public Health 70:133–141.

HIBBARD, JUDITH H., and CLYDE R. POPE
1983 "Gender roles, illness orientation and use of medical services." Social Science and Medicine 17:129–137.

HING, ESTHER, MARY GRACE KOVAR, and DOROTHY P. RICE
1983 Sex Differences in Health and Use of Medical Care: United States, 1979. Vital and Health Statistics. Series 3, No. 24. DHHS Pub. No. PHS 83–1408. Hyattsville, MD: National Center for Health Statistics.

HOUSE, JAMES S.
1981 Work Stress and Social Support. Reading, MA: Addison-Wesley.

IBRAHIM, MICHEL A.
1980 "The changing health state of women." American Journal of Public Health 70:120–121.

KAPLAN, BERTON H., JOHN C. CASSEL, and SUSAN GORE
1977 "Social support and health." Medical Care 15 (Supplement):47–58.

KASPER, JUDITH A.
1982 Prescribed Medicines: Use, Expenditures, and Sources of Payment. Data Preview 9. National Medical Care Expenditures Survey. DHHS Pub. No. PHS 82–3320. [Rockville, MD]: National Center for Health Services Research.

LEWIS, CHARLES E., and MARY ANN LEWIS
1977 "The potential impact of sexual equality on health." New England Journal of Medicine 297:863–869.

LEWIS, CHARLES E., MARY ANN LEWIS, and ANN LORIMER
1977 "Child-initiated care: The use of school nursing services by children in an 'adult-free' system." Pediatrics 60:499–507.

MADDOX, GEORGE L., and ELIZABETH B. DOUGLASS
1974 "Aging and individual differences: A longitudinal analysis of social, psychological, and physiological indicators." Journal of Gerontology 21:555–563.

MANTON, KENNETH G.
1982 "Changing concepts of morbidity and mortality in the elderly population." Milbank Memorial Fund Quarterly/Health and Society 60:183–244.

MANTON, KENNETH G., and ERIC STALLARD
1982 "The use of mortality time series data to produce hypothetical morbidity distributions and project mortality trends." Demography 19:223–240.

MARCUS, ALFRED C., and TERESA E. SEEMAN
1981a "Sex differences in health status: A reexamination of the nurturant role hypothesis. Comment on Gove and Hughes, 1979." American Sociological Review 46:119–123.

1981b "Sex differences in reports of illness and disability: A preliminary test of the 'fixed role obligations' hypothesis." Journal of Health and Social Behavior 22:174–182.

MARCUS, ALFRED C., and JUDITH M. SIEGEL
1982 "Sex differences in the use of physician services: A preliminary test of the fixed role hypothesis." Journal of Health and Social Behavior 23:186–197.

MARCUS, ALFRED C., TERESA E. SEEMAN, and CAROL W. TELESKY
1983 "Sex differences in reports of illness and disability: A further test of the fixed role hypothesis." Social Science and Medicine 17:993–1002.

1985 "Comment on Gove, 1985." Social Science and Medicine 19:84–88.

MARSHALL, JAMES R., DAVID I. GREGORIO, and DEBRA WALSH
1982 "Sex differences in illness behavior: Care seeking among cancer patients." Journal of Health and Social Behavior 23:197–204.

MATHIOWETZ, NANCY A., and ROBERT M. GROVES
1985 "The effects of respondent rules on health survey reports." American Journal of Public Health 75:639–644.

McCRANIE, EDWARD W., ALAN J. HOROWITZ, and RICHARD M. MARTIN
1978 "Alleged sex-role stereotyping in the assessment of women's physical complaints: A study of general practitioners." Social Science and Medicine 12:111–116.

McMILLEN, MARILYN M.
1984 "Twentieth century trends in United States mortality." Paper presented at the Population Association of America meetings. (McMillen: National Center for Health Statistics, 3700 East-West Highway, Hyattsville, MD 20782.)

McMILLEN, MARILYN M., and HARRY M. ROSENBERG
1983 "Trends in United States mortality." Proceedings of the American Statistical Association (Social Statistics Section) 88–92.

MECHANIC, DAVID
1964 "The influence of mothers on their children's health attitudes and behavior." Pediatrics 33:444–453.

1976 "Sex, illness, illness behavior, and the use of health services." Social Science and Medicine 12B:207–214.

1980 "Comment on Gove and Hughes, 1979." American Sociological Review 45:513–514.

MECHANIC, DAVID, and PAUL D. CLEARY.
1980 "Factors associated with the maintenance of positive health behavior." Preventive Medicine 9:805–814.

MELLINGER, GLEN D., and MITCHELL B. BALTER
1981 "Prevalence and patterns of use of psychotherapeutic drugs: Results from a 1979 national survey of American adults." Pp. 117–135 in Gianni Tognoni, Cesario Bellantuono, and Malcolm H. Lader (eds.), Epidemiological Impact of Psychotropic Drugs. New York: Elsevier Scientific Pub. Co./North Holland Biomedical Press.

NADER, PHILIP R., and SUSAN G. BRINK
1981 "Does visiting the school health room teach appropriate or inappropriate use of health services? Children's use of school health rooms." American Journal of Public Health 71:416–419.

NATHANSON, CONSTANCE A.
1975 "Illness and the feminine role: A theoretical review." Social Science and Medicine 9:57–62.

1977a "Sex, illness, and medical care: A review of data, theory, and method." Social Science and Medicine 11:13–25.

1977b "Sex roles as variables in preventive health behavior." Journal of Community Health 3:142–155.

1978 "Sex roles as variables in the interpretation of morbidity data: A methodological critique." International Journal of Epidemiology 7:253–262.

1980 "Social roles and health status among women: The significance of employment." Social Science and Medicine 14A:463–471.

1984 "Sex differences in mortality." Pp. 191–213 in Ralph H. Turner and James F. Short (eds.), Annual Review of Sociology. Volume 10. Palo Alto, CA: Annual Reviews Inc.

NATHANSON, CONSTANCE A., and GERDA LORENZ
1982 "Women and health: The social dimensions of biomedical data." Pp. 37–87 in Janet Z. Giele (ed.), Women in the Middle Years. New York: Wiley.

NATIONAL ANALYSTS INC.
1972 A Study of Health Practices and Opinions. Final Report to the Food and Drug Administration NTIS Pub. No. PB-210–978. (National Technical Information Service, U.S. Department of Commerce, Springfield, VA 22151.)

ORTMEYER, LINDA E.
1979 "Females' natural advantage? Or, the unhealthy environment of males? The status of sex mortality differentials." Women and Health 42:121–133.

PALMORE, ERDMAN B.
1969a "Physical, mental, and social factors in predicting longevity." The Gerontologist 9:103–108.

1969b "Predicting longevity: A follow-up controlling for age." The Gerontologist 9:247–250.

PENNEBAKER, JAMES W.
1982 The Psychology of Physical Symptoms. New York: Springer-Verlag.

RABKIN, JUDITH G., and ELMER L. STRUENING
1976 "Life events, stress, and illness." Science 194:1013–1020.

RETHERFORD, ROBERT D.
1972 "Tobacco smoking and the sex mortality differential." Demography 9:203–216.

ROSSITER, LOUIS F.
1983 "Prescribed medicines: Findings from the National Medical Care Expenditure [sic] Survey." American Journal of Public Health 73:1312–1315.

SCHOENBORN, CHARLOTTE A., KATHLEEN M. DANCHIK, and JACK ELINSON
1981 Basic Data from Wave I of the National Survey of Personal Health Practices and Consequences. Vital and Health Statistics. Series 15, No. 2. DHHS Pub. No. PHS 81–1163. Hyattsville, MD: National Center for Health Statistics.

SORENSEN, GLORIAN, and JEYLAN T. MORTIMER
1985 "Work and health among women: Models from the literature." Unpublished manuscript under review for publication. (Sorensen: Division of Epidemiol-

ogy. School of Public Health, The University of Minnesota, Minneapolis MN 55455.)

STELLMAN, JEANNE M.
1977 Women's Work, Women's Health: Myths and Realities. New York: Pantheon.
1978 "Occupational health hazards of women: An overview." Preventive Medicine 7:281–293.

STROEBE, MARGARET S., and WOLFGANG STROEBE
1983 "Who suffers more? Sex differences in health risks of the widowed." Psychological Bulletin 93:279–301.

SVARSTAD, BONNIE L.
1983 "Stress and the use of nonprescription drugs: An epidemiological study." Research in Community and Mental Health 3:233–254.

SVARSTAD, BONNIE L., PAUL D. CLEARY, DAVID MECHANIC, and PAMELA A. ROBERS
1985 "Why do women use more prescribed drugs? A study of biomedical factors." Unpublished manuscript under review for publication. (Svarstad: School of Pharmacy, University of Wisconsin, Madison, WI 53706.)

VERBRUGGE, LOIS M.
1976a "Females and illness: Recent trends in sex differences in the United States." Journal of Health and Social Behavior 17:387–403.-02
1976b "Sex differentials in morbidity and mortality in the United States." Social Biology 23:275–296.
1979 "Female illness rates and illness behavior: Testing hypotheses about sex differences in health." Women and Health 4:61–79.
1980a "Comment on Gove and Hughes, 1979." American Sociological Review 45:507–513.
1980b "Sex differences in complaints and diagnoses." Journal of Behavioral Medicine 3:327–355.
1980c "Recent trends in sex mortality differentials in the United States." Women and Health 5:17–37.
1982a "Sex differentials in health." Public Health Reports 97:417–437.
1982b "Work satisfaction and physical health." Journal of Community Health 7:262–283.
1982c "Sex differences in legal drug use." Journal of Social Issues 38:59–76.
1983a "Women and men: Mortality and health of older people." Pp. 139–174 in Matilda W. Riley, Beth B. Hess, and Kathleen Bond (eds.), Aging in Society: Selected Reviews of Recent Research. Hillsdale, NJ: Lawrence Erlbaum Assoc.
1983b "Multiple roles and physical health of women and men." Journal of Health and Social Behavior 24:16–30.
1983c "The social roles of the sexes and their relative health and mortality." Pp. 221–245 in Alan D. Lopez and Lado T. Ruzicka (eds.), Sex Differentials in Mortality: Trends, Determinants, and Consequences. Canberra, Australia: Department of Demography, Australian National University.
1984a "A health profile of older women with comparisons to older men." Research on Aging 6:291–322.
1984b "Longer life but worsening health? Trends in health and mortality of middle-aged and older persons." Milbank Memorial Fund Quarterly/Health and Society 62:475–519.
1985 "From sneezes to adieux: Stages of health for American men and women." Unpublished manuscript under review for publication.

VERBRUGGE, LOIS M., and RICHARD P. STEINER
1980 "Sex differences in health—Testing sociological hypotheses." Paper presented at the American Sociological Association meetings. (Available from first author.)

VERBRUGGE, LOIS M., and RICHARD P. STEINER
1981 "Physician treatment of men and women patients—Sex bias or appropriate care?" Medical Care 19:609–632.
1985 "Prescribing drugs to men and women." Health Psychology 4:79–98.

VERBRUGGE, LOIS M., and JENNIFER H. MADANS
1985 "Social roles and health trends of American women." Milbank Memorial Fund Quarterly/Health and Society 63(Fall issue).

VERBRUGGE, LOIS M., and DEBORAH L. WINGARD
1986 "Sex differentials in health and mortality." In Ann H. Stromberg (ed.), Women, Health, and Medicine. Palo Alto, CA: Mayfield Pub. Co.

VEROFF, JOSEPH, ELIZABETH DOUVAN, and RICHARD A. KULKA
1981 The Inner American—A Self-Portrait from 1957 to 1976. New York: Basic Books Inc.

WALDRON, INGRID
1976 "Why do women live longer than men?" Social Science and Medicine 10:349–362.
1980 "Employment and women's health: An analysis of causal relationships." International Journal of Health Services 10:434–454.

1982   "An analysis of causes of sex differences in mortality and morbidity." Pp. 69–115 in Walter R. Gove and G. Russell Carpenter (eds.), The Fundamental Connection Between Nature and Nurture. Lexington Books, D.C. Heath and Co.

1983a   "Sex differences in illness incidence, prognosis and mortality: Issues and evidence." Social Science and Medicine 17:1107–1123.

1983b   "Sex differences in human mortality: The role of genetic factors." Social Science and Medicine 17:321–333.

1985   "The contribution of smoking to sex differences in mortality." Paper presented at the Population Association of American meetings. (Waldron: Department of Biology, University of Pennsylvania, Philadelphia, PA 19104.)

WALDRON, INGRID, JOAN HEROLD, DENNIS DUNN, and ROGER STAUM
1982   "Reciprocal effects of health and labor force participation in women—Evidence from two longitudinal studies." Journal of Occupational Medicine 24:126–132.

WALLEN, JACQUELINE, HOWARD WAITZKIN, and JOHN D. STOECKLE
1979   "Physician stereotypes about female health and illness: A study of patient's sex and the informative process during medical interviews." Women and Health 4:135–146.

WHITE, KERR L., T. FRANKLIN WILLIAMS, and BERNARD G. GREENBERG
1961   "The ecology of medical care." New England Journal of Medicine 265:885–892.

WILEY, JAMES A. and TERRY C. CAMACHO
1980   "Life-style and future health: Evidence from the Alameda County Study." Preventive Medicine 9:1–21.

WINGARD, DEBORAH L.
1982   "The sex differential in mortality rates." American Journal of Epidemiology 115:205–216.

1984   "The sex differential in morbidity, mortality, and lifestyle." Pp. 433–458 in Lester Breslow, Jonathan E. Fielding, and Lester B. Lave (eds.), Annual Review of Public Health. Volume 5. Palo Alto, CA: Annual Reviews Inc.

WINGARD, DEBORAH L., LUCINA SUAREZ, and ELIZABETH BARRETT-CONNOR
1983   "The sex differential in mortality from all causes and ischemic heart disease." American Journal of Epidemiology 117:165–172.

Prevention

As is noted in the brief discussion of Light's comparison of the "professional" and "state" models of a health care system, found in the introduction to Chapter 13, in societies characterized by the professional model—where the perogatives of physicians determine the strategies to maintain good health and combat disease—prevention receives relatively little attention. There may be, however, one light at the end of the tunnel. Americans are certainly paying greater attention to the ills of such things as bad diet, smoking, excessive tanning, stress, and incautious driving as the term "wellness" is beginning to be heard throughout the land.

Changes in the diet of Americans provide one very good example of the important relationship between social epidemiological research and prevention. Epidemiological research has shown how diet is associated with cancer, heart disease, and a long list of other debilitating chronic diseases (Winikoff 1983). This knowledge of the health hazards of some of our traditional foodstuffs has apparently encouraged many Americans to modify their diets. For example, from 1982 to 1985 consumption of refined sugar and sugary foods dropped by 29%; salty foods and bacon and sausage, by 21%; hot dogs, luncheon meats, eggs, and beef, by 16%; fresh pork and soft drinks, by 14%; other fats and oils, by 11%; bread, by 10%; and butter, by 5%. Meanwhile, Americans increased their consumption of fruits and vegetables by 25%; poultry by 17%; fish by 15%; cheese by 8%; margarine by 6%; and shellfish by 4% (American Institute for Cancer Research 1985).

There is another light that is far less visible. Many environmental factors over which individuals have no control put them at risk. Just to name one, health risks in the workplace have received a great deal of attention within the last two decades. A number of studies have shown, for example, that black workers are far more at risk from their jobs than are white workers. Due to opposition from business and industry, public health measures directed at alleviating environmental sources of ill health in the workplace have not been developed in proportion to what needs to be done.

In the initial article, John B. and Sonja M. McKinlay present an argument that modern medicine has been far less important in the decline in disease-related mortality than have been preventative, public health measures. Looking at data for 10 major killer infectious diseases, the authors note that the decline in deaths from these diseases occurred well before the development of modern medical interventions, such as vaccines for the measles and influenza. After providing statistical evidence for their position, the authors conclude that "in general, medical measures have contributed little to the overall decline in mortality in the United States since 1900." An addendum to the McKinlay and McKinlay article illustrates the complexity of medical and public health measures influencing the decline in mortality in Milwaukee. The chronological listing of events and their relationship to the decline in mortality comes from the book *The Healthiest City: Milwaukee and the Politics of Health Reform* written by Judith Walzer Leavitt.

In the second article in this chapter, Carlos Castillo-Salgado presents a frequently expressed criticism of health prevention and promotion strategies, which are centered around the theme of the individual's responsibility for his or her health. In his view, this often amounts to "victim blaming" in a society in which the individual is consistently exposed to a vast number of societal influences encouraging unhealthy lifestyle practices. Unlike some writers, however, Castillo-Salgado does not completely reject attempts to change lifestyles for the purpose of better health. Rather, using the workplace as his context, he argues for a more comprehensive health promotion agenda where an emphasis is placed on improving those aspects of the environment that are damaging to the individual's health.

References

AMERICAN INSTITUTE FOR CANCER RESEARCH 1985. Trends in Food Consumption. *American Institute for Cancer Research Newsletter,* 8:8.

WINIKOFF, B. 1983. Nutritional Patterns, Social Choices and Health. In D. Mechanic (ed.), *Handbook of Health, Health Care, and the Health Professions.* New York: The Free Press, pp. 81–98.

Medical Measures and the Decline of Mortality

John B. McKinlay
Sonja M. McKinlay

. . . by the time laboratory medicine came effectively into the picture the job had been carried far toward completion by the humanitarians and social reformers of the nineteenth century. Their doctrine that nature is holy and healthful was scientifically naive but proved highly effective in dealing with the most important health problems of their age. When the tide is receding from the beach it is easy to have the illusion that one can empty the ocean by removing water with a pail.

R. Dubos, Mirage of Health, *New York: Perennial Library, 1959, p. 23*

INTRODUCING A MEDICAL HERESY

The modern "heresy" that medical care (as it is traditionally conceived) is generally unrelated to improvements in the health of populations (as distinct from individuals) is still dismissed as unthinkable in much the same way as the so-called heresies of former times. And this is despite a long history of support in popular and scientific writings as well as from able minds in a variety of disciplines. History is replete with examples of how, understandably enough, self-interested individuals and groups denounced popular customs and beliefs which appeared to threaten their own domains of practice, thereby ren-

This article originally appeared under the title "The Questionable Contribution of Medical Measures to the Decline of Mortality in the United States in the Twentieth Century" in the *Milbank Memorial Fund Quarterly/Health and Society*, vol. 55, no. 3, 1977, pp. 405–428. Copyright © 1977 by Milbank Memorial Fund Quarterly.

dering them heresies (for example, physicians' denunciation of midwives as witches, during the Middle Ages). We also know that vast institutional resources have often been deployed to neutralize challenges to the assumptions upon which everyday organizational activities were founded and legitimated (for example, the Spanish Inquisition). And since it is usually difficult for organizations themselves to directly combat threatening "heresies," we often find otherwise credible practitioners, perhaps unwittingly, serving the interests of organizations in this capacity. These historical responses may find a modern parallel in the way everyday practitioners of medicine, on their own altruistic or "scientific" grounds and still perhaps unwittingly, serve present-day institutions (hospital complexes, university medical centers, pharmaceutical houses, and insurance companies) by spearheading an assault on a most fundamental challenging heresy of our time: *that the introduction of specific medical measures and/ or the expansion of medical services are generally not responsible for most of the modern decline in mortality.*

In different historical epochs and cultures, there appear to be characteristic ways of explaining the arrival and departure of natural viscissitudes. For salvation from some plague, it may be that the gods were appeased, good works rewarded, or some imbalance in nature corrected. And there always seems to be some person or group (witch doctors, priests, medicine men) able to persuade others, sometimes on the basis of acceptable evidence for most people at that time, that they have *the* explanation for the phenomenon in question and may even claim responsibility for it. They also seem to benefit most from common acceptance of the explanations they offer. It is not uncommon today for biotechnological knowledge and specific medical interventions to be invoked as *the major reason* for most of the modern (twentieth century) decline in mortality.[1] Responsibility for this decline is often claimed by, or ascribed to, the present-day major beneficiaries of this prevailing explanation. But both in terms of the history of knowledge and on the basis of data presented in this paper, one can reasonably wonder whether the supposedly more sophisticated explanations proffered in our own time (while seemingly distinguishable from those accepted in the past) are really all that different from those of other cultures and earlier times, or any more reliable. Is medicine, the physician, or the medical profession any more entitled to claim responsibility for the decline in mortality that obviously has occurred in this century than, say, some folk hero or aristocracy of priests sometime in the past?

AIMS

Our general intention in this paper is to sustain the ongoing debate on the questionable contribution of specific medical measures and/or the expansion of medical services to the observable decline in mortality in the twentieth century. More specifically, the following three tasks are addressed: (a) selected studies are reviewed which illustrate that, far from being idiosyncratic and/or heretical, the issue addressed in this paper has a long history, is the subject of considerable attention elsewhere, attracts able minds from a variety of disciplines, and remains a timely issue for concern and research; (b) age- and sex-adjusted mortality rates (standardized to the population of 1900) for the United States, 1900–1973, are presented and then considered in relation to a number of specific and supposedly effective medical interventions (both chemotherapeutic and prophylactic). So far as we know, this is the first time such data have been employed for this particular purpose in the United States, although reference will be made to a similar study for England and Wales; and (c) some policy implications are outlined.

BACKGROUND TO THE ISSUE

The beginning of the serious debate on the questionable contribution of medical measures is commonly associated with the appearance, in Britain, of Talbot Griffith's (1967) *Population Problems in the Age of Malthus*. After examining certain medical activities associated with the eighteenth century—particularly the growth of hospital, dispensary, and midwifery services, additions to knowledge of physiology and anatomy, and the introduction of smallpox inoculation—Griffith concluded that they made important contributions to the observable decline in mortality at that time. Since then, in Britain and more recently in the United States, this debate has continued, regularly engaging scholars from economic history, demography, epidemiology, statistics, and other disciplines. Habakkuk (1953), an economic historian, was probably the first to seriously challenge the prevailing view that the modern increase in population was due to a fall in the death rate attributable to medical interventions. His view was that this rise in population resulted from an increase in the birth rate, which, in turn, was associated with social, economic, and industrial changes in the eighteenth century.

McKeown, without doubt, has pursued the argument more consistently and with greater effect than any other researcher, and the reader is referred to his recent work for more detailed background information. Employing the data and techniques of historical demography, McKeown (a physician by training) has provided a detailed and convincing analysis of the major reasons for the decline of mortality in England and Wales during the eighteenth, nineteenth, and twentieth centuries (McKeown et al., 1955, 1962, 1975). For the eighteenth century, he concludes that the decline was largely attributable to improvements in the environment. His findings for the nineteenth century are summarized as follows:

> . . . the decline of mortality in the second half of the nineteenth century was due wholly to a reduction of deaths from infectious diseases; there was no evidence of a decline in other causes of death. Examination of the diseases which contributed to the decline suggested that the main influences were (a) rising standards of living, of which the most significant feature was a better diet; (b) improvements in hygiene; and (c) a favorable trend in the relationship between some micro-organisms and the human host. Therapy made no contributions, and the effect of immunization was restricted to smallpox which ac-

counted for only about one-twentieth of the reduction of the death rate. (*Emphasis added. McKeown et al., 1975, p. 391*)

While McKeown's interpretation is based on the experience of England and Wales, he has examined its credibility in the light of the very different circumstances which existed in four other European countries: Sweden, France, Ireland, and Hungary (McKeown et al., 1972). His interpretation appears to withstand this cross-examination. As for the twentieth century (1901–1971 is the period actually considered), McKeown argues that about three-quarters of the decline was associated with control of infectious diseases and the remainder with conditions not attributable to microorganisms. He distinguishes the infections according to their modes of transmission (air- water- or food-borne) and isolates three types of influences which figure during the period considered: medical measures (specific therapies and immunization), reduced exposure to infection, and improved nutrition. His conclusion is that:

> *The main influences on the decline in mortality were improved nutrition on air-borne infections, reduced exposure (from better hygiene) on water- and food-borne diseases and, less certainly, immunization and therapy on the large number of conditions included in the miscellaneous group. Since these three classes were responsible respectively for nearly half, one-sixth, and one-tenth of the fall in the death rate, it is probable that the advancement in nutrition was the major influence. (McKeown, et al., 1975, p. 422)*

More than twenty years of research by McKeown and his colleagues recently culminated in two books—*The Modern Rise of Population* (1976a) and *The Role of Medicine: Dream, Mirage or Nemesis* (1976b)—in which he draws together his many excellent contributions. That the thesis he advances remains highly newsworthy is evidenced by recent editorial reaction in *The Times* of London (1977).

No one in the United States has pursued this thesis with the rigor and consistency which characterize the work by McKeown and his colleagues in Britain. Around 1930, there were several limited discussions of the questionable effect of medical measures on selected infectious diseases like diphtheria (Lee, 1931; Wilson and Miles, 1946; Bolduan, 1930)

and pneumonia (Pfizer and Co., 1953). In a presidential address to the American Association of Immunologists in 1954 (frequently referred to by McKeown), Magill (1955) marshalled an assortment of data then available—some from England and Wales—to cast doubt on the plausibility of existing accounts of the decline in mortality for several conditions. Probably the most influential work in the United States is that of Dubos who, principally in *Mirage of Health* (1959), *Man Adapting* (1965), and *Man, Medicine and Environment* (1968), focused on the nonmedical reasons for changes in the health of overall populations. In another presidential address, this time to the Infectious Diseases Society of America, Kass (1971), again employing data from England and Wales, argued that most of the decline in mortality for most infectious conditions occurred prior to the discovery of either "the cause" of the disease or some purported "treatment" for it. Before the same society and largely on the basis of clinical experience with infectious diseases and data from a single state (Massachusetts), Weinstein (1974), while conceding there are some effective treatments which seem to yield a favorable outcome (e.g., for poliomyelitis, tuberculosis, and possibly smallpox), argued that despite the presence of supposedly effective treatments some conditions may have increased (e.g., subacute bacterial endocarditis, streptococcal pharyngitis, pneumococcal pneumonia, gonorrhea, and syphilis) and also that mortality for yet other conditions shows improvement in the absence of any treatment (e.g., chickenpox). With the appearance of his book, *Who Shall Live?* (1974), Fuchs, a health economist, contributed to the resurgence of interest in the relative contribution of medical care to the modern decline in mortality in the United States. He believes there has been an unprecedented improvement in health in the United States since about the middle of the eighteenth century, associated primarily with a rise in real income. While agreeing with much of Fuchs' thesis, we will present evidence which seriously questions his belief that "beginning in the mid '30s, major therapeutic discoveries made significant contributions independently of the rise in real income."

Although neither representative nor exhaustive, this brief and selective background should serve to introduce the analysis which follows. Our intention is to highlight the following: (a) the debate over the questionable contribution of medical measures to the modern decline of mortality has a long history and remains topical; (b) although sometimes popularly associated with dilettantes such as Ivan Illich (1976), the debate continues to preoccupy able scholars from a variety of disciplines and remains a matter of concern to the most learned societies; (c) although of emerging interest in the United States, the issue is already a matter of concern and considerable research elsewhere; (d) to the extent that the subject has been pursued in the United States, there has been a restrictive tendency to focus on a few selected diseases, or to employ only statewide data, or to apply evidence from England and Wales directly to the United States situation.

HOW RELIABLE ARE MORTALITY STATISTICS?

We have argued elsewhere that mortality statistics are inadequate and can be misleading as indicators of a nation's overall health status (McKinlay and McKinlay, forthcoming). Unfortunately, these are the only types of data which are readily accessible for the examination of time trends, simply because comparable morbidity and disability data have not been available. Apart from this overriding problem, several additional caveats in the use of mortality statistics are: (a) difficulties introduced by changes in the registration area in the United States in the early twentieth century; (b) that often no single disease, but a complex of conditions, may be responsible for death (Krueger, 1966); (c) that studies reveal considerable inaccuracies in recording the cause of death (Moriyama et al., 1958); (d) that there are changes over time in what it is fashionable to diagnose (for example, ischaemic heart disease and cerebrovascular disease); (e) that changes in disease classifications (Dunn and Shackley, 1945) make it difficult to compare some conditions over time and between countries (Reid and Rose, 1964); (f) that some conditions result in immediate death while others have an extended period of latency; and (g) that many conditions are severely debilitating and consume vast medical resources but are now generally non-fatal (e.g., arthritis and diabetes). Other obvious limitations could be added to this list.

However, it would be foolhardy indeed to dismiss all studies based on mortality measures simply because they are possibly beset *with known limitations*. Such data are preferable to those the limitations of which are either unknown or, if known, cannot be estimated. Because of an overawareness of potential inaccuracies, there is a timorous tendency to disregard or devalue studies based on mortality evidence, even though there are innumerable examples of their fruitful use as a basis for planning and informed social action (Alderson, 1976). Sir Austin Bradford Hill (1955) considers one of the most important features of Snow's work on cholera to be his adept use of mortality statistics. A more recent notable example is the study by Inman and Adelstein (1969) of the circumstantial link between the excessive absorption of bronchodilators from pressurized aerosols and the epidemic rise in asthma mortality in children aged ten to fourteen years. Moreover, there is evidence that some of the known inaccuracies of mortality data tend to cancel each other out.[2] Consequently, while mortality statistics may be unreliable for use in individual cases, when pooled for a country and employed in population studies, they can reveal important trends and generate fruitful hypotheses. They have already resulted in informed social action (for example, the use of geographical distributions of mortality in the field of environmental pollution).

Whatever limitations and risks may be associated with the use of mortality statistics, they obviously apply equally to all studies which employ them—both those which attribute the decline in mortality to medical measures and those which argue the converse, or something else entirely. And, if such data constitute acceptable evidence in support of the presence of medicine, then it is not unreasonable, or illogical, to employ them in support of some opposing position. One difficulty is that, depending on the nature of the results, double standards of rigor seem to operate in the evaluation of different studies. Not surprisingly, those which challenge prevailing myths or beliefs are subject to the most stringent methodological and statistical scrutiny, while supportive studies, which frequently employ the flimsiest impressionistic data and inappropriate techniques of analysis, receive general and uncritical acceptance. Even if all possible "ideal" data were available (which they never will be) and if, after appropriate analysis, they happened to support the viewpoint of this paper, we are doubtful that medicine's protagonists would find our thesis any more acceptable.

THE MODERN DECLINE IN MORTALITY

Despite the fact that mortality rates for certain conditions, for selected age and sex categories, continue to fluctuate, or even increase (U.S. Dept. HEW, 1964; Moriyama and Gustavus, 1972; Lilienfeld, 1976), there can be little doubt that a marked decline in overall mortality for the United States has occurred since about 1900 (the earliest point for which reliable national data are available).

Just how dramatic this decline has been in the United States is illustrated in Fig. 1 which shows age-adjusted mortality rates for males and females separately.[3] Both sexes experienced a marked decline in mortality since 1900. The female decline began to level off by about 1950, while 1960 witnessed the beginning of a slight increase for males. Figure 1 also reveals a slight but increasing divergence between male and female mortality since about 1920.

Figure 2 depicts the decline in the overall age- and sex-adjusted rate since the beginning of this century. Between 1900 and 1973, there was a 69.2 percent decrease in overall mortality. The average annual rate of decline from 1900 until 1950 was .22 per 1,000, after which it became an almost negligible decline of .04 per 1,000 annually. Of the total fall in the standardized death rate between 1900 and 1973, 92.3 percent occurred prior to 1950. Figure 2 also plots the decline in the standardized death rate *after* the total number of deaths in each age and sex category has been reduced by the number of deaths attributed to the eleven major infectious conditions (typhoid, smallpox, scarlet fever, measles, whooping cough, diphtheria, influenza, tuberculosis, pneumonia, diseases of the digestive system, and poliomyelitis). It should be noted that, although this latter rate also shows a decline (at least until 1960), its slope is much more shallow than that for the overall standardized death rate. A major part of the decline in deaths from these causes since about 1900 may be attributed to the virtual disappearance of these infectious diseases.

An absurdity is reflected in the third broken line in Fig. 2 which also plots the increase in the proportion of Gross National Product expended annually for medical care. *It is evident that the begin-*

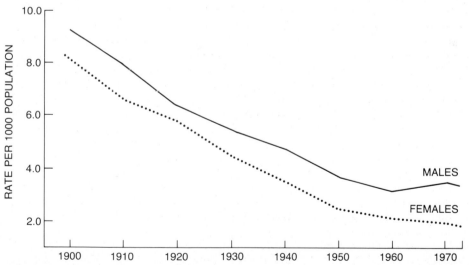

Figure 1 The Trend in Mortality for Males and Females Separately (Using Age-Adjusted Rates) for the United States, 1900–1973.*

* For these and all other age- and sex-adjusted rates in this paper, the standard population is that of 1900.

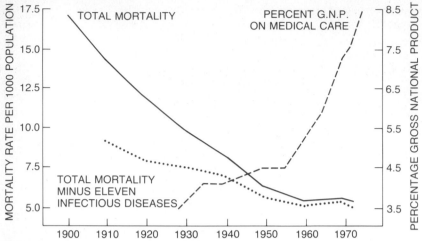

Figure 2   Age- and Sex-Adjusted Mortality Rates for the United States 1900–1973, Including and Excluding Eleven Major Infectious Diseases, Contrasted with the Proportion of the Gross National Product Expended on Medical Care.

ning of the precipitate and still unrestrained rise in medical care expenditures began when nearly all (92 percent) of the modern decline in mortality this century had already occurred.[4]

Figure 3 illustrates how the proportion of deaths contributed by the infectious and chronic conditions has changed in the United States since the beginning of the twentieth century. In 1900, about 40 percent of all deaths were accounted for by eleven major infectious diseases, 16 percent by three chronic conditions, 4 percent by accidents, and the remainder (37 percent) by all other causes. By 1973, only 6 percent of all deaths were due to these eleven infectious diseases, 58 percent to the same three chronic conditions, 9 percent to accidents, and 27 percent were contributed by other causes.[5]

Now to what phenomenon, or combination of events can we attribute this modern decline in overall mortality? Who (if anyone), or what group, can claim to have been instrumental in effecting this reduction? Can anything be gleaned from an analysis of mortality experience to date that will inform health care policy for the future?

It should be reiterated that a major concern of this paper is to determine the effect, if any, of specific medical measures (both chemotherapeutic and pro-

phylactic) on the decline of mortality. It is clear from Figs. 2 and 3 that most of the observable decline is due to the rapid disappearance of some of the major infectious diseases. Since this is where most of the decline has occurred, it is logical to focus a study of the effect of medical measures on this category of conditions. Moreover, for these eleven conditions, there exist clearly identifiable medical interventions to which the decline in mortality has been popularly ascribed. No analogous interventions exist for the major chronic diseases such as heart disease, cancer, and stroke. Therefore, even where a decline in mortality from these chronic conditions may have occurred, this cannot be ascribed to any specific measure.

THE EFFECT OF MEDICAL MEASURES ON TEN INFECTIOUS DISEASES WHICH HAVE DECLINED

Table 1 summarizes data on the effect of major medical interventions (both chemotherapeutic and prophylactic) on the decline in the age- and sex-adjusted death rates in the United States, 1900–1973, for ten of the eleven major infectious diseases listed

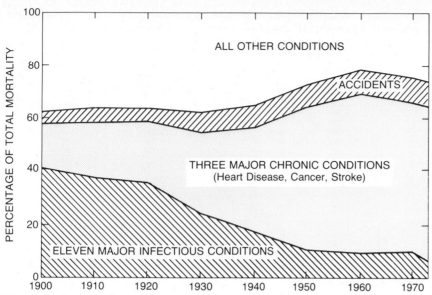

Figure 3 Pictorial Representation of the Changing Contribution of Chronic and Infectious Conditions to Total Mortality (Age- and Sex-Adjusted), in the United States, 1900–1973.

above. Together, these diseases accounted for approximately 30 percent of all deaths at the turn of the century and nearly 40 percent of the total decline in the mortality rate since then. The ten diseases were selected on the following criteria: (a) some decline in the death rate had occurred in the period 1900–1973; (b) significant decline in the death rate is commonly attributed to some specific medical measure for the disease; and (c) adequate data for the disease over the period 1900–1973 are available. The diseases of the digestive system were omitted primarily because of lack of clarity in diagnosis of specific diseases such as gastritis and enteritis.

Some additional points of explanation should be noted in relation to Table 1. First, the year of medical intervention coincides (as nearly as can be determined) with the first year of widespread or commercial use of the appropriate drug or vaccine.[6] This date does *not* necessarily coincide with the date the measure was either first discovered, or subject to clinical trial. Second, the decline in the death rate for smallpox was calculated using the death rate for 1902 as being the earliest year for which this

statistic is readily available (U.S. Bureau of the Census, 1906). For the same reasons, the decline in the death rate from poliomyelitis was calculated from 1910. Third, the table shows the contribution of the decline in each disease to the total decline in mortality over the period 1900–1973 (column b). The overall decline during this period was 12.14 per 1,000 population (17.54 in 1900 to 5.39 in 1973). Fourth, in order to place the experience for each disease in some perspective, Table 1 also shows the contribution of the relative fall in mortality after the intervention to the overall fall in mortality since 1900 (column e). In other words, the figures in this last column represent the percentage of the total fall in mortality contributed by each disease after the date of medical intervention.

It is clear from column b that only reductions in mortality from tuberculosis and pneumonia contributed substantially to the decline in total mortality between 1900 and 1973 (16.5 percent and 11.7 percent, respectively). The remaining eight conditions *together* accounted for less than 12 percent of the total decline over this period. Disregarding smallpox

TABLE 1 The contribution of medical measures (both chemotherapeutic and prophylactic) to the fall in the age- and sex-adjusted death rates (S.D.R.) of ten common infectious diseases, and to the overall decline in the S.D.R., for the United States, 1900–1973

DISEASE	FALL IN S.D.R. PER 1,000 POPULATION, 1900–1973 (a)	FALL IN S.D.R. AS % OF THE TOTAL FALL IN S.D.R. $(b) = \dfrac{(a)}{12.14} \times 100\%$	YEAR OF MEDICAL INTERVENTION (EITHER CHEMO- THERAPY OR PRO- PHYLAXIS)	FALL IN S.D.R. PER 1,000 POP- ULATION AFTER YEAR OF INTER- VENTION (c)	FALL IN S.D.R. AFTER INTER- VENTION AS % OF TOTAL FALL FOR THE DISEASE $(d) = \dfrac{(c)}{(a)} \times 100\%$	FALL IN S.D.R. AFTER INTER- VENTION AS % OF TOTAL FALL IN S.D.R. FOR ALL CAUSES $(e) = \dfrac{(b)(c)\%}{(a)}$
Tuberculosis	2.00	16.48	Izoniazid/ Streptomycin, 1950	0.17	8.36	1.38
Scarlet Fever	0.10	0.84	Penicillin, 1946	0.00	1.75	0.01
Influenza	0.22	1.78	Vaccine, 1943	0.05	25.33	0.45
Pneumonia	1.42	11.74	Sulphonamide, 1935	0.24	17.19	2.02
Diphtheria	0.43	3.57	Toxoid, 1930	0.06	13.49	0.48
Whooping Cough	0.12	1.00	Vaccine, 1930	0.06	51.00	0.51
Measles	0.12	1.04	Vaccine, 1963	0.00	1.38	0.01
Smallpox	0.02	0.16	Vaccine, 1800	0.02	100.00	0.16
Typhoid	0.36	2.95	Chloramphenicol, 1948	0.00	0.29	0.01
Poliomyelitis	0.03	0.23	Vaccine, Salk/ Sabin, 1955	0.01	25.87	0.06

(for which the only effective measure had been introduced about 1800), only influenza, whooping cough, and poliomyelitis show what could be considered substantial declines of 25 percent or more after the date of medical intervention. However, even under the somewhat unrealistic assumption of a constant (linear) rate of decline in the mortality rates, only whooping cough and poliomyelitis even approach the percentage which would have been expected. The remaining six conditions (tuberculosis, scarlet fever, pneumonia, diphtheria, measles, and typhoid) showed negligible declines in their mortality rates subsequent to the date of medical intervention. The seemingly quite large percentages for pneumonia and diphtheria (17.2 and 13.5, respectively) must of course be viewed in the context of relatively early interventions—1935 and 1930.

In order to examine more closely the relation of mortality trends for these diseases to the medical interventions, graphs are presented for each disease in Fig. 4. Clearly, for tuberculosis, typhoid, measles, and scarlet fever, the medical measures considered were introduced at the point when the death rate for each of these diseases was already negligible. Any change in the rates of decline which may have occurred subsequent to the interventions could only be minute. Of the remaining five diseases (excluding smallpox with its negligible contribution), it is only for poliomyelitis that the medical measure appears to have produced any noticeable change in the trends. Given peaks in the death rate for 1930, 1950 (and possibly for 1910), a comparable peak could have been expected in 1970. Instead, the death rate dropped to the point of disappearance after 1950 and has remained negligible. The four other diseases (pneumonia, influenza, whooping cough, and diphtheria) exhibit relatively smooth mortality trends which are unaffected by the medical measures, even though these were introduced relatively early, when the death rates were still notable.

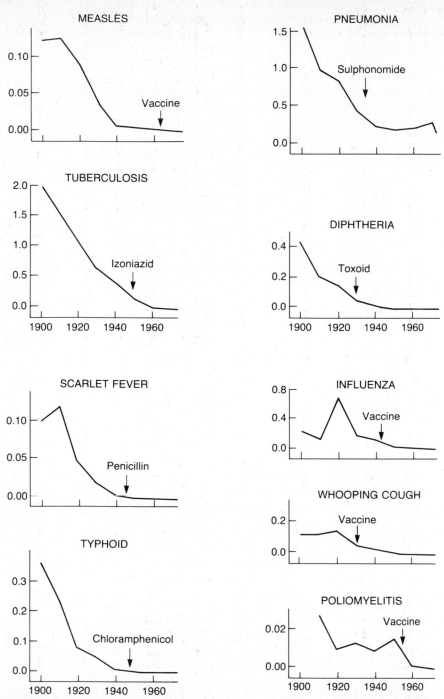

Figure 4 The Fall in the Standardized Death Rate (per 1,000 Population) for Nine Common Infectious Diseases in Relation to Specific Medical Measures, for the United States, 1900–1973.

It may be useful at this point to briefly consider the common and dubious practice of projecting estimated mortality trends (Witte and Axnick, 1975). In order to show the beneficial (or even detrimental) effect of some medical measure, a line, estimated on a set of points observed prior to the introduction of the measure, is projected over the period subsequent to the point of intervention. Any resulting discrepancy between the projected line and the observed trend is then used as some kind of "evidence" of an effective or beneficial intervention. According to statistical theory on least squares estimation, an estimated line can serve as a useful predictor, but the prediction is only valid, and its error calculable, within the range of the points used to estimate the line. Moreover, those predicted values which lie at the extremes of the range are subject to much larger errors than those nearer the center. It is, therefore, probable that, even if the projected line was a reasonable estimate of the trend after the intervention (which, of course, it is not), the divergent observed trend is probably well within reasonable error limits of the estimated line (assuming the error could be calculated), as the error will be relatively large. In other words, this technique is of dubious value as no valid conclusions are possible from its application, and a relatively large prediction error cannot be estimated, which is required in order to objectively judge the extent of divergence of an observed trend.

With regard to the ten infectious diseases considered in this paper, when lines were fitted to the nine or ten points available over the entire period (1900–1973), four exhibited a reasonably good fit to a straight line (scarlet fever, measles, whooping cough, and poliomyelitis), while another four (typhoid, diphtheria, tuberculosis, and pneumonia) showed a very good quadratic fit (to a curved line). Of the remaining two diseases, smallpox showed a negligible decline, as it was already a minor cause of death in 1900 (only 0.1 percent), and influenza showed a poor fit because of the extremely high death rate in 1920. From Fig. 4 it is clear, however, that the rate of decline slowed in more recent years for most of the diseases considered—a trend which could be anticipated as rates approach zero.[7]

Now it is possible to argue that, given the few data points available, the fit is somewhat crude and may be insensitive to any changes subsequent to a point of intervention. However, this can be countered with the observation that, given the relatively low death rates for these diseases, any change would have to be extremely marked in order to be detected in the overall mortality experience. Certainly, from the evidence considered here, only poliomyelitis appears to have had a noticeably changed death rate subsequent to intervention. Even if it were assumed that this change was entirely due to the vaccines, then only about one percent of the decline following interventions for the diseases considered here (column d of Table 1) could be attributed to medical measures. Rather more conservatively, if we attribute some of the subsequent fall in the death rates for pneumonia, influenza, whooping cough, and diphtheria to medical measures, then perhaps 3.5 percent of the fall in the overall death rate can be explained through medical intervention in the major infectious diseases considered here. Indeed, given that it is precisely for these diseases that medicine claims most success in lowering mortality, 3.5 percent probably represents a reasonable upper-limit estimate of the total contribution of medical measures to the decline in mortality in the United States since 1900.

CONCLUSIONS

Without claiming they are definitive findings, and eschewing pretentions to an analysis as sophisticated as McKeown's for England and Wales, one can reasonably draw the following conclusions from the analysis presented in this paper:

In general, medical measures (both chemotherapeutic and prophylactic) appear to have contributed little to the overall decline in mortality in the United States since about 1900—having in many instances been introduced several decades after a marked decline had already set in and having no detectable influence in most instances. More specifically, with reference to those five conditions (influenza, pneumonia, diphtheria, whooping cough, and poliomyelitis) for which the decline in mortality appears substantial after the point of intervention—and on the unlikely assumption that all of this decline is attributable to the intervention—it is estimated that at most 3.5 percent of the total decline in mortality since 1900 could be ascribed to medical measures introduced for the diseases considered here.

These conclusions, in support of the thesis introduced earlier, suggest issues of the most strategic significance for researchers and health care legislators. Profound policy implications follow from either a confirmation or a rejection of the thesis. If one subscribes to the view that we are slowly but surely eliminating one disease after another because of medical interventions, then there may be little commitment to social change and even resistance to some reordering of priorities in medical expenditures. If a disease X is disappearing primarily because of the presence of a particular intervention or service Y, then clearly Y should be left intact, or, more preferably, be expanded. Its demonstrable contribution justifies its presence. But, if it can be shown convincingly, and on commonly accepted grounds, that the major part of the decline in mortality is unrelated to medical care activities, then some commitment to social change and a reordering of priorities may ensue. For, if the disappearance of X is largely unrelated to the presence of Y, or even occurs in the absence of Y, then clearly the expansion and even the continuance of Y can be reasonably questioned. Its demonstrable ineffectiveness justifies some reappraisal of its significance and the wisdom of expanding it in its existing form.

In this paper we have attempted to dispel the myth that medical measures and the presence of medical services were primarily responsible for the modern decline of mortality. The question now remains: if they were not primarily responsible for it, then how is it to be explained? An adequate answer to this further question would require a more substantial research effort than that reported here, but is likely to be along the lines suggested by McKeown which were referred to early in this paper. Hopefully, this paper will serve as a catalyst for such research, incorporating adequate data and appropriate methods of analysis, in an effort to arrive at a more viable alternative explanation.

Notes

1. It is obviously important to distinguish between (a) advances in knowledge of the cause and natural course of some condition and (b) improvements in our ability to effectively treat some condition (that is, to alter its natural course). In many instances these two areas are disjoint and appear at different stages of development. There are, on the one hand, disease processes about which considerable knowledge has been accrued, yet this has not resulted (nor necessarily will) in the development of effective treatments. On the other hand, there are conditions for which demonstrably effective treatments have been devised in the absence of knowledge of the disease process and/or its causes.

2. Barker and Rose cite one study which compared the ante-mortem and autopsy diagnoses in 9,501 deaths which occurred in 75 different hospitals. Despite lack of a concurrence on *individual* cases, the *overall* frequency was very similar in diagnoses obtained on either an ante-mortem or post-mortem basis. As an example they note that clinical diagnoses of carcinoma of the rectum were confirmed at autopsy in only 67 percent of cases, but the incorrect clinical diagnoses were balanced by an almost identical number of lesions diagnosed for the first time at autopsy (Barker and Rose, 1976).

3. All age and sex adjustments were made by the "direct" method using the population of 1900 as the standard. For further information on this method of adjustment, see Hill (1971) and Shryock et al. (1971).

4. Rutstein (1967), although fervently espousing the traditional view that medical advances have been largely responsible for the decline in mortality, discussed this disjunction and termed it "The Paradox of Modern Medicine." More recently, and from a perspective that is generally consistent with that advanced here, Powles (1973) noted the same phenomenon in England and Wales.

5. Deaths in the category of chronic respiratory diseases (chronic bronchitis, asthma, emphysema, and other chronic obstructive lung diseases) could not be included in the group of chronic conditions because of insurmountable difficulties inherent in the many changes in disease classification and in the tabulation of statistics.

6. In determining the dates of intervention we relied upon: (a) standard epidemiology and public health texts; (b) the recollections of authorities in the field of infectious diseases; and (c) recent publications on the same subject.

7. For this reason, a negative exponential model is sometimes used to fit a curved line to such data. This was not presented here as the number of points available was small and the difference between a simple quadratic and negative exponential fit was not, upon investigation, able to be detected.

References

ALDERSON, M. 1976. *An Introduction to Epidemiology.* London: Macmillan Press, pp. 7–27.

BARKER, D.J.P., and ROSE, G. 1976. *Epidemiology in Medical Practice*. Churchill Livingstone, p. 6.

BOLDUAN, C.F. 1930. *How to Protect Children From Diphtheria*. New York: N.Y.C. Health Department.

DUBOS, R. 1959. *Mirage of Health*. New York: Harper & Row.

Dubos, R. 1965. *Man Adapting*. New Haven, Connecticut: Yale University Press.

Dubos, R. 1968. *Man, Medicine and Environment*. London: Pall Mall Press.

DUNN, H.L., and SHACKLEY, W. 1945. *Comparison of cause of death assignments by the 1929 and 1938 revisions of the International List: Deaths in the United States, 1940 Vital Statistics—Special Reports* 19:153–277, 1944, Washington, D.C.: U.S. Department of Commerce, Bureau of the Census.

FUCHS, V.R. 1974. *Who Shall Live?* New York: Basic Books, p. 54.

GRIFFITH, T. 1967. *Population Problems in the Age of Malthus*. 2nd ed. London: Frank Cass.

HABAKKUK, H.J. 1953. English Population in the Eighteenth Century. *Economic History Review,* 6.

HILL, A.B. 1971. *Principles of Medical Statistics*. 9th ed. London: Oxford University Press.

HILL, A.B. 1955. Snow—An Appreciation. *Proceedings of the Royal Society of Medicine* 48:1008–1012.

ILLICH, I. 1976. *Medical Nemesis*. New York: Pantheon Books.

INMAN, W.H.W., and ADELSTEIN, A.M. 1969. Rise and fall of asthma mortality in England and Wales, in relation to use of pressurized aerosols. *Lancet* 2:278–285.

KASS, E.H. 1971. Infectious diseases and social change. *The Journal of Infectious Diseases* 123 (1):110–114.

KRUEGER, D.E. 1966. New enumerators for old denominators—multiple causes of death. In *Epidemiological Approaches to the Study of Cancer and Other Chronic Diseases,* edited by W. Haenszel. National Cancer Printing Office, pp. 431–443.

LEE, W.W. 1931. Diphtheria Immunization in Philadelphia and New York City. *Journal of Preventive Medicine* (Baltimore) 5:211–220.

LILIENFELD, A.M. 1976. *Foundations of Epidemiology*. New York: Oxford University Press, pp. 51–111.

McKEOWN, T. 1976a. *The Modern Rise of Population*. London: Edward Arnold.

McKEOWN, T. 1976b. *The Role of Medicine: Dream, Mirage or Nemesis*. London: Nuffield Provincial Hospitals Trust.

McKEOWN, T.; BROWN, R.G.; and RECORD, R.G. 1972. An interpretation of the modern rise of population in Europe. *Population Studies* 26:345–382.

McKEOWN, T., and RECORD, R.G. 1955. Medical evidence related to English population changes in the eighteenth century. *Population Studies* 9:119–141.

McKEOWN, T., and RECORD, R.G. 1962. Reasons for the decline in mortality in England and Wales during the nineteenth century. *Population Studies* 16:94–122.

McKEOWN, T.; RECORD, R.G.; and TURNER, R.D. 1975. An interpretation of the decline of mortality in England and Wales during the twentieth century, *Population Studies* 29:391–422.

McKINLAY, J.B., and McKINLAY, S.M. *A refutation of the thesis that the health of the nation is improving*. Forthcoming.

MAGILL, T.P. 1955. The immunologist and the evil spirits. *Journal of Immunology* 74:1–8.

MORIYAMA, I.M.; BAUM, W.S.; HAENSZEL, W.M.; and MATTISON, B.F. 1958. Inquiry into diagnostic evidence supporting medical certifications of death. *American Journal of Public Health* 48:1376–1387.

MORIYAMA, I.M., and GUSTAVUS, S.O. 1972. *Cohort Mortality and Survivorship: United States Death—Registration States, 1900–1968*. National Center for Health Statistics, Series 3, No. 16. Washington, D.C.: U.S. Government Printing Office.

PFIZER, C. and COMPANY. 1953. *The Pneumonias, Management with Antibiotic Therapy*. Brooklyn.

POWLES, J. 1973. On the limitations of modern medicine. *Science, Medicine and Man* 1:2–3.

REID, O.D., and ROSE, G.A. 1964. Assessing the comparability of mortality statistics. *British Medical Journal* 2:1437–1439.

RUTSTEIN, D. 1967. *The Coming Revolution in Medicine*. Cambridge, Massachusetts: MIT Press.

SHRYOCK, H., et al. 1971. *The Methods and Materials of Demography*. Washington, D.C.: U.S. Government Printing Office.

THE TIMES (London). 1977. The Doctors Dilemma: How to Cure Society of a Life Style That Makes People Sick. Friday, January 21.

U.S. DEPARTMENT OF HEALTH, EDUCATION AND WELFARE. 1964. *The Change in Mortality Trend in the United States*. National Center for Health Statistics, Series 3, No. 1. Washington D.C.: U.S. Government Printing Office.

U.S. BUREAU OF THE CENSUS. 1906. *Mortality Statistics 1900–1904*. Washington, D.C.: Government Printing Office.

WEINSTEIN, L. 1974. Infectious Disease: Retrospect and Reminiscence. *The Journal of Infectious Diseases* 129 (4):480–492.

WILSON, G.S., and MILES, A.A. 1946. In Topley and Wilson's *Principles of Bacteriology and Immunity*. Baltimore: Williams and Wilkins.

WITTE, J.J., and AXNICK, N.W. 1975. The benefits from ten years of measles immunization in the United States. *Public Health Reports* 90 (3):205–207.

Addendum: A Chronological Outline of Public Health History in Milwaukee

Judith Walzer Leavitt

1837	Milwaukee incorporated as a village
1843	Smallpox epidemic
1845	Milwaukee Medical Association formed
1846	Milwaukee incorporated as a city consolidating three sections
	Smallpox epidemic
1849	Cholera epidemic
1850	Population: 20,061
	More than one-third of Milwaukee's population German
1860	Population: 45,246
1862	Anti-hog ordinance
1864	Citizen petition to state legislature to establish an independent Board of Health
1867	Permanent Board of Health established by state legislature

	Dr. James Johnson appointed President of the Board of Health
1868	Smallpox epidemic; vaccination campaign
	Passavant Hospital accepts city smallpox patients
	Schools closed due to smallpox in second, sixth, and ninth wards
	E. S. Chesbrough survey for city water works
1870	Population: 71,440
	Death Rate: 20.93
1871	Appropriation to begin construction of Chesbrough's water works
	Sewer pipes laid
	Milwaukee City dispensary opened
	Smallpox epidemic; vaccination campaign
1872	Smallpox epidemic hits German population most severely
	61 percent of all deaths under five years of age

1874   Health officer attempts slaughter house regulation

City water works opened

1875   "Swill children" replaced as garbage collectors by ward contracts

1876   Smallpox epidemic, hits immigrant Poles and Germans hardest

Push for city hospital

Wisconsin State Board of Health established (tenth in nation)

1877   Dr. Isaac H. Stearns appointed health officer

Prohibition on cutting ice below sewers

Health officer requests asphalt pavement for health reasons; ignored. Milwaukee streets paved with wood

Housing recommendations ignored by council

Purchase of land in eleventh ward for city hospital

Placard ordinance

Vaccination required for children to be admitted to public schools

1878   Dr. Orlando W. Wight appointed Milwaukee's first health commissioner

Board of Health becomes department of health

Health survey of public schools

Garbage contract let for whole city; disposal by feed and land fill

General milk ordinance prohibiting sale of impure milk; no enforcement provision

1879   Public suspicion of contamination in water supply

River nuisance

Night scavengers licensed and inspected by health department

City Isolation Hospital opened; no sewer or water connections

Crisis in garbage collection; six weeks with none

Survey of dairies conducted by health department

Milk ordinance rejected

1880   Population: 115,587

Death Rate: 20.68

Two assistants added to health commissioner's staff

Restrictions put on slaughtering process

Report of expert engineers—E. S. Chesbrough, George Waring and Moses Lane—submitted on intercepting sewers

1881   Dr. Robert Martin appointed health commissioner

Smallpox "scare"

1882   Milk survey conducted by health department; *Sentinel* exposes foul conditions of urban dairies

1883   Milk legislation fails to pass

1886   Health commissioner collected and disposed of city garbage; dumped in Lake Michigan

1887   River nuisance leads to appropriation for Milwaukee River Flushing Tunnel

Contract let to cremate city garbage

Milk ordinance passed to inspect milk and license vendors

1888   Ordinance restricts cattle slaughter to proscribed limits

American Public Health Association holds annual meeting in Milwaukee

Milwaukee River Flushing Tunnel completed

Storing of pure and polluted ice in same ice house prohibited

Compromise milk ordinance passed requiring registration in lieu of licensing; no inspections

Milk price jumps from 5¢ to 7¢ a quart

1889   Merz rendering plant disposes of city garbage

1890   Population: 204,468

Death Rate: 18.33

Dr. U.O.B. Wingate appointed health commissioner

Garbage "temporarily" dumped into Lake Michigan

1891   New water intake

Health commissioner recommends school medical inspections; no action

Milwaukee Anti-Vaccination Society established

Milk ordinance provides for licensure

of milk dealers, inspections, and out-
laws sale of swill milk

1892   Butchering within city proscribed; required to connect to city's sewer system

Privy vault construction limited and
regulated

Johnston Emergency Hospital opened

Cholera threat

Health commissioner given power to
remove to hospital anyone suffering
from contagious disease who is dangerous to the public health

"Garbage campaign" led to contract
with the Wisconsin Rendering Company to operate Merz plant in
Mequon

1893   City Isolation Hospital remodeled

Wisconsin College of Physicians and
Surgeons opened

State law provided for appointment of
Registrar of Vital Statistics

1894   Dr. Walter Kempster appointed health
commissioner

Smallpox epidemic; riots

Diphtheria antitoxin available in city

Repeal of forcible removal ordinance

Milwaukee Medical College opens

1895   Dr. Kempster impeached and removed
from office

Dr. H. E. Bradley appointed acting
health commissioner

Diphtheria stations around the city
distribute free antitoxin

1896   Dr. Kempster reinstated as health
commissioner

Five assistants and food analyst added
to staff

Laboratory begins functioning systematically

Public school nuisances corrected

Daily inspection of milk samples begins

Gridley Dairy pasteurizes milk

Civil Service legislation governs health
department appointments

1897   State Supreme Court decision, *Adams
v. Burdge,* limited authority to vacci-
nate schoolchildren without state
legislation

Garbage contract with Wisconsin Rendering Company expired; garbage
crisis results

First vote on municipal ownership of
garbage disposal plant passed

1898   Dr. F. M. Schulz appointed health commissioner

Bacteriologist and chemist added to
staff

Second vote on municipal ownership
of garbage disposal plant passed

Strong milk and cream regulation ordinance fails to pass

1900   Population: 285,315

Death Rate: 13.88

Privy vault construction prohibited on
streets having water and sewer pipes

Health department began medical inspection of schools to control spread
of infectious diseases (temporary)

Ordinance regulating sale of horse and
dog meat and sale of exposed food

1901   City Isolation Hospital #2 opened for
diseases other than smallpox

Governor vetoed bill providing for compulsory vaccination

Contract let for building municipal garbage plant

1902   Jones Island Crematory, city owned
and operated garbage incineration
plant, opened

1903   Milwaukee Medical Society Milk Commission formed

Straus Depot opened in Milwaukee under auspices of Babies Free Hospital
Association

1904   Movement to build a new city hospital

Anti-spitting ordinance

Smallpox epidemic

Certified milk sold at 14¢ a quart

Milwaukee County Medical Society appointed Tuberculosis Commission
(precursor to the Wisconsin Anti-Tu-
berculosis Association, 1908)

1905   City water contaminated; boiling urged

Milwaukee Medical Society urged systematic school medical inspections

1906   Dr. Gerhard A. Bading appointed
health commissioner

Bad meat scandal; meat markets to be licensed

Tenement law restricted ill-ventilated living conditions

City Building Inspector condemned City Isolation Hospital #2 as a fire trap

Milwaukee Medical Society executed trial medical inspection of schools

State legislation required vaccination of schoolchildren during an epidemic in their district

Bacterial inspections of milk begun

1907   Kinnickinnic Flushing Tunnel opened

Rudolph Hering report on garbage disposal in Milwaukee

Ordinance passed requiring milk to be bottled and sealed before sale

Visiting Nurse Association incorporated

1908   Ordinance on tuberculin testing of cattle passed; not enforced until 1926

1909   School medical inspection officially began under the School Board

Common Council adopted Hering's plans for garbage disposal

1910   Emil Seidel elected mayor with Socialist majority in the common council on platform that included free medical care for all

Population: 373,857

Death Rate: 13.90

78 percent of population foreign-born or foreign stock

Erie Street Garbage Incineration Plant opened; Jones Island Plant closed

Dr. F. A. Kraft appointed health commissioner

1911   Rendering within city limits prohibited; ordinance not enforced

Sewerage Commission report found city's water contaminated; filtration plant recommended

Construction begun on new city hospital

Blue Mound Sanatorium for tuberculosis patients

Medical inspection of private school-

children instituted under the health department

Responsibility for garbage collection and disposal shifted from the health department to the department of public works

Approximately 50 percent of Milwaukee's milk pasteurized

Milk plants scored by health department—only two receive "excellent" rating

Attack on "Hokey Pokey" ice-cream vendor

Child Welfare Commission opened fourteenth-ward demonstration project for free consultation on the care and feeding of infants

1912   City water treated with hypochlorite of lime

South View Hospital (new city isolation hospital) opened

Division of Tuberculosis created within health department

Child Welfare Division created within health department

Gerhard Bading, former health commissioner, elected mayor, non-partisan

1913   *Adams v. Milwaukee*, United States Supreme Court sustained tuberculin testing of cattle, also giving the city jurisdiction outside its boundaries

City financially supported Babies Fresh Air Pavilion

1914   Smallpox epidemic

Dr. George C. Ruhland appointed health commissioner

"Milk war" led to compromises on tuberculin test enforcement

1916   Chlorinating apparatus breakdown led to referendum for sewage treatment plant

Housing survey marked beginning of campaign against unhealthy housing

City Club Sickness Survey showed 10 percent of Milwaukeeans sick

Old Isolation Hospital razed

Pasteurization ordinance on all milk but certified

Ordinance prohibiting people with communicable diseases from working in establishments where food was prepared

Tuberculosis diagnostic clinics opened by health department (formerly under auspices of Society for the Care of the Sick)

1918 Flu hits Milwaukee; successful campaign launched to fight it

1919 School medical inspections unified for public and private schools under the health department

Health department decentralized with sub-stations on the north side and the south side

"Care of Baby and Young Child" pamphlet distributed to the homes of new-borns

1920 Pasteurization upheld in *Pfeffer v. City of Milwaukee*

Population: 457,147

Death Rate: 11.6

Venereal disease division created within health department

Visiting Nurse Association started its maternity service

1921 Dental Clinic opened by health department

Anti-noise ordinance

1924 Dr. John P. Koehler appointed health commissioner

1925 Virulent smallpox epidemic arrested by vigorous health department action; 427,959 people vaccinated

1926 Intensive diphtheria prevention campaign began using toxin-antitoxin and the Schick test

Tuberculin test enforced for cows producing for the Milwaukee market

1930 Population: 578,249

Death Rate: 9.6

All milk, except certified milk, pasteurized

Certificates of Merit issued by health department for eating establishments

Milwaukee awarded first prize for cities over 500,000 population in national health conservation contest

1931 Milwaukee received second place in national health contest

1932 Milwaukee won first place in national health contest

1933 Common council borrowed WPA money to construct a water purification plant

Milwaukee won second place in national health contest

1934 Scarlet Fever immunization program

Milwaukee received Special Certificate of Merit in national health conservation contest

1936 Milwaukee again awarded first prize in national health contest

1938 County Medical Society, Visiting Nurse Association, and St. Joseph's Hospital began community program for the care of premature babies

1939 New city water purification plant opened

Health department evening venereal disease clinic begun

Milwaukee won first prize in the national health contest for the fourth time

1940 Population: 587,472

Death Rate: 9.5

Dr. Edward R. Krumbiegel appointed health commissioner

1941 Milwaukee placed on the National Health Honor Roll in the national health contest

1942 Pamphlet "Baby's Care" issued by health department to replace 1919 publication; distributed to home of all newborns

Milwaukee placed on National Health Honor Roll

Convalescent homes and homes for the aged licensed and supervised by the health department

1943 "The March of Health" weekly radio dramatizations produced by the health department

Milwaukee again placed on National Health Honor Roll; contest discontinued

1944   Whooping cough and diphtheria immunization of all children started

Penicillin therapy for gonorrhea begun at city hospital

1945   School Hygiene Clinic opened

1946   "Rapid treatment center" started for syphilis patients at city hospital

1947   City-wide chest X-ray program

Tuberculosis Control Center established

1948   Benjamin Spock's *Baby and Child Care* replaced city pamphlet for distribution to families of newborn babies

Mobile child welfare clinic for outlying areas of the city

1949   Improved child immunization program used tri-immunol combined vaccine against whooping cough, diphtheria, and tetanus

Blue Cross hospital insurance began payment at city hospital

1950   Population: 637,392

Death Rate: 9.6

First woman, Margaret E. Hatfield, M.D., M.P.H., appointed as Deputy Commissioner of Health. She left in 1953 to join state Board of Health and in 1960 became health commissioner of Kenosha

Milwaukee Cancer Diagnostic Clinic, a cooperative venture with the health department, Marquette University Medical School, and the Milwaukee Chapter of the American Cancer Society, opened

Promotion of Health in the Workplace: The Relative Worth of Lifestyle and Environmental Approaches

Carlos Castillo-Salgado

INTRODUCTION

During the last 5 years in the United States there has been a growing interest in disease prevention and promotion of health. Disease prevention and health promotion have been designated as major health initiatives in important documents: The National Health Information and Health Promotion Act of 1976 [1], the 1978 Report of the HEW Departmental Task Force on Prevention [2], the 1979 Surgeon General's Report entitled *Healthy People* [3] and the 1980 *Promoting Health, Preventing Disease; Objectives for the Nation* [4].

In the fall of 1980, under the auspices of the First Surgeon General's Report of Health Promotion and Disease, the document, 'Objectives for the Nation,' set out specific and measurable objectives for 15 areas. Five of those areas related specifically to health promotion: Smoking Cessation; Reducing Misuse of Alcohol and Drugs; Improved Nutrition; Exercise and Fitness; and Stress Control [4].

In addition, American public health institutions and private corporations have shown a recent interest in primary prevention, self-care and self-help activities as valuable alternatives for implementing health promotion in the workplace.

Of great importance is the emerging interest in health promotion, with an 'apparent' major shift from the medical model to a rediscovery of the importance of prevention. While there are many laudable elements about this emphasis on prevention, the current 'lifestyle' health promotion model has an inherent 'blaming the victim' perspective.

I have reviewed recent developments and opportunities in the promotion of health. Since the issues covered on this matter are many and varied, this presentation will focus on the current approaches for the promotion of health in the workplace, and, also highlight some of the major implications of the lifestyle approach.

Under the emerging health promotion trend, important conceptual changes about health are arising. Lifestyle and individual behavior are considered the main forces in the development of chronic diseases [5]. Recognition of the health-illness process as a linear consequence of the individual's behavior is the central feature of this approach. The implication of this conceptual shift is the explicit emphasis on the role and responsibility of the individual in the genesis of disease and maintenance of health. Consequently, problems over which the individual has little direct control, such as those involving unemployment and occupational environment are minimized. Under this paradigm, health action must be concentrated on individual behavior, which becomes the major focus and target for intervention. This shift of responsibility from social, economic and environmental forces to individual behavior provides the illusion that profit-oriented corporations can be transformed into health-oriented corporations.

The following sections will review some of the major strategies for health promotion. In addition, it will analyze some of the major implications and

This article originally appeared under the title "Assessing Recent Developments in the Promotion of Health in the American Workplace" in *Social Science and Medicine*, vol. 19 (1984), pp. 349–358.

social consequences of the modification of the lifestyle approach of prevention and health promotion on the overall health status of the working population. A more comprehensive approach for promoting health in the work site, also, will be discussed.

WHAT IS HEALTH PROMOTION?

There are several interpretations as to what constitutes the meaning and scope of health promotion. Under the model of the 'natural history of disease' of Leavell and Clark [6], health promotion is defined as any intervention directed to maintain the health status of individuals and groups. This model suggests that promotion of health is a broad concept in which the basic categorical entities are: adequate housing; healthy and secure conditions at work; education; nutrition; recreation; marriage counseling; etc. In addition, the model recognizes health promotion and specific protection as dual entities that comprise primary prevention. This approach tends to integrate health promotional categories as specific activities for maintaining and improving the general status of individuals and groups. Nevertheless, health promotion activities are not necessarily related to a particular disease(s).

In general terms, health promotion can be seen as a combination of non-specific disease oriented activities (environmental, political, educational, economic, recreational) designed to provide a healthy condition and prevent the activation and/or emergence of any disease process in individuals and groups.

Health promotion activities are basically carried out on two levels: the environmental level and the individual-lifestyle level. Both environmental and individual strategies can have important roles in the promotion of health and the control of disease at different sites, i.e. community, home, educational institutions and workplace.

STRATEGIES FOR HEALTH PROMOTION

In recent years comparable terminology has been used in classifying health strategies: environmental vs lifestyle; individual vs community; and passive vs active measures. The passive vs active approach for improving health is defined in terms of "the amount of action required by individuals in order for them to be protected" [7]. At one pole are the 'passive' measures which automatically cover or protect individuals without any effort or actions from them. Examples of these measures are: iodination of salt, pasteurization of milk; fluoridation of water, 'childproof' caps on medicine bottles, etc. At the other pole are interventions which demand or impose individual action each time the person is protected. Examples of active measures are boiling water before using it, fastening a seat belt on each trip, monitoring intake of sugar, cholesterol, salt, fat and chemical additives, etc.

According to Williams and other authors [8–10], the advantage of passive interventions is that, once they are implemented, they apply to virtually everyone. Active measures, on the other hand, to be protective and effective must be implemented by each individual. Historically, the results of active measures have been substantially less successful in providing protection and being effective. Williams [8] recognizes that most health problems could be reduced by a combined strategy of both active and passive interventions. However, when effective and feasible passive approaches are available, their adoption and implementation should be encouraged. The author also remarks that the practice of effective active interventions by individuals should also be promoted, in cases where passive measures are not available, or when the incorporation of the active interventions would provide additional protection.

The efficacy of selected environmental or individual-lifestyle strategies is determined primarily by their impact on the health status, as reflected in morbidity and mortality patterns. It is important to keep in mind that the selection of a particular intervention or strategy should depend on its effectiveness compared to alternate interventions.

There is debate and controversy as to what level of environmental or individual-lifestyle strategies should be selected for protective action. Although environmental and individual levels are not mutually exclusive categories, each strategy has a different impact on health and social matters.

Tracing some historical results of these strategies for controlling disease and promoting health, Terris points out that during the period covered by the 'First Epidemiological Revolution' [11], approximately three-fifths of all deaths in the United States were caused by infectious diseases. Terris and other investigators [12–14] remark that medical care *per se* has played a secondary role in decreasing morbidity and mortality from infectious diseases. Successful control of the infectious diseases was achieved largely as a result of environmental control interventions directed at water, sanitation, milk, food supplies, as well as by immunizations. Presently, the leading causes of death in the United States are the chronic diseases. During the past few decades, epidemiologic studies have shown the role of the major risk factors in the genesis of the leading causes of death: heart disease; cancer; cerebrovascular diseases; accidents; cirrhosis of the liver; etc. Those major risk factors are: hypertension; cigarette smoking; high serum cholesterol; and occupational exposure to toxic substances and harmful processes. Each of these factors is amenable to change. However, the crucial question is what are the specific determinants of such factors, and what are the most efficient and effective means to eliminate them. Controversy arises at this point. The lifestyle and environmental approaches give different alternatives and solutions.

LIFESTYLE MODELING

Terris [11] defines this health policy controversy in two directions: the direction presented by the lifestyle approach, and the direction generated by epidemiological knowledge. Under the first direction, one important question to be asked concerns the ideological obstacles created by powerful industrial and other private interests on rejecting any government action and regulatory control. At present, the tobacco, liquor and food industries have the freedom to spread their message without serious restrictions. Terris remarks that it is difficult to accept that smoking is an individual matter when it is well known that cigarette advertising, costing more than $300 million a year, transformed smoking from a minor to a major addiction. A similar situation is present in the alcohol and food industries. An illustrative example of the external influence on food habits is presented by Green and Iverson [15]. The authors, drawing from several studies [16–18], reported that a child under the age of 12 may be exposed to over 22,000 commercials per year, of which 25% are for cereals (mostly high sugar cereals); 25% are for candy, gum and other sweets; 10% are for eating places, mostly fast-food restaurants; and 18% are for toys, many of questionable safety.

In relation to the economical and social pressures involved in public health issues, an important discussion has been presented by McKinlay [19]. He highlights the activities of the 'manufacturers of illness', defined as "those individuals, interest groups, and organizations which, in addition to producing material goods and services, also produce, as inevitable by products, widespread morbidity and mortality" [20]. This research recognizes the enormous influential power that these groups have in the creation of disease-inducing behavior. Of special concern to McKinlay is the paradox of the effective use of behavioral science knowledge to create at-risk behaviors, and the less than effective application of the same knowledge to eliminate such behavior. He also observes that in many instances, by the time health workers intervene, 'real damage' has already been done by the 'manufacturers of illness.' In addition, he notes that these groups create unnecessary and artificially perceived 'needs' (i.e. the need for sweet food, or extra vitamin intake).

The success of the activities promoted by these groups, according to McKinlay, lies in the way they are engineered and bound with essential elements of the existent dominant culture. The binding of 'risk-behavior' to culture is accomplished in several forms [21]: (a) exhortations for risk-behavior are based on those legitimized values, norms and principles which are extensively recognized in the social and cultural system, e.g. cigarette smoking portrayed as a pleasurable, relaxing activity associated with social success, virility and feminity [22]; (b) appeals which imply that certain dimensions of at-risk actions are subscribed to by cultural heroes and/or by technical experts, e.g. the use of sport's champions, movie stars or physicians and nurses to endorse the use of a specific drug product, cigarette brand, alcoholic beverage, food, etc.

In this context, it seems appropriate to review some aspects of regulation. In the United States, the major regulatory agency for the 'control' of the advertising industry is the Federal Trade Commission (FTC). In a 1981 report [23] the Commission presented several important facts on smoking advertisements: "Cigarettes are the most heavily advertised product in America. It has been estimated that the six major cigarette companies spent one billion dollars in 1980 to sell their product. The figure is several hundred times greater than the amount government spends on public service announcements on smoking hazards. The National Commission on Smoking and Public Policy reported in 1978 that the tobacco industry spent more on advertising cigarettes in one day than the (then) National Clearing House on Smoking and Health, the government's primary agency working on this area, spent in one year. . . . In 1979 cigarettes also continued to be the product most heavily advertised in newspapers. . . . The top five outdoor advertisers in 1979 were the five largest cigarette companies."

Under these conditions, the economic expenditure of the tobacco industry represents a real threat to any health promotional program seeking smoking cessation. These marketing and economical forces cannot be eliminated or neutralized by giving the individual the entire responsibility. Strong regulatory action as well as additional interventions are required. However, resistance and hostility to any regulatory action are the prevailing attitudes and actions within the political arena. As a consequence of taking some strong stands for controlling advertising, the FTC was recently forced by the Congress to back away from its regulatory efforts in relation to the advertising industry, and instead to substitute with an educational approach. Reviewing this problem, Green [24] noted that education could be seen as "an empowering strategy to give people power to resist the marketing forces of the industry." It would be difficult to argue the contrary and reject the importance of education; however, in this context, education as an opposite strategy to regulation may have little or no impact on controlling smoking patterns. Breslow [25] noted that by 1980, thirteen nations banned all advertising of cigarettes, and another nine had adopted stringent control.

In an extensive analysis, Breslow [26] presented the major forces and conflicts involved in public policy for smoking prevention and control. He mentions that "there can be no doubt that among all present-day disease-causing agents, cigarette smoking does the greatest day-to-day harm to the health of the people in industrialized society." The magnitude of the problem has been quantified in hundreds of studies. However, the tobacco issue is not a simple problem. Strong economic interests are behind the conflict. During 1975, in the United States tobacco sales rose to 15.7 billion dollars [27]. In this milieu, serious attempts to reduce and/or eliminate cigarette smoking cannot ignore the restrictions and barriers imposed by these strong interests. Insisting upon individual responsibility disregarding other forces is not an appropriate public health decision. Breslow [28] reports straightforwardly on the forces involved in this matter: ". . . Pressures to initiate, to quit smoking are largely social in nature. Even pressures to continue smoking cigarettes, or not to, come mainly from one's social milieu. . . . Cigarette smoking in a literal, important sense is a matter of individual choice. Each person who can have access to cigarettes personally decides each day whether or not to smoke them. In a larger perspective, however, the decision is not made so purely and simply. Habit, including social, psychological, and physiological addictive elements, largely determines the daily decision. . . . Individual decisions about cigarette smoking are not made in a vacuum, but in a highly structured social situation where pressures favoring or opposing cigarette smoking exert strong influences."

It seems evident that routine day-by-day behavior and response patterns of individuals and groups are greatly influenced by external forces, i.e. economic interests, mass media. This is especially true in the major target areas subject to behavioral modification strategies such as smoking, nutrition and drinking.

At first glance individual behavior modification seems an appropriate strategy for promoting healthy lifestyles. However, given the complex social matrix in which individual behaviors are articulated, this strategy is not likely to be successful. One of the more powerful influences on individual behavior is social pressure [29]. A more comprehensive strategy incorporating occupational and social environmental control actions, in addition to lifestyle modification, is a more realistic and effective approach.

In relation to the social control of smoking, Syme and Alcalay [30] recognize that "health education campaigns usually occur in sporadic and isolated contexts; they rarely take into account that smoking is part of an accepted and valued way of life; they assume that health is the most important priority for people—an assumption rarely supported by empirical evidence." Social values are articulated in an economic and social matrix that must be fully understood. Recently an innovative health research model has been proposed [31]. The focus of attention is the study of the 'etiologies of lifestyle.' This model is based upon the analysis of behavioral data, and attempts to develop the reconstruction of the 'natural history of habit formation' and 'lifestyle development.' The model suggests that recognition of 'developmental patterns' will provide information of critical transitions and experiences that may have altered or precipitated such behavioral patterns. Although this model has not been applied and still is in the process of elaboration, to effectively reach the goals, socioeconomic and environmental components must be emphasized in the framework. As long as the questions are posed in behavioral and individual terms, the answers will be expressed by individual responsibility and behavioral strategies.

In sum, underlying the behavioral modification-health promotion model is the postulate that health and illness are largely a matter of individual choice and will. Further, it suggests that by encouraging healthy lifestyles among individuals and groups, and stressing the individual responsibility in health problems, the goal of decreasing current morbidity and mortality indices can be achieved. Indeed, no one can diminish the importance of the individual dimension of the health-illness process, and of the role the individual has in determining part of the quality of his or her health. Moreover, it may be true that individuals and groups cannot achieve healthy patterns if their behavior corresponds to unhealthy practices. The promotion of healthy lifestyles, however, is but one of the activities needed to assure health and prevent disease. In promoting health and preventing disease, no single measure will suffice. Considering the complexity of the social, economic, cultural and political forces involved, a more comprehensive health strategy is essential.

ENVIRONMENTAL APPROACH

Significant health changes have emerged during the past half-century in industrialized countries. The social, physical and work environment has created a synergistic effect that has contributed to the rapid development of chronic diseases, accidents and premature deaths. During this period, epidemiologic studies have identified the multicausal nature of the chronic diseases as well as the recognition of these diseases as leading causes of mortality and morbidity in the United States.

As the health status of the population has mainly been influenced by deleterious social and environmental factors, measures for coping with those influences should include corresponding environmental and social interventions. For the direction of these interventions, Terris [32] suggests the use of the preventive model which incorporates both environmental and individual factors. Under this model, he mentions, public health action will reach the 'second epidemiological revolution' [33] controlling chronic disease and accidents. Three basic components have been presented by Terris as alternatives to preventive programs [34]: control of the environment, screening and health education. This model separates the available measures for control of the environment into those which are regulatory in nature, and those which are based on financial considerations. Among those socio-environmental actions are: imposition of financial barriers against tobacco, alcohol and other harmful substances; regulations to prevent air and water pollution, accidents, and exposure to radiation and other toxic substances in places such as industry, medical care facilities, home and in the general community; regulations requiring installation of safety features in motor vehicles; laws requiring that only unsaturated fats can be used in commercial baking, and that labels specify the amount and degree of saturation of the fats contained in packaged food. In addition, he proposes some financial measures, such as increase in taxation of harmful substances and subsidies and additional support to promote changes in the agricultural and industrial production patterns.

Similar criteria for health promotion intervention have been suggested by Nelson et al. [35]. These investigators present a set of four 'incentives' or 'tools' to be used for intervention and health promotion:

(1) Education: this category provides individuals and groups with the knowledge and motivation required to make an informed decision, taking into account health risks and benefits.
(2) Subsidization: this category provides indi-

viduals and groups with tangible rewards for engaging in an activity judged to be healthful.

(3) Taxation: this category includes actions taken to provide individuals and groups with financial sanctions for engaging in an activity judged to be health-aversive.

(4) Regulation: this category includes legislation designed to compel or force individuals and groups to engage in activity judged to be healthful or to refrain from activity judged to be health-aversive.

In addition, to achieve the final objective of reducing the risk of developing chronic diseases and premature death, a comprehensive effort towards environmental control action needs to be accomplished. The pursuit of this effort follows two directions. The first considers the direct health consequences of major forces operating in both social and work environments, while the second concerns the influence of those forces on individual behavior and decisions that characterize one's lifestyle. Representative of the first direction is the negative health impact of air pollution, or the presence of multiple toxic substances: pesticides, such as organochlorine insecticides; food additives, such as cyclamates, artificial flavoring and coloring agents; metals, such as lead, mercury; drugs, such as nicotine, psychotropic agents, alcohol, tranquilizers; radiation; multiple untested industrial chemicals; and subtherapeutic doses of antibiotic drugs and hormonal products used for feeding animals to promote growth and which are finally consumed by humans. One of the most dramatic relationships of these forces occurs between the work environment and carcinogenesis [36]. The characteristic effect of health hazards in the workplace is its insidious nature: slow, cumulative, irreversible and complicated by non-occupational factors, but also, destructive, disabling and fatal. The likelihood of a toxic substance having a carcinogenic effect on an individual is heightened by two variables: the concentration of the substance absorbed and the duration of exposure to it. The target group logically is the working population who spend eight hours a day throughout a working life exposed to such a toxic and harmful environment [37].

On the other hand, one of the most potent forces influencing lifestyle is the workplace, because it is the one place where much time is spent, where the greatest functional activity occurs, and where the closest social contact exists [38]. At work, processes of production as well as formal and informal systems are crucial determinants of health-related problems.

With these concepts in mind, multiple steps must be accomplished to effectively reduce the risk of developing disease and to promote health at the work site. Environmental and behavioral changes conducive to health must be identified and interventions for promoting these changes encouraged. In the next section a review of the health promotion strategies at the workplace considering those aspects and concerns will be presented.

HEALTH PROMOTION PROGRAMS IN THE AMERICAN WORKPLACE

Recently, the idea of developing programs within work settings for health promotion and disease prevention has begun to receive special consideration among American business groups, government officials and health professionals. Among the locations in which health promotion strategies can be implemented, the workplace has been judged to be an ideal setting to accomplish a high degree of effectiveness. Gainor and Guillory [39] state that one or more of the following elements can be used as suitable criteria for selecting a potential effective location:

(a) potential for addressing one or more of the seven risk factors (smoking, alcohol use, obesity, exercise, stress, hypertension and accident prevention and injury control);

(b) presence of high-risk groups;

(c) amount of time target groups remain in setting;

(d) potential for reaching underserved, hard-to-reach populations;

(e) potential for influencing personal behavior modification;

(f) potential for accomplishing environment modification;

(g) potential for both inducing and maintaining change;

(h) credibility in eyes of consumer public;

(i) potential for contributing to needed research in health promotive methods and maintenance of behavior change.

Following this criteria, the workplace has been mentioned as a convenient setting for several reasons: (a) cigarette smoking, alcohol consumption and elevated blood pressure are referred to as the three most important determinants of mortality in the adult population in industrialized countries [40]. More than half of the adult population in the United States are in the working population—a total of some 85 million persons. At least 10% of these individuals are known to suffer from high blood pressure or some form of cardiovascular disease [41]; (b) men and women who are employed spend nearly 30% of his or her waking hours there [42]; (c) the worksite provides a well defined population and offers accessibility to large groups of people [43]; (d) the number of work-related injuries, deaths and illnesses in the United States documents the existence of a significant social problem [44]. For 1979 the Bureau of Labor Statistics (BLS) reported 5.96 million occupationally related injuries [45]. The Public Health Service estimates that 390,000 new cases of occupational disease occur annually and that occupational diseases cause over 100,000 deaths each year [46]; (e) in addition, the periodic gathering of health information on workers can be used for (47): (1) study of the natural history of health and disease; (2) tracking of individual health behavior against expected norms and against program objectives; and (3) evaluation of individual programs and/or complete operating health systems. In this context, the workplace has been referred to as "one of the most promising and challenging sites for health behavior change" [48].

According to former Deputy Assistant Secretary for Health J. M. McGinnis [49], corporate interest in health promotion activities is based upon three premises: (1) the total cost of medical care in the U.S.A. has risen dramatically. In 1960 the costs were $26.9 billion (5.3% of the Gross National Product). By 1970 those costs increased to $75 billion (7.6% of the GNP), and by 1980 the costs were reported at $243.4 billion (9.4% of the GNP), with business paying over half of the national health care costs; (2) investment in health promotion activities will allow an increment in worker productivity and substantial long-term cost savings (through reducing costs associated with absenteeism, disability, job turnover, hospitalization, and premature death); (3) it is a feasible way to reduce the risks of major disease and premature death among employees.

Corporate Medical Director at New York Telephone G. H. Collings [50] has expressed: because of the "disenchantment with Medicare, Medicaid, and other recent programs, it is unlikely that comprehensive health improvement will rise from the federal level." Also, in his opinion, the medical care system has shown its inability to broaden its focus and incorporate more health promotion functions. These conditions "leave business as the principal remaining structure in which the desired health objectives can be reached." This attitude of business about health promotion, however, is based mainly upon economic considerations. In Collings' words: "As a result of these economic pressures (escalating cost of health benefit plans), business is overcoming its natural reluctance to get involved in health care matters and is finding that corporate opportunity in the health arena transcends the original issue of cost-containment. Among the advantages are less absenteeism and more productivity on the job; reducing coping problems among employees (both management and non-management); and enhanced functional efficiency of the corporate organism as a whole" [51].

In the workers' opinion, "Health practices should not be promoted primarily on the basis of more productivity or less absenteeism and turnover. Those are secondary products. The main concern of occupational health programs should be with human lives saved—not with man-hours lost" [52].

Both views of the problem require serious consideration. The cost of medical care is obviously a critical issue. For example, it has been reported that General Motors spends more on health care than on steel from its principal supplier. Victor Zink of G.M. declared that the cost of health insurance and health care accounted for $142 of the cost of every automobile released from the assembly line [53]. On the other hand, there is a danger, as J. K. Iglehart [54] points out, when conflicting interests between health care providers and private business, as sellers and buyers of health care services, transform health care as more nearly an economic product, than a social good.

The high human cost of deleterious processes of production also has been raised as a prominent issue. Growing interest and concern have been expressed in the long-neglected area of occupational health. The work environment has been primarily responsible for increasing the risk and likelihood of developing multiple diseases and premature deaths in the working population. It has been widely reported that several injury and health hazards are inherent of the job. Consequently, health promotion programs should be designed to modify work environment as well as to provide the workers information and support systems to improve their health and security.

CURRENT PERSPECTIVES ON HEALTH PROMOTION

In a recent editorial in *Family and Community Health* (The Journal of Health Promotion and Maintenance) entitled: 'Change and Health Promoting Activities for the 1980s,' A. M. Reinhardt and M. D. Quinn stated: "For health promotion to be effective, each individual must assume a major share of responsibility of their own well-being. . . . Self-responsibility is the *key* to wellness maintenance and enhancement, along with an emphasis on physical fitness, awareness and practice of healthy nutritional habits, coping effectively with stressors on a daily basis, and *environmental sensitivity* including psychological health" (emphasis added). It seems to be clear that the message transmitted by this health strategy is solidly grounded in the tradition of individualism, self-help and self-responsibility: The primary and ultimate responsibility for health and illness lies in the realm of individuals. Furthermore, environmental influences could be dissipated with 'environmental sensitivity,' defined as the "individual's sensitivity to their own physical and emotional needs . . ." [55].

The model postulated for health promotion in occupational settings is based upon two fundamental premises: (1) the focus on the worker's health behavior change; and (2) the placement of responsibility for health on the worker—'where it belongs,' as described by a special report from the U.S. Chamber of Commerce's Foundation for Public Health [56]. R. N. Beck, Executive Vice President of Bank of America, following these premises, has presented recently the corporate interpretation of health promotion programs. The primary principle described by Beck is the acceptance of the 'individual responsibility' of each worker for his or her health. In this respect, Beck remarks: "Responsibility for good health belongs to the individual, not the doctor, not the company, not the government" [57]. The role of the companies, in this perspective, is mentioned as 'company assistance,' arguing that "since it is the individual's responsibility for good health, the company should not take over full care" [58]. Instead, he suggests, it should provide support to assist workers to choose healthy lifestyles. A major problem with the 'fundamental' principle of this approach is the allocation of the entire responsibility for health to the individuals, and as a contrapart elimination of the responsibility of social institutions and private structures. The corporate conceptualization of health promotion not only is inconsistent with the reality of the workplace, but also reflects a paternalistic view whereby means of the 'generous assistance' from the private sector, profit-oriented corporations are transformed to health-oriented corporations.

This unidimensional strategy applied to the workplace offers rather limited opportunities for promoting health and preventing disease in the working population. It is difficult to accept the elimination of environmental factors in any model or strategy for health promotion in the workplace, primarily because strong evidence has been generated from epidemiological studies acknowledging occupational risks associated with multiple chemical products and harmful industrial processes. Based on information released by the International Association for Research on Cancer, a division of the World Health Organization, Tomatis *et al.* [59] report that at least 26 substances have been identified as carcinogenic to humans, and that 221 chemicals have been proved to be carcinogenic in animal experiments. It is important to point out that most of these 221 chemicals can be found in the worksite, but only a small number of them have been regulated as hazardous or carcinogenic materials [60]. Also, in recent years, epidemiological and experimental research in cancer etiology has provided information to identify several environmental factors [61] as major carcinogenic determinants in man. Higginson and Muir [62] report that at least 80% of all cancer can be attributed to environmental influences. These studies provide insight into the basic relationship between social, biological and work environment and lifestyle practices. Lifestyle practices are highly dependent upon the social matrix, work structure and organization, and upon cultural values. Based on these important consider-ations, serious attempts to promote health at the workplace should move to actions directed to modify hazardous working conditions, limiting stressful job demands and changing at-risk work structures. The focus of attention, however, is placed in the behav-ioral model. For those involved in health program evaluation it should be noted that there are several characteristics of the behavioral model that make it difficult to achieve the final objective of reducing the risk of developing chronic disease and premature death. A major problem is the linear identification between health process and health behavior. Conse-quently, the model reduces its scope to the behavioral dimension of the process. The continuum of the be-havioral model, thus, is expressed in different indi-vidual levels according to the complexity of the inter-vention: (1) increase in awareness; (2) increase in knowledge; (3) change in attitudes; (4) change in behavior; and finally (5) reduction of risk [63]. The model assumes that these changes can be done in a vacuum. In essence, the socio-environmental com-ponent (which independently plays a crucial role and creates an intermediary influence on behavior life-style) is delineated as a residual category.

It has been suggested that the following are four major components of an effective health promotion program [64]: (1) assessment of risk; (2) risk reduc-tion; (3) evaluation; and (4) environmental and social support. Because of the multiple-risk nature of any chronic disease, between identifying a risk factor for a particular disease, and reducing the risk of developing disease, multiple actions need to be im-plemented and environmental and social networks must be supportive and reinforcing. The technique most widely used for risk assessment in health pro-motion programs is the health hazard/health risk appraisal (HHA/HRA). A recent evaluation of the scientific basis of this technique, and of its predictive value, has reported many problems in relation to its validity—both internal and external. The conclu-sion of this report emphasizes caution and concern because of the ineffectiveness of this technique. Also, the authors expressed concern that "HHA/HRA pro-grams may constitute 'blaming the victim' or may pay insufficient regard to the influence of environ-mental and social factors on health and health re-lated behaviors" [65].

DesJardin *et al.* [66] have indicated that several

options can be incorporated into educational pro-grams to promote workplace safety and health: (a) training workers to identify specific occupational hazards and to use legal resources in having them corrected; (b) developing contact between workers and occupational health specialists; (c) stimulating understanding of and interest in job health by help-ing workers write leaflets and hazard information sheets; (d) establishing accident and health hazard reporting systems; and (e) facilitating links among union or worker groups facing similar problems. In addition to monitoring and controlling environmen-tal work conditions, worker education in safety and accident prevention, and in the recognition of poten-tial health hazards is essential for the success of any occupational health program.

One area that continuously has been neglected in health promotion activities, and in which the be-havioral model lacks effectiveness, is that which re-lates to shift workers. Because of the importance of this sector of the working population, a brief discus-sion on health, work structure and health promotion will be presented.

HEALTH PROMOTION LIFESTYLE CHANGES IN SHIFT WORKERS

The nature and requirements of the process of pro-duction in industrialized societies have generated in the workplace the application of a model in which increased productivity can be achieved through tech-nological changes and reorganization of the work process. An example of the latter is shift work. In addition to various physical, biological and chemical hazards, the social and structural organization of work and job demands directly affect the health of shift workers and their families.

The proportion of workers in the United States doing shift work in 1975 was 26.8% [67, 68]. This accounts for more than 22 million workers.

Some of the health consequences of shift work are related to physiological, social and psychologic problems. Some of the disturbances are generated by alteration of 24-hour circadian rhythms and the 28-day ovarian cycle in women.

The major problems found in shift workers in-clude: disturbances in sleep, disturbances of the ali-mentary tract, nervous system problems, sexual problems, isolation from family and friends and disruptions in social life [69, 70]. Several studies have reported that night shift workers show an increase in caffeine and tobacco consumption [71]. Also important to point out is the insufficient attention that this sector of the working population has received by health investigators. There is a lack of experimental and epidemiological studies evaluating the health status, and the at-risk conditions of the work structure and job demands on shift workers. The evaluation of the physiological impact of shift work through the circadian rhythms and the body's ability to metabolize toxic chemicals and drugs are areas suggested to be investigated [72, 73].

The current behavioral strategy for health promotion disregards the enormous impact that work structure and job demands impose on the health of the shift workers. Individual behaviors are highly dependent on the work environment. The model has restrictions in several of its postulates. Nutrition, for example, is an area in which blaming the victim will not be an effective approach, particularly for night shift and rotative shift workers, since digestive disorders among these workers are related to a lack of adequate eating facilities at night. Real options need to be in the worker's hands. Promoting health in shift work conditions needs to incorporate a multifaceted approach in which work structure changes, environment changes and supporting social network should have central importance. . . .

SUMMARY AND CONCLUSIONS

During the last few years, the individual-based lifestyle approach has gained momentum in the area of health promotion and disease prevention. This approach has been adopted extensively in health promotion programs for different target groups. Of critical importance is the incorporation of this approach into the field of occupational health.

This document aims to provide a characterization of the present directions of health promotion. Two major strategies for promoting health at the workplace were identified and discussed: (a) the individual-based lifestyle model, and (b) the environmental-social approach.

The most salient feature of the individual-based lifestyle approach is the orientation and reactivation of the traditional medical model towards an individualistic and fragmented vision of health. To a large extent health and disease are identified as phenomena dependent mainly on individual behaviors and individual decisions. This approach limits the spectrum of health promotion in the workplace to a series of activities centralized in the modification of the worker's health behavior and promoting the placement of responsibility for health on each individual worker. The behavioral activities promoted range from changes in awareness, knowledge and attitudes to changes in behavior and finally changes in health status. These steps are supposed to lead workers to informed choices for changing their 'disease behavior' to a more health oriented behavior. Although the individual's behavioral elements are important mediating factors in the genesis of health-illness conditions, it is quite evident that the generation of the process of health-illness, particularly in the workplace, is much more than just workers' behaviors.

Consequently, this concept provides an incomplete and partial picture of health by belittling the economic, social, ecological and environmental conditions of life and work which play a crucial role as mediating and determinant structures of both health and lifestyle [73].

Beyond individual behaviors, environmental and working conditions, social structure and organization of the process of work and production have a determinant influence in the creation and maintenance of health and illness in the working population. Besides this critical point, it is important to consider that individuals and groups' behaviors (including 'health risk behavior') are articulated internally to a social network of behavior patterns which are accepted in the social environment. Moreover, those behaviors are promoted and strongly maintained by powerful societal forces such as mass media and the advertising industry. Therefore, efforts and programs directed to influence individuals and groups to transform their disease behavior into a healthier practice have to take into consideration the fact that the current behavior patterns are not solely a matter of individual choice and will, but, to a greater extent, a societal structure of multiple determinants. At this point, it is questionable whether the individual-lifestyle approach will ever be able to improve the working and living conditions and health opportunities essential to reach a healthy status for the working population. . . .

After reviewing the lifestyle approach, this document emphasizes the importance of the environmental approach. The conceptualization of this health perspective embodies and recognizes the socioeconomic and environmental factors as main determinants of the lifestyle, the work structure and of the patterns and distribution of health-illness in the population. The health promotion interventions at the workplace suggested by this strategy include the modification of the hazardous working conditions, limiting stressful job demands, and changing at-risk work structures. The sphere of action under this comprehensive approach should include interventions through four incentives: taxation, regulation, subsidization and education.

Under this health alternative it is crucial that workers or their representatives be included as full participants in the overall process of planning, organization and implementation of the activities of promotion of health in the workplace.

References

1. The National Health Information and Health Promotion Act of 1976.

2. U.S. Department of Health, Education and Welfare. Departmental Task Force on Disease Prevention and Health Promotion: Federal Programs and Prospects. Government Printing Office, Washington, DC, 1978.

3. Office of Assistant Secretary for Health and Surgeon General: *Healthy People:* The Surgeon General's Report on Health Promotion and Disease Prevention, DHEW Publication No. (PHS) 79–50071, Public Health Service, U.S. Government Printing Office, Washington, DC, 1979.

4. Department of Health and Human Services. *Public Health Service: Promoting Health/Preventing Disease, Objectives for the Nation.* U.S. Government Printing Office, Washington, DC, 1980.

5. Lalonde M. A new perspective of the health of Canadians. A Working Document. Government of Canada, 1974.

6. Leavell H. R. and Clark E. G. *Preventive Medicine for the Doctor in his Community. An Epidemiological Approach,* Chap. 2, pp. 14–38. McGraw-Hill, New York, 1965.

7. Williams A. F. Passive and active measures for controlling disease and injury: the role of health psychologists. *Hlth Psychol.* **1**, 399, 1982.

8. *Ibid.,* pp. 399–409.

9. Baker S. P. Childhood injuries: the community approach to prevention. *J. Publ. Hlth Policy* **2**, 235–246, 1981.

10. Halddon Jr W. Strategy in preventive medicine: passive versus active approaches to reducing human wastage. *J. Trauma* **14**, 353–355, 1974.

11. Terris M. Epidemiology as a guide to health policy. *A. Rev. Publ. Hlth* **1**, 323–344, 1980.

12. McKeown T. *The Modern Rise of Population.* Academic Press, New York, 1976.

13. McKinlay J. B. and McKinlay S. M. The questionable contribution of medical measures to the decline of mortality in the United States in the twentieth century. *Milbank Meml. Fund Q.* **55**, 405–428, 1977.

14. Rosen G. The bacteriological, immunologic, and chemotherapeutic period 1875–1950. *Bull. N.Y. Acad. Med.* **40**, 483–493, 1964.

15. Green L. and Iversen D. C. School health education. *A. Rev. Publ. Hlth* 321–338, 1982.

16. Winnick C., Williamson L. G., Chuzmir S. F. and Winnick M. P. *Children's Television Commercials: A Content Analysis.* Praeger, New York, 1973.

17. NSF Report. Research on the effects of television advertising to children. *Nat. Sci. Fund.*, Washington, DC, 1977.

18. Barcus F. E. Weekend commercial children's television. Action for Children's Television, Newton, MA, 1975.

19. McKinlay J. B. A case for refocussing upstream—the political economy of illness. In: *Applying Behavioral Science to Cardiovascular Risk.* Proceedings of a Conference (Edited by Enrlow A. J. and Henderson J. B.), pp. 7–16. American Heart Association, Seattle, WA, 1975.

20. *Ibid.,* p. 7.

21. *Ibid.,* p. 9.

22. Breslow L. Control of cigarette smoking from a public policy perspective. *A. Rev. Publ. Hlth* **3**, 143, 1982.

23. Federal Trade Commission. Staff Report on the Cigarette Advertising Investigation, pp. 2–4. FTC, Washington, DC, 1981.

24. Green L. W. Emerging Federal Perspectives on Health Promotion. Monograph No. 1, pp. 22. Teachers College, Columbia University, 1981.

25. Breslow L. Control of cigarette smoking from a public policy perspective. *A. Rev. publ. Hlth* **3**, 135, 1982.

26. Breslow L. *op. cit.,* pp. 129–151.

27. Luce B. R. and Schwiezer S. The economic consequences of smoking. *New Engl. J. Med.* **298,** 569–571, 1978.

28. Breslow L. *op. cit.,* p. 132.

29. Syme L. S. and Alcalay R. Control of cigarette smoking from a social perspective. *A. Rev. Publ. Hlth* **3,** 196, 1982.

30. Syme L. S. and Alcalay R. *Ibid.,* p. 189.

31. Green L. W. Cross-cutting issues in the study of health behavior and health promotion. Unpublished Document, presented at Montreal, Canada, 1982.

32. Terris M. The complex tasks of the second epidemiologic revolution: the Joseph W. Mountin Lecture. *J. Publ. Hlth Policy* **3,** 8–24, 1983.

33. Terris M. The epidemiologic revolution, national health insurance and the role of health departments. *Am. J. Publ. Hlth* **66,** 1155–1165, 1976.

34. Terris M. *op. cit.,* pp. 334–335, 1980.

35. Nelson E. C., Keller A. M. and Zubkoff M. Incentives for health promotion: the Government's role. In *Strategies for Public Health, Promoting Health and Preventing Disease* (Edited by Ng L. K. Y. and Davis D. L.), pp. 218–231. Von Nostrand Reinhold, New York, 1981.

36. Grozuczak J. Health promotion strategies for unionized workers. In *Strategies for Public Health, Promoting Health and Preventing Disease* (Edited by Ng L. K. Y. and Davis D. L.), pp. 235–247. Van Nostrand Reinhold, New York, 1981.

37. *Ibid.,* p. 239.

38. Nelson E. C. *et al. op cit.,* p. 225.

39. Gainor A. K. and Guillory M. Arenas for practicing health promotion. *Fam. Communit. Hlth* **5,** No. 4, 30–31, 1983.

40. Kuller L., Meilahn E., Townsend M. and Weinberg G. Control of cigarette smoking from a medical perspective. *A. Rev. Publ. Hlth* **3,** 153–178, 1982.

41. High Blood Pressure Control in the Work Setting: Issues, Models and Resources. *Proceedings of the National Conference,* p. 4. Merck, Sharpe & Dohme, West Point, PA, 1976.

42. McGinnis J. M. and Duval M. K. Foreword. In *Managing Health Promotion in the Workplace. Guidelines for Implementation and Evaluation* (Edited by Parkinson R. S. *et al.*), p. 1. Mayfield, Palo Alto, CA, 1982.

43. McGinnis J. M. and Duval M. K. *op. cit.,* p. 2.

44. Desjardins R. B., Bigoness W. J. and Harris L. R. Labor-management aspects of occupational risk. *A. Rev. Publ. Hlth* **3,** 201–224, 1982.

45. Bureau of Statistics, *Occupational Injury and Death Statistics.* Washington, DC, 1980.

46. Cited in Asford N. *Crisis in the Workplace: Occupational Disease and Injury.* A report to the Ford Foundation. MIT Press, Cambridge, MA.

47. Collins G. H. Perspectives of industry regarding health promotion. In *Managing Health Promotion in the Workplace. Guidelines for Implementation and Evaluation* (Edited by Parkinson, R. S. *et al.*), p. 120. Mayfield, Palo Alto, CA, 1982.

48. McGinnis J. M. and Duval M. K. *op. cit.,* p. 1.

49. *Ibid.,* p. 2.

50. Collins G. H. *op cit.,* p. 119.

51. *Ibid.,* p. 120.

52. High Blood Pressure Control in the Work Setting: Issues, Models and Resources. *Proceedings of the National Conference,* p. 8. Merck, Sharpe & Dohme, West Point, PA, 1976.

53. *Ibid.,* p. 18; and Brennan A. J. Health promotion: what's in it for business and industry. *Hlth Educ. Q.* **9,** Special Suppl., 9–19, 1982.

54. Inglehart J. K. Health policy report. Health care and American business. *New Engl. J. Med.* 120–124, 1982.

55. Reinhardt A. D. and Quinn M. D. From the Editors. "Change and health promoting activities for the 1980s." *Fam. Communit. Hlth.* **5,** No. 4, viii, 1983.

56. U.S. Chamber of Commerce Foundation. *A National Health Care Strategy: How Business can Promote Good Health for Employees and their Families.* National Chamber Foundation, U.S. Chamber of Commerce. Government Printing Office, Washington, DC, 1978.

57. Beck R. N. IBMs plan for life: toward a comprehensive health care strategy (Worksite Health Promotion). *Hlth Educ. Q.* **9,** Special Suppl. p. 55, 1982.

58. Beck R. N. *op. cit.,* p. 56, 1982.

59. Tomatis L., Agthe C., Bartsch H., Huff J., Montesano R., Saracci R., Walker E. and Wilbourne J. Evaluation of the carcinogenicity of chemicals: a review of the IARC monograph programme. *Cancer Res.* **38,** 877–885, 1978.

60. Davis D. L. and Rall D. P. Risk assessment for disease prevention. In *Promoting Health and Preventing Disease* (Edited by Ng L. K. Y. and Davis D. L.), p. 134, Van Nostrand Reinhold, New York, 1981.

61. For a complete list of those environmental causes of human cancer, see Fraumeni J. F. Epidemiologic approaches to cancer etiology. *A. Rev. Publ. Hlth* **3,** 88, 1982.

62. Higginson J. and Muir C. S. Epidemiology. In *Cancer Medicine* (Edited by Hollander J. F. and Frei E. III), pp. 241–306. Lea & Febiger, Philadelphia, 1973.

63. Parkinson R. S. (Ed.) A hierarchy of program needs and objectives. In *Managing Health Promotion in the*

Workplace. Guidelines for Implementation and Evaluation, pp. 17–21. Mayfield, Palo Alto, CA, 1982.

64. *Ibid.,* pp. 8–9.

65. Wagner E. H., Beery W. L., Schoenbach V. J. and Graham A. M. An assessment of health hazard health risk appraisal. *Am. J. Publ. Hlth* **74,** 351, 1982.

66. Desjardin R. B. *et al. op. cit.,* p. 220, 1982.

67. Tasto D. and Colligan M. *Shift Work Practices in the United States.* U.S. Department of Health, Education and Welfare, Publication No. 77–148, Washington, DC, 1977.

68. Baker D. The use of health consequences of shift work. *Int. J. Hlth Serv.* **10,** 405–420, 1980.

69. Rutenfranz J., Colguhoun W., Knauth P. and Ghata J. Biomedical and psychosocial aspects of shift work: a review. *Scand. J. Work Envir. Hlth* **3,** 165–162, 1977.

70. Baker D. *op. cit.,* p. 414, 1980.

71. Cited in Baker D. *op. cit.,* p. 414, 1980.

72. Ede M. C. Circadian rhythms in drug effectiveness and toxicity in shift workers. In *Shift Work and Health,* pp. 140–141. U.S. Department of Health, Education and Welfare, Publication No. 76–203, Washington, DC, 1976.

73. See: Wenzel E. Perspectives of the W.H.O. regional office for Europe: health promotion and lifestyles. *Int. J. Hlth Educ.* **1,** Nos 3/4, 57–60, 1983.